Davis's Comprehensive Handbook of Laboratory and Diagnostic Tests— *with Nursing Implications*

Zoanne Burgess Schnell, PhD, RN
Anne M. Van Leeuwen, MA, BS, MT(ASCP)
Todd R. Kranpitz, MS, BS, NMT, ARRT

F. A. DAVIS COMPANY • PHILADELPHIA

F. A. Davis Company
1915 Arch Street
Philadelphia, PA 19103
www.fadavis.com

Printed in Canada

Last digit indicates print number: 10 9 8 7 6 5 4 3

Acquisitions Editor: Lisa B. Deitch
Developmental Editor: Gett Services
Production Editor: Lisa J. Collins
Cover Designer: Louis J. Forgione

As new scientific information becomes available through basic and clinical research, recommended treatments and drug therapies undergo changes. The authors and publisher have done everything possible to make this book accurate, up to date, and in accord with accepted standards at the time of publication. The authors, editors, and publisher are not responsible for errors or omissions or for consequences from application of the book, and make no warranty, expressed or implied, in regard to the contents of the book. Any practice described in this book should be applied by the reader in accordance with professional standards of care used in regard to the unique circumstances that may apply in each situation. The reader is advised always to check product information (package inserts) for changes and new information regarding dose and contraindications before administering any drug. Caution is especially urged when using new or infrequently ordered drugs.

ISBN 0-8036-1042-4

DEDICATION

To my parents, Eugene and Edith Burgess, whose love and nurturing gave me confidence to pursue my goals. To my husband, Rich, and sons, Richard, Patrick, and Shey, who have added immeasurable joy to my life and support during work on "the book." To my colleagues and friends for their interest and encouragement throughout the writing process. Especially to Dr. Rachel Pollow, whose use of flow charts as a teaching tool inspired some of the activities suggested in the accompanying *Instructor's Guide* and Student Workbook. To Anne and Todd, whose wit, wisdom, and perseverance made this project happen and whose friendship I will always cherish. To Lisa Deitch, Acquisitions Editor, who shared our vision of this book. And, finally, to the patients, family members, students, and friends who have shared their laboratory and diagnostic testing experiences, keeping me in touch with the "human" side of it all.

Zoanne Burgess Schnell, PhD, RN
Professor
Department of Nursing, Food and Nutrition
Plattsburgh State University of New York
Plattsburgh, New York

To my parents, James and Marceline, who always told me I could do or be anything I wished as long as I believed in myself. To my husband, Don, and daughters, Sarah and Margaret, for their humor, patience, support, and love throughout the entire project. I could not have done this without them. To my writing partners, Todd and Zoanne, for their friendship, creativity, commitment, and professional skills. To Lisa Deitch, Acquisitions Editor, for her excellent direction and unwavering encouragement. To Lisa Collins, Production Editor, for her outstanding editorial guidance and support. To my medical technology and nursing friends and colleagues, Bev, Cathy, Evelyn, Ruth, and Lynda, for their interest, support, and advice. And to Rudy and Winston, my favorite and loyal canines, who always snoozed by my feet during countless predawn writing sessions.

Anne M. Van Leeuwen, MA, BS, MT (ASCP)
Administrator
Eye Care for the Adirondacks, P.C.
Plattsburgh, New York

To my wife, Mindy, who never once thought I could not succeed, and my son, Jake, for their support throughout the entire project. I could not have done this without them. To my coauthors, Zoanne and Anne, for their direction, endless commitment, and organizational skills, but most of all for their friendship. To Lisa Deitch, for her immeasurable faith in and support for this project, and to my friends and colleagues, Fay and Dr. De Lise, for their encouragement and ongoing advice.

Todd R. Kranpitz, MS, BS, ARRT (R) (N), NM (NMTCB), ASCP (N)
Director of Imaging Services
King's Daughters Medical Center
Ashland, Kentucky

ABOUT THIS BOOK

Laboratory and diagnostic studies are essential components of a complete patient assessment. Examined in conjunction with an individual's history and physical examination, laboratory and diagnostic data provide clues about health status. Nurses are increasingly expected to integrate an understanding of laboratory and diagnostic procedures and expected outcomes in assessment, planning, implementation, and evaluation of nursing care. The data help develop and support nursing diagnoses, interventions, and outcomes.

Nurses may interface with laboratory and diagnostic testing on several levels, including:

- Interacting with patients and families of patients undergoing diagnostic tests or procedures, and providing pretest, intratest, and post-test information and support
- Maintaining quality control to prevent or eliminate problems that may interfere with the accuracy and reliability of test results
- Ensuring completion of testing in a timely and accurate manner
- Collaborating with other health care professionals in interpreting findings as they relate to planning and implementing total patient care
- Communicating significant alterations in test outcomes to other appropriate health care team members
- Coordinating interdisciplinary efforts

Whether the nurse's role at each level is direct or indirect, the underlying responsibility to the patient, family, and community remains the same.

This book is a reference for nurses, nursing students, and other health care professionals. It is useful as a clinical tool as well as a supportive text to supplement clinical courses. It guides the nurse in planning what needs to be assessed, monitored, treated, and taught regarding pretest requirements, intratest procedures, and post-test care. It can be used by nursing students at all levels as a textbook in theory classes, integrating laboratory and diagnostic data as one aspect of nursing care; by practicing nurses, to update information; and in clinical settings as a quick reference. Designed for use in academic and clinical settings, *Davis's Comprehensive Handbook of Laboratory and Diagnostic Procedures—with Nursing Implications* provides the user with a comprehensive reference that allows easy access to information about laboratory and diagnostic tests and procedures. A general overview of how all the tests and procedures included

vii

in this book relate to body systems can be found in tables following the monographs. All tests and procedures are listed in alphabetical order by their complete name, allowing the user to locate information quickly without having to place tests in a specific category or body system. Each monograph is presented in a consistent format for easy identification of specific information at a glance. The following information is provided for each laboratory and diagnostic test:

- *Test Name* for each monograph is given as a commonly used designation, and all test monographs in the book are organized in alphabetical order by name.
- *Synonyms/Acronyms* for each test are listed where appropriate.
- *Specimen Type* includes the amount of specimen usually collected and where appropriate the type of collection tube or container commonly recommended. Specimen requirements vary from laboratory to laboratory. The amount of specimen collected is usually more than what is minimally required so that additional specimen is available, if needed, for repeat testing (quality control failure, dilutions, or confirmation of unexpected results). In the case of diagnostic tests, the *type of test* procedure (e.g., nuclear medicine, x-ray) is given.
- *Reference Values* for each monograph include age-specific and gender-specific variations, when indicated. It is important to give consideration to the normal variation of laboratory values over life span and across cultures; sometimes what might be considered an abnormal value in one circumstance is actually what is expected in another. Reference values for laboratory tests are given in conventional and standard international (SI) units. The factor used to convert conventional to SI units is also given. Because laboratory values can vary by method, each laboratory reference range is listed along with the associated methodology.
- *Description* of the study's purpose and insight into how and why the test results can affect health are included.
- *Indications* are a list of what the test is used for in terms of assessment, evaluation, monitoring, screening, identifying, or assisting in the diagnosis of a clinical condition.
- *Results* present a list of conditions in which values may be increased or decreased and in some cases an explanation of variations that may be encountered.
- *Critical Values* or findings that may be life-threatening or for which particular concern may be indicated are given along with age span considerations where applicable. This section also includes signs and symptoms associated with a critical value as well as possible nursing interventions.
- *Interfering Factors* are substances or circumstances that may influence the results of the test, rendering the results invalid or unreliable. Knowledge of interfering factors is an important aspect of quality assurance and includes pharmaceuticals, foods, natural and additive therapies, timing of test in relation to other tests or procedures, collection site, handling of specimen, and underlying patient conditions.
- *Nursing Implications and Procedure* provides an outline of pretest, intratest, and post-test concerns.

- *Pretest* section addresses the need to
  - Obtain pertinent clinical, laboratory, dietary, and therapeutic history of the patient, especially as it pertains to comparison of previous test results, preparation for the test, and identification of potentially interfering factors.
  - Understand the interrelationship between various body systems. In this section the reader is informed of the body systems that may be involved in the study of interest and is referred to system tables where related studies are alphabetically cross-referenced.
  - Explain the requirements and restrictions related to the procedure as well as what to expect; provide the education necessary for the patient to be properly informed.
  - Anticipate and allay patient concerns or anxieties.
  - Provide for patient safety.
- *Intratest* section can be used in a quality control assessment by the nurse or as a guide to the nurse who may be called on to participate in specimen collection or perform preparatory procedures and gives
  - Specific directions for specimen collection and test performance.
  - Important information such as patient sensation and expected duration of the procedure.
  - Precautions to be taken by the nurse and patient.
- *Post-test* section provides guidelines regarding
  - Specific monitoring and therapeutic measures that should be performed after the procedure (e.g., maintaining bed rest, obtaining vital signs to compare with baseline values, signs and symptoms of complications).
  - Specific instructions for the patient and family, such as when to resume usual diet, medications, and activity.
  - General nutritional guidelines related to excess or deficit as well as common food sources for dietary replacement.
  - Indications for interventions from public health representatives or for special counseling related to test outcomes.
  - Indications for follow-up testing that may be required within specific time frames.
  - Related tests for consideration and evaluation is an alphabetical listing of related laboratory and/or diagnostic tests that is intended to provoke a deeper and broader investigation of multiple pieces of information; the tests provide related data that when combined can form a more complete picture of health or illness.

Color and icons have been used to facilitate locating critical information at a glance.

The nursing process is evident throughout the laboratory and diagnostic monographs. Within each phase of the testing procedure, the nurse has certain potential roles and responsibilities. These should be evident in reading each monograph. A summary list of nursing diagnoses associated with each phase of the testing procedure is provided in the appendices for ease of reference.

Information provided in the appendices includes a summary of specimen collection procedures and materials, describing specific tube tops used for various blood tests; a list of common laboratory panels, the tests in them, and the minimum specimen requirements; a summary chart that details suggested approaches to persons at various developmental stages to assist the provider in facilitating cooperation and understanding; a list of some of the herbs and nutraceuticals that have been associated with adverse clinical reactions or have been associated with drug interactions related to the affected body system; and guidelines for standard and universal precautions.

Finally, additional supportive materials are provided for the instructor and student in an *Instructor's Guide*. Presentations and case studies with emphasis on laboratory and diagnostic test–related information and nursing implications have been developed for selected conditions and body systems. Open-ended and NCLEX-type, multiple-choice questions are provided as well as suggested critical thinking activities. This supplemental material will aid the instructor in integrating laboratory and diagnostic materials in assessment and clinical courses and provide examples of activities to enhance student learning.

PREFACE

L aboratory and diagnostic testing. The words themselves often conjure up cold and impersonal images of needles, specimens lined up in collection containers, and high-tech electronic equipment. But they do not stand alone. They are tied to, bound with, and tell of health or disease in the blood and tissue of a person. Laboratory and diagnostic studies augment the health care provider's assessment of the quality of an individual's physical being. Test results guide the plans and interventions geared toward strengthening life's quality and endurance. Beyond the pounding noise of the MRI, the cold steel of the x-ray table, the sting of the needle, the invasive collection of fluids and tissue, and the probing and inspection is the gathering of evidence that supports the health care provider's ability to discern the course of a disease and the progression of its treatment. Laboratory and diagnostic data must be viewed with thought and compassion, however, as well as with microscopes and machines. We must remember that behind the specimen and test result is the person from whom it came, a person who is someone's son, daughter, mother, father, husband, wife, friend.

This book is written to help health care providers in their understanding and interpretation of laboratory and diagnostic procedures and their outcomes. Just as important, it is dedicated to all health care professionals who experience the wonders in the science of laboratory and diagnostic testing, performed and interpreted in a caring and efficient manner.

CONTENTS

ACETYLCHOLINE RECEPTOR ANTIBODY

SYNONYM/ACRONYM: AChR.

SPECIMEN: Serum (1 mL) collected in a red-top tube.

REFERENCE VALUE: (Method: Radioimmunoassay) Less than 0.03 nmol/L.

DESCRIPTION: When present, acetylcholine receptor antibody (AChR) blocks acetylcholine from binding to receptor sites on the muscle membrane. AChR destroys acetylcholine receptor sites, interfering with neuromuscular transmission and causing muscle weakness. Antibodies to acetylcholine receptor sites are present in 90 percent of patients with myasthenia gravis (MG) and in 75 to 80 percent of patients who either have ocular forms of MG or are in remission. ■

INDICATIONS:
- Confirm the presence, but not the severity, of MG
- Differentiate between generalized and ocular forms of MG, because patients with the ocular form have lower titers
- Monitor the effectiveness of immunosuppressive therapy for MG
- Monitor the remission stage of MG

RESULT

Increased in:
- Amyotrophic lateral sclerosis
- MG (4.8 nmol/L indicates generalized MG, 1.2 nmol/L indicates ocular MG, and 0.9 nmol/L indicates remission)

- Thymoma associated with MG

Decreased in: N/A

CRITICAL VALUES: N/A

INTERFERING FACTORS:
- Drugs that may produce false-positive results include muscle relaxants, such as metocurine and succinylcholine.
- Drugs that may increase AChR levels include penicillamine.
- Immunosuppressive therapy is the recommended treatment for MG; prior immunosuppressive drug administration may result in negative test results.
- Recent radioactive scans or radiation within 1 week of the test can interfere with test results when radioimmunoassay is the test method.

Nursing Implications and Procedure

Pretest:

➤ Obtain a history of the patient's complaints, including a list of known allergens.

➤ Obtain a history of the patient's musculoskeletal system and results of previously performed tests and

1

procedures. For related tests, refer to the musculoskeletal system table.

➤ Obtain a list of the medications the patient is taking, especially immunosuppressive drugs. Include herbs, nutritional supplements, and nutraceuticals. The requesting health care practitioner and laboratory should be advised if the patient regularly uses these products so that their effects can be taken into consideration when reviewing results.

➤ Note any recent procedures that can interfere with test results.

➤ There are no food, fluid, or medication restrictions unless by medical direction.

➤ Review the procedure with the patient.

➤ Inform the patient that specimen collection takes approximately 5 to 10 minutes.

Intratest: ■

➤ Direct the patient to breathe normally and to avoid unnecessary movement.

➤ Observe standard precautions and follow the general guidelines in Appendix A. Perform a venipuncture; collect the specimen in a 5-mL red-top tube.

➤ Label the specimen, and promptly transport it to the laboratory.

Post-test: ■

➤ Observe venipuncture site for bleeding or hematoma formation. Apply pressure bandage.

➤ Evaluate test results in relation to the patient's symptoms and other tests performed. Related laboratory tests include antinuclear antibodies, antithyroglobulin and antithyroid peroxidase antibodies, myoglobin, rheumatoid factor, thyroid-stimulating hormone, and thyroxine.

ACID PHOSPHATASE, PROSTATIC

· ·

SYNONYMS/ACRONYM: Prostatic acid phosphatase, o-phosphoric monoester phosphohydrolase, PAP.

SPECIMEN: Plasma (1 mL) collected in lavender-top (ethylenediaminetetraacetic acid [EDTA]) tube. Serum (1 mL) collected in a red-top tube is also acceptable, but care must be taken to use the same type of collection container for serial measurements.

Swab with vaginal secretions may be submitted in the appropriate transfer container. Other material such as clothing may be submitted for analysis. Consult the laboratory or emergency services department for the proper specimen collection instructions and containers.

REFERENCE VALUE: (Method: Enzyme immunoassay)

Conventional Units	SI Units (Conversion Factor: ×1.0)
Less than 2.5 ng/mL	Less than 2.5 µg/L

DESCRIPTION: Acid phosphatases are enzymes found in many tissues, including the prostate gland, bone, spleen, liver, and kidney, as well as in red blood cells and platelets. Seminal fluid also contains high concentrations of acid phosphatase, and detection of this enzyme in vaginal swabs or from other physical evidence is used to investigate rape. Acid phosphatase activity is highest in the prostate gland; however, prostatic acid phosphatase (PAP) levels are not significantly increased in the early stages of prostatic cancer, so this test is not recommended as a screening tool. Prostate-specific antigen has replaced PAP for the staging of carcinoma of the prostate and diagnosis of metastatic adenocarcinoma of the prostate. ■

INDICATIONS:
- Assist in the investigation of sexual assault and rape.
- Assist with differential diagnosis of other disorders associated with elevated PAP, red blood cell phosphatase, or platelet acid phosphatase, such as leukemia.
- Evaluate the effectiveness of treatment for prostatic cancer (recurrence after prostatectomy). Levels decrease with effective treatment. Rising levels are associated with a poor prognosis.
- Investigate or evaluate an enlarged prostate gland, especially if prostatic carcinoma is suspected.

RESULT

Increased in:

- Acute myelogenous leukemia
- Benign prostatic hypertrophy
- Gaucher's disease
- Liver disease
- Metastatic bone cancer
- Niemann-Pick disease
- Paget's disease
- After prostate surgery, biopsy, or manipulation
- Prostatic cancer
- Prostatic infarct
- Prostatitis
- Sickle cell crisis
- Thrombocytosis

Decreased in: N/A

CRITICAL VALUES: N/A

INTERFERING FACTORS:
- Drugs that may increase PAP levels include alglucerase, androgens (females), buserelin, and clofibrate.
- Drugs that may decrease PAP levels include alcohol, fluorides, ketoconazole, oxalates, and phosphates.
- Prostatic massage, rectal examination, or urinary catheterization within 48 hours of the test can cause elevated PAP levels.
- Specimens should be drawn in the morning because PAP exhibits diurnal variation.

Nursing Implications and Procedure • • • • • • • • • • •

Pretest:

➤ Obtain a history of the patient's complaints, especially alterations in urinary elimination. Obtain a list of known allergens.

➤ Obtain a history of the patient's genitourinary, immune, and reproductive system and results of previously performed tests and procedures. For related tests, refer to the genitourinary, immune, and reproductive system tables.

➤ Obtain a list of the medications the patient is taking, including herbs, nutritional supplements, and nutraceuticals. The requesting health care practitioner and laboratory should be advised if the patient regularly uses these products so that their effects can be taken into consideration when reviewing results.

➤ Note any recent procedures that can interfere with test results.

➤ There are no food, fluid, or medication restrictions unless by medical direction.

➤ Review the procedure with the patient.

➤ Inform the patient that blood specimen collection takes approximately 5 to 10 minutes.

Intratest:

➤ Direct the patient to breathe normally and to avoid unnecessary movement.

➤ Observe standard precautions and follow the general guidelines in Appendix A. Perform a venipuncture, and collect the specimen in a 5-mL lavender-top tube.

➤ Label the specimen, and promptly transport it to the laboratory, because results can be altered within 1 hour.

Post-test:

➤ Observe venipuncture site for bleeding or hematoma formation. Apply pressure bandage.

➤ Recognize anxiety related to test results and offer support. Provide teaching and disease information, as appropriate. Counsel the male patient, as appropriate, that sexual dysfunction related to altered body function, drugs, or radiation may occur. Educate the patient regarding counseling services, as appropriate.

➤ Offer support, as appropriate, to patients who may be the victim of rape or sexual assault. Educate the patient regarding access to counseling services. Provide a nonjudgmental, nonthreatening atmosphere for discussing the risks of sexually transmitted diseases. Discuss problems the patient may experience (e.g., guilt, depression, anger) if test results indicate the presence of semen.

➤ Evaluate test results in relation to the patient's symptoms and other tests performed. Related laboratory tests include prostate biopsy, prostate-specific antigen, and semen analysis.

ADRENAL GLAND SCAN
• •

SYNONYM/ACRONYM: Adrenal scintiscan.

AREA OF APPLICATION: Adrenal gland.

CONTRAST: Radioactive NP-59 (iodomethyl-19-norcholesterol) or metaiodobenzylguanidine (MIBG).

DESCRIPTION: This nuclear medicine study evaluates function of the adrenal glands. The secretory function of the adrenal glands is controlled primarily by the anterior pituitary, which produces adrenocorticotropic hormone (ACTH). ACTH stimulates the adrenal cortex to produce cortisone and secrete aldosterone. Adrenal imaging is most useful in differentiation of hyperplasia versus adenoma in primary aldosteronism when computed tomography (CT) and magnetic resonance imaging (MRI) findings are equivocal. High concentrations of cholesterol (the precursor in the synthesis of adrenocorticosteroids, including aldosterone) are stored in the adrenal cortex. This allows the radionuclide, which attaches to the cholesterol, to be used in identifying pathology in the secretory function of the adrenal cortex. The uptake of the radionuclide occurs gradually over time; imaging is performed within 24 to 48 hours of injection of the radionuclide dose and continued daily for 3 to 5 days. Imaging reveals increased uptake, unilateral or bilateral uptake, or absence of uptake in the detection of pathologic processes. Suppression studies can be done to differentiate the presence of tumor from hyperplasia of the glands followed by prescanning treatment with corticosteroids. ■

INDICATIONS:
- Aid in the diagnosis of Cushing's syndrome and aldosteronism

- Differentiate between asymmetric hyperplasia and asymmetry from aldosteronism with dexamethasone suppression test

- Determine adrenal suppressibility with prescan administration of corticosteroid to diagnose and localize adrenal adenoma, aldosteronomas, androgen excess, and low-renin hypertension

- Aid in the diagnosis of gland tissue destruction caused by infection, infarction, neoplasm, or suppression

- Aid in locating adrenergic tumors

RESULT

Normal Findings:
- Normal bilateral uptake of radionuclide and secretory function of adrenal cortex

- No evidence of tumors, infection, infarction, or suppression

- Normal salivary glands and urinary bladder, and vague shape of the liver and spleen sometimes seen

Abnormal Findings:
- Adrenal gland suppression

- Adrenal infarction

- Adrenal tumor

- Hyperplasia

- Infection

- Pheochromocytoma

INTERFERING FACTORS

This procedure is contraindicated for:
- Patients who are pregnant or suspected

of being pregnant, unless the potential benefits of the procedure far outweigh the risks to the fetus and mother.

Factors that may impair clear imaging:

• Inability of the patient to cooperate or remain still during the procedure because of age, significant pain, or mental status

• Retained barium from a previous radiologic procedure

• Obesity, because patients may exceed the weight limit for the equipment

• Incorrect positioning of the patient, which may produce poor visualization of the area to be examined

Other considerations:

• Consultation with a physician before the procedure regarding radiation safety concerns for infants of patients who are lactating.

• Risks associated with radiographic overexposure that can result from frequent radiologic procedures. Personnel in the room with the patient should stand away from the patient or leave the area while the examination is being done. Badges that reveal the level of exposure to radiation should be worn by personnel working in the areas where the examination is being done.

Nursing Implications and Procedure · · · · · · · · · · ·

Pretest: ■

➤ Inform the patient that the procedure detects adrenal gland function.

➤ Inform the patient that a special nuclear medicine department technologist performs the test. The test usually involves a prolonged scanning schedule over a period of days.

➤ Obtain a history of the patient's complaints, including a list of known allergens.

➤ Obtain a history of the patient's adrenal system and results of previously performed laboratory tests, surgical procedures, medical therapy for adrenal pathology, and other diagnostic procedures. For related tests, refer to the endocrine system table.

➤ Obtain a list of the medications the patient is taking.

➤ All adrenal blood tests should be done before doing this test.

➤ Determine date of last menstrual period and possibility of pregnancy in perimenopausal women.

➤ Ask the patient to lie still during the procedure because movement produces unreliable results.

➤ Administer saturated solution of potassium iodide (SSKI) 24 hours before the study to prevent thyroid uptake of the free radioactive iodine.

➤ *An informed consent needs to be obtained and witnessed.*

Intratest: ■

➤ Ask patient to remove jewelry and any other metallic objects from the area to be scanned.

➤ Have the patient put on a hospital gown and void before scanning.

➤ Insert an intravenous line and inject the radionuclide intravenously on day 1; images are done on days 1, 2, and 3. Imaging is done from the urinary bladder to the base of the skull to scan for a primary tumor. Each image takes 20 minutes, and total imaging time is 1 to 2 hours per day.

➤ Ask the patient to hold still during the procedure because movement produces unreliable results.

➤ The images are recorded on film or stored electronically for recall and postprocedure interpretation by a physician.

Post-test: ■

➤ Unless contraindicated, advise the patient to drink increased amounts of fluids for 48 to 72 hours to eliminate the radionuclide from the body.

➤ Advise the patient that SSKI (120 mg/day) will be administered for 10 days after the injection of the radionuclide.

➤ A written report of the examination will be completed by a physician specializing in this branch of medicine. The report will be sent to the ordering provider, who will discuss this report with the patient.

➤ Depending on the results of this procedure, additional testing may be performed.

➤ Inform the patient to flush the toilet immediately after each voiding following the procedure and to meticulously wash hands with soap and water after each voiding for 72 hours after the procedure.

➤ Tell all caregivers to wear gloves when discarding urine for 48 hours after the procedure. Wash gloved hands with soap and water before removing gloves. Then wash hands after the gloves are removed.

➤ Evaluate test results in relation to the patient's symptoms and other tests performed. Related diagnostic tests include adrenal angiography, CT, MRI, and positron emission tomography scans of the abdomen.

ADRENOCORTICOTROPIC HORMONE (AND CHALLENGE TESTS)

SYNONYM/ACRONYM: Corticotropin, ACTH.

SPECIMEN: Plasma (2 mL) from lavender-top (ethylenediaminetetra-acetic acid [EDTA]) tube for adrenocorticotropic hormone (ACTH), and serum (1 mL) from a red-top tube for cortisol. Collect specimens in a prechilled heparinized plastic syringe, and carefully transfer into collection containers by gentle injection to avoid hemolysis. Alternatively, specimens can be collected in prechilled lavender- and red-top tubes. Tiger- and green-top (heparin) tubes are also acceptable for cortisol, but take care to use the same type of collection container for serial measurements. Immediately transport specimen tightly capped and in an ice slurry to the laboratory. The specimens should be immediately processed. Plasma for ACTH analysis should be transferred to a plastic container.

Procedure	Medication Administered, Adult Dosage	Recommended Collection Times
zACTH stimulation, rapid test	250 µg cosyntropin IM or IV bolus after overnight fast	3 cortisol levels: baseline immediately before bolus, 30 min after bolus, and 60 min after bolus

(Continued on the following page)

Procedure	Medication Administered, Adult Dosage	Recommended Collection Times
Corticotropin-releasing hormone (CRH) stimulation	IV dose of 1 μg/kg ovine CRH between 9 a.m. and 8 p.m.	3 cortisol and 3 ACTH levels: baseline before injection, 30 min after injection, and 60 min after injection
Dexamethasone suppression (overnight)	Oral dose of 1 mg dexamethasone (Decadron) at 11 p.m.	Collect cortisol at 8 a.m. on the morning after the dexamethasone dose
Metyrapone stimulation (overnight)	Oral dose of 30 mg/kg metyrapone with snack at midnight	Collect cortisol and ACTH at 8 a.m. on the morning after the metyrapone dose

REFERENCE VALUE: (Method: Immunoradiometric assay)

ACTH

Age	Conventional Units	SI Units (Conversion Factor ×0.22)
Cord blood	50–570 pg/mL	11–125 pmol/L
Newborn	10–185 pg/mL	2–41 pmol/L
Adult supine specimen collected in morning	9–52 pg/mL	2–11 pmol/L
Women on oral contraceptives	5–29 pg/mL	1–6 pmol/L

ACTH Challenge Tests

ACTH (Cosyntropin) Stimulated, Rapid Test	Conventional Units	SI Units (Conversion Factor ×27.6)
Baseline	Cortisol greater than 5 μg/dL	Greater than 138 nmol/L
Peak response	Cortisol greater than 20 μg/dL	Greater than 552 nmol/L

Corticotropin-Releasing Hormone Stimulated	2–4-fold increase over baseline ACTH or cortisol level	2–4-fold increase over baseline values

	Conventional Units	SI Units (Conversion Factor ×27.6)
Dexamethasone Suppressed, Overnight Test	Cortisol less than 3 µg/dL next day	Less than 83 nmol/L

	Conventional Units	SI Units (Conversion Factor ×0.22)
Metyrapone Stimulated, Overnight Test	ACTH greater than 150 pg/mL	Greater than 33 pmol/L

	Conventional Units	SI Units (Conversion Factor ×27.6)
	Cortisol less than 3 µg/dL next day	Less than 83 nmol/L

DESCRIPTION: The anterior pituitary gland secretes ACTH. This hormone stimulates adrenal cortex secretion of glucocorticoids, androgens, and to a lesser degree, mineralocorticoids. Hypothalamic-releasing factor stimulates ACTH release. Cortisol and ACTH test results are evaluated together because any change in one causes a change in the other. ACTH levels exhibit a diurnal variation, peaking between 6 and 8 a.m. and reaching the lowest point between 6 and 11 p.m. Evening levels are generally one half to two thirds lower than morning levels. Cortisol levels also vary diurnally, with the lowest values occurring during the morning hours and peak levels occurring in the evening. ■

INDICATIONS:
• Determine adequacy of replacement therapy in congenital adrenal hyperplasia

• Determine adrenocortical dysfunction

• Differentiate between increased ACTH release with decreased cortisol levels and decreased ACTH release with increased cortisol levels

RESULT: ACTH secretion exhibits diurnal variation with values being highest in the morning. A lack of change in values from morning to evening is clinically significant. In hypopituitarism, concentrations of hormones secreted by the pituitary gland and hormones secreted by its target organs decrease.

The cosyntropin test is used when adrenal insufficiency is suspected. Cosyntropin is a synthetic form of ACTH. A baseline cortisol level is collected before the injection of cosyntropin. Specimens are subsequently collected at 30- and 60-minute intervals. If the adrenal glands function normally, cortisol levels rise significantly after administration of cosyntropin.

The CRH stimulation test works as well as the dexamethasone suppression test (DST) in distinguishing Cushing's disease from conditions in which ACTH is secreted ectopically (e.g., tumors not located in the pituitary gland that secrete ACTH). In the cosyntropin test, cortisol levels are measured after intravenous administration of CRH. A fourfold increase in cortisol levels above baseline is seen in Cushing's disease. No increase in cortisol is seen if ectopic ACTH secretion is the cause.

The DST is useful in differentiating the causes of increased cortisol levels. Dexamethasone is a synthetic steroid that suppresses secretion of ACTH. With the DST, a baseline morning cortisol level is collected, and the patient is given a 1-mg dose of dexamethasone at bedtime. A second specimen is collected the following morning. If cortisol levels have not been suppressed, adrenal adenoma is suspected. The DST also produces abnormal results in the presence of certain psychiatric illnesses (e.g., endogenous depression).

The metyrapone stimulation test is used to distinguish corticotropin-dependent causes (pituitary Cushing's disease and ectopic Cushing's disease) from corticotropin-independent causes (e.g., carcinoma of the lung or thyroid) of increased cortisol levels. Metyrapone inhibits the conversion of 11-deoxycortisol to cortisol. Cortisol levels should decrease to less than 3 µg/dL if normal pituitary

stimulation by ACTH occurs after an oral dose of metyrapone. Specimen collection and administration of the medication are performed as with the overnight dexamethasone test.

Increased in:

- Addison's disease (primary adrenocortical hypofunction)

- Congenital adrenal hyperplasia

- Cushing's disease (pituitary dependent)

- Ectopic ACTH-producing tumors

- Menstruation

- Nelson's syndrome

- Pregnancy

- Stress

Decreased in:

- Adenoma

- Adrenal carcinoma

- Hypopituitarism

- Secondary adrenocortical insufficiency

CRITICAL VALUES: N/A

INTERFERING FACTORS:

- Drugs that may increase ACTH levels include aminoglutethimide, amphetamines, insulin, levodopa, metoclopramide, metyrapone, pyrogens, mifepristone (RU 486), and vasopressin.

- Drugs that may decrease ACTH levels include adrenal corticosteroids and dexamethasone.

- Test results are affected by the time the test is done because ACTH levels vary diurnally, with the highest values occurring between 6 and 8 a.m. and the lowest values occurring at night. Samples should be collected at the same time of day, between 6 and 8 a.m.

- Excessive physical activity can produce elevated levels.

- Recent radioactive scans or radiation within 1 week before the test can interfere with test results when immunoradiometric assay is the test method.

- The metyrapone stimulation test is ⚠ contraindicated in patients with suspected adrenal insufficiency.

- ⚠ Metyrapone may cause gastrointestinal distress and/or confusion.

Nursing Implications and Procedure · · · · · · · · · · ·

Pretest: ▮

➤ Obtain a history of the patient's complaints, including a list of known allergens.

➤ Obtain a history of the patient's endocrine system and results of previously performed tests and procedures. For related tests, refer to the endocrine system table.

➤ Obtain a list of the medications the patient is taking, including herbs, nutritional supplements, and nutraceuticals. The requesting health care practitioner and laboratory should be advised if the patient regularly uses these products so that their effects can be taken into consideration when reviewing results.

➤ Note any recent procedures that can interfere with test results.

➤ No food, fluid, or medication restrictions exist unless by medical direction.

➤ Review the procedure with the patient. Inform the patient that more than one sample may be necessary to ensure accurate results and that the samples are obtained at specific times to determine high and low levels of the hormone.

➤ Tell the patient to refrain from strenuous exercise for 12 hours before the test and to remain in bed or at rest for 1 hour immediately before the test.

➤ Inform the patient that each specimen collection takes approximately 5 to 10 minutes.

➤ Prepare an ice slurry in a cup or plastic bag to have on hand for immediate transport of the specimen to the laboratory.

Intratest: ▮

➤ Ensure that strenuous exercise was avoided for 12 hours before the test and that 1 hour of bed rest was taken immediately before the test. Specimens should be collected between 6 and 8 a.m.

➤ Direct the patient to breathe normally and to avoid unnecessary movement.

➤ Observe standard precautions and follow the general guidelines in Appendix A. Perform a venipuncture, and collect the specimen in a prechilled plastic heparinized syringe or in prechilled collection containers listed under "Specimen."

➤ Label, note the time of collection, and promptly transport the specimen to the laboratory. The tightly capped sample should be placed in an ice slurry immediately after collection. Information on the specimen label can be protected from water in the ice slurry if the specimen is first placed in a protective plastic bag.

➤ When ACTH hypersecretion is suspected, a second sample may be requested between 6 and 8 p.m. to determine if changes are the result of diurnal variation in ACTH levels.

Post-test: ▮

➤ Observe venipuncture site for bleeding or hematoma formation. Apply pressure bandage.

➤ Evaluate test results in relation to the patient's symptoms and other tests performed. Related laboratory tests include cortisol, follicle-stimulating hormone, growth hormone, luteinizing hormone, testosterone, thyroid-stimulating hormone, and thyroxine.

ALANINE AMINOTRANSFERASE

SYNONYMS/ACRONYMS: Serum glutamic pyruvate transaminase (SGPT), ALT.

SPECIMEN: Serum (1 mL) collected in a red- or tiger-top tube. Plasma (1 mL) collected in a green-top (heparin) tube is also acceptable.

REFERENCE VALUE: (Method: Spectrophotometry)

Age	Conventional Units	SI Units (Conversion Factor ×0.017)
Newborn–1 y	13–45 U/L	0.22–0.77 µKat/L
2 y–adult		
Male	10–40 U/L	0.17–0.68 µKat/L
Female	7–35 U/L	0.12–0.60 µKat/L

DESCRIPTION: Alanine aminotransferase (ALT), formerly known as serum glutamic pyruvic transaminase (SGPT), is an enzyme produced by the liver. It acts as a catalyst in the reversible transfer of an amino group between alanine and α-ketoglutarate. The highest concentration of ALT is found in liver cells, moderate amounts are found in kidney cells, and smaller amounts are found in heart and skeletal muscle. When liver damage occurs, serum levels of ALT rise to 50 times normal, making this a useful test in evaluating liver injury. ALT is also used to screen donated blood before transfusion because the enzyme may be elevated in the absence of detectable serologic markers of hepatitis. ∎

INDICATIONS:

• Compare serially with aspartate aminotransferase (AST) levels to track the course of liver disease.

• Monitor liver damage resulting from hepatotoxic drugs.

• Monitor response to treatment of liver disease, with tissue repair indicated by gradually declining levels.

• In blood banks, use as a routine screen for hepatitis in donor blood samples. Samples are rejected if levels are greater than 1.5 times the upper limits of normal.

RESULT

Increased in:

• Acute pancreatitis

• Biliary tract obstruction

- Burns (severe)
- Chronic alcohol abuse
- Cirrhosis
- Fatty liver
- Hepatic carcinoma
- Hepatitis
- Infectious mononucleosis
- Muscle injury from intramuscular injections, trauma, infection, and seizures (recent)
- Muscular dystrophy
- Myocardial infarction
- Myositis
- Preeclampsia
- Shock (severe)

Decreased in:
- Pyridoxal phosphate deficiency

CRITICAL VALUES: N/A

INTERFERING FACTORS:
- Drugs that may increase ALT levels by causing cholestasis include amitriptyline, anabolic steroids, androgens, benzodiazepines, chlorothiazide, chlorpropamide, dapsone, erythromycin, estrogens, ethionamide, gold salts, imipramine, mercaptopurine, nitrofurans, oral contraceptives, penicillins, phenothiazines, progesterone, propoxyphene, sulfonamides, tamoxifen, and tolbutamide.
- Drugs that may increase ALT levels by causing hepatocellular damage include acetaminophen (toxic), acetylsalicylic acid, allopurinol, amiodarone, anabolic steroids, anticonvulsants, asparaginase, azithromycin, bromocriptine, captopril, cephalosporins, chloramphenicol, clindamycin, clofibrate, danazol, enflurane, ethambutol, ethionamide, fenofibrate, fluconazole, fluoroquinolones, foscarnet, gentamicin, indomethacin, interferon, interleukin-2, levamisole, levodopa, lincomycin, low-molecular-weight heparin, methyldopa, monoamine oxidase inhibitors, naproxen, nifedipine, nitrofurans, oral contraceptives, probenecid, procainamide, quinine, ranitidine, retinol, ritodrine, sulfonylureas, tetracyclines, tobramycin, and verapamil.
- Drugs that may decrease ALT levels include cyclosporine and interferon.

Nursing Implications and Procedure • • • • • • • • • • •

Pretest:

➤ Obtain a history of the patient's complaints, including a list of known allergens.

➤ Obtain a history of the patient's hepatobiliary system and results of previously performed tests and procedures. For related tests, refer to the hepatobiliary system table.

➤ Obtain a list of the medications the patient is taking, including herbs, nutritional supplements, and nutraceuticals. The requesting health care practitioner and laboratory should be advised if the patient regularly uses these products so that their effects can be taken into consideration when reviewing results.

➤ There are no food, fluid, or medication restrictions unless by medical direction.

➤ Review the procedure with the patient.

➤ Inform the patient that specimen collection takes approximately 5 to 10 minutes.

Intratest:

➤ Direct the patient to breathe normally and to avoid unnecessary movement.

➤ Observe standard precautions and follow the general guidelines in Appendix A. Perform a venipuncture, and collect the specimen in a 5-mL red- or tiger-top tube.

➤ Label the specimen, and promptly transport it to the laboratory.

Post-test:

➤ Observe venipuncture site for bleeding or hematoma formation. Apply pressure bandage.

➤ Increased ALT levels may be associated with liver disease. Dietary recommendations may be indicated and vary depending on the severity of the condition. A low-protein diet may be in order if the patient's liver has lost the ability to process the end products of protein metabolism. A diet of soft foods may be required if esophageal varices have developed. Ammonia levels may be used to determine whether protein should be added to or reduced from the diet. Patients should be encouraged to eat simple carbohydrates and emulsified fats (as in homogenized milk or eggs), as opposed to complex carbohyderates (e.g., starch, fiber, and glycogen [animal carbohydrates]) and complex fats, which would require additional bile to emulsify it so that it can be used. The cirrhotic patient should be carefully observed for the development of ascites, in which case fluid and electrolyte balance requires strict attention.

➤ Evaluate test results in relation to the patient's symptoms and other tests performed. Related laboratory tests include acetaminophen, ammonia, AST, bilirubin, electrolytes, γ-glutamyl transpeptidase, hepatitis antigens and antibodies, lactate dehydrogenase, and liver biopsy.

ALBUMIN AND ALBUMIN/ GLOBULIN RATIO

• •

SYNONYM/ACRONYM: Alb, A/G ratio.

SPECIMEN: Serum (1 mL) collected in a red- or tiger-top tube. Plasma (1 mL) collected in green-top (heparin) tube is also acceptable.

REFERENCE VALUE: (Method: Spectrophotometry) Normally the albumin/globulin (A/G) ratio is greater than 1.

Age	Conventional Units	SI Units (Conversion Factor ×10)
Newborn–4 d	2.8–4.4 g/dL	28–44 g/L
5 d–14 y	3.8–5.4 g/dL	38–54 g/L
15–18 y	3.2–4.5 g/dL	32–45 g/L
19–60 y	3.4–4.8 g/dL	34–48 g/L
61–90 y	3.2–4.6 g/dL	32–46 g/L
Greater than 90 y	2.9–4.5 g/dL	29–45 g/L

DESCRIPTION: Most of the body's total protein is a combination of albumin and globulins. Albumin, the protein present in the highest concentrations, is the main transport protein in the body. Albumin also maintains plasma oncotic pressure. Serum albumin values are affected by the process of synthesis, distribution, and degradation. Low levels may be the result of either inadequate production or excessive loss. Albumin levels are more useful as an indicator of chronic deficiency than of short-term deficiency.

Albumin levels are affected by posture. Results from specimens collected in an upright posture are higher than results from specimens collected in a supine position.

The A/G ratio is useful in the evaluation of liver and kidney disease. The ratio is calculated using the following formula:

albumin/(total protein − albumin), where globulin is the difference between the total protein value and the albumin value. For example, with a total protein of 7 g/dL and albumin of 4 g/dL, the A/G ratio is calculated as 4/(7 − 4) or 4/3 = 1.33. A reversal in the ratio where globulin exceeds albumin (i.e., ratio less than 1.0) is clinically significant.■

INDICATIONS:

- Assess nutritional status of hospitalized patients, especially geriatric patients
- Evaluate chronic illness
- Evaluate liver disease

RESULT

Increased in:

- Any condition that results in a decrease of plasma water (e.g., dehydration)
- Hyperinfusion of albumin

Decreased in:

- Insufficient intake:
  Malabsorption
  Malnutrition

- Decreased synthesis by the liver:
  Acute and chronic liver disease
  (e.g., alcoholism, cirrhosis,
  hepatitis)

- Inflammation and chronic diseases:
  Amyloidosis
  Bacterial infections
  Monoclonal gammopathies (e.g.,
  multiple myeloma,
  Waldenström's
  macroglobulinemia)
  Neoplasm
  Parasitic infestations
  Peptic ulcer
  Prolonged immobilization
  Rheumatic diseases
  Severe skin disease

- Increased loss over body surface:
  Rapid hydration or overhydration
  Burns
  Enteropathies related to sensitivity
  to ingested substances (e.g.,
  gluten sensitivity, Crohn's
  disease, ulcerative colitis)
  Fistula (gastrointestinal or
  lymphatic)
  Hemorrhage
  Kidney disease
  Renal protein loss
  Repeated thoracentesis or
  paracentesis
  Trauma and crush injuries

- Increased catabolism:
  Fever
  Cushing's disease
  Preeclampsia
  Thyroid dysfunction

- Increased blood volume (hypervolemia):
  Congestive heart failure
  Pregnancy
  Monoclonal gammopathies
  (Waldenström's disease, myeloma)

CRITICAL VALUES: N/A

INTERFERING FACTORS:
- Drugs that may increase albumin levels include enalapril.

- Drugs that may decrease albumin levels include acetaminophen (poisoning), dapsone, dextran, estrogens, ibuprofen, nitrofurantoin, oral contraceptives, phenytoin, prednisone (high doses), trazodone, and valproic acid.

- Availability of administered drugs is affected by variations in albumin levels.

Nursing Implications and Procedure

Pretest:

➤ Obtain a history of the patient's complaints, including a list of known allergens.

➤ Obtain a history of the patient's gastrointestinal, genitourinary, and hepatobiliary system and results of previously performed tests and procedures. For related tests, refer to the gastrointestinal, genitourinary, hepatobiliary system, and therapeutic/toxicology tables.

➤ Obtain a list of the medications the patient is taking, including herbs, nutritional supplements, and nutraceuticals. The requesting health care practitioner and laboratory should be advised if the patient regularly uses these products so that their effects can be taken into consideration when reviewing results.

➤ There are no food, fluid, or medication restrictions unless by medical direction.

➤ Review the procedure with the patient.

➤ Inform the patient that specimen collection takes approximately 5 to 10 minutes.

Intratest:

➤ Direct the patient to breathe normally and to avoid unnecessary movement.

➤ Observe standard precautions and follow the general guidelines in Appendix A.

➤ Perform a venipuncture, and collect the specimen in a 5-mL red- or tiger-top tube.

➤ Label the specimen, and promptly transport it to the laboratory.

Post-test:

➤ Observe venipuncture site for bleeding or hematoma formation. Apply pressure bandage.

➤ Dietary recommendations may be indicated and vary depending on the severity of the condition. Ammonia levels may be used to determine whether protein should be added to or reduced from the diet.

➤ Evaluate test results in relation to the patient's symptoms and other tests performed. Related laboratory tests include alanine aminotransferase, alkaline phosphatase, ammonia, aspartate aminotransferase, bilirubin, electrolytes, γ-glutamyl transpeptidase, hemoglobin, hematocrit, hepatitis antibodies and antigens, liver biopsy, osmolality, prealbumin, protein, protein electrophoresis, and smooth muscle antibody.

ALDOLASE

SYNONYM/ACRONYM: ALD.

SPECIMEN: Serum (1 mL) collected in a red- or tiger-top tube.

REFERENCE VALUE: (Method: Spectrophotometry)

Age	Conventional Units	SI Units (Conversion Factor ×0.017)
Newborn–2 y	3.4–11.8 U/L	0.06–0.20 µKat/L
25 m–16 y	1.2–8.8 U/L	0.02–0.15 µKat/L
Adult	Less than 7.4 U/L	Less than 0.13 µKat/L

DESCRIPTION: Aldolase (ALD), an enzyme found throughout the body, catalyzes the breakdown of glucose to lactate. Highest concentrations of this enzyme are found in skeletal and cardiac muscle, liver, and pancreas. When trauma or disease causes cellular breakdown of these muscles or organs, large amounts of ALD are released into the blood. Measuring serum levels helps to determine the presence, and in some cases the progress, of disease. This test is not commonly requested because the assay of other liver enzymes and creatine kinase is generally sufficient to provide the necessary information. ∎

INDICATIONS:
- Assist in the diagnosis of Duchenne's muscular dystrophy
- Differentiate neuromuscular disorders from neurologic disorders, such as multiple sclerosis or myasthenia gravis

RESULT

Increased in:
- Carcinoma (lung, breast, and genitourinary tract, and metastasis to liver)
- Central nervous system tumors
- Delirium tremens
- Dermatomyositis
- Duchenne's muscular dystrophy
- Gangrene
- Hemolytic anemias
- Hepatitis (acute viral or toxic)
- Infectious mononucleosis
- Leukemia (granulocytic and megaloblastic)
- Limb girdle muscular dystrophy
- Myocardial infarction
- Pancreatitis (acute)
- Polymyositis
- Psychoses and schizophrenia (acute)

• Severe crush injuries

• Tetanus

• Trichinosis

Decreased in:
• Hereditary fructose intolerance

CRITICAL VALUES: N/A

INTERFERING FACTORS:
• Drugs that may increase aldolase levels include aminocaproic acid, carbenoxolone, clofibrate, chlorinated and organophosphorus insecticides, labetalol, and thiabendazole.

• Drugs that may decrease aldolase levels include phenothiazines (in schizophrenic patients with high initial values) and probucol.

• Intramuscular injections may increase aldolase levels as a result of muscle trauma.

• Red blood cells contain aldolase; hemolysis may cause a false elevation in values.

Nursing Implications and Procedure

Pretest:

➤ Obtain a history of the patient's complaints, including a list of known allergens.

➤ Obtain history of neuromuscular disorders, related treatments, and complaints of muscle fatigue or loss of strength.

➤ Obtain a history of the patient's hepatobiliary and musculoskeletal system and results of previously performed tests and procedures. For related tests, refer to the hepatobil-

iary and musculoskeletal system tables.

➤ Obtain a list of the medications the patient is taking, including herbs, nutritional supplements, and nutraceuticals. The requesting health care practitioner and laboratory should be advised if the patient regularly uses these products so that their effects can be taken into consideration when reviewing results.

➤ There are no food, fluid, or medication restrictions unless by medical direction.

➤ Review the procedure with the patient.

➤ Inform the patient that specimen collection takes approximately 5 to 10 minutes.

Intratest:

➤ Direct the patient to breathe normally and to avoid unnecessary movement.

➤ Observe standard precautions and follow the general guidelines in Appendix A. Perform a venipuncture, and collect the specimen in a 5-mL red- or tiger-top tube.

➤ Label the specimen, and promptly transport it to the laboratory.

Post-test:

➤ Observe venipuncture site for bleeding or hematoma formation. Apply pressure bandage.

➤ Evaluate test results in relation to the patient's symptoms and other test results. Related laboratory tests include alkaline phosphatase, antimitochondrial antibody, aspartate aminotransferase, creatine kinase and isoenzymes, Jo-1 antibody, lactate dehydrogenase and isoenzymes, liver biopsy, muscle biopsy, and myoglobin.

ALDOSTERONE

SYNONYM/ACRONYM: N/A.

SPECIMEN: Serum (1 mL) collected in a red- or tiger-top tube. Plasma (1 mL) collected in green-top (heparin) or lavender-top (ethylenediaminetetra-acetic acid [EDTA]) tube is also acceptable.

REFERENCE VALUE: (Method: Radioimmunoassay)

Age	Conventional Units	SI Units (Conversion Factor ×0.0277)
Cord blood	40–200 ng/dL	1.11–5.54 nmol/L
3 d–1 wk	7–184 ng/dL	0.19–5.10 nmol/L
1 mo–1 y	5–90 ng/dL	0.14–2.49 nmol/L
13–23 mo	7–54 ng/dL	0.19–1.50 nmol/L
2–10 y		
Supine	3–35 ng/dL	0.08–0.97 nmol/L
Upright	5–80 ng/dL	0.14–2.22 nmol/L
11–15 y		
Supine	2–22 ng/dL	0.06–0.61 nmol/L
Upright	4–48 ng/dL	0.11–1.33 nmol/L
Adult		
Supine	3–16 ng/dL	0.08–0.44 nmol/L
Upright	7–30 ng/dL	0.19–0.83 nmol/L

These values reflect a normal-sodium diet. Values for a low-sodium diet are three to five times higher.

DESCRIPTION: Aldosterone is a mineralocorticoid secreted by the zona glomerulosa of the adrenal cortex in response to decreased serum sodium, decreased blood volume, and increased serum potassium. Aldosterone increases sodium reabsorption in the renal tubules, resulting in potassium excretion and increased water retention, blood volume, and blood pressure. A variety of factors influence serum aldosterone levels, including sodium intake, certain medications, and activity. This test is of little diagnostic value unless plasma renin activity is measured simultaneously (see chapter titled "Renin"). Patients with serum potassium less than 3.6 mEq/L and 24-hour urine potassium greater than 40mEq/L fit the general criteria to test for aldosteronism. Renin is low in primary aldosteronism and high in secondary aldosteronism. A ratio of plasma aldosterone to plasma renin activity greater than 50 is significant. ∎

INDICATIONS:
- Evaluate hypertension of unknown cause, especially with hypokalemia not induced by diuretics
- Investigate suspected hyperaldosteronism, as indicated by elevated levels
- Investigate suspected hypoaldosteronism, as indicated by decreased levels

RESULT

Increased with Decreased Renin Levels

Primary hyperaldosteronism:
- Adenomas (Conn's syndrome)
- Bilateral hyperplasia of the aldosterone-secreting zona glomerulosa cells

Increased with Increased Renin Levels

Secondary hyperaldosteronism:
- Bartter's syndrome
- Cardiac failure
- Chronic obstructive pulmonary disease
- Cirrhosis with ascites formation
- Diuretic abuse
- Hypovolemia secondary to hemorrhage and transudation
- Laxative abuse
- Nephrotic syndrome
- Starvation (after 10 days)
- Thermal stress
- Toxemia of pregnancy

Decreased

Without hypertension:
- Addison's disease
- Hypoaldosteronism secondary to renin deficiency
- Isolated aldosterone deficiency

With hypertension:
- Acute alcohol intoxication
- Diabetes
- Excess secretion of deoxycorticosterone
- Turner's syndrome (25 percent of cases)

CRITICAL VALUES: N/A

INTERFERING FACTORS:
- Drugs that may increase aldosterone levels include amiloride, ammonium chloride, angiotensin, angiotensin II, dobutamine, dopamine, endralazine, fenoldopam, hydralazine, hydrochlorothiazide, laxatives (abuse), metoclopramide, nifedipine, opiates, potassium, spironolactone, and zacopride.

- Drugs that may decrease aldosterone levels include atenolol, captopril, carvedilol, cilazapril, enalapril, fadrozole, glycyrrhiza, ibopamine, indomethacin, lisinopril, nicardipine, nonsteroidal anti-inflammatory drugs, perindopril, ranitidine, saline, sinorphan, and verapamil. Prolonged heparin therapy also decreases aldosterone levels.

- Upright body posture, stress, strenuous exercise, and late pregnancy can lead to increased levels.

- Recent radioactive scans or radiation within 1 week before the test can interfere with test results when radioimmunoassay is the test method.

- Diet can significantly affect results. A low-sodium diet can increase serum aldosterone, whereas a high-sodium diet can decrease levels. Decreased serum sodium and elevated serum potassium increase aldosterone secretion. Elevated serum sodium and decreased serum potassium suppress aldosterone secretion.

Nursing Implications and Procedure • • • • • • • • • • •

Pretest: ◼

➤ Obtain a history of the patient's complaints, including a list of known allergens.

➤ Obtain a history of known or suspected fluid or electrolyte imbalance, hypertension, renal function, or stage of pregnancy. Note the amount of sodium ingested in the diet over the past 2 weeks.

➤ Obtain a history of the patient's endocrine and genitourinary system and results of previously performed tests and procedures. For related tests, refer to the endocrine and genitourinary system tables.

➤ Obtain a list of the medications the patient is taking, including herbs, nutritional supplements, and nutraceuticals. The requesting health care practitioner and laboratory should be advised if the patient is regularly using these products so that their effects can be taken into consideration when reviewing results.

➤ Note any recent procedures that can interfere with test results.

➤ The patient should be on a normal-sodium diet (1 to 2 g of sodium per day) for 2 to 4 weeks before the test.

➤ Under medical direction, the patient should avoid diuretics, antihypertensive drugs and herbals, and cyclic progestogens and estrogens for 2 to 4 weeks before the test.

➤ Review the procedure with the patient. Inform the patient that multiple specimens may be required.

➤ Inform the patient that the required position, supine/lying down or upright/sitting up, must be maintained for 2 hours before specimen collection.

➤ Inform the patient that each specimen collection takes approximately 5 to 10 minutes.

Intratest: ◼

➤ Ensure that the patient has complied with dietary preparations and other pretesting restrictions.

➤ Direct the patient to breathe normally and to avoid unnecessary movement.

➤ Observe standard precautions and follow the general guidelines in Appendix A. Perform a venipuncture after the patient has been in the upright (sitting or standing) position for 2 hours. If a supine specimen is requested on an inpatient, the specimen should be collected early in the morning before rising. Collect the specimen in a 5-mL red- or tiger-top tube.

➤ Label the specimen, and promptly transport it to the laboratory on ice. Specify patient position (upright or supine) and exact source of specimen (peripheral versus arterial).

Post-test: ◼

➤ Observe venipuncture site for bleeding or hematoma formation. Apply pressure bandage.

➤ Instruct the patient to resume usual diet and medication as directed by the health care practitioner.

➤ Instruct the patient to notify the health care practitioner of any signs and symptoms of dehydration or fluid overload related to elevated aldosterone levels or compromised sodium regulatory mechanisms.

➤ Aldosterone levels are involved in the regulation of body fluid volume. Educate patients about the importance of proper water balance. Although there is no recommended dietary allowance (RDA) for water, adults need 1 mL/kcal per day. Infants need more water because their basal metabolic heat production is much higher than in adults. Tap water may also contain other nutrients. Water-softening systems replace minerals (e.g., calcium, magnesium, iron) with sodium, so caution should be used if a low-sodium diet is prescribed.

➤ Because aldosterone levels have an effect on sodium levels, some consideration may be given to dietary adjustment if sodium allowances need to be regulated. Educate patients with low sodium levels that the major source of dietary sodium is table salt. Many foods, such as milk and other dairy products, are also good sources of dietary sodium. Most other dietary sodium is available through consumption of processed foods. Patients who need to follow low-sodium diets should avoid beverages such as colas, ginger ale, Gatorade, lemon-lime sodas, and root beer. Many over-the-counter medications, including antacids, laxatives, analgesics, sedatives, and antitussives, contain significant amounts of sodium. The best advice is to emphasize the importance of reading all food, beverage, and medicine labels. In 1989, the Subcommittee on the 10th Edition of the RDAs established 500 mg as the recommended minimum limit for dietary intake of sodium. There are no RDAs established for potassium, but the estimated minimum intake for adults is 200 mEq/d. Potassium is present in all plant and animal cells, making dietary replacement simple. A health care practitioner or nutritionist should be consulted before considering the use of salt substitutes.

➤ Evaluate test results in relation to the patient's symptoms and other tests performed. Related laboratory tests include catecholamines, urine catecholamines, cortisol, creatinine, urine creatinine, glucose, kidney biopsy, magnesium, urine magnesium, osmolality, urine osmolality, potassium, urine potassium, urine protein, renin, sodium, urine sodium, urea nitrogen, and urinalysis.

ALKALINE PHOSPHATASE AND ISOENZYMES

. . . .

SYNONYMS/ACRONYM: Alk Phos, ALP and fractionation, heat-stabile ALP.

SPECIMEN: Serum (1 mL) collected in a red- or tiger-top tube. Plasma (1 mL) collected in green-top (heparin) tube is also acceptable.

REFERENCE VALUE: (Method: Spectrophotometry for total alkaline phosphatase, inhibition/electrophoresis for fractionation)

Total ALP	Conventional Units	SI Units (Conversion Factor $\times 0.017$)	Bone Fraction	Liver Fraction
1–5 y				
Male	56–350 U/L	0.95–5.95 µKat/L	39–308 U/L	Less than 8–101 U/L
Female	73–378 U/L	1.24–6.43 µKat/L	56–300 U/L	Less than 8–53 U/L
6–7 y				
Male	70–364 U/L	1.19–6.19 µKat/L	50–319 U/L	Less than 8–76 U/L
Female	73–378 U/L	1.24–6.43 µKat/L	56–300 U/L	Less than 8–53 U/L
8 y				
Male	70–364 U/L	1.19–6.19 µKat/L	50–258 U/L	Less than 8–62 U/L
Female	98–448 U/L	1.67–7.62 µKat/L	78–353 U/L	Less than 8–62 U/L
9–12 y				
Male	112–476 U/L	1.90–8.09 µKat/L	78–339 U/L	Less than 8–81 U/L
Female	98–448 U/L	1.67–7.62 µKat/L	78–353 U/L	Less than 8–62 U/L
13 y				
Male	112–476 U/L	1.90–8.09 µKat/L	78–389 U/L	Less than 8–48 U/L
Female	56–350 U/L	0.95–5.95 µKat/L	28–252 U/L	Less than 8–50 U/L
14 y				
Male	112–476 U/L	1.90–8.09 µKat/L	78–389 U/L	Less than 8–48 U/L
Female	56–266 U/L	0.95–4.52 µKat/L	31–190 U/L	Less than 8–48 U/L
15 y				
Male	70–378 U/L	1.19–6.43 µKat/L	48–311 U/L	Less than 8–39 U/L
	42–168 U/L	0.71–2.86 µKat/L	20–115 U/L	
Female				Less than 8–53 U/L
16 y				
Male	70–378 U/L	1.19–6.43 µKat/L	48–311 U/L	Less than 8–39 U/L
Female	28–126 U/L	0.48–2.14 µKat/L	14–87 U/L	Less than 8–50 U/L
17 y				
Male	56–238 U/L	0.95–4.05 µKat/L	34–190 U/L	Less than 8–39 U/L
Female	28–126 U/L	0.48–2.14 µKat/L	17–84 U/L	Less than 8–53 U/L

(Continued on the following page)

Total ALP	Conventional Units	SI Units (Conversion Factor ×0.017)	Bone Fraction	Liver Fraction
18 y				
Male	56–182 U/L	0.95–3.09 µKat/L	34–146 U/L	Less than 8–39 U/L
Female	28–126 U/L	0.48–2.14 µKat/L	17–84 U/L	Less than 8–53 U/L
19 y				
Male	42–154 U/L	0.71–2.62 µKat/L	25–123 U/L	Less than 8–39 U/L
Female	28–126 U/L	0.48–2.14 µKat/L	17–84 U/L	Less than 8–53 U/L
20 y				
Male	45–138 U/L	0.76–2.35 µKat/L	25–73 U/L	Less than 8–48 U/L
Female	33–118 U/L	0.56–2.01 µKat/L	17–56 U/L	Less than 8–50 U/L
Adult				
Male	35–142 U/L	0.60–2.41 µKat/L	11–73 U/L	0–93 U/L
Female	25–125 U/L	0.42–2.12 µKat/L		

DESCRIPTION: ALP is an enzyme found in the liver, in Kupffer cells lining the biliary tract, and in bones, intestines, and placenta. Additional sources of ALP include the proximal tubules of the kidneys, pulmonary alveolar cells, germ cells, vascular bed, lactating mammary glands, and granulocytes of circulating blood. ALP is referred to as alkaline because it functions optimally at a pH of 9.0. This test is most useful for determining the presence of liver or bone disease.

Isoelectric focusing methods can identify 12 isoenzymes of ALP. Certain cancers produce small amounts of distinctive Regan and Nagao ALP isoenzymes. Four main ALP isoenzymes, however, are of clinical significance: ALP_1 of liver origin, ALP_2 of bone origin, ALP_3 of intestinal origin (occasionally present in individuals with blood type O and B), and ALP_4 of placental origin (third trimester). ALP levels vary by age and gender. Values in children are higher than in adults because of the level of bone growth and development. An immunoassay method is available for measuring bone-specific ALP as an indicator of increased bone turnover and estrogen deficiency in postmenopausal women. ■

INDICATIONS:

• Evaluate signs and symptoms of various disorders associated with elevated ALP levels, such as biliary obstruction, hepatobiliary disease, and bone disease, including malignant processes

• Differentiate obstructive hepatobiliary tract disorders from hepatocellular disease; greater elevations of ALP are seen in the former

- Determine effects of renal disease on bone metabolism
- Determine bone growth or destruction in children with abnormal growth patterns

RESULT

Increased in:
- Liver disease:
  Biliary atresia
  Biliary obstruction
  Chronic active hepatitis
  Cirrhosis
  Diabetes mellitus (diabetic hepatic lipidosis)
  Extrahepatic duct obstruction
  Granulomatous or infiltrative liver diseases
  Infectious mononucleosis
  Viral hepatitis
- Bone disease:
  Healing fractures
  Metabolic bone diseases (rickets, osteomalacia)
  Metastatic tumors in bone
  Osteogenic sarcoma
  Osteoporosis
  Paget's disease (osteitis deformans)
- Other conditions:
  Advanced pregnancy
  Amyloidosis
  Cancer of the lung or pancreas
  Chronic renal failure
  Congestive heart failure
  Growing children
  Hodgkin's disease
  Hyperparathyroidism (primary or secondary to chronic renal disease)
  Perforated bowel
  Pulmonary and myocardial infarctions
  Sarcoidosis

Ulcerative colitis

Decreased in:
- Anemia (severe)
- Cretinism
- Hypophosphatasia (congenital, rare)
- Hypothyroidism
- Kwashiorkor
- Nutritional deficiency of zinc or magnesium
- Scurvy

CRITICAL VALUES: N/A

INTERFERING FACTORS:
- Drugs that may increase ALP levels by causing cholestasis include amitryptyline, anabolic steroids, androgens, benzodiazepines, chlorothiazide, chlorpropamide, dapsone, erythromycin, estrogens, ethionamide, gold salts, imipramine, mercaptopurine, nitrofurans, oral contraceptives, penicillins, phenothiazines, progesterone, propoxyphene, sulfonamides, tamoxifen, and tolbutamide.

- Drugs that may increase ALP levels by causing hepatocellular damage include acetaminophen (toxic), acetylsalicylic acid, allopurinol, amiodarone, anabolic steroids, anticonvulsants, asparaginase, azithromycin, bromocriptine, captopril, cephalosporins, chloramphenicol, clindamycin, clofibrate, danazol, enflurane, ethambutol, ethionamide, fenofibrate, fluconazole, fluoroquinolones, foscarnet, gentamicin, indomethacin, interferon, interleukin-2, levamisole, levodopa, lincomycin, low-molecular-weight heparin, methyldopa, monoamine oxidase inhibitors, naproxen, nifedipine, nitrofurans, oral contraceptives, probenecid, procainamide, quinine, ranitidine, retinol, ritodrine, sulfonylureas, tetracyclines, tobramycin, and verapamil.

- Drugs that may cause an overall decrease in ALP levels include calcitriol, clodronate, clofibrate, cyclosporine, etidronate, ipriflavone, norethisterone, oral contraceptives, pamidronate, tamoxifen, theophylline, and ursodiol.

- Hemolyzed specimens may cause falsely elevated results.

Nursing Implications and Procedure • • • • • • • • • • •

Pretest:

➤ Obtain a history of the patient's complaints, including a list of known allergens.

➤ Obtain a history of the patient's hepatobiliary and musculoskeletal system and results of previously performed tests and procedures. For related tests, refer to the hepatobiliary and musculoskeletal system tables.

➤ Obtain a list of the medications the patient is taking, including herbs, nutritional supplements, and nutraceuticals. The requesting health care practitioner and laboratory should be advised if the patient is regularly using these products so that their effects can be taken into consideration when reviewing results.

➤ There are no food, fluid, or medication restrictions unless by medical direction.

➤ Review the procedure with the patient.

➤ Inform the patient that specimen collection takes approximately 5 to 10 minutes.

Intratest:

➤ Direct the patient to breathe normally and to avoid unnecessary movement.

➤ Observe standard precautions and follow the general guidelines in Appendix A. Perform a venipuncture, and collect the specimen in a 5-mL red- or tiger-top tube.

➤ Label the specimen, and promptly transport it to the laboratory.

Post-test:

➤ Observe venipuncture site for bleeding or hematoma formation. Apply pressure bandage.

➤ Increased ALP levels may be associated with liver disease. Dietary recommendations may be indicated and vary depending on the severity of the condition. A low-protein diet may be in order if the patient's liver has lost the ability to process the end products of protein metabolism. A diet of soft foods may be required if esophageal varices have developed. Ammonia levels may be used to determine whether protein should be added to or reduced from the diet. Patients should be encouraged to eat simple carbohydrates and emulsified fats (as in homogenized milk or eggs), as opposed to complex carbohydrates (e.g., starch, fiber, and glycogen [animal carbohydrates]) and complex fats, which would require additional bile to emulsify it so that it can be used. The cirrhotic patient should be carefully observed for the development of ascites, in which case fluid and electrolyte balance requires strict attention.

➤ Evaluate test results in relation to the patient's symptoms and other tests performed. Related laboratory tests include acetaminophen, ammonia, alanine aminotransferase, albumin, α_1-antitrypsin, α_1-antitrypsin phenotyping, ammonia, anti-DNA antibodies, antimitochondrial antibodies, antinuclear antibodies, anti–smooth muscle antibodies, aspartate aminotransferase, bilirubin (total, direct, and indirect), bone biopsy, calcium, ceruloplasmin, C3 complement, C4 complement, copper, electrolytes, γ-glutamyl transpeptidase, hepatitis antigens and antibodies, liver biopsy, magnesium, parathyroid hormone, phosphorus, protein, protein electrophoresis, prothrombin time, salicylate, vitamin D, and zinc.

ALLERGEN-SPECIFIC IMMUNOGLOBULIN E

SYNONYMS/ACRONYM: Allergen profile, radioallergosorbent test (RAST).

SPECIMEN: Serum (2 mL per group of six allergens, 0.5 mL for each additional individual allergen) collected in a red- or tiger-top tube.

REFERENCE VALUE: (Method: Radioimmunoassay)

RAST Scoring Method		Alternate Scoring Method (ASM): Increasing Levels of Allergy Sensitivity	
Specific IgE Antibody Level	kIU/L	ASM Class	ASM % Reference
Absent or undetectable	Less than 0.35	0	Less than 70
Low	0.35–0.70	1	70–109
Moderate	0.71–3.50	2	110–219
High	3.51–17.50	3	220–599
Very high	Greater than 17.50	4	600–1999
		5	2000–5999
		6	Greater than 5999

DESCRIPTION: Allergen-specific immunoglobulin E (IgE) or RAST is generally requested for groups of allergens commonly known to incite an allergic response in the affected individual. The test is based on the use of a radiolabeled anti-IgE reagent to detect IgE in the patient's serum, produced in response to specific allergens. The panels include allergens such as animal dander, antibiotics, dust, foods, grasses, insects, trees, mites, molds, venom, and weeds. Allergen testing is useful for evaluating the cause of hay fever, extrinsic asthma, atopic eczema, respiratory allergies, and potentially fatal reactions to insect venom, penicillin, and other drugs or chemicals. RAST has replaced skin tests and provocation procedures, which were inconvenient, painful, and hazardous to patients. ■

INDICATIONS:
• Test for specific allergic sensitivity before initiating immunotherapy or desensitization shots

- Test for specific allergic sensitivity, when skin testing is unreliable
- Test for allergens when there is a known history of severe allergic reaction to skin testing
- Evaluate patients who refuse to submit to skin testing or who have generalized dermatitis or other dermatopathic conditions
- Test for allergens when skin testing is inappropriate, such as in infants
- Monitor response to desensitization procedures

RESULT: Different scoring systems are used in the interpretation of RAST results.

Increased in:
- Allergic rhinitis
- Anaphylaxis
- Asthma (exogenous)
- Atopic dermatitis
- *Echinococcus* infection
- Eczema
- Hay fever
- Hookworm infection
- Schistosomiasis
- Visceral larva migrans

Decreased in:
- Asthma (endogenous)
- Pregnancy
- Radiation therapy

CRITICAL VALUES: N/A

INTERFERING FACTORS: Recent radioactive scans or radiation within 1 week of the test can interfere with test results when radioimmunoassay is the test method.

Nursing Implications and Procedure

Pretest:

➤ Obtain a history of the patient's complaints, including a list of known allergens.

➤ Obtain a history of the patient's immune and respiratory system and results of previously performed tests and procedures. For related tests, refer to the immune and respiratory system table.

➤ Obtain a list of the medications the patient is taking, including herbs, nutritional supplements, and nutraceuticals. The requesting health care practitioner and laboratory should be advised if the patient regularly uses these products so that their effects can be taken into consideration when reviewing results.

➤ Note any recent procedures that can interfere with test results.

➤ There are no food, fluid, or medication restrictions unless by medical direction.

➤ Review the procedure with the patient.

➤ Inform the patient that specimen collection takes approximately 5 to 10 minutes.

Intratest:

➤ Direct the patient to breathe normally and to avoid unnecessary movement.

➤ Observe standard precautions and follow the general guidelines in Appendix A. Perform a venipuncture, and collect the specimen in a 5-mL red- or tiger-top tube.

➤ The allergy panel desired should be indicated as part of the laboratory requisition process. Label the specimen, and promptly transport it to the laboratory.

➤ Observe venipuncture site for bleeding or hematoma formation. Apply pressure bandage.

➤ Consideration should be given to diet if food allergies are present. Lifestyle adjustments may be necessary depending on the specific allergens identified.

➤ Evaluate test results in relation to the patient's symptoms and other tests performed. Related laboratory tests include arterial/alveolar oxygen ratio, blood gases, complete blood count, eosinophil count, hypersensitivity pneumonitis, IgE, ova and parasites, and theophylline.

ALVEOLAR/ARTERIAL GRADIENT AND ARTERIAL/ALVEOLAR OXYGEN RATIO

SYNONYM/ACRONYMS: Alveolar-arterial difference, A/a gradient, a/A ratio.

SPECIMEN: Arterial blood (1 mL) collected in a heparinized syringe. Specimen should be transported tightly capped and in an ice slurry.

REFERENCE VALUE: (Method: Selective electrodes that measure pO_2 and pCO_2)

Alveolar/arterial gradient	Less than 10 mm Hg at rest (room air) 20–30 mm Hg at maximum exercise activity (room air)
Arterial/alveolar oxygen ratio	Greater than 0.75 (75%)

DESCRIPTION: The ability of oxygen to diffuse from the alveoli into the lungs is of use when assessing a patient's level of oxygenation. This test can help identify the cause of hypoxemia (low oxygen levels in the blood) and intrapulmonary shunting that might result from one of the following three situations: ventilated alveoli without perfusion, unventilated alveoli with perfusion, or collapse of alveoli and associated blood vessels. Information regarding the alveolar/arterial (A/a) gradient can be estimated indirectly using the partial pressure of oxygen (pO_2) (obtained from blood gas analysis) in a simple mathematical formula:

A/a gradient $=$ pO_2 in alveolar air (estimated) $-$ pO_2 in arterial blood (measured)

An estimate of alveolar pO_2 is accomplished by subtracting the water vapor pressure from the barometric pressure, multiplying the resulting pressure by the fraction of inspired oxygen (FIO_2; percentage of oxygen the patient is breathing), and subtracting this from $1^1/_4$ times the arterial partial pressure of carbon dioxide (pCO_2). The gradient is obtained by subtracting the patient's arterial pO_2 from the calculated alveolar pO_2.

Alveolar $pO_2 = [(\text{barometric pressure} - \text{water vapor pressure}) \times FIO_2] - [1^1/_4 \times pCO_2]$

A/a gradient $=$ arterial pO_2 (measured) $-$ alveolar pO_2 (estimated)

The arterial/alveolar (a/A) ratio reflects the percentage of alveolar pO_2 that is contained in arterial pO_2. It is calculated by dividing the arterial pO_2 by the alveolar pO_2:

$$a/A = paO_2/paO_2.$$

The A/a gradient increases as the concentration of oxygen the patient inspires increases. If the gradient is abnormally high, either there is a problem with the ability of oxygen to pass across the alveolar membrane or oxygenated blood is being mixed with nonoxygenated blood. The a/A ratio is not dependent on FIO_2; it does not increase with a corresponding increase in inhaled oxygen. For patients on a mechanical ventilator with a changing FIO_2, the a/A ratio can be used to determine if oxygen diffusion is improving. ∎

INDICATIONS:
• Assist in identifying the cause of hypoxemia

• Assess intrapulmonary or coronary artery shunting

RESULT

Increased in:
• Acute respiratory distress syndrome

• Atelectasis

• Atrial venous shunts

• Bronchospasm

• Chronic obstructive pulmonary disease

• Congenital cardiac septal defects

• Underventilated alveoli (mucus plugs)

• Pneumothorax

• Pulmonary edema

• Pulmonary embolus

• Pulmonary fibrosis

CRITICAL VALUES: N/A

INTERFERING FACTORS:
• Specimens should be collected before administration of oxygen therapy.

• The temperature of the patient should be noted and reported to the laboratory if significantly elevated or depressed so that measured values can be corrected to actual body temperature.

• Exposure of sample to room air affects test results.

• Values normally increase with increasing age (see monograph titled "Blood Gases").

• Samples for A/a gradient evaluation are obtained by arterial puncture, which carries a risk of bleeding, especially in patients with bleeding disorders or who are taking medications for a bleeding disorder.

• Prompt and proper specimen processing, storage, and analysis are important to achieve accurate results. Specimens should always be transported to the laboratory as quickly as possible after collection. Delay in transport of the sample or transportation without ice may affect test results.

Nursing Implications and Procedure · · · · · · · · · · ·

Pretest:

➤ Obtain a history of the patient's complaints, including a list of known allergens.

➤ Obtain a history of the patient's respiratory system and any bleeding disorders as well as results of previously performed tests and procedures, especially bleeding time, coagulation time, complete blood count, platelets, partial thromboplastin time, and prothrombin time. For related tests, refer to the respiratory system table.

➤ Obtain a list of medications the patient is taking, including anticoagulants, acetylsalicylic acid, herbals, and nutraceuticals; take particular note of any products that are known to affect coagulation. It is recommended that use of such products be discontinued 14 days before dental or surgical procedures. The requesting health care practitioner and laboratory should be advised if the patient regularly uses these products so that their effects can be taken into consideration when reviewing results.

➤ Note any recent procedures that can interfere with test results.

➤ There are no food, fluid, or medication restrictions unless by medical direction.

➤ Review the procedure with the patient.

➤ Perform the Allen test (see monograph titled "Blood Gases").

➤ Inform the patient that specimen collection usually takes approximately 15 to 20 minutes.

Intratest:

➤ Direct the patient to breathe normally and to avoid unnecessary movement.

➤ Observe standard precautions and follow the general guidelines in Appendix A.

➤ Perform an arterial puncture and collect the specimen in a heparinized syringe. There has been no difference in values noted when samples are collected in plastic versus glass syringes.

➤ Label the specimen, and promptly transport it to the laboratory. The tightly capped sample should be placed in an ice slurry immediately after collection. Information on the specimen label can be protected from water in the ice slurry if the specimen is first placed in a protective plastic bag.

Post-test:

➤ Observe arterial puncture site for bleeding or hematoma formation. Apply pressure bandage.

➤ Intervene appropriately for hypoxia and ventilatory disturbances.

➤ Evaluate test results in relation to the patient's symptoms and other tests performed. Related laboratory tests include allergen-specific immunoglobulin E (IgE), α_1-antitrypsin, α_1-antitrypsin phenotyping, blood gases, D-dimer, electrolytes, eosinophil count, fibrinogen, hypersensitivity pneumonitis, IgE, and theophylline.

ALZHEIMER'S DISEASE MARKERS

SYNONYMS/ACRONYMS: CSF tau protein and β-amyloid 42, AD.

SPECIMEN: Cerebrospinal fluid (CSF) (1 to 2 mL) collected in a plain plastic conical tube.

REFERENCE VALUE: (Method: Enzyme-linked immunosorbent assay) Tau protein and β-amyloid 42 measurements in CSF are used in conjunction as biochemical markers of Alzheimer's disease (AD). Scientific studies indicate that a combination of elevated tau protein and decreased β-amyloid 42 protein levels are consistent with the presence of AD. Values are highly dependent on the reagents and standards used in the assay. Ranges vary among laboratories; the testing laboratory should be consulted for interpretation of results.

DESCRIPTION: AD is the most common cause of dementia in the elderly population. AD is a disorder of the central nervous system that results in progressive and profound memory loss followed by loss of cognitive abilities and death. It may follow years of progressive formation of amyloid plaques and brain tangles, or it may appear as an early-onset form of the disease. Two recognized pathological features of AD are neurofibrillary tangles and amyloid plaques found in the brain. Abnormal forms of the microtubule-associated tau protein are the main component of the classic neurofibrillary tangles found in patients with AD. Tau protein concentration is believed to reflect the number of neurofibrillary tangles and may be an indication of the severity of the disease. β-Amyloid 42 is a free-floating protein normally present in CSF. It is believed to accumulate in the central nervous system of patients with AD, causing the formation of amyloid plaques on brain tissue. The result is that these patients have lower CSF values compared to age-matched non-AD control subjects. ∎

INDICATIONS:
• Assist in establishing a diagnosis of AD

RESULT

Increased in:

• Acquired immunodeficiency syndrome
• AD
• Cerebrovascular disease
• Creutzfeldt-Jakob disease
• Meningoencephalitis
• Pick's disease

CRITICAL VALUES: N/A

INTERFERING FACTORS:
- Some patients with AD may have normal levels of tau protein because of an insufficient number of neurofibrillary tangles.

Nursing Implications and Procedure • • • • • • • • • • •

Pretest:

➤ Obtain a history of the patient's complaints, including a list of known allergens.

➤ Review results of tests and procedures previously performed.

➤ Obtain a list of the medications the patient is taking, including herbs, nutritional supplements, and nutraceuticals. The requesting health care practitioner and laboratory should be advised if the patient regularly uses these products so that their effects can be taken into consideration when reviewing results.

➤ There are no food, fluid, or medication restrictions unless by medical direction.

➤ Inform the patient that the position required for the lumbar puncture may be awkward but that someone will assist. Stress the importance of remaining still and breathing normally throughout the procedure.

➤ Inform the patient that a stinging sensation may be felt as the local anesthetic is injected. Tell the patient to report any pain or other sensations that may require repositioning of the spinal needle.

➤ Review the procedure with the patient.

➤ Inform the patient that the procedure will be performed by a health care practitioner and will take approximately 20 minutes.

➤ Determine whether the patient has an allergy to local anesthetics and

inform the health care practitioner accordingly.

➤ *Obtain written and informed consent before administering any medication before the procedure.*

Intratest:

➤ Direct the patient to breathe normally and to avoid unnecessary movement.

➤ Observe standard precautions and follow the general guidelines in Appendix A.

➤ To perform a lumbar puncture, position the patient in the knee-chest position at the side of the bed. Provide pillows to support the spine or for the patient to grasp. The sitting position is an alternative. In this position, the patient must bend the neck and chest to the knees.

➤ Prepare the site (usually between L3 and L4 or L4 and L5) with povidone-iodine, and drape the area.

➤ A local anesthetic is injected. Using sterile technique, the health care practitioner inserts the spinal needle through the spinous processes of the vertebrae and into the subarachnoid space. The stylet is removed. CSF drips from the needle if it is properly placed.

➤ Attach the stopcock and manometer, and measure initial CSF pressure. Normal pressure for an adult in the lateral recumbent position is 90 to 180 mm H_2O. These values depend on the body position and are different in a horizontal or sitting position.

➤ If the initial pressure is elevated, the health care practitioner may perform Queckenstedt's test. To perform this test, apply pressure to the jugular vein for about 10 seconds. CSF pressure usually rises in response to the occlusion, then rapidly returns to normal within 10 seconds after the pressure is released. Sluggish response may indicate CSF obstruction.

➤ Obtain CSF. Take a final pressure reading and remove the needle. Clean the puncture site with an antiseptic solution, and apply a small bandage.

➤ Label the specimen, and promptly transport it to the laboratory.

Post-test: ∎

➤ Administer fluids, if permitted, to replace lost CSF and help prevent or relieve headache, which is a side effect of lumbar puncture.

➤ Position the patient flat, either on the back or abdomen, although some health care practitioners allow 30° elevation. Maintain this position for 8 hours. Changing position is acceptable as long as the body remains horizontal.

➤ Check the puncture site for leakage, and frequently monitor body signs, such as temperature and blood pressure.

➤ Observe the patient for neurologic changes, such as altered level of consciousness, change in pupils, reports of tingling or numbness, and irritability.

➤ Recognize anxiety related to test results. Provide teaching and information regarding the clinical implications of the test results, as appropriate. Reassure family members and offer access to appropriate counseling and other supportive services.

➤ Evaluate test results in relation to the patient's symptoms and other tests performed.

AMINO ACID SCREEN, BLOOD

SYNONYM/ACRONYM: N/A.

SPECIMEN: Serum (1 mL) collected in a red- or tiger-top tube. Plasma (1 mL) collected in green-top (heparin) tube is also acceptable.

REFERENCE VALUE: (Method: Chromatography) There are numerous amino acids. The following tables include the most frequently screened. All units are nanomoles per milliliter (nmol/mL).

Age	Alanine	β-Alanine	Anserine	α-Amino-adipic Acid	α-Amino-n-butyric Acid
Premature	212–504	0	—	0	14–52
Newborn–1 mo	131–710	0–10	0	0	8–24
2 mo–2 y	143–439	0–7	0	0	3–26
2–18 y	152–547	0–7	0	0	4–31
Adult	177–583	0–12	0	0–6	5–41

Age	γ-Amino-butyric Acid	β-Aminoiso-butyric Acid	Arginine	Asparagine	Aspartic Acid
Premature	0	0	34–96	90–295	24–50
Newborn–1 mo	0–2	0	6–140	29–132	20–129
2 mo–2 y	0	0	12–133	21–95	0–23
2–18 y	0	0	10–140	23–112	1–24
Adult	0	0	15–128	35–74	1–25

Age	Carnosine	Citrulline	Cysta-thionine	Cystine	Ethanol-amine
Premature	—	20–87	5–10	15–70	—
Newborn–1 mo	0–19	10–45	0–3	17–98	0–115
2 mo–2 y	0	3–35	0–5	16–84	0–4
2–18 y	0	1–46	0–3	5–45	0–7
Adult	0	12–55	0–3	5–82	0–153

Age	Glutamic Acid	Glutamine	Glycine	Histidine	Homo-cystine
Premature	107–276	248–850	298–602	72–134	3–20
Newborn–1 mo	62–620	376–709	232–740	30–138	0
2 mo–2 y	10–133	246–1182	81–436	41–101	0
2–18 y	5–150	254–823	127–341	41–125	0–5
Adult	10–131	205–756	151–490	72–124	0

Age	Hydroxy-lysine	Hydroxy-proline	Isoleucine	Leucine	Lysine
Premature	0	0–80	23–85	151–220	128–255
Newborn–1 mo	0–7	0–91	26–91	48–160	92–325
2 mo–2 y	0–7	0–63	31–86	47–155	52–196
2–18 y	0–2	3–45	22–107	49–216	48–284
Adult	0	0–53	30–108	72–201	116–296

Age	Methionine	1-Methyl-histidine	3-Methyl-histidine	Ornithine	Phenyl-alanine
Premature	37–91	4–28	5–33	77–212	98–213
Newborn–1 mo	10–60	0–43	0–5	48–211	38–137
2 mo–2 y	9–42	0–44	0–5	22–103	31–75
2–18 y	7–47	0–42	0–5	10–163	26–91
Adult	10–42	0–39	0–8	48–195	35–85

(Continued on the following page)

Age	Phospho-ethanolamine	Phospho-serine	Proline	Sarcosine	Serine
Premature	5–35	10–45	92–310	0	127–248
Newborn–1 mo	3–27	7–47	110–417	0–625	99–395
2 mo–2 y	0–6	1–20	52–298	0	71–186
2–18 y	0–69	1–30	59–369	0–9	69–187
Adult	0–40	2–14	97–329	0	58–181

Age	Taurine	Threonine	Tryptophan	Tyrosine	Valine
Premature	151–411	150–330	28–136	147–420	99–220
Newborn–1 mo	46–492	90–329	0–60	55–147	86–190
2 mo–2 y	15–143	24–174	23–71	22–108	64–294
2–18 y	10–170	35–226	0–79	24–115	74–321
Adult	54–210	60–225	10–140	34–112	119–336

DESCRIPTION: Screening for inborn errors of amino acid metabolism is generally performed on infants after an initial urine test comes back positive. Certain congenital enzyme deficiencies interfere with normal amino acid metabolism and cause excessive accumulation of or deficiencies in amino acid levels. Reduced growth rates, mental retardation, or various unexplained symptoms can result unless the abnormality is identified and corrected early in life. ∎

INDICATIONS:
- Assist in the detection of noninherited disorders evidenced by elevated amino acid levels
- Detect inborn errors of amino acid metabolism

RESULT

Increased (total amino acids) in:
- Aminoacidopathies (usually inherited; specific amino acids are implicated)
- Brain damage (severe)
- Burns
- Diabetes
- Eclampsia
- Fructose intolerance (hereditary)
- Malabsorption
- Renal failure (acute or chronic)
- Reye's syndrome
- Severe liver damage
- Shock

Decreased (total amino acids) in:
- Adrenocortical hyperfunction
- Carcinoid syndrome
- Fever
- Glomerulonephritis
- Hartnup disease
- Huntington's chorea
- Malnutrition
- Nephrotic syndrome
- Pancreatitis (acute)
- Polycystic kidney disease
- Rheumatoid arthritis

CRITICAL VALUES: N/A

INTERFERING FACTORS:

- Drugs that may increase plasma amino acid levels include bismuth salts, glucocorticoids, levarterenol, 11-oxysteroids, and testosterone (elderly).

- Drugs that may decrease plasma amino acid levels include cerulein, estrogens (males), epinephrine, glucose, oral contraceptives, progesterone (males), and secretin.

- Amino acids exhibit a strong circadian rhythm; values are highest in the afternoon and lowest in the morning. Protein intake does not influence diurnal variation but significantly affects absolute concentrations. A 12-hour fast before specimen collection is required.

Nursing Implications and Procedure · · · · · · · · · · ·

Pretest: ■

➤ Obtain a history of the patient's complaints, including a list of known allergens.

➤ Obtain a history of the patient's reproductive system as it relates to genetic disease, as well as results of previously performed tests and procedures. For related tests, refer to the reproductive system table.

➤ Obtain a list of the medications the patient is taking, including herbs, nutritional supplements, and nutraceuticals. The requesting health care practitioner and laboratory should be advised if the patient regularly uses these products so that their effects can be taken into consideration when reviewing results.

➤ There are no fluid or medication restrictions unless by medical direction.

➤ Instruct the patient to fast for at least 12 hours before specimen collection.

➤ Review the procedure with the patient.

➤ Inform the patient that specimen collection takes approximately 5 to 10 minutes.

Intratest: ■

➤ Ensure that the patient has complied with dietary and other pretesting restrictions.

➤ Direct the patient to breathe normally and to avoid unnecessary movement.

➤ Observe standard precautions and follow the general guidelines in Appendix A. Perform a venipuncture, and collect the specimen in a 5-mL red- or tiger-top tube.

➤ Label the specimen, and promptly transport it to the laboratory.

Post-test: ■

➤ Observe venipuncture site for bleeding or hematoma formation. Apply pressure bandage.

➤ Instruct the patient to resume usual diet, as directed by the health care practitioner.

➤ Instruct caregiver in special dietary modifications, as appropriate to treat deficiency, or refer caregiver to a qualified nutritionist. Amino acids are classified as essential (i.e., must be present simultaneously in sufficient quantities); conditionally or acquired essential (i.e., under certain stressful conditions, they become essential); and nonessential (i.e., can be produced by the body, when needed, if diet does not provide them). Essential amino acids include lysine, threonine, histidine, isoleucine, methionine, phenylalanine, tryptophan, and valine. Conditionally essential amino acids include cysteine, tyrosine, arginine, citrulline, taurine, and carnitine. Nonessential amino acids include alanine, glutamic acid, aspartic acid, glycine, serine, proline, glutamine, and asparagine. A high intake of specific amino acids can cause other amino acids to become essential.

➤ Recognize anxiety related to test results and offer support, as appropriate. Provide teaching and disease information, as appropriate. Educate the patient regarding access to genetic or other counseling services.

➤ Evaluate test results in relation to the patient's symptoms and other tests performed. Related laboratory tests include ammonia and urine amino acid screen.

AMINO ACID SCREEN, URINE

SYNONYM/ACRONYM: N/A.

SPECIMEN: Urine (10 mL) from a random or timed specimen collected in a clean plastic collection container with hydrochloric acid as a preservative.

REFERENCE VALUE: (Method: Chromatography) There are numerous amino acids. The following tables include the most frequently screened. All units are nanomoles per milligram (nmol/mg) creatinine.

Age	Alanine	β-Alanine	Anserine	α-Amino-adipic Acid	α-Amino-n-butyric Acid
Premature	1320–4040	1020–3500	—	70–460	50–710
Newborn–1 mo	982–3055	25–288	0–3	0–180	8–65
2 mo–2 y	767–6090	0–297	0–5	45–268	30–136
2–18 y	231–915	0–65	0	2–88	0–77
Adult	240–670	0–130	0	40–110	0–90

Age	γ-Amino-butyric Acid	β-Aminoiso-butyric Acid	Arginine	Asparagine	Aspartic Acid
Premature	20–260	50–470	190–820	1350–5250	580–1520
Newborn–1 mo	0–15	421–3133	35–214	185–1550	336–810
2 mo–2 y	0–105	802–4160	38–165	252–1280	230–685
2–18 y	15–30	291–1482	31–109	72–332	0–120
Adult	15–30	10–510	10–90	99–470	60–240

Age	Carnosine	Citrulline	Cysta-thionine	Cystine	Ethanol-amine
Premature	260–370	240–1320	260–1160	480–1690	—
Newborn–1	97–665	27–181	16–147	212–668	840–3400
mo	203–635	22–180	33–470	68–710	0–2230
2 mo–2 y	72–402	10–99	0–26	25–125	0–530
2–18 y	10–90	8–50	20–50	43–210	0–520
Adult					

Age	Glutamic Acid	Glutamine	Glycine	Histidine	Homo-cystine
Premature	380–3760	520–1700	7840–23,600	1240–7240	580–2230
Newborn–1	70–1058	393–1042	5749–16,423	908–2528	0–88
mo					
2 mo–2 y	54–590	670–1562	3023–11,148	815–7090	6–67
2–18 y	0–176	369–1014	897–4500	644–2430	0–32
Adult	39–330	190–510	730–4160	460–1430	0–32

Age	Hydroxy-lysine	Hydroxy-proline	Isoleucine	Leucine	Lysine
Premature	—	560–5640	250–640	190–790	1860–15,460
Newborn–1	10–125	40–440	125–390	78–195	270–1850
mo					
2 mo–2 y	0–97	0–4010	38–342	70–570	189–850
2–18 y	40–102	0–3300	10–126	30–500	153–634
Adult	40–90	0–26	16–180	30–150	145–634

Age	Methionine	1-Methyl-histidine	3-Methyl-histidine	Ornithine	Phenyl-alanine
Premature	500–1230	170–880	420–1340	260–3350	920–2280
Newborn–1	342–880	96–499	189–680	118–554	91–457
mo					
2 mo–2 y	174–1090	106–1275	147–391	55–364	175–1340
2–18 y	16–114	170–1688	182–365	31–91	61–314
Adult	38–210	170–1680	160–520	20–80	51–250

Age	Phospho-ethanolamine	Phospho-serine	Proline	Sarcosine	Serine
Premature	80–340	500–1690	1350–10,460	0	1680–6000
Newborn–1	0–155	150–339	370–2323	0–56	1444–3661
mo					
2 mo–2 y	108–533	112–304	254–2195	30–358	845–3190
2–18 y	18–150	70–138	0	0–26	362–1100
Adult	20–100	40–510	0	0–80	240–670

(Continued on the following page)

Age	Taurine	Threonine	Tryptophan	Tyrosine	Valine
Premature	5190–23,620	840–5700	0	1090–6780	180–890
Newborn–1 mo	1650–6220	445–1122	0	220–1650	113–369
2 mo–2 y	545–3790	252–1528	0–93	333–1550	99–316
2–18 y	639–1866	121–389	0–108	122–517	58–143
Adult	380–1850	130–370	0–70	90–290	27–260

DESCRIPTION: Urine amino acid testing is used in the initial screening for congenital defects and disorders of amino acid metabolism. The major genetic disorders include phenylketonuria, tyrosinuria, and alcaptonuria, a defect in the phenylalanine-tyrosine conversion pathway. Renal aminoaciduria is also associated with conditions marked by defective tubular reabsorption from congenital disorders, such as hereditary fructose intolerance, cystinuria, and Hartnup disease. Early diagnosis and treatment of certain aminoacidurias can prevent mental retardation, reduced growth rates, or various unexplained symptoms. Values are age dependent. A positive screen on a random sample should be followed up with a timed collection. ■

INDICATIONS:
• Assist in the detection of noninherited disorders evidenced by elevated amino acid levels

• Screen for inborn errors of amino acid metabolism

RESULT

Increased (total amino acids) in:
• Primary causes (inherited):
Aminoaciduria (specific)
Cystinosis
Fanconi's syndrome
Fructose intolerance
Galactosemia
Hartnup disease
Lactose intolerance
Lowe's syndrome
Maple syrup disease
Tyrosinosis
Wilson's disease

• Secondary causes (noninherited):
Chronic renal failure
Diabetic ketosis
Hyperparathyroidism
Hyperthyroidism
Multiple myeloma
Osteomalacia
Liver necrosis and cirrhosis
Muscular dystrophy (progressive)
Thalassemia major
Vitamin deficiency (B, C, and D)
Viral hepatitis

Decreased in: N/A

CRITICAL VALUES: N/A

INTERFERING FACTORS:
• Drugs that may increase urine amino acid levels include acetaminophen, amikacin, aminocaproic acid, amphetamine, ampicillin, cephalexin, colistin, corticotropin, dopamine, ephedrine, epinephrine, erythromycin, ethylenediamine, gentamicin, hydrocortisone, hydroxyaminobutyric acid, kanamycin, levarterenol, levodopa, mafenide, metanephrine, methamphetamine, methyldopa, neomycin, normetanephrine, penicillamine,

phenacetin, phenobarbital, phenyl-ephrine, phenylpropanolamine, poly-myxin, primidone, proSobee, pseudo-ephedrine, streptozocin, tetracycline, triamcinolone, and vigabatrin.

• Drugs that may decrease urine amino acid levels include insulin.

• Amino acids exhibit a strong circadian rhythm; values are highest in the afternoon and lowest in the morning. Protein intake does not influence diurnal variation but significantly affects absolute concentrations; a 12-hour fast before specimen collection is required.

• Dilute urine (specific gravity less than 1.010) should be rejected for analysis.

Nursing Implications and Procedure • • • • • • • • • • •

Pretest: ■

➤ Obtain a history of the patient's complaints, including a list of known allergens.

➤ Obtain a history of the patient's reproductive system as it relates to genetic disease, as well as results of previously performed tests and procedures. For related tests, refer to the reproductive system table.

➤ Obtain a list of the medications the patient is taking, including herbs, nutritional supplements, and nutraceuticals. The requesting health care practitioner and laboratory should be advised if the patient regularly uses these products so that their effects can be taken into consideration when reviewing results.

➤ There are no fluid or medication restrictions unless by medical direction.

➤ Instruct the patient to fast for at least 12 hours before specimen collection.

➤ Instruct the patient to avoid exces-sive exercise and stress during the 24-hour collection of urine.

➤ Review the procedure with the patient. Provide a nonmetallic urinal, bedpan, or toilet-mounted collection device.

➤ If a timed collection is requested, inform the patient that all urine collected over a 24-hour period must be saved; if a preservative has been added to the container, instruct the patient not to discard the preserva-tive. Instruct the patient not to void directly into the laboratory collection container. Instruct the patient to avoid defecating in the collection device and to keep toilet tissue out of the collection device to prevent contamination of the specimen. Place a sign in the bathroom as a reminder to save all urine.

➤ Instruct the patient to void all urine into the collection device and pour the urine into the laboratory collec-tion container. Alternatively, the specimen can be left in the collec-tion device for a health care staff member to add to the laboratory collection container.

Intratest: ■

➤ Ensure that the patient has complied with dietary preparations and other pretesting restrictions.

➤ Observe standard precautions and follow the general guidelines in Appendix A.

Random specimen (collect in early morning):

➤ *Infant:* Clean and dry the genital area, attach the collection device securely to prevent leakage, and observe for voiding. Remove collec-tion device carefully from the skin to prevent irritation. Transfer the urine into a specimen container. For dipstick method, place dipstick or reagent pad into the urine specimen or on the diaper saturated with urine. Remove, compare with color chart, and record results.

➤ *Adult:* Instruct the patient to obtain

a clean-catch specimen as described in Appendix A. If an indwelling catheter is in place, it may be necessary to clamp off the catheter for 15 to 30 minutes before specimen collection. Cleanse specimen port with antiseptic swab, and then aspirate 5 mL of urine with a 21- to 25-gauge needle and syringe. Transfer urine to a plastic container.

Timed specimen:

➤ Obtain a clean 3-L urine specimen container, toilet-mounted collection device, and plastic bag (for transport of the specimen container). The specimen must be refrigerated or kept on ice throughout the entire collection period. If an indwelling urinary catheter is in place, the drainage bag must be kept on ice.

➤ Begin the test between 6 and 8 a.m., if possible. Collect first voiding and discard. Record the time the specimen was discarded as the beginning of the timed collection period. The next morning, ask the patient to void at the same time the collection was started and add this last voiding to the container.

➤ If an indwelling catheter is in place, replace the tubing and container system at the start of the collection time. Keep the container system on ice during the collection period or empty the urine into a larger container periodically during the collection period; monitor to ensure continued drainage, and conclude the test the next morning at the same hour the collection started.

➤ At the conclusion of the test, compare the quantity of urine with the urinary output record for the collection; if the specimen contains less than what was recorded as output, some urine may have been discarded, invalidating the test.

➤ Label the specimen, and promptly transport it to the laboratory. Include on the label the amount of urine, test start and stop times, and age of the patient.

Post-test:

➤ Instruct the patient to resume usual diet as directed by the health care practitioner.

➤ Instruct caregiver in special dietary modifications, as appropriate, to treat deficiency, or refer caregiver to a qualified nutritionist. Amino acids are classified as essential (i.e., must be present simultaneously in sufficient quantities); conditionally or acquired essential (i.e., under certain stressful conditions, they become essential); and nonessential (i.e., can be produced by the body, when needed, if diet does not provide them). Essential amino acids include lysine, threonine, histidine, isoleucine, methionine, phenylalanine, tryptophan, and valine. Conditionally essential amino acids include cysteine, tyrosine, arginine, citrulline, taurine, and carnitine. Nonessential amino acids include alanine, glutamic acid, aspartic acid, glycine, serine, proline, glutamine, and asparagine. A high intake of specific amino acids can cause other amino acids to become essential.

➤ Recognize anxiety related to test results and offer support, as appropriate. Provide teaching and disease information, as appropriate. Educate the patient regarding access to genetic or other counseling services.

➤ Evaluate test results in relation to the patient's symptoms and other tests performed. Related laboratory tests include ammonia and blood amino acid screen.

δ-AMINOLEVULINIC ACID

. . . .

SYNONYM/ACRONYM: δ-ALA.

SPECIMEN: Urine (25 mL) from a timed specimen collected in a dark plastic container with hydrochloric acid as a preservative.

REFERENCE VALUE: (Method: Spectrophotometry)

Conventional Units	SI Units (Conversion Factor ×7.626)
1.5–7.5 mg/24 h	11.4–57.2 μmol/24 h

DESCRIPTION: δ-Aminolevulinic acid (δ-ALA) is involved in the formation of porphyrins. Disturbances in porphyrin metabolism can cause an increase in δ-ALA excretion in urine. Although lead poisoning can cause increased urinary excretion, the measurement of δ-ALA is not useful to indicate lead toxicity because it is not detectable in the urine until the blood lead level approaches and exceeds 40 μg/dL. ■

INDICATIONS:
• Assist in the diagnosis of porphyrias

RESULT

Increased in:
• Acute porphyrias
• Aminolevulinic acid dehydrase deficiency
• Hereditary tyrosinemia

• Lead poisoning

Decreased in:
• Liver disease (alcoholic)

CRITICAL VALUES: N/A

INTERFERING FACTORS:
• Drugs that may increase δ-ALA levels include ammonia, glucosamine, and penicillins.

• Cisplatin may decrease δ-ALA levels.

• Numerous drugs are suspected as potential initiators of attacks of acute porphyria, but those classified as unsafe for high-risk individuals include antipyrine, aminopyrine, aminoglutethimide, barbiturates, carbamazepine, carbromal, chlorpropamide, danazol, dapsone, diclofenac, diphenylhydantoin, ergot preparations, ethchlorvynol, ethinamate, glutethimide, griseofulvin, mephenytoin, meprobamate, methyprylone, N-isopropyl meprobamate, novobiocin, phenylbutazone, primidone, pyrazolone preparations, succinimides, sulfonamides, sulfonethylmethane, sulfomethane, synthetic estrogens and progestins, tolazamide, tolbutamide, trimethadione, and valproic acid.

Nursing Implications and Procedure • • • • • • • • • •

Pretest:

➤ Obtain a history of the patient's complaints, including a list of known allergens.

➤ Obtain a history of the patient's hematopoietic system and results of previously performed tests and procedures. For related tests, refer to the hematopoietic system table.

➤ Obtain a list of the medications the patient is taking, including herbs, nutritional supplements, and nutraceuticals. The requesting health care practitioner and laboratory should be advised if the patient regularly uses these products so that their effects can be taken into consideration when reviewing results.

➤ There are no food, fluid, or medication restrictions unless by medical direction.

➤ Review the procedure with the patient. Provide a nonmetallic urinal, bedpan, or toilet-mounted collection device.

➤ Usually a 24-hour time frame for urine collection is ordered. Inform the patient that all urine must be saved during that 24-hour period. Instruct the patient not to void directly into the laboratory collection container. Instruct the patient to avoid defacating in the collection device and to keep toilet tissue out of the collection device to prevent contamination of the specimen. Place a sign in the bathroom to remind the patient to save all urine.

➤ Instruct the patient to void all urine into the collection device and then to pour the urine into the laboratory collection container. Alternatively, the specimen can be left in the collection device for a health care staff member to add to the laboratory collection container.

Intratest:

➤ Observe standard precautions and follow the general guidelines in Appendix A.

➤ Obtain a clean 3-L urine specimen container, toilet-mounted collection device, and plastic bag (for transport of the specimen container). The specimen must be refrigerated or kept on ice throughout the entire collection period. If an indwelling urinary catheter is in place, the drainage bag must be kept on ice.

➤ Begin the test between 6 and 8 a.m., if possible. Collect first voiding and discard. Record the time the specimen was discarded as the beginning of the timed collection period. The next morning, ask the patient to void at the same time the collection was started, and add this last voiding to the container.

➤ If an indwelling catheter is in place, replace the tubing and container system at the start of the collection time. Keep the container system on ice during the collection period, or empty the urine into a larger container periodically during the collection period. Monitor to ensure continued drainage, and conclude the test the next morning at the same hour the collection was begun.

➤ At the conclusion of the test, compare the quantity of urine with the urinary output record for the collection; if the specimen contains less than what was recorded as output, some urine may have been discarded, invalidating the test.

> Label the specimen, and promptly transport it to the laboratory. Include on the label the amount of urine as well as test start and stop times. On the label, note the ingestion of any medications that may affect test results.

> Evaluate test results in relation to the patient's symptoms and other tests performed. Related laboratory tests include lead and urine porphyrins.

AMMONIA

· ·

SYNONYM/ACRONYM: NH_3.

SPECIMEN: Plasma (1 mL) collected in completely filled green-top (heparin) tube. Specimen should be transported tightly capped and in an ice slurry.

REFERENCE VALUE: (Method: Spectrophotometry)

Age	Conventional Units	SI Units (Conversion Factor ×0.587)
Newborn	170–341 µg/dL	100–200 µmol/L
Adult	19–60 µg/dL	11–35 µmol/L

DESCRIPTION: Blood ammonia (NH_3) comes from two sources: deamination of amino acids during protein metabolism and degradation of proteins by colon bacteria. The liver converts ammonia in the portal blood to urea, which is excreted by the kidneys. When liver function is severely compromised, especially in situations in which decreased hepatocellular function is combined with impaired portal blood flow, ammonia levels rise. Ammonia is potentially toxic to the central nervous system. ■

INDICATIONS:

• Evaluate advanced liver disease or other disorders associated with altered serum ammonia levels

• Identify impending hepatic encephalopathy with known liver disease

• Monitor the effectiveness of treatment for hepatic encephalopathy, indicated by declining levels

• Monitor patients receiving hyperalimentation therapy

RESULT

Increased in:

- Gastrointestinal hemorrhage

- Genitourinary tract infection with distention and stasis

- Inborn enzyme deficiency

- Hepatic coma

- Liver failure, late cirrhosis

- Reye's syndrome

- Total parenteral nutrition

Decreased in: N/A

CRITICAL VALUES: N/A

INTERFERING FACTORS:

- Drugs that may increase ammonia levels include ammonium salts, asparaginase, barbiturates, diuretics, ethanol, fibrin hydrolysate, fluorides, furosemide, thiazides, and valproic acid.

- Drugs/organisms that may decrease ammonia levels include diphenhydramine, kanamycin, neomycin, tetracycline, and *Lactobacillus acidophilus.*

- Hemolysis falsely increases ammonia levels.

- Prompt and proper specimen processing, storage, and analysis are important to achieve accurate results. The specimen should be collected on ice; the collection tube should be filled completely, and then kept tightly stoppered. Ammonia increases rapidly in the collected specimen, so analysis should be performed within 20 minutes of collection.

Nursing Implications and Procedure · · · · · · · · · · ·

Pretest:

➤ Obtain a history of the patient's complaints, including a list of known allergens.

➤ Obtain a history of the patient's gastrointestinal, genitourinary, and hepatobiliary systems, as well as results of previously performed tests and procedures. For related tests, refer to the gastrointestinal, genitourinary, and hepatobiliary system tables.

➤ Obtain a list of the medications the patient is taking, including herbs, nutritional supplements, and nutraceuticals. The requesting health care practitioner and laboratory should be advised if the patient regularly uses these products so that their effects can be taken into consideration when reviewing results.

➤ There are no food, fluid, or medication restrictions unless by medical direction.

➤ Review the procedure with the patient.

➤ Inform the patient that specimen collection takes approximately 5 to 10 minutes.

Intratest:

➤ Direct the patient to breathe normally and to avoid unnecessary movement.

➤ Observe standard precautions and follow the general guidelines in Appendix A.

➤ Perform a venipuncture, and collect the specimen in a 5-mL green-top tube.

➤ Label the specimen, and promptly transport it to the laboratory. The tightly capped sample should be placed in an ice slurry immediately after collection. Information on the specimen label can be protected from water in the ice slurry by first placing the specimen in a protective plastic bag.

Post-test:

➤ Observe venipuncture site for bleeding or hematoma formation. Apply pressure bandage.

➤ Increased ammonia levels may be associated with liver disease. Dietary recommendations may be indicated, depending on the severity of the condition. A low-protein diet may be in order if the patient's liver has lost the ability to process the end products of protein metabolism. A diet of soft foods may be required if esophageal varices have developed. Ammonia levels may be used to determine whether protein should be added to or reduced from the diet. Patients should be encouraged to eat simple carbohydrates and emulsified fats (as in homogenized milk or eggs), as opposed to complex carbohydrates (e.g., starch, fiber, and glycogen [animal carbohydrates]) and complex fats, which would require additional bile to emulsify it so that it could be used. The cirrhotic patient should be carefully observed for the development of ascites, in which case fluid and electrolyte balance requires strict attention.

➤ Evaluate test results in relation to the patient's symptoms and other tests performed. Related laboratory tests include acetaminophen, alanine aminotransferase, albumin, anion gap, aspartate aminotransferase, bilirubin, blood gases, calcium, complete blood count, electrolytes, glucose, lactic acid, ketones, osmolality, protein, prothrombin time, urea nitrogen, and uric acid.

AMNIOTIC FLUID ANALYSIS

SYNONYM/ACRONYM: N/A.

SPECIMEN: Amniotic fluid (10 – 20 mL) collected in a clean amber glass or plastic container.

REFERENCE VALUE: (Method: Macroscopic observation of fluid for color and appearance, radioimmunoassay for α-fetoprotein, electrophoresis for acetylcholinesterase, spectrophotometry for creatinine and bilirubin, chromatography for lecithin/sphingomyelin [L/S] ratio and phosphatidylglycerol, tissue culture for chromosome analysis, dipstick for leukocyte esterase, and automated cell counter for white blood cell count and lamellar bodies)

Test	Reference Value
Color	Colorless to pale yellow
Appearance	Clear
α-Fetoprotein	Less than 2.0 MoM
Acetylcholinesterase	Absent
Creatinine	1.8–4.0 mg/dL at term
Bilirubin	Less than 0.075 mg/dL in early pregnancy
	Less than 0.025 mg/dL at term
L/S ratio	Greater than 2:1 at term
Phosphatidylglycerol	Present at term
Chromosome analysis	Normal karyotype
White blood cell count	None seen
Leukocyte esterase	Negative
Lamellar bodies	30,000–50,000 platelet equivalents

DESCRIPTION: Amniotic fluid is formed in the membranous sac that surrounds the fetus. The total volume of fluid at term is 500 to 2500 mL. In amniocentesis, fluid is obtained by ultrasound-guided needle aspiration from the amniotic sac. This procedure is generally performed between 14 and 16 weeks' gestation, but it also can be done between 26 and 35 weeks' gestation if fetal distress is suspected. Amniotic fluid is tested to identify genetic and neural tube defects, hemolytic diseases of the newborn, fetal infection, fetal renal malfunction, or maturity of the fetal lungs (see monograph titled "Lecithin/Sphingomyelin Ratio") ■

INDICATIONS:
- Assist in the diagnosis of (in utero) metabolic disorders, such as cystic fibrosis; or errors of lipid, carbohydrate, or amino acid metabolism
- Evaluate fetus in families with a history of genetic disorders, such as Down syndrome, Tay-Sachs disease, chromosome or enzyme anomalies, or inherited hemoglobinopathies
- Evaluate fetus in mothers of advanced maternal age (some of the aforementioned tests are routinely requested in mothers aged 35 years and older)
- Evaluate fetus in mothers with a history of miscarriage or stillbirth
- Evaluate known or suspected hemolytic disease involving the fetus in an Rh-sensitized pregnancy, indicated by rising bilirubin levels, especially after the 30th week of gestation
- Evaluate suspected neural tube defects, such as spina bifida or myelomeningocele, as indicated by elevated α-fetoprotein (see monograph titled "$α_1$-Fetoprotein" for information related to triple-marker testing)
- Detect infection secondary to ruptured membranes
- Determine fetal maturity when preterm delivery is being considered. Fetal maturity is indicated by an L/S ratio of 2:1 or greater (see monograph titled "Lecithin/Sphingomyelin Ratio")
- Determine fetal sex when the mother is a known carrier of a sex-linked abnormal gene that could be transmitted to male offspring, such as hemophilia or Duchenne's muscular dystrophy

• Determine the presence of fetal distress in late-stage pregnancy

RESULT:

• Yellow, green, red, or brown fluid indicates the presence of bilirubin, blood (fetal or maternal), or meconium, which indicate fetal distress or death, hemolytic disease, or growth retardation.

• Elevated bilirubin levels indicate fetal hemolytic disease or intestinal obstruction. Measurement of bilirubin is not usually performed before 20 to 24 weeks' gestation because no action can be taken before then. The severity of hemolytic disease is graded by optical density (OD) zones: A value of 0.28 to 0.46 OD at 28 to 31 weeks' gestation indicates mild hemolytic disease, which probably will not affect the fetus; 0.47 to 0.90 OD indicates a moderate effect on the fetus; and 0.91 to 1.0 OD indicates a significant effect on the fetus. A trend of increasing values with serial measurements may indicate the need for intrauterine transfusion or early delivery, depending on the fetal age. After 32 to 33 weeks' gestation, early delivery is preferred over intrauterine transfusion, because early delivery is more effective in providing the required care to the neonate.

• Creatinine concentration greater than 2.0 mg/dL indicates fetal maturity (at 36 to 37 weeks) if maternal creatinine is also within the expected range. This value should be interpreted in conjunction with other parameters evaluated in amniotic fluid and especially with the L/S ratio because normal lung development depends on normal kidney development.

• L/S ratio less than 2:1 and absence of phosphatidylglycerol at term indicate fetal lung immaturity and possible respiratory distress syndrome. The expected L/S ratio for the fetus of an insulin-dependent diabetic mother is higher (3.5:1). (See monograph titled "Lecithin/Sphingomyelin Ratio.")

• Lamellar bodies are specialized alveolar cells in which lung surfactant is stored. They are approximately the size of platelets. Their presence in sufficient quantities is an indicator of fetal lung maturity.

• Elevated α-fetoprotein levels and presence of acetylcholinesterase indicates a neural tube defect (see monograph titled "α$_1$-Fetoprotein").

• Abnormal karyotype indicates genetic abnormality (e.g., Tay-Sachs disease, mental retardation, chromosome or enzyme anomalies, and inherited hemoglobinopathies). (See monograph titled "Chromosome Analysis, Blood.")

• Elevated white blood cell count and positive leukocyte esterase are indicators of infection.

CRITICAL VALUES: N/A

INTERFERING FACTORS:

• Bilirubin may be falsely elevated if maternal hemoglobin or meconium is present in the sample; fetal acidosis may also lead to falsely elevated bilirubin levels.

• Bilirubin may be falsely decreased if the sample is exposed to light or if amniotic fluid volume is excessive.

• Maternal serum creatinine should be measured simultaneously for comparison with amniotic fluid creatinine for proper interpretation. Even in circumstances in which the maternal serum value is normal, the results of the amniotic fluid creatinine may be misleading. A high fluid creatinine value in the fetus of a diabetic mother may reflect the increased muscle mass of a larger fetus. If the fetus is big, the creatinine may be high and the fetus may still have immature kidneys.

- Contamination of the sample with blood or meconium or complications in pregnancy may yield inaccurate L/S ratios.

- α-Fetoprotein and acetylcholinesterase may be falsely elevated if the sample is contaminated with fetal blood.

- Karyotyping cannot be performed under the following conditions: (1) failure to promptly deliver samples for chromosomal analysis to the laboratory performing the test, or (2) improper incubation of the sample, which causes cellular death.

- Recent radioactive scans or radiation within 1 week before the test can interfere with test results when radioimmunoassay is the test method.

- Amniocentesis is contraindicated in ⚠ women with a history of premature labor or incompetent cervix. It is also contraindicated in the presence of placenta previa or abruptio placentae.

Nursing Implications and Procedure • • • • • • • • • • • •

Pretest: ■

➤ Obtain a history of the patient's complaints, including a list of known allergens.

➤ Obtain a history of the patient's reproductive system and previous pregnancies, as well as other tests and procedures previously performed. For related tests, refer to the reproductive system table.

➤ Obtain a list of medications the patient is taking, including herbs, nutritional supplements, and nutraceuticals. The requesting health care practitioner and laboratory should be advised if the patient is regularly using these products so that their effects can be taken into consideration when reviewing results.

➤ Note any recent procedures that can interfere with test results.

➤ There are no food, fluid, or medication restrictions unless by medical direction.

➤ Review the procedure with the patient. Sensitivity to cultural and social issues and concern for modesty is important in providing psychological support.

➤ Explain the purpose of the study and how the procedure is performed. Address concerns about pain related to the procedure. Inform the patient that a health care practitioner performs the test, which takes 20 to 30 minutes to complete.

➤ Warn the patient that normal results do not guarantee a normal fetus.

➤ Explain the necessity of remaining still during the procedure.

➤ Determine whether the patient has an allergy to local anesthetics, and inform the health care practitioner accordingly.

➤ *Obtain written and informed consent before administering any medications prior to the procedure.*

Intratest: ■

➤ Direct the patient to breathe normally and to avoid unnecessary movement.

➤ Record maternal and fetal baseline vital signs. Monitor for uterine contractions.

➤ Observe standard precautions and follow the general guidelines in Appendix A.

➤ Assemble the necessary equipment, including an amniocentesis tray with solution for skin preparation, local anesthetic, 10- or 20-mL syringe, needles of various sizes (including a 22-gauge, 5-inch spinal needle), sterile drapes, sterile gloves, and foil-covered or amber specimen collection containers.

➤ Ensure that the patient has a full bladder before the procedure if gestation is 20 weeks or less; have patient void before procedure if gestation is 21 weeks or more.

➤ Assist the patient to a supine position. Raise the head or legs slightly to promote comfort and to relax abdominal muscles. If the uterus is large, place a pillow or rolled blanket under the patient's right side to prevent hypertension resulting from great-vessel compression.

➤ Note fetal position and pocket of amniotic fluid as determined by ultrasound and palpation.

➤ Cleanse suprapubic area with an antiseptic solution and protect with sterile drapes. A local anesthetic is injected. Explain that this may cause a stinging sensation.

➤ A 22-gauge, 5-inch spinal needle is inserted through the abdominal and uterine walls. Explain that a sensation of pressure may be experienced when the needle is inserted. Explain to the patient how to use focusing and controlled breathing for relaxation during the procedure.

➤ After the fluid is collected and the needle is withdrawn, apply slight pressure to the site. If there is no evidence of bleeding or other drainage, apply a sterile adhesive bandage to the site.

➤ Label the specimen, and promptly transport it to the laboratory.

Post-test:

➤ Fetal heart rate and maternal life signs (heart rate, blood pressure, pulse, and respiration) should be compared with baseline values and closely monitored every 15 minutes for 30 to 60 minutes after the amniocentesis procedure.

➤ Explain that slight cramping can occur after the procedure.

➤ Tell the patient to report fever, leaking amniotic fluid, vaginal bleeding, uterine contractions, or changes in fetal activity (either an increase or a decrease) to a health care practitioner.

➤ Inform the patient that it may be 2 to 4 weeks before all results are available.

➤ Recognize anxiety related to test results and offer support. Provide teaching and information regarding the clinical implications of the test results, as appropriate. Encourage the family to seek appropriate counseling if concerned with pregnancy termination, and to seek genetic counseling if a chromosomal abnormality is determined. Decisions regarding elective abortion should take place in the presence of both parents. Provide a nonjudgmental, nonthreatening atmosphere for discussing the risks and difficulties of delivering and raising an abnormal infant, as well as exploring other options (termination of pregnancy or adoption). It is also important to discuss problems the mother and father may experience (guilt, depression, anger) if fetal abnormalities are detected.

➤ Evaluate test results in relation to the patient's symptoms and other tests performed. Related laboratory tests include α-fetoprotein, chromosome analysis, and L/S ratio.

AMYLASE

SYNONYM/ACRONYM: N/A.

SPECIMEN: Serum (1 mL) collected in a red- or tiger-top tube. Plasma (1 mL) collected in green-top (heparin) tube is also acceptable.

REFERENCE VALUE: (Method: Spectrophotometry)

Conventional Units	SI Units (Conversion Factor ×0.017)
30–110 U/L	0.51–1.87 μKat/L

DESCRIPTION: Amylase, a digestive enzyme, splits starch into disaccharides. Although many cells have amylase activity (e.g., liver, small intestine, ovaries, skeletal muscles), circulating amylase is derived from the parotid glands and the pancreas. Amylase is a sensitive indicator of pancreatic acinar cell damage and pancreatic obstruction. Newborns and children up to 2 years old have little measurable serum amylase. Most of this enzyme in the early years of life is produced by the salivary glands. ∎

INDICATIONS:

- Assist in the diagnosis of early acute pancreatitis; serum amylase begins to rise within 6 to 24 hours after onset and returns to normal in 2 to 7 days

- Assist in the diagnosis of macroamylasemia, a disorder seen in alcoholism, malabsorption syndrome, and other digestive problems

- Assist in the diagnosis of pancreatic duct obstruction, which causes serum levels to remain elevated

- Detect blunt trauma or inadvertent surgical trauma to the pancreas

- Differentiate between acute pancreatitis and other causes of abdominal pain that require surgery

RESULT

Increased in:

- Abdominal trauma

- Alcoholism

- Carcinoma of the head of the pancreas (advanced)

- Common bile duct obstruction

- Diabetic ketoacidosis

- Duodenal obstruction

- Ectopic pregnancy

- Gastric resection

- Macroamylasemia

- Mumps

- Pancreatitis

- Pancreatic cyst and pseudocyst

- Parotitis

- Perforated peptic ulcer involving the pancreas

- Peritonitis

- Postoperative period

- Some tumors of the lung and ovaries

- Viral infections

Decreased in:

- Cystic fibrosis (advanced)

- Hepatic disease (severe)

- Pancreatic insufficiency

- Pancreatectomy

CRITICAL VALUES: N/A

INTERFERING FACTORS:

- Drugs and substances that may increase amylase levels include asparaginase, captopril, cimetidine, clofibrate, corticosteroids, estrogens, ethacrynic acid, furosemide, ibuprofen, methyldopa, nitrofurantoin, oral contraceptives, pentamidine, sulfonamides, tetracycline, thiazide diuretics, valproic acid, zalcitabine, and alcohol.

- Drugs that may decrease amylase levels include anabolic steroids, citrates, and fluorides.

Nursing Implications and Procedure • • • • • • • • • • •

Pretest: ■

➤ Obtain a history of the patient's complaints, including a list of known allergens.

➤ Obtain a history of the patient's endocrine, gastrointestinal, and hepatobiliary systems, as well as results of previously performed tests and procedures. For related tests, refer to the endocrine, gastrointestinal, and hepatobiliary system tables.

➤ Obtain a list of the medications the patient is taking, including herbs, nutritional supplements, and nutraceuticals. The requesting health care practitioner and laboratory should be advised if the patient regularly uses these products so that their effects can be taken into consideration when reviewing results.

➤ There are no food, fluid, or medication restrictions unless by medical direction.

➤ Review the procedure with the patient.

➤ Inform the patient that specimen collection takes approximately 5 to 10 minutes.

Intratest: ■

➤ Direct the patient to breathe normally and to avoid unnecessary movement.

➤ Observe standard precautions and follow the general guidelines in Appendix A. Perform a venipuncture, and collect the specimen in a 5-mL red- or tiger-top tube.

➤ Label the specimen, and promptly transport it to the laboratory.

Post-test: ■

➤ Observe venipuncture site for bleeding or hematoma formation. Apply pressure bandage.

➤ Increased amylase levels may be associated with gastrointestinal disease or alcoholism. Small, frequent meals work best for patients with gastrointestinal disorders. Consideration should be given to dietary alterations in the case of gastrointestinal disorders. Usually after acute symptoms subside and bowel sounds return, patients are given a clear liquid diet, progressing to a low-fat, high-carbohydrate diet. Vitamin B_{12} may be ordered for parenteral administration to patients with decreased levels, especially if their disease prevents adequate absorption of the vitamin. The alcoholic patient should be encouraged to avoid alcohol and to seek appropriate counseling for substance abuse.

➤ Evaluate test results in relation to the patient's symptoms and other tests performed. Related laboratory tests include alanine aminotransferase, alkaline phosphatase, aspartate aminotransferase, fluid amylase, bilirubin, CA 19-9, calcium, fecal fat, γ-glutamyl transpeptidase, lipase, magnesium, mumps serology, triglycerides, and white blood cell count.

ANALGESIC AND ANTIPYRETIC DRUGS: ACETAMINOPHEN, ACETYLSALICYLIC ACID

SYNONYMS/ACRONYM: *Acetaminophen* (Acephen, Aspirin Free Anacin, Apacet, Banesin, Dapa, Datril, Dorcol, Gebapap, Halenol, Liquiprin, Meda Cap, Panadol, Redutemp, Tempra, Tylenol, Ty-Pap, Uni-Ace); *Acetylsalicylic acid* (salicylate, aspirin, Anacin, Aspergum, Bufferin, Ecotrin, Empirin, Measurin, Synalgos, ZORprin, ASA).

SPECIMEN: Serum (1 mL) collected in a red-top tube.

REFERENCE VALUE: (Method: Immunoassay)

Drug	Therapeutic Dose*	SI Units	Half-Life	Volume of Distribution	Protein Binding	Excretion
		(Conversion Factor ×6.62)				
Acetaminophen	10–30 µg/mL	66–199 µmol/L	1–3 h	0.95 L/kg	20–50%	85–95% hepatic, metabolites, renal
		(Conversion Factor ×0.073)				
Salicylate	15–20 mg/dL	1.1–1.4 mmol/L	2–3 h	0.1–0.3 L/kg	90–95%	1° hepatic, metabolites, renal

* Conventional units.

DESCRIPTION: Acetaminophen is used for headache, fever, and pain relief, especially for individuals unable to take salicylate products or who have bleeding conditions. It is the analgesic of choice for children less than 13 years of age; salicylates are avoided in this age group because of the association between aspirin and Reye's syndrome. Acetaminophen is rapidly absorbed from the gastrointestinal tract and reaches peak concentration within 30 to 60 minutes after administration of a therapeutic dose. It can be a silent killer because by the time symptoms of intoxication appear 24 to 48 hours after ingestion, the antidote is ineffective. Acetylsalicylic acid (ASA) is also used for headache, fever, and pain relief. Some patients with cardiovascular disease take small prophylactic doses. The main site of toxicity for both drugs is the liver, particularly in the presence of liver disease or decreased drug metabolism and excretion.

Many factors must be considered in interpreting drug levels, including patient age, patient weight, interacting medications, electrolyte balance, protein levels, water balance, conditions that affect absorption and excretion, and foods, herbals, vitamins, and minerals that can potentiate or inhibit the intended target concentration. ∎

INDICATIONS:

• Suspected overdose

• Suspected toxicity

• Therapeutic monitoring

RESULT

Increased in:
• Acetaminophen
  Alcoholic cirrhosis
  Liver disease
  Toxicity

• ASA
  Toxicity

Decreased in:
• Noncompliance with therapeutic regimen

CRITICAL VALUES: ⚠ *Note:* The adverse effects of subtherapeutic levels are also important. Care should be taken to investigate signs and symptoms of too little and too much medication.

Acetaminophen: Greater than 150 mg/mL

Signs and symptoms of acetaminophen intoxication occur in stages over a period of time. In stage I (0 to 24 hours after ingestion), symptoms may include gastrointestinal irritation, pallor, lethargy, diaphoresis, metabolic acidosis, and possibly coma. In stage II (24 to 48 hours after ingestion), signs and symptoms may include right upper quadrant abdominal pain; elevated liver enzymes, aspartate aminotransferase (AST) and alanine aminotransferase (ALT); and possible decreased renal function. In stage III (72 to 96 hours after ingestion), signs and symptoms may include nausea, vomiting, jaundice, confusion, coagulation disorders, continued elevation of AST and ALT, decreased renal function, and coma. Intervention may include gastrointestinal decontamination (stomach pumping) if the patient presents within 6 hours of ingestion or administration of acetylcysteine in the case of an acute intoxication in which the patient presents more than 6 hours after ingestion.

ASA: Greater than 50 mg/dL

Signs and symptoms of salicylate intoxication include ketosis, convulsions, dizziness, nausea, vomiting, hyperactivity, hyperglycemia, hyperthermia, respiratory arrest, and tinnitus. Possible interventions include emesis, gastric lavage followed by administration of activated charcoal, alkalinization of the urine with bicarbonate, and a single dose of vitamin K (for rare instances of hypoprothrombinemia).

INTERFERING FACTORS:

• Drugs that may increase acetaminophen levels include diflunisal, metoclopramide, and probenecid.

• Drugs that may decrease acetaminophen levels include cholestyramine, iron, oral contraceptives, and propantheline.

- Drugs that increase ASA levels include sulfinpyrazone.

- Drugs that decrease ASA levels include activated charcoal, antacids (aluminum hydroxide), and iron.

Nursing Implications and Procedure • • • • • • • • • •

Pretest:

➤ Obtain a history of the patient's complaints, including a list of known allergens.

➤ Review results of previously performed tests and procedures. For related tests, refer to the genitourinary, hepatobiliary, and therapeutic/toxicology system tables.

➤ Obtain a list of the medications the patient is taking, including herbs, nutritional supplements, and nutraceuticals. The requesting health care practitioner and laboratory should be advised if the patient is regularly using these products so that their effects can be taken into consideration when reviewing results.

➤ There are no food, fluid, or medication restrictions unless by medical direction.

➤ Review the procedure with the patient.

➤ Inform the patient that specimen collection takes approximately 5 to 10 minutes.

Intratest:

➤ Direct the patient to breathe normally and to avoid unnecessary movement.

➤ Observe standard precautions and follow the general guidelines in Appendix A. Perform a venipuncture, and collect the specimen in a 5-mL red-top tube.

➤ Label the specimen, and promptly transport it to the laboratory.

Post-test:

➤ Observe venipuncture site for bleeding or hematoma formation. Apply pressure bandage.

➤ Explain to the patient the importance of following the medication regimen and instructions regarding food and drug interactions.

➤ Instruct the patient to be prepared to list to the pharmacist any other medications he or she is already taking in the event that the requesting health care practitioner gives the patient a prescription to be filled.

➤ Evaluate test results in relation to the patient's symptoms and other tests performed. Related laboratory tests include ALT, AST, bilirubin, complete blood count, creatinine, electrolytes, glucose, lactic acid, liver biopsy, activated partial thromboplastin time, prothrombin time, and blood urea nitrogen.

ANGIOGRAPHY, ABDOMEN

• •

SYNONYMS/ACRONYM: Abdominal angiogram, abdominal arteriography.

AREA OF APPLICATION: Abdomen.

CONTRAST: Iodine based.

DESCRIPTION: Angiography allows x-ray visualization of the large and small arteries, veins, and their associated branches of the abdominal vasculature and organ parenchyma after contrast-medium injection. This visualization is accomplished by the injection of contrast medium through a catheter, which most commonly has been inserted into the femoral artery or vein and advanced through the iliac artery and aorta into the organ-specific artery or vein. Images of the organ under study and associated vessels are displayed on a monitor and recorded on film or stored electronically for future viewing and evaluation. Patterns of circulation, organ function, and changes in vessel wall appearance can be viewed to help diagnose the presence of vascular abnormalities, aneurysm, tumor, trauma, or lesions. The catheter used to administer the contrast medium to confirm the diagnosis of organ lesions may be used to deliver chemotherapeutic drugs or different types of media to stop bleeding. Catheters with attached inflatable balloons and wire mesh stents are used to widen areas of stenosis and to keep the vessels open, frequently replacing surgery. Angiography is one of the definitive tests for organ disease and may be used to evaluate chronic disease, evaluate organ failure, treat arterial stenosis, differentiate a vascular cyst from hypervascular cancers, and evaluate the effectiveness of medical or surgical treatment. ■

INDICATIONS:

- Detect tumors and arterial supply, extent of venous invasion, and tumor vascularity

- Differentiate between tumors and cysts

- Detect nonmalignant tumors before surgical resection

- Allow infusion of thrombolytic drugs into an occluded artery

- Aid in angioplasty, atherectomy, or stent placement

- Detect artery stenosis, evidenced by vessel dilation, collateral vessels, or increased vascular pressure

- Detect arterial occlusion, which may be evidenced by a transection of the artery caused by trauma or penetrating injury

- Evaluate tumor vascularity before surgery or embolization

- Evaluate the vascular system of prospective organ donors before surgery

- Detect thrombosis, arteriovenous fistula, aneurysms, or emboli in abdominal vessels

- Evaluate organ transplantation for function or organ rejection

- Evaluate placement of a shunt or stent

RESULT

Normal Findings:
- Normal structure, function, and patency of abdominal organ vessels

- Contrast medium normally circulates

throughout abdomen symmetrically and without interruption

- No evidence of obstruction, variations in number and size of vessels and organs, malformations, cysts, or tumors

Abnormal Findings:

- Abscess or inflammation

- Arterial aneurysm

- Arterial stenosis, dysplasia, or organ infarction

- Arteriovenous fistula or other abnormalities

- Congenital anomalies

- Cysts or tumors

- Organ hematoma

- Trauma causing tears or other disruption

INTERFERING FACTORS

This procedure is contraindicated for:

- Patients with allergies to shellfish or ⚠ iodinated dye. The contrast medium used may cause a life-threatening allergic reaction. Patients with a known hypersensitivity to contrast medium may benefit from premedication with corticosteroids or the use of nonionic contrast medium.

- Patients with bleeding disorders.

- Patients who are pregnant or suspected of being pregnant, unless the potential benefits of the procedure far outweigh the risks to the fetus and mother.

- Elderly and other patients who are ⚠ chronically dehydrated before the test, because of their risk of contrast-induced renal failure.

- ⚠ Patients who are in renal failure.

Factors that may impair clear imaging:

- Gas or feces in the gastrointestinal tract resulting from inadequate cleansing or failure to restrict food intake before the study

- Retained barium from a previous radiologic procedure

- Metallic objects within the examination field (e.g., jewelry, earrings, dental amalgams), which may inhibit organ visualization and can produce unclear images

- Improper adjustment of the radiographic equipment to accommodate obese or thin patients, which can cause overexposure or underexposure and a poor-quality study

- Patients who are very obese, who may exceed the weight limit for the equipment

- Incorrect positioning of the patient, which may produce poor visualization of the area to be examined

- Inability of the patient to cooperate or remain still during the procedure because of age, significant pain, or mental status

Other considerations:

- Failure to follow dietary restrictions before the procedure may cause the procedure to be canceled or repeated.

- Consultation with a physician should occur before the procedure for radiation safety concerns regarding infants of patients who are lactating.

- Risks associated with radiographic overexposure can result from frequent x-ray procedures. Personnel in the room with the patient should wear a protective lead apron, stand behind a shield, or leave the area while the examination is being done. Personnel working in the area where the examination is being done should wear badges that reveal their level of exposure to radiation.

Nursing Implications and Procedure • • • • • • • • • • •

Pretest:

➤ Inform the patient that the procedure will be performed by a physician and will take 1 to 2 hours.

➤ Inform the patient that the procedure will not be painful, but there may be moments of discomfort.

➤ Inform the patient that a burning and flushing sensation may be felt throughout the body during injection of the contrast medium. After injection of the contrast medium, the patient may experience an urge to cough, flushing, nausea, or a salty or metallic taste.

➤ *An informed consent needs to be obtained and witnessed.*

➤ Instruct the patient regarding the importance of lying motionless throughout the procedure.

➤ Instruct the patient to avoid taking anticoagulant medication or to reduce dosage as ordered before undergoing the procedure.

➤ Determine the date of last menstrual period and the possibility of pregnancy in perimenopausal women.

➤ Patients receiving metformin (Glucophage) for non–insulin-dependent (type 2) diabetes should discontinue the drug on the day of the test and continue to withhold it for 48 hours after the test. Failure to do so may result in lactic acidosis.

➤ Ensure that food has been restricted for at least 8 hours before the procedure.

➤ Instruct the patient to remove metallic objects and valuables before the test.

➤ Obtain a history of known hypersensitivity to iodine, seafood, or contrast medium from previous x-ray procedures.

➤ Obtain a history of the patient's complaints, medication usage, and known allergens.

➤ Obtain a history of the patient's abdominal organs and the results of previous performed tests, treatment, surgeries, and procedures. For related tests, refer to the cardiovascular system table.

➤ Ascertain recent coagulation times and other laboratory test results.

➤ Take baseline vital signs and assess neurologic status.

➤ Complications of the procedure include hemorrhage, infection at the insertion site, cardiac arrhythmias, and embolism caused by the inadvertent dislodgment of an atherosclerotic plaque.

➤ This procedure may be terminated if chest pain, severe cardiac arrhythmias, or signs of a cerebrovascular accident occur.

Intratest:

➤ Have emergency equipment readily accessible.

➤ If the patient has a history of severe allergic reactions to any substance or drug, administer ordered prophylactic steroids or antihistamines before the procedure. Use nonionic contrast medium for the procedure.

➤ Using a pen, mark the site of the patient's peripheral pulses before angiography; this allows quicker and more consistent assessment of the pulses after the procedure.

➤ Place electrocardiographic electrodes on the patient for cardiac monitoring. Establish baseline rhythm; determine if the patient has ventricular arrhythmias.

➤ Establish intravenous fluid line for the injection of contrast medium, emergency drugs, and sedatives.

➤ Administer a mild sedative, as ordered.

➤ Place the patient in the supine position on an x-ray table. Cleanse the selected vein, and cover with a sterile drape.

➤ A local anesthetic is injected at the site, and a small incision is made or a needle inserted. The femoral artery or vein is punctured and the guidewire inserted. The catheter is inserted over the guidewire and threaded into the aorta and the specific organ artery under fluoroscopy.

➤ The contrast medium is injected, and a rapid series of images is taken during and after the filling of the vessels to be examined. Delayed images may be taken to examine the vessels after time has elapsed and to monitor the venous phase of the procedure.

➤ Ask the patient to breathe deeply to relieve nausea.

➤ Monitor the patient for complications related to the contrast medium (e.g., allergic reaction, anaphylaxis, bronchospasm).

➤ The catheter is removed, and a pressure dressing is applied over the puncture site.

➤ Assess extremities for signs of ischemia caused by a catheter-induced thrombus.

Post-test:

➤ Instruct the patient to resume taking ordered medications that were discontinued before the procedure. Renal function should be assessed before metformin is restarted.

➤ Instruct the patient to maintain bed rest for 4 to 6 hours after the procedure or as ordered, to resume previous diet, and to increase fluid intake to counteract the diuretic effects of the contrast medium.

➤ Advise the patient to immediately report symptoms such as fast heart rate, difficulty breathing, skin rash, itching, or decreased urinary output.

➤ Observe the catheter insertion site for bleeding, inflammation, or hematoma formation.

➤ Instruct the patient to apply cold compresses to the puncture site, as needed, to reduce discomfort or edema.

➤ Monitor for absence of pulse distal to catheter insertion site.

➤ Assess neurologic status and vital signs every 15 minutes or as directed.

➤ Observe for a delayed allergic reaction to contrast medium.

➤ A written report of the examination is completed by a physician who specializes in this branch of medicine. The report is sent to the ordering provider, who discusses the results with the patient.

➤ Evaluate test results in relation to the patient's symptoms and other tests performed. Related diagnostic tests include computed tomography and magnetic resonance angiography.

ANGIOGRAPHY, ADRENAL

SYNONYMS/ACRONYM: Adrenal angiogram, adrenal arteriography.

AREA OF APPLICATION: Adrenal gland.

CONTRAST: Iodine based.

DESCRIPTION: Adrenal angiography evaluates adrenal dysfunction by allowing x-ray visualization of the large and small arteries of the adrenal gland vasculature and parenchyma. This visualization is accomplished by the injection of contrast medium through a catheter that has been inserted into the femoral artery for viewing the artery (arteriography) or into the femoral vein for viewing the veins (venography). After the catheter is in place, a blood sample may be taken from the vein of each gland to assess cortisol levels in determining a diagnosis of Cushing's syndrome or the presence of pheochromocytoma. After injection of the contrast medium through the catheter, images of the adrenal glands and associated vessels surrounding the adrenal tissue are displayed on a monitor and are recorded on film or electronically. Patterns of circulation, adrenal function, and changes in vessel wall appearance can be viewed to help diagnose the presence of vascular abnormalities, trauma, or lesions. This definitive test for adrenal disease may be used to evaluate chronic adrenal disease, evaluate arterial or venous stenosis, differentiate an adrenal cyst from adrenal tumors, and evaluate medical therapy or surgery of the adrenal glands. ■

INDICATIONS:

- Detect and determine the location of adrenal tumors evidenced by arterial supply, extent of venous invasion, and tumor vascularity

- Differentiate between adrenal tumors and adrenal cysts

- Detect nonmalignant tumors before surgical resection

- Allow infusion of thrombolytic drugs into an occluded artery

- Perform angioplasty, perform atherectomy, or place a stent

- Detect arterial stenosis, evidenced by vessel dilation, collateral vessels, or increased vascular pressure

- Detect arterial occlusion, evidenced by a transection of the artery caused by trauma or a penetrating injury

- Evaluate tumor vascularity before surgery or embolization

- Detect thrombosis, arteriovenous fistula, aneurysms, or emboli in vessels

- Detect adrenal hyperplasia

- Collect blood samples from the vein for laboratory analysis

RESULT

Normal Findings:
- Normal structure, function, and patency of adrenal vessels

- Contrast medium circulating throughout the adrenal gland symmetrically and without interruption

- No evidence of obstruction, variations in number and size of vessels and organs, malformations, cysts, or tumors

Abnormal Findings:
- Adrenal adenoma

- Adrenal carcinoma

- Bilateral adrenal hyperplasia

- Pheochromocytoma

INTERFERING FACTORS

This procedure is contraindicated for:
- Patients with allergies to shellfish or iodinated contrast medium. The contrast medium used may cause

a life-threatening allergic reaction. Patients with a known hyper-sensitivity to contrast medium may benefit from premedication with corticosteroids or the use of nonionic contrast medium.

• Patients with bleeding disorders.

• Patients who are pregnant or suspected of being pregnant, unless the potential benefits of the procedure far outweigh the risks to the fetus and mother.

• Elderly and other patients who are ⚠ chronically dehydrated before the test, because of their risk of contrast-induced renal failure.

• ⚠ Patients who are in renal failure.

Factors that may impair clear imaging:

• Gas or feces in the gastrointestinal tract resulting from inadequate cleansing or failure to restrict food intake before the study

• Retained barium from a previous radiologic procedure

• Metallic objects within the examination field (e.g., jewelry, earrings, dental amalgams), which may inhibit organ visualization and can produce unclear images

• Improper adjustment of the radiographic equipment to accommodate obese or thin patients, which can cause overexposure or underexposure and a poor-quality study

• Patients who are very obese, who may exceed the weight limit for the equipment

• Incorrect positioning of the patient, which may produce poor visualization of the area to be examined

• Inability of the patient to cooperate or remain still during the procedure because of age, significant pain, or mental status

Other considerations:

• Failure to follow dietary restrictions before the procedure may cause the procedure to be canceled or repeated.

• Consultation with a physician should occur before the procedure for radiation safety concerns regarding infants of patients who are lactating.

• Risks associated with radiographic overexposure can result from frequent x-ray procedures. Personnel in the room with the patient should wear a protective lead apron, stand behind a shield, or leave the area while the examination is being done. Personnel working in the area where the examination is being done should wear badges that reveal their level of exposure to radiation.

Nursing Implications and Procedure • • • • • • • • • • •

Pretest: ■

➤ Inform the patient that the procedure will be performed by a physician and will take 1 to 2 hours.

➤ Inform the patient that the procedure is not painful, but there may be moments of discomfort.

➤ Inform the patient that a burning and flushing sensation may be felt throughout the body during the injection of contrast medium. After the injection of the contrast medium, the patient may experience an urge to cough, flushing, nausea, or a salty or metallic taste.

➤ *An informed consent needs to be obtained and witnessed.*

➤ Instruct the patient regarding the importance of lying motionless throughout the procedure.

➤ Instruct patient to avoid taking anticoagulant medication or to reduce the dosage as ordered before undergoing the procedure.

➤ Patients receiving metformin

(Glucophage) for non–insulin-dependent (type 2) diabetes should discontinue the drug on the day of the test and continue to withhold it for 48 hours after the test. Failure to do so may result in lactic acidosis.

➤ Determine date of last menstrual period and possibility of pregnancy in perimenopausal women.

➤ Ensure that food has been restricted for at least 8 hours before the procedure.

➤ Instruct the patient to remove dentures and metallic objects, including jewelry, before the test.

➤ Obtain a history of known hypersensitivity to iodine, seafood, or contrast medium from previous x-ray procedures.

➤ Obtain a history of the patient's complaints, medication usage, and known allergens.

➤ Obtain a history of the patient's adrenal system and tests, treatments, surgeries, and procedures previously performed. For other related tests, refer to the cardiovascular and endocrine system tables.

➤ Ascertain recent coagulation times, and obtain the results of other laboratory tests as ordered.

➤ Take baseline vital signs and assess neurologic status and peripheral pulses.

➤ The test is contraindicated in the presence of atherosclerosis.

➤ Adrenal hemorrhage may occur from the pressure of the contrast medium on the gland tissue, leading to adrenal insufficiency.

➤ In arteriography, severe hypertensive crisis leading to death may occur if the patient has a pheochromocytoma. Premedication may be administered for several days before the procedure to prevent life-threatening complications.

➤ Potential complications of the procedure are hemorrhage, infection at the insertion site, cardiac arrhythmias, embolism caused by the inadvertent dislodgment of an ather-osclerotic plaque, and thrombophlebitis depending on the vessel used.

Intratest: ■

➤ Have emergency life support equipment readily accessible.

➤ Have the patient void and put on a gown without metallic closures. Remove all metallic objects, but allow the patient to wear dentures and hearing aid.

➤ If the patient has a history of severe allergic reactions to any substance or drug, administer ordered prophylactic steroids or antihistamines before the procedure, and use nonionic contrast medium for the procedure.

➤ Using a pen, mark the site of the patient's peripheral pulses before angiography; this allows quicker and more consistent assessment of the pulses after the procedure.

➤ Place electrocardiographic electrodes on the patient for cardiac monitoring. Establish baseline rhythm; determine if the patient has ventricular arrhythmias.

➤ Establish intravenous fluid line for the injection of contrast medium, emergency drugs, and sedatives.

➤ Administer a mild sedative as ordered.

➤ If the patient is suspected of having a pheochromocytoma, administer medication as ordered to prevent a potentially fatal hypertensive episode.

➤ Place the patient in the supine position on an x-ray table. Cleanse and drape the groin to create a sterile field.

➤ A local anesthetic is injected at the site, and a small incision is made or a needle inserted. The femoral artery is punctured and the guidewire inserted. The catheter is inserted over the guidewire and threaded into the aorta and into the renal arteries under fluoroscopy. For venography, the vein is punctured, and the catheter is advanced into the adrenal vein under fluoroscopic visualization.

➤ The contrast medium is injected, and a rapid series of images is taken during and after the filling of the vessels to be examined. Delayed images may be taken to examine the vessels after a time and to monitor the venous phase of the procedure. Blood samples are obtained through the catheter for laboratory examination in venographic studies.

➤ Ask the patient to breathe deeply to relieve nausea.

➤ Monitor the patient for complications related to the contrast medium (e.g., allergic reaction, anaphylaxis, bronchospasm).

➤ The catheter is removed and a pressure dressing applied over the puncture site for 5 to 10 minutes or longer until bleeding has stopped.

➤ Assess extremities for signs of ischemia caused by a catheter-induced thrombus.

ᵉ Post-test:

➤ Instruct the patient to resume taking ordered medications that were discontinued before the procedure. Renal function should be assessed before metformin is restarted.

➤ Instruct the patient to maintain bed rest for 4 to 6 hours after the procedure or as ordered, to resume previous diet, and to increase fluid intake

to counteract the diuretic effects of contrast medium.

➤ Advise the patient to immediately report symptoms such as fast heart rate, difficulty breathing, skin rash, itching, or decreased urinary output.

➤ Observe the catheter insertion site for bleeding, inflammation, or hematoma formation.

➤ Instruct the patient to apply cold compresses to the puncture site, as needed, to reduce discomfort or edema.

➤ Monitor for absence of pulse distal to catheter insertion site.

➤ Assess neurologic status and vital signs every 15 minutes for 2 hours or as directed.

➤ Observe for a delayed allergic reaction to contrast medium.

➤ A written report of the examination is completed by a physician who specializes in this branch of medicine. The report is sent to the ordering provider, who discusses the results with the patient.

➤ Evaluate test results in relation to the patient's symptoms and other tests performed. Related diagnostic tests include computed tomography, magnetic resonance imaging, positron emission tomography, and magnetic resonance angiography of the abdomen; and adrenal imaging done by nuclear medicine.

ANGIOGRAPHY, CORONARY

SYNONYMS/ACRONYM: Angiocardiography, cardiac angiography, cardiac catheterization, cineangiocardiography, coronary arteriography.

AREA OF APPLICATION: Heart.

CONTRAST: Iodine based.

DESCRIPTION: Angiography allows x-ray visualization of the heart, aorta, inferior vena cava, pulmonary artery and vein, and coronary arteries after injection of contrast medium. Contrast medium is injected through a catheter, which has been inserted into a peripheral vein for a right heart catheterization or an artery for a left heart catheterization; through the same catheter, cardiac pressures are recorded. Images of the heart and associated vessels are displayed on a monitor and are recorded on film or electronically. Patterns of circulation, cardiac output, cardiac functions, and changes in vessel wall appearance can be viewed to help diagnose the presence of vascular abnormalities or lesions. Pulmonary artery abnormalities are seen with right heart views, and coronary artery and thoracic aorta abnormalities are seen with left heart views. Coronary angiography is a definitive test for coronary artery disease, and it is useful for evaluating other types of cardiac abnormalities. ∎

INDICATIONS:
• Detect narrowing of coronary vessels or abnormalities of the great vessels in patients with angina, syncope, abnormal electrocardiogram, hypercholesteremia with chest pain, and persistent chest pain after revascularization

• Quantify the severity of atherosclerotic, occlusive coronary artery disease

• Evaluate cardiac valvular and septal defects

• Evaluate previous cardiac surgery or other interventional procedures

• Evaluate cardiac muscle function

• Evaluate ventricular aneurysms

• Evaluate disease associated with the aortic arch

• Allow infusion of thrombolytic drugs into an occluded coronary artery

• Monitor pulmonary pressures and cardiac output

• Perform angioplasty, perform atherectomy, or place a stent

RESULT

Normal Findings:
• Normal great vessels and coronary arteries

Abnormal Findings:
• Aortic atherosclerosis
• Aortic dissection
• Aortitis
• Aneurysms
• Cardiomyopathy
• Congenital anomalies
• Coronary artery atherosclerosis and degree of obstruction
• Graft occlusion
• Pulmonary artery abnormalities
• Septal defects
• Trauma causing tears or other disruption
• Tumors
• Valvular disease

CRITICAL VALUES: N/A

INTERFERING FACTORS

This procedure is contraindicated for:
• Patients with allergies to shellfish or iodinated dye. The contrast medium used may cause a life-threatening allergic reaction. Patients

with a known hypersensitivity to contrast medium may benefit from premedication with corticosteroids or the use of nonionic contrast medium.

• Patients with bleeding disorders.

• Patients who are pregnant or suspected of being pregnant, unless the potential benefits of the procedure far outweigh the risk of radiation exposure to the fetus.

• Elderly and compromised patients who ⚠ are chronically dehydrated before the test, because of their risk of contrast-induced renal failure.

• ⚠ Patients who are in renal failure.

Factors that may impair clear imaging:
• Inability of the patient to cooperate or remain still during the procedure because of age, significant pain, or mental status

• Metallic objects within the examination field (e.g., jewelry or body rings), which may inhibit organ visualization and can produce unclear images

• Improper adjustment of the radiographic equipment to accommodate obese or thin patients, which can cause overexposure or underexposure and a poor-quality study

• Patients who are very obese, who may exceed the weight limit for the equipment

• Incorrect positioning of the patient, which may produce poor visualization of the area to be examined

Other considerations:
• Failure to follow dietary restrictions before the procedure may cause the procedure to be canceled or repeated.

• Consultation with the radiologist should occur before the procedure for radiation safety concerns regarding infants and patients who are lactating.

• Risks associated with radiographic overexposure can result from frequent x-ray procedures. Personnel in the room with the patient should wear a protective lead apron, stand behind a shield, or leave the area while the examination is being done. Personnel working in the area where the examination is being done should wear badges that reveal their level of exposure to radiation.

Nursing Implications and Procedure • • • • • • • • • • •

Pretest: ■

➤ Inform the patient that the procedure will be performed by a physician and will take 1 to 2 hours.

➤ Inform the patient that the procedure is not painful, but there may be moments of discomfort.

➤ Inform the patient that a burning and flushing sensation may be felt throughout the body during the injection of contrast medium. For 5 minutes after the injection of the contrast medium, the patient may experience an urge to cough, flushing, nausea, or a salty or metallic taste.

➤ *An informed consent needs to be obtained and witnessed.*

➤ Instruct the patient regarding the importance of lying motionless throughout the procedure.

➤ Instruct patient to avoid taking anticoagulant medication or to reduce the dosage as ordered before the procedure.

➤ Patients receiving metformin (Glucophage) for non–insulin-dependent (type 2) diabetes should discontinue the drug on the day of the test and continue to withhold it for 48 hours after the test. Failure to do so may result in lactic acidosis.

➤ Ensure that food and fluids have been restricted for at least 8 hours before the procedure.

➤ Instruct the patient to remove dentures, metallic objects, and valuables before the test.

➤ Obtain a history of known hypersensitivity to iodine, seafood, or contrast medium from previous x-ray procedures. Also obtain a history of ventricular arrhythmias or asthma. For other related tests, refer to the cardiovascular system table.

➤ Ascertain recent coagulation times and other laboratory tests as ordered.

➤ Take baseline vital signs, and assess neurologic status.

➤ Complications of this procedure ⚠ include cardiac arrhythmias, reaction to the iodinated contrast medium, bleeding, infection, arterial thrombosis or embolism, pulmonary or cerebral embolism, vascular perforation, renal failure, and pneumothorax.

➤ This procedure may be terminated if chest pain, severe cardiac arrhythmias, or signs of a cerebrovascular accident occur.

Intratest: ■

➤ Have emergency equipment readily accessible.

➤ If the patient has a history of severe allergic reactions to any substance or drug, administer ordered prophylactic steroids or antihistamines before the procedure. Use nonionic contrast medium for the procedure.

➤ Ask the patient to remove his or her clothes and put on a hospital gown.

➤ Using a pen, mark the site of the patient's peripheral pulses before angiography; this allows quicker and more consistent assessment of the pulses after the procedure.

➤ Place electrocardiographic electrodes on the patient for cardiac monitoring. Establish a baseline rhythm; determine if the patient has ventricular arrhythmias.

➤ Establish an intravenous fluid line for the injection of contrast medium, emergency drugs, or sedatives.

➤ Administer a mild sedative as ordered.

➤ Place the patient in the supine position on an x-ray table. Cleanse the selected vein, and cover with a sterile drape.

➤ A local anesthetic is injected at the site, and a small incision is made or a needle inserted. The catheter is inserted into the femoral or brachial artery for the left side of the heart and the femoral or anticubital vein for the right side of the heart under fluoroscopy. A rapid series of images is obtained after the dye injection. The table may be tilted in various positions to facilitate different views of the heart.

➤ Ask the patient to breathe deeply to relieve nausea; to cough or breathe deeply to permit entry of the catheter into the pulmonary artery; and to move the diaphragm in a downward position, allowing clearer visualization of the heart. Coughing can also correct some arrhythmias.

➤ Monitor the patient for complications related to the contrast medium (e.g., allergic reaction, anaphylaxis, bronchospasm) or to catheterization (e.g., arrhythmias, cardiac or vessel perforation).

➤ The catheter is removed, and a pressure dressing is applied over the puncture site.

➤ Assess extremities for signs of ischemia caused by a catheter-induced thrombus.

Post-test: ■

➤ Instruct the patient to resume taking ordered medications that were discontinued before the procedure. Renal function should be assessed before metformin is restarted.

➤ Instruct the patient to maintain bed rest for 6 to 8 hours after the procedure or as ordered, to resume previous diet, and to increase fluid intake to counteract the diuretic effects of contrast medium.

➤ Advise the patient to immediately report symptoms such as fast heart rate, difficulty breathing, skin rash, itching, or decreased urinary output.

➤ Observe the catheter insertion site for bleeding, inflammation, or hematoma formation.

➤ Monitor for absence of pulse distal to catheter insertion site.

➤ Assess neurologic status and vital signs every 15 minutes for 2 hours or as directed.

➤ Observe for a delayed allergic reaction to contrast medium.

➤ A physician who specializes in this branch of medicine sends a written report to the ordering provider, who discusses the results with the patient.

➤ Evaluate test results in relation to the patient's symptoms and other tests performed. Related diagnostic tests include nuclear imaging, computed tomography, magnetic resonance imaging, and positron emission tomography of the heart.

ANGIOGRAPHY, MAGNETIC RESONANCE

· ·

SYNONYM/ACRONYM: MRA.

AREA OF APPLICATION: Vascular.

CONTRAST: Can be done with or without contrast (gadolinium).

DESCRIPTION: Magnetic resonance imaging (MRI) uses a magnet and radio waves to produce an energy field that can be displayed as an image. The magnetic field causes the hydrogen atoms in tissue to line up, and when radio waves are directed toward the magnetic field, the atoms absorb the radio waves and change their position. When the radio waves are turned off, the atoms go back to their original position, this change in the energy field is sensed by the equipment, and an image is generated by the attached computer system. MRI produces cross-sectional images of the vessels in multiple planes with-out the use of ionizing radiation or the interference of bone or surrounding tissue.

Magnetic resonance angiography (MRA) is an application of MRI that provides images of blood flow and diseased and normal blood vessels. In patients who are allergic to iodinated contrast medium, MRA is used in place of angiography. MRA is particularly useful for visualizing vascular abnormalities, dissections, and other pathology. Special imaging sequences allow the visualization of moving blood within the vascular system. Two common techniques to obtain images of flowing blood are time-of-flight and phase-contrast MRA. In time-of-flight imaging, incoming blood makes the vessels appear bright and surrounding tissue is suppressed. Phase-contrast images are produced by subtracting the stationary tissue surrounding the vessels where the blood is moving through vessels during the imaging, producing high-contrast images. MRA is the most accurate technique for imaging blood flowing in veins and small arteries (*laminar flow*), but it does not accurately depict blood flow in tortuous sections of vessels and distal to bifurcations and stenosis. Swirling blood may cause a signal loss and result in inadequate images, and the degree of vessel stenosis may be overestimated. Images can be obtained in two-dimensional (series of slices) or three-dimensional sequences. ∎

INDICATIONS:
- Detect thoracic and abdominal vascular diseases
- Identify congenital vascular diseases
- Determine renal artery stenosis
- Evaluate postoperative angioplasty sites and bypass grafts
- Detect pericardial abnormalities
- Detect peripheral vascular disease
- Differentiate aortic aneurysms from tumors near the aorta
- Evaluate cardiac chambers and pulmonary vessels
- Monitor and evaluate the effectiveness of medical or surgical treatment

RESULT

Normal Findings:
- Normal blood flow in the area being examined, including blood flow rate

Abnormal Findings:
- Coarctations
- Dissections
- Thrombosis within a vessel
- Tumor invasion of a vessel
- Vascular abnormalities
- Vessel stenosis
- Vessel occlusion

CRITICAL VALUES: N/A

INTERFERING FACTORS

This procedure is contraindicated for:
- Patients with certain ferrous metal prosthetics, valves, aneurysm clips, inner ear prostheses, or other metallic objects
- Patients with metal in their body, such as shrapnel or ferrous metal in the eye
- Patients with cardiac pacemakers, because the pacemaker can be deactivated by MRI
- Patients who are claustrophobic
- Patients who are pregnant or suspected of being pregnant, unless the potential benefits of the procedure far outweigh the risks to the fetus and mother

Factors that may impair clear imaging:
- Inability of the patient to cooperate or remain still during the procedure because of age, significant pain, or mental status
- Patients with extreme cases of claustrophobia, unless sedation is given before the study
- Patients who are very obese, who may exceed the weight limit for the equipment
- Incorrect positioning of the patient,

which may produce poor visualization of the area to be examined

- Metallic objects within the examination field (e.g., jewelry or body rings), which may inhibit organ visualization and can produce unclear images

Other considerations:

- Improper injection of the contrast medium. If contrast medium is allowed to seep deep into the muscle tissue, vascular visualization will be impossible.

Nursing Implications and Procedure · · · · · · · · · · ·

Pretest:

➤ Inform the patient that the test permits assessment of the vascular system.

➤ Inform the patient that the procedure is performed in a special department by a technologist and a physician and takes approximately 30 to 60 minutes.

➤ Obtain a history of allergies or sensitivities to contrast medium.

➤ Obtain pertinent history of vascular findings. For related tests, refer to the cardiovascular system table.

➤ Ensure that the patient and staff have removed all external metallic objects before entering the scanning room.

➤ Obtain a history of previous surgeries and determine if the patient has ever had any device implanted into his or her body.

➤ Inform the patient that intravenous contrast medium may be injected after the first series of images, with a second series of scans following.

➤ Inform the patient that the technologist will place him or her in a supine position on a flat table in a large cylindrical scanner.

➤ Ask the patient to lie still during the procedure because movement produces unclear images.

➤ Tell the patient to expect to hear loud banging from the scanner and possibly to see magneto-phosphenes (flickering lights in the visual field); these will stop when the procedure is over.

➤ Instruct the patient to take slow, deep breaths if nausea occurs during the procedure.

➤ Do not restrict food and fluids.

Intratest:

➤ Ask the patient to remove jewelry, including watches, hairpins, and other metallic objects, and credit cards.

➤ Ask the patient to void before the procedure.

➤ Administer a sedative to a child or to an uncooperative adult, as ordered.

➤ Administer an antianxiety agent, as ordered, if the patient has claustrophobia.

➤ Place the patient in a supine position on a flat table; use foam wedges to help maintain position and immobilization. Ask the patient to lie still during the procedure because movement produces unclear images, thus affecting the results and making interpretation difficult.

➤ Supply earplugs to the patient to block out the loud, banging sounds that occur during the test.

➤ The table is moved into the scanner. Instruct the patient to remain still. The scanner makes noises as it acquires images of the body. The patient may be asked to hold his or her breath to facilitate visualization. A number of images are taken. These images are reconstructed by a computer and reviewed.

➤ Administer the contrast medium, if ordered. A second series of images is obtained.

Post-test:

➤ A physician who specializes in this branch of medicine sends a written report to the ordering provider, who discusses the results with the patient.

➤ Evaluate test results in relation to the patient's symptoms and other tests performed. Related diagnostic tests include computed tomography, angiogram, and Doppler ultrasound.

ANGIOGRAPHY, PULMONARY

SYNONYMS/ACRONYM: Pulmonary angiography, pulmonary arteriography.

AREA OF APPLICATION: Pulmonary vasculature.

CONTRAST: Iodine based.

DESCRIPTION: Pulmonary angiography allows x-ray visualization of the pulmonary vasculature after injection of an iodinated contrast medium into the pulmonary artery or a branch of this great vessel. Contrast medium is injected through a catheter that has been inserted into the vascular system, usually through the femoral vein. It is one of the definitive tests for pulmonary embolism, but it is also useful for evaluating other types of pulmonary vascular abnormalities. It is definitive for peripheral pulmonary artery stenosis, anomalous pulmonary venous drainage, and pulmonary fistulae. Hemodynamic measurements during pulmonary angiography can assist in the diagnosis of pulmonary hypertension and cor pulmonale. ■

INDICATIONS:
• Detect acute pulmonary embolism

• Detect tumors; aneurysms; congenital defects; vascular changes associated with emphysema, blebs, and bullae; and heart abnormalities

• Evaluate pulmonary circulation

• Determine the cause of recurrent or severe hemoptysis

• Detect arteriovenous malformations or aneurysms

RESULT

Normal Findings:
• Normal pulmonary vasculature; radiopaque iodine contrast medium should circulate symmetrically and without interruption through the pulmonary circulatory system.

Abnormal Findings:
• Aneurysms

• Arterial hypoplasia or stenosis

• Arteriovenous malformations

- Bleeding caused by tuberculosis, bronchiectasis, sarcoidosis, or aspergilloma
- Inflammatory diseases
- Pulmonary embolism (acute or chronic)
- Pulmonary sequestration
- Tumors

CRITICAL VALUES: N/A

INTERFERING FACTORS

This procedure is contraindicated for:

- Patients with allergies to shellfish or ⚠ iodinated dye. The contrast medium used may cause a life-threatening allergic reaction. Patients with a known hypersensitivity to contrast medium may benefit from premedication with corticosteroids or the use of nonionic contrast medium.
- Patients who are pregnant or suspected of being pregnant, unless the potential benefits of the procedure far outweigh the risks to the fetus and mother.
- Elderly and other patients who are ⚠ chronically dehydrated before the test, because of their risk of contrast-induced renal failure.
- ⚠ Patients who are in renal failure.

Factors that may impair clear imaging:

- Inability of the patient to cooperate or remain still during the procedure because of age, significant pain, or mental status
- Improper adjustment of the radiographic equipment to accommodate obese or thin patients, which can cause overexposure or underexposure and a poor-quality study
- Patients who are very obese, who may exceed the weight limit for the equipment

- Incorrect positioning of the patient, which may produce poor visualization of the area to be examined
- Metallic objects within the examination field (e.g., jewelry or body rings), which may inhibit organ visualization and can produce unclear images

Other considerations:

- Failure to follow dietary restrictions before the procedure may cause the procedure to be canceled or repeated.
- Consultation with a physician should occur before the procedure for radiation safety concerns regarding infants of patients who are lactating.
- Risks associated with radiographic overexposure can result from frequent x-ray procedures. Personnel in the room with the patient should wear a protective lead apron, stand behind a shield, or leave the area while the examination is being done. Personnel working in the area where the examination is being done should wear badges that reveal their level of exposure to radiation.

Nursing Implications and Procedure • • • • • • • • • • •

Pretest:

➤ Inform the patient that the procedure will be performed by a physician and will take 60 minutes.

➤ Inform the patient that the procedure is not painful, but there may be moments of discomfort.

➤ Inform the patient that a burning and flushing sensation may be felt throughout the body during the injection of the contrast medium. Also, for 5 minutes after the injection of the contrast medium, the patient may experience an urge to cough, flushing, nausea, or a salty or metallic taste.

➤ *An informed consent needs to be obtained and witnessed.*

➤ Instruct the patient regarding the importance of lying motionless throughout the procedure.

➤ Obtain a list of medications the patient is taking.

➤ Instruct the patient to avoid taking anticoagulant medication or to reduce the dosage as ordered before the procedure.

➤ Patients receiving metformin (Glucophage) for non–insulin-dependent (type 2) diabetes should discontinue the drug on the day of the test and continue to withhold it for 48 hours after the test. Failure to do so may result in lactic acidosis.

➤ Ensure that food and fluids have been restricted for at least 8 hours before the procedure.

➤ Instruct the patient to remove dentures, metallic objects, and valuables before the test.

➤ Obtain a history of known hypersensitivity to iodine, seafood, or contrast medium from previous x-ray procedures. Obtain a history of ventricular arrhythmias or asthma. For other tests, refer to the respiratory system table.

➤ Ascertain recent coagulation times, blood urea nitrogen, and creatinine values, as ordered.

➤ Complications of this procedure may include cardiac arrhythmias, reaction to the iodinated contrast medium, vascular perforation, and arterial infarct.

➤ Obtain and record baseline vital signs.

Intratest: ■

➤ Have emergency equipment readily accessible.

➤ If the patient has a history of severe allergic reactions to any substance or drug, administer ordered prophylactic steroids or antihistamines before the procedure. Use nonionic contrast medium for the procedure.

➤ Using a pen, mark the site of the patient's peripheral pulses before angiography; this allows quicker and more consistent assessment of the pulses after the procedure.

➤ Place electrocardiographic electrodes on the patient for cardiac monitoring. Establish baseline rhythm; determine if the patient has ventricular arrhythmias.

➤ Establish intravenous fluid line for the injection of contrast medium, emergency drugs, and sedatives.

➤ Administer a mild sedative as ordered.

➤ Place the patient in the supine position on an x-ray table. Cleanse the selected vein, and cover with a sterile drape.

➤ A local anesthetic is injected at the site, and a small incision is made or a needle inserted. The catheter is inserted into the femoral, brachial, or jugular vein and threaded into the inferior vena cava and right side of the heart under fluoroscopy. From the right ventricle, the catheter is threaded into the pulmonary circulation. A rapid series of images is obtained, with at least two views of each lung obtained after the contrast-medium injection.

➤ Monitor the patient for complications related to the contrast medium (e.g., allergic reaction, anaphylaxis, bronchospasm) or to catheterization (e.g., arrhythmias, cardiac or vessel perforation).

➤ The catheter is removed, and a pressure dressing is applied over the puncture site.

➤ Assess extremities for signs of ischemia caused by a catheter-induced thrombus.

Post-test: ■

➤ Instruct the patient to resume ordered medications that were discontinued before the procedure. Renal function should be assessed before metformin is restarted.

➤ Instruct the patient to maintain bed

rest for 6 to 8 hours after the procedure or as ordered, to resume previous diet, and to increase fluid intake to counteract the diuretic effects of contrast medium.

➤ Advise the patient to immediately report symptoms such as fast heart rate, difficulty breathing, skin rash, itching, or decreased urinary output.

➤ Observe the catheter insertion site for bleeding, inflammation, or hematoma formation.

➤ Observe for a delayed allergic reaction to contrast medium.

➤ A physician who specializes in this branch of medicine sends a written report to the ordering provider, who discusses the results with the patient.

➤ Evaluate test results in relation to patient's symptoms and other tests performed. Related diagnostic tests include chest radiograph, electrocardiogram, lung scan, computed tomography of the chest, echocardiogram, and magnetic resonance imaging of the chest.

ANGIOGRAPHY, RENAL

· ·

SYNONYMS/ACRONYM: Renal angiogram, renal arteriography.

AREA OF APPLICATION: Kidney.

CONTRAST: Iodine based.

DESCRIPTION: Renal angiography allows x-ray visualization of the large and small arteries of the renal vasculature and parenchyma or the renal veins and their branches. Contrast medium is injected through a catheter that has been inserted into the femoral artery or vein and advanced through the iliac artery and aorta into the renal artery or the inferior vena cava into the renal vein. Images of the kidneys and associated vessels are displayed on a monitor and recorded on film or electronically. Patterns of circulation, renal function, or changes in vessel wall appearance can be viewed to help diagnose the presence of vascular abnormalities, trauma, or lesions. This definitive test for renal disease may be used to evaluate chronic renal disease, renal failure, and renal artery stenosis; differentiate a vascular renal cyst from hypervascular renal cancers; and evaluate renal transplant donors, recipients, and the kidney after transplantation. ■

INDICATIONS:

• Detect renal tumors as evidenced by arterial supply, extent of venous invasion, and tumor vascularity

- Differentiate between renal tumors and renal cysts

- Detect nonmalignant tumors before surgical resection

- Allow infusion of thrombolytic drugs into an occluded artery

- Perform angioplasty, perform atherectomy, or place a stent

- Detect renal artery stenosis as evidenced by vessel dilation, collateral vessels, or increased renovascular pressure

- Detect arterial occlusion as evidenced by a transection of the renal artery caused by trauma or a penetrating injury

- Evaluate tumor vascularity before surgery or embolization

- Evaluate the renal vascular system of prospective kidney donors before surgery

- Detect thrombosis, arteriovenous fistulae, aneurysms, or emboli in renal vessels

- Evaluate postoperative renal transplantation for function or organ rejection

- Detect small kidney or absence of a kidney

- Evaluate renal function in chronic renal failure or end-stage renal disease or hydronephrosis

- Collect blood samples from renal vein for renin analysis

RESULT

Normal Findings:

- Normal structure, function, and patency of renal vessels

- Contrast medium circulating throughout the kidneys symmetrically and without interruption

- No evidence of obstruction, variations in number and size of vessels and organs, malformations, cysts, or tumors

Abnormal Findings:

- Abscess or inflammation

- Arterial stenosis, dysplasia, or infarction

- Arteriovenous fistula or other abnormalities

- Congenital anomalies

- Intrarenal hematoma

- Renal artery aneurysm

- Renal cysts or tumors

- Trauma causing tears or other disruption

CRITICAL VALUES: N/A

INTERFERING FACTORS

This procedure is contraindicated for:

- Patients with allergies to shellfish or iodinated dye. The contrast medium used may cause a life-threatening allergic reaction. Patients with a known hypersensitivity to contrast medium may benefit from premedication with corticosteroids or the use of nonionic contrast medium.

- Patients with bleeding disorders.

- Patients who are pregnant or suspected of being pregnant, unless the potential benefits of the procedure far outweigh the risks to the fetus and mother.

- Elderly and other patients who are chronically dehydrated before the test, because of their risk of contrast-induced renal failure.

- Patients who are in renal failure.

Factors that may impair clear imaging:

- Gas or feces in the gastrointestinal tract

resulting from inadequate cleansing or failure to restrict food intake before the study

• Retained barium from a previous radiologic procedure

• Inability of the patient to cooperate or remain still during the procedure because of age, significant pain, or mental status

• Metallic objects within the examination field (e.g., jewelry, earrings, dental amalgams), which may inhibit organ visualization and can produce unclear images

• Improper adjustment of the radiographic equipment to accommodate obese or thin patients, which can cause overexposure or underexposure and a poor-quality study

• Patients who are very obese, who may exceed the weight limit for the equipment

• Incorrect positioning of the patient, which may produce poor visualization of the area to be examined

Other considerations:
• Failure to follow dietary restrictions before the procedure may cause the procedure to be canceled or repeated. Failure to withhold dietary sodium or medications may interfere with accurate analysis of blood sample for renin when done during renal venography.

• Consultation with a physician should occur before the procedure for radiation safety concerns regarding infants of patients who are lactating.

• Risks associated with radiographic overexposure can result from frequent x-ray procedures. Personnel in the room with the patient should wear a protective lead apron, stand behind a shield, or leave the area while the examination is being done. Personnel working in the area where the examination is being done should wear badges that reveal their level of exposure to radiation.

Nursing Implications and Procedure • • • • • • • • • •

Pretest:

➤ Inform the patient that the physician will take 1 to 2 hours to perform the procedure.

➤ Inform the patient that the procedure is not painful, but there may be moments of discomfort.

➤ Inform the patient that a burning and flushing sensation may be felt throughout the body during injection of the contrast medium. After the injection of the contrast medium, the patient may experience an urge to cough, flushing, nausea, or a salty or metallic taste.

➤ *An informed consent needs to be obtained and witnessed.*

➤ Determine date of last menstrual period and possibility of pregnancy in perimenopausal women.

➤ Instruct the patient regarding the importance of lying motionless throughout the procedure.

➤ Instruct patient to avoid taking anticoagulant medication or to reduce the dosage as ordered before the procedure.

➤ Patients receiving metformin (Glucophage) for non–insulin-dependent (type 2) diabetes should discontinue the drug on the day of the test and continue to withhold it for 48 hours after the test. Failure to do so may result in lactic acidosis.

➤ Ensure that food has been restricted for at least 8 hours before the procedure.

➤ Instruct the patient to remove dentures, metallic objects, and valuables before the test.

➤ Obtain a history of known hypersensitivity to iodine, seafood, or contrast medium from previous x-ray procedures.

➤ Obtain a history of the patient's complaints, medication usage, and known allergens.

➤ Obtain a history of the patient's renal system as well as tests and procedures previously performed.

➤ Ascertain recent coagulation times and other laboratory tests as ordered. For related tests, refer to the cardiovascular and genitourinary/renal systems tables.

➤ Take baseline vital signs and assess neurologic status.

➤ Complications of the procedure include hemorrhage, infection at the insertion site, cardiac arrhythmias, and embolism caused by the inadvertent dislodgment of an atherosclerotic plaque.

➤ This procedure may be terminated if chest pain, severe cardiac arrhythmias, or signs of a cerebrovascular accident occur.

Intratest:

➤ Have emergency equipment readily accessible.

➤ If the patient has a history of severe allergic reactions to various substances or drugs, administer ordered prophylactic steroids or antihistamines before the procedure. Use nonionic contrast medium for the procedure.

➤ Using a pen, mark the site of the patient's peripheral pulses before angiography; this allows quicker and more consistent assessment of the pulses after the procedure.

➤ Place electrocardiographic electrodes on the patient for cardiac monitoring. Establish baseline rhythm; determine if the patient has ventricular arrhythmias.

➤ Establish intravenous fluid line for the injection of contrast medium, emergency drugs, and sedatives.

➤ Administer a mild sedative as ordered.

➤ Place the patient in the supine position on an x-ray table. Cleanse the selected vein, and cover with a sterile drape.

➤ A local anesthetic is injected at the site, and a small incision is made or a needle inserted. The femoral artery or vein is punctured and the guidewire inserted. The catheter is inserted over the guidewire and threaded up into the aorta and into the renal arteries under fluoroscopy.

➤ The contrast medium is injected, and a rapid series of images is taken during and after the filling of the vessels to be examined. Delayed images may be taken to examine the vessels after time has elapsed and to monitor the venous phase of the procedure.

➤ Ask the patient to breathe deeply to relieve nausea.

➤ Monitor the patient for complications related to the contrast medium (allergic reaction, anaphylaxis, bronchospasm).

➤ The catheter is removed, and a pressure dressing is applied over the puncture site.

➤ Assess extremities for signs of ischemia caused by a catheter-induced thrombus.

Post-test:

➤ Instruct the patient to resume taking ordered medications that were discontinued before the procedure. Renal function should be assessed before metformin is restarted.

➤ Instruct the patient to maintain bed rest for 4 to 6 hours after the procedure or as ordered, to resume previous diet, and to increase fluid intake to counteract the diuretic effects of contrast medium.

➤ Advise the patient to immediately report symptoms such as fast heart rate, difficulty breathing, skin rash, itching, or decreased urinary output.

➤ Observe the catheter insertion site for bleeding, inflammation, or hematoma formation.

➤ Instruct the patient to apply cold compresses to the puncture site, as needed, to reduce discomfort or edema.

➤ Monitor for absence of pulse distal to catheter insertion site.

➤ Assess neurologic status and vital signs every 15 minutes for 2 hours or as directed.

➤ Observe for a delayed allergic reaction to contrast medium.

➤ A physician who specializes in this branch of medicine prepares a writ-ten report that is sent to the ordering provider, who discusses the results with the patient.

➤ Evaluate test results in relation to the patient's symptoms and other tests performed. Related diagnostic tests include computed tomography (CT) and magnetic resonance angiography of the kidneys; and positron emission tomography, CT, and magnetic resonance imaging of the abdomen.

ANGIOTENSIN-CONVERTING ENZYME

· ·

SYNONYM/ACRONYM: Angiotensin-I-converting enzyme (ACE).

SPECIMEN: Serum (1 mL) collected in a red- or tiger-top tube.

REFERENCE VALUE: (Method: Spectrophotometry)

Age	Conventional Units	SI Units (Conversion Factor ×0.017)
0–2 y	5–83 U/L	0.09–1.41 μKat/L
3–7 y	8–76 U/L	0.14–1.29 μKat/L
8–14 y	6–89 U/L	0.10–1.51 μKat/L
Greater than 14 y	8–52 U/L	0.14–0.88 μKat/L

DESCRIPTION: Angiotensin-converting enzyme (ACE) production occurs mainly in the epithelial cells of the pulmonary bed. Smaller amounts are found in blood vessels and renal tissue, where ACE converts angiotensin I to angiotensin II; this conversion helps regulate arterial blood pressure. Angiotensin II stimulates the adrenal cortex to produce aldosterone. Aldosterone is a hormone that helps the kidneys maintain water balance by retaining sodium and promoting the excretion of potassium.

ACE levels are used primarily in the evaluation of hypertension and active sarcoidosis, a granulomatous disease that can affect many organs, including the lungs. Serial levels are useful in correlating the therapeutic response to corticosteroid treatment. Increasing ACE levels with positive gallium scans in sarcoidosis patients receiving steroids indicate a poor response to therapy. Monitoring ACE levels may also have some utility in assessing the risk of pulmonary damage in affected patients receiving antineoplastic agents. Thyroid hormones may play a role in regulating ACE levels: decreased levels have been noted in patients with clinical hypothyroidism and anorexia nervosa, whereas increased levels have been noted in patients with hyperthyroidism. Elevations of serum ACE have been reported in 20 to 30 percent of patients with abnormal α_1-antitrypsin variants. ACE levels are sometimes ordered on cerebrospinal fluid to evaluate patients with neurosarcoidosis. Results must be interpreted with care because of the nonspecificity of increased and decreased ACE levels. ACE is normally elevated in pediatric patients and therefore is not a useful marker in the evaluation of disease for patients less than 20 years of age. ■

INDICATIONS:

• Assist in establishing a diagnosis of sarcoidosis

• Assist in the evaluation of Gaucher's disease

• Assist in the treatment of sarcoidosis

• Evaluate hypertension

• Evaluate the severity and activity of sarcoidosis

RESULT

Increased in:
• Bronchitis (acute and chronic)

• Connective tissue disease

• Gaucher's disease

• Hansen's disease (leprosy)

• Histoplasmosis and other fungal diseases

• Hyperthyroidism (untreated)

• Pulmonary fibrosis

• Rheumatoid arthritis

• Sarcoidosis

Decreased in:
• Advanced pulmonary carcinoma

• The period following corticosteroid therapy for sarcoidosis

CRITICAL VALUES: N/A

INTERFERING FACTORS:

• Drugs that may increase serum ACE levels include triiodothyronine.

• Drugs that may decrease serum ACE levels include captopril, cilazapril, enalapril, fosinopril, lisinopril, nicardipine, pentopril, perindopril, propranolol, quinapril, ramipril, and trandolapril.

• Prompt and proper specimen processing, storage, and analysis are important to achieve accurate results. Failure to freeze sample if not tested immediately may cause falsely decreased values because ACE degrades rapidly.

Nursing Implications and Procedure · · · · · · · · · · ·

Pretest:

➤ Obtain a history of the patient's complaints, including a list of known allergens.

➤ Obtain a history of the patient's endocrine, immune, musculoskeletal, and respiratory systems, as well as results of previously performed tests and procedures. For related tests, refer to the endocrine, immune, musculoskeletal, and respiratory system tables.

➤ Obtain a list of the medications the patient is taking, including herbs, nutritional supplements, and nutraceuticals. The requesting health care practitioner and laboratory should be advised if the patient regularly uses these products so that their effects can be taken into consideration when reviewing results.

➤ There are no food, fluid, or medication restrictions unless by medical direction.

➤ Note the patient's age. This test is rarely ordered on patients less than 20 years old.

➤ Review the procedure with the patient.

➤ Inform the patient that specimen collection usually takes 5 to 10 minutes.

Intratest:

➤ Direct the patient to breathe normally and to avoid unnecessary movement.

➤ Observe standard precautions and follow the general guidelines in Appendix A.

➤ Perform a venipuncture, and collect the specimen in a 5-mL red- or tiger-top tube.

➤ Label the specimen, and promptly transport it to the laboratory.

Post-test:

➤ Observe venipuncture site for bleeding or hematoma formation. Apply pressure bandage.

➤ ACE levels affect the regulation of fluid balance and electrolytes. Dietary adjustment may be considered if sodium allowances need to be regulated. Educate patients with low sodium levels that the major source of dietary sodium is found in table salt. Many foods such as milk and other dairy products are also good sources of dietary sodium. Most other dietary sodium is available through consumption of processed foods. Patients who need to follow low-sodium diets should be advised to avoid beverages such as colas, ginger ale, Gatorade, lemon-lime sodas, and root beer. Many over-the-counter medications, including antacids, laxatives, analgesics, sedatives, and antitussives, contain significant amounts of sodium. The best advice is to emphasize the importance of reading all food, beverage, and medicine labels. In 1989, the Subcommittee on the 10th Edition of the Recommended Dietary Allowances (RDAs) established 500 mg as the recommended minimum limit for dietary intake of sodium. There are no RDAs established for potassium, but the estimated minimum intake for adults is 200 mEq/d. Potassium is present in all plant and animal cells, making dietary replacement fairly simple. A health care practitioner or nutritionist should be consulted before considering the use of salt substitutes.

➤ Evaluate test results in relation to the patient's symptoms and other tests performed. Related laboratory tests include aldosterone, alkaline phosphatase, α_1-antitrypsin, α_1-antitrypsin phenotyping, arterial/alveolar oxygen ratio, anion gap, blood gases, serum and urine calcium, electrolytes, erythrocyte sedimentation rate, urine protein, liver biopsy, lymph node biopsy, phosphorus, potassium, protein electrophoresis, renin, rheumatoid factor, skin biopsy, sodium, and thyroid hormone levels.

ANION GAP

. . . . ■ . . . . . .

SYNONYM/ACRONYM: AG, Agap.

SPECIMEN: Serum (1 mL) for electrolytes collected in a red- or tiger-top tube. Plasma (1 mL) collected in green-top (heparin) tube is also acceptable.

REFERENCE VALUE: (Method: Anion gap is derived mathematically from the direct measurement of sodium, chloride, and total carbon dioxide.) There are differences between serum and plasma values for some electrolytes. The reference ranges listed are based on serum values.

Age	Conventional Units	SI Units (Conversion Factor ×1)
Child	8–16 mEq/L	8–16 mmol/L
Adult	8–16 mEq/L	8–16 mmol/L

DESCRIPTION: The anion gap is used most frequently as a clinical indicator of metabolic acidosis. It does not include measurement of important cations, such as calcium, potassium (usually), and magnesium; or anions, such as proteins, forms of phosphorus, sulfur, and organic acids. The anion gap is calculated as follows:

(sodium − [chloride + HCO₃⁻])

Because HCO_3^- is not directly measured on most multichannel chemistry analyzers, HCO_3^- is estimated by substitution of total carbon dioxide value in the calculation. Some laboratories may include potassium in the calculation of anion gap. Calculations including potassium can be invalidated because minor amounts of hemolysis can contribute significant levels of potassium leaked into the serum as a result of cell rupture. The anion gap is also widely used as a laboratory quality control measure because low gaps usually indicate a reagent, calibration, or instrument error. ■

INDICATIONS:
• Evaluate metabolic acidosis

• Indicate the presence of a disturbance in electrolyte balance

• Indicate the need for laboratory instrument recalibration or review of electrolyte reagent preparation and stability

RESULT

Increased in:
• Dehydration (severe)

• Excessive exercise

- Ketoacidosis caused by starvation, high-protein/low-carbohydrate diet, diabetes, and alcoholism

- Lactic acidosis

- Poisoning (salicylate, methanol, ethylene glycol, or paraldehyde)

- Renal failure

- Uremia

Decreased in:

- Hyperchloremia

- Hypergammaglobulinemia (multiple myeloma)

- Hypoalbuminemia

- Hyponatremia (hyperviscosity syndromes)

TCO_2 is commonly substituted for HCO_3^- in anion gap calculations. It is important to note the clinical significance of excessive HCO_3^-, which occurs in renal alkalosis, gastrointestinal alkalosis, and excessive ingestion of exogenous sources of alkali, the effects of which may not be accurately reflected by the calculated anion gap.

CRITICAL VALUES: N/A

INTERFERING FACTORS

- Drugs that can increase or decrease the anion gap include those listed in the individual electrolyte (i.e., sodium, chloride, calcium, magnesium, and total carbon dioxide), total protein, lactic acid, and phosphorus monographs.

- Specimens should never be collected above an intravenous line because of the potential for dilution when the specimen and the intravenous solution combine in the collection container, falsely decreasing the result. There is also the potential of contaminating the sample with the substance of interest, contained in the intravenous solution, falsely increasing the result.

Nursing Implications and Procedure

Pretest:

➤ Obtain a history of the patient's complaints, including a list of known allergens.

➤ Obtain a history of the patient's cardiovascular, endocrine, gastrointestinal, genitourinary, hematopoietic, immune, and respiratory systems, as well as results of previously performed tests and procedures. For other related tests, refer to the cardiovascular, endocrine, gastrointestinal, genitourinary, hematopoietic, immune, and respiratory system tables.

➤ Obtain a list of the medications the patient is taking, including herbs, nutritional supplements, and nutraceuticals. The requesting health care practitioner and laboratory should be advised if the patient regularly uses these products so that their effects can be taken into consideration when reviewing results.

➤ There are no food, fluid, or medication restrictions unless by medical direction.

➤ Review the procedure with the patient.

➤ Inform the patient that specimen collection takes approximately 5 to 10 minutes.

Intratest:

➤ Direct the patient to breathe normally and to avoid unnecessary movement.

➤ Observe standard precautions and follow the general guidelines in Appendix A. Perform a venipuncture, and collect the specimen in a 5-mL red- or tiger-top tube.

➤ Label the specimen, and promptly transport it to the laboratory.

Post-test:

➤ Observe venipuncture site for bleeding or hematoma formation. Apply pressure bandage.

➤ Specific dietary considerations are listed in the monographs on individual electrolytes (i.e., sodium, chloride, calcium, and magnesium), total protein, and phosphorus.

➤ The anion gap can be used to indicate the presence of dehydration. Evaluate the patient for signs and symptoms of dehydration. Dehydration is a significant and common finding in geriatric patients and patients with decreased renal function.

➤ Evaluate test results in relation to the patient's symptoms and other tests performed. Related laboratory tests include albumin, blood gases, creatinine, electrolytes, ethanol, glucose, ketones, lactic acid, osmolality, protein, protein electrophoresis, salicylate, blood urea nitrogen, and urinalysis.

ANTIARRHYTHMIC DRUGS: DIGOXIN, DISOPYRAMIDE, FLECAINIDE, LIDOCAINE, PROCAINAMIDE, QUINIDINE

SYNONYMS/ACRONYMS: *Digoxin* (Allocar, Cardioreg, Digacin, Lanocor, Lanoxicaps, Lanoxin, Lenoxin, Purgoxin); *disopyramide* (Dicorynan, Napamide, Norpace, Rhythmodan, Ritmilen); *flecainide* (Almartyn, Tambocor); *lidocaine* (Anestacon, Baylocaine, Dalcaine, Dilocaine, Duo-Trach, LidoPen, Lignocaine, Nervocaine, Norocaine, Octocaine, Xylocaine); *procainamide* (Biocoryl, Novocainamidum, Novocamid, Procaine Amide Hydrochloride, Procan SR, Pronestyl, Pronestyl SR, Retard, Rhythmin); *quinidine* (Biquin, Cardioquin, Cin-Quin, Kiditard, Kinidin, Quinaglute, Dura-Tabs, Quinalan, Quinidex, Extentabs, Quini, Durules, Quinora, Systodin).

SPECIMEN: Serum (1 mL) collected in a red-top tube.

Drug	Route of Administration	Recommended Collection Time
Digoxin	Oral	Trough: 12–24 h after dose
		Never draw peak samples
Disopyramide	Oral	Trough: immediately before next dose
		Peak: 2–5 h after dose
Flecainide	Oral	Trough: immediately before next dose
		Peak: 3 h after dose
Lidocaine	IV	15 min, 1 h, then every 24 h
Procainamide	IV	15 min; 2, 6, 12 hours; then every 24 h
Procainamide	Oral	Trough: immediately before next dose
		Peak: 75 min after dose
Quinidine sulfate	Oral	Trough: immediately before next dose
		Peak: 1 h after dose
Quinidine gluconate	Oral	Trough: immediately before next dose
		Peak: 5 h after dose
Quinidine polygalacturonate	Oral	Trough: immediately before next dose
		Peak: 2 h after dose

IV = intravenous.

Drug (Indication)	Therapeutic Dose*	SI Units	Half-Life (h)	Volume of Distribution (L/kg)	Protein Binding (%)	Excretion
Digoxin (arrhythmias)	1.5–2.0 ng/mL	*(Conversion Factor × 1.28)* 1.9–2.6 nmol/L	20–60	7	20–30	60% renal 40% hepatic
Digoxin (CHF)	0.8–1.5 ng/mL	1.0–1.9 nmol/L				
Disopyramide (atrial arrhythmias)	2.8–3.2 µg/mL	*(Conversion Factor × 2.95)* 8.3–9.4 µmol/L	4–10	0.7–0.9	50–80	50% renal 50% hepatic
Disopyramide (ventricular arrhythmias)	3.3–7.5 µg/mL	9.7–22.1 µmol/L				
Flecainide	0.2–1.0 µg/mL	*(Conversion Factor × 2.41)* 0.5–2.4 µmol/L	7–27	5–13	30–60	30% renal 70% hepatic
Lidocaine	1.5–6.0 µg/mL	*(Conversion Factor × 4.27)* 6.4–26 µmol/L	1.5–2	1–1.5	60–70	90% hepatic
Procainamide	4–10 µg/mL	*(Conversion Factor × 4.23)* 17–42 µmol/L	2–6	2–4	10–20	50% renal 50% hepatic
N-acetyl procainamide	5–30 µg/mL	*(Conversion Factor × 3.61)* 18–108 µmol/L	8			
Quinidine	2–5 µg/mL	*(Conversion Factor × 3.08)* 6–15 µmol/L	6–8	2–3	80–90	10–30% renal 60–80% hepatic

* Conventional units.
CHF = congestive heart failure.

DESCRIPTION: Cardiac glycosides are used in the prophylactic management and treatment of heart failure and ventricular and atrial arrhythmias. Because these drugs have narrow therapeutic windows, they must be monitored closely. The signs and symptoms of toxicity are often difficult to distinguish from those of cardiac disease. Patients with toxic levels may show gastrointestinal, ocular, and central nervous system effects and disturbances in potassium balance.

Many factors must be considered in effective dosing and monitoring of therapeutic drugs, including patient age, patient weight, interacting medications, electrolyte balance, protein levels, water balance, conditions that affect absorption and excretion, and the ingestion of substances (e.g., foods, herbals, vitamins, and minerals) that can either potentiate or inhibit the intended target concentration. Peak and trough collection times should be documented carefully in relation to the time of medication administration. ■

IMPORTANT NOTE: This information must be communicated clearly and accurately to avoid misunderstanding of the dose time in relation to the collection time. Miscommunication between the individual administering the medication and the individual collecting the specimen is the most frequent cause of subtherapeutic levels, toxic levels, and misleading information used in the calculation of future doses.

INDICATIONS:

• Assist in the diagnosis and prevention of toxicity

• Monitor compliance to therapeutic regimen

• Monitor patients who have a pacemaker, who have impaired renal or hepatic function, or who are taking interacting drugs

RESULT

Level	Result
Normal levels	Therapeutic effect
Subtherapeutic levels	Adjust dose as indicated
Toxic levels	Adjust dose as indicated
Digoxin	Renal impairment, CHF, elderly patients
Disopyramide	Renal or hepatic impairment
Flecainide	Renal or hepatic impairment, CHF
Lidocaine	Hepatic impairment, CHF
Procainamide	Renal impairment
Quinidine	Hepatic impairment, CHF, elderly patients

CHF = congestive heart failure.

CRITICAL VALUES: ⚠ Adverse effects of subtherapeutic levels are important. Care should be taken to investigate the signs and symptoms of too little and too much medication.

Digoxin: Greater Than 2.5 ng/mL

Signs and symptoms of digoxin toxicity include arrhythmias, anorexia, hyperkalemia, nausea, vomiting, diarrhea, changes in mental status, and visual disturbances (objects appear yellow or have halos around them). Possible interventions include discontinuing the medication, continuous electrocardiogram (ECG) monitoring (prolonged P-R interval, widening QRS interval, lengthening Q-Tc, and atrioventricular block), transcutaneous pacing, administration of activated charcoal (if the patient has a gag reflex and central nervous system function), support and treatment of electrolyte disturbance, and administration of Digibind (digoxin immune Fab). The amount of Digibind given depends on the level of digoxin to be neutralized. Digoxin levels must be measured before the administration of Digibind. Digoxin levels should not be measured for several days after administration of Digibind in patients with normal renal function (1 week or longer in patients with decreased renal function). Digibind cross-reacts in the digoxin assay and may provide misleading elevations or decreases in values depending on the particular assay in use by the laboratory.

Disopyramide: Greater Than 7 µg/mL

Signs and symptoms of disopyramide toxicity include prolonged Q-T interval, ventricular tachycardia, hypotension, and heart failure. Possible interventions include discontinuing the medication, airway support, and ECG and blood pressure monitoring.

Flecainide: Greater than 1 µg/mL

Signs and symptoms of flecainide toxicity include exaggerated pharmacologic effects resulting in arrhythmia. Possible interventions include discontinuing the medication as well as continuous ECG, respiratory, and blood pressure monitoring.

Lidocaine: Greater Than 9 µg/mL

Signs and symptoms of lidocaine toxicity include slurred speech, central nervous system depression, cardiovascular depression, convulsions, muscle twitches, and possible coma. Possible interventions include continuous ECG monitoring, airway support, seizure precautions, and hourly monitoring of temperature for hyperthermia.

Procainamide: Greater Than 12 µg/mL; Procainamide + N-acetyl Procainamide: Greater Than 30 µg/mL

The active metabolite of procainamide is N-acetyl procainamide (NAPA). Signs and symptoms of procainamide toxicity include torsades de pointes (ventricular tachycardia), nausea, vomiting, agranulocytosis, and hepatic disturbances. Possible interventions include airway protection, emesis, gastric lavage, and administration of sodium lactate.

Quinidine: Greater Than 8 µg/mL

Signs and symptoms of quinidine toxicity include ataxia, nausea, vomiting, diarrhea, respiratory system depression, hypotension, syncope, anuria, arrhythmias (heart block, widening of QRS and Q-T intervals), asystole, hallucinations, paresthesia, and irritability. Possible interventions include airway support, emesis, gastric lavage, administration of activated charcoal, administration of sodium lactate, and temporary transcutaneous or transvenous pacemaker.

INTERFERING FACTORS:

- Drugs that may increase digoxin levels or increase risk of toxicity include amiodarone, amphotericin B, diltiazem, diclofenac, erythromycin, propantheline, quinidine, spironolactone, tetracycline, and verapamil.

- Drugs that may decrease digoxin levels include aluminum hydroxide (antacids), cholestyramine, colestipol, kaolin-pectin, metoclopramide, neomycin, phenytoin, and sulfasalazine.

- Drugs that may increase disopyramide levels or increase risk of toxicity include amiodarone and troleandomycin.

- Drugs that may decrease disopyramide levels include rifampin.

- Drugs that may increase flecainide levels or increase risk of toxicity include amiodarone and cimetidine.

- Drugs that may increase lidocaine levels or increase risk of toxicity include anticonvulsants, beta blockers, cimetidine, metoprolol, nadolol, and propranolol.

- Drugs that may increase procainamide levels or increase risk of toxicity include amiodarone, other antiarrhythmics, cimetidine, ranitidine, and trimethoprim.

- Drugs that may increase quinidine levels or increase risk of toxicity include amiodarone, cimetidine, verapamil, and thiazide diuretics.

- Drugs that may decrease quinidine levels include disopyramide, nifedipine, phenobarbital, phenytoin, and rifampin.

- Digitoxin cross-reacts with digoxin; results are falsely elevated if digoxin is measured when the patient is taking digitoxin.

- Digitalis-like immunoreactive substances are found in the sera of some patients who are not taking digoxin, causing false-positive results. Patients whose sera contain digitalis-like immunoreactive substances usually have a condition related to salt and fluid retention, such as renal failure, hepatic failure, low renin hypertension, and pregnancy.

- Unexpectedly low digoxin levels may be found in patients with thyroid disease.

- Disopyramide may cause a decrease in glucose levels. It may also potentiate the anticoagulating effects of warfarin.

- Long-term administration of procainamide can cause false-positive antinuclear antibody results and development of a lupus-like syndrome in some patients.

- Quinidine may potentiate the effects of neuromuscular blocking medications and warfarin anticoagulants.

- Concomitant administration of quinidine and digoxin can rapidly raise digoxin to toxic levels. If both drugs are to be given together, the digoxin level should be measured before the first dose of quinidine and again in 4 to 6 days.

Nursing Implications and Procedure

Pretest:

➤ Obtain a history of the patient's complaints, including a list of known allergens.

➤ Review results of previously performed tests and procedures. For related tests, refer to the cardiovascular system and therapeutic/toxicology tables.

➤ Obtain a list of the medications the patient is taking, including herbs, nutritional supplements, and nutraceuticals. The requesting health care practitioner and laboratory should be advised if the patient regularly uses these products so that their effects can be taken into consideration when reviewing results.

➤ There are no food, fluid, or medication restrictions unless by medical direction.

➤ Review the procedure with the patient.

➤ Inform the patient that specimen collection takes approximately 5 to 10 minutes.

Intratest:

➤ Direct the patient to breathe normally and to avoid unnecessary movement.

➤ Observe standard precautions and follow the general guidelines in Appendix A. Consider recommended collection time around dosing schedule. Perform a venipuncture, and collect the specimen in a 5-mL red-top tube.

➤ Label the specimen, and promptly transport it to the laboratory.

Post-test:

➤ Observe venipuncture site for bleeding or hematoma formation. Apply pressure bandage.

➤ Explain to the patient the impor-

tance of following the medication regimen and instructions regarding drug interactions. Instruct the patient to report any unusual sensations, such as dizziness or blurry vision, immediately to his or her health care practitioner.

➤ Instruct the patient to be prepared to provide the pharmacist with a list of other medications he or she is already taking in the event that the requesting health care practitioner prescribes a medication.

➤ Evaluate test results in relation to the patient's symptoms and other tests performed. Related laboratory tests include alanine aminotransferase, albumin, alkaline phosphatase, aspartate aminotransferase, creatinine, electrolytes, and urea nitrogen.

ANTIBIOTIC DRUGS— AMINOGLYCOSIDES: AMIKACIN, GENTAMICIN, TOBRAMYCIN; TRICYCLIC GLYCOPEPTIDE: VANCOMYCIN

SYNONYMS: *Amikacin* (Amikin); *gentamicin* (Garamycin, Genoptic, Gentacidin, Gentafair, Gentak, Gentamar, Gentrasul, G-myticin, Oco-Mycin, Spectro-Genta); *tobramycin* (Nebcin, Tobrex); *vancomycin* (Lyphocin, Vancocin, Vancoled).

SPECIMEN: Serum (1 mL) collected in a red-top tube.

Antibiotic Type	Route of Administration	Recommended Collection Time*
Aminoglycosides		
Amikacin	IV, IM	Trough: immediately before next dose
		Peak: 30 min after 30-min IV
Gentamicin	IV, IM	Trough: immediately before next dose
		Peak: 30 min after 30-min IV infusion
Tobramycin	IV, IM	Trough: immediately before next dose
		Peak: 30 min after 30-min IV infusion
Tricyclic glycopeptide		
Vancomycin	IV, PO	Trough: immediately before next dose
		Peak: 2 h after dose

* Usually after fifth dose if given every 8 h or third dose if given every 12 h.
IV = intravenous; IM = intramuscular; PO = by mouth.

Drug	Therapeutic Dose*	SI Units	Half-Life (h)	Volume of Distribution (L/kg)	Protein Binding (%)	Excretion
Amikacin		*(Conversion Factor × 1.71)*				
Peak	20–30 µg/mL	34–51 µmol/L	4–8	0.4–1.3	50	90% renal
Trough	4–8 µg/mL	7–14 µmol/L				
Gentamicin		*(Conversion Factor × 2.09)*				
Peak	6–10 µg/mL	12–21 µmol/L	4–8	0.4–1.3	50	90% renal
Trough	Less than 2 µg/mL	Less than 4 µmol/L				
Tobramycin		*(Conversion Factor × 2.14)*				
Peak	6–10 µg/mL	13–21 µmol/L	4–8	0.4–1.3	50	90% renal
Trough	Less than 2 µg/mL	Less than 4 µmol/L				
Vancomycin		*(Conversion Factor × 0.69)*				
Peak	20–40 µg/mL	14–28 µmol/L	4–8	0.4–1.3	50	90% renal
Trough	5–10 µg/mL	3–7 µmol/L				

* Conventional units.

91

DESCRIPTION: The aminoglycoside antibiotics amikacin, gentamicin, and tobramycin are used against many gram-negative (*Acinetobacter, Citrobacter, Enterobacter, Escherichia coli, Klebsiella, Proteus, Providencia, Pseudomonas, Salmonella, Serratia,* and *Shigella*) and some gram-positive (*Staphylococcus aureus*) pathogenic microorganisms. Aminoglycosides are poorly absorbed through the gastrointestinal tract and are most frequently administered intravenously.

Vancomycin is a tricyclic glycopeptide antibiotic used against many gram-positive microorganisms, such as staphylococci, *Streptococcus pneumoniae,* group A β-hemolytic streptococci, enterococci, *Corynebacterium,* and *Clostridium.* Vancomycin has also been used in an oral form for the treatment of pseudomembranous colitis resulting from *Clostridium difficile* infection. This approach is less frequently used because of the emergence of vancomycin-resistant enterococci.

Many factors must be considered in effective dosing and monitoring of therapeutic drugs, including patient age, patient weight, interacting medications, electrolyte balance, protein levels, water balance, conditions that affect absorption and excretion, and ingestion of substances (e.g., foods, herbals, vitamins, and minerals) that can either potentiate or inhibit the intended target concentration. The most serious side effects of the aminoglycosides and vancomycin are renal impairment and irreversible ototoxicity (uncommon). Peak and trough collection times should be documented carefully in relation to the time of medication administration. ∎

IMPORTANT NOTE: This information must be clearly and accurately communicated to avoid misunderstanding of the dose time in relation to the collection time. Miscommunication between the individual administering the medication and the individual collecting the specimen is the most frequent cause of subtherapeutic levels, toxic levels, and misleading information used in the calculation of future doses. Some pharmacies use a computerized pharmacokinetic approach to dosing that eliminates the need to be concerned about peak and trough collections; random specimens are adequate.

INDICATIONS:
- Assist in the diagnosis and prevention of toxicity
- Monitor renal dialysis patients or patients with rapidly changing renal function
- Monitor therapeutic regimen

RESULT

Level	Result
Normal levels	Therapeutic effect
Subtherapeutic levels	Adjust dose as indicated
Toxic levels	Adjust dose as indicated
Amikacin	Renal, hearing impairment
Gentamicin	Renal, hearing impairment
Tobramycin	Renal, hearing impairment
Vancomycin	Renal, hearing impairment

CRITICAL VALUES: ⚠ The adverse effects of subtherapeutic levels are important. Care should be taken to investigate signs and symptoms of too little and too much medication.

Signs and symptoms of toxic levels of these antibiotics are similar and include loss of hearing and decreased renal function. The most important intervention is accurate therapeutic drug monitoring so the medication can be discontinued before irreversible damage is done.

Drug Name	Toxic Levels
Amikacin	Peak greater than 35 μg/mL, trough greater than 10 μg/mL
Gentamicin	Peak greater than 10 μg/mL, trough greater than 2 μg/mL
Tobramycin	Peak greater than 10 μg/mL, trough greater than 2 μg/mL
Vancomycin	Peak greater than 40 μg/mL, trough greater than 10 μg/mL

INTERFERING FACTORS

- Drugs that may decrease aminoglycoside efficacy include bleomycin, daunorubicin, doxorubicin, and penicillins (e.g., carbenicillin, piperacillin).

- Obtain a culture before and after the first dose of aminoglycosides.

- The risks of ototoxicity and nephrotoxicity are increased by the concomitant administration of aminoglycosides.

Nursing Implications and Procedure ● ● ● ● ● ● ● ● ● ● ●

Pretest: ■

➤ Obtain a history of the patient's complaints, including a list of known allergens.

➤ Review results of previously performed tests and procedures. For related tests, refer to the genitourinary and immune system and therapeutic/toxicology tables.

➤ Obtain a list of the medications the patient is taking, including herbs, nutritional supplements, and nutraceuticals. The requesting health care practitioner and laboratory should be advised if the patient regularly uses such products so that their effects can be taken into consideration when reviewing results.

➤ There are no food, fluid, or medica-

tion restrictions unless by medical direction.

➤ Review the procedure with the patient.

➤ Inform the patient that specimen collection takes approximately 5 to 10 minutes.

Intratest: ■

➤ Direct the patient to breathe normally and to avoid unnecessary movement.

➤ Observe standard precautions and follow the general guidelines in Appendix A. Consider recommended collection time around dosing schedule. Perform a venipuncture, and collect the specimen in a 5-mL red-top tube.

➤ Label the specimen, and promptly transport it to the laboratory.

Post-test: ■

➤ Observe venipuncture site for bleeding or hematoma formation. Apply pressure bandage.

➤ Explain to the patient the importance of following the medication regimen and instructions regarding food and drug interactions.

➤ Evaluate test results in relation to the patient's symptoms and other tests performed. Related laboratory tests include albumin, creatinine, creatinine clearance, blood urea nitrogen, and urinalysis.

ANTIBODIES, ANTICYTOPLASMIC NEUTROPHILIC

• •

SYNONYMS/ACRONYMS: Cytoplasmic antineutrophil cytoplasmic antibody (c-ANCA), perinuclear antineutrophil cytoplasmic antibody (p-ANCA).

SPECIMEN: Serum (1 mL) collected in a red-top tube.

REFERENCE VALUE: (Method: Indirect immunofluorescence) Negative.

DESCRIPTION: There are two types of cytoplasmic neutrophil antibodies identified by their cellular staining characteristics. c-ANCA (cytoplasmic) is specific for proteinase 3 in neutrophils and monocytes and is found in the sera of patients with Wegener's granulomatosis. Wegener's disease includes granulomatous inflammation of the upper and lower respiratory tract and vasculitis. p-ANCA (perinuclear) is specific for myeloperoxidase, elastase, and lactoferrin, as well as other enzymes in neutrophils. p-ANCA is present in the sera of patients with pauci-immune necrotizing glomerulonephritis. ■

INDICATIONS:
• Distinguish between vasculitic disease and the effects of therapy

• Assist in the diagnosis of Wegener's granulomatosis and its variants

• Distinguish between biliary cirrhosis and sclerosing cholangitis

• Differential diagnosis of ulcerative colitis

RESULT

Increased in:
• c-ANCA
  Wegener's granulomatosis and its variants

• p-ANCA
  Alveolar hemorrhage
  Angiitis and polyangiitis
  Autoimmune liver disease
  Capillaritis
  Churg-Strauss syndrome
  Felty's syndrome
  Inflammatory bowel disease
  Leukocytoclastic skin vasculitis
  Necrotizing-crescentic
    glomerulonephritis
  Rheumatoid arthritis
  Vasculitis

Decreased in: N/A

CRITICAL VALUES: N/A

INTERFERING FACTORS: N/A

Nursing Implications and Procedure . . . .

Pretest: ■

➤ Obtain a history of the patient's complaints, including a list of known allergens.

➤ Obtain a history of the patient's gastrointestinal, genitourinary, hepatobiliary, immune, and musculoskeletal system and results of previously performed tests and procedures. For related tests, refer to the gastrointestinal, genitourinary, hepatobiliary, immune, and musculoskeletal system tables.

➤ Obtain a list of the medications the patient is taking, including herbs, nutritional supplements, and nutraceuticals. The requesting health care practitioner and laboratory should be advised if the patient regularly uses these products so that their effects can be taken into consideration when reviewing results.

➤ There are no food, fluid, or medication restrictions unless by medical direction.

➤ Review the procedure with the patient.

➤ Inform the patient that specimen collection takes approximately 5 to 10 minutes.

Intratest: ■

➤ Direct the patient to breathe normally and to avoid unnecessary movement.

➤ Observe standard precautions and follow the general guidelines in Appendix A. Perform a venipuncture, and collect the specimen in a 5-mL red-top tube.

➤ Label the specimen, and promptly transport it to the laboratory.

Post-test: ■

➤ Observe venipuncture site for bleeding or hematoma formation. Apply pressure bandage.

➤ Evaluate test results in relation to the patient's symptoms and other tests performed. Related laboratory tests include anti–glomerular basement membrane antibody, antimitochondrial antibody, eosinophil count, kidney biopsy, rheumatoid factor, and urinalysis.

ANTIBODIES, ANTI–GLOMERULAR BASEMENT MEMBRANE

. . . .

SYNONYMS/ACRONYM: Goodpasture's antibody, anti-GBM.

SPECIMEN: Serum (1 mL) collected in a red- or tiger-top tube. Lung or kidney tissue also may be submitted for testing. Refer to related biopsy monographs for specimen collection instructions.

REFERENCE VALUE: (Method: Direct or indirect immunofluorescence) Negative.

DESCRIPTION: Autoimmune kidney disease can result from the presence of antibodies to renal glomerular basement membrane (GBM). Of patients with anti-GBM, 10 to 20 percent show false-negative results. ■

INDICATIONS:

• Detect the presence of anti-GBM antibodies to differentiate glomerulonephritis caused by anti-GBM from other causes of glomerulonephritis

RESULT

Increased in:

• Glomerulonephritis

• Goodpasture's disease

• Idiopathic pulmonary hemosiderosis

Decreased in: N/A

CRITICAL VALUES: N/A

INTERFERING FACTORS: N/A

Nursing Implications and Procedure • • • • • • • • • • •

Pretest: ■

➤ Obtain a history of the patient's complaints, including a list of known allergens.

➤ Obtain a history of the patient's genitourinary, immune, and respiratory systems and results of previously performed tests and procedures. For related tests, refer to the genitourinary, immune, and respiratory system tables.

➤ Obtain a list of the medications the patient is taking, including herbs, nutritional supplements, and nutraceuticals. The requesting health care practitioner and laboratory should be advised if the patient regularly uses such products so that their effects can be taken into consideration when reviewing results.

➤ There are no food, fluid, or medication restrictions unless by medical direction.

➤ Review the procedure with the patient.

➤ Inform the patient that specimen collection takes approximately 5 to 10 minutes.

Intratest: ■

➤ Direct the patient to breathe normally and to avoid unnecessary movement.

➤ Observe standard precautions and follow the general guidelines in Appendix A. Perform a venipuncture, and collect the specimen in a 5-mL red-top tube.

➤ Label the specimen, and promptly transport it to the laboratory.

Post-test: ■

➤ Observe venipuncture site for bleeding or hematoma formation. Apply pressure bandage.

➤ Evaluate test results in relation to the patient's symptoms and other tests performed. Related laboratory tests include antineutrophilic cytoplasmic antibody, kidney biopsy, lung biopsy, and urinalysis.

ANTIBODIES, ANTINUCLEAR, ANTI-DNA, AND ANTICENTROMERE

SYNONYMS/ACRONYMS: ANA, Anti-DNA (Anti-ds DNA).

SPECIMEN: Serum (2 mL) collected in a red-top tube.

REFERENCE VALUE: (Method: Indirect fluorescent antibody for ANA and anticentromere; enzyme-linked immunosorbent assay [ELISA] for Anti-DNA)
ANA and anticentromere: titer of 1:40 or less
Anti-DNA: titer of less than 1:10

DESCRIPTION: Antinuclear antibodies (ANA) are autoantibodies mainly located in the nucleus of affected cells. The presence of ANA indicates systemic lupus erythematosus (SLE), related collagen vascular diseases, and immune complex diseases. Antibodies against cellular DNA are strongly associated with SLE. Anticentromere antibodies are a subset of ANA. Their presence is strongly associated with CREST syndrome (*c*alcinosis, *R*aynaud's phenomenon, *e*sophageal dysfunction, *s*clerodactyly, *t*elangiectasia). ANA and anticentromere antibodies are detected using Hep-2 (human epithelial cultured cells). Anti-DNA antibodies can be detected using a *Crithidia luciliae* substrate. Women are much more likely than men to be diagnosed with SLE. ■

INDICATIONS:
• Assist in the diagnosis and evaluation of SLE

• Evaluate suspected immune disorders, such as rheumatoid arthritis, systemic sclerosis, polymyosis, Sjögren's syndrome, and mixed connective tissue disease

RESULT

ANA Pattern	Associated Antibody
Rim and/or homogeneous	Double-stranded DNA Single- or double-stranded DNA

(Continued on following page)

ANA Pattern	Associated Antibody
Homogeneous	Histones
Speckled	Sm (Smith) antibody
	RNP
	SS-B/La, SS-A/Ro
Diffuse speckled with positive mitotic figures	Centromere
Nucleolar	Nucleolar, RNP

ANA patterns are helpful in that certain conditions are frequently associated with specific patterns, but the patterns are not diagnostic for a particular disease. RNP = ribonucleoprotein.

Increased in:

- Drug-induced lupus erythematosus
- Lupoid hepatitis
- Mixed connective tissue disease
- Polymyositis
- Progressive systemic sclerosis
- Rheumatoid arthritis
- Sjögren's disease
- SLE

Decreased in: N/A

CRITICAL VALUES: N/A

INTERFERING FACTORS:

- Drugs that may cause positive results include carbamazepine, chlorpromazine, ethosuximide, hydralazine, isoniazid, mephenytoin, methyldopa, penicillins, phenytoin, primidone, procainamide, and quinidine.

- A patient can have lupus and test ANA negative.

Nursing Implications and Procedure • • • • • • • • • • •

Pretest:

➤ Obtain a history of the patient's complaints, including a list of known allergens.

➤ Obtain a history of the patient's im-
mune and musculoskeletal systems and results of previously performed tests and procedures. For related tests, refer to the immune and musculoskeletal system tables.

➤ Obtain a list of the medications the patient is taking, including herbs, nutritional supplements, and nutraceuticals. The requesting health care practitioner and laboratory should be advised if the patient regularly uses these products so that their effects can be taken into consideration when reviewing results.

➤ There are no food, fluid, or medication restrictions unless by medical direction.

➤ Review the procedure with the patient.

➤ Inform the patient that specimen collection takes approximately 5 to 10 minutes.

Intratest:

➤ Direct the patient to breathe normally and to avoid unnecessary movement.

➤ Observe standard precautions and follow the general guidelines in Appendix A. Perform a venipuncture, and collect the specimen in a 5-mL red-top tube.

➤ Label the specimen, and promptly transport it to the laboratory.

Post-test:

➤ Observe venipuncture site for bleeding or hematoma formation. Apply pressure bandage.

➤ Educate the patient, as appropriate, regarding the importance of preventing infection, which is a significant cause of death in immunosuppressed individuals.

➤ Recognize anxiety related to test results and offer support, as appropriate. Provide teaching and disease information, as appropriate. Educate the patient regarding access to counseling services. Collagen and connective tissue diseases are chronic. As such, they must be addressed on a continuous basis and may require significant changes in lifestyle.

➤ Evaluate test results in relation to the patient's symptoms and other tests performed. Related laboratory tests include anticardiolipin antibody, antiscleroderma antibodies, C3, C4, total complement, erythrocyte sedimentation rate, extractable nuclear antibodies, Jo-1 antibody, kidney biopsy, procainamide, rheumatoid factor, and skin biopsy.

ANTIBODIES, ANTISCLERODERMA

SYNONYMS/ACRONYM: Progressive systemic sclerosis antibody, Scl-70 antibody.

SPECIMEN: Serum (1 mL) collected in a red-top tube.

REFERENCE VALUE: (Method: Indirect fluorescent antibody) Negative.

DESCRIPTION: Antiscleroderma antibodies are associated with progressive systemic sclerosis, a condition that affects multiple systems, including the skin, gastrointestinal tract, lungs, blood vessels, heart, and kidneys. These antibodies are present in the sera of patients with CREST syndrome (*c*alcinosis, *R*aynaud's phenomenon, *e*sophageal dysfunction, *s*clerodactyly, *t*elangiectasia). ∎

INDICATIONS:
• Assist in the diagnosis of scleroderma

RESULT

Increased in:

• CREST syndrome

• Progressive diffuse scleroderma

Decreased in: N/A

CRITICAL VALUES: N/A

INTERFERING FACTORS: N/A

Nursing Implications and Procedure

Pretest:

➤ Obtain a history of the patient's complaints, including a list of known allergens.

➤ Obtain a history of the patient's

immune and musculoskeletal systems and results of previously performed tests and procedures. For related tests, refer to the immune and musculoskeletal system tables.

➤ Obtain a list of the medications the patient is taking, including herbs, nutritional supplements, and nutraceuticals. The requesting health care practitioner and laboratory should be advised if the patient regularly uses these products so that their effects can be taken into consideration when reviewing results.

➤ There are no food, fluid, or medication restrictions unless by medical direction.

➤ Review the procedure with the patient.

➤ Inform the patient that specimen collection takes approximately 5 to 10 minutes.

Intratest:

➤ Direct the patient to breathe normally and to avoid unnecessary movement.

➤ Observe standard precautions and follow the general guidelines in Appendix A. Perform a venipuncture, and collect the specimen in a 5-mL red-top tube.

➤ Label the specimen, and promptly transport it to the laboratory.

Post-test:

➤ Observe venipuncture site for bleeding or hematoma formation. Apply pressure bandage.

➤ Collagen diseases are chronic and must be addressed on a continuous basis. Significant changes in lifestyle may be required. Recognize anxiety related to test results and offer support, as appropriate. Educate the patient regarding access to counseling services.

➤ Evaluate test results in relation to the patient's symptoms and other tests performed. Related laboratory tests include anticentromere antibodies, anti-DNA antibodies, antinuclear antibodies, Jo-1 antibody, Sjögren's antibody, kidney biopsy, skin biopsy, extractable nuclear antibodies, and rheumatoid factor.

ANTIBODIES, ANTISPERM

• •

SYNONYMS/ACRONYM: N/A.

SPECIMEN: Serum (1 mL) collected in a red-top tube.

REFERENCE VALUE: (Method: Immunoassay)

Result	Sperm Bound by Immunobead (%)
Negative	0–15
Weak positive	16–30
Moderate positive	31–50
Strong positive	51–100

DESCRIPTION: A major cause of infertility in men is blocked efferent testicular ducts. As a result of the reabsorption of sperm from the blocked ducts, antibodies against the sperm may be produced over time and thereby may lower the patient's fertility. Semen and cervical mucus can also be tested for antisperm antibodies. ■

INDICATIONS:
• Evaluation of infertility

RESULT

Increased in:
• Blocked testicular efferent duct

• Postvasectomy

Decreased in: N/A

CRITICAL VALUES: N/A

INTERFERING FACTORS:
• The patient should not ejaculate for 3 to 4 days before specimen collection if semen will be evaluated.

• Sperm antibodies have been detected in pregnant women and in women with primary infertility.

Nursing Implications and Procedure • • • • • • • • • • •

Pretest: ■

➤ Obtain a history of the patient's complaints, including a list of known allergens.

➤ Obtain a history of the patient's immune and reproductive systems and results of previously performed tests and procedures. For related tests, refer to the immune and reproductive system tables.

➤ Obtain a list of the medications the patient is taking, including herbs, nu-tritional supplements, and nutraceuticals. The requesting health care practitioner and laboratory should be advised if the patient regularly uses these products so that their effects can be taken into consideration when reviewing results.

➤ There are no food, fluid, or medication restrictions unless by medical direction.

➤ Review the procedure with the patient. Inform the patient that additional specimens may be required. Sensitivity to cultural and social issues, as well as concern for modesty, is important in providing psychological support.

➤ Inform the patient that specimen collection takes approximately 5 to 10 minutes.

Intratest: ■

➤ Direct the patient to breathe normally and to avoid unnecessary movement.

➤ Observe standard precautions and follow the general guidelines in Appendix A. Perform a venipuncture, and collect the specimen in a 5-mL red-top tube.

➤ Label the specimen, and promptly transport it to the laboratory.

Post-test: ■

➤ Observe venipuncture site for bleeding or hematoma formation. Apply pressure bandage.

➤ Recognize anxiety related to test results. Provide teaching and information regarding the clinical implications of the test results, as appropriate. Provide a supportive, nonjudgmental environment when assisting a patient through the process of fertility testing. Educate the patient regarding access to counseling services, as appropriate.

➤ Evaluate test results in relation to the patient's symptoms and other tests performed. Related laboratory tests include luteinizing hormone, progesterone, semen analysis, and testosterone.

ANTIBODIES, ANTISTREPTOLYSIN O

SYNONYM/ACRONYM: Streptozyme, ASO.

SPECIMEN: Serum (1 mL) collected in a red-top tube.

REFERENCE VALUE: (Method: Nephelometry) Less than 200 IU/mL.

DESCRIPTION: Group A β-hemolytic streptococci secrete the enzyme streptolysin O, which can destroy red blood cells. The enzyme acts as an antigen and stimulates the immune system to develop streptolysin O antibodies. These antibodies occur within 1 month after the onset of a streptococcal infection. Detection of the antibody over several weeks strongly suggests exposure to group A β-hemolytic streptococci. ■

INDICATIONS:

• Assist in establishing a diagnosis of streptococcal infection

• Evaluate patients with streptococcal infections for the development of acute rheumatic fever or nephritis

• Monitor response to therapy in streptococcal illnesses

RESULT

Increased in:

• Endocarditis

• Glomerulonephritis

• Rheumatic fever

• Scarlet fever

Decreased in: N/A

CRITICAL VALUES: N/A

INTERFERING FACTORS:

• Drugs that may decrease ASO titers include antibiotics and corticosteroids because therapy suppresses antibody response.

Nursing Implications and Procedure

Pretest:

➤ Obtain a history of the patient's complaints, including a list of known allergens.

➤ Obtain a history of the patient's immune system and results of previously performed tests and procedures. For related tests, refer to the immune system table.

➤ Obtain a list of the medications the patient is taking, including herbs, nutritional supplements, and nutraceuticals. The requesting health care practitioner and laboratory should be advised if the patient regularly uses these products so that their effects can be taken into consideration when reviewing results.

➤ There are no food, fluid, or medication restrictions unless by medical direction.

➤ Review the procedure with the patient.

➤ Inform the patient that specimen collection takes approximately 5 to 10 minutes.

Intratest: ■

➤ Direct the patient to breathe normally and to avoid unnecessary movement.

➤ Observe standard precautions and follow the general guidelines in Appendix A. Perform a venipuncture, and collect the specimen in a 5-mL red-top tube.

➤ Label the specimen, and promptly transport it to the laboratory.

Post-test: ■

➤ Observe venipuncture site for bleeding or hematoma formation. Apply pressure bandage.

➤ Administer antibiotics as ordered, and instruct the patient in the importance of completing the entire course of antibiotic therapy even if no symptoms are present.

➤ Evaluate test results in relation to the patient's symptoms and other tests performed. Related laboratory tests include anti-DNAse streptococcal, rapid streptococcal screen, and throat culture.

ANTIBODIES, ANTITHYROGLOBULIN AND ANTITHYROID PEROXIDASE

· ·

SYNONYMS/ACRONYM: Thyroid antibodies, antithyroid peroxidase antibodies (TPO antibodies were previously called thyroid antimicrosomal antibodies).

SPECIMEN: Serum (1 mL) collected in a red-top tube.

REFERENCE VALUE: (Method: Radioimmunoassay)

Antibody	Conventional Units	SI Units (Conversion Factor ×1)
Antithyroglobulin antibody	Less than 0.3 U/mL	Less than 0.3 kU/L
Antiperoxidase antibody	Less than 0.3 U/mL	Less than 0.3 kU/L

DESCRIPTION: Thyroid antibodies are mainly immunoglobulin G–type antibodies. Antithyroid peroxidase antibodies bind with microsomal antigens on cells lining the microsomal membrane. They are thought to destroy thyroid tissue as a result of stimulation by lymphocytic killer cells. These antibodies are present in hypothyroid and hyperthyroid conditions. Antithyroglobulin antibodies are autoantibodies directed against thyroglobulin. The function of this antibody is unclear. Both tests are normally requested together. ■

INDICATIONS:

• Assist in confirming suspected inflammation of thyroid gland

• Assist in the diagnosis of suspected hypothyroidism caused by thyroid tissue destruction

• Assist in the diagnosis of suspected thyroid autoimmunity in patients with other autoimmune disorders

RESULT

Increased in:

• Autoimmune disorders

• Graves' disease

• Goiter

• Hashimoto's thyroiditis

• Idiopathic myxedema

• Pernicious anemia

• Thyroid carcinoma

Decreased in: N/A

CRITICAL VALUES: N/A

INTERFERING FACTORS:

• Lithium may increase thyroid antibody levels.

• Recent radioactive scans or radiation within 1 week before the test can interfere with test results when radioimmunoassay is the test method.

Nursing Implications and Procedure • • • • • • • • • • •

Pretest: ■

➤ Obtain a history of the patient's complaints, including a list of known allergens.

➤ Obtain a history of the patient's endocrine and immune system and results of previously performed tests and procedures. For related tests, refer to the endocrine and immune system tables.

➤ Obtain a list of the medications the patient is taking, including herbs, nutritional supplements, and nutraceuticals. The requesting health care practitioner and laboratory should be advised if the patient regularly uses these products so that their effects can be taken into consideration when reviewing results.

➤ Note any recent procedures that can interfere with test results.

➤ There are no food, fluid, or medication restrictions unless by medical direction.

➤ Review the procedure with the patient.

➤ Inform the patient that specimen collection takes approximately 5 to 10 minutes.

Intratest: ■

➤ Direct the patient to breathe normally and to avoid unnecessary movement.

➤ Observe standard precautions and follow the general guidelines in Appendix A. Perform a venipuncture, and collect the specimen in a 5-mL red-top tube.

➤ Label the specimen, and promptly transport it to the laboratory.

Post-test: ■

➤ Observe venipuncture site for bleeding or hematoma formation. Apply pressure bandage.

➤ Evaluate test results in relation to the patient's symptoms and other tests performed. Related laboratory tests include complete blood count, thyroid biopsy, thyroid-stimulating hormone, free thyroxine, thyroxine, and triiodothyronine.

ANTIBODIES, CARDIOLIPIN, IMMUNOGLOBULIN G, AND IMMUNOGLOBULIN M

SYNONYMS/ACRONYMS: Antiphospholipid antibody, lupus anticoagulant, LA, ACA.

SPECIMEN: Serum (1 mL) collected in a red-top tube.

REFERENCE VALUE: (Method: Immunoassay, enzyme-linked immunosorbent assay [ELISA]) Negative.

DESCRIPTION: Cardiolipin antibody is one of several identified antiphospholipid antibodies. Antiphospholipid antibody syndrome is characterized by noninflammatory thrombosis of blood vessels. These antibodies are found in individuals with lupus erythematosus, lupus-related conditions, infectious diseases, drug reactions, and sometimes fetal loss. Cardiolipin antibodies are often found in association with lupus anticoagulant. ■

INDICATIONS:
• Assist in the diagnosis of antiphospholipid antibody syndrome

RESULT

Increased in:
• Chorea
• Drug reactions
• Epilepsy
• Infectious diseases
• Mitral valve endocarditis

• Patients with lupus-like symptoms (often ANA negative)
• Placental infarction
• Recurrent fetal loss (strong association with two or more occurrences)
• Recurrent venous and arterial thromboses

Decreased in: N/A

CRITICAL VALUES: N/A

INTERFERING FACTORS: Cardiolipin antibody is partially cross-reactive with syphilis reagin antibody and lupus anticoagulant. False-positive rapid plasma reagin results may occur.

Nursing Implications and Procedure

Pretest:

➤ Obtain a history of the patient's complaints, including a list of known allergens.

➤ Obtain a history of the patient's hematopoietic, immune, and reproductive systems and results of previously performed tests and procedures. For related tests, refer to the hematopoietic, immune, and reproductive system tables.

➤ Obtain a list of the medications the patient is taking, including herbs, nutritional supplements, and nutraceuticals. The requesting health care practitioner and laboratory should be advised if the patient regularly uses these products so that their effects can be taken into consideration when reviewing results.

➤ There are no food, fluid, or medication restrictions unless by medical direction.

➤ Review the procedure with the patient.

➤ Inform the patient that specimen collection takes approximately 5 to 10 minutes.

Intratest:

➤ Direct the patient to breathe normally and to avoid unnecessary movement.

➤ Observe standard precautions and follow the general guidelines in Appendix A. Perform a venipuncture, and collect the specimen in a 5-mL red-top tube.

➤ Label the specimen, and promptly transport it to the laboratory.

Post-test:

➤ Observe venipuncture site for bleeding or hematoma formation. Apply pressure bandage.

➤ Evaluate test results in relation to the patient's symptoms and other tests performed. Related laboratory tests include antinuclear antibodies, complete blood count, fibrinogen, protein C, protein S, syphilis serology, and Sjögren antibodies.

ANTIBODIES, GLIADIN (IMMUNOGLOBULIN G AND IMMUNOGLOBULIN A)

SYNONYMS/ACRONYMS: Endomysial antibodies, gliadin (IgG and IgA) antibodies, EMA.

SPECIMEN: Serum (1 mL) collected in a red-top tube.

REFERENCE VALUE: (Method: Immunoassay)

Gliadin Antibody	Conventional Units
IgA	Less than 5 U
IgG	Less than 57 U

DESCRIPTION: Gliadin is a water-soluble protein found in the gluten of wheat, rye, oats, and barley. The intestinal mucosa of certain individuals does not digest gluten, allowing a toxic buildup of gliadin. Antibodies to gliadin form and result in damage to the intestinal mucosa. In severe cases, intestinal mucosa can be lost; lactose intolerance compounds the condition. Immunoglobulin G (IgG) and immunoglobulin A (IgA) gliadin antibodies are detectable in the serum of patients with gluten-sensitive enteropathy. ■

INDICATIONS:
• Assist in the diagnosis of asymptomatic gluten-sensitive enteropathy in some patients with dermatitis herpetiformis
• Assist in the diagnosis of gluten-sensitive enteropathies
• Assist in the diagnosis of nontropical sprue
• Monitor dietary compliance of patients with gluten-sensitive enteropathies

RESULT

Increased in:
• Asymptomatic gluten-sensitive enteropathy
• Celiac disease
• Dermatitis herpetiformis
• Nontropical sprue

Decreased in: N/A

CRITICAL VALUES: N/A

INTERFERING FACTORS:
• Conditions other than gluten-sensitive enteropathy can result in elevated antibody levels without corresponding histologic evidence. These conditions include Crohn's disease, postinfection malabsorption, and food protein intolerance.
• A negative IgA gliadin result, especially with a positive IgG gliadin result in an untreated patient, does not rule out active gluten-sensitive enteropathy.

Nursing Implications and Procedure ● ● ● ● ● ● ● ● ● ● ●

Pretest: ■
➤ Obtain a history of the patient's complaints, including a list of known allergens.
➤ Obtain a history of the patient's gastrointestinal and immune systems and results of previously performed tests and procedures. For related tests, refer to the gastrointestinal and immune system tables.
➤ Obtain a list of foods and medications the patient is taking, including herbs, nutritional supplements, and nutraceuticals. The requesting health care practitioner and laboratory should be advised if the patient regularly uses these products so that their effects can be taken into consideration when reviewing results.
➤ There are no food, fluid, or medication restrictions unless by medical direction.
➤ Review the procedure with the patient.
➤ Inform the patient that specimen collection takes approximately 5 to 10 minutes.

Intratest: ■
➤ Direct the patient to breathe normally and to avoid unnecessary movement.
➤ Observe standard precautions and follow the general guidelines in Appendix A. Perform a venipuncture, and collect the specimen in a 5-mL red-top tube.
➤ Label the specimen, and promptly transport it to the laboratory.

Post-test: ■
➤ Observe venipuncture site for bleeding or hematoma formation. Apply pressure bandage.
➤ Recognize anxiety related to test results and offer support. Provide teaching and information regarding

the clinical implications of the test results, as appropriate. Educate the patient regarding access to appropriate counseling services.

➤ Encourage the patient with abnormal findings to consult with a qualified nutritionist to plan a lactose- and gluten-free diet. This dietary planning is complex because patients are often malnourished and have other related nutritional problems.

➤ Evaluate test results in relation to the patient's symptoms and other tests performed. Related laboratory tests include albumin, calcium, skin biopsy, D-xylose tolerance test, electrolytes, fecal analysis, fecal fat, folic acid, iron, and lactose tolerance test.

ANTIBODY, ANTIMITOCHONDRIAL

SYNONYM/ACRONYM: AMA.

SPECIMEN: Serum (1 mL) collected in a red-top tube.

REFERENCE VALUE: (Method: Indirect fluorescent antibody) Negative or titer less than 1:20.

DESCRIPTION: Antimitochondrial antibodies are found in 90 percent of patients with primary biliary cirrhosis (PBC). PBC is identified most frequently in women age 35 to 60 years. ■

INDICATIONS:
• Assist in the diagnosis of PBC

• Assist in the differential diagnosis of chronic liver disease

RESULT

Increased in:
• PBC

• Hepatitis (alcoholic, viral)

• Rheumatoid arthritis (occasionally)

• Systemic lupus erythematosus (occasionally)

• Thyroid disease (occasionally)

Decreased in: N/A

CRITICAL VALUES: N/A

INTERFERING FACTORS: N/A

Nursing Implications and Procedure

Pretest:

➤ Obtain a history of the patient's complaints, including a list of known allergens.

➤ Obtain a history of the patient's hepatobiliary and immune systems, as well as results of previously performed tests and procedures. For related tests, refer to the hepatobiliary and immune system tables.

➤ Obtain a list of the medications the patient is taking, including herbs, nutritional supplements, and nutraceuticals. The requesting health care practitioner and laboratory should be advised if the patient regularly uses these products so that their effects can be taken into consideration when reviewing results.

➤ There are no food, fluid, or medication restrictions unless by medical direction.

➤ Review the procedure with the patient.

➤ Inform the patient that specimen collection takes approximately 5 to 10 minutes.

Intratest:

➤ Direct the patient to breathe normally and to avoid unnecessary movement.

➤ Observe standard precautions and follow the general guidelines in Appendix A. Perform a venipuncture, and collect the specimen in a 5-mL red-top tube.

➤ Label the specimen, and promptly transport it to the laboratory.

Post-test:

➤ Observe venipuncture site for bleeding or hematoma formation. Apply pressure bandage.

➤ The presence of antimitochondrial antibodies may be associated with liver disease. Dietary recommendations may be indicated and vary depending on the severity of the condition. A low-protein diet may be in order if the liver cannot process the end products of protein metabolism. A diet of soft foods may be required if esophageal varices have developed. Ammonia levels may be used to determine whether protein should be added to or reduced from the diet. Patients should be encouraged to eat simple carbohydrates and emulsified fats (as in homogenized milk or eggs), as opposed to complex carbohydrates (e.g., starch, fiber, and glycogen [animal carbohydrates]) and complex fats, which would require additional bile to emulsify it so that it could be used. Observe the cirrhotic patient carefully for the development of ascites; if ascites develops, pay strict attention to fluid and electrolyte balance.

➤ Evaluate test results in relation to the patient's symptoms and other tests performed. Related laboratory tests include albumin, alkaline phosphatase, ammonia, anticytoplasmic neutrophilic antibodies, antinuclear antibodies, anti–smooth muscle antibodies, bilirubin, electrolytes, liver biopsy, and γ-glutamyl transpeptidase.

ANTIBODY, ANTI–SMOOTH MUSCLE

• •

SYNONYM/ACRONYM: ASMA.

SPECIMEN: Serum (1 mL) collected in a red-top tube.

REFERENCE VALUE: (Method: Indirect fluorescent antibody) Negative.

DESCRIPTION: Anti–smooth muscle antibodies are autoantibodies found in high titers in the sera of patients with autoimmune diseases of the liver and bile duct. ∎

INDICATIONS:

• Differential diagnosis of liver disease

RESULT

Increased in:

• Autoimmune hepatitis

• Chronic active viral hepatitis

• Infectious mononucleosis

Decreased in: N/A

CRITICAL VALUES: N/A

INTERFERING FACTORS: N/A

Nursing Implications and Procedure • • • • • • • • • • • •

Pretest: ∎

➤ Obtain a history of the patient's complaints, including a list of known allergens.

➤ Obtain a history of the patient's hepatobiliary and immune systems, as well as results of previously performed tests and procedures. For related tests, refer to the hepatobiliary and immune system tables.

➤ Obtain a list of the medications the patient is taking, including herbs, nutritional supplements, and nutraceuticals. The requesting health care practitioner and laboratory should be advised if the patient regularly uses these products so that their effects can be taken into consideration when reviewing results.

➤ There are no food, fluid, or medication restrictions unless by medical direction.

➤ Review the procedure with the patient.

➤ Inform the patient that specimen collection takes approximately 5 to 10 minutes.

Intratest: ∎

➤ Direct the patient to breathe normally and to avoid unnecessary movement.

➤ Observe standard precautions and follow the general guidelines in Appendix A. Perform a venipuncture, and collect the specimen in a 5-mL red-top tube.

➤ Label the specimen, and promptly transport it to the laboratory.

Post-test: ∎

➤ Observe venipuncture site for bleeding or hematoma formation. Apply pressure bandage.

➤ The presence of anti–smooth muscle antibodies may be associated with liver disease. Dietary recommendations may be indicated and vary depending on the severity of the condition. A low-protein diet may be in order if the liver cannot process the end products of protein metabolism. A diet of soft foods may be required if esophageal varices have developed. Ammonia levels may be used to determine whether protein should be added to or reduced from the diet. Patients should be encouraged to eat simple carbohydrates and emulsified fats (as in homogenized milk or eggs), as opposed to complex carbohydrates (e.g., starch, fiber, and glycogen [animal carbohydrates]) and complex fats, which would require additional bile to emulsify it so that it could be used. Observe the cirrhotic patient carefully for the development of ascites; if ascites develops, pay strict attention to fluid and electrolyte balance.

➤ Evaluate test results in relation to the patient's symptoms and other tests performed. Related laboratory tests include alkaline phosphatase, ammonia, antimitochondrial antibody, antinuclear antibody, aspartate aminotransferase, liver biopsy, bilirubin, hepatitis serology, serum protein electrophoresis, and prothrombin time.

ANTIBODY, Jo-1

SYNONYM/ACRONYM: Antihistidyl transfer tRNA synthase.

SPECIMEN: Serum (1 mL) collected in a red-top tube.

REFERENCE VALUE: (Method: Immunoassay) Negative.

DESCRIPTION: Jo-1 is an autoantibody found in the sera of some antinuclear antibody–positive patients. Compared to the presence of other autoantibodies, the presence of Jo-1 suggests a more aggressive disease course and a higher risk of mortality. The clinical effects of this autoantibody include acute onset, fever, dry and cracked skin on the hands, Raynaud's phenomenon, and arthritis. ▪

INDICATIONS:
• Test for idiopathic inflammatory myopathies

RESULT

Increased in:
• Dermatomyositis
• Polymyositis

Decreased in: N/A

CRITICAL VALUES: N/A

INTERFERING FACTORS: N/A

Nursing Implications and Procedure

Pretest:

➤ Obtain a history of the patient's complaints, including a list of known allergens.

➤ Obtain a history of the patient's immune and musculoskeletal systems, as well as results of previously performed tests and procedures. For related tests, refer to the immune and musculoskeletal system tables.

➤ Obtain a list of the medications the patient is taking, including herbs, nutritional supplements, and nutraceuticals. The requesting health care practitioner and laboratory should be advised if the patient regularly uses these products so that their effects can be taken into consideration when reviewing results.

➤ There are no food, fluid, or medication restrictions unless by medical direction.

➤ Review the procedure with the patient.

➤ Inform the patient that specimen collection takes approximately 5 to 10 minutes.

Intratest:

➤ Direct the patient to breathe normally and to avoid unnecessary movement.

➤ Observe standard precautions and follow the general guidelines in Appendix A. Perform a venipuncture, and collect the specimen in a 5-mL red-top tube.

➤ Label the specimen, and promptly transport it to the laboratory.

Post-test:

➤ Observe venipuncture site for bleed-

ing or hematoma formation. Apply pressure bandage.

➤ Evaluate test results in relation to the patient's symptoms and other tests performed. Related laboratory tests include alanine aminotransferase, aldolase, antinuclear antibody, aspartate aminotransferase, creatine kinase, urine creatinine, erythrocyte sedimentation rate, extractable nuclear antibodies, lactate dehydrogenase and isoenzymes, muscle biopsy, myoglobin, rheumatoid factor, scleroderma antibody, Sjögren's antibodies, and skin biopsy.

ANTICONVULSANT DRUGS: CARBAMAZEPINE, ETHOSUXIMIDE, PHENOBARBITAL, PHENYTOIN, PRIMIDONE, VALPROIC ACID

SYNONYMS/ACRONYM: *Carbamazepine* (Carbategretal, Carbazep, Epitrol, Tegretol); *ethosuximide* (Suxinutin, Zarontin, Zartalin); *phenobarbital* (Barbita, Comizial, Fenilcal, Gardenal, Luminal, Phenemal, Phenobarb, phenobarbitone, Stental Extentabs); *phenytoin* (Antisacer, Dilantin, Dintoina, Diphenylan Sodium, Ditan, Epanutin, Epinal, Fenytoin); *primidone* (Desoxyphenobarbital, Hexamidinum, Majsolin, Mylepsin, Mysoline, Primaclone, Prysolin); *valproic acid* (Depakene, Depakote, Depamide, dipropylacetic acid, Epilim, Ergenyl, Leptilan, Valkote).

SPECIMEN: Serum (1 mL) collected in a red-top tube.

Drug	Route of Administration
Carbamazepine*	Oral
Ethosuximide*	Oral
Phenobarbital*	Oral
Phenytoin*	Oral
Primidone*	Oral
Valproic Acid*	Oral

* Recommended collection time = trough: immediately before next dose (at steady state) or at a consistent sampling time.

Drug	Therapeutic Dose*	SI Units	Half-Life (h)	Volume of Distribution (L/kg)	Protein Binding (%)	Excretion
		(Conversion Factor × 4.23)				
Carbamazepine	4–12 µg/mL	17–51 µmol/L	15–40	0.8–1.8	60–80	Hepatic
		(Conversion Factor × 7.08)				
Ethosuximide	40–100 µg/mL	283–708 µmol/L	25–70	0.7	0–5	Renal
		(Conversion Factor × 4.31)				
Phenobarbital	Adult: 20–40 µg/mL Child: 15–30 µg/mL	Adult: 86–172 µmol/L Child: 65–129 µmol/L	50–140	0.5–1.0 L/kg	40–50	80% Hepatic 20% Renal
		(Conversion Factor × 3.96)				
Phenytoin	10–20 µg/mL	40–79 µmol/L	Adult: 20–40 Child: 10	0.6–0.7	85–95	Hepatic
		(Conversion Factor × 4.58)				
Primidone	Adult: 5–12 µg/mL Child: 7–10 µg/mL	Adult: 23–55 µmol/L Child: 32–46 µmol/L	4–12	0.5–1.0	0–20	Hepatic
		(Conversion Factor × 6.93)				
Valproic Acid	50–100 µg/mL	347–693 µmol/L	8–15	0.1–0.5	85–95	Renal

* Conventional units.

113

DESCRIPTION: Anticonvulsants are used to reduce the frequency and severity of seizures for patients with epilepsy. Carbamazepine is also used for controlling neurogenic pain in trigeminal neuralgia and diabetic neuropathy and for treating for bipolar disease and other neurologic and psychiatric conditions.

Many factors must be considered in effective dosing and monitoring of therapeutic drugs, including patient age, patient weight, interacting medications, electrolyte balance, protein levels, water balance, conditions that affect absorption and excretion, and foods, herbals, vitamins, and minerals that can either potentiate or inhibit the intended target concentration. ∎

INDICATIONS:

• Assist in the diagnosis of and prevention of toxicity

• Monitor compliance to therapeutic regimen

RESULT

Level	Response
Normal levels	Therapeutic effect
Subtherapeutic levels	Adjust dose as indicated
Toxic levels	Adjust dose as indicated
Carbamazepine	Hepatic impairment
Ethosuximide	Hepatic impairment
Phenobarbital	Hepatic impairment
Phenytoin	Hepatic impairment
Primidone	Hepatic impairment
Valproic acid	Renal impairment

CRITICAL VALUES: ⚠ It is important to note the adverse effects of subtherapeutic levels. Care must be taken to investigate the signs and symptoms of too little and too much medication.

Carbamazepine: Greater than 12 μg/mL

Signs and symptoms of carbamazepine toxicity include respiratory depression, seizures, stupor, and possible coma. Possible interventions include gastric lavage (contraindicated if ileus is present); airway protection; administration of fluids and vasopressors for hypotension; treatment of seizures with diazepam, phenobarbital, or phenytoin; cardiac monitoring; monitoring of vital signs; and discontinuing the medication. Emetics are contraindicated.

Ethosuximide: Greater than 150 μg/mL

Signs and symptoms of ethosuximide toxicity include nausea, vomiting, and lethargy. Possible interventions include administration of activated charcoal, administration of saline cathartic and gastric lavage (contraindicated if ileus is present), airway protection, hourly assessment of neurologic function, and discontinuing the medication.

Phenobarbital: Greater than 40 μg/mL

Signs and symptoms of phenobarbital toxicity include cold, clammy skin; ataxia; central nervous system depression; hypothermia; hypotension; cyanosis; Cheyne-Stokes respiration; tachycardia; possible coma; and possible renal impairment. Possible interventions include gastric lavage, administration of activated charcoal with cathartic, airway protection, possible intubation and mechanical ventilation (especially during gastric lavage if there is no gag reflex), monitoring for hypotension, and discontinuing the medication.

Phenytoin: Greater than 40 μg/mL

Signs and symptoms of phenytoin toxicity include double vision, nystagmus, lethargy, central nervous system depression, and possible coma. Possible interventions include airway support, electrocardiographic monitoring, administration of activated charcoal, gastric lavage with warm saline or tap water, administration of saline or sorbitol cathartic, and discontinuing the medication.

Primidone: Greater than 12 μg/mL

Signs and symptoms of primidone toxicity include ataxia, anemia, and central nervous system depression. Possible interventions include airway protection, treatment of anemia with vitamin B_{12} and folate, and discontinuing the medication.

Valproic Acid: Greater than 200 μg/mL

Signs and symptoms of valproic acid toxicity include numbness, tingling, weakness, and mental changes. Possible interventions include administration of activated charcoal and naloxone and discontinuing the medication.

INTERFERING FACTORS

- Drugs that may increase carbamazepine levels or increase risk of toxicity include cimetidine, danazol, diltiazem, erythromycin, isoniazid, propoxyphene, triacetyloleandomycin, valproic acid, and verapamil.

- Drugs that may decrease carbamazepine levels include phenobarbital, phenytoin, and primidone.

- Drugs that may increase phenobarbital levels or increase risk of toxicity include

barbital drugs, furosemide, primidone, salicylates, and valproic acid.

- Phenobarbital may affect the metabolism of other drugs, increasing their effectiveness, such as beta blockers, chloramphenicol, corticosteroids, doxycycline, griseofulvin, haloperidol, methylphenidate, phenothiazines, phenylbutazone, propoxyphene, quinidine, theophylline, tricyclic antidepressants, and valproic acid.

- Phenobarbital may affect the metabolism of other drugs, decreasing their effectiveness, such as chloramphenicol, cyclosporine, ethosuximide, oral anticoagulants, oral contraceptives, phenytoin, and theophylline.

- Phenobarbital is an active metabolite of primidone, and both drug levels should be monitored while the patient is receiving primidone to avoid either toxic or subtherapeutic levels of both medications.

- Drugs that may increase phenytoin levels or increase the risk of phenytoin toxicity include amiodarone, azapropazone, carbamazepine, cimetidine, chloramphenicol, disulfiram, ethanol, fluconazole, halothane, ibuprofen, imipramine, levodopa, miconazole, metronidazole, nifedipine, phenylbutazone, sulfonamides, tricyclic antidepressants, trazodone, and trimethoprim. Small changes in formulation (i.e., changes in brand) also may increase phenytoin levels or increase the risk of phenytoin toxicity.

- Drugs that may decrease phenytoin levels include bleomycin, carbamazepine, cisplatin, disulfiram, folic acid, intravenous fluids containing glucose, nitrofurantoin, oxacillin, rifampin, salicylates, and vinblastine.

- Primidone decreases the effectiveness of oral anticoagulants.

- Drugs that may increase valproic acid

levels or increase risk of toxicity include dicumarol, phenylbutazone, and high doses of salicylate.

• Drugs that may decrease valproic acid levels include carbamazepine, phenobarbital, phenytoin, and primidone

Nursing Implications and Procedure • • • • • • • • • • •

Pretest:

➤ Obtain a history of the patient's complaints, including a list of known allergens.

➤ Review results of previously performed tests and procedures. For related tests, refer to the hepatobiliary system and therapeutic/toxicology tables.

➤ Obtain a list of medications the patient is taking, including herbs, nutritional supplements, and nutraceuticals. The requesting health care practitioner and laboratory should be advised if the patient regularly uses these products so that their effects can be taken into consideration when reviewing results.

➤ There are no food, fluid, or medication restrictions unless by medical direction.

➤ Review the procedure with the patient.

➤ Inform the patient that specimen collection takes approximately 5 to 10 minutes.

Intratest:

➤ Direct the patient to breathe normally and to avoid unnecessary movement.

➤ Observe standard precautions and follow the general guidelines in Appendix A. Review dosing schedule to ensure that peak and trough specimens are ordered to be collected at the appropriate time. Perform a venipuncture, and collect the specimen in a 5-mL red-top tube.

➤ Label the specimen, and promptly transport it to the laboratory.

Post-test:

➤ Observe venipuncture site for bleeding or hematoma formation. Apply pressure bandage.

➤ Explain to the patient the importance of following the medication regimen and instructions regarding food and drug interactions.

➤ Instruct the patient to immediately report any unusual sensations, such as dizziness or disturbances in vision, to his or her health care practitioner.

➤ Instruct the patient to be prepared to list to the pharmacist the other medications he or she is already taking in the event that the requesting health care practitioner gives the patient a prescription to be filled.

➤ Evaluate test results in relation to the patient's symptoms and other tests performed. Related laboratory tests include albumin, electrolytes, and protein.

ANTIDEOXYRIBONUCLEASE-B, STREPTOCOCCAL

• •

SYNONYMS/ACRONYM: ADNase-B, AntiDNase-B titer, antistreptococcal DNase-B titer, streptodornase.

SPECIMEN: Serum (1 mL) collected in a red-top tube.

REFERENCE VALUE: (Method: Spectrophotometry)

Age	Normal Results
Preschoolers	Less than 61 U
School-age children	Less than 171 U
Adults	Less than 86 U

DESCRIPTION: The presence of streptococcal DNase antibodies is an indicator of recent infection, especially if a rise in antibody titer can be shown. This test is more sensitive than the antistreptolysin-O test. A rise in titer of two or more dilution increments between acute and convalescent specimens is clinically significant. ■

INDICATIONS:
- Investigate the presence of streptococcal antibodies as a source of recent infection

RESULT

Increased in:
- Streptococcal infections (systemic)

Decreased in: N/A

CRITICAL VALUES: N/A

INTERFERING FACTORS: N/A

Nursing Implications and Procedure • • • • • • • • • • •

Pretest: ■

➤ Obtain a history of the patient's complaints, including a list of known allergens.

➤ Obtain a history of the patient's immune system and results of previously performed tests and procedures. For related tests, refer to the immune system table.

➤ Obtain a list of the medications the patient is taking, including herbs, nutritional supplements, and nutraceuticals. The requesting health care practitioner and laboratory should be advised if the patient regularly uses these products so that their effects can be taken into consideration when reviewing results.

➤ There are no food, fluid, or medication restrictions unless by medical direction.

➤ Review the procedure with the patient.

➤ Inform the patient that each specimen collection takes approximately 5 to 10 minutes.

Intratest: ■

➤ Direct the patient to breathe normally and to avoid unnecessary movement.

➤ Observe standard precautions and follow the general guidelines in Appendix A. Perform a venipuncture, and collect the specimen in a 5-mL red-top tube.

➤ Label the specimen, and promptly transport it to the laboratory.

Post-test: ■

➤ Observe venipuncture site for bleeding or hematoma formation. Apply pressure bandage.

➤ Administer analgesics and antibiotics as ordered, and instruct the patient in the importance of completing the entire course of antibiotic therapy even if no symptoms are present.

➤ Inform the patient that a convalescent specimen may be requested in 7 to 10 days.

> Evaluate test results in relation to the patient's symptoms and other tests performed. Related laboratory tests include antistreptolysin-O antibody, rapid streptococcal screen, and throat culture.

ANTIDEPRESSANT DRUGS: AMITRYPTYLINE, NORTRIPTYLINE, DOXEPIN, IMIPRAMINE, DESIPRAMINE

SYNONYMS/ACRONYM: Tricyclic antidepressants: *amitryptyline* (Elavil, Endep, Etrafon, Limbitrol, Triavil); *nortriptyline* (Allegron, Aventyl, Norval, Pamelor); *doxepin* (Adapin, Co-Dax, Novoxapin, Sinequan, Triadapin); *imipramine* (Berkomine, Dimipressin, Iprogen, Janimine, Presamine, Tofranil); *desipramine* (Norpramin).

SPECIMEN: Serum (1 mL) collected in a red-top tube.

Drug	Route of Administration	Recommended Collection Time
Amitriptyline	Oral	Trough: immediately before next dose (at steady state)
Nortriptyline	Oral	Trough: immediately before next dose (at steady state)
Doxepin	Oral	Trough: immediately before next dose (at steady state)
Imipramine	Oral	Trough: immediately before next dose (at steady state)
Desipramine	Oral	Trough: immediately before next dose (at steady state)

REFERENCE VALUE: (Method: Chromatography for amitryptyline, nortriptyline, and doxepin; immunoassay for imipramine and desipramine)

Drug	Therapeutic Dose*	SI Units	Half-Life (h)	Volume of Distribution (L/kg)	Protein Binding (%)	Excretion
			(Conversion Factor ×3.61)			
Amitryptyline	120–250 ng/mL	433–903 nmol/L	17–40	10–36	85–95	Hepatic
			(Conversion Factor ×3.8)			
Nortriptyline	50–150 ng/mL	190–570 nmol/L	20–90	15–23	90–95	Hepatic
			(Conversion Factor ×3.58)			
Combined doxepin and desmethyl-doxepin	150–251 ng/mL	540–900 nmol/L	10–25	10–30	75–85	Hepatic
			(Conversion Factor ×3.57)			
Imipramine	150–250 ng/mL	536–892 nmol/L	6–28	9–23	60–95	Hepatic
			(Conversion Factor ×3.75)			
Desipramine	75–300 ng/mL	281–1125 nmol/L	6–28	9–23	60–95	Hepatic

* Conventional units.

DESCRIPTION: Tricyclic antidepressants are used in the treatment of major depression. They have also been used effectively to treat bipolar disorder, panic disorder, attention deficit hyperactivity disorder (ADHD), obsessive compulsive disorder (OCD), enuresis, eating disorders (bulimia nervosa in particular), nicotine dependence (tobacco), and cocaine dependence.

Many factors must be considered in effective dosing and monitoring of therapeutic drugs, including patient age, patient weight, interacting medications, electrolyte balance, protein levels, water balance, conditions that affect absorption and excretion, and foods, herbals, vitamins, and minerals that can either potentiate or inhibit the intended target concentration. Peak and trough collection times should be documented carefully in relation to the time of medication administration. ∎

IMPORTANT NOTE: This information must be clearly and accurately communicated to avoid misunderstanding of the dose time in relation to the collection time. Miscommunication between the individual administering the medication and the individual collecting the specimen is the most frequent cause of subtherapeutic levels, toxic levels, and misleading information used in calculation of future doses.

INDICATIONS:
- Assist in the diagnosis and prevention of toxicity

- Evaluate overdose, especially in combination with ethanol (*Note:* Doxepin abuse is unusual)

- Monitor compliance to therapeutic regimen

RESULT

Level	Response
Normal levels	Therapeutic effect
Subtherapeutic levels	Adjust dose as indicated
Toxic levels	Adjust dose as indicated
Amitryptyline	Hepatic impairment
Nortriptyline	Hepatic impairment
Doxepin	Hepatic impairment
Imipramine	Hepatic impairment
Desipramine	Hepatic impairment

CRITICAL VALUES: ⚠ It is important to note the adverse effects of subtherapeutic levels of antidepressants. Care must be taken to investigate signs and symptoms of too little and too much medication.

Tricyclic Antidepressants:

- Amitryptyline: Greater than 500 ng/mL

- Nortriptyline: Greater than 500 ng/mL

- Combined doxepin and desmethyldoxepin: Greater than 500 ng/mL

- Imipramine: Greater than 500 ng/mL

- Desipramine: Greater than 400 ng/mL
  Signs and symptoms of tricyclic antidepressant toxicity include agitation, hallucinations, confusion, seizures, arrhythmias, hyperthermia, flushing, dilation of the pupils, and possible coma. Possible interventions include administration of activated charcoal; emesis; gastric lavage with saline; administration of physostigmine to counteract seizures, hyperten-

sion, or respiratory depression; administration of bicarbonate, propranolol, lidocaine, or phenytoin to counteract arrhythmias; and electrocardiographic monitoring.

INTERFERING FACTORS: Cyclic antidepressants may potentiate the effects of oral anticoagulants.

Nursing Implications and Procedure • • • • • • • • • •

Pretest: ■

➤ Obtain a history of the patient's complaints, including a list of known allergens.

➤ Review results of previously performed tests and procedures. For related tests, refer to the hepatobiliary system and therapeutic/toxicology tables.

➤ Obtain a list of the medications the patient is taking, including herbs, nutritional supplements, and nutraceuticals. The requesting health care practitioner and laboratory should be advised if the patient regularly uses these products so that their effects can be taken into consideration when reviewing results.

➤ There are no food, fluid, or medication restrictions unless by medical direction.

➤ Review the procedure with the patient.

➤ Inform the patient that specimen collection takes approximately 5 to 10 minutes.

Intratest: ■

➤ Direct the patient to breathe normally and to avoid unnecessary movement.

➤ Observe standard precautions and follow the general guidelines in Appendix A. Review dosing schedule to ensure that peak and trough specimens are ordered to be collected at the appropriate time. Perform a venipuncture, and collect the specimen in a 5-mL red-top tube.

➤ Label the specimen, and promptly transport it to the laboratory.

Post-test: ■

➤ Observe venipuncture site for bleeding or hematoma formation. Apply pressure bandage.

➤ Explain to the patient the importance of following the medication regimen and instructions regarding food and drug interactions.

➤ Instruct the patient to immediately report any unusual sensations (e.g., severe headache, vomiting, sweating, clammy skin, visual disturbances) to the health care practitioner. Blood pressure should be monitored regularly.

➤ Instruct the patient to be prepared to list to the pharmacist the other medications he or she is already taking in the event that the requesting health care practitioner prescribes a medication.

➤ Evaluate test results in relation to the patient's symptoms and other tests performed.

ANTIDIURETIC HORMONE

SYNONYMS/ACRONYM: Vasopressin, arginine vasopressin hormone, ADH.

SPECIMEN: Plasma (1 mL) collected in lavender-top (ethylenediaminetetraacetic acid [EDTA]) tube.

REFERENCE VALUE: (Method: Radioimmunoassay)

RECOMMENDATION: This test should be ordered and interpreted with results of a serum osmolality.

Serum Osmolality*	Antidiuretic Hormone*	SI Units (Conversion Factor ×0.926)
270–280 mOsm/kg	Less than 1.5 pg/mL	Less than 1.4 pmol/L
280–285 mOsm/kg	Less than 2.5 pg/mL	Less than 2.3 pmol/L
285–290 mOsm/kg	1–5 pg/mL	0.9–4.6 pmol/L
290–295 mOsm/kg	2–7 pg/mL	1.9–6.5 pmol/L
295–300 mOsm/kg	4–12 pg/mL	3.7–11.1 pmol/L

* Conventional units.

DESCRIPTION: Antidiuretic hormone (ADH) is formed by the hypothalamus and stored in the posterior pituitary gland. ADH is released in response to increased serum osmolality or decreased blood volume. When the hormone is active, small amounts of concentrated urine are produced; in its absence, large amounts of dilute urine are produced. Although a 1 percent change in serum osmolality stimulates ADH secretion, blood volume must decrease by approximately 10 percent for ADH secretion to be induced. Psychogenic stimuli, such as stress, pain, and anxiety, may also stimulate ADH release, but the mechanism is unclear. ∎

INDICATIONS:
- Evaluate polyuria or altered serum osmolality to identify possible alterations in ADH secretion as the cause.

- Detect central nervous system trauma, surgery, or disease that may lead to impaired ADH secretion.

- Differentiate neurogenic (central) diabetes insipidus from nephrogenic diabetes insipidus by decreased ADH levels in neurogenic diabetes insipidus or elevated levels in nephrogenic diabetes insipidus if normal feedback mechanisms are intact.

- Assist in the diagnosis of known or suspected malignancy associated with syndrome of inappropriate ADH secretion (SIADH), such as oat cell lung cancer, thymoma, lymphoma, leukemia, pancreatic carcinoma, prostate gland carcinoma, and intestinal carcinoma; elevated ADH levels indicate the presence of this syndrome.

• Assist in the diagnosis of known or suspected pulmonary conditions associated with SIADH, such as tuberculosis, pneumonia, and positive-pressure mechanical ventilation.

RESULT

Increased in:
• Acute intermittent porphyria

• Brain tumor

• Disorders involving the central nervous system, thyroid gland, and adrenal gland

• Ectopic production (systemic neoplasm)

• Guillain-Barré syndrome

• Nephrogenic diabetes insipidus

• Pain, stress, or exercise

• Pneumonia

• Pulmonary tuberculosis

• SIADH

• Tuberculosis meningitis

Decreased in:
• Nephrotic syndrome

• Pituitary (central) diabetes insipidus

• Psychogenic polydipsia

CRITICAL VALUES: Effective treatment of SIADH depends on identifying and resolving the cause of increased ADH production. Signs and symptoms of SIADH are the same as those for hyponatremia, including irritability, tremors, muscle spasms, convulsions, and neurologic changes. The patient has enough sodium, but it is diluted in excess retained water.

INTERFERING FACTORS
• Drugs that may increase ADH levels include barbiturates, carbamazepine, chlorpropamide, chlorthalidone, cisplatin, clofibrate, ether, furosemide, haloperidol, hydrochlorothiazide, lithium, methyclothiazide, narcotic analgesics, phenothiazides, polythiazide, tolbutamide, tricyclic antidepressants, vidarabine, vinblastine, and vincristine.

• Drugs that may decrease ADH levels include clonidine, demeclocycline, ethanol, lithium carbonate, and phenytoin.

• Recent radioactive scans or radiation within 1 week before the test can interfere with test results when radioimmunoassay is the test method.

• ADH exhibits diurnal variation, with highest levels of secretion occurring at night; first morning collection is recommended.

• ADH secretion is also affected by posture, with higher levels measured while upright.

Nursing Implications and Procedure

Pretest:

➤ Obtain a history of the patient's complaints, including a list of known allergens.

➤ Obtain a history of the patient's endocrine and genitourinary systems, as well as results of previously performed tests and procedures. For related tests, refer to the endocrine and genitourinary system tables.

➤ Obtain a list of the medications the patient is taking, including herbs, nutritional supplements, and nutraceuticals. The requesting health care practitioner and laboratory should be advised if the patient regularly uses these products so that their effects can be taken into consideration when reviewing results.

➤ Note any recent procedures that can interfere with test results.

➤ There are no food, fluid, or medication restrictions unless by medical direction.

➤ Review the procedure with the patient.

➤ Inform the patient that specimen collection takes approximately 5 to 10 minutes.

Intratest:

➤ The patient should be encouraged to be calm and in a sitting position for specimen collection.

➤ Direct the patient to breathe normally and to avoid unnecessary movement.

➤ Observe standard precautions and follow the general guidelines in

Appendix A. Perform a venipuncture, and collect the specimen in a 5-mL lavender-top tube.

➤ Label the specimen, and promptly transport it to the laboratory.

Post-test:

➤ Observe venipuncture site for bleeding or hematoma formation. Apply pressure bandage.

➤ Inform the patient, as appropriate, that treatment may include diuretic therapy and fluid restriction to successfully eliminate the excess water.

➤ Evaluate test results in relation to the patient's symptoms and other tests performed. Related laboratory tests include serum and urine electrolytes, serum and urine osmolality, serum and urine sodium, thyroid-stimulating hormone, urea nitrogen, uric acid, and urinalysis.

ANTIGENS/ANTIBODIES, ANTI–EXTRACTABLE NUCLEAR

• •

SYNONYMS/ACRONYMS: La antibodies, Ro antibodies, SS-A antibodies, SS-B antibodies, ENA.

SPECIMEN: Serum (1 mL) collected in a red-top tube.

REFERENCE VALUE: (Method: Immunoassay) Negative.

DESCRIPTION: The extractable nuclear antigens (ENAs) include ribonucleoprotein (RNP), Smith (Sm), SS-A/Ro, and SS-B/La antigens. ENAs and antibodies to them are found in various combinations in individuals with combinations of overlapping rheumatologic symptoms. ∎

INDICATIONS:

• Assist in the diagnosis of mixed connective tissue disease

• Assist in the diagnosis of Sjögren's syndrome

• Assist in the diagnosis of systemic lupus erythematosus (SLE)

RESULT

Increased in:

- Anti-SS-A/Ro–positive patients have photosensitivity.

- Anti-RNP is associated with mixed connective tissue disease.

- Anti-SS-A and anti-SS-B are helpful in antinuclear antibody (ANA)–negative cases of SLE.

- Anti-SS-A/ANA–positive, anti-SS-B–negative patients are likely to have nephritis.

- Anti-SS-A/anti-SS-B–positive sera are found in patients with neonatal lupus.

- Anti-SS-A–positive patients may also have antibodies associated with antiphospholipid syndrome.

- Anti-SS-A/La is associated with primary Sjögren's syndrome.

- Anti-SS-A/Ro is a predictor of congenital heart block in neonates born to mothers with SLE.

Decreased in: N/A

CRITICAL VALUES: N/A

INTERFERING FACTORS: N/A

Nursing Implications and Procedure · · · · · · · · · · · ·

Pretest:

➤ Obtain a history of the patient's complaints, including a list of known allergens.

➤ Obtain a history of the patient's immune and musculoskeletal systems, as well as results of previously performed tests and procedures. For related tests, refer to the immune and musculoskeletal system tables.

➤ Obtain a list of medications the patient is taking, including herbs, nutritional supplements, and nutraceuticals. The requesting health care practitioner and laboratory should be advised if the patient regularly uses these products so that their effects can be taken into consideration when reviewing results.

➤ There are no food, fluid, or medication restrictions unless by medical direction.

➤ Review the procedure with the patient.

➤ Inform the patient that specimen collection takes approximately 5 to 10 minutes.

Intratest:

➤ Direct the patient to breathe normally and to avoid unnecessary movement.

➤ Observe standard precautions and follow the general guidelines in Appendix A. Perform a venipuncture, and collect the specimen in a 5-mL red-top tube.

➤ Label the specimen, and promptly transport it to the laboratory.

Post-test:

➤ Observe venipuncture site for bleeding or hematoma formation. Apply pressure bandage.

➤ Educate the patient, as appropriate, in the importance of preventing infection, which is a significant cause of death in immunosuppressed individuals.

➤ Recognize anxiety related to test results and offer support. Provide teaching and disease information, as appropriate. Educate the patient regarding access to counseling services. Collagen and connective tissue diseases are chronic; as such, they must be addressed on a continuous basis and may require significant changes in lifestyle.

➤ Evaluate test results in relation to the patient's symptoms and other tests performed. Related laboratory tests include anticardiolipin antibodies, anti-DNA antibodies, ANA, and scleroderma antibody.

ANTIPSYCHOTIC DRUGS AND ANTIMANIC DRUGS: HALOPERIDOL, LITHIUM

SYNONYMS/ACRONYM: Antipsychotic drugs: *haloperidol* (Dozic, Fortunan, Haldol); **antimanic drugs:** *lithium* (Cibalith-S, Eskalith, Lithane, Lithobid, Lithonate, Lithotabs).

SPECIMEN: Serum (1 mL) collected in a red-top tube.

Drug	Route of Administration	Recommended Collection Time
Haloperidol	Oral	Peak: 3–6 h
Lithium	Oral	12 h after dose

REFERENCE VALUE: (Method: Chromatography for haloperidol; ion selective electrode for lithium)

Drug	Therapeutic Dose*	SI Units	Half-Life (h)	Volume of Distribution (L/kg)	Protein Binding (%)	Excretion
Haloperidol	5–20 ng/mL	*(Conversion Factor ×2.66)* 13–53 nmo/L	15–40	18–30	90	Hepatic
Lithium	0.6–1.2 mEq/L	*(Conversion Factor ×1)* 0.6–1.2 mmol/L	18–24	0.7–1.0	0	Renal

*Conventional units.

DESCRIPTION: Haloperidol is an antipsychotic tranquilizer used for the following indications: acute and chronic psychotic disorders, Tourette's syndrome, and hyperactive children with severe behavioral problems. Lithium is used in the treatment of manic depression.

Many factors must be considered in effective dosing and monitoring of therapeutic drugs, including patient age, patient weight, interacting medications, electrolyte balance, protein levels, water balance, conditions that affect absorption and excretion, and foods, herbals, vitamins, and minerals that can either potentiate or inhibit the intended target concentration. Peak collection times should be documented carefully in relation to the time of medication administration. ∎

IMPORTANT NOTE: This information must be clearly and accurately communicated to avoid misunderstanding of the dose time in relation to the collection time. Miscommunication between the individual administering the medication and the individual collecting the specimen is the most frequent cause of subtherapeutic levels, toxic levels, and misleading information used in calculation of future doses.

INDICATIONS:

• Assist in the diagnosis and prevention of toxicity

• Monitor compliance to therapeutic regimen

RESULT

Level	Response
Normal levels	Therapeutic effect
Subtherapeutic levels	Adjust dose as indicated
Toxic levels	Adjust dose as indicated
Haloperidol	Hepatic impairment
Lithium	Renal impairment

CRITICAL VALUES: ⚠ It is important to note the adverse effects of subtherapeutic levels. Care must be taken to investigate signs and symptoms of not enough medication and too much medication.

Haloperidol: Greater than 42 ng/mL

Signs and symptoms of haloperidol toxi-

city include hypotension, respiratory depression, and extrapyramidal neuromuscular reactions. Possible interventions include emesis (contraindicated in the absence of gag reflex or in the presence of central nervous system depression or excitation) and gastric lavage followed by administration of activated charcoal.

Lithium: Greater than 1.5 mEq/L

Signs and symptoms of lithium toxicity include ataxia, coarse tremors, muscle weakness, vomiting, diarrhea, confusion, convulsions, stupor, T-wave flattening, loss of consciousness, and possible coma. Possible interventions include administration of activated charcoal, gastric lavage, and administration of intravenous fluids with diuresis.

INTERFERING FACTORS:

• Haloperidol may increase levels of tricyclic antidepressants and increase the risk of lithium toxicity.

• Drugs that may increase lithium levels include thiazide diuretics, angiotensin-converting enzyme inhibitors, and some nonsteroidal anti-inflammatory drugs.

• Drugs and substances that may decrease lithium levels include acetazolamide, theophylline, osmotic diuretics, and caffeine.

Nursing Implications and Procedure • • • • • • • • • •

Pretest: ∎

➤ Obtain a history of the patient's complaints, including a list of known allergens.

➤ Review results of tests and procedures previously performed. For related tests, refer to the genitourinary and hepatobiliary system and therapeutic/toxicology tables.

➤ Obtain a list of medications the

patient is taking, including herbs, nutritional supplements, and nutraceuticals. The requesting health care practitioner and laboratory should be advised if the patient regularly uses these products so that their effects can be taken into consideration when reviewing results.

➤ There are no food, fluid, or medication restrictions unless by medical direction.

➤ Review the procedure with the patient.

➤ Inform the patient that specimen collection takes approximately 5 to 10 minutes.

Intratest:

➤ Direct the patient to breathe normally and to avoid unnecessary movement.

➤ Observe standard precautions and follow the general guidelines in Appendix A. Consider recommended collection time around dosing schedule. Perform a venipuncture, and collect the specimen in a 5-mL red-top tube.

➤ Label the specimen, and promptly transport it to the laboratory.

Post-test:

➤ Explain to the patient the importance of following the medication regimen and instructions regarding food and drug interactions.

➤ Instruct the patient receiving haloperidol to immediately report any unusual symptoms (e.g., blurred vision, dry eyes) to the requesting health care practitioner.

➤ Instruct the patient receiving lithium to immediately report any unusual symptoms (e.g., nausea, vomiting, diarrhea, dizziness, visual disturbances) to the requesting health care practitioner.

➤ Instruct the patient to be prepared to list to the pharmacist the other medications he or she is already taking in the event that the requesting health care practitioner prescribes a medication.

➤ Evaluate test results in relation to the patient's symptoms and other tests performed. Patients receiving lithium should be monitored especially for albumin, calcium, creatinine, glucose, magnesium, potassium, sodium, and blood urea nitrogen.

ANTITHROMBIN III

SYNONYM/ACRONYM: Heparin cofactor assay, AT-III.

SPECIMEN: Plasma (1 mL) collected in blue-top (sodium citrate) tube.

REFERENCE VALUE: (Method: Radioimmunodiffusion)

	Conventional Units	SI Units (Conversion Factor ×10)
Immunologic assay	21–30 mg/dL	210–300 mg/L

	Conventional Units	SI Units (Conversion Factor ×0.01)
Functional assay	85–115% of standard	0.85–1.15

DESCRIPTION: Antithrombin III (AT-III) can inhibit thrombin and factors IX, X, XI, and XII. It is a heparin cofactor, interacting with heparin and thrombin. AT-III acts to increase the rate of thrombin neutralized or inhibited, and it decreases the total quantity of thrombin inhibited. Patients with low levels show some level of resistance to heparin therapy. ■

INDICATIONS:
• Investigate tendency for thrombosis

RESULT

Increased in:
• Acute hepatitis
• Inflammation
• Menstruation
• Obstructive jaundice
• Renal transplant
• Vitamin K deficiency

Decreased in:
• Carcinoma
• Chronic liver failure
• Cirrhosis
• Congenital deficiency
• Disseminated intravascular coagulation
• Liver transplant or partial hepatectomy
• Nephrotic syndrome
• Pulmonary embolism

CRITICAL VALUES: N/A

INTERFERING FACTORS:

• Drugs that may increase AT-III levels include anabolic steroids, gemfibrozil, and warfarin.

• Drugs that may decrease AT-III levels include asparaginase, heparin, estrogens, gestodene, and oral contraceptives.

• Placement of the tourniquet for longer than 1 minute can result in venous stasis and changes in the concentration of the plasma proteins to be measured. Platelet activation may also occur under these conditions, resulting in erroneous measurements.

Nursing Implications and Procedure

Pretest:

➤ Obtain a history of the patient's complaints, including a list of known allergens.

➤ Obtain a history of the patient's hematopoietic system and results of previously performed tests and procedures. For other related tests, refer to the hematopoietic system table.

➤ Obtain a list of medications the patient is taking, including herbs, nutritional supplements, and nutraceuticals. The requesting health care practitioner and laboratory should be advised if the patient regularly uses these products so that their effects can be taken into consideration when reviewing results.

➤ There are no food, fluid, or medication restrictions unless by medical direction.

➤ Review the procedure with the patient.

➤ Inform the patient that specimen

collection takes approximately 5 to 10 minutes.

Intratest:

➤ Direct the patient to breathe normally and to avoid unnecessary movement.

➤ Observe standard precautions and follow the general guidelines in Appendix A. Perform a venipuncture, and collect the specimen in a 5-mL blue-top tube. When multiple specimens are drawn, the blue-top tube should be collected after sterile (i.e., blood culture) and red-top tubes. When coagulation testing is the only work to be done, an extra red-top tube should be collected before the blue-top tube to avoid contaminating the specimen with tissue thromboplastin.

➤ Label the specimen, and promptly transport it to the laboratory.

IMPORTANT NOTE: Presently two different concentrations of sodium citrate preservative are added to blue-top tubes for coagulation studies: 3.2 percent and 3.8 percent. The National Committee for Clinical Laboratory Standards (NCCLS) guideline for sodium citrate is 3.2 percent. Laboratories establish reference ranges for coagulation testing based on numerous factors, including sodium citrate concentration, test equipment, and test reagents. Inquire from the laboratory as to which concentration is used.

Post-test:

➤ Observe venipuncture site for bleeding or hematoma formation. Apply pressure bandage.

➤ Evaluate test results in relation to the patient's symptoms and other tests performed. Some related laboratory tests include partial thromboplastin time, protein C, protein S, and vitamin K.

α_1-ANTITRYPSIN AND α_1-ANTITRYPSIN PHENOTYPING

• •

SYNONYMS/ACRONYMS: α_1-antitrypsin: A_1AT, α_1-AT, AAT; α_1-antitrypsin phenotyping: A_1AT phenotype, α_1-AT phenotype, AAT phenotype, Pi phenotype.

SPECIMEN: Serum (1 mL) for α_1-antitrypsin (α_1-AT) and serum (2 mL) for α_1-AT phenotyping collected in a red- or tiger-top tube.

REFERENCE VALUE: (Method: Rate nephelometry for α_1-AT, isoelectric focusing/high-resolution electrophoresis for α_1-AT phenotyping)

α_1-Antitrypsin

Age	Conventional Units	SI Units (Conversion Factor $\times 0.01$)
0–1 mo	124–348 mg/dL	1.24–3.48 g/L
2–6 mo	111–297 mg/dL	1.11–2.97 g/L
7 mo–2 y	95–251 mg/dL	0.95–2.51 g/L
3 y–19 y	110–279 mg/dL	1.10–2.79 g/L
Adult	126–226 mg/dL	1.26–2.26 g/L

α_1-Antitrypsin Phenotyping

There are three major protease inhibitor phenotypes:

MM—Normal
SS—Intermediate; heterozygous
ZZ—Markedly abnormal; homozygous

The total level of measurable α_1-AT varies with genotype. The effects of α_1-AT deficiency depend on the patient's personal habits, but are most severe in patients who smoke tobacco.

DESCRIPTION: α_1-AT is the main glycoprotein produced by the liver. Its inhibitory function is directed against proteolytic enzymes, such as trypsin, elastin, and plasmin, released by alveolar macrophages and bacteria. In the absence of α_1-AT, functional tissue is destroyed by proteolytic enzymes and replaced with excessive connective tissue. Emphysema develops at an earlier age in α_1-AT–deficient emphysema patients than in other emphysema patients. α_1-AT deficiency is passed on as an autosomal-recessive trait. Inherited deficiencies are associated early in life with development of lung and liver disorders. In the pediatric population, the ZZ phenotype usually presents as liver disease, cholestasis, and cirrhosis. Greater than 80% of ZZ-deficient individuals ultimately develop chronic lung or liver disease. It is important to identify inherited deficiencies early in life. Typically, α_1-AT–deficient patients have circulating levels less than 50 mg/dL. Patients who have α_1-AT values less than 140 mg/dL should be phenotyped.

Elevated levels are found in normal individuals when an inflammatory process, such as rheumatoid arthritis, bacterial infection, neoplasm, and vasculitis, is present. Decreased levels are found in affected patients with chronic obstructive pulmonary disease (COPD) and in children with cirrhosis of the liver. Decreased α_1-AT levels also may be elevated into the normal range in heterozygous α_1-AT–deficient patients during concurrent infection, pregnancy, estrogen therapy, steroid therapy, cancer, and postoperative periods. Homozygous α_1-AT–deficient patients do not show such an elevation. ∎

INDICATIONS:

• Assist in establishing a diagnosis of COPD

• Assist in establishing a diagnosis of liver disease

• Detect hereditary absence or deficiency of α_1-AT

RESULT

Increased in:

* Acute and chronic inflammatory conditions

* Carcinomas

* Estrogen therapy

* Postoperative recovery

* Pregnancy

* Steroid therapy

* Stress (extreme physical)

Decreased in:

* COPD

* Homozygous α_1-AT–deficient patients

* Liver disease (severe)

* Liver cirrhosis (child)

* Malnutrition

* Nephrotic syndrome

CRITICAL VALUES: N/A

INTERFERING FACTORS:

* α_1-AT is an acute-phase reactant protein, and any inflammatory process elevates levels. If a serum C-reactive protein is performed simultaneously and is positive, the patient should be retested for α_1-AT in 10 to 14 days.

* Rheumatoid factor causes false-positive elevations.

* Drugs that may increase serum α_1-AT levels include aminocaproic acid, estrogen therapy, oral contraceptives (high-dose preparations), oxymetholone, streptokinase, tamoxifen, and typhoid vaccine.

Nursing Implications and Procedure • • • • • • • • • • •

Pretest:

➤ Obtain a history of the patient's complaints, including a list of known allergens.

➤ Obtain a history of the patient's hepatobiliary and respiratory system and results of previously performed tests and procedures. For related tests, refer to the hepatobiliary and respiratory system tables.

➤ Obtain a list of the medications the patient is taking, including herbs, nutritional supplements, and nutraceuticals. Oral contraceptives should be withheld 24 hours before the specimen is collected, although this restriction should first be confirmed with the person ordering the test. The requesting health care practitioner and laboratory should be advised if the patient regularly uses these products so that their effects can be taken into consideration when reviewing results.

➤ There are no food, fluid, or medication restrictions unless by medical direction.

➤ Review the procedure with the patient.

➤ Inform the patient that specimen collection usually takes approximately 5 to 10 minutes.

Intratest:

➤ Direct the patient to breathe normally and to avoid unnecessary movement.

➤ Observe standard precautions and follow the general guidelines in Appendix A. Perform a venipuncture, and collect the specimen in a 5-mL red- or tiger-top tube.

➤ Label the specimen, and promptly transport it to the laboratory.

Post-test:

➤ Observe venipuncture site for bleeding or hematoma formation. Apply pressure bandage.

➤ Instruct the patient to resume usual medication as directed by the health care practitioner.

➤ Educate the patient with abnormal findings in preventive measures for protection of the lungs (e.g., avoid contact with persons who have respiratory or other infections; avoid the use of tobacco; avoid areas having highly polluted air; and avoid work environments with hazards such as fumes, dust, and other respiratory pollutants).

➤ Instruct the affected patient in deep breathing and pursed-lip breathing to enhance breathing patterns as appropriate. Inform the patient of smoking cessation programs, as appropriate.

➤ Recognize anxiety related to test results and offer support. Provide teaching and information regarding the clinical implications of the test results, as appropriate. Because decreased α_1-AT can be an inherited disorder, it may be appropriate to recommend resources for genetic counseling if levels less than 140 mg/dL are reported. It may also be appropriate to inform the patient that α_1-AT phenotype testing can be performed on family members to determine the homozygous or heterozygous nature of the deficiency.

➤ Inform the patient of the importance of medical follow-up, and suggest ongoing support resources to assist the patient in coping with chronic illness and possible early death.

➤ Malnutrition is commonly seen in α_1-AT–deficient patients with severe respiratory disease for many reasons, including fatigue, lack of appetite, and gastrointestinal distress. Research has estimated that the daily caloric intake required for respiration in patients with COPD is 10 times higher than that required of normal individuals. Inadequate nutrition can result in hypophosphatemia, especially in the respirator-dependent patient. During periods of starvation, phosphorus leaves the intracellular space and moves outside the tissue, resulting in dangerously decreased phosphorus levels. Adequate intake of vitamins A and C is important to prevent pulmonary infection and to decrease the extent of lung tissue damage. The importance of following the prescribed diet should be stressed to the patient and caregiver.

➤ Water balance must be closely monitored in α_1-AT–deficient patients with COPD. Fluid retention can lead to pulmonary edema.

➤ Evaluate test results in relation to the patient's symptoms and other tests performed. Related laboratory tests include arterial/alveolar oxygen ratio, angiotensin-converting enzyme, anion gap, blood gases, electrolytes, osmolality, and phosphorus.

APOLIPOPROTEIN A

SYNONYM/ACRONYM: Apo A.

SPECIMEN: Serum (1 mL) collected in a red- or tiger-top tube.

REFERENCE VALUE: (Method: Immunonephelometry)

Sex/Age	Conventional Units	SI Units (Conversion Factor ×0.01)
Male		
Newborn	41–93 mg/dL	0.41–0.93 g/L
6 mo–4 y	67–163 mg/dL	0.67–1.63 g/L
Adult	81–166 mg/dL	0.81–1.66 g/L
Female		
Newborn	38–106 mg/dL	0.38–1.06 g/L
6 mo–4 y	60–148 mg/dL	0.60–1.48 g/L
Adult	80–214 mg/dL	0.80–2.14 g/L

DESCRIPTION: Apolipoprotein A (Apo A), the major component of high-density lipoprotein (HDL), is synthesized in the liver and intestines. Apolipoproteins assist in the regulation of lipid metabolism by activating and inhibiting enzymes required for this process. Apo A-I activates the enzyme lecithin-cholesterol acyltransferase (LCAT), whereas Apo A-II inhibits LCAT. The apolipoproteins also help keep lipids in solution as they circulate in the blood and direct the lipids toward the correct target organs and tissues in the body. It is believed that Apo A measurements may be more important than HDL cholesterol measurements as a predictor of coronary artery disease (CAD). There is an inverse relationship between Apo A levels and risk for developing CAD. Because of difficulties with method standardization, the above-listed reference ranges should be used as a rough guide in assessing abnormal conditions. Values for African-Americans are 5 to 10 mg/dL higher than values for whites. ■

INDICATIONS:
• Evaluation for risk of CAD

RESULT

Increased in:
• Familial hyper-α-lipoproteinemia
• Weight reduction

Decreased in:
• A-β-lipoproteinemia
• Cholestasis
• Chronic renal failure
• Diabetes (uncontrolled)
• Diet high in carbohydrates or polyunsaturated fats
• Familial deficiencies of related enzymes and lipoproteins
• Hepatocellular disorders
• Hypertriglyceridemia
• Nephrotic syndrome
• Premature coronary heart disease
• Smoking

CRITICAL VALUES: N/A

INTERFERING FACTORS:
• Drugs and substances that may increase Apo A levels include anticonvulsants, beclobrate, bezafibrate, ciprofibrate, estrogens, furosemide, lovastatin, pravastatin, prednisolone, simvastatin, and ethanol (abuse).
• Drugs that may decrease Apo A levels include androgens, beta blockers, diuretics, and probucol.

Nursing Implications and Procedure ∙ ∙ ∙ ∙ ∙ ∙ ∙ ∙ ∙ ∙

Pretest:

➤ Obtain a history of the patient's complaints, including a list of known allergens.

➤ Obtain a history of the patient's cardiovascular system and results of previously performed tests and procedures. For related tests, refer to the cardiovascular system table.

➤ Obtain a list of medications the patient is taking, including herbs, nutritional supplements, and nutraceuticals. The requesting health care practitioner and laboratory should be advised if the patient regularly uses these products so that their effects can be taken into consideration when reviewing results.

➤ The patient should abstain from food for 6 to 12 hours before specimen collection.

➤ There are no fluid or medication restrictions unless by medical direction.

➤ Review the procedure with the patient.

➤ Inform the patient that specimen collection takes approximately 5 to 10 minutes.

Intratest:

➤ Ensure that the patient complied with dietary pretesting restrictions.

➤ Direct the patient to breathe normally and to avoid unnecessary movement.

➤ Observe standard precautions and follow the general guidelines in Appendix A. Perform a venipuncture, and collect the specimen in a 5-mL red- or tiger-top tube.

➤ Label the specimen, and promptly transport it to the laboratory.

Post-test:

➤ Observe venipuncture site for bleeding or hematoma formation. Apply pressure bandage.

➤ Instruct the patient to resume usual diet as directed by the health care practitioner.

➤ Decreased Apo A levels may be associated with CAD. Nutritional therapy is recommended for individuals identified to be at high risk for developing CAD. Overweight patients should be encouraged to achieve a normal weight. The American Heart Association Step 1 and Step 2 diets may be helpful in achieving a goal of reducing total cholesterol and triglyceride levels. The Step 1 diet emphasizes a reduction in foods high in saturated fats and cholesterol. Red meats, eggs, and dairy products are the major sources of saturated fats and cholesterol. If triglycerides are also elevated, the patient should be advised to eliminate or reduce alcohol and simple carbohydrates from the diet. The Step 2 diet recommends stricter reductions.

➤ Evaluate test results in relation to the patient's symptoms and other tests performed. Related laboratory tests include apolipoprotein B, total cholesterol, HDL cholesterol, low-density lipoprotein cholesterol, lipoprotein electrophoresis, and triglycerides.

APOLIPOPROTEIN B

• •

SYNONYM/ACRONYM: Apo B.

SPECIMEN: Serum (1 mL) collected in a red- or tiger-top tube.

REFERENCE VALUE: (Method: Immunonephelometry)

Age	Conventional Units	SI Units (Conversion Factor ×0.01)
Newborn–5 y	11–31 mg/dL	0.11–0.31 g/L
5–17 y		
Male	47–139 mg/dL	0.47–1.39 g/L
Female	41–96 mg/dL	0.41–0.96 g/L
Adult		
Male	46–174 mg/dL	0.46–1.74 g/L
Female	46–142 mg/dL	0.46–1.42 g/L

DESCRIPTION: Apolipoprotein B (Apo B), the major component of the low-density lipoproteins (chylomicrons, LDL, and very-low-density lipoprotein), is synthesized in the liver and intestines. Apolipoproteins assist in the regulation of lipid metabolism by activating and inhibiting enzymes required for this process. The apolipoproteins also help keep lipids in solution as they circulate in the blood and direct the lipids toward the correct target organs and tissues in the body. ■

INDICATIONS:
• Evaluation for risk of coronary artery disease (CAD)

RESULT

Increased in:
• Anorexia nervosa
• Cushing's syndrome
• Diabetes
• Dysglobulinemia
• Emotional stress
• Hepatic disease
• Hepatic obstruction
• Hyperlipoproteinemias
• Hypothyroidism
• Infantile hypercalcemia
• Nephrotic syndrome
• Porphyria
• Pregnancy
• Premature CAD

- Renal failure

- Werner's syndrome

Decreased in:

- Alpha lipoprotein deficiency (Tangier disease)

- Acute stress (burns, illness)

- Chronic anemias

- Chronic pulmonary disease

- Familial deficiencies of related enzymes and lipoproteins

- Hyperthyroidism

- Inflammatory joint disease

- Intestinal malabsorption

- Malnutrition

- Myeloma

- Reye's syndrome

- Weight reduction

CRITICAL VALUES: N/A

INTERFERING FACTORS:

- Drugs that may increase Apo B levels include amiodarone, androgens, beta blockers, catecholamines, cyclosporine, diuretics, ethanol (abuse), etretinate, glucogenic corticosteroids, oral contraceptives, and phenobarbital.

- Drugs that may decrease Apo B levels include fibrates, beclobrate, cholestyramine, captopril, ketanserin, lovastatin, niacin, nifedipine, pravastatin, prazosin, probucol, and simvastatin.

Nursing Implications and Procedure · · · · · · · · · ·

Pretest:

➤ Obtain a history of the patient's complaints, including a list of known allergens.

➤ Obtain a history of the patient's cardiovascular system and results of previously performed tests and procedures. For related tests, refer to the cardiovascular system table.

➤ Obtain a list of medications the patient is taking, including herbs, nutritional supplements, and nutraceuticals. The requesting health care practitioner and laboratory should be advised if the patient regularly uses these products so that their effects can be taken into consideration when reviewing results.

➤ The patient should abstain from food for 6 to 12 hours before specimen collection.

➤ There are no fluid or medication restrictions unless by medical direction.

➤ Review the procedure with the patient.

➤ Inform the patient that specimen collection takes approximately 5 to 10 minutes.

Intratest:

➤ Ensure that the patient complied with dietary pretesting restrictions.

➤ Direct the patient to breathe normally and to avoid unnecessary movement.

➤ Observe standard precautions and follow the general guidelines in Appendix A. Perform a venipuncture, and collect the specimen in a 5-mL red- or tiger-top tube.

➤ Label the specimen, and promptly transport it to the laboratory.

Post-test:

➤ Observe venipuncture site for bleeding or hematoma formation. Apply pressure bandage.

➤ Instruct the patient to resume usual diet as directed by the health care practitioner.

➤ Increased Apo B levels may be associated with CAD. Nutritional therapy is recommended for individuals identified to be at high risk for developing

CAD. Overweight patients should be encouraged to achieve a normal weight. The American Heart Association Step 1 and Step 2 diets may be helpful in achieving a goal of reducing total cholesterol and triglyceride levels. The Step 1 diet emphasizes a reduction in foods high in saturated fats and cholesterol. Red meats, eggs, and dairy products are the major sources of saturated fats and cholesterol. If triglycerides are also elevated, the patient should be advised to eliminate or reduce alcohol and simple carbohydrates from the diet. The Step 2 diet recommends stricter reductions.

➤ Evaluate test results in relation to the patient's symptoms and other tests performed. Related laboratory tests include apolipoprotein A, total cholesterol, high-density lipoprotein cholesterol, LDL cholesterol, lipoprotein electrophoresis, and triglycerides.

ARTHROGRAM

SYNONYM/ACRONYM: Joint study.

AREA OF APPLICATION: Shoulder, elbow, wrist, hip, knee, ankle, temporomandibular joint.

CONTRAST: Iodinated or gadolinium.

DESCRIPTION: An arthrogram evaluates the cartilage, ligaments, and bony structures that compose a joint. After local anesthesia is administered to the area of interest, a fluoroscopically guided small-gauge needle is inserted into the joint space. Fluid in the joint space is aspirated and sent to the laboratory for analysis. Contrast medium is inserted into the joint space to outline the soft tissue structures and the contour of the joint. After brief exercise of the joint, radiographs or magnetic resonance images (MRIs) are obtained. Arthrograms are used primarily for assessment of persistent, unexplained joint discomfort. ■

INDICATIONS:
• Evaluate pain, swelling, or dysfunction of a joint

• Monitor disease progression

RESULT

Normal Findings:

- Normal bursae, menisci, ligaments, and articular cartilage of the joint (*note*: the cartilaginous surfaces and menisci should be smooth, without evidence of erosion, tears, or disintegration)

Abnormal Findings:

- Arthritis

- Cysts

- Diseases of the cartilage (chondromalacia)

- Injury to the ligaments

- Joint derangement

- Meniscal tears or laceration

- Muscle tears

- Osteochondral fractures

- Osteochondritis dissecans

- Synovitis

- Synovial tumor

INTERFERING FACTORS

This procedure is contraindicated for:

- Patients who are pregnant or suspected of being pregnant, unless the potential benefits of the procedure far outweigh the risks to the fetus and mother.

- Patients with bleeding disorders, active arthritis, or joint infections.

- Patients with allergies to shellfish or ⚠ iodinated dye. The contrast medium used may cause a life-threatening allergic reaction. Patients with a known hypersensitivity to the medium may benefit from premedication with corticosteroids or the use of a nonionic contrast medium.

Factors that may impair clear imaging:

- Inability of the patient to cooperate or remain still during the procedure because of age, significant pain, or mental status

- Metallic objects within the examination field (e.g., jewelry, earrings, dental amalgams), which may inhibit organ visualization and can produce unclear images

- Improper adjustment of the radiographic equipment to accommodate obese or thin patients, which can cause overexposure or underexposure and a poor-quality study

- Patients who are very obese, who may exceed the weight limit for the equipment

- Incorrect positioning of the patient, which may produce poor visualization of the area to be examined

Other considerations:

- Consultation with a physician should occur before the procedure for radiation safety concerns regarding infants of patients who are lactating.

- Risks associated with radiographic overexposure can result from frequent x-ray procedures. Personnel in the room with the patient should wear a protective lead apron, stand behind a shield, or leave the area while the examination is being done. Personnel working in the area where the examination is being done should wear badges that reveal their level of exposure to radiation.

Nursing Implications and Procedure • • • • • • • • • • •

Pretest: ▉

➤ Inform the patient about the purpose of the procedure, various positions to assume, and the need for the patient to hold his or her breath periodically.

➤ Obtain a history of the patient's joint problems and the results of previously performed tests, surgery, therapy, injury, medication usage, and procedures. For related tests, refer to the musculoskeletal system table.

➤ A physician performs this procedure, which lasts 30 minutes.

➤ There are no food, fluid, or medication restrictions.

➤ Inform the patient that discomfort may be experienced when the contrast medium is injected.

➤ *An informed consent needs to be obtained and witnessed.*

Intratest:

➤ Clothing and metallic objects are removed from the joint to be examined.

➤ Patients are given a gown and robe to wear.

➤ When x-rays are used, lead protection is placed over the gonads to prevent their irradiation.

➤ Place the patient on the table in a supine position.

➤ The skin surrounding the joint is aseptically cleaned and anesthetized.

➤ A small-gauge needle is inserted into the joint space.

➤ Any fluid in the space is aspirated and sent to the laboratory for analysis.

➤ Contrast medium is inserted into the joint space with fluoroscopic guidance.

➤ The needle is removed, and the joint

is exercised to help distribute the contrast medium.

➤ X-rays or MRIs are taken of the joint.

➤ The patient is instructed to inhale deeply and hold his or her breath while the x-ray film is taken, and then to exhale after the film is taken.

Post-test:

➤ Inform the patient that further examinations may be needed to evaluate disease progression and to determine the need for a change in therapy.

➤ Answer any questions or concerns voiced by the patient or family.

➤ Assess the joint for swelling after the test. Apply ice as needed.

➤ Instruct the patient to use a mild analgesic (aspirin, acetaminophen), as ordered, if there is discomfort.

➤ Advise the patient to avoid strenuous activity until approved by the physician.

➤ Instruct the patient to notify the health care provider if he or she experiences fever or increased pain, drainage, warmth, edema, or swelling of the joint.

➤ Inform the patient that noises from the joint after the procedure are common and should disappear 24 to 48 hours after the procedure.

➤ A physician who specializes in this branch of medicine sends a written report to the ordering health care provider, who discusses the results with the patient.

➤ Evaluate test results in relation to the patient's symptoms and other tests performed. Related diagnostic tests include MRIs, x-rays, and bone scans of the joint in question.

ARTHROSCOPY

· ·

SYNONYM/ACRONYM: N/A.

AREA OF APPLICATION: Joints.

CONTRAST: None.

DESCRIPTION: Arthroscopy provides direct visualization of a joint through the use of a fiberoptic endoscope. The arthroscope has a light, fiberoptics, and lenses; it connects to a monitor, and the images are recorded for future study and comparison. This procedure is used for inspection of joint structures, performance of a biopsy, and surgical repairs to the joint. Meniscus removal, spur removal, and ligamentous repair are some of the surgical procedures that may be performed. This procedure is most commonly performed to diagnose athletic injuries and acute or chronic joint disorders. Because arthroscopy allows direct visualization, degenerative processes can be accurately differentiated from injuries. A local anesthetic allows the arthroscope to be inserted through the skin with minimal discomfort. This procedure may also be done under a spinal or general anesthetic, especially if surgery is anticipated. ■

INDICATIONS:

- Evaluate the presence of gout

- Evaluate the extent of arthritis

- Evaluate joint pain and damaged cartilage

- Remove loose objects

- Evaluate meniscal, patellar, condylar, extrasynovial, and synovial injuries or diseases of the knee

- Detect torn ligament or tendon

- Monitor effectiveness of therapy

RESULT

Normal Findings:

- Normal muscle, ligament, cartilage, synovial, and tendon structures of the joint

Abnormal Findings:

- Arthritis

- Chondromalacia

- Cysts

- Degenerative joint changes

- Ganglion or Baker's cyst

- Gout or pseudogout

- Joint tumors

- Loose bodies

- Meniscal disease

- Osteoarthritis

- Osteochondritis

- Rheumatoid arthritis

- Subluxation, fracture, or dislocation

- Synovitis
- Torn cartilage
- Torn ligament
- Torn rotator cuff
- Trapped synovium

INTERFERING FACTORS

This procedure is contraindicated for:

- Patients with bleeding disorders, active arthritis, or cardiac conditions
- Patients with joint infection or skin infection near proposed arthroscopic site
- Patients who have had an arthrogram within the last 14 days

Factors that may impair clear imaging:

- Inability of the patient to cooperate or remain still during the procedure because of age, significant pain, or mental status
- Metallic objects within the examination field (e.g., jewelry, earrings, dental amalgams), which may inhibit organ visualization and can produce unclear images
- Improper adjustment of the radiographic equipment to accommodate obese or thin patients, which can cause overexposure or underexposure and a poor-quality study
- Patients who are very obese, who may exceed the weight limit for the equipment
- Incorrect positioning of the patient, which may produce poor visualization of the area to be examined
- Fibrous ankylosis of the joint preventing effective use of the arthroscope
- Joints with flexion of less than 50°
- Failure to follow dietary restrictions before the procedure may cause the procedure to be canceled or repeated.

Nursing Implications and Procedure ● ● ● ● ● ● ● ● ● ● ●

Pretest: ■

➤ Inform the patient that the procedure is generally performed under local anesthesia in an endoscopy or surgical suite by a physician. The procedure takes approximately 15 to 45 minutes.

➤ Instruct the patient not to eat or drink 6 to 8 hours before the test.

➤ Obtain a history of allergies or sensitivities to anesthetics, symptoms, and use of analgesics, medications, and antibiotics. Obtain a history of known or suspected musculoskeletal or joint disorders and results of previously performed tests and procedures. For related tests, refer to the musculoskeletal system table.

➤ An informed consent needs to be obtained and witnessed before administration of medications.

➤ Determine previous abnormalities in laboratory test results, particularly hematologic or coagulation tests.

➤ Crutch walking should be taught before the procedure if it is anticipated postoperatively.

➤ The joint area and areas 5 to 6 inches above and below the joint are shaved and prepared for the procedure.

➤ The patient is given a preprocedure sedative, as ordered.

Intratest: ■

➤ Resuscitation equipment and patient monitoring equipment must be available.

➤ Have the patient remove dentures, contact lenses, eyeglasses, and jewelry. Notify the physician if the patient has crownwork that could affect the examination. Have the patient remove clothing and change into a gown for the procedure.

➤ The extremity is scrubbed, elevated, and wrapped with an elastic bandage from the distal portion of the extremity to the proximal portion to drain as much blood from the limb as possible.

➤ A pneumatic tourniquet placed around the proximal portion of the limb is inflated, and the elastic bandage is removed.

➤ As an alternative to a tourniquet, a mixture of lidocaine with epinephrine and sterile normal saline may be instilled into the joint to help reduce bleeding.

➤ The joint is placed in a 45° angle, and a local anesthetic is administered.

➤ A small incision is made in the skin in the lateral or medial aspect of the joint.

➤ The arthroscope is inserted into the joint spaces. The joint is manipulated as it is visualized. Added puncture sites may be needed to provide a full view of the joint.

➤ Biopsy or treatment can be performed at this time, and photographs should be taken for future reference.

➤ After inspection, specimens may be obtained for cytologic and microbiologic study. All specimens are placed in appropriate containers, labeled properly, and promptly sent to the laboratory.

➤ The joint is irrigated, and the arthroscope is removed. Manual pressure is applied to the joint to remove remaining irrigation solution.

➤ The incision sites are sutured, and a pressure dressing is applied.

➤ Gloves and gowns are worn throughout the procedure.

Post-test:

➤ Advise the patient to avoid strenuous activity involving the joint until approved by the physician.

➤ Inform the patient to resume normal diet and medications.

➤ Instruct the patient to take an analgesic for joint discomfort after the procedure; ice bags may be used to reduce postprocedure swelling.

➤ Monitor the patient's circulation and sensations in the joint area.

➤ Emphasize that any fever as well as excessive bleeding, difficulty breathing, incision site redness, swelling, and tenderness must be reported to the physician.

➤ To reduce swelling, instruct the patient to elevate the joint when sitting and to avoid overbending of the joint.

➤ Inform the patient to shower after 48 hours but to avoid a tub bath until after his or her appointment with the physician.

➤ A physician who specializes in this branch of medicine provides a written report to the ordering health care provider, who discusses the results with the patient.

➤ Evaluate procedure results in relation to the patient's symptoms and other tests performed. Related diagnostic tests include magnetic resonance imaging, x-rays, and bone scans of the joint.

ASPARTATE AMINOTRANSPEPTIDASE

· ·

SYNONYM/ACRONYMS: Serum glutamic-oxaloacetic transaminase, AST, SGOT.

SPECIMEN: Serum (1 mL) collected in a red- or tiger-top tube.

REFERENCE VALUE: (Method: Spectrophotometry, enzymatic at 37°C)

Age	Conventional Units	SI Units (Conversion Factor ×0.17)
Newborn	47–150 U/L	0.80–2.55 μKat/L
10 d–23 m	9–80 U/L	0.15–1.36 μKat/L
2–59 y		
Male	15–40 U/L	0.26–0.68 μKat/L
Female	13–35 U/L	0.22–0.60 μKat/L
60–90 y		
Male	19–48 U/L	0.32–0.82 μKat/L
Female	9–36 U/L	0.15–0.61 μKat/L

DESCRIPTION: Aspartate amino-transferase (AST) is an enzyme that catalyzes the reversible transfer of an amino between aspartate and α-ketoglutaric acid. It was formerly known as serum glutamic-oxaloacetic transaminase (SGOT). AST exists in large amounts in liver and myocardial cells and in smaller but significant amounts in skeletal muscle, kidneys, pancreas, and the brain. Serum AST rises when there is cellular damage to the tissues where the enzyme is found. AST values greater than 500 U/L are usually associated with hepatitis and other hepatocellular diseases in an acute phase. AST levels are very elevated at birth and decrease with age. *Note:* Measurement of AST in evaluation of myocardial infarction has been replaced by more sensitive tests, such as creatine kinase–MB fraction (CK-MB) and troponin. ∎

INDICATIONS:

- Assist in the diagnosis of disorders or injuries involving the tissues where AST is normally found
- Assist (formerly) in the diagnosis of myocardial infarction (*note:* AST rises within 6 to 8 hours, peaks at 24 to 48 hours, and declines to normal within 72 to 96 hours)
- Compare serially with alanine amino-transferase levels to track the course of hepatitis
- Monitor response to therapy with potentially hepatotoxic or nephrotoxic drugs
- Monitor response to treatment for various disorders in which AST may be elevated, with tissue repair indicated by declining levels

RESULT

Significantly increased in (greater than five times normal levels):
- Acute hepatitis
- Acute hepatocellular disease
- Acute pancreatitis
- Shock

Moderately increased in (three to five times normal levels):
- Biliary tract obstruction
- Cardiac arrhythmias

- Chronic hepatitis

- Congestive heart failure

- Dermatomyositis

- Liver tumors

- Muscular dystrophy

Slightly increased in (two to three times normal):

- Cerebrovascular accident

- Cirrhosis, fatty liver

- Delirium tremens

- Hemolytic anemia

- Pericarditis

- Pulmonary infarction

CRITICAL VALUES: N/A

INTERFERING FACTORS:
- Drugs that may increase AST levels by causing cholestasis include amitriptyline, anabolic steroids, androgens, benzodiazepines, chlorothiazide, chlorpropamide, dapsone, erythromycin, estrogens, ethionamide, gold salts, imipramine, mercaptopurine, nitrofurans, oral contraceptives, penicillins, phenothiazines, progesterone, propoxyphene, sulfonamides, tamoxifen, and tolbutamide.

- Drugs that may increase AST levels by causing hepatocellular damage include acetaminophen (toxic), acetylsalicylic acid, allopurinol, amiodarone, anabolic steroids, anticonvulsants, asparaginase, azithromycin, bromocriptine, captopril, cephalosporins, chloramphenicol, clindamycin, clofibrate, danazol, enflurane, ethambutol, ethionamide, fenofibrate, fluconazole, fluoroquinolones, foscarnet, gentamicin, indomethacin, interferon, interleukin-2, levamisole, levodopa, lincomycin, low-molecular-weight heparin, methyldopa, monoamine oxidase inhibitors, naproxen, nifedipine, nitrofurans, oral contraceptives, probenecid, procainamide, qui-

nine, ranitidine, retinol, ritodrine, sulfonylureas, tetracyclines, tobramycin, and verapamil.

- Hemolysis falsely increases AST values.

Nursing Implications and Procedure • • • • • • • • •

Pretest: ▮

➤ Obtain a history of the patient's complaints, including pain related to ischemia or inflammation. Obtain a list of known allergens.

➤ Obtain a history of the patient's cardiovascular and hepatobiliary systems, as well as results of previously performed tests and procedures. For related tests, refer to the cardiovascular and hepatobiliary system tables.

➤ Obtain a list of medications the patient is taking, including herbs, nutritional supplements, and nutraceuticals. The requesting health care practitioner and laboratory should be advised if the patient regularly uses these products so that their effects can be taken into consideration when reviewing results.

➤ There are no food, fluid, or medication restrictions unless by medical direction.

➤ Review the procedure with the patient.

➤ Inform the patient that specimen collection takes approximately 5 to 10 minutes.

Intratest: ▮

➤ Direct the patient to breathe normally and to avoid unnecessary movement.

➤ Observe standard precautions and follow the general guidelines in Appendix A. Perform a venipuncture, and collect the specimen in a 5-mL red- or tiger-top tube. Handle the specimen gently to avoid hemolysis.

➤ Label the specimen, and promptly transport it to the laboratory.

Post-test:

➤ Observe venipuncture site for bleeding or hematoma formation. Apply pressure bandage.

➤ Increased AST levels may be associated with liver disease. Dietary recommendations may be indicated and vary depending on the condition and its severity. Currently, there are no specific medications that can be given to cure hepatitis, but elimination of alcohol ingestion and a diet optimized for convalescence are commonly included in the treatment plan. A high-calorie, high-protein, moderate-fat diet with a high fluid intake is often recommended for patients with hepatitis. Treatment of cirrhosis is different; a low-protein diet may be in order if the patient's liver can no longer process the end products of protein metabolism. A diet of soft foods may be required if esophageal varices have developed. Ammonia levels may be used to determine whether protein should be added to or reduced from the diet. Patients should be encouraged to eat simple carbohydrates and emulsified fats (as in homogenized milk or eggs), as opposed to complex carbohydrates (e.g., starch, fiber, and glycogen [animal carbohydrates]) and complex fats, which would require additional bile to emulsify it so that it could be used. The cirrhotic patient should be observed carefully for the development of ascites, in which case fluid and electrolyte balance requires strict attention.

➤ Increased AST levels may be associated with coronary artery disease (CAD). Nutritional therapy is recommended for individuals identified to be at high risk for CAD. Overweight patients should be encouraged to achieve a normal weight. The American Heart Association Step 1 and Step 2 diets may be helpful in achieving a goal of reducing total cholesterol and triglyceride levels. The Step 1 diet emphasizes a reduction in foods high in saturated fats and cholesterol. Red meats, eggs, and dairy products are the major sources of saturated fats and cholesterol. If triglycerides are also elevated, the patient should be advised to eliminate or reduce alcohol and simple carbohydrates from the diet. The Step 2 diet recommends stricter reductions.

➤ Instruct the patient to immediately report chest pain and changes in breathing pattern to the health care practitioner.

➤ Evaluate test results in relation to the patient's symptoms and other tests performed. Related laboratory tests include acetaminophen, albumin, alkaline phosphatase, alanine aminotransferase, α_1-antitrypsin/phenotyping, ammonia, antimitochondrial antibody, bilirubin, liver biopsy, ethanol, ferritin, γ-glutamyltransferase, hepatitis antigens and antibodies, iron/total iron-binding capacity, protein, and prothrombin time if liver disease is suspected; and creatine kinase, lactate dehydrogenase, magnesium, and troponin I if myocardial infarction is suspected.

ATRIAL NATRIURETIC FACTOR

SYNONYMS/ACRONYMS: Atrial natriuretic hormone, atrial natriuretic peptide, ANF, ANH.

SPECIMEN: Plasma (1 mL) collected in a chilled, lavender-top tube. Specimen should be transported tightly capped and in an ice slurry.

REFERENCE VALUE: (Method: Radioimmunoassay)

Conventional Units	SI Units (Conversion Factor ×1)
20–77 pg/mL	20–77 ng/L

DESCRIPTION: Atrial natriuretic factor (ANF) is a hormone secreted from cells in the right atrium of the heart when right atrial pressure increases. The release of this cardiac peptide is stimulated by increases in the stretch of the atrial wall caused by an increase in blood pressure or blood volume. ANF receptors are also stimulated by elevated sodium levels. This extremely potent hormone enhances salt and water excretions by blocking aldosterone and renin secretion. ANF inhibits angiotensin II and vasopressin, resulting in vasodilation and a decrease in blood volume and blood pressure. ■

INDICATIONS:
• Assist in the confirmation of congestive heart failure (CHF), as indicated by increased level
• Identify asymptomatic cardiac volume overload, as indicated by increased level

RESULT

Increased in:
• Asymptomatic cardiac volume overload
• CHF
• Elevated cardiac filling pressure
• Paroxysmal atrial tachycardia

Decreased in: N/A

CRITICAL VALUES: N/A

INTERFERING FACTORS:
• Drugs that may increase ANF levels include atenolol, candoxatril, captopril, carteolol, dopamine, morphine, oral contraceptives, vasopressin, and verapamil.

• Drugs that may decrease ANF levels include clonidine, prazosin, and urapidil.

• Recent radioactive scans or radiation within 1 week before the test can interfere with test results when radioimmunoassay is the test method.

Nursing Implications and Procedure · · · · · · · · · · ·

Pretest: ■

➤ Obtain a history of the patient's complaints, including a list of known allergens. Be alert to signs and symptoms of altered cardiopulmonary tissue perfusion related to ventilation-perfusion imbalance, decreased cardiac output related to altered muscle contractility, and fluid-volume excess related to glomerular filtration rate.

➤ Obtain a history of the patient's cardiovascular system and results of previously performed tests and procedures. For related tests, refer to the cardiovascular system table.

➤ Obtain a list of medications the patient is taking, including herbs, nutritional supplements, and nutraceuticals. The requesting health care practitioner and laboratory should be advised if the patient regularly uses these products so that their effects can be taken into consideration when reviewing results.

➤ Instruct the patient to fast for 6 to 12 hours before the test and to avoid taking medications that interfere with test results, as directed by the health care practitioner. *Note:* Drugs such as beta-blocking agents, calcium antagonists, cardiac glycosides, and vasodilators can affect results.

➤ Note any recent procedures that may interfere with test results.

➤ Review the procedure with the patient.

➤ Inform the patient that specimen collection takes approximately 5 to 10 minutes.

➤ Prepare an ice slurry in a cup or plastic bag to have on hand for immediate transport of the specimen to the laboratory.

Intratest:

➤ Ensure that the patient complied with dietary preparation and other pretesting restrictions.

➤ Direct the patient to breathe normally and to avoid unnecessary movement.

➤ Observe standard precautions and follow the general guidelines in Appendix A. Perform a venipuncture,

and collect the specimen in a chilled, 5-mL lavender-top tube.

➤ Label the specimen, and promptly transport it to the laboratory. The tightly capped sample should be placed in an ice slurry immediately after collection. Information on the specimen label can be protected from water in the ice slurry if the specimen is first placed in a protective plastic bag.

Post-test:

➤ Observe venipuncture site for bleeding or hematoma formation. Apply pressure bandage.

➤ Overweight patients with high blood pressure should be encouraged to achieve a normal weight. Other changeable risk factors warranting patient education include strategies to safely decrease sodium intake, increase physical activity, decrease alcohol consumption, eliminate tobacco use, and decrease cholesterol levels.

➤ Evaluate test results in relation to the patient's symptoms and other tests performed. Related laboratory tests include aldosterone, antiarrhythmic drugs, antidiuretic hormone, calcium, electrolytes, and renin.

BACTERIAL CULTURE, ANAL/ GENITAL, EAR, EYE, SKIN, AND WOUND

. . . .

SYNONYM/ACRONYM: N/A.

SPECIMEN: Sterile fluid or swab from affected area placed in transport media tube provided by laboratory.

REFERENCE VALUE: (Method: Culture aerobic and/or anaerobic on selected media; DNA probe assays are available for identification of *Neisseria gonorrhoeae.*) Negative: no growth of pathogens.

DESCRIPTION: When indicated by patient history, anal cultures may be performed to isolate the organism responsible for sexually transmitted disease.

Ear and eye cultures are performed to isolate the organism responsible for chronic or acute infectious disease of the ear and eye.

Skin and soft tissue samples from infected sites must be collected carefully to avoid contamination from the surrounding normal skin flora. Skin and tissue infections may be caused by both aerobic and anaerobic organisms. Therefore, a portion of the sample should be placed in aerobic and anaerobic transport media. Care must be taken to use transport media that is approved by the laboratory performing the testing.

A wound culture involves collecting a specimen of exudates, drainage, or tissue so that the causative organism can be isolated and pathogens identified. Specimens can be obtained from superficial and deep wounds.

Optimally, specimens should be obtained before antibiotic use. The method used to culture and grow the organism depends on the suspected infectious organism. There are transport media specifically for bacterial agents. The laboratory will select the appropriate media for suspect organisms. The laboratory will initiate antibiotic sensitivity testing if indicated by test results. Sensitivity testing identifies the antibiotics to which organisms are susceptible to ensure an effective treatment plan. ∎

INDICATIONS

Anal/genital:

- Assist in the diagnosis of sexually transmitted diseases

- Determine the cause of genital itching or purulent drainage

- Determine effective antimicrobial therapy specific to the identified pathogen

Ear:

- Isolate and identify organisms responsible for ear pain, drainage, or changes in hearing

- Isolate and identify organisms responsible for outer-, middle-, or inner-ear infection

- Determine effective antimicrobial therapy specific to the identified pathogen

Eye:

- Isolate and identify pathogenic microorganisms responsible for infection of the eye

- Determine effective antimicrobial therapy specific to identified pathogen

Skin:

- Isolate and identify organisms responsible for skin eruptions, drainage, or other evidence of infection

- Determine effective antimicrobial therapy specific to the identified pathogen

Sterile fluids:

- Isolate and identify organisms before surrounding tissue becomes infected
- Determine effective antimicrobial therapy specific to the identified pathogen

Wound:

- Detect abscess or deep-wound infectious process
- Determine if an infectious agent is the cause of wound redness, warmth, or edema with drainage at a site
- Determine presence of infectious agents in a stage 3 and stage 4 decubitus ulcer
- Isolate and identify organisms responsible for the presence of pus or other exudate in an open wound
- Determine effective antimicrobial therapy specific to the identified pathogen

RESULT

Positive findings in:

Anal/Endocervical/Genital

Infections or carrier states caused by the following organisms: *Gardnerella vaginalis, N. gonorrhoeae,* toxin-producing strains of *Staphylococcus aureus,* and *Treponema pallidum.*

Ear

Commonly identified organisms include *Escherichia coli, Proteus* spp., *Pseudomonas aeruginosa, Staphylococcus aureus,* and β-hemolytic *Streptococcus.*

Eye

Commonly identified organisms include *Haemophilus influenzae, H. aegyptius, N. gonorrhoeae, Pseudomonas aeruginosa, Staphylococcus aureus,* and *Streptococcus pneumoniae.*

Skin

Commonly identified organisms include *Bacteroides, Clostridium, Corynebacterium, Pseudomonas, Staphylococci,* and group A *Streptococci.*

Sterile fluids

Commonly identified pathogens include *Bacteroides, Enterococcus* spp., *E. coli, Pseudomonas aeruginosa,* and *Peptostreptococcus* spp.

Wound

Aerobic and anaerobic microorganisms can be identified in wound culture specimens. Commonly identified organisms include *Clostridium perfringens, Klebsiella, Proteus, Pseudomonas, Staphylococcus aureus, and group A* Streptococcus.

CRITICAL VALUES: N/A

INTERFERING FACTORS:

- Failure to collect adequate specimen, improper collection or storage technique, and failure to transport specimen in a timely fashion are causes for specimen rejection.
- Pretest antimicrobial therapy will delay or inhibit the growth of pathogens.
- Testing specimens more than 1 hour after collection may result in decreased growth or nongrowth of organisms.

Nursing Implications and Procedure • • • • • • • • • •

Pretest:

➤ Obtain a history of the patient's complaints, including a list of known allergens.

➤ Obtain a history of the patient's immune system and, as appropriate, a history of sexual activity, as well as results of previously performed tests and procedures. For related tests, refer to the immune and reproductive system tables.

➤ Obtain a list of the medications the patient is taking, including herbs, nutritional supplements, and nutraceuticals. The requesting health care practitioner and laboratory should be advised if the patient regularly uses these products so that their effects can be taken into consideration when reviewing results.

➤ Note any recent procedures that can interfere with test results.

➤ There are no food or fluid restrictions unless by medical direction.

➤ Review the procedure with the patient. Sensitivity to cultural and social issues, as well as concern for modesty, is important in providing psychological support.

➤ Instruct female patients not to douche for 24 hours before a cervical or vaginal specimen is to be obtained.

➤ Inform the patient that specimen collection takes approximately 5 to 10 minutes.

Intratest: ■

➤ Direct the patient to breathe normally and to avoid unnecessary movement.

➤ Observe standard precautions and follow the general guidelines in Appendix A.

Anal

➤ Place the patient in a lithotomy or side-lying position and drape for privacy. Insert the swab 1 inch into the anal canal and rotate, move it from side-to-side to allow it to come into contact with the microorganisms. Remove the swab. Place the swab in the Culturette tube, and squeeze the bottom of the tube to release the transport medium. Ensure that the end of the swab is immersed in the medium. Repeat with a clean swab if the swab is pushed into feces.

Genital

Female patient

➤ Position the patient on the gynecologic examination table with the feet up in stirrups. Drape the patient's legs to provide privacy and reduce chilling.

➤ Cleanse the external genitalia and perineum from front to back with towelettes provided in culture kit. Using a Culturette swab, obtain a sample of the lesion or discharge from the urethra or vulva. Place the swab in the Culturette tube, and squeeze the bottom of the tube to release the transport medium. Ensure that the end of the swab is immersed in the medium.

➤ To obtain a vaginal and endocervical culture, insert a water-lubricated vaginal speculum, and apply pressure to the speculum to express exudate from the cervix. Insert the swab into the cervical orifice and rotate the swab to collect the secretions containing the microorganisms. Remove and place in the appropriate culture medium. Material from the vagina can be collected by moving a swab along the sides of the vaginal mucosa. The swab is removed and then placed in a tube of saline medium.

Male patient

➤ To obtain a urethral culture, cleanse the penis (retracting the foreskin), compress to express discharge from the urethra, and insert a swab into the urethral orifice to obtain a sample of the discharge. Place the swab in the Culturette tube, and squeeze the bottom of the tube to release the transport medium. Ensure that the end of the swab is immersed in the medium.

Ear

➤ Cleanse the area surrounding the site with a swab containing cleaning solution to remove any contaminating material or flora that have collected in the ear canal. If needed, remove any cerumen that has collected.

➤ Insert a Culturette swab approximately 1/4 inch into the external ear canal. Rotate the swab in the area containing the exudate. Carefully remove the swab, ensuring that it does not touch the side or opening of the ear canal.

➤ Place the swab in the Culturette tube, and squeeze the bottom of the tube to release the transport medium. Ensure that the end of the swab is immersed in the medium.

Eye

➤ Pass a moistened swab over the appropriate site, avoiding eyelid and eyelashes unless those areas are selected for study. Collect any visible pus or other exudate. Place the swab in the Culturette tube, and squeeze the bottom of the tube to release the transport medium. Ensure that the end of the swab is immersed in the medium.

➤ An appropriate health care practitioner should perform procedures requiring eye scrapings.

Skin

➤ Using a sterile scalpel, scrape the skin from several areas of the affected site. If indicated, select the dark, moist areas of the folds of the skin and outer growing edges of the infection where microorganisms are most likely to flourish. Place the scrapings in a Petri dish or spread on a slide. Aspirate any fluid from a pustule or vesicle using a sterile needle and tuberculin syringe. Flush the exudate into a Petri dish or sterile collection tube. If the lesion is not fluid filled, open the lesion with a scalpel and swab the area with a sterile cotton-tipped swab. Place the swab in the Culturette tube, and squeeze the bottom of the tube to release the transport medium. Ensure that the end of the swab is immersed in the medium.

Sterile fluid

➤ Refer to related body fluid monographs (i.e., amniotic fluid, cerebrospinal fluid, pericardial fluid, peritoneal fluid, pleural fluid, synovial fluid) for specimen collection.

Wound

➤ Place the patient in a comfortable position, and drape the site to be cultured. Cleanse the area around the wound to remove flora indigenous to the skin.

➤ Place a Culturette swab in a superficial wound where the exudate is the most excessive without touching the wound edges. Place the swab in the Culturette tube, and squeeze the bottom of the tube to release the transport medium. Ensure that the end of the swab is immersed in the medium. Use more than one swab and Culturette tube to obtain specimens from other areas of the wound.

➤ To obtain a deep wound specimen, insert a sterile syringe and needle into the wound and aspirate the drainage. Following aspiration, inject the material into a tube containing an anaerobic culture medium.

General

➤ Label the specimen, including specimen source (left or right as appropriate), patient age and gender, date and time of collection, and current antibiotic therapy (if any). Promptly transport the specimen to the laboratory. Do not freeze the specimen or allow it to dry.

Post-test: ■

Anal/endocervical/genital

➤ Inform the patient that final results may take from 24 hours to 4 weeks, depending on the test performed.

➤ Advise the patient to avoid sexual contact until test results are available.

➤ Instruct in vaginal suppository and

douche procedures and administration of topical medication to treat specific conditions, as indicated.

➤ Inform infected patients that all sexual partners must be tested for the microorganism.

➤ Inform the patient that positive culture findings for certain organisms must be reported to a local health department official, who will question him or her regarding sexual partners.

➤ Offer support, as appropriate, to patients who may be the victims of rape or sexual assault. Educate the patient regarding access to counseling services. Provide a nonjudgmental, nonthreatening atmosphere for discussing the risks of sexually transmitted diseases. It is also important to discuss problems the patient may experience (e.g., guilt, depression, anger).

Wound

➤ Instruct in wound care and nutritional requirements (e.g., protein, vitamin C) to promote wound healing.

General

➤ Emphasize the importance of reporting continued signs and symptoms of the infection.

➤ Inform the patient that a repeat culture may be needed in 1 week after completion of the antimicrobial regimen.

➤ Advise the patient that final test results may take 24 to 72 hours depending on the organism suspected, but that antibiotic therapy may be started immediately. Administer antibiotics as ordered, and instruct the patient in the importance of completing the entire course of antibiotic therapy even if no symptoms are present.

➤ Evaluate test results in relation to the patient's symptoms and other tests performed. Related laboratory tests include relevant tissue biopsies and Gram stain.

BACTERIAL CULTURE, BLOOD

SYNONYM/ACRONYM: N/A.

SPECIMEN: Whole blood collected in bottles containing standard aerobic and anaerobic culture media; 10 to 20 mL for adult patients or 1 to 5 mL for pediatric patients.

REFERENCE VALUE: (Method: Growth of organisms in standard culture media identified by radiometric or infrared automation, or by manual reading of subculture.) Negative: no growth of pathogens.

DESCRIPTION: Blood cultures are collected whenever bacteremia or septicemia is suspected. Although mild bacteremia is found in many infectious diseases, a persistent, continuous, or recurrent bacteremia indicates a more serious condition that may require immediate treatment. Early detection of pathogens in the blood may aid in making clinical and etiologic diagnoses.

Blood culture involves the introduction of a specimen of blood into artificial aerobic and anaerobic growth culture medium. The culture is incubated for a specific length of time, at a specific temperature, and under other conditions suitable for the growth of pathogenic microorganisms. Pathogens enter the bloodstream from soft-tissue infection sites, contaminated intravenous lines, or invasive procedures (e.g., surgery, tooth extraction, cystoscopy). A blood culture may also be done with an antimicrobial removal device (ARD). This involves transferring some of the blood sample into a special vial containing absorbent resins that remove antibiotics from the sample before the culture is performed. The laboratory will initiate antibiotic sensitivity testing if indicated by test results. Sensitivity testing identifies the antibiotics to which the organisms are susceptible to ensure an effective treatment plan. ■

INDICATIONS:

- Determine sepsis in the newborn as a result of prolonged labor, early rupture of membranes, maternal infection, or neonatal aspiration

- Evaluate chills and fever in patients with infected burns, urinary tract infections, rapidly progressing tissue infection, postoperative wound sepsis, and indwelling venous or arterial catheter

- Evaluate intermittent or continuous temperature elevation of unknown origin

- Evaluate persistent, intermittent fever associated with a heart murmur

- Evaluate a sudden change in pulse and temperature with or without chills and diaphoresis

- Evaluate suspected bacteremia after invasive procedures

- Identify the cause of shock in the postoperative period

RESULT

Positive findings in:

- Bacteremia or septicemia: *Aerobacter, Bacteroides, Brucella, Clostridium perfringens,* enterococci, *Escherichia coli* and other coliform bacilli, *Haemophilus influenzae, Klebsiella, Listeria monocytogenes, Pseudomonas aeruginosa, Salmonella, Staphylococcus aureus, Staphylococcus epidermidis,* and β-hemolytic *Streptococcus.*

- Plague

- Malaria (by special request, a stained capillary smear would be examined)

- Typhoid fever

Note: *Candida albicans* is a yeast that can cause disease and can be isolated by blood culture.

CRITICAL VALUES: ⚠ Positive findings must be immediately communicated to the primary health care practitioner.

INTERFERING FACTORS:

- Pretest antimicrobial therapy will delay or inhibit growth of pathogens.

• Contamination of the specimen by the skin's resident flora may invalidate interpretation of test results.

• An inadequate amount of blood or number of blood specimens drawn for examination may invalidate interpretation of results.

• Specimens that are tested more than 1 hour after collection may result in decreased growth or nongrowth of organisms.

• Negative findings do not ensure the absence of infection.

Nursing Implications and Procedure • • • • • • • • • • •

Pretest: ■

➤ Obtain a history of the patient's complaints, including a list of known allergens.

➤ Obtain a history of the patient's immune system, as well as results of previously performed tests and procedures. For related tests, refer to the immune system table.

➤ Obtain a list of the medications the patient is taking, including herbs, nutritional supplements and nutraceuticals. The requesting health care practitioner and laboratory should be advised if the patient regularly uses these products so that their effects can be taken into consideration when reviewing results.

➤ There are no food or fluid restrictions unless by medical direction.

➤ Establish whether the patient is sensitive to iodine.

➤ Review the procedure with the patient. Inform the patient that multiple specimens may be required at timed intervals.

➤ Inform the patient that specimen collection takes approximately 5 to 10 minutes.

Intratest: ■

➤ Direct the patient to breathe normally and to avoid unnecessary movement.

➤ Observe standard precautions and follow the general guidelines in Appendix A.

➤ The high risk for infecting a patient by venipuncture can be decreased by using an aseptic technique during specimen collection.

➤ The contamination of blood cultures by skin and other flora can also be dramatically reduced by careful preparation of the puncture site and collection containers before specimen collection. Cleanse the rubber stoppers of the collection containers with the appropriate disinfectant as recommended by the laboratory, allow to air-dry, and cleanse with 70% alcohol. Once the vein has been located by palpation, cleanse the site with 70% alcohol followed by swabbing with an iodine solution. The iodine should be swabbed in a circular concentric motion, moving outward or away from the puncture site. The iodine should be allowed to completely dry before the sample is collected. If the patient is sensitive to iodine, a double alcohol scrub or green soap may be substituted.

➤ If collection is performed by directly drawing the sample into a culture tube, fill the aerobic culture tube first.

➤ If collection is performed using a syringe, transfer the blood sample directly into each culture bottle.

➤ More than three sets of cultures per day do not significantly add to the likelihood of pathogen capture. Capture rates are more likely affected by obtaining a sufficient volume of blood per culture.

➤ The use of ARDs or resin bottles is costly and controversial with respect to their effectiveness versus standard culture techniques. They may be useful in selected cases, such as when septicemia or bacteremia is

Disease Suspected	Recommended Collection
Bacterial pneumonia, fever of unknown origin, meningitis, osteomyelitis, sepsis	2 sets of cultures; each collected from a separate site, 30 minutes apart
Acute or subacute endocarditis	3 sets of cultures; each collected from a separate site, 60 minutes apart. If cultures are negative after 24 to 48 hours, repeat collections
Septicemia, fungal or mycobacterial infection in immunocompromised patient	2 sets of cultures; each collected from a separate site, 30 to 60 minutes apart (laboratory may use a lysis concentration technique to enhance recovery)
Septicemia, bacteremia after therapy has been initiated or request to monitor effectiveness of antimicrobial therapy	2 sets of cultures; each collected from a separate site, 30 to 60 minutes apart (consider use of ARD to enhance recovery)

suspected after antimicrobial therapy has been initiated.

➤ Label the specimen, and promptly transport it to the laboratory.

Post-test:

➤ Cleanse the iodine from the collection site.

➤ Observe the venipuncture site for bleeding or hematoma formation. Apply a pressure bandage.

➤ Instruct the patient to resume usual medication as directed by the health care practitioner.

➤ Instruct the patient in the antimicrobial regimen and in the importance of completing the entire course of antibiotic therapy even if no symptoms are present.

➤ Inform the patient that preliminary results should be available in 24 to 72 hours, but final results are not available for 5 to 7 days.

➤ Instruct the patient to report fever, chills, and other signs and symptoms of acute infection to the health care practitioner.

➤ Evaluate test results in relation to the patient's symptoms and other tests performed. A related laboratory test is the complete blood count.

BACTERIAL CULTURE, SPUTUM

SYNONYM/ACRONYM: Routine culture of sputum.

SPECIMEN: Sputum (10 to 15 mL).

REFERENCE VALUE: (Method: Aerobic culture on selective and enriched media; microscopic examination of sputum by Gram stain.) The presence of normal upper respiratory flora should be expected. Tracheal aspirates and bronchoscopy samples can be contaminated with normal flora, but transtracheal aspiration specimens should show no growth. Normal respiratory flora include *Neisseria catarrhalis, Candida albicans,*diphtheroids, α-hemolytic *Streptococcus,* and some staphylococci. The presence of normal flora does not rule out infection. A normal Gram stain of sputum contains polymorphonuclear leukocytes, alveolar macrophages, and a few squamous epithelial cells.

DESCRIPTION: This test involves collecting a sputum specimen so the pathogen can be isolated and identified. The test results will reflect the type and number of organisms present in the specimen, as well as the antibiotics to which the identified pathogenic organisms are susceptible. Sputum collected by expectoration or suctioning with catheters and by bronchoscopy cannot be cultured for anaerobic organisms; instead transtracheal aspiration or lung biopsy must be used. The laboratory will initiate antibiotic sensitivity testing if indicated by test results. Sensitivity testing identifies antibiotics to which the organisms are susceptible to ensure an effective treatment plan. ■

INDICATIONS:

Culture:

• Assist in the diagnosis of respiratory infections, as indicated by the presence or absence of organisms in culture

Gram Stain:

• Assist in the differentiation of grampositive from gram-negative bacteria in respiratory infection

• Assist in the differentiation of sputum from upper respiratory tract secretions, the latter being indicated by excessive squamous cells or absence of polymorphonuclear leukocytes

RESULT:

• The major difficulty in evaluating results is in distinguishing organisms infecting the lower respiratory tract from organisms that have colonized but not infected the lower respiratory tract. Review of the Gram stain assists in this process. The presence of greater than 25 squamous epithelial cells per low-power field (lpf) indicates oral contamination, and the specimen should be rejected. The presence of many polymorphonuclear neutrophils and few squamous epithelial cells indicates that the specimen was collected from an area of infection and is satisfactory for further analysis.

• Bacterial pneumonia can be caused by *Streptococcus pneumoniae, Haemophilus influenzae,* staphylococci, and some gram-negative bacteria. Other pathogens that can be identified by culture are *Corynebacterium diphtheriae, Klebsiella pneumoniae,* and *Pseudomonas aeruginosa.* Some infectious agents, such as *C. diphtheriae,* are more fastidious in their growth requirements and cannot be cultured and identified without special treatment. Suspicion of infection by less commonly identified and/or fastidious organisms must be communicated to the laboratory to ensure selection of the proper procedure required for identification.

CRITICAL VALUES: N/A

INTERFERING FACTORS:
• Contamination with oral flora may invalidate results.

• Specimen collection after antibiotic therapy has been initiated may result in inhibited or no growth of organisms.

Nursing Implications and Procedure • • • • • • • • • •

Pretest: ■

➤ Obtain a history of the patient's complaints, including a list of known allergens.

➤ Obtain a history of the patient's immune and respiratory system, as well as results of previously performed tests and procedures. For related tests, refer to the immune and respiratory system tables.

➤ Obtain a list of the medications the patient is taking, including herbs, nutritional supplements and nutraceuticals. The requesting health care practitioner and laboratory should be advised if the patient is regularly using these products so their effects can be taken into consideration when reviewing results.

➤ Note any recent procedures that can interfere with test results.

➤ Ensure that the patient has fasted and refrained from consuming liquids since midnight the previous night if bronchoscopy is to be performed.

➤ If the specimen is collected by expectoration or tracheal suctioning, there are no food, fluid, or medication restrictions (except antibiotics) unless by medical direction.

➤ Reassure the patient that he or she will be able to breathe during the procedure if specimen collected is accomplished via suction method. Ensure that oxygen has been administered 20 to 30 minutes before the procedure if the specimen is to be obtained by tracheal suctioning.

➤ Address concerns about pain related to the procedure. Explain that a sedative and/or anesthetic will be administered before the procedure to promote relaxation and reduce discomfort during the procedure, and that general anesthesia will be administered for open biopsy. Atropine is usually given before bronchoscopy examinations to reduce bronchial secretions and prevent vagally induced bradycardia. Meperidine (Demerol) or morphine may be given as a sedative. Lidocaine is sprayed in the patient's throat to reduce discomfort caused by the presence of the tube.

➤ Assess if the patient has an allergy to local anesthetics, and inform the health care practitioner accordingly.

➤ Ensure that the patient is not allergic to anesthesia before bronchoscopy procedure is performed under general anesthesia.

➤ *Obtain written and informed consent before administering any medications prior to the biopsy or bronchoscopy procedure.*

➤ Assist with mouth care (i.e., rinsing mouth with water), if needed, before collection so as not to contaminate the specimen by oral secretions.

➤ Inform the patient that the test helps identify organisms that cause respiratory tract infections. Emphasize that sputum and saliva are not the same.

➤ Assist in providing extra fluids, unless contraindicated, and proper humidification to decrease tenacious secretions. Inform the patient that increasing fluid intake before retiring on the night before the test aids in liquefying secretions and may make it easier to expectorate in the morning. Also explain that humidifying inspired air also helps liquefy secretions.

➤ Instruct the patient to brush the teeth or rinse the mouth before obtaining the specimen, to avoid excessive contamination of the specimen with organisms normally found in the mouth.

➤ Instruct the patient not to touch the edge or inside of the container with the hands or mouth.

➤ Review the procedure with the patient.

➤ The time it takes to collect a proper specimen varies according to the level of patient cooperation and the specimen collection site.

Intratest: ■

➤ Ensure that the patient has complied with dietary restrictions before bronchoscopy.

➤ Observe standard precautions and follow the general guidelines in Appendix A.

Bronchoscopy:

➤ Record baseline vital signs. The patient is positioned in relation to the type of anesthesia being used. For general anesthesia the patient is placed in a supine position with the neck hyperextended. If local anesthesia is used, the patient is seated and the tongue and oropharynx are sprayed and swabbed with anesthetic. The patient is then helped to a supine or side-lying position and the bronchoscope is inserted. After inspection, the samples are collected from suspicious sites by bronchial brush or biopsy forceps.

Expectorated specimen:

➤ Request the patient to sit upright, with assistance and support (such as with an overbed table) as needed. Ask the patient to take two or three deep breaths and to cough deeply. Any sputum raised should be expectorated directly into a sterile sputum collection container. If the patient is unable to produce the desired amount of sputum, several strategies may be attempted. One approach is to have the patient drink two glasses of water and then assume the positions for postural drainage of the upper and middle lung segments. Support for effective coughing may be provided by placement of the hands or a pillow over

the diaphragmatic area and application of slight pressure. Another approach is to place a vaporizer or other humidifying device at the bedside. After sufficient exposure to adequate humidification, postural drainage of the upper and middle lung segments may be repeated before attempting to obtain the specimen. Other methods may include obtaining an order for an expectorant and administering it along with additional water approximately 2 hours before attempting to obtain the specimen. In addition, chest percussion and postural drainage of all lung segments may be employed. If the patient is still unable to raise sputum, the use of an ultrasonic nebulizer ("induced sputum") may be necessary and is usually performed by a respiratory therapist.

Tracheal suctioning:

➤ Obtain the necessary equipment, including a suction device, a suction kit, and a Lukens tube or in-line trap. Position the patient with head elevated as high as tolerated. Put on sterile gloves, with the dominant hand maintained as sterile and the nondominant hand as clean. Using the sterile hand, attach the suction catheter to the rubber tubing of the Lukens tube or in-line trap. Then attach the suction tubing to the male adapter of the trap with the clean hand. Lubricate the suction catheter with sterile saline. Tell nonintubated patients to protrude the tongue and take a deep breath as the suction catheter is passed through the nostril. When the catheter enters the trachea, a reflex cough will be stimulated; immediately advance the catheter into the trachea and apply suction. Maintain suction for approximately 10 seconds and never for longer than 15 seconds. Then withdraw the catheter without applying suction. Separate the suction catheter and suction tubing from the trap, and place the rubber tubing over the male adapter to seal the unit. For intubated patients or those with a tracheostomy, the previous procedure is followed except that the suction catheter is passed through the existing endotracheal or tracheostomy tube rather than through the nostril. The patient should be hyperoxygenated before and after the procedure in accordance with usual protocols for suctioning these patients.

➤ Provide sterile sputum collection containers. Label the specimen, and promptly transport it to the laboratory. It is advisable to note antimicrobial therapy on the collection container.

Post-test:

➤ Monitor vital signs and compare with baseline values.

➤ Note the color, consistency, and volume of the specimen collected.

➤ Instruct the patient to resume usual diet and medication as directed by the health care practitioner.

➤ If bronchoscopy has been performed, inform the patient to drink liquids or eat food only after the gag reflex returns.

➤ Instruct the patient to perform mouth care after the specimen has been obtained.

➤ Provide comfort measures and treatment as needed, such as antiseptic gargles, inhalants, and warm moist applications. A cool beverage may aid in relieving throat irritation caused by coughing or suctioning.

➤ Instruct the patient to notify someone immediately if difficulty in breathing or swallowing or if bleeding occurs.

➤ Observe the patient's color and respiratory rate. Administer oxygen, as necessary.

➤ Administer analgesics and antibiotics as ordered and instruct the patient in the importance of completing the entire course of antibiotic therapy even if no symptoms are present.

➤ Evaluate test results in relation to the patient's symptoms and other tests performed. Related laboratory tests include acid-fast culture and smear, arterial/alveolar oxygen ratio, lung biopsy, blood gases, complete blood count, and Gram stain.

BACTERIAL CULTURE, STOOL

SYNONYM/ACRONYM: N/A.

SPECIMEN: Fresh random stool collected in a clean plastic container.

REFERENCE VALUE: (Method: Culture on selective media for identification of pathogens usually to include *Salmonella, Shigella, Escherichia coli* O157:H7, *Yersinia enterocolitica,* and *Campylobacter*; latex agglutination or enzyme immunoassay for *Clostridium* A and B toxins) Negative: No growth of pathogens. Normal fecal flora is 96 to 99 percent anaerobes and 1 to 4 percent aerobes. Normal flora present may include *Bacteroides, Candida albicans, Clostridium, Enterococcus, E. coli, Proteus, Pseudomonas,* and *Staphylococcus aureus.*

DESCRIPTION: Stool culture involves collecting a sample of feces so that organisms present can be isolated and identified. Certain bacteria are normally found in feces. However, when overgrowth of these organisms occurs or pathologic organisms are present, diarrhea or other signs and symptoms of systemic infection occur. These symptoms are the result of damage to the intestinal tissue by the pathogenic organisms. Routine stool culture normally screens for a small number of common pathogens, such as *Campylobacter, Salmonella,* and *Shigella.* Identification of other bacteria is initiated by special request or upon consultation with a microbiologist when there is knowledge of special circumstances. The laboratory will initiate antibiotic sensitivity testing if indicated by test results. Sensitivity testing identifies the antibiotics to which organisms are susceptible to ensure an effective treatment plan. ■

INDICATIONS:
• Assist in establishing a diagnosis for diarrhea of unknown etiology

• Identify pathogenic organisms causing gastrointestinal disease and carrier states

RESULT

Positive findings in:
• Bacterial infection: *Aeromonas* spp., *Bacillus cereus, Campylobacter, Clostridium, E. coli* including serotype O157:H7, *Plesiomonas shigelloides, Salmonella, Shigella, Yersinia,* and *Vibrio.* Isolation of *Staphylococcus aureus* may indicate infection or a carrier state.

• Botulism: *Clostridium botulinum* (the bacteria must also be isolated from the food or the presence of toxin confirmed in the stool specimen).

CRITICAL VALUES: N/A

INTERFERING FACTORS:
• A rectal swab does not provide an adequate amount of specimen for evaluating the carrier state and should be avoided in favor of a standard stool specimen.

• A rectal swab should never be submitted for *Clostridium* toxin studies. Specimens for *Clostridium* toxins should be refrigerated if they are not immediately transported to the laboratory as toxins degrade rapidly.

• A rectal swab should never be submitted for *Campylobacter* culture. Excessive exposure of the sample to air or room temperature may damage this type of bacteria so that they will not grow in the culture.

• Therapy with antibiotics before specimen collection may decrease the type and the amount of bacteria.

• Failure to transport the culture within 1 hour of collection or urine contamination of the sample may affect results.

• Barium and laxatives used less than 1 week before the test may reduce bacterial growth.

Nursing Implications and Procedure • • • • • • • • • •

Pretest: ■

➤ Obtain a history of the patient's complaints, including a list of known allergens.

➤ Obtain a history of the patient's travel to foreign countries.

➤ Obtain a history of the patient's gastrointestinal and immune systems, recent dietary history, and results of previously performed tests and procedures. For related tests, refer to the gastrointestinal and immune system tables.

➤ Obtain a list of the medications the patient is taking (especially antibiotics), including herbs, nutritional supplements, and nutraceuticals. The requesting health care practitioner and laboratory should be advised if the patient regularly uses these products so that their effects can be taken into consideration when reviewing results.

➤ Note any recent procedures that can interfere with test results. Hold antibiotics, by medical direction, until after specimen has been collected.

➤ There are no food or fluid restrictions unless by medical direction.

➤ Review the procedure with the patient.

Intratest:

➤ Observe standard precautions and follow the general guidelines in Appendix A.

➤ Collect a stool specimen directly into a clean container. If the patient requires a bedpan, make sure it is clean and dry and use a tongue blade to transfer the specimen to the container. Make sure representative portions of the stool are sent for analysis.

➤ If collecting the specimen by rectal swab, insert swab past the patient's anal sphincter. Rotate the swab, allowing 15 to 30 seconds for the specimen to absorb on the swab, withdraw it, and place in media container provided by the laboratory.

➤ Label the specimen, note any antibiotics the patient may be taking and the appearance of the specimen on the label, and promptly transport the specimen to the laboratory.

Post-test:

➤ Instruct the patient to resume usual medication as directed by the health care practitioner.

➤ Advise the patient that final test results may take up to 72 hours but that antibiotic therapy may be started immediately. Instruct the patient about the importance of completing the entire course of antibiotic therapy even if no symptoms are present. *Note*: antibiotic therapy is frequently contraindicated for *Salmonella* infection unless the infection has progressed to a systemic state.

➤ Evaluate test results in relation to the patient's symptoms and other tests performed. Related laboratory tests include fecal analysis, and ova and parasites.

BACTERIAL CULTURE, THROAT OR NASAL PHARYNGEAL

• •

SYNONYM/ACRONYM: Routine throat culture.

SPECIMEN: Throat or nasal pharyngeal swab.

REFERENCE VALUE: (Method: Aerobic culture) No growth.

DESCRIPTION: The routine throat culture is a commonly ordered test to screen for the presence of Group A β-hemolytic *Streptococci*. *S. pyogenes* is the organism that most commonly causes acute pharyngitis. The more dangerous sequelae of scarlet fever, rheumatic heart disease, and glomerulonephritis are less frequently seen because of the early treatment of infection at the pharyngitis stage. There are a number of other bacterial agents responsible for pharyngitis. Specific cultures can be set up to detect other pathogens such as *Bordetella, Corynebacteria, Haemophilus,* or *Neisseria* if they are suspected or by special request from the health care practitioner. *Corynebacterium diphtheriae* is the causative agent of diphtheria. *Neisseria gonorrhoeae* is a sexually transmitted pathogen. In children, a positive throat culture for *Neisseria* usually indicates sexual abuse. The laboratory will initiate antibiotic sensitivity testing if indicated by test results. Sensitivity testing identifies the antibiotics to which the organisms are susceptible to ensure an effective treatment plan. ■

INDICATIONS:

• Assist in the diagnosis of bacterial infections such as tonsillitis, diphtheria, gonorrhea, or pertussis

• Assist in the diagnosis of upper respiratory infections resulting in bronchitis, pharyngitis, croup, and influenza

• Isolate and identify Group A β-hemolytic *Streptococci* as the cause of strep throat, acute glomerulonephritis, scarlet fever, or rheumatic fever

RESULT: Reports on cultures that are positive for Group A β-hemolytic

Streptococci are generally available within 24 to 48 hours. Cultures that report of normal respiratory flora are issued after 48 hours. Culture results of no growth for *Corynebacterium* require 72 hours to report; 48 hours are required to report negative *Neisseria* cultures.

CRITICAL VALUES: N/A

INTERFERING FACTORS:

• Contamination with oral flora may invalidate results.

• Specimen collection after antibiotic therapy has been initiated may result in inhibited or nongrowth of organisms.

Nursing Implications and Procedure . . . .

Pretest:

➤ Obtain a history of the patient's complaints, including a list of known allergens.

➤ Obtain a history of the patient's immune and respiratory system, as well as results of previously performed tests and procedures. For related tests, refer to the immune and respiratory system tables.

➤ Obtain a list of the medications the patient is taking, including herbs, nutritional supplements, and nutraceuticals. The requesting health care practitioner and laboratory should be advised if the patient regularly uses these products so that their effects can be taken into consideration when reviewing results.

➤ Note any recent therapies or procedures that can interfere with test results.

➤ There are no food, fluid, or medication restrictions (except antibiotics) unless by medical direction.

➤ Review the procedure with the patient. In cases of acute epiglottitis, do not swab the throat unless you are equipped to establish an alternative airway if needed.

➤ The time it takes to collect a proper specimen varies according to the level of cooperation of the patient.

Intratest:

➤ Observe standard precautions and follow the general guidelines in Appendix A.

➤ To collect the throat culture, tilt the patient's head back. Swab both tonsillar pillars and oropharynx with the sterile Culturette. A tongue depressor can be used to ensure that contact with the tongue and uvula is avoided.

➤ A nasopharyngeal specimen is collected through the use of a flexible probe inserted through the nose and directed toward the back of the throat.

➤ Place the swab in the Culturette tube and squeeze the bottom of the Culturette tube to release the liquid transport medium. Ensure that the end of the swab is immersed in the liquid transport medium.

➤ Label the collection container and include the specimen site. It is advisable to note antimicrobial therapy on the collection container. Promptly transport the specimen to the laboratory.

Post-test:

➤ Instruct the patient to resume usual medication as directed by the health care practitioner.

➤ Instruct the patient to perform mouth care after the specimen has been obtained.

➤ Provide comfort measures and treatment such as antiseptic gargles, inhalants, and warm moist applications as needed. A cool beverage may aid in relieving throat irritation caused by coughing or suctioning.

➤ Instruct the patient to notify someone immediately if difficulty in breathing or swallowing or if bleeding occurs.

➤ Administer analgesics and antibiotics as ordered and instruct the patient in the importance of completing the entire course of antibiotic therapy even if no symptoms are present.

➤ Evaluate test results in relation to the patient's symptoms and other tests performed. Related laboratory tests include complete blood count and group A streptococcal screen.

BACTERIAL CULTURE, URINE

SYNONYM/ACRONYM: N/A.

SPECIMEN: Urine (5 mL) collected in a sterile plastic collection container.

REFERENCE VALUE: (Method: Culture on selective and enriched media)
Negative: no growth.

DESCRIPTION: A urine culture involves collecting a urine specimen so that the organism causing disease can be isolated and identified. Urine can be collected by clean catch, urinary catheterization, or suprapubic aspiration. The severity of the infection or contamination of the specimen can be determined by knowing the type and number of organisms (colonies) present in the specimen. The laboratory will initiate sensitivity testing if indicated by test results. Sensitivity testing identifies the antibiotics to which the organisms are susceptible to ensure an effective treatment plan.

Commonly detected organisms are those normally found in the genitourinary tract, including enterococci, *Escherichia coli, Klebsiella, Proteus,* and *Pseudomonas.* A culture showing multiple organisms indicates a contaminated specimen.

Colony counts of 100,000/mL or more indicate urinary tract infection (UTI).

Colony counts of 1000/mL or less suggest contamination resulting from poor collection technique.

Colony counts between 1000 and 10,000/mL may be significant depending on a variety of factors including patient's age, gender, number of types of organisms present, method of specimen collection, and presence of antibiotics. ∎

INDICATIONS:

• Assist in the diagnosis of suspected UTI

• Determine the sensitivity of significant organisms to antibiotics

• Monitor the response to UTI treatment

RESULT

Positive findings in:

• UTIs

Negative findings in:

• N/A

CRITICAL VALUES: N/A

INTERFERING FACTORS:

• Antibiotic therapy initiated before specimen collection may produce false-negative results.

• Improper collection techniques may result in specimen contamination.

• Specimen storage for longer than 30 minutes at room temperature or 24 hours at refrigerated temperature may result in overgrowth of bacteria and false-positive results.

• Results of urine culture are often interpreted along with routine urinalysis findings.

• Discrepancies between culture and urinalysis may be reason to recollect the specimen.

Nursing Implications and Procedure • • • • • • • • • •

Pretest: ∎

➤ Obtain a history of the patient's complaints, including a list of known allergens.

➤ Obtain a history of the patient's genitourinary and immune systems, as well as results of previously performed tests and procedures. For related tests, refer to the genitourinary and immune system tables.

➤ Obtain a list of the medications the patient is taking, including herbs, nutritional supplements, and nutraceuticals. The requesting health care practitioner and laboratory should be advised if the patient regularly uses these products so that their effects can be taken into consideration when reviewing results.

➤ Hold antibiotics, by medical direction, until after specimen has been collected.

➤ There are no food or fluid restrictions unless by medical direction.

➤ Review the procedure with the patient. Instruct the patient on clean-catch procedure and provide necessary supplies.

➤ Inform the patient that specimen collection depends on patient cooperation and usually takes approximately 5 to 10 minutes.

Intratest: ■

➤ Observe standard precautions and follow the general guidelines in Appendix A.

Clean-catch specimen:

➤ Instruct the male patient to (1) thoroughly wash his hands, (2) cleanse the meatus, (3) void a small amount into the toilet, and (4) void directly into the specimen container.

➤ Instruct the female patient to (1) thoroughly wash her hands; (2) cleanse the labia from front to back; (3) while keeping the labia separated, void a small amount into the toilet; and (4) without interrupting the urine stream, void directly into the specimen container.

Pediatric urine collector:

➤ Appropriately cleanse the genital area and allow the area to dry. Remove the covering over the adhesive strips on the collector bag and apply over the genital area. Diaper the child. When specimen is obtained, place the entire collection bag in a sterile urine container.

Indwelling catheter:

➤ Empty drainage tube of urine. It may be necessary to clamp off the catheter for 15 to 30 minutes before specimen collection. Cleanse specimen port with antiseptic swab, and then aspirate 5 mL of urine with a 21- to 25-gauge needle and syringe. Transfer urine to a sterile container.

Urinary catheterization:

➤ Place female patient in lithotomy position or male patient in supine position. Using sterile technique, open the straight urinary catheterization kit and perform urinary catheterization. Place the retained urine in a sterile specimen container.

Suprapubic aspiration:

➤ Place the patient in a supine position. Cleanse the area with antiseptic and drape with sterile drapes. Using sterile technique, insert needle and remove sterile sample. Place the returned sample in a sterile specimen container. Place a dry, sterile dressing over the site.

➤ Do not collect urine from the pouch from the patient with a urinary diversion (e.g., ileal conduit). Instead, perform catheterization through the stoma.

General:

➤ Label the specimen, and promptly transport it to the laboratory. Indicate on the label the date and time of collection, method of specimen collection, and any medications the patient has taken that may interfere with test results.

Post-test: ■

➤ Instruct the patient to resume usual medication as directed by the health care practitioner.

➤ Instruct the patient to report symptoms such as pain related to tissue inflammation, pain or irritation during void, bladder spasms, or alterations in urinary elimination.

> Observe for signs of inflammation if the specimen is obtained by suprapubic aspiration.

> Instruct patient to begin antibiotic therapy, as prescribed and instruct the patient in the importance of completing the entire course of antibiotic therapy even if no symptoms are present.

> Instruct patient on the proper technique for wiping the perineal area (front to back) after a bowel movement.

> UTIs are more common in women who use diaphragm–spermicide contraception. These patients can be educated, as appropriate, in the proper insertion and removal of the contraceptive device to avoid recurrent UTI.

> Evaluate test results in relation to the patient's symptoms and other tests performed. Related laboratory tests include Gram stain, urinalysis, and white blood cell count.

BARIUM ENEMA

· ·

SYNONYMS/ACRONYMS: Air-contrast barium enema, double-contrast barium enema, lower GI series, BE.

AREA OF APPLICATION: Colon.

CONTRAST: Barium sulfate, air, iodine mixture.

DESCRIPTION: This radiologic examination of the colon, distal small bowel, and occasionally the appendix follows installation of barium using a rectal tube inserted into the rectum or an existing ostomy. The patient must retain the barium while a series of radiographs are obtained. Visualization can be improved by using air or barium as the contrast medium (double-contrast study). A combination of x-ray and fluoroscopy techniques is used to complete the study. This test is especially useful in the evaluation of patients experiencing lower abdominal pain, changes in bowel habits, or the passage of stools containing blood or mucus, and for visualizing polyps, diverticula, and tumors. A barium enema may be therapeutic; it may reduce an obstruction caused by intussusception, or telescoping of the intestine. Barium enema should be performed before an upper gastrointestinal study or barium swallow. ■

INDICATIONS:

• Determine the cause of rectal bleeding, blood, pus, or mucus in feces

• Evaluate unexplained weight loss, anemia, or a change in bowel pattern

• Identify and locate benign or malignant polyps or tumors

- Evaluate suspected inflammatory process, congenital anomaly, motility disorder, or structural change

RESULT:

Normal Findings:

- Normal size, filling, shape, position, and motility of the colon

- Normal filling of the appendix and terminal ileum

Abnormal Findings:

- Appendicitis
- Colorectal cancer
- Congenital anomalies
- Crohn's disease
- Diverticular disease
- Fistulas
- Gastroenteritis
- Granulomatous colitis
- Hirschsprung's disease
- Intussusception
- Perforation of the colon
- Polyps
- Sarcoma
- Sigmoid torsion
- Sigmoid volvulus
- Stenosis
- Tumors
- Ulcerative colitis

INTERFERING FACTORS:

This procedure is contraindicated for:

- Patients that are pregnant or suspected of being pregnant, unless the potential benefits of the procedure far outweigh the risks to the fetus and mother.

- Patients with intestinal obstruction, acute ulcerative colitis, acute diverticulitis, megacolon, or suspected rupture of the colon.

Factors that may impair clear imaging:

- Inability of the patient to cooperate or remain still during the procedure because of age, significant pain, or mental status

- Metallic objects within the examination field (e.g., jewelry or body rings), which may inhibit organ visualization and can produce unclear images

- Improper adjustment of the radiographic equipment to accommodate obese or thin patients, causing overexposure or underexposure and poorquality study

- Inability of the patient to tolerate introduction of or retention of barium, air, or both in the bowel

- Gas or feces in the gastrointestinal tract resulting from inadequate cleansing or failure to restrict food intake before the study

- Retained barium from a previous radiological procedure

- Spasm of the colon, which can mimic the radiographic signs of cancer (*note*: the use of IV glucagon minimizes spasm)

- Patients who are very obese, who may exceed the weight limit for the equipment

- Incorrect positioning of the patient, which may produce poor visualization of the area to be examined

Other considerations:

- Ensure that this procedure is performed before an upper gastrointestinal study or barium swallow.

- Ensure that the patient followed dietary restrictions before the procedure; failure to do so may cause the procedure to be canceled or repeated.

• Consultation with a physician should occur before the procedure for radiation safety concerns regarding infants of patients who are lactating.

• Risks associated with radiographic overexposure can result from frequent x-ray procedures. Personnel in the room with the patient should wear a protective lead apron, stand behind a shield, or leave the area while the examination is being done. Badges that reveal the level of exposure to radiation should be worn by persons working in the area where the examination is being done.

• Possible complications of barium enema include perforation of the colon, water intoxication, barium granulomas, and rarely, intraperitoneal and extraperitoneal extravasation of barium and barium embolism.

Nursing Implications and Procedure • • • • • • • • • •

Pretest:

➤ Inform the patient about the purpose of the procedure, and the need to have contrast medium instilled into the rectum. The procedure is not painful, but the patient may experience cramping, abdominal fullness, or an urge to defecate.

➤ Obtain a history of the patient's complaints and a list of any medications the patient is taking.

➤ Obtain a history of the patient's lower gastrointestinal system and the results of previously performed tests, surgery, therapy, and procedures. For related tests, refer to the gastrointestinal system table.

➤ Determine patient's allergies, including barium and latex.

➤ Assess for iodine allergy, including allergies to shellfish, if iodinated contrast medium is to be used.

➤ The 30- to 60-minute procedure is done by a physician and/or technologist.

➤ Instruct the patient to eat a low-residue diet for several days before the procedure, to consume only clear liquids the evening before the test, and to withhold food and fluids for 8 hours before the test.

➤ Inform the patient that a laxative and cleansing enema may be needed the day before the procedure, with cleansing enemas on the morning of the procedure, depending on the institution's policy.

➤ Determine date of last menstrual period and possibility of pregnancy in perimenopausal women.

➤ Instruct patients with a colostomy to follow the same dietary preparation, take laxatives the evening before, and perform colostomy irrigation before the study.

➤ Assess for completion of bowel preparation according to the institution's procedure.

Intratest:

➤ Remove clothing and metallic objects from the pelvic area.

➤ Provide patient with a gown with tie closures and a robe to wear.

➤ If appropriate, remove any wires connected to electrodes.

➤ Place the patient on the x-ray table in a supine position or have the patient stand in front of an x-ray fluoroscopy screen.

➤ An initial image is taken. The patient is helped to a side-lying position (Sims' position). A rectal tube is inserted into the anus while an attached balloon is inflated after it is situated against the anal sphincter.

➤ Barium is instilled into the colon and then the movement is observed through the colon by fluoroscopy.

➤ Images are taken at different angles and positions to aid in the evaluation of the patient's problem.

➤ For patients with a colostomy, an indwelling urinary catheter is inserted into the stoma and barium is administered.

➤ The patient is returned to a position of comfort, and is placed on a bedpan or helped to the bathroom to expel the barium.

➤ After the expulsion of the barium, an additional film is taken of the intestine.

➤ If a double-contrast barium enema has been ordered, air is then instilled in the intestine and additional films are taken.

Post-test:

➤ Instruct the patient to resume food, fluids, and medications withheld before the procedure.

➤ Inform the patient of the possible need for further examinations to evaluate and determine the need for a change in therapy or progression of the disease process.

➤ If iodine is used, monitor for reaction to iodinated contrast medium including rash, urticaria, tachycardia, hyperpnea, hypertension, or palpitations.

➤ Instruct the patient to take a mild laxative and increase fluid intake (four glasses) to aid in elimination of barium, unless contraindicated.

➤ Instruct the patient that stools will be white or light in color for 2 to 3 days. If the patient is unable to eliminate the barium, or if stools do not return to normal color, the patient should notify the physician.

➤ Advise patients with a colostomy to administer tap water colostomy irrigation to aid in barium removal.

➤ Carefully monitor the patient for fatigue and fluid and electrolyte imbalance.

➤ Determine if the patient or patient's family has any further questions or concerns.

➤ A physician specializing in this branch of medicine will send a report to the ordering health care provider who will discuss the results with the patient.

➤ Evaluate test results in relation to the patient's symptoms and other tests performed. Related diagnostic tests include colonoscopy, as well as computed tomography and magnetic resonance imaging of the abdomen.

BARIUM SWALLOW

SYNONYMS/ACRONYM: Esophagram, video swallow, esophagus x-ray, swallowing function, esophagography.

AREA OF APPLICATION: Esophagus.

CONTRAST: Barium sulfate, water-soluble iodinated contrast.

DESCRIPTION: This radiologic examination of the esophagus evaluates motion and anatomic structures of the esophageal lumen by recording images of the lumen while the patient swallows a barium solution of milkshake consistency and chalky taste. The procedure uses fluoroscopic and cineradiographic techniques. The barium swallow is often performed as part of an upper gastrointestinal series or cardiac series and is indicated for patients with a history of dysphagia and regurgitation. In patients with esophageal reflux, the radiologist may identify reflux of the barium from the stomach back into the esophagus. Muscular abnormalities such as achalasia, as well as diffuse esophageal spasm, can be easily detected with this procedure. ▪

INDICATIONS:
- Determine the cause of dysphagia, heartburn, or regurgitation

- Evaluate suspected esophageal motility disorders

- Detect esophageal reflux, tracheoesophageal fistulas, and varices

- Evaluate suspected polyps, strictures, Zenker's diverticula, tumor, or inflammation

- Determine the type and location of foreign bodies within the pharynx and esophagus

- Confirm the integrity of esophageal anastomoses in the postoperative patient

RESULT

Normal Findings:
- Normal peristalsis through the esophagus into the stomach with normal size, filling, patency, and shape of the esophagus

Abnormal Findings:
- Acute or chronic esophagitis

- Achalasia

- Benign or malignant tumors

- Chalasia

- Diverticula

- Esophageal ulcers

- Esophageal varices

- Hiatal hernia

- Perforation of the esophagus

- Strictures or polyps

INTERFERING FACTORS:

This procedure is contraindicated for:
- Patients who are pregnant or suspected of being pregnant, unless the potential benefits of the procedure far outweigh the risks to the fetus and mother

- Patients with intestinal obstruction or suspected esophageal rupture, unless water-soluble iodinated contrast medium is used

- Patients with suspected tracheoesophageal fistula, unless barium is used

Factors that may impair clear imaging:

- Inability of the patient to cooperate or remain still during the procedure because of age, significant pain, or mental status

- Metallic objects within the examination field (e.g., jewelry, earrings, and/or dental amalgams), which may inhibit organ visualization and can produce unclear images

- Improper adjustment of the radiographic equipment to accommodate obese or thin patients, which can cause overexposure or underexposure and poor-quality study

• Patients who are very obese, who may exceed the weight limit for the equipment

• Incorrect positioning of the patient, which may produce poor visualization of the area to be examined

Other considerations:

• A potential complication of a barium swallow is barium-induced fecal impaction.

• Ensure that the procedure is done after cholangiography and barium enema.

• Consultation with a physician should occur before the procedure for radiation safety concerns regarding infants of patients who are lactating.

• Risks associated with radiographic overexposure can result from frequent x-ray procedures. Personnel in the room with the patient should wear a protective lead apron, stand behind a shield, or leave the area while the examination is being done. Badges that reveal the level of exposure to radiation should be worn by persons working in the area where the examination is being done.

Nursing Implications and Procedure

Pretest:

➤ Inform the patient about the purpose of the procedure and the need to swallow contrast medium.

➤ Obtain a history of the patient's complaints and a list of medications taken.

➤ Obtain a history of the patient's esophageal and gastrointestinal systems, as well as the results of previously performed tests, surgeries, therapies, and procedures. For re-

lated tests, refer to the gastrointestinal system table.

➤ A physician and/or technologist performs the procedure, which lasts 15 to 30 minutes.

➤ Instruct the patient to withhold food and fluids for 8 hours before the test.

➤ No pain is associated with the study.

➤ Determine date of last menstrual period and possibility of pregnancy in perimenopausal women.

Intratest:

➤ Remove any clothing and metallic objects from the esophageal area.

➤ Give the patient a gown and robe to wear.

➤ Remove any wires connected to electrodes, if allowed.

➤ Place the patient on the x-ray table in a supine position or have the patient stand in front of an x-ray fluoroscopy screen.

➤ An initial image is taken and the patient is stood in front of a fluoroscopy screen and is asked to swallow a barium solution with or without a straw.

➤ Images are taken at different angles and positions to aid in the evaluation of patient's problem.

➤ The patient may be asked to drink additional barium to complete the study. Swallowing the additional barium evaluates the passage of barium from the esophagus into the stomach.

➤ Return the patient to a comfortable position; help the patient from the x-ray table to a chair or stretcher.

Post-test:

➤ Instruct the patient to resume food, fluids, and medications withheld before the procedure.

➤ Inform the patient of the possible need for further examinations to evaluate and determine the need for a change in therapy or progression of the disease process.

➤ Unless contraindicated, instruct the patient to take a mild laxative and increase fluid intake (four glasses) to aid in elimination of barium.

➤ Instruct the patient that stools will be white or light in color for 2 to 3 days. If the patient is unable to eliminate the barium, or if stools do not return to normal color, the patient should notify the physician.

➤ Determine if the patient or family members have any further questions or concerns.

➤ A physician specializing in this branch of medicine will send a report to the ordering health care provider, who will discuss the results with the patient.

➤ Evaluate test results in relation to the patient's symptoms and other tests performed. Related diagnostic tests include endoscopy, computed tomography and magnetic resonance imaging of the neck, and thyroid scan.

BILIRUBIN AND BILIRUBIN FRACTIONS

SYNONYMS/ACRONYM: Conjugated/direct bilirubin, unconjugated/indirect bilirubin, delta bilirubin, TBil.

SPECIMEN: Serum (1 mL) collected in a red- or tiger-top tube. Plasma (1 mL) collected in green-top (heparin) tube or in a heparinized microtainer is also acceptable.

REFERENCE VALUE: (Method: Spectrophotometry) Total bilirubin levels in infants should decrease to adult levels by day 10 as the development of the hepatic circulatory system matures. Values in breastfed infants may take longer to reach normal adult levels. Values in premature infants may initially be higher than in full-term infants and also take longer to decrease to normal levels.

Bilirubin	Conventional Units	SI Units (Conversion Factor ×17.1)
Total bilirubin		
Newborn–1 d	1.4–8.7 mg/dL	24–149 μmol/L
1–2 d	3.4–11.5 mg/dL	58–97 μmol/L
3–5 d	1.5–12.0 mg/dL	26–205 μmol/L
1 mo–adult	0.3–1.2 mg/dL	5–21 μmol/L
Unconjugated bilirubin	Less than 1.1 mg/dL	Less than 19 μmol/L
Conjugated bilirubin	Less than 0.3 mg/dL	Less than 5 μmol/L
Delta bilirubin	Less than 0.2 mg/dL	Less than 3 μmol/L

DESCRIPTION: Bilirubin is a byproduct of heme catabolism from aged red blood cells. Bilirubin is primarily produced in the liver, spleen, and bone marrow. Total bilirubin is the sum of unconjugated bilirubin, monoglucuronide and diglucuronide, conjugated bilirubin, and albumin-bound delta bilirubin. Unconjugated bilirubin is carried to the liver by albumin, where it becomes conjugated. In the small intestine, conjugated bilirubin converts to urobilinogen and then to urobilin. Urobilin is then excreted in the feces. Increases in bilirubin levels can result from prehepatic and/or posthepatic conditions, making fractionation useful in determining the cause of the increase in total bilirubin levels. Delta bilirubin has a longer half-life than the other bilirubin fractions and therefore remains elevated during convalescence after the other fractions have decreased to normal levels. When bilirubin concentration increases the yellowish pigment deposits in skin and sclera. This increase in yellow pigmentation is termed *jaundice* or *icterus*. ∎

INDICATIONS:
- Assist in the differential diagnosis of obstructive jaundice

- Assist in the evaluation of liver and biliary disease

- Monitor the effects of drug reactions on liver function

- Monitor jaundice in newborn patients

- Monitor the effects of phototherapy on jaundiced newborns

RESULT

Increased in:
- Prehepatic (hemolytic) jaundice

Erythroblastosis fetalis
The post–blood transfusion period, when a number of units are rapidly infused or in the case of a delayed transfusion reaction
Hematoma
Hemolytic anemias
Pernicious anemia
Physiologic jaundice of the newborn
Red blood cell enzyme abnormalities (i.e., G-6-PD, pyruvate kinase, spherocytosis)

- Hepatic jaundice—bilirubin conjugation failure
Crigler-Najjar syndrome

- Hepatic jaundice—disturbance in bilirubin transport
Dubin-Johnson syndrome (preconjugation transport failure)
Gilbert's disease (postconjugation transport failure)

- Hepatic jaundice—liver damage or necrosis
Alcoholism
Cholangitis
Cholestatic drug reactions
Cholecystitis
Cirrhosis
Hepatitis
Hepatocellular damage
Infectious mononucleosis

- Posthepatic jaundice
Advanced tumors of the liver
Biliary obstruction

- Other conditions
Anorexia or starvation
Breast milk jaundice
Hypothyroidism

Decreased in: N/A

CRITICAL VALUES: ⚠ Sustained hyperbilirubinemia can result in brain damage. *Kernicterus* refers to the deposition of bilirubin in the basal ganglia and brainstem nuclei. There is no exact level of bilirubin that puts infants at risk for developing kernicterus. Symptoms of kernicterus in infants include lethargy, poor feeding, upward deviation of the eyes, and seizures. Generally, levels in excess of 15 to 20 mg/dL are reason for intervention. Intervention may include early frequent feedings to stimulate gastrointestinal motility, phototherapy, and exchange transfusion.

INTERFERING FACTORS:

• Drugs that may increase bilirubin levels by causing cholestasis include amitryptyline, anabolic steroids, androgens, benzodiazepines, chlorothiazide, chlorpropamide, dapsone, erythromycin, estrogens, ethionamide, gold salts, imipramine, mercaptopurine, nitrofurans, oral contraceptives, penicillins, phenothiazines, progesterone, propoxyphene, sulfonamides, tamoxifen, and tolbutamide.

• Drugs that may increase bilirubin levels by causing hepatocellular damage include acetaminophen (toxic), acetylsalicylic acid, allopurinol, amiodarone, anabolic steroids, anticonvulsants, asparaginase, azithromycin, bromocriptine, captopril, cephalosporins, chloramphenicol, clindamycin, clofibrate, danazol, enflurane, ethambutol, ethionamide, fenofibrate, fluconazole, fluoroquinolones, foscarnet, gentamicin, indomethacin, interferon, interleukin-2, low-molecular-weight heparin, levamisole, levodopa, lincomycin, monoamine oxidase inhibitors, methyldopa, naproxen, nifedipine, nitrofurans, oral contraceptives, probenecid, procainamide, quinine, ranitidine, retinol, ritodrine, sulfonylureas, tetracyclines, tobramycin, and verapamil.

• Drugs that may increase bilirubin levels by causing hemolysis include amphotericin B, carbamazepine, carbutamide, cephaloridine, cephalothin, chlorpromazine, chlorpropamide, dinitrophenol, ibuprofen, insulin, isoniazid, levodopa, mefenamic acid, melphalan, methotrexate, methyldopa, penicillins, phenacetin, procainamide, quinidine, quinine, rifampin, stibophen, sulfonamides, and tolbutamide.

• Bilirubin is light sensitive. Therefore, the collection container should be suitably covered to protect the specimen from light between the time of collection and analysis.

Nursing Implications and Procedure • • • • • • • • • •

Pretest:

➤ Obtain a history of the patient's complaints, including a list of known allergens.

➤ Obtain a history of the patient's hepatobiliary system, as well as results of previously performed tests and procedures. For related tests, refer to the hepatobiliary system table.

➤ Obtain a list of the medications the patient is taking, including herbs, nutritional supplements, and nutraceuticals. The requesting health care practitioner and laboratory should be advised if the patient regularly uses these products so their effects can be taken into consideration when reviewing results.

➤ There are no food, fluid, or medication restrictions unless by medical direction.

➤ Review the procedure with the patient.

➤ Inform the patient that specimen collection takes approximately 5 to 10 minutes.

Intratest:

➤ Direct the patient to breathe normally and to avoid unnecessary movement.

➤ Observe standard precautions and follow the general guidelines in Appendix A. Perform a venipuncture, and collect the specimen in a 5-mL red- or tiger-top tube.

➤ Label, protect from light, and promptly transport the specimen to the laboratory.

Post-test:

➤ Observe venipuncture site for bleeding or hematoma formation. Apply pressure bandage.

➤ Increased bilirubin levels may be associated with liver disease. Dietary recommendations may be indicated depending on the condition and severity of the condition. Currently, for example, there are no specific medications that can be given to cure hepatitis, but elimination of alcohol ingestion and a diet optimized for convalescence are commonly included in the treatment plan. A high-calorie, high-protein, moderate-fat diet with a high fluid intake is often recommended for the patient with hepatitis. Treatment of cirrhosis is different because a low-protein diet may be in order if the patient's liver has lost the ability to process the end products of protein metabolism. A diet of soft foods may also be required if esophageal varices have developed. Ammonia levels may be used to determine whether protein should be added or reduced from the diet. Patients should be encouraged to eat simple carbohydrates and emulsified fats (as in homogenized milk or eggs), as opposed to complex carbohydrates (e.g., starch, fiber, and glycogen [animal carbohydrates]) and complex fats, which would require additional bile to emulsify it so that it could be used. The cirrhotic patient should be carefully observed for the development of ascites, in which case, fluid and electrolyte balance requires strict attention. The alcoholic patient should be encouraged to avoid alcohol and also to seek appropriate counseling for substance abuse.

➤ Intervention for hyperbilirubinemia in the neonatal patient may include early frequent feedings (to stimulate gastrointestinal motility), phototherapy, and exchange transfusion.

➤ Evaluate test results in relation to the patient's symptoms and other tests performed. Related laboratory tests include alanine aminotransferase, albumin, alkaline phosphatase, α_1-antitrypsin/phenotyping, ammonia, amylase, antimitochondrial antibody, anti–smooth muscle antibody, aspartate aminotransferase, cholesterol, coagulation factor assays, complete blood count, copper, γ-glutamyl transpeptidase, hepatitis serologies, infectious mononucleosis screen, lipase, liver biopsy, protein, prothrombin time, and urinalysis.

BIOPSY, BLADDER

SYNONYM/ACRONYM: N/A.

SPECIMEN: Bladder tissue or cells.

REFERENCE VALUE: (Method: Macroscopic and microscopic examination of tissue) No abnormal tissue or cells.

DESCRIPTION: A urologist performs a biopsy of the bladder during cystoscopic examination. The procedure is usually carried out under general anesthesia. After the bladder is filled with saline for irrigation, the bladder and urethra are examined by direct and lighted visualization using a cystoscope. A sample of suspicious bladder tissue is then excised and examined macroscopically and microscopically to determine the presence of cell morphology and tissue abnormalities. ■

INDICATIONS:

• Assist in confirmation of malignant lesions of the bladder or ureter, especially if tumor is seen by radiological examination

• Assist in the evaluation of cases in which symptoms such as hematuria persist after previous treatment (e.g., removal of polyps or kidney stones)

• Monitor existing recurrent benign lesions for malignant changes

RESULT: Positive findings in neoplasm of the bladder or ureter.

CRITICAL VALUES: N/A

INTERFERING FACTORS:

• This test is contraindicated in patients ⚠ with an acute infection of the bladder, urethra, or prostate.

• ⚠ This test is contraindicated in patients with bleeding disorders.

Nursing Implications and Procedure • • • • • • • • • •

Pretest: ■

 ➤ Obtain a history of the patient's complaints, including a list of known allergens.

➤ Obtain a history of the patient's genitourinary and immune systems, any bleeding disorders, and results of previously performed tests and procedures, especially bleeding time, clotting time, complete blood count, partial thromboplastin time, platelets, and prothrombin time. For related tests, refer to the genitourinary and immune system tables.

➤ Obtain a list of the medications the patient is taking, including anticoagulant therapy drugs, acetylsalicylic acid, herbs, and nutraceuticals known to affect coagulation. These products should be discontinued 14 days before dental or surgical procedures. The requesting health care practitioner and laboratory should be advised if the patient regularly uses these products so their effects can be taken into consideration when reviewing results.

➤ There are no medication restrictions unless by medical direction. Prophylactic antibiotics may be administered before or after the procedure in certain cases.

➤ Instruct the patient that nothing should be taken by mouth if general or spinal anesthesia will be used. Clear liquids may be permitted, by medical direction, if a local anesthetic will be used for the procedure.

➤ Review the procedure with the patient. Sensitivity to cultural and social issues, as well as concern for modesty, is important in providing psychological support.

➤ Inform patients that they may experience back pain and burning or pressure in the genital area during and after the procedure.

➤ Address concerns about pain related to the procedure. Explain that a sedative may be administered to promote relaxation during the procedure.

➤ Inform the patient that if a local anesthetic is used, the patient may experience the urge to urinate.

➤ Assess if the patient has an allergy to local anesthetics, and inform the health care practitioner accordingly.

➤ Confirm nonallergy to anesthesia before the procedure is performed under general anesthesia.

➤ *Obtain written and informed consent before administering any medications prior to the procedure.*

➤ Inform the patient that the procedure is performed under sterile conditions by a surgeon. Specimen collection takes approximately 30 to 45 minutes.

Intratest:

➤ Record baseline vital signs.

➤ Ensure that the patient has complied with pretesting dietary restrictions.

➤ Observe standard precautions and follow the general guidelines in Appendix A.

➤ Direct the patient to breathe normally and to avoid unnecessary movement while a local anesthetic is administered into the urethra, before insertion of the cystoscope.

➤ Place the patient in a lithotomy position on the examination table (with the feet up in stirrups). Drape the patient's legs. Clean the external genitalia with a suitable antiseptic solution.

➤ Once the cystoscope is inserted, the bladder is irrigated with saline. A tissue sample is removed using a cytology brush or biopsy forceps. Catheters may be used to obtain samples from the ureter.

➤ Place the specimens in the appropriate containers. Label the specimen, indicating site location, and promptly transport it to the laboratory.

Post-test:

➤ Instruct the patient to resume usual diet as directed by the health care practitioner.

➤ After open biopsy, monitor vital signs every 15 minutes for 1 hour, then every 2 hours for 4 hours, and as ordered. Take temperature every 4 hours for 24 hours.

➤ After local anesthesia, monitor vital signs and compare with baseline values.

➤ Monitor fluid intake and output for 24 hours. Instruct the patient how to do this if the patient is an outpatient.

➤ Encourage fluid intake of 3000 mL in 24 hours, unless contraindicated by another medical condition.

➤ Apply heat to the lower abdomen to relieve pain and muscle spasms if approved by medical direction.

➤ Inform the patient that blood may be seen in the urine after the first or second postprocedural voiding.

➤ Instruct the patient to report any further changes in urinary pattern, volume, or appearance.

➤ Instruct the patient to immediately report pain, chills, or fever indicative of risk of infection, hemorrhage, or perforation of the bladder as a result of cystoscopy.

➤ If ordered, administer analgesic and prophylactic antibiotic.

➤ Assist the patient in alleviating discomfort by administering warm sitz bath or hip bath.

➤ Recognize anxiety related to test results and offer support. Provide teaching and information regarding the clinical implications of the test results, as appropriate. Educate the patient regarding access to counseling services.

➤ Evaluate test results in relation to the patient's symptoms and other tests performed. Related laboratory tests include routine urinalysis and urine bladder cancer test.

BIOPSY, BONE

SYNONYM/ACRONYM: N/A.

SPECIMEN: Bone tissue.

REFERENCE VALUE: (Method: Microscopic study of bone samples) No abnormal tissue or cells.

DESCRIPTION: Biopsy is the excision of a sample of tissue that can be analyzed microscopically to determine cell morphology and the presence of tissue abnormalities. This test is used to assist in confirming the diagnosis of cancer when clinical symptoms or x-rays are suspicious. After surgical incision to reveal the affected area, bone biopsy is obtained. An alternative collection method is needle biopsy, in which a plug of bone is removed using a special serrated needle. ■

INDICATIONS:
• Differentiation of a benign from a malignant bone lesion

• Radiographic evidence of a bone lesion

RESULT

Abnormal findings in:
• Ewing's sarcoma

• Multiple myeloma

• Osteoma

• Osteosarcoma

CRITICAL VALUES: N/A

INTERFERING FACTORS: This procedure is contraindicated in patients with bleeding disorders.

Nursing Implications and Procedure

Pretest: ■

➤ Obtain a history of the patient's complaints, including a list of known allergens.

➤ Obtain a history of the patient's immune and musculoskeletal systems, any bleeding disorders, and results of previously performed tests and procedures, especially complete bleeding time, complete blood count, clotting time, partial thromboplastin time, platelets, and prothrombin time. For related tests, refer to the immune and musculoskeletal system tables.

➤ Obtain a list of the medications the patient is taking, including anticoagulant therapy, acetylsalicylic acid, herbs, and nutraceuticals known to affect coagulation. These products should be discontinued 14 days before dental or surgical procedures. The requesting health care practitioner and laboratory should be advised that the patient regularly uses these products so their effects can be taken into consideration when reviewing results.

➤ *Open biopsy:* Explain that foods and

fluids are restricted after midnight the day before the open biopsy surgery.

➤ *Needle biopsy:* There are usually no restrictions on food or fluids before needle biopsy.

➤ There are no medication restrictions unless by medical direction.

➤ Review the procedure with the patient. Sensitivity to cultural and social issues, as well as concern for modesty, is important in providing psychological support.

➤ Assess if the patient has an allergy to local anesthetics, and inform the health care practitioner accordingly.

➤ Inform the patient that a general anesthetic will be administered before the open biopsy. Ensure nonallergy to anesthesia is confirmed before procedure performed under general anesthesia.

➤ *Obtain written and informed consent before administering any medications prior to the procedure.*

➤ Inform the patient that the procedure is performed by a surgeon, that it usually takes about 30 minutes to complete, and that sutures may be necessary to close the site.

Intratest:

➤ Ensure that the patient has complied with pretesting dietary restrictions before the open biopsy procedure.

➤ Observe standard precautions and follow the general guidelines in Appendix A.

➤ It may be necessary to shave and perform an orthopedic skin preparation before needle biopsy.

➤ Administer premedication as directed.

Open biopsy:

➤ Record baseline vital signs. After a surgical incision is complete, the surgeon locates the suspected lesion and removes sufficient tissue for analysis.

Needle biopsy:

➤ Assist the patient into a comfortable position in which the biopsy site can be supported and exposed. Cleanse the skin with an antiseptic solution. Administer local anesthetic and protect the site with sterile drapes. A small incision is made and the biopsy needle is inserted to remove the specimen.

➤ Place tissue samples in formalin solution. Ensure that the specimen is properly labeled, indicating site location, especially left or right; promptly transport the specimen to the laboratory.

Post-test:

➤ Instruct the patient to resume usual diet as directed by the health care practitioner.

➤ After open biopsy, monitor vital signs every 15 minutes for 1 hour, then every 2 hours for 4 hours, and as ordered. Take temperature every 4 hours for 24 hours.

➤ After local anesthesia, monitor vital signs and compare with baseline values.

➤ Inspect biopsy site for excessive bleeding.

➤ Instruct the patient in the care and assessment of the site. Instruct the patient to report any redness, edema, bleeding, or pain at the biopsy site. Instruct the patient to keep the site clean and change the dressing as needed.

➤ Administer mild analgesic and antibiotic therapy as ordered. Remind the patient of the importance of completing the entire course of antibiotic therapy, even if signs and symptoms disappear before completion of therapy.

➤ Inform the patient of a follow-up appointment for removal of sutures, if indicated.

➤ Recognize anxiety related to test results and offer support. Provide teaching and information regarding the clinical implications of the test results, as appropriate. Educate the patient regarding access to counseling services.

➤ Evaluate test results in relation to the patient's symptoms and other tests performed. Related laboratory tests include alkaline phosphatase; β_2-microglobulin; bone marrow biopsy; calcium; urine calcium; complete blood count; cortisol; immunofixation electrophoresis; immunoglobulin A, G, and M; parathyroid hormone; phosphorus; urine and serum protein electrophoresis; urine and serum total protein; urinalysis; and vitamin D.

BIOPSY, BONE MARROW

· ·

SYNONYM/ACRONYM: N/A.

SPECIMEN: Bone marrow aspirate, bone core biopsy, marrow and peripheral smears.

REFERENCE VALUE: (Method: Microscopic study of bone and bone marrow samples, flow cytometry) Reference ranges are subject to many variables and therefore the laboratory should be consulted for their specific interpretation. Some generalities may be commented on regarding findings as follows:

- Ratio of marrow fat to cellular elements is related to age, with the amount of fat increasing with increasing age.
- Normal cellularity, cellular distribution, presence of megakaryocytes, and absence of fibrosis or tumor cells.
- The myeloid-to-erythrocyte ratio (M:E) is 2:1 to 4:1 in adults. It may be slightly higher in children.

Differential Parameter	Conventional Units
Erythrocyte precursors	18–32%
Myeloblasts	0–2%
Promyelocytes	2–6%
Myelocytes	9–17%
Metamyelocytes	7–25%
Bands	10–16%
Neutrophils	18–28%
Eosinophils and precursors	1–5%
Basophils and precursors	0–1%
Monocytes and precursors	1–5%
Lymphocytes	9–19%
Plasma cells	0–1%

DESCRIPTION: This test involves the removal of a small sample of bone marrow by aspiration, needle biopsy, or open surgical biopsy for a complete hematological analysis. The marrow is a suspension of blood, fat, and developing blood cells, which is evaluated for morphology and examined for all stages of maturation; iron stores; and M:E cells. Sudan B and periodic acid–Schiff (PAS) stains can be performed for microscopic examination to differentiate the types of leukemia, although flow cytometry and cytogenetics have become more commonly used techniques for this purpose. ■

INDICATIONS:
- Determine marrow differential (proportion of the various types of cells present in the marrow) and M:E
- Evaluate abnormal results of complete blood count or white blood cell count with differential showing increased numbers of leukocyte precursors
- Evaluate hepatomegaly or splenomegaly
- Identify bone marrow hyperplasia or hypoplasia
- Monitor effects of exposure to bone marrow depressants
- Monitor bone marrow response to chemotherapy or radiation therapy

RESULT

Increased reticulocytes:
- Compensated red blood cell (RBC) loss
- Response to vitamin B_{12} therapy

Decreased reticulocytes:
- Aplastic crisis of sickle-cell disease or hereditary spherocytosis

Increased neutrophils (total):
- Acute myeloblastic leukemia
- Myeloid (chronic) leukemias

Decreased neutrophils (total):
- Aplastic anemia
- Leukemias (monocytic and lymphoblastic)

Increased lymphocytes:
- Aplastic anemia
- Lymphatic leukemia
- Lymphomas
- Lymphosarcoma
- Mononucleosis
- Viral infections

Increased plasma cells:
- Cancer
- Cirrhosis of the liver
- Connective tissue disorders
- Hypersensitivity reactions
- Infections
- Macroglobulinemia
- Ulcerative colitis

Increased megakaryocytes:
- Hemorrhage
- Infections
- Increasing age
- Megakaryocytic myelosis
- Myeloid leukemia
- Pneumonia
- Polycythemia vera
- Thrombocytopenia

Decreased megakaryocytes:

- Agranulocytosis
- Cirrhosis of the liver
- Pernicious aplastic anemia
- Radiation therapy
- Thrombocytopenia purpura

Increased M:E:

- Bone marrow failure
- Infections
- Leukemoid reactions
- Myeloid leukemia

Decreased M:E:

- Anemias
- Hepatic disease
- Polycythemia vera
- Posthemorrhagic hematopoiesis

Increased normoblasts:

- Anemias
- Chronic blood loss
- Polycythemia vera

Decreased normoblasts:

- Aplastic anemia
- Folic acid or vitamin B_{12} deficiency
- Hemolytic anemia

Increased eosinophils:

- Bone marrow cancer
- Lymphadenoma
- Myeloid leukemia

CRITICAL VALUES: N/A

INTERFERING FACTORS:

- Recent blood transfusions, iron therapy, or administration of cytotoxic agents may alter test results.

- This procedure is contraindicated in patients with known bleeding disorders.

Nursing Implications and Procedure • • • • • • • • • • •

Pretest: ◼

➤ Obtain a history of the patient's complaints, including a list of known allergens.

➤ Obtain a history of the patient's hematopoietic and immune system and any bleeding disorders, as well as results of previously performed tests and procedures, especially bleeding time, clotting time, complete blood count, partial thromboplastin time, platelets, and prothrombin time. For related tests, refer to the hematopoietic and immune system tables.

➤ Obtain a list of the medications the patient takes, including anticoagulant therapy, acetylsalicylic acid, herbals, and nutraceuticals known to affect coagulation. These products should be discontinued 14 days before dental or surgical procedures. The requesting health care practitioner and laboratory should be advised if the patient regularly uses such products so their effect can be taken into consideration when reviewing results.

➤ Note any recent procedures that can interfere with test results.

➤ There are no food, fluid, or medication restrictions unless by medical direction.

➤ Review the procedure with the patient. Sensitivity to cultural and social issues, as well as concern for modesty, is important in providing psychological support. Explain that discomfort of the puncture will be minimized with local anesthetics or systemic analgesics and that the site may remain tender for several weeks. For children, provide equipment and a doll with which to role-play a simulated procedure. Inform the patient that bed rest for 10 to 30 minutes (depending on the test site) is required after the procedure.

➤ Assess if the patient has an allergy to local anesthetics and inform the health care practitioner accordingly.

➤ *Obtain written and informed consent before administering any medications prior to the procedure.*

➤ Explain that the test is done at the bedside or in a treatment room by a health care practitioner and requires about 20 minutes.

Intratest:

➤ Record baseline vital signs.

➤ Observe standard precautions and follow the general guidelines in Appendix A.

➤ Administer premedication prescribed for pain or anxiety. Direct the patient to breathe normally and to avoid unnecessary movement.

➤ Assist the patient to the desired position depending on the test site to be used. In young children, the most frequently chosen site is the proximal tibia. Vertebral bodies T10 through L4 are preferred in older children. In adults, the sternum or iliac crests are the preferred sites.

➤ Place the patient in the prone, sitting, or side-lying position for the vertebral bodies; the side-lying position for iliac crest or tibial sites; or the supine position for the sternum.

Needle aspiration:

➤ Prepare the skin with an antiseptic solution and drape the site. Record baseline vital signs. The health care practitioner will anesthetize the site with procaine or lidocaine, and then insert a needle with stylet into the marrow. The stylet is removed, a syringe attached, and a 0.5-mL aliquot of marrow withdrawn. The needle is removed and pressure applied to the site. The aspirate is applied to slides, and when dry, a fixative is applied.

Needle biopsy:

➤ Record baseline vital signs. Local anesthetic is introduced deeply enough to include periosteum. A cutting biopsy needle is introduced through a small skin incision and bored into the marrow cavity. A core needle is introduced through the cutting needle, and a plug of marrow is removed. The needles are withdrawn, and the specimen is placed in a preservative solution. Pressure is applied to the site for 5 to 10 minutes, and a dressing is applied.

➤ Label the specimen, and promptly transport it to the laboratory.

Post-test:

➤ After local anesthesia, monitor vital signs and compare with baseline values.

➤ Advise the patient or caregiver to keep ice on the site and not to remove the bandage for 24 hours.

➤ Instruct the patient to immediately report any signs of infections or excessive bleeding.

➤ Recognize anxiety related to test results and offer support. Provide teaching and information regarding the clinical implications of the test results, as appropriate. Educate the patient regarding access to counseling services.

➤ Evaluate test results in relation to the patient's symptoms and other tests performed. Related laboratory tests include complete blood count, serum and urine immunofixation electrophoresis, leukocyte alkaline phosphatase, lymph node biopsy, and vitamin B_{12}.

BIOPSY, BREAST

SYNONYM/ACRONYM: N/A.

SPECIMEN: Breast tissue or cells.

REFERENCE VALUE: (Method: Macroscopic and microscopic examination of tissue) No abnormal cells or tissue.

DESCRIPTION: Fine-needle and open biopsies of the breast have become more commonly ordered in recent years as increasing emphasis on early detection of breast cancer has become stronger. Breast biopsies are used to assist in the identification and prognosis of breast cancer. ∎

INDICATIONS:
• Evidence of breast lesion by palpation, mammography, or ultrasound

• Observable breast changes such as "peau d'orange" skin, scaly skin of the areola, drainage from the nipple, or ulceration of the skin

RESULT: Positive findings in carcinoma of the breast.

CRITICAL VALUES: N/A

INTERFERING FACTORS: This procedure is contraindicated in patients with bleeding disorders.

Nursing Implications and Procedure

Pretest:

➤ Obtain a history of the patient's complaints, including a list of known allergens.

➤ Obtain a history of the patient's immune and reproductive systems, any bleeding disorders, and results of previously performed tests and procedures, especially bleeding time, clotting time, complete blood count, partial thromboplastin time, platelets, and prothrombin time. For related tests, refer to the immune and reproductive system tables.

➤ Obtain a list of the medications the patient is taking, including anticoagulant therapy, acetylsalicylic acid, herbs, and nutraceuticals known to affect coagulation. It is recommended that use be discontinued 14 days before dental or surgical procedures. The requesting health care practitioner and laboratory should be advised if the patient regularly uses these products so their effects can be taken into consideration when reviewing results.

➤ *Needle biopsy:* There are no food, fluid, or medication restrictions before needle biopsy unless by medical direction.

➤ *Open biopsy:* Food and fluids are restricted for at least 12 hours before an open biopsy.

➤ Review the procedure with the patient. Sensitivity to cultural and social issues, as well as concern for modesty, is important in providing psychological support.

➤ Address concerns about pain related to the procedure and discuss the possibility of administering a sedative to promote relaxation during the procedure.

➤ Assess if the patient has an allergy to local anesthetics, and inform the health care practitioner accordingly.

➤ Ensure nonallergy to anesthesia before the open biopsy procedure is performed under general anesthesia.

➤ *Obtain written and informed consent before administering any medications prior to the procedure.*

➤ In certain cases, administer prophylactic antibiotics before or after the procedure.

➤ Inform the patient that specimen collection takes approximately 20 to 30 minutes.

Intratest:

➤ Observe standard precautions and follow the general guidelines in Appendix A.

Open biopsy:

➤ Ensure that the patient has complied with pretesting dietary restrictions before open biopsy. Record baseline vital signs. The specimen is obtained by surgical excision.

Needle biopsy:

➤ Assist the patient into a supine position and cleanse the biopsy site with an antiseptic. Record baseline vital signs. Inject the local anesthetic and protect the biopsy site with sterile drapes. Direct the patient to breathe normally and to avoid unnecessary movement. A needle is inserted into the mass and tissue, and fluid is aspirated.

➤ Apply a sterile dressing to the site.

➤ Place the specimens in the appropriate containers. Ensure that the spec-

imen is properly labeled, indicating location, especially left or right breast; promptly transport the specimen to the laboratory.

Post-test:

➤ Instruct the patient to resume usual diet and medication, if withheld, as directed by the health care practitioner.

➤ After open biopsy, monitor vital signs every 15 minutes for 1 hour, then every 2 hours for 4 hours, and as ordered. Take temperature every 4 hours for 24 hours.

➤ After local anesthesia, monitor vital signs, and compare with baseline values.

➤ Instruct the patient in proper cleansing of the site. Stress the importance of a follow-up appointment for suture removal.

➤ Instruct the patient to report excessive bleeding, redness, edema, or pain at the biopsy site.

➤ Administer analgesics and antibiotics as ordered, and instruct the patient in the importance of completing the entire course of antibiotic therapy, even if no symptoms are present.

➤ Instruct and educate the patient how to perform monthly breast self-examination and emphasize, as appropriate, the importance of having a mammogram performed annually.

➤ Recognize anxiety related to test results and offer support. Provide teaching and information regarding the clinical implications of the test results, as appropriate. Educate the patient regarding access to counseling services.

➤ Evaluate test results in relation to the patient's symptoms and other tests performed. Related laboratory tests include cancer antigen 15-3, HER-2/neu oncoprotein, estrogen and progesterone receptors, and carcinoembryonic antigen.

BIOPSY, CERVICAL

SYNONYM/ACRONYM: N/A.

SPECIMEN: Cervical tissue.

REFERENCE VALUE: (Method: Microscopic examination of tissue cells) No abnormal cells or tissue.

DESCRIPTION: Biopsy is the excision of a sample of tissue that can be analyzed microscopically to determine cell morphology and the presence of tissue abnormalities. The cervical biopsy is used to assist in confirmation of cancer when screening tests are positive. Cervical biopsy is obtained using an instrument that punches into the tissue and retrieves a tissue sample. Schiller's test entails applying an iodine solution to the cervix. Normal cells pick up the iodine and stain brown. Abnormal cells do not pick up any color. Punch biopsy results may indicate the need for a cone biopsy of the cervix. Cone biopsy is a surgical procedure requiring general anesthesia. ■

INDICATIONS:

- Follow-up to abnormal Papanicolaou (Pap) smear, Schiller's test, or colposcopy
- Suspected cervical malignancy

RESULT

Positive findings in:

- Carcinoma in situ
- Cervical dysplasia
- Cervical polyps

CRITICAL VALUES: N/A

INTERFERING FACTORS:

- The test is contraindicated in cases of acute pelvic inflammatory disease, cervicitis, or bleeding disorders.
- This test should not be performed while the patient is menstruating.

Nursing Implications and Procedure

Pretest:

➤ Obtain a history of the patient's complaints, including a list of known allergens.

➤ Obtain a history of the patient's immune and reproductive systems, any bleeding disorders, and results of previously performed tests and procedures, especially bleeding time, clotting time, complete blood count, partial thromboplastin time, platelets, and prothrombin time. For related tests, refer to the immune and reproductive system tables.

➤ Obtain a list of the medications the

patient is taking, including anticoagulant therapy, acetylsalicylic acid, herbs, and nutraceuticals known to affect coagulation. These products should be discontinued 14 days before dental or surgical procedures. The requesting health care practitioner and laboratory should be advised if the patient regularly uses these products so their effects can be taken into consideration when reviewing results.

➤ *Cervical biopsy:* There are no food, fluid, or medication restrictions before needle biopsy unless by medical direction.

➤ *Cone biopsy:* Food and fluids are restricted for at least 12 hours before an open biopsy.

➤ Review the procedure with the patient. Sensitivity to cultural and social issues, as well as concern for modesty, is important in providing psychological support.

➤ Address concerns about pain related to the procedure.

➤ Encourage the use of relaxation and controlled breathing during the procedure to aid in reducing discomfort.

➤ Confirm nonallergy to anesthesia before the cone biopsy procedure is performed under general anesthesia.

➤ *Obtain written and informed consent before administering any medications prior to the procedure.*

➤ Inform the patient that specimen collection takes approximately 20 to 30 minutes. Specimen collection will be performed by a health care practitioner.

Intratest: ■

➤ Have patient remove clothes below the waist. Assist the patient into a lithotomy position on a gynecologic examination table with feet in stirrups. Drape the patient's legs.

➤ Observe standard precautions and follow the general guidelines in Appendix A.

Cone biopsy:

➤ Ensure that the patient has complied with dietary preparation and other pretesting restrictions before open biopsy. Record baseline vital signs. The specimen is obtained by surgical excision.

Cervical biopsy:

➤ Cleanse the external genitalia with an antiseptic solution. Direct the patient to breathe normally and to avoid unnecessary movement. Swab the cervix with 3% acetic acid before insertion of the colposcope. Biopsy forceps are inserted and the tissue samples are obtained.

➤ Place the specimens in the appropriate containers containing formalin solution. Label the specimen, indicating site location, and promptly transport it to the laboratory.

➤ Bleeding is common and is controlled by cautery or silver nitrate application. The health care practitioner may insert a tampon after the speculum is removed if bleeding persists.

Post-test: ■

➤ After general anesthesia for cone biopsy, monitor vital signs and compare with baseline values.

➤ Observe for bleeding.

➤ Instruct the patient to expect a gray-green vaginal discharge for several days, to avoid strenuous activity for 8 to 24 hours, to avoid douching or intercourse for 2 weeks or as instructed by the health care practitioner, and to report excessive bleeding to the health care practitioner.

➤ Recognize anxiety related to test results and offer support. Provide teaching and information regarding the clinical implications of the test results, as appropriate. Educate the patient regarding access to counseling services.

➤ Evaluate test results in relation to the patient's symptoms and other tests performed. A related laboratory test is the Pap smear.

BIOPSY, CHORIONIC VILLUS

SYNONYM/ACRONYM: N/A.

SPECIMEN: Chorionic villus tissue.

REFERENCE VALUE: (Method: Tissue culture) Normal karyotype.

DESCRIPTION: This test is used to detect fetal abnormalities caused by numerous genetic disorders. The advantage over amniocentesis is that it can be performed as early as the eighth week of pregnancy, permitting earlier decisions regarding termination of pregnancy. However, unlike amniocentesis this test will not detect neural tube defects. ∎

INDICATIONS:
- Assist in the diagnosis of in utero metabolic disorders such as cystic fibrosis or other errors of lipid, carbohydrate, or amino acid metabolism
- Detect abnormalities in the fetus of women of advanced maternal age
- Determine fetal gender when the mother is a known carrier of a sex-linked abnormal gene that could be transmitted to male offspring, such as hemophilia or Duchenne's muscular dystrophy
- Evaluate fetus in families with a history of genetic disorders, such as Down syndrome, Tay-Sachs disease, chromosome or enzyme anomalies, or inherited hemoglobinopathies

RESULT

Abnormal karyotype: Numerous

genetic disorders. Generally, the laboratory provides detailed interpretive information regarding the specific chromosome abnormality detected.

CRITICAL VALUES: N/A

INTERFERING FACTORS:
- The test is contraindicated in the patient with a history of or in the presence of incompetent cervix.

Nursing Implications and Procedure

Pretest: ∎

➤ Obtain a history of the patient's complaints, including a list of known allergens.

➤ Obtain a history of the patient's reproductive system, as well as results of previously performed tests and procedures. For related tests, refer to the reproductive system table.

➤ Obtain a list of the medications the patient takes, including herbs, nutritional supplements, and nutraceuticals. The requesting health care practitioner and laboratory should be advised if the patient regularly uses such products so their effect can be taken into consideration when reviewing results.

➤ There are no food, fluid, or medication restrictions unless by medical direction.

➤ Review the procedure with the patient. Sensitivity to cultural and social issues, as well as concern for modesty, is important in providing psychological support.

➤ Address concerns about pain related to the procedure and that relaxation and controlled breathing during the procedure will aid in reducing discomfort.

➤ Have the patient void before the procedure.

➤ Warn the patient that normal results do not guarantee a normal fetus. Assure the patient that precautions to avoid injury to the fetus will be taken by localizing the fetus with ultrasound. Inform the patient that specimen collection takes approximately 10 to 15 minutes.

➤ *Obtain written and informed consent before administering any medications prior to the procedure.*

Intratest:

➤ Position the patient in a lithotomy position on a gynecologic examination table with feet in stirrups. Drape the patient's legs.

➤ Record maternal and fetal baseline vital signs.

➤ Observe standard precautions and follow the general guidelines in Appendix A.

➤ Cleanse the external genitalia with an antiseptic solution. Direct the patient to breathe normally and avoid unnecessary movement.

➤ The speculum is inserted and a suction catheter is inserted via the speculum to the biopsy site. A syringe is connected to the catheter and the specimen is withdrawn.

➤ Place the specimens in the appropriate containers. Label indicating site location and promptly transport the specimen to the laboratory.

Post-test:

➤ Monitor maternal and fetal vital signs and compare with baseline values.

➤ Observe for bleeding and instruct patient to immediately report excessive bleeding, abdominal pain, temperature, or chills.

➤ Instruct the patient to expect a gray-green vaginal discharge for several days, to avoid strenuous activity for 8 to 24 hours, to avoid douching or intercourse for 2 weeks or as instructed by the health care practitioner, and to report excessive bleeding to the health care practitioner.

➤ Recognize anxiety related to test results and provide support. Provide teaching and information regarding the clinical implications of the test results, as appropriate. Encourage family to seek counseling if concerned with pregnancy termination or to seek genetic counseling if chromosomal abnormality is determined. Decisions regarding elective abortion should take place in the presence of both parents. Provide a nonjudgmental, nonthreatening atmosphere for a discussion during which risks of delivering an abnormal infant are discussed with options (termination of pregnancy or adoption). It is also important to discuss problems the mother and father may experience (guilt, depression, anger) if fetal abnormalities are detected. Evaluate test results in relation to the patient's symptoms and other tests performed. Related laboratory tests include amniotic fluid analysis, α-fetoprotein, chromosome analysis, hexosaminidase A and B, and lecithin/sphingomyelin ratio.

BIOPSY, INTESTINAL

SYNONYM/ACRONYM: N/A.

SPECIMEN: Intestinal tissue or cells.

REFERENCE VALUE: (Method: Macroscopic and microscopic examination of tissue) No abnormal tissue or cells.

DESCRIPTION: Intestinal biopsy is the excision of a tissue sample from the small intestine for microscopic analysis to determine cell morphology and the presence of tissue abnormalities. This test assists in confirming the diagnosis of cancer or intestinal disorders. Biopsy specimen is usually obtained during endoscopic examination. ■

INDICATIONS:
• Assist in the diagnosis of various intestinal disorders, such as lactose and other enzyme deficiencies, celiac disease, and parasitic infections

• Confirm suspected intestinal malignancy

• Confirm suspicious findings during endoscopic visualization of the intestinal wall

RESULT

Abnormal findings in:
• Cancer

• Celiac disease

• Lactose deficiency

• Parasitic infestation

• Tropical sprue

CRITICAL VALUES: N/A

INTERFERING FACTORS:
• Barium swallow within 48 hours of small intestine biopsy affects results.

• This procedure is contraindicated in patients with bleeding disorders and aortic arch aneurysm.

Nursing Implications and Procedure

Pretest:

➤ Obtain a history of the patient's complaints, including a list of known allergens.

➤ Obtain a history of the patient's gastrointestinal and immune systems, any bleeding disorders, and results of previously performed tests and procedures, especially bleeding time, clotting time, complete blood count, partial thromboplastin time, platelets, and prothrombin time. For related tests, refer to the gastrointestinal and immune system tables.

➤ Obtain a list of the medications the patient is taking, including anticoagulant therapy, acetylsalicylic acid, herbs, and nutraceuticals known to affect coagulation. These products should be discontinued 14 days before dental or surgical procedures. The requesting health care practitioner and laboratory should be advised if the patient regularly uses these products so their effects can be taken into consideration when reviewing results.

➤ Note any recent procedures that can interfere with test results.

➤ There are no medication restrictions unless by medical direction.

➤ Explain that food and fluids are restricted for 6 to 8 hours before the test.

➤ Review the procedure with the patient. Sensitivity to cultural and social issues, as well as concern for modesty, is important in providing psychological support.

➤ Address concerns about pain related to the procedure. Explain that a sedative may be administered to promote relaxation during the procedure.

➤ Determine if the patient has an allergy to local anesthetics, and inform the health care practitioner accordingly.

➤ *Obtain written and informed consent before administering any medications prior to the procedure.*

➤ Remove full or partial dentures. Inform the health care practitioner if the patient has any crowns or caps on the teeth.

➤ Inform the patient that the procedure is performed by a surgeon and usually takes about 60 minutes to complete.

Intratest:

➤ Ensure that the patient has complied with pretesting dietary restrictions.

➤ Record baseline vital signs.

➤ Observe standard precautions and follow the general guidelines in Appendix A.

➤ Administer ordered premedication.

➤ Assist the patient into a semireclining position. Direct the patient to

breathe normally and to avoid unnecessary movement.

➤ A local anesthetic is sprayed into the throat. A protective tooth guard and a bite block may be placed in the mouth.

➤ The flexible endoscope is passed into and through the mouth, and the patient is asked to swallow. Once the endoscope passes into the esophagus, assist the patient into the left lateral position. A suction device is used to drain saliva.

➤ The esophagus, stomach, and duodenum are visually examined as the endoscope passes through each section. A biopsy specimen can be taken from any suspicious sites.

➤ Tissue samples are obtained by inserting a cytology brush or biopsy forceps through the endoscope.

➤ When the examination and tissue removal are complete, the endoscope and suction device are withdrawn and the tooth guard and bite block are removed.

➤ Place tissue samples in formalin solution. Label the specimen, indicating site location, and promptly transport it to the laboratory.

Post-test:

➤ Instruct the patient to resume usual diet as directed by the health care practitioner.

➤ After local anesthesia, monitor vital signs and compare with baseline values. Assess and record breath sounds and characteristics of respiration.

➤ Note any chest pain, upper abdominal pain, pain on swallowing, difficulty breathing, or expectoration of blood. Report these to the health care practitioner immediately.

➤ Instruct the patient not to eat or drink until the anesthesia has worn off. Assess the patient's ability to swallow before allowing liquids or solid foods.

➤ Instruct the patient to maintain a

side-lying position for 2 hours after the procedure to prevent aspiration of secretions.

➤ Recognize anxiety related to test results and offer support. Provide teaching and information regarding the clinical implications of the test results, as appropriate. Educate the patient regarding access to counseling services.

➤ Evaluate test results in relation to the patient's symptoms and other tests performed. Related laboratory tests include albumin, calcium, electrolytes, D-xylose tolerance, gliadin antibodies, fecal analysis, fecal fat, folic acid, iron/total iron-binding capacity, lactose tolerance, ova and parasites, prothrombin time, vitamin B_{12}, and vitamin D.

BIOPSY, KIDNEY

· ·

SYNONYM/ACRONYM: Renal biopsy.

SPECIMEN: Kidney tissue or cells.

REFERENCE VALUE: (Method: Macroscopic and microscopic examination of tissue) No abnormal cells or tissue.

DESCRIPTION: Kidney or renal biopsy is the excision of a tissue sample from the kidney for microscopic analysis to determine cell morphology and the presence of tissue abnormalities. This test assists in confirming a diagnosis of cancer found on x-ray or ultrasound or to diagnose certain inflammatory or immunologic conditions. Biopsy specimen is usually obtained either percutaneously or after surgical incision. ■

INDICATIONS:

• Assist in confirming suspected renal malignancy

• Assist in the diagnosis of the cause of renal disease

• Determine extent of involvement in systemic lupus erythematosus or other immunologic disorders

• Monitor progression of nephrotic syndrome

• Monitor renal function after transplantation

RESULT

Positive findings in:

• Acute and chronic poststreptococcal glomerulonephritis

• Amyloidosis infiltration

• Cancer

• Disseminated lupus erythematosus

• Goodpasture's syndrome

• Immunologic rejection of transplanted kidney

- Nephrotic syndrome

- Pyelonephritis

- Renal venous thrombosis

CRITICAL VALUES: N/A

INTERFERING FACTORS:

- This procedure is contraindicated in ⚠ bleeding disorders, advanced renal disease, uncontrolled hypertension, or solitary kidney (except transplanted kidney).

- Obesity and severe spinal deformity can make percutaneous biopsy impossible.

Nursing Implications and Procedure • • • • • • • • • • •

Pretest: ■

➤ Obtain a history of the patient's genitourinary and immune system including a list of known allergens.

➤ Obtain a history of bleeding disorders, as well as results of previously performed tests and procedures, especially bleeding time, clotting time, complete blood count, partial thromboplastin time, platelets, and prothrombin time. For related tests, refer to the genitourinary and immune system tables.

➤ Obtain a list of the medications the patient takes, including anticoagulant therapy, acetylsalicylic acid, herbals, and nutraceuticals known to affect coagulation. These products should be discontinued 14 days before dental or surgical procedures. The requesting health care practitioner and laboratory should be advised if the patient regularly uses such products so their effect can be taken into consideration when reviewing results.

➤ There are no medication restrictions unless by medical direction.

➤ Instruct the patient that nothing should be taken by mouth beginning the night before the procedure.

➤ Review the procedure with the patient. Sensitivity to cultural and social issues, as well as concern for modesty is important in providing psychological support.

➤ Address concerns about pain related to the procedure. Explain that a sedative may be administered to promote relaxation during the procedure.

➤ Assess if the patient has an allergy to local anesthetics and inform the health care practitioner accordingly.

➤ Confirm nonallergy to anesthesia before open biopsy procedure performed under general anesthesia.

➤ *Obtain written and informed consent before administering any medications prior to the procedure.*

➤ Inform the patient that the procedure is performed by a surgeon under sterile conditions using a local anesthetic (e.g., lidocaine) and that specimen collection takes approximately 40 to 60 minutes.

Intratest: ■

➤ Ensure that the patient has complied with dietary restrictions before open biopsy.

➤ Direct the patient to breathe normally and to avoid unnecessary movement.

➤ Observe standard precautions and follow the general guidelines in Appendix A.

➤ Administer ordered premedication.

Open biopsy:

➤ Record baseline vital signs. After administration of anesthesia, a surgical incision is made, suspicious areas located, and tissue samples collected.

Percutaneous needle biopsy:

➤ Assist the patient into a prone position. Cleanse the site with antiseptic. A local anesthetic is injected and a sterile field is prepared. A sandbag may be placed under the abdomen to aid in moving the kidneys to the desired position. Instruct the patient to take a deep breath and hold it while the needle is inserted. As the needle enters the kidney, instruct the patient to exhale. The needle is rotated to obtain a plug of tissue, and then removed.

➤ Place the specimens in the appropriate containers. Label the specimen, indicating site location, especially left or right; promptly transport the specimen to the laboratory.

➤ Apply manual pressure for 5 to 20 minutes, and then apply a pressure dressing.

Post-test:

➤ Instruct the patient to resume usual diet as directed by the health care practitioner.

➤ After open biopsy, monitor vital signs every 15 minutes for 1 hour, then every 2 hours for 4 hours, and as ordered. Take temperature every 4 hours for 24 hours.

➤ After local anesthesia, monitor vital signs and compare with baseline values.

➤ Inform the patient that blood may be seen in the urine after the first or second postprocedural voiding.

➤ Monitor fluid intake and output for 24 hours. Instruct the patient how to do this if the patient is an outpatient.

➤ Instruct the patient to report any changes in urinary pattern or volume or any unusual appearance of the urine. If urinary volume is less than 200 mL in the first 8 hours, encourage the patient to increase fluid intake unless contraindicated by another medical condition.

➤ Instruct the patient to immediately report symptoms such as backache, flank pain, shoulder pain, lightheadedness, burning on urination, hematuria, chills, or fever, which may indicate the presence of infection, hemorrhage, or inadvertent puncture of other internal organs.

➤ Observe the needle site or incision for bleeding.

➤ Observe the patient for other signs of distress including hypotension and tachycardia.

➤ After percutaneous biopsy, instruct the patient to stay in bed lying on the affected side for at least 30 minutes with a pillow or sandbag under the site to prevent bleeding. The patient also needs to remain on bed rest for 24 hours.

➤ Instruct the patient to avoid strenuous activity, sports, and heavy lifting for 2 weeks after the procedure.

➤ Recognize anxiety related to test results and offer support. Provide teaching and information regarding the clinical implications of the test results, as appropriate. Educate the patient regarding access to counseling services.

➤ Evaluate test results in relation to the patient's symptoms and other tests performed. Related laboratory tests include albumin, aldosterone, antiglomerular basement membrane antibody, β_2-microglobulin, creatinine, creatinine clearance, osmolality, urine osmolality, potassium, urine potassium, protein, urine protein, renin, sodium, urine sodium, urea nitrogen, urinalysis, and urine cytology.

BIOPSY, LIVER

SYNONYM/ACRONYM: N/A.

SPECIMEN: Liver tissue or cells.

REFERENCE VALUE: (Method: Macroscopic and microscopic examination of tissue) No abnormal cells or tissue.

DESCRIPTION: Liver biopsy is the excision of a tissue sample from the liver for microscopic analysis to determine cell morphology and the presence of tissue abnormalities. This test is used to assist in confirming a diagnosis of cancer or certain disorders of the hepatic parenchyma. Biopsy specimen is usually obtained either percutaneously or after surgical incision. ∎

INDICATIONS:
• Assist in confirming suspected hepatic malignancy
• Assist in confirming suspected hepatic parenchymal disease
• Assist in diagnosing the cause of persistently elevated liver enzymes, hepatomegaly, or jaundice

RESULT

Positive findings in:
• Benign tumor
• Cancer
• Cholesterol ester storage disease
• Cirrhosis
• Galactosemia
• Hemochromatosis

• Hepatic involvement with systemic lupus erythematosus, sarcoidosis, or amyloidosis
• Hepatitis
• Parasitic infestations (e.g., amebiasis, malaria, visceral larva migrans)
• Reye's syndrome
• Wilson's disease

CRITICAL VALUES: N/A

INTERFERING FACTORS: This procedure is contraindicated in patients with bleeding disorders, suspected vascular tumor of the liver, ascites that may obscure proper insertion site for needle biopsy, subdiaphragmatic or right hemothoracic infection, or biliary tract infection.

Nursing Implications and Procedure

Pretest:

➤ Obtain a history of the patient's complaints especially fatigue and pain related to inflammation and swelling of the liver.

➤ Obtain a list of known allergens.

➤ Obtain a history of the patient's

hepatobiliary and immune system, any bleeding disorders, and results of previously performed tests and procedures, especially bleeding time, clotting time, complete blood count, partial thromboplastin time, platelets, and prothrombin time. For related tests, refer to the hepatobiliary and immune system tables.

➤ Obtain a list of the medications the patient is taking, including anticoagulant therapy, acetylsalicylic acid, herbs, and nutraceuticals known to affect coagulation. These products should be discontinued 14 days before dental or surgical procedures. The requesting health care practitioner and laboratory should be advised if the patient regularly uses these products so their effects can be taken into consideration when reviewing results.

➤ There are no medication restrictions unless by medical direction.

➤ Explain that food and fluids are restricted beginning midnight of the day before the test.

➤ Review the procedure with the patient. Sensitivity to cultural and social issues, as well as concern for modesty, is important in providing psychological support.

➤ Address concerns about pain related to the procedure. Explain that a sedative and/or anesthetic will be administered before the procedure to promote relaxation during the percutaneous biopsy, and that general anesthesia will be administered for open biopsy.

➤ Assess if the patient has an allergy to local anesthetics, and inform the health care practitioner accordingly.

➤ Ensure that nonallergy to anesthesia is confirmed before the open biopsy procedure is performed under general anesthesia.

➤ *Obtain written and informed consent before administering any medications prior to the procedure.*

➤ Inform the patient that the procedure is performed by a surgeon under sterile conditions and usually takes about 90 minutes to complete.

Needle biopsy should take about 15 minutes.

Intratest:

➤ Ensure that the patient has complied with dietary restrictions before open biopsy.

➤ Instruct the patient to avoid coughing or straining, as this may increase intra-abdominal pressure.

➤ Administer ordered premedication 30 to 60 minutes before the procedure.

➤ Observe standard precautions and follow the general guidelines in Appendix A.

Open biopsy:

➤ Record baseline vital signs. After administration of anesthesia, a surgical incision is made, suspicious areas are located, and tissue samples collected.

Percutaneous needle biopsy:

➤ Help the patient to a supine or left lateral position with the right hand under the head. Record baseline vital signs. After the site has been cleansed with antiseptic, a local anesthetic is injected and a sterile field is prepared. The patient is instructed to take a deep breath, exhale forcefully, and hold the breath while the needle is inserted under sterile conditions. The needle is rotated to obtain a core of liver tissue and then removed. Once the needle is removed, the patient may breathe. A pressure dressing is then applied.

➤ Place tissue samples in formalin solution. Label the specimen, indicating site location, and promptly transport it to the laboratory.

Post-test:

➤ Instruct the patient to resume usual diet as directed by the health care practitioner.

➤ After open biopsy, monitor vital signs every 15 minutes for 1 hour, then every 2 hours for 4 hours, and as ordered. Take temperature every 4 hours for 24 hours.

➤ After local anesthesia, monitor vital signs and compare with baseline values.

➤ After percutaneous biopsy, instruct the patient to stay in bed lying on the affected side for at least 2 hours with a pillow or rolled towel under the site to prevent bleeding. The patient will also need to remain on bed rest for 24 hours.

➤ Instruct the patient in the care and assessment of the site, observe for bleeding, hematoma formation, bile leakage, and inflammation. Note any pleuritic pain, persistent right shoulder pain, or abdominal pain.

➤ Recognize anxiety related to test results and offer support. Provide teaching and information regarding the clinical implications of the test results, as appropriate. Educate the patient regarding access to counseling services.

➤ Evaluate test results in relation to the patient's symptoms and other tests performed. Related laboratory tests include alanine aminotransferase, albumin, alkaline phosphatase, α_1-antitrypsin/phenotyping, ammonia, amylase, antimitochondrial antibody, anti–smooth muscle antibody, aspartate aminotransferase, bilirubin, bilirubin fractions, cholesterol, coagulation factor assays, complete blood count, copper, γ-glutamyl transpeptidase, infectious mononucleosis screen, lipase, prothrombin time, and urinalysis.

BIOPSY, LUNG

SYNONYM/ACRONYM: Transbronchial lung biopsy, open lung biopsy.

SPECIMEN: Lung tissue or cells.

REFERENCE VALUE: (Method: Macroscopic and microscopic examination of tissue) No abnormal tissue or cells; no growth in culture.

DESCRIPTION: A biopsy of the lung is performed to obtain lung tissue for examination of pathologic features. The specimen can be obtained transbronchially or by open lung biopsy. In a transbronchial biopsy, forceps pass through the bronchoscope to obtain the specimen. In a transbronchial needle aspiration biopsy, a needle passes through a bronchoscope to obtain the specimen. In a transcatheter bronchial brushing, a brush is inserted through the bronchoscope. In an open lung biopsy, the chest is opened and a small thoracic incision is made to remove tissue from the chest wall. Lung biopsies are used to differentiate between infection and other sources of disease indicated by initial radiology studies, computed tomography scans, or sputum analysis. Specimens are cultured to detect pathogenic organisms or directly examined for the presence of malignant cells. ■

INDICATIONS:

• Assist in the diagnosis of lung cancer

• Assist in the diagnosis of fibrosis and degenerative or inflammatory diseases of the lung

• Assist in the diagnosis of sarcoidosis

RESULT

Abnormal findings in:

• Amyloidosis

• Cancer

• Granulomas

• Infections caused by *Blastomyces, Histoplasma, Legionella* spp., and *Pneumocystis carinii*

• Sarcoidosis

• Systemic lupus erythematosus

• Tuberculosis

CRITICAL VALUES:

• Shortness of breath, cyanosis, or rapid pulse during the procedure must be reported immediately.

• Any postprocedural decrease in breath sounds noted at the biopsy site should be reported immediately.

INTERFERING FACTORS:

• Conditions such as vascular anomalies of the lung, bleeding abnormalities, or pulmonary hypertension may increase the risk of bleeding.

• Conditions such as bullae or cysts and respiratory insufficiency increase the risk of pneumothorax.

Nursing Implications and Procedure • • • • • • • • • •

Pretest:

➤ Obtain a history of the patient's complaints, including a list of known allergens.

➤ Obtain a history of the patient's immune and respiratory systems, any bleeding disorders, and results of previously performed tests and procedures, especially bleeding time, clotting time, complete blood count, partial thromboplastin time, platelets, and prothrombin time. For related tests, refer to the immune and respiratory system tables.

➤ Obtain a list of the medications the patient is taking, including anticoagulant therapy, acetylsalicylic acid, herbs, and nutraceuticals known to affect coagulation. These products should be discontinued 14 days before dental or surgical procedures. The requesting health care practitioner and laboratory should be advised if the patient regularly uses these products so their effects can be taken into consideration when reviewing results.

➤ There are no medication restrictions unless by medical direction.

➤ Instruct the patient to fast and refrain from taking liquids beginning midnight of the day before the bronchoscopy or open lung biopsy procedure is to be performed.

➤ Review the procedure with the patient. Sensitivity to cultural and social issues, as well as concern for modesty, is important in providing psychological support.

➤ Address concerns about pain related to the procedure. Explain that a sedative and/or anesthetic will be administered before the procedure to promote relaxation and reduce discomfort during the procedure. General anesthesia will be administered for open biopsy. Atropine is usually given before bronchoscopy examinations to reduce bronchial secretions and prevent vagally induced bradycardia. Meperidine (Demerol) or morphine may be given as a sedative. Lidocaine is sprayed in the patient's throat to reduce discomfort caused by the presence of the tube.

➤ Assess if the patient has an allergy to local anesthetics, and inform the health care practitioner accordingly.

➤ Ensure that nonallergy to anesthesia is confirmed before the open biopsy procedure is performed under general anesthesia.

➤ *Obtain written and informed consent before administering any medications prior to the procedure.*

➤ Inform the patient that the fine-needle biopsy procedure will be performed by a surgeon under sterile conditions and will take approximately 30 minutes. A bronchoscopy usually takes 15 to 30 minutes.

Intratest:

➤ Ensure that the patient is in compliance with pretesting dietary restrictions. Direct the patient to breathe normally and to avoid unnecessary movement, because coughing or sudden movements could result in perforation of the lung.

➤ Observe standard precautions and follow the general guidelines in Appendix A.

➤ Administer any ordered premedication 30 to 60 minutes before the procedure.

Needle biopsy:

➤ Assist patient to a sitting position with arms on a pillow over a bed table. Record baseline vital signs. Clean site with antiseptic, administer anesthesia, and drape area with sterile towels. Instruct patient to remain still and to avoid coughing during the procedure. The needle is inserted through the posterior chest wall and into the intercostal space. The needle is rotated to obtain the sample and then withdrawn. Pressure is applied to the site, and a pressure dressing is applied.

Bronchoscopy:

➤ Record baseline vital signs. The patient is positioned in relation to the type of anesthesia being used. For general anesthesia, the patient is placed in a supine position with the neck hyperextended. If local anesthesia is used, the patient is seated while the tongue and oropharynx are sprayed and swabbed with anesthetic. The patient is then helped to a supine or side-lying position and the bronchoscope is inserted. After inspection, the tissue samples are collected from suspicious sites by bronchial brush or biopsy forceps.

Open biopsy:

➤ Record baseline vital signs. The patient is prepared for thoracotomy under general anesthesia in the operating room. Tissue specimens are collected from suspicious sites. A chest tube is inserted after the procedure.

➤ Carefully observe the patient for any signs of respiratory distress during the procedure.

➤ Place specimen from needle aspiration or brushing on clean glass microscope slides. Place tissue or aspirate specimens in appropriate sterile container for culture or appropriate fixative container for histologic studies.

➤ Label the specimen, indicating site location, especially left or right; promptly transport the specimen to the laboratory.

Post-test:

➤ After general anesthesia, monitor vital signs every 15 minutes for 1 hour, then every 2 hours for 4 hours, and as ordered. Take temperature every 4 hours for 24 hours.

➤ After local anesthesia, monitor vital signs and compare with baseline values.

➤ Instruct the patient not to eat or drink until the effects of the anesthesia have worn off and the gag reflex has returned to avoid accidental aspiration.

➤ Instruct the patient to resume usual diet as directed by the health care practitioner.

➤ Observe the patient for hemoptysis, difficulty breathing, cough, air hunger, or absent breathing sounds over the affected area. Monitor chest tube patency and drainage after a thoracotomy.

➤ Evaluate the patient for symptoms indicating the development of pneumothorax, such as dyspnea, tachypnea, anxiety, decreased breathing sounds, or restlessness. A chest x-ray may be ordered to check for the presence of this complication.

➤ Evaluate the patient for symptoms of empyema, such as fever, tachycardia, malaise, or elevated white blood cell count.

➤ Observe the patient's sputum for blood if a biopsy was taken, because large amounts of blood may indicate the development of a problem; a small amount of streaking is expected. Evaluate the patient for signs of bleeding such as tachycardia, hypotension, or restlessness.

➤ Instruct the patient to remain in a semi-Fowler's position after bronchoscopy or fine needle aspiration to maximize ventilation. Semi-Fowler's position is a semisitting position with the knees flexed and supported by pillows on the bed or examination table.

➤ Emergency resuscitation equipment should be readily available if the vocal cords become spastic after intubation. Some hoarseness is expected after intubation.

➤ Instruct the patient to use lozenges or gargle for throat discomfort.

➤ Inform the patient of smoking cessation programs as appropriate.

➤ Inform the patient of the importance of medical follow-up. Recognize anxiety related to test results and provide support. Provide teaching and information regarding the clinical implications of the test results. Educate the patient regarding access to counseling services, as appropriate. Malnutrition is commonly seen in patients with severe respiratory disease for numerous reasons including fatigue, lack of appetite, and gastrointestinal distress. Adequate intake of vitamins A and C are also important to prevent pulmonary infection and to decrease the extent of lung tissue damage. The importance of following the prescribed diet should be stressed to the patient/caregiver.

➤ Evaluate test results in relation to the patient's symptoms and other tests performed. Related laboratory tests include arterial/alveolar oxygen ratio, antiglomerular basement membrane antibody, blood gases, complete blood count, culture and Gram/acid-fast stain, cytology, and sputum findings.

BIOPSY, LYMPH NODE

Synonym/Acronym: N/A.

Specimen: Lymph node tissue or cells.

REFERENCE VALUE: (Method: Macroscopic and microscopic examination of tissue) No abnormal tissue or cells.

DESCRIPTION: Lymph node biopsy is the excision of a tissue sample from one or more lymph nodes for microscopic analysis to determine cell morphology and the presence of tissue abnormalities. This test assists in confirming a diagnosis of cancer, diagnosing disorders causing systemic illness, or determining the stage of metastatic cancer. A biopsy specimen is usually obtained either by needle biopsy or after surgical incision. Biopsies are most commonly performed on the following types of lymph nodes: cervical nodes, which drain the face and scalp; axillary nodes, which drain the arms, breasts, and upper chest; and inguinal nodes, which drain the legs, external genitalia, and lower abdominal wall. ■

INDICATIONS:

• Assist in confirming suspected fungal or parasitic infections of the lymphatics

• Assist in confirming suspected malignant involvement of the lymphatics

• Determine the stage of metastatic cancer

• Differentiate between benign and malignant disorders that may cause lymph node enlargement

• Evaluate persistent enlargement of one or more lymph nodes for unknown reasons

RESULT

Abnormal findings in:

• Chancroid

• Fungal infection (e.g., cat scratch disease)

• Immunodeficiency

• Infectious mononucleosis

• Lymph involvement of systemic diseases (e.g., systemic lupus erythematosus, sarcoidosis)

• Lymphangitis

• Lymphogranuloma venereum

• Malignancy (e.g., lymphomas, leukemias)

• Metastatic disease

• Parasitic infestation (e.g., pneumoconiosis)

CRITICAL VALUES: N/A

INTERFERING FACTORS: This procedure is contraindicated in patients with bleeding disorders.

Nursing Implications and Procedure

Pretest:

➤ Obtain a history of the patient's complaints, including a list of known allergens.

➤ Obtain a history of the patient's immune and musculoskeletal systems, any bleeding disorders, and results of previously performed tests and procedures, especially bleeding time, clotting time, complete blood count, partial thromboplastin time, platelets, and prothrombin time. For related tests, refer to the immune and musculoskeletal system tables.

➤ Obtain a list of the medications that the patient is taking, including anticoagulant therapy, acetylsalicylic acid, herbs, and nutraceuticals known to affect coagulation. These products should be discontinued 14 days before dental or surgical procedures. The requesting health care practitioner and laboratory should be advised if the patient regularly uses these products so their effects can be taken into consideration when reviewing results.

➤ There are no medication restrictions unless by medical direction.

➤ Explain that food and fluids are restricted beginning at midnight of the day before the open biopsy procedure. There are usually no such restrictions before needle biopsy.

➤ Review the procedure with the patient. Sensitivity to cultural and social issues, as well as concern for modesty, is important in providing psychological support.

➤ Address concerns about pain related to the procedure. Explain that a sedative will be administered to promote relaxation and reduce discomfort during percutaneous needle biopsy, and a general anesthetic will be administered before the open biopsy.

➤ Assess if the patient has an allergy to local anesthetics, and inform the health care practitioner accordingly.

➤ Confirm nonallergy to anesthesia before the open biopsy procedure is performed under general anesthesia.

➤ *Obtain written and informed consent before administering any medications prior to the procedure.*

➤ Inform the patient that it may be necessary to shave the site before specimen collection.

➤ Inform the patient that the procedure is performed under sterile conditions by a surgeon and usually takes about 30 minutes to complete. Needle biopsy should take about 15 minutes.

Intratest:

➤ Ensure that the patient has complied with pretesting dietary restrictions.

➤ Observe standard precautions and follow the general guidelines in Appendix A.

➤ Administer ordered premedication.

Open biopsy:

➤ Record baseline vital signs. After administration of local anesthetic (for surface nodes) or general anesthesia (for deeper nodes), a surgical incision is made; the suspicious nodes are then located, grasped with forceps, and removed. The site is closed and a sterile dressing is applied.

Percutaneous needle biopsy:

➤ Assist the patient to a position that exposes the affected node. Record baseline vital signs. After the site has been cleansed with antiseptic solution, a local anesthetic is injected and a sterile field is prepared. The node is grasped with the fingers, and a needle (with attached syringe) is inserted directly into the node. The node is aspirated to collect the specimen. A sterile dressing is applied.

➤ Label the specimen, indicating site location, and promptly transport it to the laboratory.

Post-test:

➤ Instruct the patient to resume usual diet as directed by the health care practitioner.

➤ After open biopsy, monitor vital signs every 15 minutes for 1 hour, and then every 2 hours for 4 hours, and as ordered. Take temperature every 4 hours for 24 hours.

➤ After local anesthesia, monitor vital signs and compare with baseline values.

➤ Inspect biopsy site for excessive bleeding.

➤ Instruct the patient in the care and assessment of the site. Instruct the patient to keep the site clean and change the dressing as needed to avoid risk of infection resulting from altered skin integrity.

➤ Instruct the patient to report any redness, edema, bleeding, or pain at the biopsy site.

➤ Administer a mild analgesic as ordered.

➤ Recognize anxiety related to test

results and offer support. Provide teaching and information regarding the clinical implications of the test results, as appropriate. Educate the patient regarding access to counseling services.

➤ Evaluate test results in relation to the patient's symptoms and other tests performed. Related laboratory tests include CD4/CD8 enumeration; cerebrospinal fluid analysis; *Chlamydia* serology; culture for bacteria/fungus; complete blood count; cytomegalovirus serology; Gram stain; HIV-1/HIV-2 serology; immunofixation electrophoresis; immunoglobulins A, G, and M; infectious mononucleosis screen; rheumatoid factor; total protein; total protein electrophoresis; and toxoplasmosis serology.

BIOPSY, MUSCLE

SYNONYM/ACRONYM: N/A.

SPECIMEN: Muscle tissue or cells.

REFERENCE VALUE: (Method: Macroscopic and microscopic examination of tissue) No abnormal tissue or cells.

DESCRIPTION: Muscle biopsy is the excision of a tissue sample from one of many muscles for microscopic analysis to determine cell morphology and the presence of tissue abnormalities. This test is used to confirm a diagnosis of neuropathy or myopathy and to diagnose parasitic infestation. A biopsy specimen is usually obtained from the deltoid or gastrocnemius muscle after a surgical incision. ■

INDICATIONS:
• Assist in confirming suspected fungal infection or parasitic infestation of the muscle

• Assist in diagnosing the cause of neuropathy or myopathy

• Assist in the diagnosis of Duchenne's muscular dystrophy

RESULT

Abnormal findings in:
• Alcoholic myopathy

• Amyotrophic lateral sclerosis

• Duchenne's muscular dystrophy

• Fungal infection

• Myasthenia gravis

• Myotonia congenita

• Parasitic infestation

• Polymyalgia rheumatica

• Polymyositis

CRITICAL VALUES: N/A

INTERFERING FACTORS:
• If electromyography is performed

before muscle biopsy, residual inflammation may lead to false-positive biopsy results.

• This procedure is contraindicated ⚠ in patients with bleeding disorders.

Nursing Implications and Procedure • • • • • • • • • • •

Pretest: ■

➤ Obtain a history of the patient's complaints, including a list of known allergens.

➤ Obtain a history of the patient's immune and musculoskeletal systems, any bleeding disorders, and results of previously performed tests and procedures, especially bleeding time, clotting time, complete blood count, partial thromboplastin time, platelets, and prothrombin time. For related tests, refer to the immune and musculoskeletal system tables.

➤ Obtain a list of the medications the patient is taking, including anticoagulant therapy, acetylsalicylic acid, herbs, and nutraceuticals known to affect coagulation. These products should be discontinued 14 days before dental or surgical procedures. The requesting health care practitioner and laboratory should be advised if the patient regularly uses these products so their effects can be taken into consideration when reviewing results.

➤ Note any recent procedures that can interfere with test results.

➤ There are no food, fluid, or medication restrictions unless by medical direction.

➤ Review the procedure with the patient. Sensitivity to cultural and social issues, as well as concern for modesty, is important in providing psychological support.

➤ Address concerns about pain related to the procedure. Inform the patient that a sedative will be administered to promote relaxation and reduce discomfort during the procedure.

➤ Assess if the patient has an allergy to local anesthetics, and inform the health care practitioner accordingly.

➤ *Obtain written and informed consent before administering any medications prior to the procedure.*

➤ Inform the patient that it may be necessary to shave the site before specimen collection.

➤ Inform the patient the procedure will be performed under sterile conditions by a surgeon and that it usually takes about 15 minutes to complete. Sutures may be necessary to close the site.

Intratest: ■

➤ Record baseline vital signs.

➤ Direct the patient to breathe normally and to avoid unnecessary movement.

➤ Observe standard precautions and follow the general guidelines in Appendix A.

➤ Administer ordered premedication.

➤ Assist the patient to a supine position (for deltoid biopsy) or prone position (for gastrocnemius biopsy).

➤ Cleanse the site with antiseptic solution and drape with sterile drapes. After infiltration with local anesthetic, a small incision is made over the muscle and a small bit of muscle is grasped with forceps. The area is closed with sutures or similar material and a sterile dressing is applied.

➤ Place tissue samples in normal saline solution. Label the specimen, indicating site location, and promptly transport it to the laboratory.

Post-test: ■

➤ After local anesthesia, monitor vital signs and compare with baseline values.

➤ Inspect biopsy site for excessive bleeding.

➤ Instruct the patient in the care and assessment of the site. Instruct the patient to report any redness, edema, bleeding, or pain at the biopsy site. Instruct the patient to keep the site clean and change the dressing as needed to avoid risk of infection resulting from altered skin integrity.

➤ Inform the patient that the site will be sore and tender and that movement will be difficult for several days.

➤ Administer mild analgesic and antibiotic therapy as ordered. Remind the patient of the importance of completing the entire course of antibiotic therapy, even if signs and symptoms disappear before completion of therapy.

➤ Inform the patient of a follow-up appointment for removal of sutures, if indicated.

➤ Recognize anxiety related to test results and offer support. Provide teaching and information regarding the test results, as appropriate. Educate the patient regarding access to counseling services.

➤ Evaluate test results in relation to the patient's symptoms and other tests performed. Related laboratory tests include acetylcholine receptor antibody, aldolase, antinuclear antibodies, antithyroglobulin antibodies, creatine kinase and isoenzymes, Jo-1 antibody, myoglobin, and rheumatoid factor.

BIOPSY, PROSTATE

· ·

SYNONYM/ACRONYM: N/A.

SPECIMEN: Prostate tissue.

REFERENCE VALUE: (Method: Microscopic examination of tissue cells) No abnormal cells or tissue.

DESCRIPTION: Biopsy of the prostate gland is performed to identify cancerous cells, especially if serum prostate-specific antigen is increased. ■

INDICATIONS:

• Evaluate prostatic hypertrophy of unknown etiology

• Investigate suspected cancer of the prostate

RESULT: Positive findings in prostate cancer.

CRITICAL VALUES: N/A

INTERFERING FACTORS:

• This test is contraindicated in patients with bleeding disorders.

• The various sampling approaches have individual drawbacks that should be considered: transurethral sampling does not always ensure that malignant cells will be included in the specimen, whereas transrectal sampling carries the risk of perforating the rectum and creating a channel through which malignant cells can seed normal tissue.

Nursing Implications and Procedure • • • • • • • • • •

Pretest: ▪

➤ Obtain a history of the patient's complaints, including a list of known allergens.

➤ Obtain a history of the patient's immune and reproductive systems, any bleeding disorders, and results of previously performed tests and procedures, especially bleeding time, clotting time, complete blood count, partial thromboplastin time, platelets, and prothrombin time. For related tests, refer to the immune and reproductive system tables.

➤ Obtain a list of the medications the patient is taking, including anticoagulant therapy, acetylsalicylic acid, herbs, and nutraceuticals known to affect coagulation. These products should be discontinued 14 days before dental or surgical procedures. The requesting health care practitioner and laboratory should be advised if the patient regularly uses these products so their effects can be taken into consideration when reviewing results.

➤ There are no food, fluid, or medication restrictions unless by medical direction.

➤ Review the procedure with the patient. Sensitivity to cultural and social issues, as well as concern for modesty is important in providing psychological support.

➤ Address concerns about pain related to the procedure. Explain that a local anesthetic will be administered before the procedure and that some discomfort during and after the procedure may be experienced.

➤ Assess if the patient has an allergy to local anesthetics, and inform the health care practitioner accordingly.

➤ *Obtain written and informed consent before administering any medications prior to the procedure.*

➤ In certain cases prophylactic antibiotics may be administered before or after the procedure.

➤ Have the patient void before the procedure. Administer enemas if ordered.

➤ Inform the patient that specimen collection will be performed by a health care practitioner. The specimen collection takes approximately 20 to 30 minutes.

Intratest: ▪

➤ Direct the patient to breathe normally and to avoid unnecessary movement.

➤ Observe standard precautions and follow the general guidelines in Appendix A.

➤ Record baseline vital signs.

Transurethral approach:

➤ Position patient on a urologic examination table with the feet in stirrups. Clean external genitalia with antiseptic solution. Local anesthetic is administered into the urethra and the endoscope is inserted. The tissue is excised with a cutting loop and is placed in formalin solution.

Transrectal approach:

➤ Assist the patient into a Sims' position. A rectal examination is performed to locate suspicious nodules. A biopsy needle guide is placed at the biopsy site, and the biopsy needle is inserted through the needle guide. The cells are aspirated, the needle is withdrawn, and the sample is placed in formalin solution.

Perineal approach:

➤ Position the patient in a jackknife or lithotomy position. Clean the perineum with an antiseptic solution, administer the local anesthetic, and protect the biopsy site with sterile drapes. A small incision is made and the sample is removed by needle biopsy or biopsy punch.

➤ Apply digital pressure to the biopsy site. If there is no bleeding, place a sterile dressing on the biopsy site.

➤ Place tissue samples in formalin solution. Label the specimen, indicating site location, and promptly transport it to the laboratory.

Post-test:

➤ After local anesthesia, monitor vital signs and compare with baseline values.

➤ Monitor urinary output and voiding pattern for 24 hours. Observe appearance of urine.

➤ If the perineal approach was used, observe biopsy site for bleeding or drainage.

➤ Instruct the patient to report any

rectal pain or bleeding, blood in the urine, or fever.

➤ Administer analgesics and antibiotics as ordered, and instruct the patient in the importance of completing the entire course of antibiotic therapy, even if no symptoms are present.

➤ Recognize anxiety related to test results and provide support. Provide teaching and information regarding the test results, as appropriate. Counsel the patient, as appropriate, that sexual dysfunction related to altered body function, drugs, or radiation may occur. Educate the patient regarding access to counseling services, as appropriate.

➤ Evaluate test results in relation to the patient's symptoms and other tests performed. Related laboratory tests include prostate-specific antigen and prostatic acid phosphatase.

BIOPSY, SKIN

SYNONYM/ACRONYM: N/A.

SPECIMEN: Skin tissue or cells.

REFERENCE VALUE: (Method: Macroscopic and microscopic examination of tissue) No abnormal tissue or cells.

DESCRIPTION: Skin biopsy is the excision of a tissue sample from suspicious skin lesions. The microscopic analysis can determine cell morphology and the presence of tissue abnormalities. This test assists in confirming the diagnosis of malignant or benign skin lesions. A skin biopsy can be obtained

by any of these four ways: curettage, shaving, excision, or punch. ■

INDICATIONS:
• Assist in the diagnosis of keratoses, warts, moles, keloids, fibromas, cysts, or inflamed lesions

• Assist in the diagnosis of skin cancer

• Evaluate suspicious skin lesions

RESULT

Abnormal findings in:

• Basal cell carcinoma

• Cysts

• Dermatitis

• Dermatofibroma

• Keloids

• Malignant melanoma

• Pemphigus

• Pigmented nevi

• Neurofibroma

• Seborrheic keratosis

• Skin involvement in systemic lupus erythematosus, discoid lupus erythematosus, and scleroderma

• Squamous cell carcinoma

• Warts

CRITICAL VALUES: N/A

INTERFERING FACTORS: This procedure is contraindicated in patients with bleeding disorders.

Nursing Implications and Procedure • • • • • • • • • •

Pretest:

➤ Obtain a history of the patient's complaints, including a list of known allergens.

➤ Obtain a history of the patient's immune and musculoskeletal systems, any bleeding disorders, and results of previously performed tests and procedures, especially bleeding time, clotting time, complete blood count, partial thromboplastin time, platelets, and prothrombin time. For related tests, refer to the immune and musculoskeletal system tables.

➤ Obtain a list of the medications the patient is taking, including anticoagulant therapy, acetylsalicylic acid, herbs, and nutraceuticals known to affect coagulation. These products should be discontinued 14 days before dental or surgical procedures. The requesting health care practitioner and laboratory should be advised if the patient regularly uses these products so their effects can be taken into consideration when reviewing results.

➤ There are no food, fluid, or medication restrictions unless by medical direction.

➤ Review the procedure with the patient. Sensitivity to cultural and social issues, as well as concern for modesty, is important in providing psychological support.

➤ Address concerns about pain related to the procedure. Inform the patient that a local anesthetic will be administered before the procedure.

➤ Assess if the patient has an allergy to local anesthetics, and inform the health care practitioner accordingly.

➤ *Obtain written and informed consent before administering any medications prior to the procedure.*

➤ Inform the patient that it may be necessary to shave the site before specimen collection.

➤ Inform the patient that the procedure is performed under sterile conditions by a surgeon, that it usually takes about 30 minutes to complete, and that sutures may be necessary to close the site.

Intratest:

➤ Record baseline vital signs.

➤ Assist the patient into a comfortable position in which the biopsy site can be supported and exposed.

➤ Observe standard precautions and follow the general guidelines in Appendix A.

➤ Cleanse the skin with an antiseptic solution. Direct the patient to breathe normally and to avoid unnecessary movement. Administer local anesthetic and protect the site with sterile drapes.

➤ *Curettage:* The skin is scraped with a curette to obtain specimen.

➤ *Shaving or excision:* A scalpel is used to remove a portion of the lesion that protrudes above the epidermis. If the lesion is to be excised, the incision is made as wide and as deep as needed to ensure that the entire lesion is removed. Bleeding is controlled with external pressure to the site. Large wounds are closed with sutures. An adhesive bandage is applied when excision is complete.

➤ *Punch biopsy:* A small, round punch about 4 to 6 mm in diameter is rotated into the skin to the desired depth. The cylinder of skin is pulled upward with forceps and separated at its base with a scalpel or scissors. If needed, sutures are applied. A sterile dressing is applied over the site.

➤ Place tissue samples in formalin solution. Label the specimen, indicating site location, and promptly transport it to the laboratory.

Post-test:

➤ After local anesthesia, monitor vital signs and compare with baseline values.

➤ Inspect biopsy site for excessive bleeding.

➤ Instruct the patient in the care and assessment of the site. Instruct the patient to report any redness, edema, bleeding, or pain at the biopsy site. Instruct the patient to keep the site clean and to change the dressing as needed to avoid risk of infection resulting from altered skin integrity.

➤ Administer mild analgesic and antibiotic therapy as ordered. Remind the patient of the importance of completing the entire course of antibiotic therapy, even if signs and symptoms disappear before completion of therapy.

➤ If indicated, inform the patient of a follow-up appointment for the removal of sutures.

➤ Recognize anxiety related to test results and offer support. Provide teaching and information regarding the clinical implications of the test results, as appropriate. Educate the patient regarding access to counseling services.

➤ Evaluate test results in relation to the patient's symptoms and other tests performed. Related laboratory tests include allergen-specific immunoglobulin E (IgE), IgE, antinuclear antibody, skin culture, eosinophil count, and erythrocyte sedimentation rate.

BIOPSY, THYROID

SYNONYM/ACRONYM: N/A.

SPECIMEN: Thyroid gland tissue or cells.

REFERENCE VALUE: (Method: Macroscopic and microscopic examination of tissue) No abnormal cells or tissue.

DESCRIPTION: Thyroid biopsy is the excision of a tissue sample for microscopic analysis to determine cell morphology and the presence of tissue abnormalities. This test assists in confirming a diagnosis of cancer or determining the cause of persistent thyroid symptoms. A biopsy specimen can be obtained by needle aspiration or by surgical excision. ■

INDICATIONS:

• Assist in the diagnosis of thyroid cancer or benign cysts or tumors

• Determine the cause of inflammatory thyroid disease

• Determine the cause of hyperthyroidism

• Evaluate enlargement of the thyroid gland

RESULT

Positive findings in:

• Benign thyroid cyst

• Granulomatous thyroiditis

• Hashimoto's thyroiditis

• Nontoxic nodular goiter

• Thyroid cancer

CRITICAL VALUES: N/A

INTERFERING FACTORS: This procedure is contraindicated in patients with bleeding disorders.

Nursing Implications and Procedure • • • • • • • • • • •

Pretest:

➤ Obtain a history of the patient's complaints, including a list of known allergens.

➤ Obtain a history of the patient's endocrine and immune systems, any bleeding disorders, and results of previously performed tests and procedures, especially bleeding time, clotting time, complete blood count, partial thromboplastin time, platelets, and prothrombin time. For related tests, refer to the endocrine and immune system tables.

➤ Obtain a list of the medications the patient is taking, including anticoagulant therapy, acetylsalicylic acid, herbs, and nutraceuticals known to affect coagulation. These products should be discontinued 14 days before dental or surgical procedures. The requesting health care practitioner and laboratory should be advised if the patient regularly uses these products so their effects can be taken into consideration when reviewing results.

➤ There are no medication restrictions unless by medical direction.

➤ Explain that food and fluids are not usually restricted for a needle biopsy but are restricted for 6 to 8 hours before open biopsy.

➤ Review the procedure with the patient.

➤ Assess if the patient has an allergy to local anesthetics, and inform the health care practitioner accordingly.

➤ Inform the patient that open biopsy is performed under sterile conditions by a surgeon. Ensure nonallergy to anesthesia is confirmed before the open biopsy procedure is performed under general anesthesia.

➤ *Obtain written and informed consent before administering any medications prior to the procedure.*

➤ Inform the patient that specimen collection by needle biopsy takes approximately 15 minutes. Specimens collected by open biopsy take about 30 minutes.

Intratest:

➤ Ensure that the patient has complied

with dietary restrictions before open biopsy.

➤ Administer ordered sedation. Assist the patient to a comfortable position.

➤ Observe standard precautions and follow the general guidelines in Appendix A.

➤ Cleanse the biopsy site with an antiseptic solution, and drape the area with sterile towels.

Open biopsy:

➤ Record baseline vital signs. After administration of general anesthesia, a surgical incision is made, suspicious areas are located, and tissue samples are collected.

Needle biopsy:

➤ Direct the patient to breathe normally and to avoid unnecessary movement. Instruct the patient not to swallow when the local anesthetic is injected. The biopsy needle is inserted and a sample is obtained. Pressure is applied to the site, and a sterile dressing is applied.

➤ Place tissue samples in formalin solution. Label the specimen, indicating site location, and promptly transport it to the laboratory.

Post-test:

➤ Instruct the patient to resume usual diet as directed by the health care practitioner.

➤ After open biopsy, monitor vital signs every 15 minutes for 1 hour, and then every 2 hours for 4 hours, and as ordered. Take temperature every 4 hours for 24 hours.

➤ After local anesthesia, monitor vital signs and compare with baseline values.

➤ Instruct the patient in the care and assessment of the site. Instruct the patient to report any bleeding, redness, edema, or pain at the site.

➤ Instruct the patient to return for suture removal as indicated.

➤ Recognize anxiety related to test results and offer support. Provide teaching and information regarding the clinical implications of the test results, as appropriate. Educate the patient regarding access to counseling services.

➤ Evaluate test results in relation to the patient's symptoms and other tests performed. Related laboratory tests include antithyroglobulin antibodies, thyroid-stimulating hormone, and free thyroxine.

BLADDER CANCER MARKERS, URINE

• •

SYNONYMS/ACRONYMS: NMP22, Bard BTA.

SPECIMEN: Urine (5 mL), unpreserved random specimen collected in a clean plastic collection container.

REFERENCE VALUE: (Method: Enzyme immunoassay for NMP22, immunochromatographic for Bard BTA)

NMP22: Less than 10 units/mL

Bard BTA: Negative

DESCRIPTION: Cystoscopy is still considered the gold standard for detection of bladder cancer, but other noninvasive tests are being developed including several urine assays approved by the Food and Drug Administration. Compared to cytologic studies, these assays are believed to be more sensitive but less specific for detecting transitional cell carcinoma.

NMP22: Nuclear matrix proteins (NMPs) are involved in the regulation and expression of various genes. The NMP identified as NuMA is abundant in bladder tumor cells. The dying tumor cells release the soluble NMP into the urine. This assay is quantitative.

Bladder tumor antigen (BTA): A human complement factor H–related protein (hCFHrp) is thought to be produced by bladder tumor cells as protection from the body's natural immune response. The bladder tumor antigen is released from tumor cells into the urine. This assay is qualitative. ∎

INDICATIONS:

• Detection of bladder carcinoma

• Management of recurrent bladder cancer

RESULT: Increased in bladder carcinoma.

CRITICAL VALUES: N/A

INTERFERING FACTORS:

• *NMP22:* Any condition that results in inflammation of the bladder or urinary tract may cause falsely elevated values.

• *Bard BTA:* Recent surgery, biopsy, or other trauma to the bladder or urinary tract may cause falsely elevated values. Active urinary tract infection, renal or bladder calculi, gross hemolysis, and positive leukocyte dipstick may also cause false-positive results.

Nursing Implications and Procedure ● ● ● ● ● ● ● ● ● ● ●

Pretest: ■

➤ Obtain a history of the patient's complaints, including a list of known allergens.

➤ Obtain a history of the patient's genitourinary and immune systems, as well as results of previously performed tests and procedures. For related tests, refer to the genitourinary and immune system tables.

➤ Obtain a list of the medications the patient is taking, including herbs, nutritional supplements, and nutraceuticals. The requesting health care practitioner and laboratory should be advised if the patient regularly uses these products so their effects can be taken into consideration when reviewing results.

➤ There are no food, fluid, or medication restrictions unless by medical direction.

➤ Review the procedure with the patient.

➤ Inform the patient that specimen collection takes approximately 5 minutes.

Intratest: ■

➤ Observe standard precautions and follow the general guidelines in Appendix A.

➤ Obtain urine specimen in a clean plastic collection container. Label the specimen, and promptly transport it to the laboratory.

Post-test: ■

➤ Recognize anxiety related to test

results and offer support. Provide teaching and information regarding the clinical implications of the test results, as appropriate. Educate the patient regarding access to counseling services.

➤ Evaluate test results in relation to the patient's symptoms and other tests performed. Related laboratory tests include bladder biopsy and urine cytology.

BLEEDING TIME

· ·

SYNONYM/ACRONYM: Mielke bleeding time, Simplate bleeding time, Template bleeding time, Surgicutt, Ivy bleeding time.

SPECIMEN: Whole blood.

REFERENCE VALUE: (Method: Timed observation of incision)

Template: 2.5 to 10 minutes
Ivy: 2 to 7 minutes
There are slight differences in the disposable devices used to make the incision. Although the Mielke or Template bleeding time is believed to offer greater standardization to a fairly subjective procedure, both methods are thought to be of equal sensitivity and reproducibility.

DESCRIPTION: Bleeding time assesses platelet and capillary function. ■

INDICATIONS:
• Assess platelet and capillary function

• Evaluate ecchymosis, unexplained bleeding or bruising, and tendency to bleed

• Screen for coagulopathy

RESULT:
This test does not predict excessive bleeding during a surgical procedure.

Prolonged in:
• Bernard-Soulier syndrome

• Fibrinogen disorders

• Glanzmann's thrombasthenia

• Hereditary telangiectasia

• Liver disease

• Macroglobulinemia

• Some myeloproliferative disorders

• Renal disease

• Thrombocytopenia

• von Willebrand's disease

Decreased in: N/A

CRITICAL VALUES: N/A

INTERFERING FACTORS:
• Drugs that may prolong bleeding time include acetylsalicylic acid, aminocaproic acid, ampicillin, asparaginase, carbenicillin, cefoperazone, cilostazol, dextran, diltiazem, ethanol, flurbiprofen, fluroxene, halothane, heparin, ketorolac, mezlocillin, mox-

alactam, nafcillin, naproxen, nifedipine, nonsteroidal anti-inflammatory drugs, penicillin, piroxicam, plicamycin, propranolol, streptokinase, sulindac, ticarcillin, tolmetin, urokinase, valproic acid, and warfarin.

• Drugs that may decrease bleeding time include desmopressin and erythropoietin.

• The test should not be performed on ⚠ patients who must be restrained, have excessively cold or edematous arms, have a platelet count less than 50,000/mm^3, have an infectious skin disease, or cannot have a blood pressure cuff placed on the arm.

Nursing Implications and Procedure • • • • • • • • • •

Pretest: ∎

➤ Obtain a history of the patient's complaints, including a list of known allergens.

➤ Obtain a history of the patient's hematopoietic system, as well as results of previously performed tests and procedures. For related tests, refer to the hematopoietic system table.

➤ Obtain a list of the medications the patient is taking, including herbs, nutritional supplements, and nutraceuticals. The requesting health care practitioner and laboratory should be advised if the patient regularly uses these products so their effects can be taken into consideration when reviewing results.

➤ There are no food or fluid restrictions unless by medical direction.

➤ The test should not be performed until a minimum of 10 days after the last dose of any medication containing acetylsalicylic acid.

➤ Review the procedure with the patient. Inform the patient that scarring, keloid formation, or infection may occur.

➤ Inform the patient that specimen collection takes approximately 2 to 15 minutes.

Intratest: ∎

➤ Direct the patient to breathe normally and to avoid unnecessary movement.

➤ Ensure that the patient has complied with pretesting restrictions.

➤ Observe standard precautions and follow the general guidelines in Appendix A.

➤ Place a blood pressure cuff on the arm above the elbow and inflate to 40 mm Hg. Cleanse the site with alcohol and wait until it is air-dry. Hold skin taut. Avoid superficial veins and use bleeding time device to make a parallel incision about 3 mm deep into the muscular outside area of the forearm distal to the antecubital fossa (in the direction of wrist to elbow). Start stopwatch immediately. At 30-second intervals, blot the incision site, in a clockwise fashion, on the edge of a piece of filter paper. The test concludes when the bleeding stops or if bleeding continues longer than 15 minutes. Bleeding time is determined by adding the total number of blots on the filter paper (30 seconds or 0.5 minutes.

Post-test: ∎

➤ Instruct the patient to resume usual medication as directed by the health care practitioner.

➤ Observe the incision site for bleeding. It may be necessary to place a dressing or butterfly bandage on the site after the test.

➤ Inform the patient with a bleeding disorder of the importance of taking precautions against bruising and bleeding. These precautions may include the use of soft-bristle toothbrush, use of an electric razor, avoidance of constipation, avoidance of acetylsalicylic acid and similar products, and avoidance of intramuscular injections.

➤ Evaluate test results in relation to the patient's symptoms and other tests.

▌ Related laboratory tests include clot retraction and platelet count.

BLOOD GASES

SYNONYMS/ACRONYM: Arterial blood gases (ABGs), venous blood gases, capillary blood gases, cord blood gases.

SPECIMEN: Whole blood. Specimen volume and collection container may vary with collection method. See Intratest section for specific collection instructions. Specimen should be tightly capped and transported in an ice slurry.

REFERENCE VALUE: (Method: Selective electrodes for pH, pCO_2 and pO_2)

Blood Gas Value (pH)	Birth, Cord, Full Term	Adult/Child
Arterial	7.11–7.36	7.35–7.45
Venous	7.25–7.45	7.32–7.43
Capillary	7.32–7.49	7.35–7.45
Scalp	7.25–7.40	N/A

SI units (conversion factor ×1).

pCO_2	Arterial	SI Units (Conversion Factor ×0.133)	Venous	SI Units (Conversion Factor ×0.133)	Capillary	SI Units (Conversion Factor ×0.133)
Birth, cord, full term	32–66 mm Hg	4.3–8.8 kPa	27–49 mm Hg	3.6–6.5 kPa	—	—
Adult/child	35–45 mm Hg	4.66–5.98 kPa	41–51 mm Hg	5.4–6.8 kPa	26–41 mm Hg	3.5–5.4 kPa

pO_2	Arterial	SI Units (Conversion Factor ×0.133)	Venous	SI Units (Conversion Factor ×0.133)	Capillary	SI Units (Conversion Factor ×0.133)
Birth, cord, full term	8–24 mm Hg	1.1–3.2 kPa	17–41 mm Hg	2.3–5.4 kPa	—	—
Adult/child	80–95 mm Hg	10.6–12.6 kPa	20–49 mm Hg	2.6–6.5 kPa	80–95 mm Hg	10.6–12.6 kPa

HCO$_3^-$	Arterial SI Units mmol/L (Conversion Factor ×1)	Venous SI Units mmol/L (Conversion Factor ×1)	Capillary SI Units mmol/L (Conversion Factor ×1)
Birth, cord, full term	17–24 mEq/L	17–24 mEq/L	N/A
Adult/child	18–23 mEq/L	24–28 mEq/L	18–23 mEq/L

O$_2$ Sat	Arterial	Venous	Capillary
Birth, cord, full term	40–90%	40–70%	—
Adult/child	95–99%	70–75%	95–98%

SI Units (conversion factor ×.01)

tCO$_2$	Arterial SI Units mmol/L (Conversion Factor ×1)	Venous SI Units mmol/L (Conversion Factor ×1)
Birth, cord, full term	13–22 mEq/L	14–22 mEq/L
Adult/child	22–29 mEq/L	25–30 mEq/L

BE Arterial	SI Units mmol/L (Conversion Factor ×1)
Birth, cord, full term	(−10)–(−2) mEq/L
Adult/child	(−2)–(+3) mEq/L

DESCRIPTION: Blood gas analysis is used to evaluate respiratory function and provide a measure for determining acid-base balance. Respiratory, renal, and cardiovascular system functions are integrated in order to maintain normal acid-base balance. Therefore, respiratory or metabolic disorders may cause abnormal blood gas findings. The blood gas measurements commonly reported are pH, partial pressure of carbon dioxide in the blood (pCO$_2$), partial pressure of oxygen in the blood (pO$_2$), bicarbonate (HCO$_3^-$), O$_2$ saturation, and base excess (BE) or base deficit (BD). pH reflects the number of free hydrogen ions (H$^+$) in the body. A pH less than 7.35 indicates acidosis. A pH greater than 7.45 indicates alkalosis. Changes in the ratio of free hydrogen ions to bicarbonate will result in a compensatory response from the lungs or kidneys to restore proper acid-base balance.

pCO$_2$ is an important indicator of ventilation. The level of pCO$_2$ is controlled primarily by the lungs and is referred to as the respiratory component of acid-base balance. The main buffer system in the body is the bicarbonate–carbonic acid system. Bicarbonate (HCO$_3^-$) is an important alkaline ion that participates along with other anions such as hemoglobin, proteins, and phosphates to neutralize acids. For the body to maintain proper balance, there must be a ratio of 20 parts bicarbonate to one part carbonic acid (20:1). Carbonic acid level is indirectly measured by pCO_2. Bicarbonate level is indirectly measured by the total carbon dioxide content (tCO_2). Carbonic acid levels are not measured directly, but can be estimated because it is 3 percent of the pCO_2. Bicarbonate can also be calculated from these numbers once the carbonic acid value has been obtained because of the 20:1 ratio. For example, if the pCO_2 was 40, the carbonic acid would be 1.2 ($3\% \times 40$) and the HCO_3^- would be 24 (20×1.2). The main acid in the acid-base system is carbonic acid. It is the metabolic or nonrespiratory component of the acid-base system and is controlled by the kidney. Bicarbonate levels can either be measured directly or estimated from the tCO_2 in the blood. BE/BD reflects the amount of anions available in the blood to help buffer changes in pH. A BD (negative BE) indicates metabolic acidosis, whereas positive BE indicates metabolic alkalosis.

Extremes in acidosis are generally more life threatening than alkalosis. Acidosis can develop either very quickly (e.g., cardiac arrest) or over a longer period of time (e.g., renal failure). Infants can develop acidosis very quickly if they are not kept warm and given enough calories. Children with diabetes tend to go into acidosis more quickly than do adults who have been dealing with the disease over a longer period of time. In many cases a venous or capillary specimen is satisfactory to obtain the necessary information regarding acid-base balance

without subjecting the patient to an arterial puncture with its associated risks.

As seen in the table of reference ranges, pO_2 is lower in infants than in children and adults owing to the respective level of maturation of the lungs at birth. pO_2 tends to trail off after age 30 years, by approximately 3 to 5 mm Hg per decade as the organs age and begin to lose elasticity. There is a formula that can be used to approximate the relationship between age and pO_2:

$$pO_2 = 104 - (\text{age} \times 0.27).$$

Like carbon dioxide, oxygen is carried in the body in a dissolved and combined (oxyhemoglobin) form. Oxygen content is the sum of the dissolved and combined oxygen. The oxygen-carrying capacity of the blood indicates how much oxygen could be carried if all the hemoglobin were saturated with oxygen. Percent oxygen saturation is oxygen content divided by oxygen content times 100.

Specimens other than arterial specimen are often ordered when oxygen measurements are not needed or when the information regarding oxygen can be obtained by noninvasive techniques such as pulse oximetry. Capillary blood is satisfactory for most purposes for pH and pCO_2; the use of capillary pO_2 is limited to the exclusion of hypoxia. Measurements involving oxygen are usually not useful when performed on venous samples; arterial blood is required to accurately measure pO_2 and oxygen saturation. There is considerable evidence that prolonged exposure to high levels of oxygen can result in injury, such as retinopathy of prematurity in infants or the drying of airways in any patient. Monitoring pO_2 from blood gases is especially appropriate under such circumstances. ■

INDICATIONS:

This group of tests is used to assess conditions such as asthma, chronic obstructive pulmonary disease (COPD), embolism (e.g., fatty or other embolism) during coronary arterial bypass surgery, and hypoxia. It is also used to assist in the diagnosis of respiratory failure, which is defined as a pO_2 less than 50 mm Hg and pCO_2 greater than 50 mm Hg. Blood gases can be valuable in the management of patients on ventilators or being weaned from ventilators. Blood gas values are used to determine acid-base status, the type of imbalance, and the degree of compensation as summarized in the following section. Restoration of pH to near-normal values is referred to as fully compensated balance. When pH values are moving in the same direction (i.e., increasing or decreasing) as the pCO_2 or HCO_3^-, the imbalance is metabolic. When the pH values are moving in the opposite direction from the pCO_2 or HCO_3^-, the imbalance is caused by respiratory disturbances. To remember this concept, the following mnemonic can be useful: MeTRO = *Me*tabolic *T*ogether, *R*espiratory *O*pposite.

Acid-Base Disturbance	pH	pCO_2	pO_2	BE
Respiratory Acidosis				
Uncompensated	Decreased	Increased	Normal	Normal
Compensated	Normal	Increased	Increased	Increased
Respiratory Alkalosis				
Uncompensated	Increased	Decreased	Normal	Normal
Compensated	Normal	Decreased	Decreased	Decreased
Metabolic (Nonrespiratory) Acidosis				
Uncompensated	Decreased	Normal	Decreased	Decreased
Compensated	Normal	Decreased	Decreased	Decreased
Metabolic (Nonrespiratory) Alkalosis				
Uncompensated	Increased	Normal	Increased	Increased
Compensated	Normal	Increased	Increased	Increased

RESULT:

• Acid-base imbalance is determined by evaluating pH, pCO_2, and HCO_3^- values. pH less than 7.35 reflects an acidic state, whereas pH greater than 7.45 reflects alkalosis. pCO_2 and HCO_3^- determine whether the imbalance is respiratory or nonrespiratory. Because a patient may have more than one imbalance and may also be in the process of compensating, the interpretation of blood gas values may not always seem straightforward.

• Respiratory conditions that interfere with normal breathing will cause CO_2 to be retained in the blood. This results in an increase of circulating carbonic acid and a corresponding decrease in pH (respiratory acidosis). Acute respiratory acidosis can occur in acute pulmonary edema, severe respiratory infections, bronchial obstruction, pneumothorax, hemothorax, open chest wounds, opiate poisoning, respiratory depressant drug therapy, and inhalation of air with a high CO_2 content. Chronic respiratory acidosis can be seen in patients with asthma, pulmonary fibrosis, emphysema, bronchiectasis, and respiratory depressant drug therapy. Alternately, respiratory conditions that increase the breathing rate will cause CO_2 to be removed from the alveoli more rapidly than it is being produced. This will result in an alkaline pH. Acute respiratory alkalosis may be seen in anxiety, hysteria, hyperventilation, pulmonary embolus, and an increase in artificial ventilation. Chronic respiratory alkalosis may be seen in high fever, administration of drugs (e.g., salicylate and sulfa) that stimulate the respiratory system, hepatic coma, hypoxia of high altitude, and central nervous system (CNS) lesions or injury that result in stimulation of the respiratory center.

- Metabolic (nonrespiratory) conditions that cause the excessive formation or decreased excretion of organic or inorganic acids result in metabolic acidosis. Some of these conditions include ingestion of salicylates, ethylene glycol, and methanol, as well as uncontrolled diabetes, starvation, shock, renal disease, diarrhea, and biliary or pancreatic fistula. Metabolic alkalosis results from conditions that increase pH, as can be seen in excessive intake of antacids to treat gastritis or peptic ulcer, excessive administration of HCO_3^-, loss of stomach acid caused by protracted vomiting, cystic fibrosis, or potassium and chloride deficiencies.

Increased:
- pH (metabolic alkalosis):
  Alkali ingestion (excessive)
  Gastric suctioning
  Potassium depletion: Cushing's disease, diarrhea, diuresis, excessive vomiting, excessive ingestion of licorice, inadequate potassium intake, potassium-losing nephropathy, steroid administration
- pH (respiratory alkalosis):
  CNS lesions or injuries that cause stimulation of the respiratory center

Excessive artificial ventilation
Fever
Hyperventilation
Hysteria
Salicylate intoxication

Decreased:
- pH (metabolic acidosis):
  Decreased formation of acids: diabetic ketoacidosis, high-fat/low-carbohydrate diets
  Decreased excretion of H^+: acquired (e.g., drugs, hypercalcemia), Addison's disease, Fanconi's syndrome, inherited (e.g., cystinosis, Wilson's disease), renal failure, renal tubular acidosis
  Increased acid intake
  Increased loss of alkaline body fluids: diarrhea, excess potassium, fistula

- pH (respiratory acidosis):
  Asthma
  Bronchoconstriction
  Drugs depressing the respiratory system
  Emphysema
  Pneumonia
  Pulmonary edema

Increased:
- pO_2:
  Hyperbaric oxygenation
  Hyperventilation

Decreased:
- pO_2:
  Decreased alveolar gas exchange: cancer, compression or resection of lung, respiratory distress syndrome (newborns), sarcoidosis
  Decreased ventilation or perfusion: asthma, bronchitis, bronchiectasis, cancer, croup, cystic fibrosis (mucoviscidosis), emphysema, granulomata,

pneumonia, pulmonary
infarction, shock

Hypoxemia: anesthesia, cardiac
disorders, carbon monoxide
exposure, high altitudes, near
drowning, presence of abnormal
hemoglobins

Hypoventilation: cerebrovascular
incident, drugs depressing the
respiratory system, head injury

Right to left shunt: congenital heart
disease, intrapulmonary
venoarterial shunting

Increased:
- pCO_2 (respiratory acidosis):
  Acute intermittent porphyria
  Asthma
  Bronchitis
  Cardiac disorders
  Congestive heart failure
  Cystic fibrosis
  Depression of respiratory center
  Electrolyte disturbances (severe)
  Emphysema
  Hypothyroidism (severe)
  Near drowning
  Pneumonia
  Pneumothorax
  Poliomyelitis
  Pulmonary edema
  Pulmonary tuberculosis
  Respiratory failure
  Respiratory disorders
  Tumor

- tCO_2 (metabolic alkalosis):
  Alkali ingestion (excessive)
  Hypochloremic states
  Hypokalemic states
  Salicylate intoxication
  Shock
  Vomiting

Decreased:
- pCO_2 (respiratory alkalosis):
  Anxiety

Fever
Head injury
Hyperthermia
Hyperventilation
Salicylate intoxication

- tCO_2 (metabolic acidosis):
  Diabetic ketoacidosis
  Renal disease

Increased:
- HCO_3^-:
  Anoxia
  Metabolic alkalosis
  Respiratory acidosis

Decreased:
- HCO_3^-:
  Hypocapnia
  Metabolic acidosis
  Respiratory alkalosis

Increased:
- O_2 saturation:
  Hyperbaric oxygenation
  Hypocapnia
  Hypothermia
  Oxygen therapy
  Respiratory alkalosis

Decreased:
- O_2 saturation:
  Anemia (severe)
  Anorexia
  Anoxia
  Atelectasis
  Carbon monoxide poisoning
  Cardiac disorders
  Congenital heart defects
  COPD
  Fever
  Head injury
  Hypercapnia
  Near drowning
  Pleural effusion
  Poisoning

Pneumonia
Pneumothorax
Pulmonary embolism
Respiratory distress syndrome
(adult and neonatal)
Sarcoidosis

Increased:
• Base excess: Metabolic alkalosis

Decreased:
• Base excess: Metabolic acidosis

CRITICAL VALUES:

INTERFERING FACTORS:
• Drugs that may cause an increase in pH include antacids, acetylsalicylic acid (initially), carbenicillin, carbenoxolone, ethacrynic acid, glycyrrhiza (licorice), laxatives, mafenide, and sodium bicarbonate.

• Drugs that may cause a decrease in pH include acetazolamide, acetylsalicylic acid (long term or high doses), citrates, dimethadione, ether, ethylene glycol, fluorides, mercury compounds (laxatives), methylenedioxyamphetamine, paraldehyde, and xylitol.

Arterial Blood Gas Parameter	Less Than	Greater Than
pH	7.20	7.60
HCO_3^-	10 mmol/L	40 mmol/L
pCO_2	20 mm Hg	55 mm Hg
pO_2	45 mm Hg	

• Drugs that may cause an increase in pCO_2 include acetylsalicylic acid, aldosterone bicarbonate, carbenicillin, carbenoxolone, corticosteroids, dexamethasone, ethacrynic acid, laxatives (chronic abuse), and x-ray contrast agents.

• Drugs that may cause a decrease in pCO_2 include acetazolamide, acetylsalicylic acid ethamivan, neuromuscular relaxants (secondary to postoperative hyperventilation), NSD 3004 (arterial long-acting carbonic anhydrase inhibitor), theophylline, tromethamine, and xylitol.

• Drugs that may cause an increase in pO_2 include theophylline and urokinase.

• Drugs that may cause a decrease in pO_2 include althesin, barbiturates, GM-CSF, isoproterenol, and meperidine.

• Samples for blood gases are obtained by arterial puncture, which carries a risk of bleeding, especially in patients who have bleeding disorders or are taking medications for a bleeding disorder.

• Recent blood transfusion may produce misleading values.

• Specimens with extremely elevated white blood cell counts will undergo misleading decreases in pH resulting from cellular metabolism, if transport to the laboratory is delayed.

• Specimens collected soon after a change in inspired oxygen has occurred will not accurately reflect the patient's oxygenation status.

• Specimens collected within 20 to 30 minutes of respiratory passage suctioning or other respiratory therapy will not be accurate.

• Excessive differences in actual body temperature relative to normal body temperature will not be reflected in the results. Temperature affects the amount of gas in solution. Blood gas analyzers measure samples at $37°C$ (98.6° F); therefore, if the patient is hyperthermic or hypothermic, it is important to notify the laboratory of the patient's actual body temperature at the time the specimen was collected. Fever will increase actual pO_2 and pCO_2 values; therefore the uncorrected values measured at $37°C$ will be falsely decreased. Hypothermia decreases actual pO_2 and pCO_2 values; therefore the uncorrected values measured at $37°C$ will be falsely increased.

• A falsely increased O_2 saturation may occur because of elevated levels of carbon monoxide in the blood.

• O_2 saturation is a calculated parameter based on an assumption of 100 percent hemoglobin A. Values may be misleading when hemoglobin variants with different oxygen dissociation curves are present. Hemoglobin S will cause a shift to the right, indicating decreased oxygen binding. Fetal hemoglobin and methemoglobin will cause a shift to the left, indicating increased oxygen binding.

• Excessive amounts of heparin in the sample may falsely decrease pH, pCO_2, and pO_2.

• Citrates should never be used as an anticoagulant in evacuated collection tubes for venous blood gas determinations because citrates will cause a marked analytic decrease in pH.

• Air bubbles or blood clots in the specimen are cause for rejection. Air bubbles in the specimen can falsely elevate or decrease the results depending on the patient's blood gas status. If an evacuated tube is used for venous blood gas specimen collection, the tube must be removed from the needle before the needle is withdrawn from the arm or else the sample will be contaminated with room air.

• Specimens should be placed in ice slurry immediately after collection because blood cells continue to carry out metabolic processes in the specimen after it has been removed from the patient. These natural life processes can affect pH, pO_2, pCO_2, and the other calculated values in a short period of time. The cold temperature provided by the ice slurry will slow down but not completely stop metabolic changes occurring in the sample over time. Iced specimens not analyzed within 60 minutes of collection should be rejected for analysis.

Nursing Implications and Procedure

Pretest:

➤ Obtain a history of the patient's complaints, including a list of known allergens.

➤ Obtain a history of the patient's cardiovascular and respiratory systems, any bleeding disorders, and results of tests and procedures previously performed, especially bleeding time, clotting time, complete blood count, partial thromboplastin time, platelets, and prothrombin time. For other related tests, refer to the cardiovascular and respiratory system tables.

➤ Obtain a list of the medications the patient is taking, including anticoagulant therapy, acetylsalicylic acid, herbs, and nutraceuticals known to affect coagulation. It is recommended that use of these products be discontinued 14 days before dental or surgical procedures. The requesting health care practitioner and laboratory should be advised if the patient is regularly using these products so their effects can be taken into consideration when reviewing results.

➤ Note any recent procedures that can interfere with test results.

➤ There are no food, fluid, or medication restrictions unless by medical direction.

➤ Record the patient's temperature.

➤ Indicate the type of oxygen, mode of oxygen delivery, and delivery rate as part of the test requisition process.

➤ If the sample is to be collected by radial artery puncture, perform an Allen test before puncture to ensure that the patient has adequate collateral circulation to the hand if thrombosis of the radial artery occurs after arterial puncture. The modified Allen test is performed as follows: extend the patient's wrist over a rolled towel. Ask the patient to make a fist with the hand extended over the towel. Use the second and third fingers to locate the pulses of the ulnar and radial arteries on the palmar surface of the wrist. The thumb should not be used to locate these arteries because it has a pulse. Compress both arteries and ask the patient to open and close the fist several times until the palm turns pale. Release pressure on the ulnar artery only. Color should return to the palm within 5 seconds if the ulnar artery is functioning. This is a positive Allen test, and blood gases may be drawn from the radial artery site. The Allen test should then be performed on the opposite hand. The hand to which color is restored fastest has better circulation and should be selected for specimen collection.

➤ Review the procedure with the patient and advise rest for 30 minutes before specimen collection. Be sure to explain to the patient that an arterial puncture may be painful. The site may be anesthetized with 1% to 2% lidocaine before puncture. Assess if the patient has an allergy to local anesthetics, and inform the health care practitioner accordingly.

➤ Inform the patient that specimen collection usually takes 10 to 15 minutes. The person collecting the specimen should be notified beforehand if the patient is receiving anticoagulant therapy, or taking aspirin

or other natural products that may prolong bleeding from the puncture site.

➤ Prepare an ice slurry in a cup or plastic bag to have ready for immediate transport of the specimen to the laboratory.

Intratest: ■

➤ Direct the patient to breathe normally and to avoid unnecessary movement.

➤ Observe standard precautions and follow the general guidelines in Appendix A.

Arterial

➤ Perform an arterial puncture and collect the specimen in an air-free heparinized syringe. There is no demonstrable difference in results between samples collected in plastic syringes and samples collected in glass syringes. It is very important that no room air be introduced into the collection container because the gases in the room and in the sample will begin equilibrating immediately. The end of the syringe must be stoppered immediately after the needle is withdrawn and removed. Samples should be mixed gently but thoroughly to ensure proper mixing of the heparin with the sample, which will prevent the formation of small clots leading to rejection of the sample. Label the specimen and promptly transport it to the laboratory. The tightly capped sample should be placed in an ice slurry immediately after collection. Information on the specimen label can be protected from water in the ice slurry by first placing the specimen in a protective plastic bag.

Venous

➤ Central venous blood is collected in a heparinized syringe.

➤ Venous blood collected percutaneously by venipuncture in a 5-mL green-top (heparin) tube (for adult patients) or a heparinized microtainer (for pediatric patients) may be used. Observe standard precautions and follow the general guidelines in Appendix A. The vacuum collection tube must be removed from the needle before the needle is removed from the patient's arm. Samples should be mixed gently but thoroughly to ensure proper mixing of the heparin with the sample, which will prevent the formation of small clots leading to rejection of the sample. Label the specimen, and promptly transport it to the laboratory. The tightly capped sample should be placed in an ice slurry immediately after collection. Information on the specimen label can be protected from water in the ice slurry by first placing the specimen in a protective plastic bag.

Capillary

➤ Perform a capillary puncture and collect the specimen in two 250-μL heparinized capillaries (scalp or heel for neonatal patients) or a heparinized microtainer (for pediatric patients). Observe standard precautions and follow the general guidelines in Appendix A. The capillaries should be filled as much as possible and capped on both ends. Some hospitals recommend that metal "fleas" be added to the capillary tube before the ends are capped. During transport a magnet can be moved up and down the outside of the capillary tube to facilitate mixing and prevent the formation of clots, which would cause rejection of the sample. It is important to inform the laboratory or respiratory therapy staff of the number of fleas used so the fleas can be accounted for and removed before the sample is introduced into the blood gas analyzers. Fleas left in the sample may damage the blood gas equipment if allowed to enter the analyzer. Microtainer samples should be mixed gently but thoroughly to ensure proper mixing of the heparin with the sample, which will prevent the formation of small clots leading to rejection of the sample. Label the

specimen, and promptly transport it to the laboratory.

Cord blood

➤ The sample may be collected directly from the cord, using a syringe. Label the specimen and promptly transport it to the laboratory. The tightly capped sample should be placed in an ice slurry immediately after collection. Information on the specimen label can be protected from water in the ice slurry by first placing the specimen in a protective plastic bag.

Scalp sample

➤ Samples for scalp pH may be collected anaerobically before delivery in special, scalp-sample collection capillaries and transported immediately to the laboratory for analysis. Some hospitals recommend that fleas be added to the scalp tube before the ends are capped. See preceding capillary collection for discussion of fleas.

Post-test: ■

➤ Pressure should be applied to the puncture site for at least 5 minutes in the unanticoagulated patient and for at least 15 minutes in the case of a patient receiving anticoagulant therapy. Observe puncture site for bleeding or hematoma formation. Apply pressure bandage.

➤ Observe the patient for signs or symptoms of respiratory acidosis, such as dyspnea, headache, tachycardia, pallor, diaphoresis, apprehension, drowsiness, coma, hypertension, or disorientation.

➤ Teach the patient breathing exercises to assist with the appropriate exchange of oxygen and carbon dioxide.

➤ Administer oxygen, if appropriate.

➤ Teach the patient how to properly use the incentive spirometer device or mininebulizer, if ordered.

➤ Observe the patient for signs or

symptoms of respiratory alkalosis, such as tachypnea, restlessness, agitation, tetany, numbness, seizures, muscle cramps, dizziness, or tingling fingertips.

➤ Instruct the patient to breathe deeply and slowly; performing this type of breathing exercise into a paper bag decreases hyperventilation and quickly helps the patient's breathing return to normal.

➤ Observe the patient for signs or symptoms of metabolic acidosis, such as rapid breathing, flushed skin, nausea, vomiting, dysrhythmias, coma, hypotension, hyperventilation, and restlessness.

➤ Observe the patient for signs or symptoms of metabolic alkalosis, such as shallow breathing, weakness, dysrhythmias, tetany, hypokalemia, hyperactive reflexes, and excessive vomiting.

➤ Abnormal blood gas values may be associated with diseases of the respiratory system. Malnutrition is commonly seen in patients with severe respiratory disease for reasons including fatigue, lack of appetite, and gastrointestinal distress. Research has estimated that the daily caloric intake required for respiration of patients with COPD is ten times higher than that of normal individuals. Inadequate nutrition can result in hypophosphatemia, especially in the respirator-dependent patient. During periods of starvation, phosphorus leaves the intracellular space and moves outside the tissue, resulting in dangerously decreased phosphorus levels. Adequate intake of vitamins A and C is also important to prevent pulmonary infection and to decrease the extent of lung tissue damage. The importance of following the prescribed diet should be stressed to the patient and/or caregiver.

➤ Water balance needs to be closely monitored in COPD patients. Fluid retention can lead to pulmonary edema.

➤ Evaluate test results in relation to the patient's symptoms and other tests performed. Related laboratory tests include arterial/alveolar oxygen ratio, anion gap, electrolytes, osmolality, phosphorus, and lactic acid.

BLOOD GROUPS AND ANTIBODIES

. . . .

SYNONYMS/ACRONYM: ABO group and Rh typing, blood group antibodies, type and screen, type and crossmatch.

SPECIMEN: Serum (2 mL) collected in a red-top tube. Whole blood (2 mL) collected in a lavender-top (ethylenediaminetetra-acetic acid [EDTA]) tube.

REFERENCE VALUE: (Method: FDA-licensed reagents with glass slides, glass tubes, or automated systems) Compatibility (no clumping or hemolysis).

Blood Type	Rh Type (with any ABO)	Other Antibodies That React at 37°C or with Antiglobulin	Other Antibodies That React at Room Temperature or Below
A	Positive	Kell	Lewis
B	Negative	Duffy	P
AB		Kidd	MN
O		S	Cold agglutinins
		s	
		U	

DESCRIPTION: Blood typing is a series of tests that include the ABO and Rh blood-group system performed to detect surface antigens on red blood cells by an agglutination test and compatibility tests to determine antibodies against these antigens. The major antigens in the ABO system are A and B, although AB and O are also common phenotypes. The patient with A antigens has type A blood; the patient with B antigens has type B blood. The patient with both A and B antigens has type AB blood (universal recipient); the patient with neither A nor B antigens has type O blood (universal donor). Blood type is genetically determined. After 6 months of age, individuals develop serum antibodies that react with A or B antigen absent from their own red blood cells. These are called *anti-A* and *anti-B antibodies.*

In ABO blood typing, the patient's red blood cells mix with anti-A and anti-B sera, a process known as *forward grouping.* The process then reverses, and the patient's serum mixes with type A and B cells in reverse grouping.

Generally, only blood with the same ABO and Rh group as the recipient is transfused because the anti-A and anti-B antibodies are strong agglutinins that cause a rapid, complement-mediated destruction of incompatible cells. ABO and Rh testing is also performed as a prenatal screen in pregnant women to identify the risk of hemolytic disease of the newborn. Although most of the anti-A and anti-B activity resides in the immunoglobulin M (IgM) class of immunoglobulins, some activity rests with IgG. Anti-A and anti-B antibodies of the IgG class coat the red blood cells without immediately affecting their viability and can readily cross the placenta, resulting in hemolytic disease of the newborn. Individuals with type O blood frequently have more IgG anti-A and anti-B; thus, ABO hemolytic disease of the newborn will affect infants of type O mothers almost exclusively (unless the newborn is also type O).

Major antigens of the Rh system are D (or Rh_o), C, E, c, and e. Individuals whose red blood cells possess D antigen are called Rh-positive; those who lack D antigen are called Rh-negative, no matter what other Rh antigens are present. Individuals who are Rh-negative produce anti-D antibodies when exposed to Rh-positive cells by either transfusions or pregnancy. These anti-D antibodies cross the placenta to the fetus and can cause hemolytic disease of the newborn or transfusion reactions if Rh-positive blood is administered. ∎

INDICATIONS:

- Determine ABO and Rh compatibility of donor and recipient before transfusion

- Determine anti-D antibody titer of Rh-negative mothers after sensitization by pregnancy with an Rh-positive fetus

- Determine the need for immunosuppressive therapy (e.g., with RhoGAM) when an Rh-negative woman delivers or aborts an Rh-positive fetus

- Identify donor ABO and Rh blood type for stored blood

- Identify maternal and infant ABO and Rh blood types to predict risk of hemolytic disease of the newborn

- Identify the patient's ABO and Rh blood type, especially before a procedure in which blood loss is a threat or blood replacement may be needed

RESULT:

- ABO system: A, B, AB, or O specific to person

- Rh system: positive or negative specific to person

- Cross-matching: compatibility between donor and recipient

- Incompatibility indicated by clumping (agglutination) of red blood cells

Group and Type	Incidence (%)	Alternative Transfusion Group and Type of PACKED CELL UNITS in Order of Preference If Patient's Own Group and Type Not Available
O Positive	37.4	O Negative
O Negative	6.6	None
A Positive	35.7	A Negative, O Positive, O Negative
A Negative	6.3	O Negative, O Positive, A Positive
B Positive	8.5	B Negative, O Positive, O Negative
B Negative	1.5	O Negative, O Positive, B Positive
AB Positive	3.4	AB Negative, A Positive, B Positive, A Negative, B Negative, O Positive, O Negative
AB Negative	0.6	A Negative, B Negative, O Negative, AB Positive, A Positive, B Positive, O Positive
Rh Type		
Rh Positive	85–90	
Rh Negative	10–15	

CRITICAL VALUES: ⚠ Signs and symptoms of blood transfusion reaction range from mildly febrile to anaphylactic and may include chills, dyspnea, fever, headache, nausea, vomiting, palpitations and tachycardia, chest or back pain, apprehension, flushing, hives, angioedema, diarrhea, hypotension, oliguria, hemoglobinuria, renal failure, sepsis, shock, and jaundice. Complications from disseminated intravascular coagulation (DIC) may also occur.

Possible interventions in mildly febrile reactions would include slowing the rate of infusion, then verifying and comparing patient identification, transfusion requisition, and blood bag label. The patient should be monitored closely for further development of signs and symptoms. Administration of epinephrine may be ordered.

Possible interventions in a more severe transfusion reaction may include immediate cessation of infusion, notification of the health care practitioner, keeping the intravenous (IV) line open with saline or lactated Ringer solution, collection of red- and lavender-top tubes for post-transfusion work-up, collection of urine, monitoring vital signs every 5 minutes, ordering additional testing if DIC is suspected, maintaining patent airway and blood pressure, and administering mannitol.

INTERFERING FACTORS:
• Drugs including levodopa, methyldopa, and methyldopa hydrochloride cause a false-positive in Rh typing.

• Recent administration of blood, blood products, dextran, or IV contrast medium causes cellular aggregation resembling agglutination in ABO typing.

• Abnormal proteins, cold agglutinins, and bacteremia may interfere with testing.

• Testing does not detect every antibody and may miss the presence of a weak antibody.

Nursing Implications and Procedure ● ● ● ● ● ● ● ● ● ● ●

Pretest: ◼

➤ Obtain a history of the patient's complaints, including a list of known allergens.

➤ Obtain a history of the patient's immune and hematopoietic systems, as well as results of previously performed tests and procedures. For related tests, refer to the immune and hematopoietic system tables.

➤ Obtain a list of the medications the patient is taking, including herbs, nu-

tritional supplements, and nutraceuticals. The requesting health care practitioner and laboratory should be advised if the patient regularly uses these products so their effects can be taken into consideration when reviewing results.

➤ Note any recent procedures that could interfere with test results.

➤ There are no food, fluid, or medication restrictions unless by medical direction.

➤ Although correct patient identification is important for test specimens, it is crucial when blood is collected for type and cross-match. Therefore, additional requirements are necessary, including verifying name, social security number, hospital number, date, and blood bank number on requisition and specimen labels; completing and applying a wrist band on the arm with the same information; and placing labels with the same information and blood bank number on blood sample tubes.

➤ Review the procedure with the patient.

➤ Inform the patient that specimen collection takes approximately 5 to 10 minutes.

Intratest: ◼

➤ Direct the patient to breathe normally and to avoid unnecessary movement.

➤ Observe standard precautions and follow the general guidelines in Appendix A.

➤ Perform a venipuncture, collect the specimen in a 5-mL red- and lavender-top tube.

➤ Label the specimen, and promptly transport it to the laboratory.

Post-test: ◼

➤ Observe venipuncture site for bleeding or hematoma formation. Apply pressure bandage.

➤ Inform patient of blood and Rh type, and advise the patient to record the

- information on a card or other document normally carried.
- ➤ Inform women who are Rh-negative to inform the health care practitioner of their Rh-negative status if they become pregnant or need a transfusion.

- ➤ Evaluate test results in relation to the patient's symptoms and other tests performed. Related laboratory tests include direct and indirect antiglobulin, bilirubin, cold agglutinin, haptoglobin, and urinalysis.

BLOOD POOL IMAGING

SYNONYMS/ACRONYM: Cardiac blood pool scan, ejection fraction study, gated cardiac scan, radionuclide ventriculogram, wall motion study, MUGA.

AREA OF APPLICATION: Heart.

CONTRAST: Intravenous radioactive material.

DESCRIPTION: Multigated blood pool imaging (MUGA; also known as *cardiac blood pool scan*) is used to diagnose cardiac abnormalities involving the left ventricle and myocardial wall abnormalities by imaging the blood within the cardiac chamber rather than the myocardium. The ventricular blood pool can be imaged during the initial transit of a peripherally injected, intravenous bolus of radionuclide (first-pass technique) or when the radionuclide has reached equilibrium concentration. The patient's electrocardiogram (ECG) is synchronized to the gamma camera imager and computer and thereby termed "gated." For multigated studies, technetium-99m (Tc-99m) pertechnetate is injected after an injection of pyrophosphate, allowing the labeling of circulating red blood cells; Tc-99m sulfur colloid is used for first-pass studies. Studies detect abnormalities in heart wall motion at rest or with exercise, ejection fraction, ventricular dilation, stroke volume, and cardiac output. The MUGA procedure, performed with the heart in motion, is used to obtain multiple images of the heart in contraction and relaxation during an R-to-R cardiac cycle. The resulting images can be displayed in a cinematic mode to visualize cardiac function. Repetitive data acquisitions are possible during graded levels of exercise, usually a bicycle ergometer or handgrip, to assess ventricular functional response to exercise.

After the administration of sublingual nitroglycerin; the MUGA scan can evaluate the effectiveness of the drug on ventricular function. Heart shunt imaging is done in conjunction with a resting MUGA scan to obtain ejection fraction and assess regional wall motion.

First-pass cardiac flow study is done to study heart chamber disorders including left-to-right and right-to-left shunts, determine both right and left ventricular ejection fractions, and assess blood flow through the great vessels. The study uses a jugular or antecubital vein injection of the radionuclide. ■

INDICATIONS:

- Determine ischemic coronary artery disease
- Aid in the diagnosis of myocardial infarction
- Aid in the diagnosis of true or false ventricular aneurysms
- Aid in the diagnosis of valvular heart disease and determine the optimal time for valve replacement surgery
- Quantitate cardiac output by calculating global or regional ejection fraction
- Evaluate ventricular size, function, and wall motion after an acute episode or in chronic heart disease
- Determine drug cardiotoxicity to stop therapy before development of congestive heart failure
- Determine cardiomyopathy
- Differentiate between chronic obstructive pulmonary disease and left ventricular failure
- Detect left-to-right shunts and determine pulmonary-to-systemic blood flow ratios, especially in children

RESULT

Normal Findings:

- Normal wall motion, ejection fraction (55 to 65 percent), coronary blood flow, ventricular size and function, and symmetry in contractions of the left ventricle

Abnormal Findings:

- Abnormal wall motion (akinesia or dyskinesia)
  Ischemic areas are hypokinetic
  Infarcted areas are akinetic
- Cardiac hypertrophy
- Cardiac ischemia
- Enlarged left ventricle
- Myocardial infarction

INTERFERING FACTORS:

This procedure is contraindicated for:

- Testing is contraindicated in patients with hypersensitivity to the radionuclide and in pregnancy and lactation unless the benefits of performing the test greatly outweigh the risks.
- Dipyridamole testing is not performed in patients with anginal pain at rest or in patients with severe atherosclerotic coronary vessels.
- Chemical stress with vasodilators should not be done to patients having asthma; bronchospasm can occur.

Factors that may impair clear imaging:

- Inability of the patient to cooperate or remain still during the procedure because of age, significant pain, or mental status
- Metallic objects within the examination field (e.g., jewelry, earrings, and/or dental amalgams), which may inhibit organ visualization and can produce unclear images
- Improper adjustment of the radiographic equipment to accommodate obese or thin patients, which can cause overexposure or underexposure and poor-quality study
- Patients who are very obese, who may exceed the weight limit for the equipment

• Incorrect positioning of the patient, which may produce poor visualization of the area to be examined

• Conditions such as chest wall trauma, cardiac trauma, angina that is difficult to control, significant cardiac arrhythmias, or a recent cardioversion procedure may affect test results.

Other considerations:

• Atrial fibrillation and extrasystoles invalidate the procedure.

• Suboptimal cardiac stress or patient exhaustion, preventing maximum heart rate testing, will affect results when the procedure is done in conjunction with exercise testing.

• Consultation with a physician should occur before the procedure for radiation safety concerns regarding infants of patients who are lactating.

• Risks associated with radiographic overexposure can result from frequent x-ray procedures. Personnel in the room with the patient should wear a protective lead apron, stand behind a shield, or leave the area while the examination is being done. Badges that reveal the level of exposure to radiation should be worn by persons working in the area where the examination is being done.

Nursing Implications and Procedure • • • • • • • • • •

Pretest: ■

➤ Determine the date of the last menstrual period and the possibility of pregnancy in perimenopausal women.

➤ Inform the patient that the test permits assessment of the pump action of the heart.

➤ Inform the patient that the procedure is performed in a special department by a technologist and

takes approximately 30 to 60 minutes for the examination.

➤ Reassure the patient that radioactive material poses no radioactive hazard and rarely produces side effects.

➤ Inform the patient when the procedure will be done.

➤ The results of the procedure are interpreted by a physician. The patient's physician will discuss the results with the patient.

➤ Obtain pertinent history of cardiac tests, other diagnostic procedure results, laboratory test results, medication usage, present cardiac conditions or abnormalities, and therapy received for cardiac condition. For related tests, refer to the cardiovascular system table.

➤ Obtain a history of hypersensitivity to radioactive materials injected.

➤ *Complete the informed consent document, when required.*

➤ Tell the patient to wear walking shoes for the treadmill or bicycle exercise. Emphasize to the patient the importance of reporting fatigue, pain, or shortness of breath.

➤ Ask the patient to lie very still during the procedure, as movement will produce unclear images.

➤ Restrict food for 4 hours, and medications for 24 hours before the test as ordered by the physician.

Intratest: ■

➤ Ensure that the patient has complied with dietary preparations and other pretesting restrictions.

➤ Ensure that emergency equipment is readily available during the procedure.

➤ Have the patient remove all jewelry, put on a hospital gown, and then void.

➤ The patient is placed at rest in the supine position on the scanning table.

➤ Expose the chest and attach the ECG leads.

➤ The radionuclide is administered intravenously and after 1 minute scanning is done to obtain views of the heart in the anterior, oblique, and lateral views. Between 12 and 64 images are obtained reflecting the motion of heart over the entire cardiac cycle.

➤ When done under exercise conditions, the patient is assisted onto the treadmill or bicycle ergometer and is exercised to a calculated 80 to 85 percent of the maximum heart rate as determined by the protocol selected. Images are done at each exercise level and begun immediately after injection of the radionuclide.

➤ If nitroglycerin is given, a cardiologist assessing the baseline MUGA scan injects the medication and records another scan, and then repeats this procedure until blood pressure reaches the desired level.

➤ Patients who cannot exercise are given dipyridamole before the radionuclide is injected.

➤ Patient movement during the procedure will affect the results and make interpretation difficult.

Post-test:

➤ Monitor ECG tracings and compare with baseline readings until stable.

➤ Observe the injection site for redness, swelling, or hematoma.

➤ Observe the patient for up to 60 minutes after the procedure for possible reaction to the radionuclide or complications from the procedure.

➤ Advise the patient to drink fluids to eliminate the radionuclide from the body, unless otherwise contraindicated.

➤ Instruct the patient to wash hands with soap and water after each voiding for 24 hours.

➤ Instruct the patient to resume normal activity and diet, unless otherwise indicated.

➤ A written report of the examination will be completed by a physician who specializes in this branch of medicine. The report is sent to the ordering health care provider who will discuss the results with the patient.

➤ Inform the patient that abnormalities of the heart scan can indicate the need for further studies, including cardiac catheterization and echocardiography.

➤ If possible, pregnant health care workers should avoid caring for a patient who has had a nuclear medicine procedure for the first 24 hours.

➤ Evaluate test results in relation to the patient's symptoms and other tests performed. Related diagnostic tests include echocardiography and myocardial perfusion scan.

BONE MINERAL DENSITOMETRY

• •

SYNONYM/ACRONYMS: Ultrasound densitometry, DEXA, DXA, SXA, QCT, RA.

Dual-energy x-ray absorptiometry (DEXA, DXA):
Two x-rays of different energy levels measure bone mineral density and predict risk of fracture.

Single-energy x-ray absorptiometry (SXA):
A single-energy x-ray measures bone density at peripheral sites.

Quantitative computerized tomography (QCT):
QCT is used to examine the lumbar vertebrae. It measures trabecular and cortical bone density. Results are compared to a known standard. This test is the most expensive and involves the highest radiation dose of all techniques.

Radiographic absorptiometry (RA):
A standard x-ray of the hand. Results are compared to a known standard.

Ultrasound densitometry:
Studies bone mineral content in peripheral densitometry sites such as the heel or wrist. It is not as precise as x-ray techniques, but less expensive than other techniques.

AREA OF APPLICATION:
Lumbar spine, heel, hip, wrist, whole body.

CONTRAST: None.

DESCRIPTION: Bone mineral density (BMD) can be measured at any of several body sites including spine, hip, wrist, and heel. Machines to measure BMD include computerized tomography (CT), radiographic absorptiometry, ultrasound, single-energy x-ray absorptiometry (SXA), and most commonly, dual-energy x-ray absorptiometry (DEXA). The radiation exposure from SXA and DEXA machines is approximately one-tenth that of a standard chest x-ray.

The BMD values measured by the various techniques cannot be directly compared. Therefore, they are stated in terms of standard deviation (SD) units. The patient's T-score is the number of SD units above or below the average BMD in young adults. A Z-score is the number of SD units above or below the average value for a person of the same age as the measured patient. For most BMD readings, one SD is equivalent to 10 to 12 percent of the average young-normal BMD value. A T-score of -2.5 is therefore equivalent to a bone mineral loss of 30 percent when compared to a young adult. ∎

INDICATIONS:
Osteoporosis is a condition characterized by low BMD, which results in increased risk of fracture. The National Osteoporosis Foundation (NOF) estimates that 4 to 6 million postmenopausal women in the United States have osteoporosis, and an additional 13 to 17 million (30 to 50 percent) have low bone density at the hip. It is estimated that one of every two women will experience a fracture as a result of low bone mineral content in her lifetime. The measurement of BMD gives the best indication of risk for a fracture. The lower the BMD, the greater the risk of fracture. The most common fractures are those of the hip, vertebrae, and distal forearm. Bone mineral loss is a disease of the entire skeleton and not restricted to the areas listed. The effect of the fractures has a wide range of results, from complete recovery to chronic pain, disability, and possible death.

- Determine the mineral content of bone
- Establish a diagnosis of osteoporosis
- Predict future fracture risk

- Monitor changes in BMD due to medical problems or therapeutic intervention
- Determine a possible cause of amenorrhea
- Evaluate bone demineralization associated with chronic renal failure
- Evaluate bone demineralization associated with immobilization

RESULT:

- T-score estimates the actual fracture risk compared to young adults.
- Normal bone mass is designated as a T-score value not less than −1.
- Osteoporosis is defined as a BMD T-score value less than −2.5.
- Low bone mass or osteopenia has T-scores from −1 to −2.5.
- Fracture risk increases as BMD declines from young-normal levels (low T-scores).
- Low Z-scores in older adults can be misleading because low BMD is very common.
- Z-scores estimate fracture risk compared to others of the same age (versus young-normal adults).

INTERFERING FACTORS (OR FACTORS ASSOCIATED WITH INCREASED RISK OF OSTEOPOROSIS):

This procedure is contraindicated for:
- Patients who are pregnant or suspected of being pregnant, unless the potential benefits of the procedure far outweigh the risks to the fetus and mother.

Factors that may impair clear imaging:
- Inability of the patient to cooperate or remain still during the procedure because of age, significant pain, or mental status
- Metallic objects within the examination field (e.g., jewelry, earrings, and/or dental amalgams), which may inhibit organ visualization and can produce unclear images
- Improper adjustment of the radiographic equipment to accommodate obese or thin patients, which can cause overexposure or underexposure and poor-quality study
- Patients who are very obese, who may exceed the weight limit for the equipment
- Incorrect positioning of the patient, which may produce poor visualization of the area to be examined

Other considerations:
- The use of anticonvulsant drugs, cytotoxic drugs, tamoxifen, glucocorticoid, lithium, or heparin, as well as increased alcohol intake, increased aluminum levels, excessive thyroxin, renal dialysis, or smoking, may affect the test results by either increasing or decreasing the bone mineral content.
- Consultation with a physician should occur before the procedure for radiation safety concerns regarding infants of patients who are lactating.
- Risks associated with radiographic overexposure can result from frequent x-ray procedures. Personnel in the room with the patient should wear a protective lead apron, stand behind a shield, or leave the area while the examination is being done. Badges that reveal the level of exposure to radiation should be worn by persons working in the area where the examination is being done.

Nursing Implications and Procedure • • • • • • • • • • • •

As a result of altered BMD, not the BMD testing process:

▶ Vertebral fractures may cause

complications including back pain, height loss, and kyphosis.

➤ Limited activity may result including difficulty bending and reaching.

➤ Patient may have poor self-esteem resulting from the cosmetic effects of kyphosis.

➤ Potential restricted lung function may result from fractures.

➤ Fractures may alter abdominal anatomy, resulting in constipation, pain, distention, and diminished appetite.

➤ Potential for a restricted lifestyle may result in depression and other psychological symptoms.

➤ Possible increased dependency on family for basic care may occur.

Pretest: ■

➤ Obtain a history of the patient's complaints.

➤ Obtain a list of the medications the patient is taking.

➤ Obtain a history of the patient's bone mineral status, as well as results of previously performed tests and procedures. For related tests, refer to the musculoskeletal system table.

➤ Review the procedure with the patient.

➤ Make special note of age, previous fractures, thinness, smoking, family history, fall risk, alcohol and coffee intake, age of menopause, and calcium intake.

➤ Determine date of last menstrual period and possibility of pregnancy in perimenopausal women.

➤ There are no food, fluid, or medication restrictions unless by medical direction.

➤ Inform the patient that the test usually takes 15 minutes.

Intratest: ■

➤ Clothing is not usually removed unless it contains metal or other items that would interfere with the test.

➤ Patients may want to wear a gown and robe, depending on the area to be examined.

➤ Remove all metal objects from the area to be examined.

➤ Recognize anxiety related to the testing process.

➤ Direct the patient to breathe normally and to avoid unnecessary movement.

Post-test: ■

➤ Compare new BMD values with previous value(s) to determine response to medical condition or treatment.

➤ Post-test instructions should include instructions for adequate intake of calcium and vitamin D, weight-bearing exercise, and avoidance of tobacco use and alcohol abuse.

➤ Determine if the patient or family members have any further questions or concerns.

➤ A physician specializing in this branch of medicine will send a report to the ordering health care provider who will discuss the results with the patient.

➤ Evaluate test results in relation to the patient's symptoms and other tests performed. Related tests include bone CT, magnetic resonance imaging, and x-rays.

BONE SCAN

SYNONYMS/ACRONYM: Bone imaging, radionuclide bone scan, bone scintigraphy, whole body bone scan.

AREA OF APPLICATION: Bone/skeleton.

CONTRAST: Intravenous radioactive material (diphosphonate compounds), usually combined with technetium-99m.

DESCRIPTION: This nuclear medicine scan assists in diagnosing and determining the extent of primary and metastatic bone disease and bone trauma, and monitors the progression of degenerative disorders. Abnormalities are identified by scanning 1 to 3 hours after the intravenous injection of a radionuclide such as technetium-99m methylene diphosphonate. Areas of increased uptake and activity on the bone scan represent abnormalities unless they occur in normal areas of increased activity, such as the sternum, sacroiliac, clavicle, and scapular joints in adults, and growth centers and cranial sutures in children. The radionuclide mimics calcium physiologically and therefore localizes in bone with an intensity proportional to the degree of metabolic activity. Gallium, magnetic resonance imaging (MRI), or white blood cell scanning can follow a bone scan to obtain a more sensitive study if acute inflammatory conditions such as osteomyelitis or septic arthritis are suspected. In addition, bone scan can detect fractures in patients who continue to have pain, even though x-rays have proved nega-

tive. A gamma camera detects the radiation emitted from the injected radioactive material. Whole body or representative images of the skeletal system can be obtained. ■

INDICATIONS:
- Determine the cause of unexplained bone or joint pain
- Assess degenerative joint changes or acute septic arthritis
- Confirm temporomandibular joint derangement
- Aid in the diagnosis of primary malignant bone tumors (e.g., osteogenic sarcoma, chondrosarcoma, Ewing's sarcoma, metastatic malignant tumors)
- Aid in the diagnosis of benign tumors or cysts
- Aid in the diagnosis of osteomyelitis
- Aid in the detection of traumatic or stress fractures
- Evaluate the healing process following fracture, especially if an underlying bone disease is present
- Aid in the diagnosis of metabolic bone diseases
- Detect Legg-Calvé-Perthes disease

- Evaluate prosthetic joints for infection, loosening, dislocation, or breakage
- Evaluate tumor response to radiation or chemotherapy
- Identify appropriate site for bone biopsy, lesion excision, or débridement
- Assess suspected child abuse

RESULT

Normal Findings:
- No abnormalities, as indicated by homogeneous and symmetric distribution of the radionuclide throughout all skeletal structures

Abnormal Findings:
- Bone necrosis
- Degenerative arthritis
- Fracture
- Legg-Calvé-Perthes disease
- Metastatic bone neoplasm
- Osteomyelitis
- Paget's disease
- Primary metastatic bone tumors
- Renal osteodystrophy
- Rheumatoid arthritis

INTERFERING FACTORS

This procedure is contraindicated for:
- Patients who are pregnant or suspected of being pregnant, unless the potential benefits of the procedure far outweigh the risks to the fetus and mother.

Factors that may impair clear imaging:
- Inability of the patient to cooperate or remain still during the procedure because of age, significant pain, or mental status.

- Metallic objects within the examination field (e.g., jewelry, earrings, and/or dental amalgams), which may inhibit organ visualization and can produce unclear images.
- Improper adjustment of the radiographic equipment to accommodate obese or thin patients, which can cause overexposure or underexposure and poor-quality study.
- Patients who are very obese, who may exceed the weight limit for the equipment.
- Incorrect positioning of the patient, which may produce poor visualization of the area to be examined.
- Retained barium from a previous radiologic procedure may affect the image.
- A distended bladder may obscure pelvic detail.
- Other nuclear scans done within the previous 24 to 48 hours may alter image.

Other considerations:
- The existence of multiple myeloma or thyroid cancer can result in a false-negative scan for bone abnormalities.
- Improper injection of the radionuclide may allow the tracer to seep deep into the muscle tissue, producing erroneous hot spots.
- Consultation with a physician should occur before the procedure for radiation safety concerns regarding infants of patients who are lactating.
- Risks associated with radiographic overexposure can result from frequent x-ray procedures. Personnel in the room with the patient should wear a protective lead apron, stand behind a shield, or leave the area while the examination is being done. Badges that reveal the level of exposure to radiation should be worn by persons working in

the area where the examination is being done.

Nursing Implications and Procedure • • • • • • • • • • •

➤ Inform the patient that the bone scan can detect bone disease before the disease can be detected with plain film x-rays.

➤ Inform the patient that the procedure is performed by a technologist in a special nuclear medicine department. The procedure usually takes approximately 60 minutes.

➤ Obtain a history of the patient's complaints including a list of known allergens.

➤ Obtain a history of the patient's musculoskeletal system, as well as results of previously performed tests, treatments, therapies, and surgical procedures. For related tests, refer to the musculoskeletal system table.

➤ Obtain a list of the patient's current medications.

➤ Determine date of last menstrual period and possibility of pregnancy in perimenopausal women.

➤ Inform the patient that the technologist will administer an intravenous injection of the radionuclide and that he or she will need to return 2 to 3 hours later for the scan.

➤ After the injection, the patient should be encouraged to increase fluid intake and continue normal physical activity.

➤ Instruct the patient to lie very still during the procedure because movement will produce unclear images.

➤ Sedate children who are unable to lie still.

➤ Fasting before the scan is not required unless indicated otherwise.

➤ Ask patient to remove jewelry, including watches, and any other metallic objects. Have the patient put on a hospital gown.

➤ Ask patient to void before the procedure.

➤ Place the patient in a supine position on a flat table with foam wedges to help maintain position and immobilization. The radionuclide is administered intravenously with images taken every 3 seconds for the first minute over the area to be examined. This will evaluate the blood flow to the area. A blood pool image is then obtained over the area to be examined (usually taking 2 to 3 minutes). A 2- to 3-hour delay is required between the injection and the actual bone scan to improve tumor imaging.

➤ After the delay that allows the radionuclide to be taken up by the bones, multiple images are obtained over the complete skeleton. A large field-of-view camera is used to cover the whole area. Delayed views may be taken up to 24 hours after the injection.

➤ The patient may be imaged by single photon emission computed tomography (SPECT) techniques to further clarify areas of suspicious radionuclide localization.

➤ Unless otherwise indicated, instruct the patient to resume normal activity, medications, and diet.

➤ Unless contraindicated, advise patient to drink increased amounts of fluids for 24 to 48 hours to eliminate the radionuclide from the body. Tell the patient that radionuclide is eliminated from the body within 24 to 48 hours.

➤ A physician specializing in this branch of medicine will send a report to the ordering health care provider, who will discuss the results with the patient.

➤ If a woman who is breastfeeding must have a nuclear scan, she should not breastfeed the infant until the radionuclide has been eliminated. This could take as long as 3 days. She should be instructed to express the milk and discard it during the 3-day period to prevent cessation of milk production.

➤ No other radionuclide tests should be scheduled for 24 to 48 hours after this procedure.

➤ Inform the patient to immediately flush the toilet after each voiding after the procedure and to meticulously wash hands with soap and water after each voiding for 48 hours after the procedure.

➤ Tell all caregivers to wear gloves when discarding urine for 48 hours after the procedure. Wash gloved hands with soap and water before removing gloves. Then wash ungloved hands after the gloves are removed.

➤ Evaluate test results in relation to the patient's symptoms and other tests performed. Related diagnostic tests include x-rays, CT, and MRI of the area in question.

BRONCHOSCOPY

- -

SYNONYM/ACRONYM: Flexible bronchoscopy.

AREA OF APPLICATION: Bronchial tree, larynx, trachea.

CONTRAST: None.

DESCRIPTION: This procedure provides direct visualization of the larynx, trachea, and bronchial tree by means of either a rigid or a flexible bronchoscope. A fiberoptic bronchoscope with a light incorporated is guided into the tracheobronchial tree. A local anesthetic may be used to allow the scope to be inserted through the mouth or nose into the trachea and into the bronchi. The patient must breathe during insertion and with the scope in place. The purpose of the procedure is both diagnostic and therapeutic.

The rigid bronchoscope allows visualization of the larger airways, including the lobar, segmental, and subsegmental bronchi, while maintaining effective gas exchange. Rigid bronchoscopy is preferred when large volumes of blood or secretions need to be aspirated, when foreign bodies are to be removed, when large-sized biopsy specimens are to be obtained, and for most bronchoscopies in children.

The flexible fiberoptic bronchoscope has a smaller lumen that is designed to allow for visualization of all segments of the bronchial tree. The accessory lumen of the bronchoscope is used for tissue biopsy, bronchial washings, instillation of anesthetic agents and medications, and to obtain specimens with brushes for cytologic examination. In general, fiberoptic bronchoscopy is less traumatic to the surrounding tissues than the larger rigid bronchoscopes. Fiberoptic bronchoscopy is performed under local anesthesia; patient tolerance is better for fiberoptic bronchoscopy than for rigid bronchoscopy. ∎

INDICATIONS:
• Determine etiology of persistent cough, hemoptysis, hoarseness, unexplained chest x-ray abnormalities, and/or abnormal cytologic findings in sputum

• Evaluate respiratory distress and tachypnea in an infant to rule out tracheoesophageal fistula or other congenital anomaly

• Detect end-stage bronchogenic cancer

• Treat lung cancer through instillation of chemotherapeutic agents, implantation of radioisotopes, or laser palliative therapy

• Identify hemorrhagic and inflammatory changes in Kaposi's sarcoma

• Detect lung infections and inflammation

• Remove foreign body

• Determine extent of smoke-inhalation or other traumatic injury

• Evaluate airway patency; aspirate deep or retained secretions

• Identify bleeding sites and remove clots within the tracheobronchial tree

• Evaluate possible airway obstruction in patients with known or suspected sleep apnea

• Intubate patients with cervical spine injuries or massive upper airway edema

• Evaluate endotracheal tube placement

or possible adverse sequelae to tube placement

RESULT

Normal Findings:
• Normal larynx, trachea, bronchi, bronchioles, and alveoli

Abnormal Findings:
• Abscess

• Bronchial diverticulum

• Bronchial stenosis

• Bronchogenic cancer

• Coccidioidomycosis, histoplasmosis, blastomycosis, phycomycosis

• Foreign bodies

• Inflammation

• Interstitial pulmonary disease

• Opportunistic lung infections (e.g., pneumocystitis, nocardia, cytomegalovirus)

• Strictures

• Tuberculosis

• Tumors

INTERFERING FACTORS

This procedure is contraindicated for:
• Patients with bleeding disorders, especially those associated with uremia and cytotoxic chemotherapy

• Patients with pulmonary hypertension

• Patients with cardiac conditions or dysrhythmias

• Patients with disorders that limit extension of the neck

• Patients with severe obstructive tracheal conditions

• Patients with or having the potential for respiratory failure; introduction of the bronchoscope alone may cause a 10 to 20 mm Hg drop in PaO_2

Factors that may impair a complete examination:

- Inability of the patient to cooperate or remain still during the procedure because of age, significant pain, or mental status

- Metallic objects within the examination field (e.g., jewelry, earrings, and/or dental amalgams), which may inhibit organ visualization and can produce unclear images

- Improper adjustment of the radiographic equipment to accommodate obese or thin patients, which can cause overexposure or underexposure and poor-quality study

- Patients who are very obese, who may exceed the weight limit for the equipment

- Incorrect positioning of the patient, which may produce poor visualization of the area to be examined

Other considerations:

- Hypoxemic or hypercapnic states require continuous oxygen administration.

- Failure to follow dietary restrictions before the procedure may cause the procedure to be canceled or repeated.

Nursing Implications and Procedure • • • • • • • • • • •

Pretest:

➤ Inform the patient that the procedure is performed in an endoscopy suite by a physician. The procedure is performed under local anesthesia and takes approximately 30 to 45 minutes.

➤ Instruct the patient to refrain from food and fluids for 6 to 8 hours before the test.

➤ Obtain a history of patient's complaints, including allergies or sensitivities to anesthetics, analgesics, medication usage, and antibiotics and known or suspected pulmonary disorders.

➤ Obtain a history of the patient's respiratory system, as well as results of previously performed tests, therapies, procedures, and surgeries. For related tests, refer to the respiratory system table.

➤ *Obtain a written and informed consent for the procedure before administering medication.*

➤ Determine previous abnormalities in laboratory test results, particularly hematologic or coagulation tests.

Intratest:

➤ Ensure that the patient has complied with dietary preparations and other pretesting restrictions.

➤ Keep resuscitation equipment on hand in the case of respiratory impairment or laryngospasm after the procedure.

➤ Avoid using morphine sulfate in those with asthma or other pulmonary disease. This drug can further exacerbate bronchospasms and respiratory impairment.

➤ Have patient remove dentures, contact lenses, eyeglasses, and jewelry. Notify the physician if the patient has permanent crowns on teeth. Have the patient remove clothing and change into a gown for the procedure.

➤ Provide mouth care to reduce oral bacterial flora.

Rigid bronchoscopy:

➤ The patient is placed in the supine position and a general anesthetic is administered. The patient's neck is hyperextended, and the lightly lubricated bronchoscope is inserted orally and passed through the glottis. The patient's head is turned or repositioned to aid visualization of various segments.

➤ After inspection, the bronchial brush, suction catheter, biopsy forceps, laser, and electrocautery devices are introduced to obtain specimens for cytologic or microbiologic study or for therapeutic procedures.

➤ If a bronchial washing is performed, small amounts of solution are instilled into the airways and removed. These specimens are placed in labeled containers and promptly sent to the laboratory.

➤ After the procedure, the bronchoscope is removed and the patient is placed in a side-lying position with the head slightly elevated.

Fiberoptic bronchoscopy:

➤ The patient is placed in a sitting position while the tongue and oropharynx is sprayed or swabbed with local anesthetic. When loss of sensation is adequate, the client is placed in a supine position. The fiberoptic scope can be introduced through the nose, the mouth, endotracheal tube, a tracheostomy tube, or a rigid bronchoscope. Most common insertion is through the nose. Clients with copious secretions or massive hemoptysis, or in whom airway complications are more likely, may be intubated before the bronchoscopy. Additional local anesthetic is applied through the scope as it approaches the vocal cords and the carina, eliminating reflexes in these sensitive areas. The fiberoptic approach allows visualization of airway segments without having to move the patient's head through various positions.

➤ After inspection, specimens may be obtained for cytologic and microbiologic study. All specimens are placed in appropriate containers, properly labeled, and promptly sent to the laboratory.

➤ After the procedure, the bronchoscope is removed. Patients who had local anesthesia are placed in a semi-Fowler's position to recover.

Post-test:

➤ The patient should remain in a semi-Fowler's position on either side until vital signs revert to preprocedure levels.

➤ Instruct the patient not to attempt to swallow saliva until the gag reflex has returned, but to expectorate saliva into an emesis basin.

➤ Emphasize that any excessive bleeding, difficulty breathing, changes in sputum, excessive coughing after biopsy, or pain must be reported to the physician immediately.

➤ A physician specializing in this branch of medicine will send a written report of the examination to the ordering health care provider who will discuss the results with the patient.

➤ Evaluate procedure results in relation to the patient's symptoms and other tests performed. Related diagnostic tests include chest x-ray, computed tomography and magnetic resonance imaging of the chest, and lung scan.

C-PEPTIDE

SYNONYMS/ACRONYM: Connecting peptide insulin, insulin C-peptide, proinsulin C-peptide.

SPECIMEN: Serum (1 mL) collected in a red-top tube.

REFERENCE VALUE: (Method: Radioimmunoassay)

Conventional Units	SI Units (Conversion Factor ×0.333)
0.78–1.8 ng/mL	0.26–0.63 nmol/L

DESCRIPTION: C-peptide is a biologically inactive peptide formed when beta cells of the pancreas convert proinsulin to insulin. Most of C-peptide is secreted by the kidneys. C-peptide levels usually correlate with insulin levels and provide a reliable indication of how well the beta cells secrete insulin. Release of C-peptide is not affected by exogenous insulin administration. C-peptide values double after stimulation with glucose or glucagon. An insulin–C-peptide ratio less than 1.0 indicates endogenous insulin secretion, whereas a ratio of greater than 1.0 indicates an excess of exogenous insulin. ∎

INDICATIONS:

- Assist in the diagnosis of insulinoma: Serum levels of insulin and C-peptide are elevated.

- Detect suspected factitious cause of hypoglycemia (excessive insulin administration): C-peptide levels do not increase with serum insulin levels.

- Determine beta cell function when insulin antibodies preclude accurate measurement of serum insulin production.

- Distinguish between insulin-dependent (type 1) and non–insulin-dependent (type 2) diabetes (with C-peptide–stimulating test): Patients with diabetes whose C-peptide stimulation level is greater than 18 ng/mL can be managed without insulin treatment.

- Evaluate hypoglycemia.

RESULT

Increased in:

- Endogenous hyperinsulinism
- Islet cell tumor
- Non–insulin-dependent (type 2) diabetes
- Oral hypoglycemic medication
- Pancreas or beta cell transplants
- Renal failure

Decreased in:

- Factitious hypoglycemia
- Insulin-dependent (type 1) diabetes
- Pancreatectomy

CRITICAL VALUES: N/A

INTERFERING FACTORS:

- Drugs that may increase C-peptide levels include betamethasone, chloroquine, danazol, deferoxamine, ethinyl estradiol, oral contraceptives, prednisone, and rifampin.

- Drugs that may decrease C-peptide levels include atenolol and calcitonin.

- Recent radioactive scans or radiation within 1 week before the test can interfere with test results when radioimmunoassay is the test method.

- C-peptide and endogenous insulin levels do not always correlate in obese patients.

Nursing Implications and Procedure • • • • • • • • • • •

Pretest: ■

➤ Obtain a history of the patient's complaints, including a list of known allergens.

➤ Obtain a history of the patient's endocrine system and results of previously performed tests and procedures. For related tests, refer to the endocrine system table.

➤ Obtain a list of the medications the patient is taking, including herbs, nutritional supplements, and nutraceuticals. The requesting health care practitioner and laboratory should be advised if the patient is regularly using these products so that their effects can be taken into consideration when reviewing results.

➤ Note any recent procedures that can interfere with test results.

➤ There are no fluid or medication restrictions unless by medical direction.

➤ The patient should fast for at least 10 hours before specimen collection.

➤ Review the procedure with the patient.

➤ Inform the patient that specimen collection takes approximately 5 to 10 minutes.

Intratest: ■

➤ Direct the patient to breathe normally and to avoid unnecessary movement.

➤ Ensure that the patient has complied with dietary preparations and other pretesting restrictions.

➤ Observe standard precautions and follow the general guidelines in Appendix A. Perform a venipuncture, and collect the specimen in a 5-mL red-top tube.

➤ Label the specimen, and promptly transport it to the laboratory.

Post-test: ■

➤ Observe venipuncture site for bleeding or hematoma formation. Apply pressure bandage.

➤ Instruct the patient to resume usual diet as directed by the health care practitioner.

➤ Abnormal C-peptide levels may be associated with diabetes. Instruct the diabetic patient, as appropriate, in nutritional management of the disease. Patients who adhere to dietary recommendations report a better general feeling of health, better weight management, greater control of glucose and lipid values, and improved use of insulin. There is no "diabetic diet"; however, there are many meal-planning approaches with nutritional goals endorsed by the American Dietetic Association. The nutritional requirements of each diabetic patient need to be determined individually with the appropriate health care professionals, particularly health care workers trained in nutrition.

➤ Instruct the patient and caregiver to report signs and symptoms of hypoglycemia (weakness, confusion, diaphoresis, rapid pulse) or hyperglycemia (thirst, polyuria, hunger, lethargy). Emphasize, as appropriate, that good control of glucose levels delays the onset and slows the progression of diabetic retinopathy, nephropathy, and neuropathy.

➤ Evaluate test results in relation to the patient's symptoms and other tests performed. Related laboratory tests include cortisol, glucose, glycated hemoglobin, glucose tolerance test, insulin, insulin antibodies, and microalbumin.

C-REACTIVE PROTEIN

SYNONYM/ACRONYM: CRP.

SPECIMEN: Serum (1 mL) collected in a red- or tiger-top tube.

REFERENCE VALUE: (Method: High-sensitivity immunoassay, nephelometry)

High-sensitivity immunoassay (cardiac applications)	0.08–3.10 µg/mL

Nephelometry	Conventional Units	SI Units (Conversion Factor ×10)
Cord	1–35 µg/dL	10–350 µg/L
Adult	6.8–820 µg/dL	68–8200 µg/L

DESCRIPTION: C-reactive protein (CRP) is a glycoprotein produced by the liver in response to acute inflammation. The CRP assay is a nonspecific test that determines the presence (not the cause) of inflammation; it is often ordered in conjunction with erythrocyte sedimentation rate (ESR). CRP assay is a more sensitive and rapid indicator of the presence of an inflammatory process than ESR. CRP disappears from the serum rapidly when inflammation has subsided. The inflammatory process and its association with atherosclerosis make the presence of CRP, as detected by highly sensitive CRP assays, a potential marker for coronary artery disease. It is believed that the inflammatory process may instigate the conversion of a stable plaque to a weaker one that can rupture and occlude an artery. Several major studies are in progress to confirm the correlation and to establish standardized reference ranges for this purpose. ∎

INDICATIONS:

• Assist in the differential diagnosis of appendicitis and acute pelvic inflammatory disease

• Assist in the differential diagnosis of Crohn's disease and ulcerative colitis

• Assist in the differential diagnosis of rheumatoid arthritis and uncomplicated systemic lupus erythematosus (SLE)

• Assist in the evaluation of coronary artery disease

• Detect the presence or exacerbation of inflammatory processes

• Monitor response to therapy for autoimmune disorders such as rheumatoid arthritis

RESULT

Increased in:

- Acute bacterial infections
- Crohn's disease
- Inflammatory bowel disease
- Myocardial infarction
- Pregnancy (second half)
- Rheumatic fever
- Rheumatoid arthritis
- SLE

Decreased in: N/A

CRITICAL VALUES: N/A

INTERFERING FACTORS:

- Drugs that may decrease CRP levels include aurothiomalate, methotrexate, nonsteroidal anti-inflammatory drugs, oral contraceptives (progestogen effect), penicillamine, pentopril, and sulfasalazine.

- Nonsteroidal anti-inflammatory drugs, salicylates, and steroids may cause false-negative results because of suppression of inflammation.

- Falsely elevated levels may occur with the presence of an intrauterine device.

- Lipemic samples that are turbid in appearance may be rejected for analysis when nephelometry is the test method.

Nursing Implications and Procedure

Pretest:

➤ Obtain a history of the patient's complaints, including a list of known allergens. The patient may complain of pain related to the inflammatory process in connective or other tissues.

➤ Obtain a history of the patient's cardiovascular and immune systems, as well as results of previously performed tests and procedures. For related tests, refer to the cardiovascular and immune system tables.

➤ Obtain a list of the medications the patient is taking, including herbs, nutritional supplements, and nutraceuticals. The requesting health care practitioner and laboratory should be advised if the patient regularly uses these products so that their effects can be taken into consideration when reviewing results.

➤ There are no food, fluid, or medication restrictions unless by medical direction.

➤ Review the procedure with the patient.

➤ Inform the patient that specimen collection takes approximately 5 to 10 minutes.

Intratest:

➤ Direct the patient to breathe normally and to avoid unnecessary movement.

➤ Observe standard precautions and follow the general guidelines in Appendix A. Perform a venipuncture, and collect the specimen in a 5-mL red- or tiger-top tube.

➤ Label the specimen, and promptly transport it to the laboratory.

Post-test:

➤ Observe venipuncture site for bleeding or hematoma formation. Apply pressure bandage.

➤ Evaluate test results in relation to the patient's symptoms and other tests performed. Related laboratory tests include creatine kinase and isoenzymes, ESR, homocysteine, troponin, and white blood cell count.

CA 125

SYNONYMS/ACRONYM: Carbohydrate antigen 125, cancer antigen 125.

SPECIMEN: Serum (1 mL) collected in a red-top tube.

REFERENCE VALUE: (Method: Enzyme immunoassay)

Conventional Units	SI Units (Conversion Factor ×1)
Less than 35 U/mL	Less than 35 kU/L

DESCRIPTION: CA 125, a glycoprotein present in normal endometrial tissue, appears in the blood when natural endometrial protective barriers are destroyed, as occurs in cancer or endometriosis. Persistently rising levels indicate a poor prognosis, but absence of the tumor marker does not rule out tumor presence. Levels may also rise in pancreatic, liver, colon, breast, and lung cancers. It is not useful as a screening test. ∎

INDICATIONS:

• Assist in the diagnosis of carcinoma of the cervix and endometrium

• Assist in the diagnosis of ovarian cancer

• Monitor response to treatment of ovarian cancer

RESULT

Increased in:

• Breast, colon, endometrial, liver, lung, ovarian, and pancreatic cancer

• Endometriosis

• First-trimester pregnancy

• Menses

• Ovarian abscess

• Pelvic inflammatory disease

• Peritonitis

Decreased in:

• Effective therapy or removal of the tumor

CRITICAL VALUES: N/A

INTERFERING FACTORS: N/A

Nursing Implications and Procedure

Pretest:

➤ Obtain a history of the patient's complaints, including a list of known allergens.

➤ Obtain a history of the patient's immune and reproductive systems, as well as results of previously performed tests and procedures. For related tests, refer to the immune and reproductive system tables.

➤ Obtain a list of the medications the patient is taking, including herbs, nutritional supplements, and nutraceuticals. The requesting health care practitioner and laboratory should be advised if the patient regularly uses these products so that their effects can be taken into consideration when reviewing results.

➤ There are no food, fluid, or medication restrictions unless by medical direction.

➤ Review the procedure with the patient.

➤ Inform the patient that specimen collection takes approximately 5 to 10 minutes.

Intratest:

➤ Direct the patient to breathe normally and to avoid unnecessary movement.

➤ Observe standard precautions and follow the general guidelines in Appendix A. Perform a venipuncture, and collect the specimen in a 5-mL red-top tube.

➤ Label the specimen, and promptly transport it to the laboratory.

Post-test:

➤ Observe venipuncture site for bleeding or hematoma formation. Apply pressure bandage.

➤ Recognize anxiety related to test results and offer support. Provide teaching and information regarding the clinical implications of the test results, as appropriate. Educate the patient regarding access to counseling services.

➤ Inform the patient that serial specimens may be requested at regular intervals.

➤ Evaluate test results in relation to the patient's symptoms and other tests performed. Related laboratory tests include breast biopsy, CA 19-9, and CA 15-3.

CA 15-3

• •

SYNONYMS/ACRONYM: Carbohydrate antigen 15-3, cancer antigen 15-3.

SPECIMEN: Serum (1 mL) collected in a red-top tube.

REFERENCE VALUE: (Method: Immunoradiometric)

Conventional Units	SI Units (Conversion Factor ×1)
Less than 30 U/mL	Less than 30 kU/L

DESCRIPTION: CA 15-3 monitors patients for recurrence of breast carcinoma. CA 27.29 (reference range less than 38 U/mL), a more recently approved protein marker, is replacing CA 15-3 in some reference laboratories. ∎

INDICATIONS: Monitor recurrent carcinoma of the breast

RESULT

Increased in: Recurrent carcinoma of the breast

Decreased in: Effective therapy or removal of the tumor

CRITICAL VALUES: N/A

INTERFERING FACTORS: Recent radioactive scans or radiation within 1 week before the test can interfere with test results when radioimmunoassay is the test method.

Nursing Implications and Procedure · · · · · · · · · · · ·

Pretest:

➤ Obtain a history of the patient's complaints, including a list of known allergens.

➤ Obtain a history of the patient's immune and reproductive systems, as well as results of previously performed tests and procedures. For related tests, refer to the immune and reproductive system tables.

➤ Obtain a list of the medications the patient is taking, including herbs, nutritional supplements, and nutraceuticals. Advise the requesting health care practitioner and laboratory if the patient regularly uses these products so that their effects can be taken into consideration when reviewing results.

➤ Note any recent procedures that can interfere with test results.

➤ There are no food, fluid, or medication restrictions unless by medical direction.

➤ Review the procedure with the patient.

➤ Inform the patient that specimen collection takes approximately 5 to 10 minutes.

Intratest:

➤ Direct the patient to breathe normally and to avoid unnecessary movement.

➤ Observe standard precautions and follow the general guidelines in Appendix A. Perform a venipuncture, and collect the specimen in a 5-mL red-top tube.

➤ Label the specimen, and promptly transport it to the laboratory.

Post-test:

➤ Observe venipuncture site for bleeding or hematoma formation. Apply pressure bandage.

➤ Recognize anxiety related to test results and offer support. Provide teaching and information regarding the clinical implications of the test results, as appropriate. Educate the patient regarding access to counseling services.

➤ Inform the patient that serial specimens may be requested at regular intervals.

➤ Evaluate test results in relation to the patient's symptoms and other tests performed. Related laboratory tests include breast biopsy, carcinoembryonic antigen, and CA 125.

CA 19-9

SYNONYMS/ACRONYM: Carbohydrate antigen 19-9, cancer antigen 19-9.

SPECIMEN: Serum (1 mL) collected in a red-top tube.

REFERENCE VALUE: (Method: Immunoradiometric)

Conventional Units	SI Units (Conversion Factor ×1)
Less than 37 U/mL	Less than 37 kU/L

DESCRIPTION: CA 19-9 is used to monitor patients with various types of cancer. ■

INDICATIONS:

• Monitor effectiveness of therapy

• Monitor gastrointestinal, head and neck, and gynecologic carcinomas

• Predict recurrence of cholangiocarcinoma

• Predict recurrence of stomach, pancreatic, colorectal, gallbladder, liver, and urothelial carcinomas

RESULT

Increased in:

• Gastrointestinal, head and neck, and gynecologic carcinomas

• Recurrence of stomach, pancreatic, colorectal, gallbladder, liver, and urothelial carcinomas

• Recurrence of cholangiocarcinoma

Decreased in:

• Effective therapy or removal of the tumor

CRITICAL VALUES: N/A

INTERFERING FACTORS:

• Recent radioactive scans or radiation within 1 week before the test can interfere with test results when radioimmunoassay is the test method.

Nursing Implications and Procedure

Pretest:

➤ Obtain a history of the patient's complaints, including a list of known allergens.

➤ Obtain a history of the patient's gastrointestinal and immune systems, as well as results of previously performed tests and procedures. For related tests, refer to the gastrointestinal and immune system tables.

➤ Obtain a list of the medications the patient is taking, including herbs, nutritional supplements, and nutraceuticals. The requesting health care practitioner and laboratory should be advised if the patient regularly uses these products so that their effects can be taken into consideration when reviewing results.

➤ Note any recent procedures that can interfere with test results.

➤ There are no food, fluid, or medication restrictions unless by medical direction.

➤ Review the procedure with the patient.

➤ Inform the patient that specimen collection takes approximately 5 to 10 minutes.

Intratest:

➤ Direct the patient to breathe normally and to avoid unnecessary movement.

➤ Observe standard precautions and follow the general guidelines in Appendix A. Perform a venipuncture, and collect the specimen in a 5-mL red-top tube.

➤ Label the specimen, and promptly transport it to the laboratory.

Post-test:

➤ Observe venipuncture site for bleeding or hematoma formation. Apply pressure bandage.

➤ Recognize anxiety related to test results and offer support. Provide teaching and information regarding the clinical implications of the test results, as appropriate. Educate the patient regarding access to counseling services.

➤ Inform the patient that serial specimens may be requested at regular intervals.

➤ Evaluate test results in relation to the patient's symptoms and other tests performed. Related laboratory tests include biopsy of suspect tissue, CA 15-3, CA 125, and carcinoembryonic antigen.

CALCITONIN AND CALCITONIN STIMULATION TESTS

· ·

SYNONYM/ACRONYM: Thyrocalcitonin, hCT.

SPECIMEN: Serum (3 mL) collected in a red- or tiger-top tube.

REFERENCE VALUE: (Method: Radioimmunoassay)

Procedure	Medication Administered	Recommended Collection Times
Calcium and pentagastrin stimulation	Calcium, 2 mg/kg IV for 1 min, followed by pentagastrin 0.5 µg/kg	4 calcitonin levels—baseline immediately before bolus; and 1 min, 2 min, and 5 min postbolus
Pentagastrin stimulation	Pentagastrin, 0.5 µg/kg IV push	4 calcitonin levels—baseline immediately before bolus; and 1.5 min, 2 min, and 5 min postbolus

	Conventional Units	SI Units (Conversion Factor ×1)
Calcitonin		
Male	Less than 19 pg/mL	Less than 19 ng/L
Female	Less than 14 pg/mL	Less than 14 ng/L
Maximum Response		
After Calcium and Pentagastrin Stimulation		
Male	Less than 350 pg/mL	Less than 350 ng/L
Female	Less than 94 pg/mL	Less than 94 ng/L
Maximum Response		
After Pentagastrin Stimulation		
Male	Less than 110 pg/mL	Less than 110 ng/L
Female	Less than 30 pg/mL	Less than 30 ng/L

DESCRIPTION: Calcitonin, also called thyrocalcitonin, is secreted by the parafollicular or C cells of the thyroid gland in response to elevated serum calcium levels. Calcitonin antagonizes the effects of parathyroid hormone and vitamin D so that calcium continues to be laid down in bone rather than reabsorbed into the blood. Calcitonin also increases renal clearance of magnesium and inhibits tubular reabsorption of phosphates. The net result is that calcitonin decreases the serum calcium level. The pentagastrin (Peptavlon) provocation test and the calcium pentagastrin provocation test are useful for diagnosing medullary thyroid cancer. ■

INDICATIONS:

• Assist in the diagnosis of hyperparathyroidism

• Assist in the diagnosis of medullary thyroid cancer

• Evaluate altered serum calcium levels

• Monitor response to therapy for medullary thyroid carcinoma

• Predict recurrence of medullary thyroid carcinoma

• Screen family members of patients with medullary thyroid carcinoma (20 percent have a familial pattern)

RESULT

Increased in:

• Alcoholic cirrhosis

• C-cell hyperplasia

• Cancer of the breast, lung, and pancreas

• Carcinoid syndrome

• Chronic renal failure

• Ectopic secretion (especially neuroendocrine origins)

• Hypercalcemia (any cause)

• Medullary thyroid cancer

• Pancreatitis

• Pernicious anemia

- Pregnancy (late)

- Pseudohypoparathyroidism

- Thyroiditis

- Zollinger-Ellison syndrome

Decreased in: N/A

CRITICAL VALUES: N/A

INTERFERING FACTORS:

- Drugs that may increase calcitonin levels include calcium, epinephrine, estrogens, glucagon, pentagastrin, sincalide, and oral contraceptives.

- Recent radioactive scans or radiation within 1 week before the test can interfere with test results when radioimmunoassay is the test method.

Nursing Implications and Procedure • • • • • • • • • • •

Pretest: ■

➤ Obtain a history of the patient's complaints, including a list of known allergens.

➤ Obtain a history of the patient's endocrine, genitourinary, and musculoskeletal systems, as well as results of previously performed tests and procedures. For related tests, refer to the endocrine, genitourinary, and musculoskeletal system tables.

➤ Obtain a list of medications the patient is taking, including herbs, nutritional supplements, and nutraceuticals. The requesting health care practitioner and laboratory should be advised if the patient regularly uses these products so that their effects can be taken into consideration when reviewing results.

➤ Note any recent procedures that can interfere with test results.

➤ There are no fluid or medication restrictions unless by medical direction.

➤ The patient should fast 10 to 12 hours before specimen collection.

➤ Review the procedure with the patient.

➤ Inform the patient that specimen collection takes approximately 5 to 10 minutes; a few extra minutes is required to administer the stimulation tests.

Intratest: ■

➤ Ensure that the patient has complied with dietary preparations and other pretesting restrictions.

➤ Direct the patient to breathe normally and to avoid unnecessary movement.

➤ Observe standard precautions and follow the general guidelines in Appendix A. Perform a venipuncture, and collect the specimen in a chilled 5-mL red- or tiger-top tube.

➤ Label the specimen, and promptly transport it to the laboratory.

Post-test: ■

➤ Observe venipuncture site for bleeding or hematoma formation. Apply pressure bandage.

➤ Instruct the patient to resume usual diet as directed by the health care practitioner.

➤ Evaluate test results in relation to the patient's symptoms and other tests performed. Related laboratory tests include adrenocorticotropin, calcium, catecholamines, carcinoembrionic antigen (CEA), complete blood count, magnesium, metanephrines, urine phosphorus, thyroid biopsy, and vitamin D.

CALCIUM, IONIZED

· ·

SYNONYM/ACRONYM: N/A.

SPECIMEN: Whole blood (1 mL) collected anaerobically in a heparinized syringe. Serum (1 mL) collected in a red-top tube or plasma (1 mL) collected in a green-top (heparin) tube is also acceptable. Specimen should be transported tightly capped and in an ice slurry.

REFERENCE VALUE: (Method: Ion-selective electrode)

	Conventional Units	SI Units (Conversion Factor ×0.25)
Whole blood		
Cord blood	5.20–5.84 mg/dL	1.30–1.46 mmol/L
Adult	4.60–5.08 mg/dL	1.12–1.32 mmol/L
Plasma		
Adult	4.12–4.92 mg/dL	1.03–1.23 mmol/L
Serum		
Cord blood	5.20–6.40 mg/dL	1.30–1.60 mmol/L
Adult	4.64–5.28 mg/dL	1.16–1.32 mmol/L

DESCRIPTION: Calcium is the most abundant cation in the body and participates in almost all vital body processes. (See other calcium monographs.) Circulating calcium is found in the free or ionized form; bound to organic anions such as lactate, phosphate, or citrate; and bound to proteins such as albumin. Ionized calcium is the physiologically active form of circulating calcium. About half of the total amount of calcium circulates as free ions that participate in blood coagulation, neuromuscular conduction, intracellular regulation, glandular secretion, and control of skeletal and cardiac muscle contractility. Calcium levels are regulated largely by the parathyroid glands and by vitamin D. Compared to total calcium level, ionized calcium is a better measurement of calcium metabolism. Ionized calcium levels are not influenced by protein concentrations, as seen in patients with chronic renal failure, nephrotic syndrome, malabsorption, and multiple myeloma. Levels are also not affected in patients with metabolic acid-base balance disturbances. Elevations in ionized calcium may be seen when the total calcium is normal. Measurement of ionized calcium is useful to monitor patients undergoing cardiothoracic surgery or organ transplantation. It is also useful in the evaluation of patients in cardiac arrest. ■

INDICATIONS:

- Detect ectopic parathyroid hormone–producing neoplasms
- Evaluate the effect of protein on calcium levels
- Identify individuals with hypocalcemia
- Identify individuals with toxic levels of vitamin D
- Investigate suspected hyperparathyroidism
- Monitor patients with renal failure or organ transplantation, in whom secondary hyperparathyroidism may be a complication
- Monitor patients with sepsis or magnesium deficiency

RESULT

Increased in:

- Parathyroid hormone–producing neoplasms
- Hyperparathyroidism
- Vitamin D toxicity

Decreased in:

- Burns
- Hypoparathyroidism (primary)
- Magnesium deficiency
- Multiple organ failure
- Pancreatitis
- The postdialysis period, as a result of low-calcium dialysate administration
- The post-transfusion period, as a result of the use of citrated preservative (calcium chelator)
- The postsurgical period (i.e., major surgeries)
- Premature infants with hypoproteinemia and acidosis

- Pseudohypoparathyroidism
- Sepsis
- Trauma
- Vitamin D deficiency

CRITICAL VALUES:

Less than 3.2 mg/dL
Greater than 6.4 mg/dL

Observe the patient for symptoms of critically decreased or elevated calcium levels. Hypocalcemia is evidenced by convulsions, arrhythmias, changes in electrocardiogram (ECG) in the form of prolonged ST segment and Q-T interval, facial spasms (positive Chvostek's sign), tetany, muscle cramps, numbness in extremities, tingling, and muscle twitching (positive Trousseau's sign). Possible interventions include seizure precautions, increased frequency of ECG monitoring, and administration of calcium or magnesium.

Severe hypercalcemia is manifested by polyuria, constipation, changes in ECG (shortened ST segment), lethargy, muscle weakness, apathy, anorexia, headache, and nausea, and ultimately may result in coma. Possible interventions include the administration of normal saline and diuretics to speed up excretion or administration of calcitonin or steroids to force the circulating calcium into the cells.

INTERFERING FACTORS:

- Drugs that may increase calcium levels include antacids (some), calcitriol, and lithium.
- Drugs that may decrease calcium levels include calcitonin, citrates, foscarnet, and pamidronate (initially).
- Calcium exhibits diurnal variation; serial samples should be collected at the same time of day for comparison.
- Venous hemostasis caused by prolonged use of a tourniquet during venipuncture can falsely elevate calcium levels.

• Patients on ethylenediaminetetra-acetic acid (EDTA) therapy (chelation) may show falsely decreased calcium values.

• Specimens should never be collected above an intravenous (IV) line because of the potential for dilution when the specimen and the IV solution combine in the collection container, falsely decreasing the result. There is also the potential of contaminating the sample with the substance of interest, contained in the IV solution, falsely increasing the result.

Nursing Implications and Procedure • • • • • • • • • • •

Pretest:

➤ Obtain a history of the patient's complaints, including a list of known allergens.

➤ Obtain a history of the patient's cardiovascular, endocrine, and genitourinary systems, as well as results of previously performed tests and procedures. For related tests, refer to the cardiovascular, genitourinary, and endocrine system tables.

➤ Obtain a list of the medications the patient is taking, including herbs, nutritional supplements, and nutraceuticals. The requesting health care practitioner and laboratory should be advised if the patient regularly uses these products so that their effects can be taken into consideration when reviewing results.

➤ Note any recent procedures that could interfere with test results.

➤ There are no food, fluid, or medication restrictions unless by medical direction.

➤ Review the procedure with the patient. The patient should be instructed to lie quietly for 30 minutes before specimen collection.

➤ Prepare an ice slurry for specimen transport.

➤ Inform the patient that specimen collection takes approximately 5 to 10 minutes.

Intratest:

➤ Direct the patient to breathe normally and to avoid unnecessary movement.

➤ Observe standard precautions and follow the general guidelines in Appendix A. Perform a venipuncture, and without using a tourniquet, collect the specimen in a heparinized syringe. The specimen must be maintained in an anaerobic environment; the cork should not be removed from the tube at any point in the collection process.

➤ Label the specimen, and promptly transport it to the laboratory. The tightly capped sample should be placed in an ice slurry immediately after collection. Information on the specimen label can be protected from water in the ice slurry if the specimen is first placed in a protective plastic bag.

Post-test:

➤ Observe venipuncture site for bleeding or hematoma formation. Apply pressure bandage.

➤ Patients with abnormal calcium values should be informed that daily intake of calcium is important even though body stores in the bones can be called on to supplement circulating levels. Dietary calcium can be obtained from animal or plant sources. Milk and milk products, sardines, clams, oysters, salmon, rhubarb, spinach, beet greens, broccoli, kale, tofu, legumes, and fortified orange juice are high in calcium. Milk and milk products also contain vitamin D and lactose, which assist calcium absorption. Cooked vegetables yield more absorbable calcium than raw vegetables. Patients should be informed of the substances that can inhibit calcium absorption by irreversibly binding to some of the calcium, making it unavailable for absorption, such as oxalates, which naturally occur in some vegetables; phytic acid, found in some cereals; and insoluble dietary fiber (in excessive amounts). Excessive protein intake can also negatively affect calcium absorption, especially if it is combined with foods high in phosphorus.

➤ Evaluate test results in relation to the patient's symptoms and other tests performed. Related laboratory tests include albumin, calcium, kidney stone analysis, parathyroid hormone, and vitamin D.

CALCIUM, SERUM

SYNONYM/ACRONYM: total calcium, Ca.

SPECIMEN: Serum (1 mL) collected in a red- or tiger-top tube. Plasma (1 mL) collected in green-top (heparin) tube is also acceptable.

REFERENCE VALUE: (Method: Spectrophotometry)

Age	Conventional Units	SI Units (Conversion Factor ×0.25)
Cord	8.2–11.2 mg/dL	2.05–2.80 mmol/L
0–10 d	7.6–10.4 mg/dL	1.90–2.60 mmol/L
11 d–2 y	9.0–11.0 mg/dL	2.25–2.75 mmol/L
3–12 y	8.8–10.8 mg/dL	2.20–2.70 mmol/L
13–18 y	8.4–10.2 mg/dL	2.10–2.55 mmol/L
Adult	8.2–10.2 mg/dL	2.05–2.55 mmol/L
Adult older than 90 y	8.2–9.6 mg/dL	2.05–2.40 mmol/L

DESCRIPTION: Calcium, the most abundant cation in the body, participates in almost all of the vital processes. Calcium concentration is largely regulated by the parathyroid glands and by the action of vitamin D. Of the body's calcium reserves, 98 to 99 percent is stored in the teeth and skeleton. Calcium values are higher in children because of growth and active bone formation. About 45 percent of the total amount of blood calcium circulates as free ions that participate in coagulation, neuromuscular conduction, intracellular regulation, glandular secretion, and control of skeletal and cardiac muscle contractility. The remaining calcium is bound to circulating proteins (40 percent bound mostly to albumin) and anions (15 percent bound to anions such as bicarbonate, citrate, phosphate, and lactate) and plays no physiologic role. Calcium values can be adjusted up or down by 0.8 mg/dL for every 1 g/dL that albumin is greater than or less than 4 g/dL. Calcium and phosphorus levels are inversely proportional.

Fluid and electrolyte imbalances are often seen in patients with serious illness or injury; in these clinical situations, the normal homeostatic balance of the body is altered. During surgery or in the case of a critical illness, bicarbonate, phosphate, and lactate concentrations can change dramatically. Therapeutic treatments may also cause or contribute to electrolyte imbalance. This is why total calcium values can sometimes be misleading. Abnormal calcium levels are used to indicate general malfunctions in various body systems. Ionized calcium is used in more specific conditions. (See monograph titled "Calcium, Ionized.")

Calcium values should be interpreted in conjunction with results of other tests. Normal calcium with an abnormal phosphorus value indicates impaired calcium absorption (possibly because of altered parathyroid hormone level or activity). Normal calcium with an elevated urea nitrogen value indicates possible hyperparathyroidism (primary or secondary). Normal calcium with decreased albumin value is an indication of hypercalcemia. The most common cause of hypocalcemia (low calcium levels) is hypoalbuminemia. The most common causes of hypercalcemia (high calcium levels) are hyperparathyroidism and cancer. ∎

INDICATIONS:

• Detect parathyroid gland loss after thyroid or other neck surgery, as indicated by decreased levels

• Evaluate cardiac arrhythmias and coagulation disorders to determine if altered serum calcium level is contributing to the problem

• Evaluate the effects of various disorders on calcium metabolism, especially diseases involving bone

• Monitor the effects of renal failure and various drugs on calcium levels

• Monitor the effectiveness of therapy being administered to correct abnormal calcium levels, especially calcium deficiencies

RESULT

Increased in:

• Acidosis

• Acromegaly

• Cancers (bone, Burkitt's lymphoma, Hodgkin's lymphoma, leukemia, myeloma, and metastases from other organs)

• Dehydration

• Excessive intake (milk, antacids)

• Hyperparathyroidism

• Idiopathic hypercalcemia of infancy

• Malignant disease without bone involvement (squamous cell carcinoma of the lung, kidney cancer)

• Milk alkali syndrome (Burnett's syndrome)

• Paget's disease

• Pheochromocytoma

• Polycythemia vera

• Renal transplant

• Sarcoidosis

• Thyrotoxicosis

• Vitamin D toxicity

Decreased in:

• Acute pancreatitis

- Alcoholism

- Alkalosis

- Chronic renal failure

- Cystinosis

- Hepatic cirrhosis

- Hyperphosphatemia

- Hypoalbuminemia

- Hypoparathyroidism (congenital, idiopathic, surgical)

- Inadequate nutrition

- Leprosy

- Long-term anticonvulsant therapy

- Magnesium deficiency

- Malabsorption (celiac disease, tropical sprue, pancreatic insufficiency)

- Massive blood transfusion

- Neonatal prematurity

- Osteomalacia (advanced)

- Renal tubular disease

- Vitamin D deficiency (rickets)

CRITICAL VALUES:

Less than 7 mg/dL

Greater than 12 mg/dL (some patients can tolerate higher concentrations)

Observe the patient for symptoms of critically decreased or elevated calcium levels. Hypocalcemia is evidenced by convulsions, arrhythmias, changes in electrocardiogram (ECG) in the form of prolonged ST segment and Q-T interval, facial spasms (positive Chvostek's sign), tetany, muscle cramps, numbness in extremities, tingling, and muscle twitching (positive Trousseau's sign). Possible interventions include seizure precautions, increased frequency of ECG monitoring, and administration of calcium or magnesium.

Severe hypercalcemia is manifested by polyuria, constipation, changes in ECG (shortened ST segment), lethargy, muscle weakness, apathy, anorexia, headache, and nausea and ultimately may result in coma. Possible interventions include the administration of normal saline and diuretics to speed up excretion or administration of calcitonin or steroids to force the circulating calcium into the cells.

INTERFERING FACTORS:

- Drugs that may increase calcium levels include anabolic steroids, some antacids, calcitriol, calcium salts, danazol, diuretics (long-term), ergocalciferol, isotretinoin, lithium, oral contraceptives, parathyroid extract, parathyroid hormone, prednisone, progesterone, tamoxifen, vitamin A, and vitamin D.

- Drugs that may decrease calcium levels include albuterol, alprostadil, aminoglycosides, anticonvulsants, calcitonin, diuretics (initially), glucagon, glucocorticoids, glucose, laxatives (excessive use), magnesium salts, methicillin, phosphates, plicamycin, sodium sulfate (given intravenously), tetracycline (in pregnancy), trazodone, and viomycin.

- Calcium exhibits diurnal variation; serial samples should be collected at the same time of day for comparison.

- Venous hemostasis caused by prolonged use of a tourniquet during venipuncture can falsely elevate calcium levels.

- Patients on ethylenediaminetetraacetic acid (EDTA) therapy (chelation) may show falsely decreased calcium values.

- Hemolysis and icterus cause false-positive results because of interference from biologic pigments.

- Specimens should never be collected above an intravenous (IV) line because of the potential for dilution when the specimen and the IV solution combine in the collection container, falsely decreasing the result. There is also the potential of contaminating the sample with the substance in question, contained in the IV solution, falsely increasing the result.

Nursing Implications and Procedure • • • • • • • • • • •

Pretest:

➤ Obtain a history of the patient's complaints, including a list of known allergens.

➤ Obtain a history of the patient's cardiovascular, gastrointestinal, genitourinary, hematopoietic, hepatobiliary, and musculoskeletal systems, as well as results of previously performed tests and procedures. For related tests, refer to the cardiovascular, gastrointestinal, genitourinary, hematopoietic, hepatobiliary, and musculoskeletal system tables.

➤ Obtain a list of medications the patient is taking, including herbs, nutritional supplements, and nutraceuticals. The requesting health care practitioner and laboratory should be advised if the patient regularly uses these products so that their effects can be taken into consideration when reviewing results.

➤ Note any recent procedures that can interfere with test results.

➤ There are no food, fluid, or medication restrictions unless by medical direction.

➤ Review the procedure with the patient.

➤ Inform the patient that specimen collection takes approximately 5 to 10 minutes.

Intratest:

➤ Direct the patient to breathe normally and to avoid unnecessary movement.

➤ Observe standard precautions and follow the general guidelines in Appendix A. Perform a venipuncture, and collect the specimen in a 5-mL red- or tiger-top tube.

➤ Label the specimen, and promptly transport it to the laboratory.

Post-test:

➤ Observe venipuncture site for bleeding or hematoma formation. Apply pressure bandage.

➤ Patients with abnormal calcium values should be informed that daily intake of calcium is important even though body stores in the bones can be called on to supplement circulating levels. Dietary calcium can be obtained from animal or plant sources. Milk and milk products, sardines, clams, oysters, salmon, rhubarb, spinach, beet greens, broccoli, kale, tofu, legumes, and fortified orange juice are high in calcium. Milk and milk products also contain vitamin D and lactose, which assist calcium absorption. Cooked vegetables yield more absorbable calcium than raw vegetables. Patients should be informed of the substances that can inhibit calcium absorption by irreversibly binding to some of the calcium, making it unavailable for absorption, such as oxalates, which naturally occur in some vegetables; phytic acid, found in some cereals; and insoluble dietary fiber (in excessive amounts). Excessive protein intake can also negatively affect calcium absorption, especially if it is combined with foods high in phosphorus.

➤ Evaluate test results in relation to the patient's symptoms and other tests performed. Related laboratory tests include albumin, alkaline phosphatase, calcitonin, ionized calcium, urine calcium, electrolytes, kidney stone analysis, magnesium, urine magnesium, parathyroid hormone, phosphorus, urine phosphorus, total protein, urinalysis, and vitamin D.

CALCIUM, URINE

SYNONYM/ACRONYM: N/A.

SPECIMEN: Urine (5 mL) from an unpreserved random or timed specimen collected in a clean plastic collection container.

REFERENCE VALUE: (Method: Spectrophotometry)

Age	Conventional Units*	SI Units (Conversion Factor ×0.025)*
Infant and child	Up to 6 mg/kg per 24 h	Up to 0.15 mmol/kg per 24 h
Adult on average diet	100–300 mg/24 h	2.5–7.5 mmol/24 h

* Values depend on diet. Average daily intake of calcium: 600–800 mg/24 h.

DESCRIPTION: Regulating electrolyte balance is a major function of the kidneys. In normally functioning kidneys, urine levels increase when serum levels are high and decrease when serum levels are low to maintain homeostasis. Analyzing urinary electrolyte levels can provide important clues to the functioning of the kidneys and other major organs. Tests for calcium in urine usually involve timed urine collections during a 12- or 24-hour period. Measurement of random specimens may also be requested. Urinary calcium excretion may also be expressed as calcium-to-creatinine ratio: In a healthy individual with constant muscle mass, the ratio is less than 0.14. ■

INDICATIONS:

• Assist in establishing the presence of kidney stones

• Evaluate bone disease

• Evaluate dietary intake and absorption

• Evaluate renal loss

• Monitor patients on calcium replacement

RESULT

Increased in:

• Acromegaly

• Diabetes

• Fanconi's syndrome

• Glucocorticoid excess

• Hepatolenticular degeneration

• Hyperparathyroidism

• Hyperthyroidism

• Idiopathic hypercalciuria

• Immobilization

• Kidney stones

• Some instances of leukemia and lymphoma

- Myeloma

- Neoplasm of the breast or bladder

- Osteitis deformans

- Osteolytic bone metastases (carcinoma, sarcoma)

- Osteoporosis

- Paget's disease

- Renal tubular acidosis

- Sarcoidosis

- Schistosomiasis

- Thyrotoxicosis

- Vitamin D intoxication

Decreased in:

- Hypocalcemia (other than renal disease)

- Hypocalciuric hypercalcemia (familial, nonfamilial)

- Hypoparathyroidism

- Hypothyroidism

- Malabsorption (celiac disease, tropical sprue)

- Malignant bone neoplasm

- Nephrosis and acute nephritis

- Osteoblastic metastases

- Osteomalacia

- Preeclampsia

- Pseudohypoparathyroidism

- Renal osteodystrophy

- Rickets

- Vitamin D deficiency

CRITICAL VALUES: N/A

INTERFERING FACTORS:

- Drugs that can increase urine calcium levels include acetazolamide, ammonium chloride, asparaginase, calci-

tonin, calcitriol, corticosteroids, corticotropin, dexamethasone, diuretics (initially), ergocalciferol, ethacrynic acid, mannitol (initially), meralluride, mercaptomerin, mersalyl, nandrolone, parathyroid extract, parathyroid hormone, plicamycin, sodium sulfate, sulfates, triamterene, viomycin, and vitamin D.

- Drugs that can decrease urine calcium levels include angiotensin, bicarbonate, calcitonin, citrates, diuretics (chronic), lithium, neomycin, oral contraceptives, and spironolactone.

- Failure to collect all the urine and store the specimen properly during the 24-hour test period invalidates the results.

Nursing Implications and Procedure ● ● ● ● ● ● ● ● ● ● ●

Pretest: ■

➤ Obtain a history of the patient's complaints, including a list of known allergens.

➤ Obtain a history of the patient's endocrine, genitourinary, and musculoskeletal systems, as well as results of previously performed tests and procedures. For related tests, refer to the endocrine, genitourinary, and musculoskeletal system tables.

➤ Obtain a list of the medications the patient is taking, including herbs, nutritional supplements, and nutraceuticals. The requesting health care practitioner and laboratory should be advised if the patient regularly uses these products so that their effects can be taken into consideration when reviewing results.

➤ There are no fluid or medication restrictions unless by medical direction.

➤ Instruct the patient to follow a normal calcium diet for at least 4 days before test.

➤ Review the procedure with the patient. Provide a nonmetallic urinal, bedpan, or toilet-mounted collection device.

➤ Usually a 24-hour time frame for urine collection is ordered. Inform the patient that all urine must be saved during that 24-hour period. Instruct the patient not to void directly into the laboratory collection container. Instruct the patient to avoid defecating in the collection device and to keep toilet tissue out of the collection device to prevent contamination of the specimen. Place a sign in the bathroom to remind the patient to save all urine.

➤ Instruct the patient to void all urine into the collection device and then to pour the urine into the laboratory collection container. Alternatively the specimen can be left in the collection device for a health care staff member to add to the laboratory collection container.

Intratest:

➤ Ensure that the patient has complied with dietary preparations and other pretesting restrictions.

➤ Observe standard precautions and follow the general guidelines in Appendix A.

Random specimen (collect in early morning):

➤ Obtain urine specimen in a properly labeled plastic collection container and immediately transport urine. If an indwelling catheter is in place, it may be necessary to clamp off the catheter for 15 to 30 minutes before specimen collection. Cleanse specimen port with antiseptic swab, and then aspirate 5 mL of urine with a 21- to 25-gauge needle and syringe. Transfer urine to a plastic container.

Timed specimen:

➤ Obtain a clean 3-L urine specimen container, toilet-mounted collection device, and plastic bag (for transport of the specimen container). The specimen must be refrigerated or kept on ice throughout the collection period. If an indwelling urinary catheter is in place, the drainage bag must be kept on ice.

➤ Begin the test between 6 and 8 a.m., if possible. Collect first voiding and discard. Record the time the specimen was discarded as the beginning of the timed collection period. The next morning, ask the patient to void at the same time the collection was started, and add this last voiding to the container.

➤ If an indwelling catheter is in place, replace the tubing and container system at the start of the collection time. Keep the container system on ice during the collection period or empty the urine into a larger container periodically during the collection period; monitor to ensure continued drainage, and conclude the test the next morning at the same hour the collection began.

➤ At the conclusion of the test, compare the quantity of urine with the urinary output record for the collection; if the specimen contains less than the recorded output, some urine may have been discarded, invalidating the test.

➤ Label the specimen, and promptly transport it to the laboratory. Include on the label the amount of urine collected and test start and stop times.

Post-test:

➤ Increased urine calcium levels may be associated with kidney stones. Educate the patient, if appropriate, as to the importance of drinking a sufficient amount of water when kidney stones are suspected.

➤ Evaluate test results in relation to the patient's symptoms and other tests performed. Related laboratory tests include calcium, kidney stone analysis, magnesium, urine magnesium, parathyroid hormone, urine oxalate, phosphorus, urine phosphorus, potassium, urine potassium, uric acid, urine uric acid, urinalysis, and vitamin D.

CALCULUS, KIDNEY STONE PANEL

SYNONYMS/ACRONYM: Kidney stone analysis, nephrolithiasis analysis.

SPECIMEN: Kidney stones.

REFERENCE VALUE: (Method: Infrared spectrometry) None detected.

DESCRIPTION: Renal calculi (kidney stones) are formed by the crystallization of calcium oxalate (most common), magnesium ammonium phosphate, calcium phosphate, uric acid, and cystine. Formation of stones may be due to reduced urine flow and excessive amounts of the above-mentioned insoluble substances. The presence of stones is confirmed by diagnostic visualization or passing of the stones in the urine. The chemical nature of the stones is confirmed qualitatively. ■

INDICATIONS: Identify substances present in renal calculi

RESULT

Positive findings in: Presence of renal calculi

Negative findings in: N/A

CRITICAL VALUES: N/A

INTERFERING FACTORS:

• Drugs and substances that may increase the formation of urine calculi include probenecid and vitamin D.

• Adhesive tape should not be used to attach stones to any transportation or collection container, because the adhesive interferes with infrared spectrometry.

Nursing Implications and Procedure

Pretest:

➤ Obtain a history of the patient's complaints, especially hematuria, recurrent urinary tract infection, and abdominal pain, and a list of known allergens.

➤ Obtain a history of the patient's genitourinary system and results of previously performed tests and procedures. For related tests, refer to the genitourinary system tables.

➤ Obtain a list of the medications the patient is taking, including herbs, nutritional supplements, and nutraceuticals. The requesting health care practitioner and laboratory should be advised if the patient regularly uses these products so that their effects can be taken into consideration when reviewing results.

Intratest:

➤ The patient presenting with symptoms indicating the presence of kidney stones may be provided with a device to strain the urine. The patient should be informed to transfer any particulate matter remaining in the strainer into the specimen collection container provided. Stones removed by the health care practitioner should be placed in the appropriate collection container.

➤ Label the specimen, and promptly transport it to the laboratory.

Post-test: ∎

➤ Inform the patient with kidney stones that the likelihood of recurrence is high. Educate the patient regarding risk factors that contribute to the likelihood of kidney stone formation, including family history, osteoporosis, urinary tract infections, gout, magnesium deficiency, Crohn's disease with prior resection, age, gender (males are two to three times more likely to develop stones than females), and climate.

➤ Nutritional therapy is indicated for individuals identified as being at high risk for developing kidney stones. Educate the patient that diets rich in protein, salt, and oxalates increase the risk of stone formation. Adequate fluid intake should be encouraged.

➤ Follow-up testing of urine may be requested but usually not for 1 month after the stones have passed or been removed.

➤ Evaluate test results in relation to the patient's symptoms and other tests performed. Related laboratory tests include urine calcium, urine culture, creatinine clearance, urine magnesium, urine oxalate, urine phosphorus, urine uric acid, and urinalysis.

CARBON DIOXIDE

· ·

Synonyms/Acronyms: CO_2 combining power, CO_2, tCO_2.

Specimen: Serum (1 mL) collected in a red- or tiger-top tube, plasma (1 mL) collected in a green-top (lithium or sodium heparin) tube; or whole blood (1 mL) collected in a green-top (lithium or sodium heparin) tube or heparinized syringe.

Reference Value: (Method: Colorimetry, enzyme assay, or pCO_2 electrode)

Carbon Dioxide	Conventional Units	SI Units (Conversion Factor ×1)
Plasma or serum (venous)		
Infant–2 y	13–29 mmol/L	13–29 mmol/L
2 y and older	23–29 mmol/L	23–29 mmol/L
Whole blood (venous)		
Infant–2 y	18–28 mmol/L	18–28 mmol/L
2 y and older	22–26 mmol/L	22–26 mmol/L

DESCRIPTION: Serum or plasma carbon dioxide (CO_2) measurement is usually done as part of an electrolyte panel. Total CO_2 (tCO_2) is an important component of the body's buffering capability, and measurements are used mainly in the evaluation of acid-base balance. It is important to understand the differences between tCO_2 (CO_2 content) and CO_2 gas (pCO_2). *Total CO_2* reflects the majority of CO_2 in the body mainly in the form of bicarbonate (HCO_3^-), is present as a base, and is regulated by the kidneys. *CO_2 gas* contributes little to the tCO_2 level, is acidic, and is regulated by the lungs. (See monograph titled "Blood Gases" for more information.)

CO_2 provides the basis for the principal buffering system of the extracellular fluid system, which is the bicarbonate–carbonic acid buffer system. CO_2 circulates in the body either bound to protein or physically dissolved. Constituents in the blood that contribute to tCO_2 levels are bicarbonate, carbamino compounds, and carbonic acid (carbonic acid includes undissociated carbonic acid and dissolved CO_2). Bicarbonate is the second largest group of anions in the extracellular fluid (chloride being the largest group of extracellular anions). tCO_2 levels closely reflect bicarbonate (HCO_3^-) levels in the blood, because 90 to 95 percent of CO_2 circulates as HCO_3^-. ∎

INDICATIONS:

- Evaluate decreased venous CO_2 in the case of compensated metabolic acidosis
- Evaluate increased venous CO_2 in the case of compensated metabolic alkalosis

- Monitor decreased venous CO_2 as a result of compensated respiratory alkalosis
- Monitor increased venous CO_2 as a result of compensation for respiratory acidosis secondary to significant respiratory system infection or cancer; decreased respiratory rate

RESULT

Increased in:

- Acute intermittent porphyria
- Airway obstruction
- Asthmatic shock
- Brain tumor
- Bronchitis (chronic)
- Cardiac disorders
- Depression of respiratory center
- Electrolyte disturbance (severe)
- Emphysema
- Hypothyroidism
- Hypoventilation
- Metabolic alkalosis
- Myopathy
- Poliomyelitis
- Pneumonia
- Respiratory acidosis
- Tuberculosis (pulmonary)

Decreased in:

- Acute renal failure
- Anxiety
- Dehydration
- Diabetic ketoacidosis
- Diarrhea (severe)
- High fever

- Metabolic acidosis

- Respiratory alkalosis

- Salicylate intoxication

- Starvation

CRITICAL VALUES:

Less than 15 mmol/L

Greater than 50 mmol/L

Observe the patient for signs and symptoms of excessive or insufficient CO_2 levels, and report these findings to a health care practitioner. If the patient has been vomiting for several days and is breathing shallowly, or if the patient has had gastric suctioning and is breathing shallowly, this may indicate elevated CO_2 levels. Decreased CO_2 levels are evidenced by deep, vigorous breathing and flushed skin.

INTERFERING FACTORS:

- Drugs that may cause an increase in tCO_2 levels include acetylsalicylic acid, aldosterone, bicarbonate, carbenicillin, carbenoxolone, corticosteroids, dexamethasone, ethacrinic acid, laxatives (chronic abuse), and x-ray contrast agents.

- Drugs that may cause a decrease in tCO_2 levels include acetazolamide, acetylsalicylic acid (initially), amiloride, ammonium chloride, fluorides, metformin, methicillin, nitrofurantoin, NSD 3004 (long-acting carbonic anhydrase inhibitor), paraldehyde, tetracycline, triamterene, and xylitol.

- Prompt and proper specimen processing, storage, and analysis are important to achieve accurate results. The specimen should be stored under anaerobic conditions after collection to prevent the diffusion of CO_2 gas from the specimen. Falsely decreased values result from uncovered specimens. It is estimated that CO_2 diffuses from the sample at the rate of 6 mmol/h.

Nursing Implications and Procedure • • • • • • • • • • •

➤ Obtain a history of the patient's complaints, including a list of known allergens.

➤ Obtain a history of the patient's genitourinary and respiratory systems, as well as results of previously performed tests and procedures. For related tests, refer to the genitourinary and respiratory system tables.

➤ Obtain a list of the medications the patient is taking, including herbs, nutritional supplements, and nutraceuticals. The requesting health care practitioner and laboratory should be advised if the patient regularly uses these products so that their effects can be taken into consideration when reviewing results.

➤ There are no food, fluid, or medication restrictions unless by medical direction.

➤ Review the procedure with the patient.

➤ Inform the patient that specimen collection takes approximately 5 to 10 minutes.

Intratest:

➤ Direct the patient to breathe normally and to avoid unnecessary movement.

➤ Instruct the patient to not clench and unclench the fist during specimen collection.

➤ Observe standard precautions and follow the general guidelines in Appendix A. Perform a venipuncture, and collect the specimen in a 5-mL red-, tiger-, or green-top tube.

➤ Label the specimen, and promptly transport it to the laboratory.

Post-test:

➤ Observe venipuncture site for bleeding or hematoma formation. Apply pressure bandage.

➤ Evaluate test results in relation to the patient's symptoms and other tests performed. Related laboratory tests include arterial/alveolar oxygen ratio, anion gap, blood gases, electrolytes, ketones, and salicylate.

CARBOXYHEMOGLOBIN

• •

SYNONYMS/ACRONYMS: Carbon monoxide, CO, COHb, COH.

SPECIMEN: Whole blood (1 mL) collected in a green-top (heparin) or lavender-top (ethylenediaminetetra-acetic acid [EDTA]) tube, depending on laboratory requirement. Specimen should be transported tightly capped (anaerobic) and in an ice slurry if blood gases are to be performed simultaneously. Carboxyhemoglobin is stable at room temperature.

REFERENCE VALUE: (Method: Spectrophotometry, co-oximetry)

	% Saturation of Hemoglobin	Fraction of Hemoglobin Saturation SI Units (Conversion Factor ×0.01)
Newborns	10–12%	0.1–0.12
Nonsmokers	Up to 2%	Up to 0.02
Smokers	Up to 12%	Up to 0.12

DESCRIPTION: Exogenous carbon monoxide (CO) is a colorless, odorless, tasteless byproduct of incomplete combustion derived from the exhaust of automobiles, coal and gas burning, and tobacco smoke. Endogenous CO is produced as a result of red blood cell catabolism. CO levels are elevated in newborns as a result of the combined effects of high hemoglobin turnover and the inefficiency of the infant's respiratory system. CO binds tightly to hemoglobin with an affinity 250 times greater than oxygen, competitively and dramatically reducing the oxygen-carrying capacity of hemoglobin. The increased percentage of bound CO reflects the extent to which normal transport of oxygen has been negatively affected. Overexposure causes hypoxia, which results in headache, nausea, vomiting, vertigo, collapse, or convulsions. Toxic exposure causes anoxia, increased levels of lactic acid, and irreversible tissue damage, which can result in coma or death. Acute exposure may be evidenced by a cherry red color to the lips, skin, and nail beds; this observation may not be apparent in cases of chronic exposure. A direct correlation has been implicated between carboxyhemoglobin levels and symptoms of atherosclerotic disease, angina, and myocardial infarction. ■

INDICATIONS:

• Assist in the diagnosis of suspected CO poisoning

• Evaluate exposure to fires and smoke inhalation

• Evaluate the effect of smoking on the patient

RESULT

Increased in:

• CO poisoning

• Hemolytic disease

• Tobacco smoking

Decreased in: N/A

CRITICAL VALUES:

Asymptomatic: 10 to 20 percent
Disturbance of judgment, headache, dizziness: 10 to 30 percent
Toxic concentration: greater than 20 percent
Coma, respiratory arrest, and death: greater than 50 percent

A possible intervention in moderate CO poisoning is the administration of supplemental oxygen given at atmospheric pressure. In severe CO poisoning, hyperbaric oxygen treatments may be used.

INTERFERING FACTORS: Specimen should be collected before administration of oxygen therapy.

Nursing Implications and Procedure • • • • • • • • • •

Pretest: ■

➤ Obtain a history of the patient's complaints, including a list of known allergens.

➤ Obtain a history of the patient's respiratory system and results of previously performed tests and procedures. For related tests, refer to the respiratory system table.

➤ Obtain a list of medications the patient is taking, including herbs, nutritional supplements, and nutraceuticals. The requesting health care practitioner and laboratory should be advised if the patient regularly uses these products so that their effects can be taken into consideration when reviewing results.

➤ Note any recent procedures that can interfere with test results.

➤ There are no food, fluid, or medication restrictions unless by medical direction.

➤ Review the procedure with the patient. Explain to the patient or family members that the cause of the headache, vomiting, dizziness, convulsions, or coma could be related to CO exposure.

➤ Inform the patient that specimen collection takes approximately 5 to 10 minutes.

➤ If carboxyhemoglobin measurement will be performed simultaneously with arterial blood gases, prepare an ice slurry in a cup or plastic bag and have it on hand for immediate transport of the specimen to the laboratory.

Intratest: ■

➤ Direct the patient to breathe normally and to avoid unnecessary movement.

➤ Observe standard precautions and follow the general guidelines in

Appendix A. Perform a venipuncture, and collect the specimen in a 5-mL green- or lavender-top tube.

➤ Label the specimen, and promptly transport it to the laboratory. The tightly capped sample should be placed in an ice slurry immediately after collection. Information on the specimen label can be protected from water in the ice slurry if the specimen is first placed in a protective plastic bag.

Post-test:

➤ Observe venipuncture site for bleeding or hematoma formation. Apply pressure bandage.

➤ Inform the patient of smoking cessation programs, as appropriate.

➤ Evaluate test results in relation to the patient's symptoms and other tests performed. Related laboratory tests include arterial/alveolar oxygen ratio and blood gases.

CARCINOEMBRYONIC ANTIGEN

· ·

SYNONYM/ACRONYM: CEA.

SPECIMEN: Serum (1 mL) collected in a red-top tube. Plasma (1 mL) collected in lavender-top (ethylenediaminetetra-acetic acid [EDTA]) tube is also acceptable. Care must be taken to use the same type of collection container if serial measurements are to be taken.

REFERENCE VALUE: (Method: Enzyme immunoassay)

Smoking Status	Conventional Units	SI Units (Conversion Factor ×1)
Smoker	Less than 5.0 ng/mL	Less than 5.0 µg/L
Nonsmoker	Less than 2.5 ng/mL	Less than 2.5 µg/L

DESCRIPTION: Carcinoembryonic antigen (CEA) is a glycoprotein normally produced only during early fetal life and rapid multiplication of epithelial cells, especially those of the digestive system. CEA also appears in the blood of chronic smokers. Although the test is not diagnostic for any specific disease and is not useful as a screening test for cancer, it is useful for monitoring response to antineoplastic therapy in breast and gastrointestinal cancer. ■

INDICATIONS:

• Determine stage of colorectal cancer and test for recurrence

• Monitor response to treatment of breast and gastrointestinal cancers

RESULT

Increased in:

• Benign tumors, including benign breast disease

• Colorectal, pulmonary, gastric, pancreatic, breast, head or neck, esophageal, ovarian, or prostate cancer

• Chronic tobacco smoking

• Radiation therapy (transient)

Decreased in: N/A

CRITICAL VALUES: N/A

INTERFERING FACTORS: N/A

Nursing Implications and Procedure • • • • • • • • • • •

Pretest:

➤ Obtain a history of the patient's complaints, including a list of known allergens.

➤ Obtain a history of the patient's gastrointestinal, immune, and reproductive systems, as well as results of previously performed tests and procedures. For related tests, refer to the gastrointestinal, immune, and reproductive system tables.

➤ Obtain a list of medications the patient is taking, including herbs, nutritional supplements, and nutraceuticals. The requesting health care practitioner and laboratory should be advised if the patient regularly uses these products so that their effects can be taken into consideration when reviewing results.

➤ Determine if the patient smokes,

because smokers may have false elevations.

➤ There are no food, fluid, or medication restrictions unless by medical direction.

➤ Review the procedure with the patient.

➤ Inform the patient that specimen collection takes approximately 5 to 10 minutes.

Intratest:

➤ Direct the patient to breathe normally and to avoid unnecessary movement.

➤ Observe standard precautions and follow the general guidelines in Appendix A. Perform a venipuncture, and collect the specimen in a 5-mL red-top or lavender-top tube.

➤ Label the specimen, and promptly transport it to the laboratory.

Post-test:

➤ Observe venipuncture site for bleeding or hematoma formation. Apply pressure bandage.

➤ Inform the patient that the test may be repeated monthly to monitor response to therapy.

➤ Recognize anxiety related to test results and offer support. Provide teaching and information regarding the clinical implications of the test results, as appropriate. Educate the patient regarding access to counseling services.

➤ Instruct the patient in the importance of continuing scheduled therapy or follow-up visits.

➤ Evaluate test results in relation to the patient's symptoms and other tests performed. Related laboratory tests include biopsy of suspicious tissue, CA 15-3, and CA 19-9.

CATECHOLAMINES

. . . .

SYNONYMS/ACRONYM: Epinephrine, norepinephrine, dopamine.

SPECIMEN: Plasma (2 mL) collected in green-top (heparin) tube.

REFERENCE VALUE: (Method: High-performance liquid chromatography)

	Conventional Units	SI Units
		(Conversion Factor ×5.46)
Epinephrine		
Supine, 30 min	0–110 pg/mL	0–600 pmol/L
Standing, 30 min	0–140 pg/mL	0–764 pmol/L
		(Conversion Factor ×5.91)
Norepinephrine		
Supine, 30 min	70–750 pg/mL	414–4432 pmol/L
Standing, 30 min	200–1700 pg/mL	1182–10,047 pmol/L
		(Conversion Factor ×6.53)
Dopamine		
Supine or standing	0–30 pg/mL	0–196 pmol/L

DESCRIPTION: Catecholamines are produced by the chromaffin tissue of the adrenal medulla. They are also found in sympathetic nerve endings and in the brain. The major catecholamines are epinephrine, norepinephrine, and dopamine. They prepare the body for the fight-or-flight stress response, help regulate metabolism, and are excreted from the body by the kidneys. Catecholamine levels are affected by diurnal variations, fluctuating in response to stress, postural changes, diet, smoking, drugs, and temperature changes. As a result, blood measurement is not as reliable as a 24-hour timed urine test. Results are most reliable when the specimen is collected during a hypertensive episode. Catecholamines are measured when there is high suspicion of pheochromocytoma but urine results are normal or borderline. Findings should be compared with the metabolites of epinephrine and norepinephrine, metanephrines and vanillylmandelic acid, and the product of dopamine metabolism, homovanillic acid. Use of a clonidine suppression test with measurement of plasma catecholamines may be requested.

Failure to suppress production of catecholamines after administration of clonidine supports the diagnosis of pheochromocytoma. ■

INDICATIONS:

• Assist in the diagnosis of neuroblastoma, ganglioneuroma, or dysautonomia

• Assist in the diagnosis of paragangliomas

• Assist in the diagnosis of pheochromocytoma

• Evaluate acute hypertensive episode

• Evaluate hypertension of unknown origin

• Screen for pheochromocytoma among family members with an autosomal-dominant inheritance pattern for Lindau–von Hippel disease or multiple endocrine neoplasia

RESULT

Increased in:

• Diabetic acidosis (epinephrine and norepinephrine)

• Ganglioblastoma (epinephrine, slight increase; norepinephrine, large increase)

• Ganglioneuroma (all are increased; norepinephrine, largest increase)

• Hypothyroidism (epinephrine and norepinephrine)

• Long-term manic-depressive disorders (epinephrine and norepinephrine)

• Myocardial infarction (epinephrine and norepinephrine)

• Neuroblastoma (all are increased; norepinephrine and dopamine, largest increase)

• Pheochromocytoma (epinephrine, continuous or intermittent increase; norepinephrine, slight increase)

• Shock (epinephrine and norepinephrine)

• Strenuous exercise (epinephrine and norepinephrine)

Decreased in:

• Autonomic nervous system dysfunction (norepinephrine)

• Orthostatic hypotension (norepinephrine)

• Parkinson's disease (dopamine)

CRITICAL VALUES: N/A

INTERFERING FACTORS:

• Drugs that may increase catecholamine levels include ajmaline, chlorpromazine, cyclopropane, diazoxide, ether, monoamine oxidase inhibitors, nitroglycerin, pentazocine, perphenazine, phenothiazine, promethazine, and theophylline.

• Drugs that may decrease catecholamine levels include clonidine, metyrosine, and reserpine.

• Stress, hypoglycemia, smoking, and drugs can produce elevated plasma catecholamines.

• Secretion of catecholamines exhibits diurnal variation, with the lowest levels occurring at night.

• Secretion of catecholamines varies during the menstrual cycle, with higher levels excreted during the luteal phase and lowest levels during ovulation.

• Diets high in amines (e.g., bananas, avocados, beer, aged cheese, chocolate, cocoa, coffee, fava beans, grains, tea, vanilla, walnuts, Chianti wine) can produce elevated plasma catecholamine levels, although this effect is more likely to be seen relative to certain urinary metabolites.

Nursing Implications and Procedure • • • • • • • • • • •

Pretest: ■

➤ Obtain a history of the patient's complaints, including a list of known allergens.

➤ Obtain a history of the patient's endocrine system and results of previously performed tests and procedures. For related tests, refer to the endocrine system table.

➤ Obtain a list of the medications the patient is taking, including herbs, nutritional supplements, and nutraceuticals. The requesting health care practitioner and laboratory should be advised if the patient regularly uses these products so that their effects can be taken into consideration when reviewing results.

Instruct the patient to:

➤ Follow a normal sodium diet for 3 days before testing.

➤ Abstain from smoking tobacco for 24 hours before testing.

➤ Avoid consumption of foods high in amines for 48 hours before testing.

➤ Avoid self-prescribed medications for 2 weeks before testing (especially appetite suppressants and cold and allergy medications, such as nose drops, cough suppressants, and bronchodilators).

➤ Withhold health care practitioner–prescribed medication as directed (especially methyldopa, epinephrine, levodopa, and methenamine mandelate).

➤ Fast from food and fluids for 10 to 12 hours before the test.

➤ Inform the patient that he or she may be asked to keep warm and to rest for 45 to 60 minutes before the test.

➤ Review the procedure with the patient. Inform the patient that multiple specimens may be required. Inform the patient that specimen collection takes approximately 5 to 10 minutes.

➤ Inform the patient that an intermittent infusion device may be inserted before the test because the stress of repeated venipunctures may increase catecholamine levels.

Intratest: ■

➤ Ensure that the patient complied with dietary preparations and other pretesting restrictions.

➤ Direct the patient to breathe normally and to avoid unnecessary movement.

➤ Observe standard precautions and follow the general guidelines in Appendix A. Perform a venipuncture, and collect the specimen in a chilled 5-mL green-top tube between 6 and 8 a.m.

➤ Ask the patient to stand for 10 minutes, and then obtain a second sample as previously described.

➤ Label the specimen, noting the time of collection and position of the patient, and promptly transport it to the laboratory.

Post-test: ■

➤ Observe venipuncture site for bleeding or hematoma formation. Apply pressure bandage.

➤ Instruct the patient to resume usual diet and medication as directed by the health care practitioner.

➤ Assess the patient for increased pulse and blood pressure, hyperglycemia, shakiness, and palpitations associated with increased values.

➤ Evaluate test results in relation to the patient's symptoms and other tests performed. Related laboratory tests include calcitonin, urine catecholamines, urine homovanillic acid, urine metanephrines, and urine vanillylmandelic acid.

CATECHOLAMINES, URINE

. . . .

SYNONYMS/ACRONYM: Epinephrine, norepinephrine, dopamine.

SPECIMEN: Urine (25 mL) from a timed specimen collected in a clean plastic, amber collection container with 6N hydrochloric acid as a preservative.

REFERENCE VALUE: (Method: High-performance liquid chromatography)

	Conventional Units	SI Units
		(Conversion Factor ×5.46)
Epinephrine		
1–4 y	0–6.0 μg/24 h	0–32.8 nmol/24 h
4 – 10 y	0–10.0 μg/24 h	0–54.6 nmol/24 h
10–15 y	0.5–20 μg/24 h	2.7–109 nmol/24 h
Adult	0–20 μg/24 h	0–109 nmol/24 h
		(Conversion Factor ×5.91)
Norepinephrine		
1–4 y	0–29 μg/24 h	0–171 nmol/24 h
4–10 y	8–65 μg/24 h	47–384 nmol/24 h
10 y–adult	15–80 μg/24 h	89–473 nmol/24 h
		(Conversion Factor ×6.53)
Dopamine		
1–4 y	10–260 μg/24 h	65–1698 nmol/24 h
4 y–adult	65–400 μg/24 h	424–2612 nmol/24 h

DESCRIPTION: Catecholamines are produced by the chromaffin tissue of the adrenal medulla. They also are found in sympathetic nerve endings and in the brain. The major catecholamines are epinephrine, norepinephrine, and dopamine. They prepare the body for the fight-or-flight stress response, help regulate metabolism, and are excreted from the body by the kidneys. Levels are affected by diurnal variations, fluctu-ating in response to stress, postural changes, diet, smoking, drugs, and temperature changes. As a result, blood measurement is not as reliable as a 24-hour timed urine test. For test results to be valid, all of the above-mentioned environmental variables must be controlled when the test is performed. Elevated homovanillic acid levels rule out pheochromocytoma because this tumor primarily secretes epinephrine. Elevated catecholamines without hypertension suggest neuroblastoma or ganglioneuroma. Findings should be compared with metanephrines and vanillylmandelic acid, which are the metabolites of epinephrine and norepinephrine. Findings should also be compared with homovanillic acid, which is the product of dopamine metabolism. ▪

INDICATIONS:

• Assist in the diagnosis of neuroblastoma, ganglioneuroma, or dysautonomia

• Assist in the diagnosis of pheochromocytoma

• Evaluate acute hypertensive episode

• Evaluate hypertension of unknown origin

• Screen for pheochromocytoma among family members with an autosomal-dominant inheritance pattern for Lindau–von Hippel disease or multiple endocrine neoplasia

RESULT

Increased in:

• Diabetic acidosis (epinephrine and norepinephrine)

• Ganglioblastoma (epinephrine, slight increase; norepinephrine, large increase)

• Ganglioneuroma (all are increased; norepinephrine, largest increase)

• Hypothyroidism (epinephrine and norepinephrine)

• Long-term manic-depressive disorders (epinephrine and norepinephrine)

• Myocardial infarction (epinephrine and norepinephrine)

• Neuroblastoma (all are increased; norepinephrine and dopamine, largest increase)

• Pheochromocytoma (epinephrine, continuous or intermittent increase; norepinephrine, slight increase)

• Shock (epinephrine and norepinephrine)

• Strenuous exercise (epinephrine and norepinephrine)

Decreased in:

• Autonomic nervous system dysfunction (norepinephrine)

• Orthostatic hypotension (norepinephrine)

• Parkinson's disease (dopamine)

CRITICAL VALUES: N/A

INTERFERING FACTORS:

• Drugs that may increase urine catecholamine levels include acetaminophen, atenolol, dopamine (intravenous), isoproterenol, methyldopa, niacin, nitroglycerin, prochlorperazine, rauwolfia, reserpine, syrosingopine, and theophylline.

• Drugs that may decrease urine catecholamine levels include clonidine, decaborane, guanethidine, guanfacine, methyldopa, ouabain, radiographic substances, reserpine, and bretylium tosylate.

• Stress, hypoglycemia, smoking, and drugs can produce elevated catecholamines.

• Secretion of catecholamines exhibits diurnal variation, with the lowest levels occurring at night.

• Secretion of catecholamines varies during the menstrual cycle, with higher levels excreted during the luteal phase and lowest levels during ovulation.

• Diets high in amines (e.g., bananas, avocados, beer, aged cheese, chocolate, cocoa, coffee, fava beans, grains, tea, vanilla, walnuts, Chianti wine) can produce elevated catecholamine levels.

* Failure to collect all urine and store 24-hour specimen properly will yield a falsely low result.

Nursing Implications and Procedure • • • • • • • • • • •

Pretest: ∎

➤ Obtain a history of the patient's complaints, including a list of known allergens.

➤ Obtain a history of the patient's endocrine system and results of previously performed tests and procedures. For related tests, refer to the endocrine system table.

➤ Obtain a list of medications the patient is taking, including herbs, nutritional supplements, and nutraceuticals. The requesting health care practitioner and laboratory should be advised if the patient regularly uses these products so that their effects can be taken into consideration when reviewing results.

➤ There are no fluid restrictions unless by medical direction.

Instruct the patient to:

➤ Follow a normal-sodium diet for 3 days before testing.

➤ Abstain from smoking tobacco for 24 hours before testing.

➤ Avoid consumption of foods high in amines for 48 hours before testing.

➤ Avoid self-prescribed medications for 2 weeks before testing (especially appetite suppressants and cold and allergy medications, such as nose drops, cough suppressants, and bronchodilators).

➤ Withhold health care practitioner–prescribed medication as directed (especially methyldopa, epinephrine, levodopa, and methenamine mandelate).

➤ Fast from food and fluids for 10 to 12 hours before the test.

➤ Review the procedure with the patient. Provide a nonmetallic urinal, bedpan, or toilet-mounted collection device.

➤ Usually a 24-hour time frame for urine collection is ordered. Inform the patient that all urine over a 24-hour period must be saved; if a preservative has been added to the container, instruct the patient not to discard the preservative. Instruct the patient not to void directly into the laboratory collection container. Instruct the patient to avoid defecating in the collection device and to keep toilet tissue out of the collection device to prevent contamination of the specimen. Place a sign in the bathroom as a reminder to save all urine.

➤ Instruct the patient to void all urine into the collection device, then pour the urine into the laboratory collection container. Alternatively the specimen can be left in the collection device for a health care staff member to add to the laboratory collection container.

Intratest: ∎

➤ Ensure that the patient has complied with dietary preparations and other pretesting restrictions.

➤ Instruct the patient to continue to avoid excessive exercise and stress during the 24-hour collection of urine.

➤ Observe standard precautions and follow the general guidelines in Appendix A.

Timed specimen:

➤ Obtain a clean 3-L urine specimen container, toilet-mounted collection device, and plastic bag (for transport of the specimen container). The specimen must be refrigerated or kept on ice throughout the collection period. If an indwelling urinary catheter is in place, the drainage bag must be kept on ice.

➤ Begin the test between 6 and 8 a.m., if possible. Collect first voiding and discard. Record the time the specimen was discarded as the beginning of the timed collection period. The next morning, ask the patient to void at the same time the collection was started and add this last voiding to the container.

➤ If an indwelling catheter is in place, replace the tubing and container system at the start of the collection time. Keep the container system on ice during the collection period or empty the urine into a larger container periodically during the collection period; monitor to ensure continued drainage, and conclude the test the next morning at the same hour the collection was begun.

➤ At the conclusion of the test, compare the quantity of urine with the urinary output record for the collection; if the specimen contains less than what was recorded as output, some urine may have been discarded, invalidating the test.

➤ Label the specimen and promptly transport it to the laboratory. Include on the label the amount of urine, test start and stop times, and ingestion of any foods or medications that can affect test results.

Post-test:

➤ Instruct the patient to resume usual diet and medication as directed by the health care practitioner.

➤ Evaluate test results in relation to the patient's symptoms and other tests performed. Related laboratory tests include calcitonin, plasma catecholamines, urine homovanillic acid, urine metanephrines, and urine vanillylmandelic acid.

CD4/CD8 ENUMERATION

SYNONYM/ACRONYM: T cell profile.

SPECIMEN: Whole blood (1 mL) collected in green-top (heparin) tube.

REFERENCE VALUE: (Method: Flow cytometry)

Total lymphocytes	1500–4000/mm^3
CD3	876–1900/mm^3
CD4	450–1400/mm^3
CD8	190–725/mm^3
CD20	64–475/mm^3
CD4/CD8 ratio	1.0–3.5

DESCRIPTION: Enumeration of lymphocytes, identification of cell lineage, and identification of cellular stage of development are used to diagnose and classify malignant myeloproliferative diseases and to plan treatment. T cell enumeration is also useful in the evaluation and management of immunodeficiency and autoimmune disease. A severely depressed CD4 count is an excellent predictor of imminent opportunistic infection. ▪

INDICATIONS:

• Assist in the diagnosis of AIDS and plan treatment

• Evaluate malignant myeloproliferative diseases and plan treatment

• Evaluate thymus-dependent or cellular immunocompetence

RESULT

Increased in:

• Malignant myeloproliferative diseases (e.g., acute and chronic lymphocytic leukemia, lymphoma)

Decreased in:

• AIDS

• Aplastic anemia

• Hodgkin's disease

CRITICAL VALUES: N/A

INTERFERING FACTORS:

• Drugs that may increase T cell count include interferon-γ.

• Drugs that may decrease T cell count include chlorpromazine and prednisone.

• Specimens should be stored at room temperature.

• Recent radioactive scans or radiation can decrease T cell counts.

• Values may be abnormal in patients with severe recurrent illness or after recent surgery requiring general anesthesia.

Nursing Implications and Procedure • • • • • • • • • • •

Pretest: ▪

➤ Obtain a history of the patient's complaints, including a list of known allergens.

➤ Obtain a history of the patient's immune system and results of previously performed tests and procedures. For related tests, refer to the immune system table.

➤ Obtain a list of medications the patient is taking, including herbs, nutritional supplements, and nutraceuticals. The requesting health care practitioner and laboratory should be advised if the patient regularly uses these products so that their effects can be taken into consideration when reviewing results.

➤ Note any recent procedures that can interfere with test results.

➤ There are no food, fluid, or medication restrictions unless by medical direction.

➤ Review the procedure with the patient.

➤ Inform the patient that specimen collection takes approximately 5 to 10 minutes.

Intratest: ▪

➤ Direct the patient to breathe normally and to avoid unnecessary movement.

➤ Observe standard precautions and follow the general guidelines in Appendix A. Perform a venipuncture, and collect the specimen in a 5-mL green-top tube.

➤ Label the specimen, and promptly transport it to the laboratory.

Post-test: ▪

➤ Observe venipuncture site for bleeding or hematoma formation. Apply pressure bandage.

➤ Educate the patient as to the risk of

infection related to immunosuppressed inflammatory response and fatigue related to decreased energy production.

➤ As appropriate, stress the importance of good nutrition and suggest that the patient meet with a nutritional specialist. Stress the importance of following care plan for medications and follow-up visits. Inform the patient that subsequent requests for follow-up blood work at regular intervals should be anticipated.

➤ Recognize anxiety related to test results and offer support. Provide teaching and information regarding the clinical implications of the test results, as appropriate. Educate the patient regarding access to counseling services.

➤ Evaluate test results in relation to the patient's symptoms and other tests performed. Related laboratory tests include β_2-microglobulin, bone marrow, complete blood count, and HIV-1/HIV-2 antibody.

CEREBROSPINAL FLUID ANALYSIS

SYNONYM/ACRONYM: CSF analysis.

SPECIMEN: CSF (1 to 3 mL) collected in three or four separate plastic conical tubes. Tube 1 is used for chemistry and serology testing, tube 2 is used for microbiology, tube 3 is used for cell count, and tube 4 is used for miscellaneous testing.

REFERENCE VALUE: (Method: Macroscopic evaluation of appearance; spectrophotometry for glucose, lactic acid, and protein; radioimmunoassay for myelin basic protein; nephelometry for IgG; electrophoresis for oligoclonal banding; Gram stain, India ink preparation, and culture for microbiology; microscopic examination of fluid for cell count; flocculation for Venereal Disease Research Laboratory [VDRL])

Lumbar Puncture	Conventional Units	SI Units
Color and appearance	Crystal clear	
		(Conversion Factor × 10)
Protein	15–45 mg/dL	150–450 mg/L
		(Conversion Factor × 0.0555)
Glucose		
Infant or child	60–80 mg/dL	3.3–4.4 mmol/L
Adult	40–70 mg/dL	2.2–3.9 mmol/L

(Continued on the following page)

Lumbar Puncture	Conventional Units	SI Units
		(Conversion Factor ×0.111)
Lactic acid		
Neonate	10–60 mg/dL	1.1–6.7 mmol/L
3–10 d	10–40 mg/dL	1.1–4.4 mmol/L
Adult	Less than 25.2 mg/dL	Less than 2.8 mmol/L
		(Conversion Factor × 1)
Myelin basic protein	Less than 2.5 ng/mL	Less than 2.5 µg/L
Oligoclonal bands	Absent	
		(Conversion Factor × 10)
IgG	Less than 3.4 mg/dL	Less than 34 mg/L
Gram stain	Negative	
India ink	Negative	
Culture	No growth	
RBC count	0	0
		(Conversion Factor × 1)
WBC count		
Less than 1 y	0–30/mL	0–30 × 10⁶/L
1–4 y	0–20/mL	0–20 × 10⁶/L
5–12 y	0–10/mL	0–10 × 10⁶/L
Adult	0–5/mL	0–5 × 10⁶/L

WBC Differential	Adult	Children	Adult	Children
Lymphocytes	40–80%	5–13%	0.4–0.8	0.55–0.35
Monocytes	15–45%	50–90%	0.15–0.45	0.50–0.90
Neutrophils	0–6%	0–8%	0–0.6	0–0.8
VDRL	Nonreactive			
Cytology	No abnormal cells seen			

RBC = red blood cell; VDRL = Venereal Disease Research Laboratory; WBC = white blood cell.

DESCRIPTION: Cerebrospinal fluid (CSF) circulates in the subarachnoid space and has a twofold function: to protect the brain and spinal cord from injury and to transport products of cellular metabolism andeurosecretion. CSF analysis helps determine the presence and cause of bleeding and assists in diagnosing cancer, infections, and degenerative and autoimmune diseases of the brain and spinal cord. Specimens for analysis are most frequently obtained by lumbar puncture and sometimes by ventricular or cisternal puncture. Lumbar puncture can also have therapeutic uses, including injection of drugs and anesthesia. ■

INDICATIONS:

• Assist in the diagnosis and differentiation of subarachnoid or intracranial hemorrhage

- Assist in the diagnosis and differentiation of viral or bacterial meningitis or encephalitis

- Assist in the diagnosis of diseases such as multiple sclerosis, autoimmune disorders, or degenerative brain disease

- Assist in the diagnosis of neurosyphilis and chronic central nervous system (CNS) infections

- Detect obstruction of CSF circulation due to hemorrhage, tumor, or edema

- Establish the presence of any condition decreasing the flow of oxygen to the brain

- Monitor for metastases of cancer into the CNS

- Monitor severe brain injuries

RESULT

Increases in:

- Color and appearance: bloody—hemorrhage; xanthochromic—old hemorrhage, red blood cell (RBC) breakdown, methemoglobin, bilirubin (greater than 6 mg/dL), increased protein (greater than 150 mg/dL), melanin (meningeal melanosarcoma), carotene (systemic carotenemia); hazy—meningitis; pink to dark yellow—aspiration of epidural fat; turbid—cells, microorganisms, protein, fat, or contrast medium

- Protein: meningitis, encephalitis

- Lactic acid: bacterial, tubercular, fungal meningitis

- Myelin basic protein: trauma, stroke, tumor, multiple sclerosis, subacute sclerosing panencephalitis

- IgG and oligoclonal banding: multiple sclerosis, CNS syphilis, and subacute sclerosing panencephalitis

- Gram stain: meningitis due to *Streptococcus pneumoniae, Haemophilus influenzae, Neisseria meningitidis, Cryptococcus neoformans*

- India ink preparation: meningitis due to *C. neoformans*

- Culture: encephalitis or meningitis due to herpes simplex virus, *S. pneumoniae, H. influenzae, N. meningitidis, C. neoformans*

- RBC count: hemorrhage

- White blood cell (WBC) count:

  General increase—injection of contrast media or anticancer drugs in subarachnoid space; CSF infarct; metastatic tumor in contact with CSF; reaction to repeated lumbar puncture

  Elevated WBC count with a predominance of neutrophils indicative of bacterial meningitis

  Elevated WBC count with a predominance of lymphocytes indicative of viral, tubercular, parasitic, or fungal meningitis; multiple sclerosis

  Elevated WBC count with a predominance of monocytes indicative of chronic bacterial meningitis, amebic meningitis, multiple sclerosis, toxoplasmosis

  Increased plasma cells indicative of acute viral infections, multiple sclerosis, sarcoidosis, syphilitic meningoencephalitis, subacute sclerosing panencephalitis, tubercular meningitis, parasitic infections, Guillain-Barré syndrome

  Presence of eosinophils indicative of parasitic and fungal infections, acute polyneuritis, idiopathic hypereosinophilic syndrome, reaction to drugs or a shunt in CSF

- VDRL: syphilis

Positive findings in:

- Cytology: malignant cells

Decreases in:

- Glucose: bacterial and tubercular meningitis

CRITICAL VALUES:

• Positive Gram stain, India ink preparation, or culture

• Presence of malignant cells

Any of the above-listed results should be communicated to the requesting health care practitioner immediately.

INTERFERING FACTORS:

• Drugs that may decrease CSF protein levels include cefotaxime and dexamethasone.

• Interferon-β may increase myelin basic protein levels.

• Drugs that may increase CSF glucose levels include cefotaxime and dexamethasone.

• RBC count may be falsely elevated with a traumatic spinal tap.

• This procedure is contraindicated if ⚠ infection is present at the needle insertion site.

• Recent radioactive scans or radiation within 1 week before the test can interfere with test results when radioimmunoassay is the test method.

• Note any recent procedures that can interfere with test results.

• It may also be contraindicated in ⚠ patients with degenerative joint disease or coagulation defects and in patients who are uncooperative during the procedure.

• Use with extreme caution in patients ⚠ with increased intracranial pressure because overly rapid removal of CSF can result in herniation.

Nursing Implications and Procedure • • • • • • • • • • •

Pretest: ■

➤ Obtain a history of the patient's complaints, including a list of known allergens.

➤ Obtain a history of the patient's immune and musculoskeletal systems, as well as results of previously performed tests and procedures. For related tests, refer to the immune and musculoskeletal system tables.

➤ Obtain a list of medications the patient is taking, including herbs, nutritional supplements, and nutraceuticals. The requesting health care practitioner and laboratory should be advised if the patient regularly uses these products so that their effects can be taken into consideration when reviewing results.

➤ Note any recent procedures that can interfere with test results.

➤ There are no food, fluid, or medication restrictions unless by medical direction.

➤ Review the procedure with the patient.

➤ Inform the patient that the position required may be awkward, but that someone will assist during the procedure. Stress the importance of remaining still and breathing normally throughout the procedure.

➤ Inform the patient that a stinging sensation may be felt when the local anesthetic is injected. Tell the patient to report any pain or other sensations that may require repositioning the spinal needle.

➤ Assess if the patient has an allergy to local anesthetics, and inform the health care practitioner accordingly.

➤ *Obtain written and informed consent before administering any medications prior to the procedure.*

➤ Inform the patient that the procedure is performed by a health care practitioner and takes about 20 minutes.

Intratest: ■

➤ Direct the patient to breathe normally and to avoid unnecessary movement.

➤ Record baseline vital signs.

➤ To perform a lumbar puncture, position the patient in the knee-chest position at the side of the bed. Provide pillows to support the spine or for the patient to grasp. The sitting position is an alternative. In this position, the patient must bend the neck and chest to the knees.

➤ Observe standard precautions and follow the general guidelines in Appendix A.

➤ Prepare the site—usually between L3 and L4, or between L4 and L5—with povidone-iodine and drape the area.

➤ A local anesthetic is injected. Using sterile technique, the health care practitioner inserts the spinal needle through the spinous processes of the vertebrae and into the subarachnoid space. The stylet is removed. If the needle is properly placed, CSF drips from the needle.

➤ Attach the stopcock and manometer, and measure initial pressure. Normal pressure for an adult in the lateral recumbent position is 90 to 180 mm H_2O; normal pressure for a child aged 8 years or younger is 10 to 100 mm H_2O. These values depend on the body position and are different in a horizontal or sitting position.

➤ CSF pressure may be elevated if the patient is anxious, holding his or her breath, or tensing muscles. It may also be elevated if the patient's knees are flexed too firmly against the abdomen. CSF pressure may be significantly elevated in patients with intracranial tumors. If the initial pressure is elevated, the health care practitioner may perform Queckenstedt's test. To perform this test, apply pressure to the jugular

vein for about 10 seconds. CSF pressure usually rises rapidly in response to the occlusion, and then returns to the pretest level within 10 seconds after the pressure is released. Sluggish response may indicate CSF obstruction.

➤ Obtain four vials of spinal fluid in separate tubes (1 to 3 mL in each), and label them numerically in the order they were filled.

➤ A final pressure reading is taken, and the needle is removed. Clean the puncture site with an antiseptic solution and apply a small bandage.

➤ Label the specimen, and promptly transport it to the laboratory.

Post-test: ∎

➤ If permitted, administer fluids to replace lost CSF and help prevent or relieve headache—a side effect of lumbar puncture.

➤ Position the patient flat, either on the back or abdomen; some health care practitioners allow 30° elevation. Maintain position for 8 hours. Changing position is acceptable as long as the body remains horizontal.

➤ Check the puncture site for leakage; frequently monitor vital signs such as temperature and blood pressure.

➤ Observe the patient for neurological changes, such as altered level of consciousness, change in pupils, reports of tingling or numbness, and irritability.

➤ Evaluate test results in relation to the patient's symptoms and other tests performed. Related laboratory tests include complete blood count and syphilis serology.

CERULOPLASMIN

SYNONYM/ACRONYM: Copper oxidase, Cp.

SPECIMEN: Serum (1 mL) collected in a red- or tiger-top tube.

REFERENCE VALUE: (Method: Nephelometry)

Age	Conventional Units	SI Units (Conversion Factor ×10)
Newborn–3 mo	5–18 mg/dL	50–180 mg/L
6–2 mo	33–43 mg/dL	330–430 mg/L
1–3 y	26–55 mg/dL	260–550 mg/L
4–5 y	27–56 mg/dL	270–560 mg/L
6–7 y	24–48 mg/dL	240–480 mg/L
Greater than 7 y	20–54 mg/dL	200–540 mg/L

DESCRIPTION: Ceruloplasmin is an α_2-globulin produced by the liver that binds copper for transport in the blood after it is absorbed from the gastrointestinal system. Decreased production of this globulin causes copper to be deposited in body tissues such as the brain, liver, corneas, and kidneys. ∎

INDICATIONS:

• Assist in the diagnosis of Menkes (kinky hair) syndrome

• Assist in the diagnosis of Wilson's disease

• Determine genetic predisposition to Wilson's disease

• Monitor patient response to total parenteral nutrition (hyperalimentation)

RESULT

Increased in:

• Acute infections

• Biliary cirrhosis

• Cancer of the bone, lung, stomach

• Copper intoxication

• Hodgkin's disease

• Leukemia

• Pregnancy (last trimester)

• Rheumatoid arthritis

• Tissue necrosis

Decreased in:

• Menkes syndrome

• Nutritional deficiency of copper

• Wilson's disease

CRITICAL VALUES: N/A

INTERFERING FACTORS:

• Drugs that may increase ceruloplasmin levels include anticonvulsants, norethindrone, oral contraceptives, and tamoxifen.

• Drugs that may decrease ceruloplasmin levels include asparaginase and levonorgestrel (Norplant).

• Excessive therapeutic intake of zinc may interfere with intestinal absorption of copper.

Nursing Implications and Procedure

Pretest:

➤ Obtain a history of the patient's complaints, including a list of known allergens.

➤ Obtain a history of the patient's hepatobiliary system and results of previously performed tests and procedures. For related tests, refer to the hepatobiliary system table.

➤ Obtain a list of medications the patient is taking, including herbs, nutritional supplements, and nutraceuticals. The requesting health care practitioner and laboratory should be advised if the patient regularly uses these products so that their effects can be taken into consideration when reviewing results.

➤ There are no food, fluid, or medication restrictions unless by medical direction.

➤ Review the procedure with the patient.

➤ Inform the patient that specimen collection takes approximately 5 to 10 minutes.

Intratest:

➤ Direct the patient to breathe normally and to avoid unnecessary movement.

➤ Observe standard precautions and follow the general guidelines in Appendix A. Perform a venipuncture, and collect the specimen in a 5-mL red- or tiger-top tube.

➤ Label the specimen, and promptly transport it to the laboratory.

Post-test:

➤ Observe venipuncture site for bleeding or hematoma formation. Apply pressure bandage.

➤ Instruct the patient with copper deficiency to increase intake of foods rich in copper, as appropriate. Organ meats, shellfish, nuts, and legumes are good sources of dietary copper. High intake of zinc, iron, calcium, and manganese interferes with copper absorption. Copper deficiency does not normally occur in adults; however, patients receiving long-term total parenteral nutrition should be evaluated if signs and symptoms of copper deficiency appear, such as jaundice or eye color changes. Kayser-Fleischer rings (green-gold rings) in the cornea and a liver biopsy specimen showing more than 250 μg of copper per gram confirms Wilson's disease.

➤ Inform the patient of the need for follow-up medical care as appropriate.

➤ Evaluate test results in relation to the patient's symptoms and other tests performed. Related laboratory tests include copper, liver biopsy, and zinc.

CHEST X-RAY

SYNONYM/ACRONYM: Chest radiography, CXR.

AREA OF APPLICATION: Lungs.

CONTRAST: None.

DESCRIPTION: Chest radiography, commonly called chest x-ray, is one of the most frequently performed radiologic diagnostic studies. This study yields information about the pulmonary, cardiac, and skeletal systems. X-rays penetrate air easily; areas filled with air appear dark or black on x-ray film. Bones appear near-white on the film because x-rays cannot penetrate them to reach the film. Organs and tissues appear as shades of gray because they absorb more x-ray than air but less than bone. A routine chest x-ray includes a posteroanterior and lateral view. Portable x-rays, done in more acute or critical situations, can be done at the bedside and include only the antero-posterior projection. Films may be taken with the patient supine or in a lateral decubitus position, if the presence of free pleural fluid is in question. Other projections that can be obtained are the obliques, lateral decubitus, and lordotic; in general, the part being studied is placed next to the film. Films may be taken on full inspiration and on full expiration to detect a pneumothorax. Fluoroscopic studies of the chest can also be done to evaluate movement of the chest and diaphragm during breathing and coughing. In the beginning of the disease process of tuberculosis, asthma, and chronic obstructive pulmonary disease, the results of the chest x-ray may not correlate with the clinical status of the patient and may even be normal. ■

INDICATIONS:

• Evaluate known or suspected pulmonary disorders, chest trauma, cardiovascular disorders, and skeletal disorders

• Aid in the diagnosis of diaphragmatic hernia

• Monitor resolution, progression, or maintenance of disease

• Monitor effectiveness of the treatment regimen

• Evaluate placement and position of an endotracheal tube, tracheostomy tube, nasogastric feeding tube, pacemaker wires, and intra-aortic balloon pump

RESULT

Normal Findings:

• Normal lung fields, cardiac size, mediastinal structures, thoracic spine, ribs, and diaphragm

Abnormal Findings:

- Atelectasis
- Bronchitis
- Curvature of the spinal column (scoliosis)
- Enlarged heart
- Enlarged lymph nodes
- Flattened diaphragm
- Foreign bodies lodged in the pulmonary system
- Fractures of the sternum, ribs, and spine
- Lung pathology, including tumors
- Malposition of tubes or wires
- Mediastinal tumor and pathology
- Pericardial effusion
- Pericarditis
- Pleural effusion
- Pneumonia
- Pneumothorax
- Pulmonary bases, fibrosis, infiltrates
- Tuberculosis
- Vascular abnormalities

CRITICAL VALUES: N/A

INTERFERING FACTORS:

This procedure is contraindicated for:

- Patients who are pregnant or suspected of being pregnant, unless the potential benefits of the procedure far outweigh the risks to the fetus and mother

Factors that may impair clear imaging:

- Inability of the patient to cooperate or remain still during the procedure because of age, significant pain, or mental status

- Metallic objects within the examination field (e.g., jewelry, earrings), which may inhibit organ visualization and can produce unclear images
- Improper adjustment of the radiographic equipment to accommodate obese or thin patients, which can cause overexposure or underexposure and a poor-quality study
- Patients who are very obese, who may exceed the weight limit for the equipment
- Incorrect positioning of the patient, which may produce poor visualization of the area to be examined

Other considerations:

- Consultation with a physician should occur before the procedure for radiation safety concerns regarding infants of patients who are lactating.
- Risks associated with radiographic overexposure can result from frequent x-ray procedures. Personnel in the room with the patient should wear a protective lead apron, stand behind a shield, or leave the area while the examination is being done. Badges that reveal the level of exposure to radiation should be worn by persons working in the area where the examination is being done.

Nursing Implications and Procedure

Pretest:

➤ Inform the patient about the purpose of the procedure, various positions to assume, and the need to hold his or her breath. For related tests, refer to the cardiovascular and respiratory system tables.

➤ Inform the patient that the procedure takes 5 to 10 minutes.

➤ There are no food or fluid restrictions.

> Inform the patient that no pain is associated with the study.

Intratest:

> Instruct the patient to remove clothing and metallic objects from the waist up.

> Give the patient a gown and robe to wear.

> Remove any wires connected to electrodes, if allowed.

> Place patient in a standing, sitting, or recumbent position in front of the x-ray film holder.

> For portable examinations, elevate the head of the bed to the high Fowler's position.

> Have the patient place hands on hips, extend neck, and position shoulders forward.

> Position the chest with the left side against the film holder for a lateral view.

> Instruct the patient to inhale deeply, to hold his or her breath while the x-ray is taken, and then exhale after the film is taken.

Post-test:

> Inform the patient of the possible need for additional chest x-rays to evaluate progression of the disease process or to determine the need for a change in therapy.

> Determine if the patient or family members have any further questions or concerns.

> A physician sends a written report to the ordering health care provider, who discusses the results with the patient.

> Evaluate test results in relation to the patient's symptoms and other tests performed. Related diagnostic tests include computed tomography and magnetic resonance imaging of the chest as well as a lung scan.

CHLAMYDIA GROUP ANTIBODY

· ·

SYNONYM/ACRONYM: N/A.

SPECIMEN: Serum (1 mL) collected in a red-top tube.

REFERENCE VALUE: (Method: Indirect fluorescent antibody, polymerase chain reaction) Negative or less than fourfold increase in titer.

DESCRIPTION: Chlamydia, one of the most common sexually transmitted infections, is caused by *Chlamydia trachomatis*. These gram-negative bacteria are called *obligate cell parasites* because they require living cells for growth. There are three serotypes of *C. trachomatis*: One group causes lymphogranuloma venereum, with symptoms of the first phase of the disease appearing 2 to 6 weeks after infection; another causes a genital tract infection different from lymphogranuloma venereum, in which symptoms in men appear 7 to 28 days after intercourse (women are generally asymptomatic); and the third causes the ocular disease trachoma (incubation period, 7 to 10 days). *Chlamydia psittaci* is the cause of psittacosis in birds and humans. It is increasing in prevalence as a pathogen responsible for other significant diseases of the respiratory system. The incubation period for *C. psittaci* infections in humans is 7 to 15 days, which is followed by chills, fever, and a persistent nonproductive cough.

Chlamydia is difficult to culture and grow, so antibody testing has become the technology of choice. The antigen used in many screening kits is not species specific and can confirm only the presence of *Chlamydia* spp. Newer technology using DNA probes can identify the species. Assays that can specifically identify *C. trachomatis* require special collection and transport kits. They also have specific collection instructions, and the specimens are collected on swabs. The laboratory performing this testing should be consulted before specimen collection. ∎

INDICATIONS:

• Establish *Chlamydia* as the cause of atypical pneumonia

• Establish the presence of chlamydial infection

RESULT

Positive findings in:

• Chlamydial infection

• Infantile pneumonia

• Infertility

• Lymphogranuloma venereum

• Ophthalmia neonatorum

• Pelvic inflammatory disease

• Urethritis

CRITICAL VALUES: N/A

INTERFERING FACTORS: N/A

Nursing Implications and Procedure • • • • • • • • • • •

Pretest: ∎

➤ Obtain a history of the patient's complaints, including a list of known allergens.

➤ Obtain a history of the patient's immune and reproductive systems, as well as results of previously performed tests and procedures. For related tests, refer to the immune and reproductive system tables.

➤ Obtain a list of medications the patient is taking, including herbs, nutritional supplements, and nutraceuticals. The requesting health care practitioner and laboratory should be advised if the patient regularly uses these products so that their effects can be taken into consideration when reviewing results.

➤ There are no food, fluid, or medication restrictions unless by medical direction.

➤ Review the procedure with the patient.

➤ Inform the patient that several tests may be necessary to confirm diagnosis. Any individual positive result should be repeated in 7 to 10 days to monitor a change in titer.

➤ Inform the patient that each specimen collection takes approximately 5 to 10 minutes.

Intratest: ∎

➤ Direct the patient to breathe normally and to avoid unnecessary movement.

➤ Observe standard precautions and follow the general guidelines in Appendix A. Perform a venipuncture, and collect the specimen in a 5-mL red-top tube.

► Label the specimen, and promptly transport it to the laboratory.

Post-test: ■

► Observe venipuncture site for bleeding or hematoma formation. Apply pressure bandage.

► Counsel the patient, as appropriate, as to the risk of sexual transmission and educate the patient regarding proper prophylaxis. Reinforce the importance of strict adherence to the treatment regimen.

► Inform the patient with positive *C. trachomatis* that findings must be reported to a local health department official, who will question the patient regarding his or her sexual partners.

► Recognize anxiety related to test results. Provide teaching and disease information, as appropriate.

► Offer support, as appropriate, to patients who may be the victim of rape or sexual assault. Educate the patient regarding access to counseling services. Provide a nonjudgmental, nonthreatening atmosphere for a discussion during which you explain the risks of sexually transmitted diseases. It is also important to discuss emotions the patient may experience (guilt, depression, anger) if test results indicate the presence of *Chlamydia*.

► Provide emotional support if the patient is pregnant and if results are positive. Inform the patient that *Chlamydia* infection during pregnancy places the newborn at risk for pneumonia and conjunctivitis. Educate the patient regarding access to counseling services.

► Emphasize the need to return to have a convalescent blood sample taken in 7 to 14 days.

► Evaluate test results in relation to the patient's symptoms and other tests performed. Related laboratory tests include *Chlamydia* and *Neisseria* cultures and syphilis serology.

CHLORIDE, SERUM

SYNONYM/ACRONYM: Cl⁻.

SPECIMEN: Serum (1 mL) collected in a red- or tiger-top tube. Plasma (1 mL) collected in green-top (heparin) tube is also acceptable.

REFERENCE VALUE: (Method: Ion-selective electrode)

Age	Conventional Units	SI Units (Conversion Factor ×1)
Premature	95–110 mEq/L	95–110 mmol/L
0–30 d	98–113 mEq/L	98–113 mmol/L
2 mo–adult	97–107 mEq/L	97–107mmol/L

DESCRIPTION: Chloride is the most abundant anion in the extracellular fluid. Its most important function is in the maintenance of acid-base balance, in which it competes with bicarbonate for sodium. Chloride levels generally increase and decrease proportional to sodium levels and inversely proportional to bicarbonate levels. Chloride also participates with sodium in the maintenance of water balance and aids in the regulation of osmotic pressure. Chloride contributes to gastric acid (hydrochloric acid) for digestion and activation of enzymes. The chloride content of venous blood is slightly higher than that of arterial blood because chloride ions enter red blood cells in response to absorption of carbon dioxide into the cell. As carbon dioxide enters the blood cell, bicarbonate leaves and chloride is absorbed in exchange to maintain electrical neutrality within the cell.

Chloride is provided by dietary intake, mostly in the form of sodium chloride. It is absorbed by the gastrointestinal system, filtered out by the glomeruli, and reabsorbed by the renal tubules. Excess chloride is excreted in the urine. Serum values normally remain fairly stable. A slight decrease may be detectable after meals because chloride is used to produce hydrochloric acid as part of the digestive process. Measurement of chloride levels is not as essential as measurement of other electrolytes such as sodium or potassium. Chloride is usually included in standard electrolyte panels to detect the presence of unmeasured anions via calculation of the anion gap. Chloride levels are usually not interpreted apart from sodium, potassium, carbon dioxide, and anion gap.

The patient's clinical picture needs to be considered in the evaluation of electrolytes. Fluid and electrolyte imbalances are often seen in patients with serious illness or injury because in these cases the clinical situation has affected the normal homeostatic balance of the body. It is also possible that therapeutic treatments being administered are causing or contributing to the electrolyte imbalance. Children and adults are at high risk for fluid and electrolyte imbalances when chloride levels are depleted. Children are considered to be at high risk during chloride imbalance because a positive serum chloride balance is important for expansion of the extracellular fluid compartment. Anemia, the result of decreased hemoglobin levels, is a frequent issue for elderly patients. Since hemoglobin participates in a major buffer system in the body, depleted hemoglobin levels affect the efficiency of chloride ion exchange for bicarbonate in red blood cells, which in turn affects acid-base balance. Elderly patients are also at high risk because their renal response to change in pH is slower, resulting in a more rapid development of electrolyte imbalance. ■

INDICATIONS:

- Assist in confirming a diagnosis of disorders associated with abnormal chloride values, as seen in acid-base and fluid imbalances

- Differentiate between types of acidosis (hyperchloremic versus anion gap)

- Monitor effectiveness of drug therapy to increase or decrease serum chloride levels

RESULT

Increased in:

- Acute renal failure
- Cushing's disease
- Dehydration
- Diabetes insipidus
- Excessive infusion of normal saline
- Head trauma with hypothalamic stimulation or damage
- Hyperparathyroidism (primary)
- Metabolic acidosis (associated with prolonged diarrhea)
- Renal tubular acidosis
- Respiratory alkalosis (e.g., hyperventilation)
- Salicylate intoxication

Decreased in:

- Addison's disease
- Burns
- Congestive heart failure
- Excessive sweating
- Gastrointestinal loss from vomiting (severe), diarrhea, nasogastric suction, or fistula
- Metabolic alkalosis
- Overhydration
- Respiratory acidosis (chronic)
- Salt-losing nephritis
- Syndrome of inappropriate antidiuretic hormone secretion
- Water intoxication

CRITICAL VALUES:

Less than 80 mEq/L
Greater than 115 mEq/L
Observe the patient for symptoms of critically decreased or elevated chloride levels. Proper interpretation of chloride values must be made within the context of other electrolyte values and requires clinical knowledge of the patient.

The following may be seen in hypochloremia: twitching or tremors, which may indicate excitability of the nervous system; slow and shallow breathing; and decreased blood pressure as a result of fluid loss. Possible interventions relate to treatment of the underlying cause.

Signs and symptoms associated with hyperchloremia are weakness, lethargy, and deep, rapid breathing. Proper interventions include treatments that correct the underlying cause.

INTERFERING FACTORS:

- Drugs that may cause an increase in chloride levels include acetazolamide, acetylsalicylic acid, ammonium chloride, bromide, chlorothiazide, cholestyramine, cyclosporine, guanethidine, lithium, methyldopa, oxyphenbutazone, phenylbutazone, and triamterene.

- Drugs that may cause a decrease in chloride levels include bicarbonate, corticosteroids, corticotropin, cortisone, diuretics, ethacrynic acid, furosemide, hydroflumethiazide, laxatives (if chronic abuse occurs), mannitol, meralluride, mersalyl, methyclothiazide, metolazone, and triamterene. Many of these drugs can cause a diuretic action that inhibits the tubular reabsorption of chloride. *Note:* Triamterene has nephrotoxic and azotemic effects, and when organ damage has occurred, increased serum chloride levels result.

- Elevated triglyceride or protein levels may cause a volume-displacement error in the specimen, reflecting falsely decreased chloride values when chloride measurement methods employing predilution specimens are used (e.g., indirect ion-selective electrode, flame photometry).

- Specimens should never be collected

above an intravenous (IV) line because of the potential for dilution when the specimen and the IV solution combine in the collection container, falsely decreasing the result. There is also the potential of contaminating the sample with the substance of interest, contained in the IV solution, falsely increasing the result.

Nursing Implications and Procedure ∙ ∙ ∙ ∙ ∙ ∙ ∙ ∙ ∙ ∙

Pretest:

➤ Obtain a history of the patient's complaints, including a list of known allergens.

➤ Obtain a history of the patient's cardiovascular, endocrine, gastrointestinal, genitourinary, and respiratory systems, as well as results of previously performed tests and procedures. For related tests, refer to the cardiovascular, endocrine, gastrointestinal, genitourinary, and respiratory system tables.

➤ Obtain a list of medications the patient is taking, including herbs, nutritional supplements, and nutraceuticals. The requesting health care practitioner and laboratory should be advised if the patient regularly uses these products so that their effects can be taken into consideration when reviewing results.

➤ There are no food, fluid, or medication restrictions unless by medical direction.

➤ Specimens should not be collected during hemodialysis.

➤ Review the procedure with the patient.

➤ Inform the patient that specimen collection usually takes 5 to 10 minutes.

Intratest:

➤ Direct the patient to breathe normally and to avoid unnecessary movement. Instruct the patient not to clench and unclench fist immediately before or during specimen collection.

➤ Observe standard precautions and follow the general guidelines in Appendix A. Perform a venipuncture, and collect the specimen in a 5-mL red- or tiger-top tube.

➤ Label the specimen, and promptly transport it to the laboratory.

Post-test:

➤ Observe venipuncture site for bleeding or hematoma formation. Apply pressure bandage.

➤ Observe the patient on saline IV fluid replacement therapy for signs of overhydration, especially in cases in which there is a history of cardiac or renal disease. Signs of overhydration include constant, irritable cough; chest rales; dyspnea; or engorgement of neck and hand veins.

➤ Evaluate the patient for signs and symptoms of dehydration. Dehydration is a significant and common finding in geriatric and other patients in whom renal function has deteriorated.

➤ Monitor daily weights as well as intake and output to determine whether fluid retention is occurring because of sodium and chloride excess. Patients at risk for or with a history of fluid imbalance are also at risk for electrolyte imbalance.

➤ Careful observation of the patient on IV fluid replacement therapy is important. A patient receiving a continuous 5% dextrose solution (D_5W) may not be taking in an adequate amount of chloride to meet the body's needs. The patient, if allowed, should be encouraged to drink fluids such as broths, tomato juice, or colas and to eat foods such as meats, seafood, or eggs, which contain sodium and chloride. The use of table salt may also be appropriate.

➤ Instruct patients with elevated chloride levels to avoid eating or drinking anything containing sodium chloride salt. The patient or caregiver should also be encouraged to read food labels to determine which products are suitable for a low-sodium diet.

➤ Instruct patients with low chloride levels that a decrease in iron absorption may occur as a result of less chloride available to form gastric acid, which is essential for iron absorption. In prolonged periods of chloride deficit, iron-deficiency anemia could develop.

➤ Evaluate test results in relation to the patient's symptoms and other tests performed. Related laboratory tests include anion gap, carbon dioxide, potassium, sodium, and osmolality.

CHLORIDE, SWEAT

SYNONYMS/ACRONYM: Sweat test, pilocarpine iontophoresis sweat test, sweat chloride.

SPECIMEN: Sweat (0.1 mL minimum) collected by pilocarpine iontophoresis.

REFERENCE VALUE: (Method: Ion-specific electrode or titration)

	Conventional Units	SI Units (Conversion Factor ×1)
Normal	5–40 mEq/L	5–40 mmol/L
Intermediate	40–60 mEq/L	40–60 mmol/L

DESCRIPTION: Cystic fibrosis (CF) is a genetic disease that affects normal functioning of the exocrine glands, causing them to excrete large amounts of electrolytes. Patients with CF have sweat electrolyte levels two to five times normal. Sweat test values, with family history and signs and symptoms, are required to establish a diagnosis of CF. CF is transmitted as an autosomal-recessive trait and is characterized by abnormal exocrine secretions within the lungs,

pancreas, small intestine, bile ducts, and skin. Clinical presentation may include chronic problems of the gastrointestinal and/or respiratory system. Testing of stool samples for decreased trypsin activity has been used as a screen for CF in infants and children, but this is a much less reliable method than the sweat test.

The sweat test is a noninvasive study done to assist in the diagnosis of CF when considered with other test results and physical assessments.

This test is usually performed on children, although adults may also be tested; it is not usually ordered on adults because results can be highly variable and should be interpreted with caution. Sweat for specimen collection is induced by a small electrical current carrying the drug pilocarpine. The test measures the concentration of chloride produced by the sweat glands of the skin. A high concentration of chloride in the specimen indicates the presence of CF. The sweat test is used less commonly to measure the concentration of sodium ions for the same purpose. ■

INDICATIONS:

• Assist in the diagnosis of CF

• Screen for CF in individuals with a family history of the disease

• Screen for suspected CF in children with recurring respiratory infections

• Screen for suspected CF in infants with failure to thrive and infants who pass meconium late

• Screen for suspected CF in individuals with malabsorption syndrome

RESULT

Increased in:

• Addison's disease

• Alcoholic pancreatitis

• Chronic pulmonary infections

• Congenital adrenal hyperplasia

• CF

• Familial cholestasis

• Familial hypoparathyroidism

• Fucosidosis

• Glucose-6-phosphate dehydrogenase deficiency

• Hypothyroidism

• Mucopolysaccharidosis

• Nephrogenic diabetes insipidus

Decreased in:

• Edema

• Hypoaldosteronism

• Hypoproteinemia

• Sodium depletion

CRITICAL VALUES:

20 years or younger: Greater than 60 mmol/L considered diagnostic of CF

Older than 20 years: Greater than 70 mmol/L considered diagnostic of CF

The validity of the test result is affected tremendously by proper specimen collection and handling. Before proceeding with appropriate patient education and counseling, it is important to perform duplicate testing on patients whose results are in the diagnostic or intermediate ranges. A negative test should be repeated if test results do not support the clinical picture.

INTERFERING FACTORS:

• An inadequate amount of sweat may produce inaccurate results. Sweat testing in infants less than 1 month old is not recommended because they are often incapable of producing an adequate amount of sweat sample.

• This test should not be performed on patients with skin disorders (e.g., rash, erythema, eczema).

• Improper cleaning of the skin or improper application of gauze pad or filter paper for collection affects test results.

• Hot environmental temperatures may reduce the sodium chloride concentration in sweat; cool environmental temperatures may reduce the amount of sweat collected.

- If the specimen container that stores the gauze or filter paper is handled without gloves, the test results may show a false increase in the final weight of the collection container.

- Screening for CF can be performed using a silver nitrate test paper, and a positive test can be validated by pilocarpine iontophoresis.

Nursing Implications and Procedure

Pretest:

➤ Obtain a history of the patient's complaints, including a list of known allergens.

➤ Obtain a history of the patient's endocrine and respiratory systems, especially failure to thrive or CF in other family members, as well as results of previously performed tests and procedures. For related tests, refer to the endocrine and respiratory system tables.

➤ Obtain a list of medications the patient is taking, including herbs, nutritional supplements, and nutraceuticals. The requesting health care practitioner and laboratory should be advised if the patient regularly uses these products so that their effects can be taken into consideration when reviewing results.

➤ There are no food, fluid, or medication restrictions unless by medical direction.

➤ Inform the patient and caregiver there is no pain associated with the test, but a stinging sensation may be experienced when the low electrical current is applied at the site.

➤ Review the procedure with the patient and caregiver. Encourage the caregiver to stay with and support the child during the test. The iontophoresis and specimen collec-

tion usually takes approximately 75 to 90 minutes.

➤ Explain that a positive sweat test alone is not diagnostic of CF; repetition of borderline and positive tests is generally recommended.

Intratest:

➤ The patient is placed in a position that will allow exposure of the site on the forearm or thigh. To ensure collection of an adequate amount of sweat in a small infant, two sites (right forearm and right thigh) can be used. The patient should be covered to prevent cool environmental temperatures from affecting sweat production. The site selected for iontophoresis should never be the chest or left side because of the risk of cardiac arrest from the electrical current.

➤ The site is washed with distilled water and dried. A positive electrode is attached to the site on the right forearm or right thigh and covered with a pad that is saturated with pilocarpine, a drug that stimulates sweating. A negative electrode is covered with a pad that is saturated with bicarbonate solution. Iontophoresis is achieved by supplying a low (4 to 5 mA) electrical current via the electrode for 12 to 15 minutes. Battery-powered equipment is preferred over an electrical outlet to supply the current.

➤ The electrodes are removed, revealing a red area at the site, and the site is washed with distilled water and dried to remove any possible contaminants on the skin.

➤ Preweighed disks made of filter paper are placed on the site with a forceps; to prevent evaporation of sweat collected at the site, the disks are covered with paraffin or plastic and sealed at the edges. The disks are left in place for about 1 hour. Distract the child with books or games to allay fears.

➤ After 1 hour, the paraffin covering is removed, and disks are placed in a preweighed container with forceps.

The container is sealed and sent immediately to the laboratory for weighing and analysis of chloride content. At least 100 mg of sweat is required for accurate results.

➤ Terminate the test if the patient complains of burning at the electrode site. Reposition the electrode before the test is resumed.

➤ Label the specimen, and promptly transport it to the laboratory. Do not directly handle the preweighed specimen container or filter paper.

Post-test:

➤ Observe the site for unusual color, sensation, or discomfort.

➤ Inform the patient and caregiver that redness at the site fades in 2 to 3 hours.

➤ Reinforce information regarding diagnosis and recommended treatment regimen. Provide information regarding genetic counseling and possible screening of other family members if appropriate.

➤ Help the patient and caregiver to cope with long-term implications. Recognize that anticipatory anxiety and grief related to potential lifestyle changes may be expressed when someone is faced with a chronic disorder. Provide teaching and information regarding the clinical implications of the test results, as appropriate.

➤ If appropriate, instruct the patient and caregiver that nutrition may be altered because of impaired digestive processes associated with CF. Increased viscosity of exocrine gland secretion may lead to poor absorption of digestive enzymes and fat-soluble vitamins, necessitating supplementary oral intake of digestive enzymes with each meal and

vitamin (A, D, E, and K) supplementation. Malnutrition also is seen commonly in patients with chronic, severe respiratory disease for many reasons, including fatigue, lack of appetite, and gastrointestinal distress. Research has estimated that the daily caloric intake for respiration in patients with chronic obstructive pulmonary disease (COPD) is 10 times higher than normal individuals. Inadequate nutrition can result in hypophosphatemia, especially in a respirator-dependent patient. During periods of starvation, phosphorus leaves the intracellular space and moves outside the tissue, resulting in dangerously decreased phosphorus levels. To prevent pulmonary infection and decrease the extent of lung tissue damage, adequate intake of vitamins A and C is also important. Excessive loss of sodium chloride through the sweat glands of a patient with CF may necessitate increased salt intake, especially in environments where increased sweating is induced. The importance of following the prescribed diet should be stressed to the patient and caregiver.

➤ Water balance needs to be monitored closely in patients with COPD. Fluid retention can lead to pulmonary edema.

➤ If appropriate, instruct the patient and caregiver that ineffective airway clearance related to excessive production of mucus and decreased ciliary action may result.

➤ Evaluate test results in relation to the patient's symptoms and other tests performed. Related laboratory tests include α_1-antitrypsin/phenotype, amylase, anion gap, electrolytes, fecal analysis, fecal fat, osmolality, and phosphorus.

CHOLANGIOGRAPHY, PERCUTANEOUS TRANSHEPATIC

· ·

SYNONYMS/ACRONYMS: Percutaneous cholecystogram, PTC, PTHC.

AREA OF APPLICATION: Biliary system.

CONTRAST: Radiopaque iodine-based contrast medium.

DESCRIPTION: Percutaneous transhepatic cholangiography (PTC) is a test used to the visualize the biliary system in order to evaluate persistent upper abdominal pain after cholecystectomy and to determine the presence and cause of obstructive jaundice. The liver is punctured with a thin needle under fluoroscopic guidance, and contrast medium is injected as the needle is slowly withdrawn. This test visualizes the biliary ducts without depending on the gallbladder's concentrating ability. The intrahepatic and extrahepatic biliary ducts, and occasionally the gallbladder, can be visualized to determine possible obstruction. In obstruction of the extrahepatic ducts, a catheter can be placed in the duct to allow external drainage of bile. Endoscopic retrograde cholangiopancreatography (ERCP) and PTC are the only methods available to view the biliary tree in the presence of jaundice. ERCP poses less risk and is probably done more often. PTC is an invasive procedure and has potential risks, including bleeding, septicemia, bile peritonitis, and extravasation of the contrast medium. ∎

INDICATIONS:

• Aid in the diagnosis of obstruction caused by gallstones, benign strictures, malignant tumors, congenital cysts, and anatomic variations

• Distinguish between obstructive and nonobstructive jaundice

• Determine the cause of upper abdominal pain after cholecystectomy

• Determine the cause, extent, and location of mechanical obstruction

RESULT

Normal Findings:

• Gallbladder appears normal in size and shape.

• Biliary ducts are normal in diameter, with no evidence of dilation, filling defects, duct narrowing, or extravasation.

• Contrast medium fills the ducts and flows freely.

Abnormal Findings:

• Anatomic biliary or pancreatic duct variations

• Biliary sclerosis

• Cholangiocarcinoma

- Cirrhosis

- Common bile duct cysts

- Gallbladder carcinoma

- Gallstones

- Hepatitis

- Nonobstructive jaundice

- Pancreatitis

- Sclerosing cholangitis

- Tumors, strictures, inflammation, or gallstones of the common bile duct

CRITICAL VALUES: N/A

INTERFERING FACTORS:

This procedure is contraindicated for:

- Patients with allergies to shellfish or iodinated dye. The contrast medium used may cause a life-threatening allergic reaction. Patients with a known hypersensitivity to the medium may benefit from premedication with corticosteroids or the use of nonionic contrast medium.

- Patients who are pregnant or suspected of being pregnant, unless the potential benefits of the procedure far outweigh the risks to the fetus and mother.

- Patients with cholangitis. The injection of the contrast medium can increase biliary pressure leading to bacteremia, septicemia, and shock.

- Patients with postoperative wound sepsis, hypersensitivity to iodine, or acute renal failure.

- Patients with bleeding disorders, massive ascites, or acute renal failure.

Factors that may impair clear imaging:

- Inability of the patient to cooperate or remain still during the procedure because of age, significant pain, or mental status

- Insufficient injection of contrast medium, which may produce poor-quality films

- Metallic objects within the examination field (e.g., jewelry or body rings), which may inhibit organ visualization and can produce unclear images

- Improper adjustment of the radiographic equipment to accommodate obese or thin patients, which can cause overexposure or underexposure and poor-quality study

- Patients who are very obese, who may exceed the weight limit for the equipment

- Incorrect positioning of the patient, which may produce poor visualization of the area to be examined

- Gas or feces in the gastrointestinal tract resulting from inadequate cleansing or failure to restrict food intake before the study

- Retained barium from a previous radiologic procedure

- Gas that overfills the biliary ducts

Other considerations:

- Peritonitis may occur as a result of bile extravasation.

- Failure to follow dietary restrictions before the procedure may cause the procedure to be canceled or repeated.

- Consultation with a physician should occur before the procedure for radiation safety concerns regarding infants of patients who are lactating.

- Risks associated with radiographic overexposure can result from frequent x-ray procedures. Personnel in the room with the patient should wear a protective lead apron, stand behind a shield, or leave the area while the examination is being done. Badges that reveal the level of exposure to radiation should be worn by persons working in the area where the examination is being done.

Nursing Implications and Procedure • • • • • • • • • •

Pretest: ■

➤ Inform the patient about the purpose of the procedure as well as the need to remain still and hold his or her breath for short periods of time.

➤ Obtain a history of known or suspected hypersensitivity to radiographic contrast medium, iodine, iodine-containing food, or shellfish.

➤ Obtain a history of the patient's complaints.

➤ Obtain a history of the patient's biliary and abdominal systems and the results of previously performed tests, treatments, surgeries, therapies, and procedures, especially blood urea nitrogen, creatinine, and coagulation studies. For related tests, refer to the gastrointestinal and hepatobiliary system tables.

➤ Assess date of last menstrual period to ascertain possible pregnancy in perimenopausal women.

➤ Type and screen the patient's blood for possible transfusion.

➤ Patients receiving metformin (Glucophage) for non–insulin-dependent (type 2) diabetes should discontinue the drug on the day of the test and continue to withhold it for 48 hours after the test. Failure to do so may result in lactic acidosis.

➤ *Obtain a written, informed consent for the procedure from the patient.*

➤ The procedure lasts 60 minutes.

➤ Withhold food and fluids for 8 hours before the test.

➤ Inform the patient that there may be some abdominal discomfort from the needle insertion; however, the area will have received prior anesthesia.

➤ Schedule gastrointestinal or any barium studies after this study.

➤ Obtain baseline vital signs.

➤ Instruct the patient to refrain from food and fluids for 6 to 8 hours before the test.

Intratest: ■

➤ Administer sedatives, as ordered, before the test.

➤ Review the patient's coagulation studies to determine if they are within the normal range.

➤ Administer a laxative, as ordered.

➤ Make sure clothing and metallic objects are removed from the abdominal area.

➤ Give patient a gown and robe to wear; ask patient to void before the test begins.

➤ Remove any wires connected to electrodes, if allowed.

➤ Place patient on the fluoroscopy table in a supine position.

➤ A kidney, ureter, and bladder (KUB) or plain film is taken to ensure that no barium or stool will obscure visualization of the biliary system.

➤ An area over the abdominal wall is anesthetized, and the needle is inserted and advanced under fluoroscopic guidance. Contrast medium is injected when placement is confirmed by the free flow of bile.

➤ A specimen of bile may be sent to the laboratory for culture and cytologic analysis.

➤ X-ray exposures are made, and the results are processed as soon as possible. Additional views may be necessary to visualize the area in question.

➤ At the end of the procedure, the contrast medium is aspirated from the biliary ducts, relieving pressure on the dilated ducts.

➤ If an obstruction is found during the procedure, a catheter is inserted into the bile duct to allow drainage of bile.

➤ Maintain pressure over the needle insertion site for several hours if bleeding is persistent.

➤ Establish a closed and sterile drainage system if a catheter is left in place.

Post-test:

➤ Monitor vital and neurological signs until they return to preprocedure levels.

➤ Instruct the patient to resume usual diet and medications, as directed by the physician. Renal function should be assessed before metformin is restarted.

➤ Evaluate the patient for signs of hypersensitivity or reaction to contrast medium, such as urticaria, headache, nausea, or vomiting.

➤ Observe the puncture site for signs of bleeding, hematoma formation, ecchymosis, or leakage of bile. The physician should be informed if any of these is present.

➤ Advise the patient to watch for symptoms of infection, such as pain, fever, increased pulse rate, and muscle aches.

➤ Determine if the patient or family members have any further questions or concerns.

➤ A physician specializing in this branch of medicine sends a written report to the ordering provider, who discusses the results with the patient.

➤ Inform the patient of the possible need for further examinations to evaluate and determine the need for a change in therapy.

➤ Evaluate test results in relation to the patient's symptoms and other tests performed. Related diagnostic tests include hepatobiliary scan, hepatobiliary ultrasound, computed tomography and magnetic resonance imaging of the abdomen, and KUB film.

CHOLANGIOGRAPHY, POSTOPERATIVE

· ·

SYNONYM/ACRONYM: T-tube cholangiography.

AREA OF APPLICATION: Gallbladder, bile ducts.

CONTRAST: Iodinated contrast medium.

DESCRIPTION: After cholecystectomy, a self-retaining, T-shaped tube may be inserted into the common bile duct. Postoperative (T-tube) cholangiography is a fluoroscopic and radiographic examination of the biliary tract that involves the injec-tion of a contrast medium through the T-tube inserted during surgery. This test may be performed at the time of surgery and 7 to 10 days after cholecystectomy to assess the patency of the common bile duct and to detect any remaining calculi. T-tube placement can also be done after a liver transplant because biliary duct obstruction or anastomotic leakage is possible. This test should be performed before any gastrointestinal studies using barium and after any studies involving the measurement of iodinated compounds. ▪

INDICATIONS:

• Identify the cause, extent, and location of obstruction after surgery

• Determine biliary duct patency before T-tube removal

RESULT

Normal Findings:

• Biliary ducts are normal in size.

• Contrast medium fills the ductal system and flows freely.

Abnormal Findings:

• Filling defects, dilation, or shadows within the biliary ducts, indicating calculi or neoplasm

• Appearance of channels of contrast medium outside of the biliary ducts, indicating a fistula

CRITICAL VALUES: N/A

INTERFERING FACTORS:

This procedure is contraindicated for:

• Patients who are pregnant or suspected of being pregnant, unless the potential benefits of the procedure far outweigh the risks to the fetus and mother.

• Patients with cholangitis. The injection ⚠ of the contrast medium can increase biliary pressure, leading to bacteremia, septicemia, and shock.

• Patients with postoperative wound ⚠ sepsis, hypersensitivity to iodine, or acute renal failure.

• Patients with allergies to shellfish ⚠ or iodinated dye. The contrast medium used may cause a life-threatening allergic reaction. Patients with a known hypersensitivity to the medium may benefit from premedication with corticosteroids or the use of nonionic contrast medium.

Factors that may impair clear imaging:

• Inability of the patient to cooperate or remain still during the procedure because of age, significant pain, or mental status

• Metallic objects within the examination field (e.g., jewelry or body rings), which may inhibit organ visualization and can produce unclear images

• Insufficient injection of contrast media, which may produce poor-quality films

• Improper adjustment of the radiographic equipment to accommodate obese or thin patients, which can cause overexposure or underexposure and poor-quality study

• Patients who are very obese, who may exceed the weight limit for the equipment

• Incorrect positioning of the patient, which may produce poor visualization of the area to be examined

• Presence of ascites, which may interfere with the quality of the procedure

• Gas or feces in the gastrointestinal tract resulting from inadequate cleansing or failure to restrict food intake before the study

• Retained barium from a previous radiologic procedure

Other considerations:

• Air bubbles resembling calculi may be seen if there is inadvertent injection of air.

- Peritonitis may occur as a result of bile extravasation.

- Failure to follow dietary restrictions before the procedure may cause the procedure to be canceled or repeated.

- Consultation with a physician should occur before the procedure for radiation safety concerns regarding infants of patients who are lactating.

- Risks associated with radiographic overexposure can result from frequent x-ray procedures. Personnel in the room with the patient should wear a protective lead apron, stand behind a shield, or leave the area while the examination is being done. Badges that reveal the level of exposure to radiation should be worn by persons working in the area where the examination is being done.

Nursing Implications and Procedure • • • • • • • • • •

Pretest:

➤ Explain to the patient the purpose of the study and how the procedure is performed.

➤ Determine if the patient has allergies or sensitivities to latex, anesthetics, analgesics, antibiotics, or iodine.

➤ *Obtain a written, informed consent for the procedure from the patient.*

➤ Obtain a history of suspected or existing disease of the liver, gallbladder, and duct system. For related tests, refer to the hepatobiliary system table.

➤ Assess date of last menstrual period to ascertain possible pregnancy in perimenopausal women.

➤ Explain that the procedure usually takes 30 to 60 minutes to complete and generally is performed in the operating room or the radiology suite by a physician and support staff.

➤ Inform the patient that a flushed feeling may be experienced when the contrast medium is injected.

➤ Restrict food and fluids 8 to 12 hours before the procedure.

➤ Note recent administration of barium because residual barium can obscure the organ to be examined.

➤ Ensure that a cleansing enema is administered on the morning of the procedure, if ordered, and note results.

Intratest:

➤ Have the patient remove clothing and metallic objects. Provide a gown with a tie closure.

➤ Clamp the T-tube 24 hours before and during the procedure, if ordered, to help prevent air bubbles from entering the ducts.

➤ Have the patient void before the procedure begins.

➤ An x-ray of the abdomen is obtained to determine if any residual contrast medium is present from previous studies.

➤ The patient is placed on an examination table in the supine position.

➤ The area around the T-tube is draped; the end of the T-tube is cleansed with 70% alcohol. If the T-tube site is inflamed and painful, a local anesthetic (e.g., lidocaine) may be injected around the site. A needle is inserted into the open end of the T-tube, and the clamp is removed.

➤ Contrast medium is injected, and fluoroscopy is performed to visualize contrast medium moving through the duct system.

➤ The patient may feel a bloating sensation in the upper right quadrant as the contrast medium is injected. The tube is clamped, and films are taken of the right upper quadrant in multiple positions. A delayed film may be taken 15 minutes later to visualize passage of the contrast medium into the duodenum.

➤ For procedures done after surgery, the T-tube is removed if findings are normal; a dry, sterile dressing is applied to the site.

➤ If retained calculi are identified, the T-tube is left in place for 4 to 6 weeks until the tract surrounding the T-tube is healed to perform a percutaneous removal.

Post-test:

➤ Instruct the patient to be alert for symptoms of delayed reaction to the contrast medium, such as urticaria, headache, nausea, or vomiting.

➤ Emphasize that any severe pain, fever, difficulty breathing, increased pulse rate, bile extravasation, or bleeding must be reported to the physician immediately.

➤ Instruct the patient to resume activity, medication, and diet as directed after the examination.

➤ A physician specializing in this branch of medicine sends a written report to the ordering provider, who discusses the results with the patient.

➤ Note test results in relation to other tests performed and the patient's symptoms. Inform the patient that an abnormal examination may indicate the need for additional studies. Related diagnostic tests include hepatobiliary scan; hepatobiliary ultrasound; kidney, ureter, and bladder film; and computed tomography scan of the abdomen.

CHOLANGIOPANCREATOGRAPHY, ENDOSCOPIC RETROGRADE

SYNONYM/ACRONYM: ERCP.

AREA OF APPLICATION: Gallbladder, bile ducts, pancreatic ducts.

CONTRAST: Iodinated contrast medium.

DESCRIPTION: Endoscopic retrograde cholangiopancreatography (ERCP) allows direct visualization of the pancreatic and biliary ducts with a flexible endoscope and, after injection of contrast material, with x-rays. It allows the physician to view the pancreatic, hepatic, and common bile ducts and the ampulla of Vater. ERCP and percutaneous transhepatic cholangiography (PTC) are the only procedures that allow direct visualization of the biliary and pancreatic ducts. ERCP is less invasive and has less morbidity than PTC. It is useful in the evaluation of patients with

jaundice, because the ducts can be visualized even when the patient's bilirubin level is high. (In contrast, oral cholecystography and intravenous cholangiography are not able to visualize the biliary system when the patient has high bilirubin levels.) By endoscopy, the distal end of the common bile duct can be widened, and gallstones can be removed and stents placed in narrowed bile ducts to allow bile to be drained in jaundiced patients. During endoscopy, specimens of suspicious tissue can be taken for pathologic review, and manometry pressure readings can be obtained from the bile and pancreatic ducts. ERCP is used in the diagnosis and follow-up of pancreatic disease. ■

INDICATIONS:

• Assess jaundice of unknown cause to differentiate biliary tract obstruction from liver disease

• Identify obstruction caused by calculi, cysts, ducts, strictures, stenosis, and anatomic abnormalities

• Retrieve calculi from the distal common bile duct and release strictures

• Perform therapeutic procedures, such as sphincterotomy and placement of biliary drains

• Collect specimens for cytology

RESULT

Normal Findings:

• Normal appearance of the duodenal papilla

• Patency of the pancreatic and common bile ducts

Abnormal Findings:

• Duodenal papilla tumors

• Pancreatic cancer

• Pancreatic fibrosis

• Pancreatitis

• Sclerosing cholangitis

CRITICAL VALUES: N/A

INTERFERING FACTORS:

• Inability of the patient to cooperate with the procedure because of age, significant pain, or mental status

• Failure to follow dietary restrictions before the procedure

• Previous surgery involving the stomach

or duodenum, which can make locating the duodenal papilla difficult

• Barium remaining in the stomach or bowel

• A patient with Zenker's diverticulum involving the esophagus, who may be unable to undergo ERCP

• A patient with unstable cardiopulmonary status, blood coagulation defects, or cholangitis (test may have to be rescheduled unless patient received antibiotic therapy before the test)

• A patient with known acute pancreatitis

Nursing Implications and Procedure

Pretest:

➤ Explain to the patient the purpose of the study and how the procedure is performed.

➤ *Obtain a written, informed consent for the procedure from the patient.*

➤ Obtain a history of suspected or existing disease of the pancreas, gallbladder, duct system, or other intestinal disorders. For related tests, refer to the hepatobiliary and gastrointestinal system tables.

➤ Determine if the patient has allergies or sensitivities to anesthetics, analgesics, antibiotics, or iodine.

➤ Obtain results of other tests and procedures done to diagnose disorders of or to provide treatment for the pancreas, gallbladder, biliary ducts, or intestinal system.

➤ Explain that the procedure usually takes 30 to 60 minutes to complete and generally is performed in an endoscopy suite by a physician and support staff. The physician interprets the results and sends the patient's physician a written report, to be discussed with the patient.

➤ Inform the patient that a flushed feeling may be experienced when the contrast medium is injected.

➤ Restrict food and fluids 8 to 12 hours before the procedure.

➤ Note recent administration of barium because residual barium can obscure the organ to examined.

Intratest:

➤ Have the patient put on a hospital gown and void.

➤ Administer ordered sedation.

➤ Insert an intravenous line for administration of drugs, as needed.

➤ An x-ray of the abdomen is obtained to determine if any residual contrast medium is present from previous studies.

➤ The oropharynx is sprayed or swabbed with a topical local anesthetic.

➤ The patient is placed on an examination table in the left lateral position with the left arm behind the back and right hand at the side with the neck slightly flexed. A protective guard is inserted into the mouth to cover the teeth. A bite block can also be inserted to maintain adequate opening of the mouth.

➤ The endoscope is passed through the mouth with a dental suction device in place to drain secretions. A side-viewing flexible, fiberoptic endoscope is passed into the duodenum, and a small cannula is inserted into the duodenal papilla (ampulla of Vater).

➤ The patient is placed in the prone position. The duodenal papilla is visualized and cannulated with a catheter. Occasionally the patient can be turned slightly to the right side to aid in visualization of the papilla.

➤ Intravenous glucagon or anticholinergics can be administered to minimize duodenal spasm and to facilitate visualization of the ampulla of Vater.

➤ ERCP manometry can be done at this time to measure the pressure in the bile duct, pancreatic duct, and sphincter of Oddi at the papilla area via the catheter as it is placed in the area before the contrast medium is injected.

➤ When the catheter is in place, contrast medium is injected into the pancreatic and biliary ducts via the catheter, and fluoroscopic films are taken. Biopsy specimens for cytological analysis can be obtained during the procedure.

➤ Place specimens in appropriate containers, label them properly, and promptly transport them to the laboratory.

Post-test:

➤ Tell the patient to expect some throat soreness and possible hoarseness. Advise the patient to use warm gargles, lozenges, ice packs to the neck, or cool fluids to alleviate throat discomfort.

➤ Monitor the patient for signs of respiratory depression. Resuscitation equipment should be available.

➤ Observe the patient until the effects of the sedation have worn off.

➤ Inform the patient that any belching, bloating, or flatulence is the result of air insufflation.

➤ Emphasize that any severe pain, fever, difficulty breathing, or expectoration of blood must be reported to the physician immediately.

➤ Do not allow the patient to eat or drink until the gag reflex returns, after which the patient is permitted to eat lightly for 12 to 24 hours.

➤ Instruct the patient to resume normal activity, medication, and diet 24 hours after the examination, or as tolerated, unless otherwise indicated.

➤ A physician specializing in this branch of medicine sends a written report to the ordering provider, who discusses the results with the patient.

➤ Inform the patient that an abnormal

examination may indicate the need for further studies.

➤ Evaluate test results in relation to the patient's symptoms and other tests performed. Related diag- nostic tests include ultrasound of the bile ducts, hepatobiliary scan, and computed tomography and magnetic resonance imaging of the abdomen.

CHOLESTEROL, HDL, LDL

SYNONYMS/ACRONYMS: α_1-Lipoprotein cholesterol, high-density choles- terol, HDLC, β-lipoprotein cholesterol, low-density cholesterol, LDLC.

SPECIMEN: Serum (2 mL) collected in a red- or tiger-top tube.

REFERENCE VALUE: (Method: Spectrophotometry)

HDLC	Conventional Units	SI Units (Conversion Factor ×0.0259)
Birth	6–56 mg/dL	0.16–1.45 mmol/L
Children and adults	40–65 mg/dL	0.9–1.7 mmol/L

LDLC	Conventional Units	SI Units (Conversion Factor ×0.0259)
Birth	20–56 mg/dL	0.52–1.45 mmol/L
5–19 y		
Male	65–130 mg/dL	1.68–3.37 mmol/L
Female	65–140 mg/dL	1.68–3.63 mmol/L
20–29 y		
Male	65–165 mg/dL	1.68–4.27 mmol/L
Female	55–160 mg/dL	1.42–4.14 mmol/L
30–44 y		
Male	80–185 mg/dL	2.07–4.79 mmol/L
Female	70–175 mg/dL	1.81–4.53 mmol/L
Greater than 45 y		
Male	90–185 mg/dL	2.33–4.79 mmol/L
Female	80–215 mg/dL	2.07–5.57 mmol/L

After age 10 years, values for African Americans are approximately 10 mg/dL higher than in whites in the same age group.

DESCRIPTION: High-density lipoprotein cholesterol (HDLC) and low-density lipoprotein cholesterol (LDLC) are the major transport proteins for cholesterol in the body. It is believed that HDLC may have protective properties in that its role includes transporting cholesterol from the arteries to the liver. LDLC is the major transport protein for cholesterol to the arteries from the liver. LDLC can be calculated using total cholesterol, total triglycerides, and HDLC levels.

HDLC levels less than 40 mg/dL in men and women represent a coronary risk factor. There is an inverse relationship between HDLC and risk of coronary artery disease (CAD) (i.e., lower HDLC levels represent a higher risk of CAD). Levels of LDLC in terms of risk for CAD are directly proportional to risk and vary by age group. The LDLC can be estimated using the following Friedewald formula:

$$LDLC = (Total\ Cholesterol) - (HDLC) - (VLDLC)$$

Very-low-density lipoprotein cholesterol (VLDLC) is estimated by dividing the triglycerides (conventional units) by 5. Triglycerides in SI units would be divided by 2.18 to estimate VLDLC. It is important to note that the formula is valid only if the triglycerides are less than 400 mg/dL or 4.52 mmol/L. ■

INDICATIONS:

• Determine the risk of cardiovascular disease

• Evaluate the response to dietary and drug therapy for hypercholesterolemia

• Investigate hypercholesterolemia in light of family history of cardiovascular disease

RESULT

LDLC Recommended Levels

Risk	Units Conventional	SI Units (Conversion Factor ×0.0259)
Optimal	Less than 100 mg/dL	Less than 2.59 mmol/L
Near optimal	100–129 mg/dL	2.59–3.34 mmol/L
Borderline high	130–159 mg/dL	2.67–4.11 mmol/L
High	160–189 mg/dL	4.14–4.90 mmol/L
Very high	Greater than 190 mg/dL	Greater than 4.92 mmol/L

HDLC increased in:

• Exercise

• Familial hyper-α-lipoproteinemia

• Alcoholism

• Biliary cirrhosis

• Chronic hepatitis

HDLC decreased in:

• A-β-lipoproteinemia

• Fish eye disease

• Genetic predisposition or enzyme/cofactor deficiency

• Hypertriglyceridemia

- Obesity
- Sedentary lifestyle
- Smoking
- Tangier disease
- Chronic renal failure
- Cholestasis
- Uncontrolled diabetes
- Hepatocellular disorders
- Nephrotic syndrome
- Premature CAD

LDLC increased in:

- Corneal arcus
- Hyperlipoproteinemia types IIa and IIb
- Premature CAD
- Tendon and tuberous xanthomas
- Anorexia nervosa
- Chronic renal failure
- Cushing's syndrome
- Diabetes
- Diet high in cholesterol and saturated fat
- Dysglobulinemias
- Hepatic disease
- Hepatic obstruction
- Hypothyroidism
- Nephrotic syndrome
- Porphyria
- Pregnancy

LDLC decreased in:

- Genetic predisposition or enzyme/cofactor deficiency
- Hypolipoproteinemia and a-β-lipoproteinemia
- Tangier disease
- Acute stress (severe burns, illness)

- Chronic anemias
- Chronic pulmonary disease
- Severe hepatocellular destruction or disease
- Hyperthyroidism
- Inflammatory joint disease
- Myeloma
- Reye's syndrome

CRITICAL VALUES: N/A

INTERFERING FACTORS:

- Drugs that may increase HDLC levels include albuterol, anticonvulsants, cholestyramine, cimetidine, clofibrate and other fibric acid derivatives, estrogens, ethanol (moderate use), lovastatin, niacin, oral contraceptives, pravastatin, pindolol, prazosin, and simvastatin.

- Drugs that may decrease HDLC levels include acebutolol, atenolol, nonselective β-adrenergic blocking agents, danazol, diuretics, etretinate, interferon, isotretinoin, linseed oil, metoprolol, neomycin, probucol, progesterone, thiazides, and steroids.

- Drugs that may increase LDLC levels include androgens, catecholamines, chenodiol, cyclosporine, danazol, diuretics, glucogenic corticosteroids, etretinate, and progestins.

- Drugs that may decrease LDLC levels include aminosalicylic acid, cholestyramine, colestipol, estrogens, fibric acid derivatives, interferon, lovastatin, neomycin, niacin, paravastatin, prazosin, probucol, simvastatin, terazosin, and thyroxine.

- Some of the drugs used to lower total cholesterol and LDLC or increase HDLC may cause liver damage.

- Grossly elevated triglyceride levels invalidate the Friedewald formula for mathematical estimation of LDLC, and if the triglyceride is greater than 400 mg/dL, the formula should not be used.

- Fasting before specimen collection is highly recommended. Ideally the patient should be on a stable diet for 3 weeks and fast 12 hours before specimen collection.

Nursing Implications and Procedure • • • • • • • • • • •

Pretest: ▪

➤ Obtain a history of the patient's complaints, including a list of known allergens.

➤ Obtain a history of the patient's cardiovascular system and results of previously performed tests and procedures. The presence of other risk factors, such as family history of heart disease, smoking, obesity, diet, lack of physical activity, hypertension, diabetes, previous myocardial infarction, and previous vascular disease, should be investigated. For related tests, refer to the cardiovascular system table.

➤ Obtain a list of medications the patient is taking, including herbs, nutritional supplements, and nutraceuticals. The requesting health care practitioner and laboratory should be advised if the patient regularly uses these products so that their effects can be taken into consideration when reviewing results.

➤ Instruct the patient to fast 12 hours before specimen collection.

➤ Confirm with the requesting health care practitioner that the patient should withhold medications known to influence test results, and instruct the patient accordingly.

➤ There are no fluid restrictions unless by medical direction.

➤ Review the procedure with the patient.

➤ Inform the patient that specimen collection takes approximately 5 to 10 minutes.

Intratest: ▪

➤ Ensure that the patient has complied with dietary preparations and other pretesting restrictions.

➤ Direct the patient to breathe normally and to avoid unnecessary movement.

➤ Observe standard precautions and follow the general guidelines in Appendix A. Perform a venipuncture, and collect the specimen in a 5-mL red- or tiger-top tube.

➤ Label the specimen, and promptly transport it to the laboratory.

Post-test: ▪

➤ Observe venipuncture site for bleeding or hematoma formation. Apply pressure bandage.

➤ Instruct the patient to resume usual diet and medication as directed by the health care practitioner.

➤ Decreased HDLC level and increased LDLC level may be associated with CAD. Nutritional therapy is recommended for the patient identified to be at high risk for developing CAD. If overweight, the patient should be encouraged to achieve a normal weight. The American Heart Association Step 1 and Step 2 diets may be helpful in achieving a goal of lowering total cholesterol and triglyceride levels. The Step 1 diet emphasizes a reduction in foods high in saturated fats and cholesterol. Red meats, eggs, and dairy products are the major sources of saturated fats and cholesterol. If triglycerides also are elevated, the patient should be advised to eliminate or reduce alcohol and simple carbohydrates from the diet. The Step 2 diet recommends stricter reductions.

➤ Numerous studies point to the prevalence of excess body weight in American children and adolescents. Experts estimate that obesity is present in 25 percent of the population aged 6 to 11 years. The medical, social, and emotional consequences of excess body weight are significant. Special attention should be given to instructing the child and caregiver regarding health risks and weight-control education.

➤ Evaluate test results in relation to the patient's symptoms and other tests performed. Related laboratory tests include apolipoprotein A and B, C-reactive protein, total cholesterol, homocysteine, lipoprotein electrophoresis, and triglycerides.

CHOLESTEROL, TOTAL

SYNONYM/ACRONYM: N/A.

SPECIMEN: Serum (1 mL) collected in a red- or tiger-top tube. Plasma (1 mL) collected in green-top (heparin) tube is also acceptable. It is important to use the same tube type when serial specimen collections are anticipated for consistency in testing.

REFERENCE VALUE: (Method: Spectrophotometry)

Serum

Risk	Conventional Units	SI Units (Conversion Factor ×0.0259)
Desirable	Less than 200 mg/dL	Less than 5.18 mmol/L
Borderline	200–239 mg/dL	5.18–6.19 mmol/L
High	Greater than 240 mg/dL	Greater than 6.22 mmol/L

Plasma values may be 10% lower than serum values.

DESCRIPTION: Cholesterol is a lipid needed to form cell membranes and a component of the materials that render the skin waterproof. It also helps form bile salts, adrenal corticosteroids, estrogen, and androgens. Cholesterol is obtained from the diet (exogenous cholesterol) and also synthesized in the body (endogenous cholesterol). Although most body cells can form some cholesterol, it is produced mainly by the liver and intestinal mucosa. Cholesterol is an integral component in cell membrane maintenance and hormone production. Very low cholesterol values, as is sometimes seen in critically ill patients, can be as life-threatening as very high levels.

According to the National Cholesterol Education Program, maintaining cholesterol levels less than 200 mg/dL significantly reduces the risk of coronary heart disease; no age and gender stratification is presented as part of its recommendation. Numerous studies have been done, and there are inconsistencies among the studies as to target "normals" segregated by age and gender. Beyond the total cholesterol and high-density lipoprotein cholesterol (HDLC) values, other important risk factors must be considered. Many myocardial infarctions occur even in patients whose cholesterol levels are considered to be within acceptable limits or who are in a moderate-risk category. The combination of risk factors and lipid values helps identify individuals at risk so that appropriate interventions can be taken. If the cholesterol level is greater than 200 mg/dL, repeat testing after a 12- to 24-hour fast is recommended. ▪

INDICATIONS:

• Assist in determining risk of cardiovascular disease

• Assist in the diagnosis of nephrotic syndrome, hepatic disease, pancreatitis, and thyroid disorders

• Evaluate the response to dietary and drug therapy for hypercholesterolemia

• Investigate hypercholesterolemia in light of family history of cardiovascular disease

RESULT

Increased in:

• Acute intermittent porphyria

• Alcoholism

• Anorexia nervosa

• Cholestasis

• Chronic renal failure

• Diabetes (with poor control)

• Diets high in cholesterol and fats

• Familial hyperlipoproteinemia

• Glomerulonephritis

• Glycogen storage disease (von Gierke disease)

• Gout

• Hypothyroidism (primary)

• Ischemic heart disease

• Nephrotic syndrome

• Obesity

• Pancreatic and prostatic malignancy

• Pregnancy

• Werner's syndrome

Decreased in:

• Burns

• Chronic myelocytic leukemia

• Chronic obstructive pulmonary disease

• Hyperthyroidism

• Liver disease (severe)

• Malabsorption and malnutrition syndromes

• Myeloma

• Pernicious anemia

• Polycythemia vera

• Severe illness

• Sideroblastic anemias

• Tangier disease

• Thalassemia

• Waldenström's macroglobulinemia

CRITICAL VALUES: N/A

INTERFERING FACTORS:

• Drugs that may increase cholesterol levels include amiodarone, androgens, catecholamines, cyclosporine, danazol, diclofenac, disulfiram, glucogenic corticosteroids, ibuprofen, isotretinoin, levodopa, methyclothiazide, miconazole (owing to castor oil vehicle, not the drug), nafarelin, nandrolone, some oral contraceptives, oxymetholone, phenobarbital, phenothiazine, prochlorperazine, and sotalol.

• Drugs that may decrease cholesterol levels include acebutolol, amiloride, aminosalicylic acid, ascorbic acid, asparaginase, atenolol, atorvastatin, beclobrate, bezafibrate, carbutamide, cerivastatin, cholestyramine, ciprofibrate, clofibrate, clonidine, colestipol, dextrothyroxine, doxazosin, enalapril, estrogens, fenofibrate, fenfluramine, fluvastatin, gemfibrozil, haloperidol, hydralazine, interferon, lovastatin, neomycin, niacin, pravastatin, probucol, simvastatin, tamoxifen, terazosin, thyroxine, ursodiol, and verapamil.

• Ingestion of alcohol 12 to 24 hours before the test can falsely elevate results.

• Ingestion of drugs that alter cholesterol levels within 12 hours of the test may give a false impression of cholesterol levels, unless the test is done to evaluate such effects.

• Positioning can affect results; lower levels are obtained if the specimen is from a patient who has been supine for 20 minutes.

Nursing Implications and Procedure • • • • • • • • • •

Pretest:

➤ Obtain a history of the patient's complaints, including a list of known allergens.

➤ Obtain a history of the patient's cardiovascular, gastrointestinal, hematopoietic, and hepatobiliary systems, as well as results of previously performed tests and proce-

dures. The presence of other risk factors, such as family history of heart disease, smoking, obesity, diet, lack of physical activity, hypertension, diabetes, previous myocardial infarction, and previous vascular disease, should be investigated. For related tests, refer to the cardiovascular, gastrointestinal, hematopoietic, and hepatobiliary system tables.

➤ Obtain a list of medications the patient is taking, including herbs, nutritional supplements, and nutraceuticals. The requesting health care practitioner and laboratory should be advised if the patient regularly uses these products so that their effects can be taken into consideration when reviewing results.

➤ Instruct the patient to withhold alcohol and drugs known to alter cholesterol levels for 12 to 24 hours before specimen collection, at the direction of the health care practitioner.

➤ There are no fluid or medication restrictions unless by medical direction.

➤ Fasting 6 to 12 hours before specimen collection is required if triglyceride measurements are included; it is recommended if cholesterol levels alone are measured for screening.

➤ Review the procedure with the patient.

➤ Inform the patient that specimen collection takes approximately 5 to 10 minutes.

Intratest:

➤ Ensure that the patient has complied with dietary preparations and other pretesting restrictions.

➤ Direct the patient to breathe normally and to avoid unnecessary movement.

➤ Observe standard precautions and follow the general guidelines in Appendix A. Perform a venipuncture, and collect the specimen in a 5-mL red- or tiger-top tube.

➤ Label the specimen, and promptly transport it to the laboratory.

Post-test:

➤ Observe venipuncture site for bleeding or hematoma formation. Apply pressure bandage.

➤ Instruct the patient to resume usual diet and medication as directed by the health care practitioner.

➤ Secondary causes for increased cholesterol levels should be ruled out before therapy to decrease levels is initiated by use of drugs.

➤ Increases in total cholesterol levels may be associated with coronary artery disease (CAD). Nutritional therapy is recommended for patients identified to be at high risk for developing CAD. If overweight, the patient should be encouraged to achieve a normal weight. The American Heart Association Step 1 and Step 2 diets may be helpful in achieving a goal of lowering total cholesterol and triglyceride levels. The Step 1 diet emphasizes a reduction in foods high in saturated fats and cholesterol. Red meats, eggs, and dairy products are the major sources of saturated fats and choles-

terol. If triglycerides are also elevated, the patient should be advised to eliminate or reduce alcohol and simple carbohydrates from the diet. The Step 2 diet recommends stricter reductions.

➤ Numerous studies point to the prevalence of excess body weight in American children and adolescents. Experts estimate that obesity is present in 25 percent of the population aged 6 to 11 years. The medical, social, and emotional consequences of excess body weight are significant. Special attention should be given to instructing the child and caregiver regarding health risks and weight control education.

➤ Evaluate test results in relation to the patient's symptoms and other tests performed. Related laboratory tests include apolipoprotein A and B, C-reactive protein, HDLC, low-density lipoprotein cholesterol, very-low-density lipoprotein cholesterol, chylomicrons, creatine kinase and isoenzymes, homocysteine, lipoprotein electrophoresis, myoglobin, triglycerides, and troponin.

CHROMOSOME ANALYSIS, BLOOD

SYNONYM/ACRONYM: N/A.

SPECIMEN: Whole blood (2 mL) collected in green-top (sodium heparin) tube.

REFERENCE VALUE: (Method: Tissue culture and microscopic analysis) No chromosomal abnormalities identified.

DESCRIPTION: Testing for birth defects as well as mental and physical re-

tardation can be accomplished through the use of several technologies. Chromosome analysis by phytohemagglutination assay is used to detect Down's syndrome and abnormal sexual development. Fluorescence *in situ* hybridization (FISH) testing is useful in the detection of specific microdeletion syndromes (e.g., Prader-Willi, Angelman, Beckwith-Wiedemann, Smith-Magenis, DiGeorge, Williams, Miller-Dieker) and other acquired chromosomal changes associated with hematologic disorders. Amniotic fluid, chorionic villus sampling, and cells from fetal tissue or products of conception can also be evaluated for chromosomal abnormalities. ■

INDICATIONS:

• Evaluate conditions related to cryptorchidism, hypogonadism, primary amenorrhea, and infertility

• Evaluate congenital anomaly, delayed development (physical or mental), mental retardation, and ambiguous sexual organs

• Investigate the carrier status of patients or relatives with known genetic abnormalities

• Investigate the cause of multiple miscarriages

• Provide prenatal care or genetic counseling

RESULT: The following tables list some common genetic defects:

Syndrome	Autosomal Chromosome Defect	Features
Beckwith-Wiedemann	Duplication 11p15	Macroglossia, omphalocele, ear lobe creases
Cat's eye	Trisomy 2q11	Anal atresia, coloboma
Cri du chat	Deletion 5p	Catlike cry, microcephaly, hypertelorism, mental retardation, retrognathia
Down's	Trisomy 21	Epicanthal folds, simian crease of palm, flat nasal bridge, mental retardation, congenital heart disease
Edwards'	Trisomy 18	Micrognathia, clenched third/fourth fingers with the fifth finger overlapping, rocker-bottom feet, mental retardation, congenital heart disease
Pallister-Killian	Trisomy 12p	Psychomotor delay, sparse anterior scalp hair, micrognathia, hypotonia

(Continued on the following page)

Syndrome	Autosomal Chromosome Defect	Features
Patau's	Trisomy 13	Microcephaly, cleft palate or lip, polydactyly, mental retardation, congenital heart disease
Warkam	Mosaic trisomy 8	Malformed ears, bulbous nose, deep palm creases, absent or hypoplastic patellae
Wolf-Hirschhorn	Deletion 4p	Microcephaly, growth retardation, mental retardation, carp mouth

Syndrome	Sex-Chromosome Defect	Features
XYY	47,XYY	Tall, increased risk of behavioral problems
Klinefelter's	47,XXY	Hypogonadism, infertility, underdeveloped secondary sex characteristics, learning disabilities
Triple X	47,XXX	Increased risk of infertility and learning disabilities
Ullrich-Turner	45,X	Short, gonadal dysgenesis, webbed neck, low posterior hairline, renal and cardiovascular abnormalities

CRITICAL VALUES: N/A

INTERFERING FACTORS: N/A

Nursing Implications and Procedure · · · · · · · · · · ·

Pretest: ▉

➤ Obtain a history of the patient's complaints, including a list of known allergens.

➤ Obtain a history of the patient's reproductive system, family history of known or suspected genetic disorders, and results of previously performed tests and procedures. For related tests, refer to the reproductive system table.

➤ Obtain a list of the medications the patient is taking, including herbs, nutritional supplements, and nutraceuticals. The requesting health care practitioner and laboratory should be advised if the patient regularly uses these products so that their effects can be taken into consideration when reviewing results.

➤ There are no food, fluid, or medication restrictions unless by medical direction.

➤ Review the procedure with the patient.

➤ Inform the patient that specimen collection takes approximately 5 to 10 minutes.

Intratest:

➤ Direct the patient to breathe normally and to avoid unnecessary movement.

➤ Observe standard precautions and follow the general guidelines in Appendix A. Perform a venipuncture, and collect the specimen in a 5-mL green-top tube.

➤ Label the specimen, and promptly transport it to the laboratory.

Post-test:

➤ Observe venipuncture site for bleeding or hematoma formation. Apply pressure bandage.

➤ Respond to anxiety the patient may experience because of the sensitive nature of the testing. Provide teaching and information regarding the clinical implications of the test results, as appropriate. Encourage the family to seek counseling if they are contemplating pregnancy termination or to seek genetic counseling if a chromosomal abnormality is determined. Decisions regarding elective abortion should occur in the presence of both parents. Provide a nonjudgmental, nonthreatening atmosphere for discussing the risks and difficulties of delivering and raising an abnormal infant, as well as exploring other options (termination of pregnancy or adoption). It is also important to discuss feelings the mother and father may experience (e.g., guilt, depression, anger) if fetal abnormalities are detected. Educate the patient and family regarding access to counseling services, as appropriate.

➤ Evaluate test results in relation to the patient's symptoms and other tests performed. Related laboratory tests include amniotic fluid analysis, α_1-fetoprotein, and chorionic villus biopsy.

CLOT RETRACTION

· ·

SYNONYM/ACRONYM: N/A.

SPECIMEN: Whole blood collected in a full 5-mL red-top tube.

REFERENCE VALUE: (Method: Macroscopic observation of sample) A normal clot, gently separated from the side of the test tube and incubated at 37°C, shrinks to about half of its original size within 1 hour. The result is a firm, cylindrical fibrin clot that contains red blood cells and is sharply demarcated from the clear serum. Complete clot retraction can take 6 to 24 hours.

DESCRIPTION: The clot retraction test measures the adequacy of platelet function by measuring the speed and extent of clot retraction. Normally, when blood clots in a test tube, it retracts away from the sidewalls of the tube. Platelets play a major role in the clot retraction process. When platelets are decreased or function is impaired, scant serum and a soft, plump, poorly demarcated clot form in the tube. In addition to normal platelets, clot retraction depends on the contractile protein thrombosthenin, magnesium, adenosine triphosphate (ATP), and pyruvate kinase. Clot retraction is also influenced by hematocrit and by fibrinogen structure and concentration. ∎

INDICATIONS:

- Evaluate the adequacy of platelet function
- Evaluate thrombocytopenia of unknown origin
- Investigate the possibility of Glanzmann's disease
- Investigate suspected abnormalities of fibrinogen or fibrinolytic activity

RESULT

Increased in: N/A

Decreased in: Glanzmann's thrombasthenia

CRITICAL VALUES: N/A

INTERFERING FACTORS:

- Drugs that may produce a decreased result include apronalide, carbenicillin, and plicamycin.
- Platelet count less than 100,000/μL, acetylsalicylic acid therapy, altered fibrinogen/fibrin structure, hypofibrinogenemia, polycythemia or hemoconcentration, and multiple myeloma are conditions in which abnormal clot retraction may occur, limiting the ability to form a valid assessment of platelet function.

- Prompt and proper specimen processing, storage, and analysis are important to achieve accurate results. Specimens received in the laboratory more than 1 hour after collection should be rejected.

Nursing Implications and Procedure • • • • • • • • • •

Pretest: ∎

➤ Obtain a history of the patient's complaints, including a list of known allergens.

➤ Obtain a history of the patient's hematopoietic system and results of previously performed tests and procedures. For related tests, refer to the hematopoietic system table.

➤ Obtain a list of medications the patient is taking, including herbs, nutritional supplements, and nutraceuticals. The requesting health care practitioner and laboratory should be advised if the patient regularly uses these products so that their effects can be taken into consideration when reviewing results.

➤ Note any recent procedures that can interfere with test results.

➤ There are no food, fluid, or medication restrictions unless by medical direction.

➤ Review the procedure with the patient.

➤ Inform the patient that specimen collection takes approximately 5 to 10 minutes.

Intratest: ∎

➤ Direct the patient to breathe normally and to avoid unnecessary movement.

➤ Observe standard precautions and follow the general guidelines in Appendix A. Perform a venipuncture, and collect the specimen in a 5-mL red-top tube.

➤ Label the specimen, and promptly

transport it to the laboratory within 1 hour of collection.

➤ Observe venipuncture site for bleeding or hematoma formation. Apply pressure bandage.

➤ Inform the patient with abnormal clot retraction of the importance of taking precautions against bruising and bleeding. These precautions may include the use of a soft bristle toothbrush, use of an electric razor, avoidance of constipation, avoidance of acetylsalicylic acid and similar products, and avoidance of intramuscular injections.

➤ Evaluate test results in relation to the patient's symptoms and other tests performed. Related laboratory tests include bleeding time, factor XIII, fibrinogen, and platelet count.

COAGULATION FACTORS

SYNONYMS/ACRONYMS: See table.

SPECIMEN: Whole blood in a completely filled 5-mL blue-top (sodium citrate) tube.

REFERENCE VALUE: (Method: Photo optical clot detection) Activity from 50 to 150 percent.

	Preferred Name	Synonym
Factor I	Fibrinogen	—
Factor II	Prothrombin	Prethrombin
Factor III	Tissue factor	Tissue thromboplastin
Factor IV	Calcium	Ca^{2+}
Factor V	Proaccelerin	Labile factor, accelerator globulin (AcG)
Factor VII	Proconvertin	Stabile factor, serum prothrombin conversion accelerator, autoprothrombin I
Factor VIII:C	Antihemophilic factor (AHF)	Antihemophilic globulin (AHG), antihemophilic factor A, platelet cofactor 1
Factor IX	Plasma thromboplastin component (PTC)	Christmas factor, antihemophilic factor B, platelet cofactor 2
Factor X	Stuart-Prower factor	Autoprothrombin III, thrombokinase

(Continued on the following page)

	Preferred Name	Synonym
Factor XI	Plasma thromboplastin antecedent (PTA)	Antihemophilic factor C
Factor XII	Hageman factor	Glass factor, contact factor
Factor XIII	Fibrin-stabilizing factor (FSF)	Laki-Lorand factor (LLF), fibrinase, plasma transglutinase
	Prekallikrein	Fletcher factor
	High-molecular-weight kininogen (HMWK)	Fitzgerald factor, contact activation cofactor, Williams factor, Falujenc factor

DESCRIPTION: The coagulation proteins respond to blood vessel injury in a chain of events. The intrinsic and extrinsic pathways of secondary hemostasis are a series of reactions involving the substrate protein fibrinogen, the coagulation factors (also known as *enzyme precursors* or *zymogens*), nonenzymatic cofactors (Ca^{2+}), and phospholipid. The factors were assigned Roman numerals in the order of their discovery, not their place in the coagulation sequence. Factor VI was originally thought to be a separate clotting factor. It was subsequently proved to be the same as a modified form of Factor V, and therefore the number is no longer used.

The coagulation factors are formed in the liver. They can be divided into three groups based on their common properties:

1. The contact group is activated *in vitro* by a surface such as glass and is activated *in vivo* by collagen. The contact group includes factor XI, factor XII, prekallikrein, and high-molecular-weight kininogen.
2. The prothrombin or vitamin K–dependent group includes factors II, VII, IX, and X.
3. The fibrinogen group includes

factors I, V, VIII, and XIII. They are the most labile of the factors and are consumed during the coagulation process. The factors listed in the table are the ones most commonly measured. ■

INDICATIONS:

• Identify the presence of inherited bleeding disorders

• Identify the presence of qualitative or quantitative factor deficiency

RESULT

Increased in: N/A

Decreased in:

• Congenital deficiency

• Disseminated intravascular coagulation

• Liver disease

CRITICAL VALUES: N/A

INTERFERING FACTORS:

• Drugs that may increase factor II levels include fluoxymesterone, methandrostenolone, nandrolone, and oxymetholone.

• Drugs that may decrease factor II levels include warfarin.

- Drugs that may increase factor V, VII, and X levels include anabolic steroids, fluoxymesterone, methandrostenolone, nandrolone, oral contraceptives, and oxymetholone.

- Drugs that may decrease factor V levels include streptokinase.

- Drugs that may decrease factor VII levels include asparaginase, acetylsalicylic acid, cefamandole, ceftriaxone, dextran, dicumarol, gemfibrozil, oral contraceptives, and warfarin.

- Drugs that may increase factor VIII levels include chlormadinone.

- Drugs that may decrease factor VIII levels include asparaginase.

- Drugs that may increase factor IX levels include chlormadinone and oral contraceptives.

- Drugs that may decrease factor IX levels include asparaginase and warfarin.

- Drugs that may decrease factor X levels include chlormadinone, dicumarol, oral contraceptives, and warfarin.

- Drugs that may decrease factor XI levels include asparaginase and captopril.

- Drugs that may decrease factor XII levels include captopril.

- Test results of patients on anticoagulant therapy are unreliable.

- Placement of tourniquet for longer than 1 minute can result in venous stasis and changes in the concentration of plasma proteins to be measured. Platelet activation may also occur under these conditions, causing erroneous results.

- Vascular injury during phlebotomy can activate platelets and coagulation factors, causing erroneous results.

- Hemolyzed specimens must be rejected because hemolysis is an indication of

platelet and coagulation factor activation.

- Incompletely filled tubes contaminated with heparin or clotted specimens must be rejected.

- Icteric or lipemic specimens interfere with optical testing methods, producing erroneous results.

- Incompletely filled collection tubes, specimens contaminated with heparin, clotted specimens, or unprocessed specimens not delivered to the laboratory within 1 hour of collection should be rejected.

Nursing Implications and Procedure

Pretest:

➤ Obtain a history of the patient's complaints, including a list of known allergens.

➤ Obtain a history of the patient's hematopoietic and hepatobiliary systems, any bleeding disorders, and results of previously performed tests and procedures, especially bleeding time, clotting time, complete blood count, partial thromboplastin time, platelets, and prothrombin time. For related tests, refer to the hematopoietic and hepatobiliary system tables.

➤ Obtain a list of medications the patient is taking, including anticoagulant therapy, acetylsalicylic acid, herbals, and nutraceuticals known to affect coagulation. It is recommended that use of these substances be discontinued 14 days before dental or surgical procedures. The requesting health care practitioner and laboratory should be advised if the patient regularly uses these products so that their effects can be taken into consideration when reviewing results.

➤ There are no food, fluid, or medication restrictions unless by medical direction.

➤ Review the procedure with the patient.

➤ Inform the patient that specimen collection takes approximately 5 to 10 minutes.

Intratest:

➤ Direct the patient to breathe normally and to avoid unnecessary movement.

➤ Observe standard precautions and follow the general guidelines in Appendix A. Perform a venipuncture, and collect the specimen in a 5-mL blue-top tube. *Important note:* Two different concentrations of sodium citrate preservative are currently added to blue-top tubes for coagulation studies: 3.2% and 3.8%. The National Committee for Clinical Laboratory Standards (NCCLS) guideline for sodium citrate is 3.2%. Laboratories establish reference ranges for coagulation testing based on numerous factors, including sodium citrate concentration, test equipment, and test reagents. It is important to inquire from the laboratory which concentration it recommends, because each concentration will have its own specific reference range. When multiple specimens are drawn, the blue-top tube should be collected after sterile (i.e., blood culture) and red-top tubes. When coagulation testing is the only work to be done, an extra red-top tube should be collected before the blue-top tube to avoid contaminating the specimen with tissue thromboplastin.

➤ Label the specimen, and promptly transport it to the laboratory. The NCCLS recommendation for processed and unprocessed samples stored in unopened tubes is that testing should be completed within 1 to 4 hours of collection.

Post-test:

➤ Observe venipuncture site for bleeding or hematoma formation. Apply pressure bandage.

➤ Instruct the patient to report immediately any signs of unusual bleeding or bruising.

➤ Inform the patient with decreased factor levels of the importance of taking precautions against bruising and bleeding. These precautions may include the use of a soft bristle toothbrush, use of an electric razor, avoidance of constipation, avoidance of acetylsalicylic acid and similar products, and avoidance of intramuscular injections.

➤ Evaluate test results in relation to the patient's symptoms and other tests performed. Related laboratory tests include alanine aminotransferase, alkaline phosphatase, aspartate aminotransferase, clot retraction, copper, plasminogen, protein C, prothrombin time, activated partial thromboplastin time, and vitamin K.

COLD AGGLUTININ TITER

· ·

SYNONYM/ACRONYM: Mycoplasma serology.

SPECIMEN: Serum (2 mL) collected in a red-top tube. The tube must be placed in a water bath or heat block at 37°C for 1 hour and allowed to clot before the serum is separated from the red blood cells (RBCs).

REFERENCE VALUE: (Method: Patient sera containing autoantibodies titered against type O RBCs at 2°C to 8°C. Type O cells are used because they have no antigens on the cell membrane surface. Agglutination with patient sera would not occur because of reaction between RBC blood type antigens and patient blood type antibodies.) Negative: Single titer less than 1:32 or less than a fourfold increase in titer over serial samples.

DESCRIPTION: Cold agglutinins are antibodies that cause clumping or agglutination of RBCs at cold temperatures in individuals with certain conditions or who are infected by particular organisms. Cold agglutinins are associated with *Mycoplasma pneumoniae* infection. *M. pneumoniae* has I antigen specificity to human RBC membranes. Fetal cells largely contain i antigens, but by 18 months most cells carry the I antigen. The agglutinins are usually immunoglobulin M (IgM) antibodies and cause agglutination of cells at temperatures in the range of 0°C to 10°C. The temperature of circulating blood in the extremities may be lower than core temperatures. RBCs of affected individuals may agglutinate and obstruct blood vessels in fingers, toes, and ears, or they may initiate the complement cascade. Affected cells may be lysed immediately within the capillaries and blood vessels as a result of the action of complement on the cell wall, or they may return to the circulatory system and be lysed in the spleen by macrophages.

The titer end point is the highest dilution of serum that shows a specific antigen-antibody reaction. Single titers greater than 1:64, or a fourfold increase in titer between specimens collected 5 or more days apart, are clinically significant. Patients affected with primary atypical viral pneumonia exhibit a rise in titer 8 to 10 days after the onset of illness. IgM antibodies peak in 12 to 25 days and begin to diminish 30 days after onset. ■

INDICATIONS:

- Assist in the confirmation of primary atypical pneumonia, influenza, or pulmonary embolus

- Provide additional diagnostic support for cold agglutinin disease associated with viral infections or lymphoreticular cancers

RESULT

Increased in:

- Infectious mononucleosis

- Malaria

- Multiple myeloma

- *M. pneumoniae* (primary atypical pneumonia)

- Raynaud's syndrome (severe)

- Systemic lupus erythematosus

- Trypanosomiasis

Decreased in: N/A

CRITICAL VALUES: N/A

INTERFERING FACTORS:

- Antibiotic use may interfere with or decrease antibody production.

- A high antibody titer may interfere with blood typing and crossmatching procedures.

- High titers may appear spontaneously in elderly patients and persist for many years.

• Prompt and proper specimen processing, storage, and analysis are important to achieve accurate results. Specimens should always be transported to the laboratory as quickly as possible after collection. The specimen must clot in a 37°C water bath for 1 hour before separation. Refrigeration of the sample before serum separates from the RBCs may falsely decrease the titer.

Nursing Implications and Procedure • • • • • • • • • •

Pretest:

➤ Obtain a history of the patient's complaints, including a list of known allergens.

➤ Obtain a history of the patient's immune and respiratory systems, as well as results of previously performed tests and procedures. For related tests, refer to the immune and respiratory system tables.

➤ Obtain a list of medications the patient is taking, including herbs, nutritional supplements, and nutraceuticals. The requesting health care practitioner and laboratory should be advised if the patient regularly uses these products so that their effects can be taken into consideration when reviewing results.

➤ There are no food, fluid, or medication restrictions (except antibiotics) unless by medical direction.

➤ Review the procedure with the patient. Inform the patient that multiple specimens may be required.

➤ Inform the patient that specimen collection takes approximately 5 to 10 minutes.

Intratest:

➤ Direct the patient to breathe normally and to avoid unnecessary movement.

➤ Observe standard precautions and follow the general guidelines in Appendix A. Perform a venipuncture, and collect the specimen in a 5-mL red-top tube.

➤ Inform the laboratory if the patient is receiving antibiotics.

➤ Label the specimen, and promptly transport it to the laboratory.

Post-test:

➤ Observe venipuncture site for bleeding or hematoma formation. Apply pressure bandage.

➤ Instruct the patient to resume usual medication as directed by the health care practitioner.

➤ Emphasize the need for the patient to return in 7 to 14 days for a convalescent blood sample.

➤ Evaluate test results in relation to the patient's symptoms and other tests performed. Related laboratory tests include arterial/alveolar oxygen ratio, blood gases, and complete blood count.

COLLAGEN CROSSLINKED N-TELOPEPTIDE

• •

Synonym/Acronym: NT_x.

SPECIMEN: Urine (2 mL) from a random specimen collected in a clean plastic container.

REFERENCE VALUE: (Method: Immunoassay)

Male	0–85 nmol bone collagen equivalents/mmol creatinine
Female (premenopausal)	14–76 nmol bone collagen equivalents/mmol creatinine

DESCRIPTION: Osteoporosis is the most common bone disease in the West. It is often called the "silent disease" because bone loss occurs without symptoms. The formation and maintenance of bone mass is dependent on a combination of factors that include genetics, nutrition, exercise, and hormone function. Normally the rate of bone formation is equal to the rate of bone resorption. After midlife, the rate of bone loss begins to increase. Osteoporosis is more commonly identified in women than in men. Other risk factors include thin, small-framed body structure; family history of osteoporosis; diet low in calcium; Caucasian or Asian race; excessive use of alcohol; cigarette smoking; sedentary lifestyle; long-term use of corticosteroids, thyroid replacement medications, or antiepileptics; history of bulimia, anorexia nervosa, chronic liver disease, or malabsorption disorders; and postmenopausal state. Osteoporosis is a major consequence of menopause in women owing to the decline of estrogen production. Osteoporosis is rare in premenopausal women. Estrogen replacement therapy (after menopause) is one strategy that has been commonly employed to prevent osteoporosis, although its exact protective mechanism is unknown. Results of some recently published studies indicate that there may be significant adverse side effects to estrogen replacement therapy; more research is needed to understand the long-term effects (positive and negative) of this therapy. Other treatments include raloxifene (selectively modulates estrogen receptors), calcitonin (interacts directly with osteoclasts), and bisphosphates (inhibit osteoclast-mediated bone resorption).

A noninvasive test to detect the presence of collagen crosslinked N-telopeptide (NT_x) is used to follow the progress of patients who have begun treatment for osteoporosis. NT_x is formed when collagenase acts on bone. Small NT_x fragments are excreted in the urine after bone resorption. A desirable response, 2 to 3 months after therapy is initiated, is a 30 percent reduction in NT_x and a reduction of 50 percent below baseline by 12 months. ∎

INDICATIONS:

• Assist in the evaluation of osteoporosis

• Assist in the management and treatment of osteoporosis

• Monitor effects of estrogen replacement therapy

RESULT

Increased in:

- Hyperparathyroidism
- Osteomalacia
- Osteoporosis
- Paget's disease

Decreased in:

- Effective therapy for osteoporosis

CRITICAL VALUES: N/A

INTERFERING FACTORS:

- NT_x levels are affected by urinary excretion, and values may be influenced by the presence of renal impairment or disease.

Nursing Implications and Procedure • • • • • • • • • • • •

Pretest:

➤ Obtain a history of the patient's complaints, including a list of known allergens.

➤ Obtain a history of the patient's musculoskeletal and reproductive systems, as well as results of previously performed tests and procedures. For related tests, refer to the musculoskeletal and reproductive system tables.

➤ Obtain a list of medications the patient is taking, including herbs, nutritional supplements, and nutraceuticals. The requesting health care practitioner and laboratory should be advised if the patient is regularly using these products so that their effects can be taken into consideration when reviewing results.

➤ There are no food, fluid, or medication restrictions unless by medical direction.

➤ Review the procedure with the patient.

➤ Inform the patient that specimen collection takes approximately 5 to 10 minutes.

Intratest:

➤ Observe standard precautions and follow the general guidelines in Appendix A.

➤ Instruct the patient to collect a second-void morning specimen as follows: (1) void and then drink a glass of water; (2) wait 30 minutes, and then try to void again.

➤ Label the specimen, and promptly transport it to the laboratory.

Post-test:

➤ Increased NT_x levels may be associated with osteoporosis. Nutritional therapy may be indicated for patients identified as being at high risk for developing osteoporosis. Educate the patient about the National Osteoporosis Foundation's guidelines regarding a regular regimen of weight-bearing exercises, limited alcohol intake, avoidance of tobacco products, and adequate dietary intake of vitamin D (400 to 800 IU/d) and calcium (120 mg/d). Dietary calcium can be obtained in animal or plant sources. Milk and milk products, sardines, clams, oysters, salmon, rhubarb, spinach, beet greens, broccoli, kale, tofu, legumes, and fortified orange juice are high in calcium. Milk and milk products also contain vitamin D and lactose to assist in absorption. Cooked vegetables yield more absorbable calcium than raw vegetables. Patients should also be informed of the substances that can inhibit calcium absorption by irreversibly binding to some of the calcium and making it unavailable for absorption, such as oxalates, which naturally occur in some vegetables; phytic acid, found in some cereals; and excessive intake of insoluble dietary fiber. Excessive protein intake also can affect calcium absorption negatively, especially if it is combined with foods high in phosphorus. Vitamin D is synthesized by the skin and is available in fortified dairy foods and cod liver oil.

➤ Evaluate test results in relation to the patient's symptoms and other

tests performed. Related laboratory tests include alkaline phosphatase, serum and urine calcium, phosphorus, calcitonin, parathyroid hormone, phosphorus, and vitamin D.

COLONOSCOPY

· ·

SYNONYMS/ACRONYM: Full colonoscopy, lower endoscopy, lower panendoscopy.

AREA OF APPLICATION: Colon.

CONTRAST: Air.

DESCRIPTION: Colonoscopy allows inspection of the mucosa of the entire colon, ileocecal valve, and terminal ileum using a flexible fiberoptic colonoscope inserted through the anus and advanced to the terminal ileum. The colonoscope is a multichannel instrument that allows viewing of the gastrointestinal (GI) tract lining, insufflation of air, aspiration of fluid, obtaining of tissue biopsy samples, and passage of a laser beam for obliteration of tissue and control of bleeding. Mucosal surfaces of the lower GI tract are examined for ulcerations, polyps, chronic diarrhea, hemorrhagic sites, neoplasms, and strictures. During the procedure, tissue samples may be obtained for cytology, and some therapeutic procedures may be performed, such as excision of small tumors or polyps, coagulation of bleeding sites, and removal of foreign bodies. ∎

INDICATIONS:

• Determine cause of lower GI disorders, especially when barium enema and proctosigmoidoscopy are inconclusive

• Determine source of rectal bleeding and perform hemostasis by coagulation

• Remove foreign bodies and sclerosing strictures by laser

• Confirm diagnosis of colon cancer and inflammatory bowel disease

• Follow up on previously diagnosed and treated colon cancer

• Detect Hirschsprung's disease and determine the areas affected by the disease

• Reduce volvulus and intussusception in children

• Remove colon polyps

• Investigate iron-deficiency anemia of unknown origin

• Evaluate postsurgical status of colon resection

- Evaluate stools that show a positive occult blood test, lower-GI bleeding, or change in bowel habits

- Assess GI function in a patient with a personal or family history of colon cancer, polyps, or ulcerative colitis

RESULT

Normal Findings:

- Normal intestinal mucosa with no abnormalities of structure, function, or mucosal surface in the colon or terminal ileum

Abnormal Findings:

- Bleeding sites

- Benign lesions

- Bowel distention

- Bowel infection or inflammation

- Colon cancer

- Crohn's disease

- Colitis

- Diverticula

- Foreign bodies

- Hemorrhoids

- Polyps

- Proctitis

- Tumors

- Vascular abnormalities

CRITICAL VALUES: N/A

INTERFERING FACTORS:

This procedure is contraindicated for:

- Patients with bleeding disorders or cardiac conditions

- Patients with bowel perforation, acute peritonitis, acute colitis, ischemic bowel necrosis, toxic colitis, recent bowel surgery, advanced pregnancy, severe cardiac or pulmonary disease, recent myocardial infarction, known or suspected pulmonary embolus, and large abdominal aortic or iliac aneurysm

- Patients who have had a colon anastomosis within the past 14 to 21 days, because an anastomosis may break down with gas insufflation

Factors that may impair clear imaging:

- Inability of the patient to cooperate or remain still during the procedure because of age, significant pain, or mental status

- Patients who are very obese, who may exceed the weight limit for the equipment

- Incorrect positioning of the patient, which may produce poor visualization of the area to be examined

- Strictures or other abnormalities preventing passage of the scope

- Barium swallow or upper GI series within the preceding 48 hours, which can hinder adequate visualization

- Severe lower GI bleeding or the presence of feces, barium, blood, or blood clots, which can interfere with visualization

Other considerations:

- Failure to follow dietary restrictions before the procedure may cause the procedure to be canceled or repeated.

- Bowel preparations that include laxatives or enemas should be avoided in pregnant patients or patients with inflammatory bowel disease, unless specifically directed by a physician.

Nursing Implications and Procedure • • • • • • • • • • • •

Pretest: ■

➤ Explain to the patient the purpose of the study and how the procedure is performed.

➤ *Obtain a written, informed consent for the procedure from the patient.*

➤ Obtain a history of GI disorders, noting any information relating to lower bowel, anal, rectal, or coagulation disorders.

➤ Note use of drugs that affect bleeding, such as aspirin and other salicylates.

➤ Note intake of oral iron preparations 1 week before the procedure because these cause black, sticky feces that are difficult to remove with bowel preparation.

➤ Obtain the results of other tests (particularly hematologic or coagulation tests), treatments, surgeries, medication usage, and procedures done to diagnose or treat disorders of the intestinal system. For related tests, refer to the gastrointestinal system table.

➤ Determine date of last menstrual period and possibility of pregnancy in perimenopausal women.

➤ Explain that the procedure usually takes 30 to 60 minutes to complete and is generally performed in an endoscopy suite by a physician and support staff.

➤ Restrict the diet to clear liquids for 48 hours before beginning oral bowel preparation.

➤ Ensure that ordered laxatives have been administered late in the afternoon of the day before the procedure.

➤ Inform the patient that it is important that the bowel be cleaned thoroughly so that the physician can visualize the colon and that the patient will have to receive enemas before the test.

➤ Note recent administration of barium because it can obscure the area to be examined.

➤ Resuscitation equipment should be readily available.

Intratest: ■

➤ Two hours before the procedure, administer a warm tap water or saline enema until the returns are clear or as ordered.

➤ Have the patient put on a hospital gown and void.

➤ An intravenous (IV) line may be started to allow infusion of a sedative or IV fluids.

➤ Obtain baseline vital signs.

➤ Administer ordered sedation.

➤ The patient is placed on an examination table in the left lateral decubitus position and draped with the buttocks exposed.

➤ The physician performs a visual inspection of the perianal area and a digital rectal examination.

➤ The patient is requested to bear down as if having a bowel movement as the fiberoptic tube is inserted through the rectum.

➤ The scope is advanced through the sigmoid. The patient's position is changed to supine to facilitate passage into the transverse colon. Air is insufflated through the tube during passage to aid in visualization.

➤ The patient is instructed to take deep breaths to aid in movement of the scope downward through the ascending colon to the cecum and into the terminal portion of the ileum.

➤ Air is insufflated to distend the GI tract, as needed. Biopsies, cultures, or any endoscopic surgery is performed.

➤ Foreign bodies or polyps are removed and placed in appropriate specimen containers, labeled properly, and sent to the laboratory.

➤ Photographs are obtained for future reference.

➤ At the end of the procedure, excess air and secretions are aspirated through the scope, and the colonoscope is removed.

➤ Gloves and gowns are worn by the examiner throughout the procedure.

➤ Monitor the patient for signs of respiratory depression. Resuscitation equipment should be available.

Post-test:

➤ Monitor for any rectal bleeding. Instruct the patient to expect slight rectal bleeding for 2 days after removal of polyps or biopsy specimens, but that an increasing amount of bleeding or sustained bleeding should be reported to the physician immediately.

➤ Observe the patient until the effects of the sedation have worn off.

➤ Observe the patient for indications of chest pain, abdominal pain or tenderness, or breathing problems. If these symptoms are present or increase in frequency or severity, the change should be reported to a physician immediately.

➤ Inform the patient that belching, bloating, or flatulence is the result of air insufflation.

➤ Emphasize that any severe pain, fever, difficulty breathing, or GI bleeding must be reported to the physician immediately.

➤ Resume normal activity, medication, and diet 2 hours after the procedure or as tolerated, unless otherwise indicated.

➤ Encourage the patient to drink several glasses of water to help replace fluids lost during the preparation for the test.

➤ A physician specializing in this branch of medicine sends a written report to the ordering provider, who discusses the results with the patient.

➤ Inform the patient that an abnormal examination may indicate the need for further studies.

➤ Evaluate test results in relation to the patient's symptoms and other tests performed. Related diagnostic tests include barium enema and proctosigmoidoscopy.

COLPOSCOPY

• •

SYNONYMS/ACRONYM: Endometrial biopsy, cervical biopsy.

AREA OF APPLICATION: Vagina and cervix.

CONTRAST: None.

DESCRIPTION: In this procedure, the vagina and cervix are viewed using a colposcope, a special binocular microscope and light system that magnifies the mucosal surfaces. Colposcopy is usually performed after suspicious Papanicolaou (Pap) test results or when suspected lesions cannot be visualized fully by the naked eye. The procedure is useful for identifying areas of cellular dysplasia and diagnosing cervical cancer because it provides the best view of the suspicious lesion, ensuring that the most representative area of the lesion is obtained for cytologic analysis to confirm malignant changes. Colposcopy is also valuable for assessing women with a history of exposure to diethylstilbestrol (DES) in utero. The goal is to identify precursor changes in cervical tissue before the changes advance from benign or atypical cells to cervical cancer. Photographs (cervicography) can also be taken of the cervix. ■

INDICATIONS:

- Evaluate the cervix after abnormal Pap smear

- Evaluate vaginal lesions

- Monitor women whose mothers took DES during pregnancy

- Localize the area from which cervical biopsy samples should be obtained because such areas may not be visible to the naked eye

- Monitor conservatively treated cervical intraepithelial neoplasia

RESULT

Normal Findings:

- Normal appearance of the vagina and cervix

- No abnormal cells or tissues

Abnormal Findings:

- Atrophic changes

- Cervical erosion

- Cervical intraepithelial neoplasia

- Papilloma, including condyloma

- Invasive carcinoma

- Infection

- Inflammation

- Leukoplakia

CRITICAL VALUES: N/A

INTERFERING FACTORS:

This procedure is contraindicated for:

- Patients who are pregnant or suspected of being pregnant, unless the potential benefits of the procedure far outweigh the risks to the fetus and mother

- Patients with cardiac conditions

- Patients with bleeding disorders, especially if cervical biopsy specimens are to be obtained

- Women who are currently menstruating

Factors that may impair clear imaging:

- Inability of the patient to cooperate or remain still during the procedure because of age, significant pain, or mental status

- Inadequate cleansing of the cervix of secretions and medications

- Scarring of the cervix

Nursing Implications and Procedure • • • • • • • • • •

Pretest: ■

➤ Inform the patient that the purpose of the procedure is to assess the vagina and cervix, and that it is generally performed in a physician's office by a physician or nurse practitioner.

➤ Assess whether the patient is allergic to latex.

➤ Assess date of last menstrual period to ascertain possible pregnancy in perimenopausal women. The procedure is contraindicated during menstruation; it is best performed 1 week after menses ends.

➤ Obtain a history of the patient's reproductive system and previously performed laboratory tests (especially Pap test and blood clotting times), surgeries, therapies, and procedures. For related tests, refer to the reproductive system table.

➤ Obtain a history of the patient's complaints, including a list of known allergens.

➤ Obtain a list of the medications the patient is taking, including herbs, nutritional supplements, and nutraceuticals. The requesting health care practitioner and laboratory should be advised if the patient regularly uses these products so that their effects can be taken into consideration when reviewing results.

➤ Do not restrict food or fluids before the test.

➤ Explain to the patient that if a biopsy is performed, she may feel menstrual-like cramping during the procedure and experience a minimal amount of bleeding.

➤ Gloves are worn throughout the procedure.

➤ *Obtain a written, informed consent for the procedure from the patient.*

➤ Inform the patient that the procedure lasts approximately 10 to 15 minutes.

Intratest: ■

➤ Ask the patient to remove clothing from the waist down.

➤ Give the patient a gown and robe to wear; have the patient void.

➤ Place the patient in the lithotomy position on the examining table and drape. Cleanse the external genitalia with an antiseptic solution.

➤ If a Pap smear is performed, the vaginal speculum is inserted, using water as a lubricant.

➤ The cervix is swabbed with 3% acetic acid to remove mucus or any cream medication and to improve the contrast between tissue types. The scope is positioned at the speculum and is focused on the cervix. The area is examined carefully, using light and magnification. Photographs can be taken for future reference.

➤ Tissues that appear abnormal or atypical undergo biopsy using a forceps inserted through the speculum. Bleeding, which is common after cervical biopsy, may be controlled by cautery, suturing, or application of silver nitrate or ferric subsulfate (Monsel's solution) to the site.

➤ The vagina is rinsed with sterile saline or water to remove the acetic acid and prevent burning after the procedure. If bleeding persists, a tampon may be inserted after removal of the speculum.

➤ Biopsy samples are placed in appropriate containers with special preservative solution, labeled properly, and promptly taken to the laboratory.

Post-test: ■

➤ Inform the patient to remove the vaginal tampon, if inserted, within 8 to 24 hours; after that time, the patient should wear pads if there is bleeding or drainage.

➤ Inform the patient that if a biopsy was performed, a discharge may persist for a few days to a few weeks.

➤ Advise the patient to avoid strenuous exercise 8 to 24 hours after the procedure, and to avoid douching and intercourse for about 2 weeks or as directed by the practitioner.

➤ Emphasize that persistent vaginal bleeding or abnormal vaginal discharge, abdominal pain, and fever must be reported to the physician immediately.

➤ Inform the patient that further testing may be necessary to evaluate the success of the therapy or to determine the need for a change in therapy.

➤ Evaluate for signs of infection, such as pain, fever, increased pulse rate, chills, flushing, abdominal pain, tachycardia, or muscle aches.

➤ Determine if the patient or family members have any further questions or concerns.

➤ A physician specializing in this branch of medicine sends a written report to the ordering provider, who discusses the results with the patient.

➤ Evaluate test results in relation to the patient's symptoms and any related tests performed.

COMPLEMENT C3 AND COMPLEMENT C4

· ·

SYNONYMS/ACRONYM: C3 and C4.

SPECIMEN: Serum (1 mL) collected in a red-top tube.

REFERENCE VALUE: (Method: Nephelometry)

C3

Age	Conventional Units	SI Units (Conversion Factor ×10)
Newborn	57–116 mg/dL	570–1160 mg/L
6 mo–adult	74–166 mg/dL	740–1660 mg/L
Adult	83–177 mg/dL	830–1770 mg/L

C4

Age	Conventional Units	SI Units (Conversion Factor ×10)
Newborn	10–31 mg/dL	100–310 mg/L
6 mo–6 y	15–52 mg/dL	150–520 mg/L
7–12 y	19–40 mg/dL	190–400 mg/L
13–15 y	19–57 mg/dL	190–570 mg/L
16–18 y	19–42 mg/dL	190–420 mg/L
Adult	12–36 mg/dL	120–360 mg/L

DESCRIPTION: Complement proteins act as enzymes that aid in the immunologic and inflammatory response. The complement system is an important mechanism for the destruction and removal of foreign materials. Serum complement levels are used to detect autoimmune diseases. C3 and C4 are the most frequently assayed complement proteins, along with total complement.

Circulating C3 is synthesized in the liver and comprises 70 percent of the complement system, but cells in other tissues can also produce C3. C3 is an essential activating protein in the classic and alternate complement cascades. It is decreased in patients with immunologic diseases, in whom it is consumed at an increased rate. C4 is produced primarily in the liver but can also be produced by monocytes, fibroblasts, and macrophages. C4 participates in the classic complement pathway. ■

INDICATIONS:

• Detect genetic deficiencies

• Evaluate immunologic diseases

RESULT

Normal C4 and decreased C3	Acute glomerulonephritis, membranous glomerulonephritis, immune complex diseases, SLE, C3 deficiency
Decreased C4 and normal C3	Immune complex diseases, cryoglobulinemia, C4 deficiency, hereditary angioedema
Decreased C4 and decreased C3	Immune complex diseases

Increased in:

• C3 and C4
  Acute-phase reactions

• C3
  Amyloidosis
  Cancer
  Diabetes
  Myocardial infarction
  Pneumococcal pneumonia
  Pregnancy
  Rheumatic disease
  Thyroiditis
  Viral hepatitis

• C4
  Certain malignancies

Decreased in:

• C3 and C4
  Hereditary deficiency
  Liver disease
  SLE

• C3
  Chronic infection (bacterial, parasitic, viral)
  Post–membranoproliferative glomerulonephritis
  Post–streptococcal infection
  Rheumatic arthritis

• C4
  Angioedema (hereditary and acquired)

Autoimmune hemolytic anemia
Autoimmune thyroiditis
Cryoglobulinemia
Glomerulonephritis
Juvenile dermatomyositis
Meningitis (bacterial, viral)
Pneumonia
Streptococcal or staphylococcal sepsis

CRITICAL VALUES: N/A

INTERFERING FACTORS:

• Drugs that may increase C3 levels include cimetidine and cyclophosphamide.

• Drugs that may decrease C3 levels include danazol and phenytoin.

• Drugs that may increase C4 levels include cimetidine, cyclophosphamide, and danazol.

• Drugs that may decrease C4 levels include dextran and penicillamine.

Nursing Implications and Procedure

Pretest:

➤ Obtain a history of the patient's complaints, including a list of known allergens.

➤ Obtain a history of the patient's immune system and results of previously performed tests and procedures. For related tests, refer to the immune system table.

➤ Obtain a list of medications the patient is taking, including herbs, nutritional supplements, and nutraceuticals. The requesting health care practitioner and laboratory should be advised if the patient regularly uses these products so that their effects can be taken into consideration when reviewing results.

➤ There are no food, fluid, or medication restrictions unless by medical direction.

➤ Review the procedure with the patient.

➤ Inform the patient that specimen collection takes approximately 5 to 10 minutes.

Intratest:

➤ Direct the patient to breathe normally and to avoid unnecessary movement.

➤ Observe standard precautions and follow the general guidelines in Appendix A. Perform a venipuncture, and collect the specimen in a 5-mL red-top tube.

➤ Label the specimen, and promptly transport it to the laboratory.

Post-test:

➤ Observe venipuncture site for bleeding or hematoma formation. Apply pressure bandage.

➤ Evaluate test results in relation to the patient's symptoms and other tests performed. Related laboratory tests include anticardiolipin antibody, antinuclear antibodies, total complement, and erythrocyte sedimentation rate.

COMPLEMENT, TOTAL

SYNONYM/ACRONYM: Total hemolytic complement, CH_{50}, CH_{100}.

SPECIMEN: Serum (1 mL) collected in a red-top tube.

REFERENCE VALUE: (Method: Quantitative hemolysis)

Conventional Units	SI Units (Conversion Factor (1000)
40–100 CH$_{50}$ U/mL	40–100 CH$_{50}$ kU/L

DESCRIPTION: The complement system comprises proteins that become activated and interact in a sequential cascade. The complement system is an important part of the body's natural defense against allergic and immune reactions. It is activated by plasmin and is interrelated with the coagulation and fibrinolytic systems. Activation of the complement system results in cell lysis, release of histamine, chemotaxis of white blood cells, increased vascular permeability, and contraction of smooth muscle. The activation of this system can sometimes occur with uncontrolled self-destructive effects on the body. In the serum complement assay, a patient's serum is mixed with sheep red blood cells coated with antibodies. If complement is present in sufficient quantities, 50 percent of the red blood cells are lysed. Lower amounts of lysed cells are associated with decreased complement levels. ∎

INDICATIONS:

• Evaluate complement activity in autoimmune disorders

• Assist in the diagnosis of hereditary angioedema

• Evaluate and monitor therapy for systemic lupus erythematosus

• Screen for complement deficiency

RESULT

Increased in:

• Acute-phase immune response

Decreased in:

• Autoimmune diseases

• Autoimmune hemolytic anemia

• Burns

• Cryoglobulinemia

• Hereditary deficiency

• Infections (bacterial, parasitic, viral)

• Liver disease

• Malignancy

• Membranous glomerulonephritis

• Rheumatoid arthritis

• Systemic lupus erythematosus

• Trauma

• Vasculitis

CRITICAL VALUES: N/A

INTERFERING FACTORS:

• Drugs that may increase total complement levels include cyclophosphamide and danazol.

• Specimen should not remain at room temperature longer than 1 hour.

Nursing Implications and Procedure • • • • • • • • • • •

Pretest:

➤ Obtain a history of the patient's complaints, including a list of known allergens.

➤ Obtain a history of the patient's immune system and results of previously performed tests and procedures. For related tests, refer to the immune system table.

➤ Obtain a list of medications the patient is taking, including herbs, nutritional supplements, and nutraceuticals. The requesting health care practitioner and laboratory should be advised if the patient regularly uses these products so that their effects can be taken into consideration when reviewing results.

➤ There are no food, fluid, or medication restrictions unless by medical direction.

➤ Review the procedure with the patient.

➤ Inform the patient that specimen collection takes approximately 5 to 10 minutes.

Intratest: ■

➤ Direct the patient to breathe normally and to avoid unnecessary movement.

➤ Observe standard precautions and follow the general guidelines in Appendix A. Perform a venipuncture, and collect the specimen in a 5-mL red-top tube.

➤ Label the specimen, and promptly transport it to the laboratory.

Post-test: ■

➤ Observe venipuncture site for bleeding or hematoma formation. Apply pressure bandage.

➤ Evaluate test results in relation to the patient's symptoms and other tests performed. Related laboratory tests include antinuclear antibodies, C3, C4, and erythrocyte sedimentation rate.

COMPLETE BLOOD COUNT

· ·

SYNONYM/ACRONYM: CBC.

SPECIMEN: Whole blood from one full lavender-top (ethylenediaminetetraacetic acid [EDTA]) tube or Microtainer. Whole blood from a green-top (lithium or sodium heparin) tube may be submitted, but the following automated values may not be reported: white blood cell (WBC) count, WBC differential, platelet count, and mean platelet volume.

REFERENCE VALUE: (Method: Automated, computerized multichannel analyzers that sort and size cells on the basis of changes in either electrical impedance or light pulses as the cells pass in front of a laser. Many of these analyzers are capable of determining a five-part WBC differential.) This battery of tests includes hemoglobin, hematocrit, red blood cell (RBC) count, RBC morphology, RBC indices, RBC distribution width index (RDW), platelet count, platelet size, WBC count, and WBC differential. The five-part automated WBC differential identifies and enumerates neutrophils, lymphocytes, monocytes, eosinophils, and basophils.

Hemoglobin

Age	Conventional Units	SI Units (Conversion Factor ×10)
Cord blood	13.5–20.5 g/dL	135–205 mmol/L
2 wk	13.4–19.8 g/dL	134–198 mmol/L
1 mo	10.7–17.1 g/dL	107–171 mmol/L
6 mo	11.1–14.4 g/dL	111–144 mmol/L
1 y	11.3–14.1 g/dL	113–141 mmol/L
9–14 y	12.0–14.4 g/dL	120–144 mmol/L
Adult		
Male	13.2–17.3 g/dL	132–173 mmol/L
Female	11.7–15.5 g/dL	117–155 mmol/L
Older adult (65–74 y)		
Male	12.6–17.4 g/dL	126–174 mmol/L
Female	11.7–16.1 g/dL	117–161 mmol/L

Hematocrit

Age	Conventional Units (%)	SI Units (Conversion Factor ×0.01)*
Cord blood	47–57	0.47–0.57
1 d	51–65	0.51–0.65
2 wk	47–57	0.47–0.57
1 mo	38–52	0.38–0.52
6 mo	35–41	0.35–0.41
1 y	37–41	0.37–0.41
10 y	36–42	0.36–0.42
Adult		
Male	43–49	0.43–0.49
Female	38–44	0.38–0.44

*Volume fraction.

White Blood Cell Count and Differential

Age	SI Units (Conversion Factor ×10⁹ cells/L) WBC × 10³/mm³ or cells/µL (Absolute) and %	Neutrophils Total (Absolute) and %	Bands (Absolute) and %	Segments (Absolute) and %	Lymphocytes (Absolute) and %	Monocytes (Absolute) and %	Eosinophils (Absolute) and %	Basophils (Absolute) and %
Birth	0.0–30.0	(6.0–26.0) 61%	(1.65) 9.1%	(9.4) 52%	(2.0–11) 31%	(0.4–3.1) 5.8%	(0.02–0.85) 2.2%	(0–0.64) 0.6%
1 d	9.4–34.0	(5.0–21.0) 61%	(1.75) 9.2%	(9.8) 52%	(2.0–11.5) 31%	(0.2–3.1) 5.8%	(0.02–0.95) 2.0%	(0–0.30) 0.5%
2 wk	5.0–20.0	(1.0–9.5) 40%	(0.63) 5.5%	(3.9) 34%	(2.0–17.0) 48%	(0.2–2.4) 8.8%	(0.07–1.0) 3.1%	(0–0.23) 0.4%
1 mo	5.0–19.5	(1.0–9.0) 35%	(0.49) 4.5%	(3.3) 30%	(2.5–16.5) 56%	(0.15–2.0) 6.5%	(0.07–0.90) 2.8%	(0–0.20) 0.5%
6 mo	6.0–17.5	(1.0–8.5) 32%	(0.45) 3.8%	(3.3) 28%	(4.0–13.5) 61%	(0.1– 1.3) 4.8%	(0.07–0.75) 2.5%	(0–0.20) 0.4%
1 y	6.0–17.5	(1.5–8.5) 31%	(0.35) 3.1%	(3.2) 28%	(4.0–10.5) 61%	(0.05–1.1) 4.8%	(0.05–0.70) 2.6%	(0–0.20) 0.4%
10 y	4.5–13.5	(1.8–8.0) 54%	(1.8–7.0) 3.0%	(1.8–7.0) 51%	(1.5–6.5) 38%	(0–0.8) 4.3%	(0–0.60) 2.4%	(0–0.20) 0.5%
Adult	4.5–11.0	(1.8–7.7) 59%	(0–0.7) 3.0%	(1.8–7.0) 56%	(1.0–4.8) 34%	(0–0.8) 4.0%	(0–0.45) 2.7%	(0–0.20) 0.5%

Red Blood Cell Count

Age	Conventional Units	SI Units
Cord blood	4.14–4.69×10^6 cells/mm^3	4.14–4.69×10^{12} cells /L
1 d	5.33–5.47×10^6 cells/mm^3	5.33–5.47×10^{12} cells /L
2 wk	4.32–4.98×10^6 cells/mm^3	4.32–4.98×10^{12} cells /L
1 mo	3.75–4.95×10^6 cells/mm^3	3.75–4.95×10^{12} cells /L
6 mo	3.71–4.25×10^6 cells/mm^3	3.71–4.25×10^{12} cells /L
1 y	4.40–4.48×10^6 cells/mm^3	4.40–4.48×10^{12} cells /L
10 y	4.75–4.85×10^6 cells/mm^3	4.75–4.85×10^{12} cells /L
Adult		
Male	4.71–5.14×10^6 cells/mm^3	4.71–5.14×10^{12} cells /L
Female	4.20–4.87×10^6 cells/mm^3	4.20–4.87×10^{12} cells /L

Red Blood Cell Indices

Age	MCV (fl)	MCH (pg/cell)	MCHC (g/dL)	RDW
Cord blood	107–119	35–39	32–34	14.9–18.7
1 d	104–116	35–39	32–34	14.9–18.7
2 wk	95–117	29–35	28–32	14.9–18.7
1 mo	93–115	29–35	28–34	14.9–18.7
6 mo	82–100	24–30	28–32	14.9–18.7
1 y	81–95	25–29	29–31	11.6–14.8
10 y	75–87	25–31	33–35	11.6–14.8
Adult				
Male	85–95	28–32	33–35	11.6–14.8
Female	85–95	28–32	33–35	11.6–14.8

MCV = mean corpuscular volume; MCH = mean corpuscular hemoglobin; MCHC = mean corpuscular hemoglobin concentration; RDW = RBC distribution width index.

Red Blood Cell Morphology

Morphology	Within Normal Limits	1+	2+	3+	4+
		Size			
Anisocytosis	0–5+	5–10	10–20	20–50	Greater than 50
Macrocytes	0–5+	5–10	10–20	20–50	Greater than 50
Microcytes	0–5+	5–10	10–20	20–50	Greater than 50

(*Continued on the following page*)

Morphology	Within Normal Limits	1+	2+	3+	4+
Shape					
Poikilocytes	0–2+	3–10	10–20	20–50	Greater than 50
Burr cells	0–2+	3–10	10–20	20–50	Greater than 50
Acanthocytes	Less than 1+	2–5	5–10	10–20	Greater than 20
Schistocytes	Less than 1+	2–5	5–10	10–20	Greater than 20
Dacryocytes (teardrop cells)	0–2+	2–5	5–10	10–20	Greater than 20
Codocytes (target cells)	0–2+	2–10	10–20	20–50	Greater than 50
Spherocytes	0–2+	2–10	10–20	20–50	Greater than 50
Ovalocytes	0–2+	2–10	10–20	20–50	Greater than 50
Stomatocytes	0–2+	2–10	10–20	20–50	Greater than 50
Drepanocytes (sickle cells)	Absent	Reported as present or absent			
Helmet cells	Absent	Reported as present or absent			
Agglutination	Absent	Reported as present or absent			
Rouleaux	Absent	Reported as present or absent			
Hemoglobin Content					
Hypochromia	0–2+	3–10	10–50	50–75	Greater than 75
Polychromasia					
Adult	Less than 1+	2–5	5–10	10–20	Greater than 20
Newborn	1–6+	7–15	15–20	20–50	Greater than 50

Red Blood Cell Inclusions

Inclusions	Within Normal Limits	1+	2+	3+	4+
Cabot rings	Absent	Reported as present or absent			
Basophilic stippling	0–1+	1–5	5–10	10–20	Greater than 20
Howell-Jolly bodies	Absent	1–2	3–5	5–10	Greater than 10

(Continued on the following page)

Inclusions	Within Normal Limits	1+	2+	3+	4+
Heinz bodies	Absent	Reported as present or absent			
Hemoglobin C crystals	Absent	Reported as present or absent			
Pappenheimer bodies	Absent	Reported as present or absent			
Intracellular parasites (e.g., *Plasmodium*, *Babesia*, trypanosomes)	Absent	Reported as present or absent			

Platelet Count

Age	Conventional Units	SI Units (Conversion Factor $\times 10^6$)	MPV (fl)
1–5 y	217–497 $\times 10^3/\mu L/ mm^3$	217–497 $\times 10^9/L$	7.2–10.0
Adult	150–450 $\times 10^3/\mu L/ mm^3$	181–521 $\times 10^9/L$	7.0–10.2

DESCRIPTION: A complete blood count (CBC) is a group of tests used for basic screening purposes. It is probably the most widely ordered laboratory test. Results provide the enumeration of the cellular elements of the blood, measurement of RBC indices, and determination of cell morphology by automation and evaluation of stained smears. The results can provide valuable diagnostic information regarding the overall health of the patient and the patient's response to disease and treatment. ■

INDICATIONS:

• Detect hematologic disorder, neoplasm, leukemia, or immunologic abnormality

• Determine the presence of hereditary hematologic abnormality

• Evaluate known or suspected anemia and related treatment

• Monitor the effects of physical or emotional stress

• Monitor blood loss and response to blood replacement

• Monitor fluid imbalances or treatment for fluid imbalances

• Monitor hematologic status during pregnancy

• Monitor progression of nonhematologic disorders, such as chronic obstructive pulmonary disease, malabsorption syndromes, cancer, and renal disease

• Monitor response to chemotherapy and evaluate undesired reactions to drugs that may cause blood dyscrasias

• Provide screening as part of a general physical examination, especially on admission to a health care facility or before surgery

RESULT: See monographs titled "Hemoglobin," "Hematocrit," "Red Blood Cell Indices," "Red Blood Cell Morphology and Inclusions," "Red Blood Cell Count," "Platelet Count," and "White Blood Cell Count and Differential."

Increased in: See above-listed monographs.

Decreased in: See above-listed monographs.

CRITICAL VALUES

Hemoglobin:

* Less than 6 g/dL

* Greater than 18 g/dL

Hematocrit:

* Less than 18 percent

* Greater than 54 percent

WBC count (on admission):

* Less than 2500/mm^3

* Greater than 30,000/mm^3

Platelet:

* Less than 20,000/mm^3

* Greater than 1,000,000/mm^3

The presence of abnormal cells, other morphologic characteristics, or cellular inclusions may signify a potentially life-threatening or serious health condition and should be investigated. Examples are the presence of sickle cells, moderate numbers of spherocytes, marked schisto-cytosis, oval macrocytes, basophilic stippling, eosinophil count greater than 10 percent, monocytosis greater than 15 percent, nucleated RBCs (if patient is not an infant), malarial organisms, hypersegmented neutrophils, agranular neutrophils, blasts or other immature cells, Auer rods, Döhle bodies, marked toxic granulation, or plasma cells.

INTERFERING FACTORS:

* Failure to fill the tube sufficiently (less than three-fourths full) may yield inadequate sample volume for automated analyzers and may be a reason for specimen rejection.

* Hemolyzed or clotted specimens should be rejected for analysis.

* Elevated serum glucose or sodium levels may produce elevated mean corpuscular volume values because of swelling of erythrocytes.

* Recent transfusion history should be considered when evaluating the CBC.

Nursing Implications and Procedure • • • • • • • • • • •

Pretest:

➤ Obtain a history of the patient's complaints, including a list of known allergens.

➤ Obtain a history of the patient's gastrointestinal, hematopoietic, immune, and respiratory systems, as well as results of previously performed tests and procedures. For related tests, refer to the gastrointestinal, hematopoietic, immune, and respiratory system tables.

➤ Obtain a list of medications the patient is taking, including herbs, nutritional supplements, and nutraceuticals. The requesting health care practitioner and laboratory should be advised if the patient regularly uses these products so that their effects can be taken into consideration when reviewing results.

➤ There are no food, fluid, or medication restrictions unless by medical direction.

➤ Review the procedure with the patient.

➤ Inform the patient that specimen collection takes approximately 5 to 10 minutes.

Intratest:

➤ Direct the patient to breathe normally and to avoid unnecessary movement.

➤ Observe standard precautions and follow the general guidelines in Appendix A. Perform a venipuncture, and collect the specimen in a 5-mL lavender-top (EDTA) tube. An EDTA Microtainer sample may be obtained from infants, children, and adults for whom venipuncture may not be feasible. The specimen should be analyzed within 6 hours when stored at room temperature or within 24 hours if stored at refrigerated temperature. If it is anticipated the specimen will not be analyzed within 4 to 6 hours, two blood smears should be made immediately after the venipuncture and submitted with the blood sample. Smears made from specimens older than 6 hours will contain an unacceptable number of misleading artifactual abnormalities of the RBCs, such as echinocytes and spherocytes as well as necrobiotic WBCs.

➤ Label the specimen, and promptly transport it to the laboratory.

Post-test: ■

➤ Observe venipuncture site for bleeding or hematoma formation. Apply pressure bandage.

➤ Evaluate test results in relation to the patient's symptoms and other tests performed. Related laboratory tests include erythropoietin, ferritin, iron/total iron-binding capacity, peripheral blood smear, and reticulocyte count.

COMPUTED TOMOGRAPHY, ABDOMEN

● ●

SYNONYMS/ACRONYMS: Computed axial tomography (CAT), computed transaxial tomography (CTT), abdominal CT.

AREA OF APPLICATION: Abdomen.

CONTRAST: Can be done with or without iodinated contrast medium.

DESCRIPTION: Abdominal computed tomography (CT) is a noninvasive procedure used to enhance certain anatomic views of the abdominal structures, but it becomes invasive when a contrast medium is used. The patient lies on a table and is moved in and out of a doughnut-like device called a *gantry,* which houses the x-ray tube and associated electronics. The scanner uses multiple x-ray beams and a series of detectors that rotate around the patient to produce cross-sectional views in a three-dimensional fashion by detecting and recording differences in tissue density after having an x-ray beam passed through bone and tissue. These density measurements are sent to a computer that produces a digital image of the anatomy, enabling a physician to look at slices or thin sections of certain anatomic views of the liver, biliary tract, pancreas, kidneys, spleen, intestines, and vascular system. Differentiations can be made among solid, cystic, inflammatory, or vascular lesions, and suspected hematomas and aneurysms can be identified. Iodinated contrast medium is given intravenously for blood vessel and vascular evaluation or orally for bowel and adjacent structure evaluation. Images can be recorded on photographic or x-ray film or stored in digital format as digitized computer data. Cine scanning is used to produce a series of moving images of the area scanned. The CT scan can be used to guide biopsy needles into areas of abdominal tumors to obtain tissue for laboratory analysis and placement of catheters for drainage of intra-abdominal abscesses. Tumors, before and after therapy, may be monitored with CT scanning. ■

INDICATIONS:

• Assist in differentiating between benign and malignant tumors

• Evaluation of retroperitoneal lymph nodes

• Detect tumor extension of masses and metastasis into the abdominal area

• Detect aortic aneurysms

• Differentiate aortic aneurysms from tumors near the aorta

• Differentiate between infectious and inflammatory processes

• Evaluate cysts, masses, abscesses, renal calculi, gastrointestinal (GI) bleeding and obstruction, and trauma

• Monitor and evaluate the effectiveness of medical, radiation, or surgical therapies

RESULT

Normal Findings:

• Normal size, position, and shape of abdominal organs and vascular system

Abnormal Findings:

• Adrenal tumor or hyperplasia

• Abdominal aortic aneurysm

• Abdominal abscess

• Dilation of the common hepatic duct, common bile duct, or gallbladder

• Hematomas, diverticulitis, gallstones

• Hemoperitoneum

• Hepatic cysts or abscesses

• Pancreatic pseudocyst

• Primary and metastatic neoplasms

• Renal calculi, bowel perforation, and GI bleeding and obstruction

• Splenic laceration, tumor, infiltration, and trauma

CRITICAL VALUES: N/A

INTERFERING FACTORS:

This procedure is contraindicated for:

• Patients with allergies to shellfish or iodinated dye. The contrast medium used may cause a life-threatening allergic reaction. Patients with a known hypersensitivity to the medium may benefit from premedication with corticosteroids or the use of nonionic contrast medium.

• Patients who are claustrophobic.

• Patients who are pregnant or suspected of being pregnant, unless the potential benefits of the procedure far outweigh the risks to the fetus and mother.

• Elderly and other patients who are

chronically dehydrated before the test, because of their risk of contrast-induced renal failure.

- Patients who are in renal failure.

- Young patients (17 years old and younger), unless the benefits of the x-ray diagnosis outweigh the risks of exposure to high levels of radiation.

Factors that may impair clear imaging:

- Inability of the patient to cooperate or remain still during the procedure because of age, significant pain, or mental status

- Patients with extreme claustrophobia unless sedation is given before the study

- Improper adjustment of the radiographic equipment to accommodate obese or thin patients, which can cause overexposure or underexposure and a poor-quality study

- Patients who are very obese, who may exceed the weight limit for the equipment

- Incorrect positioning of the patient, which may produce poor visualization of the area to be examined

- Gas or feces in the GI tract resulting from inadequate cleansing or failure to restrict food intake before the study

- Retained barium from a previous radiologic procedure

- Metallic objects within the examination field (e.g., jewelry or body rings), which may inhibit organ visualization and can produce unclear images

Other considerations:

- Failure to follow dietary restrictions before the procedure may cause the procedure to be canceled or repeated.

- Consultation with a physician should occur before the procedure for radia-

tion safety concerns regarding infants of patients who are lactating.

- Risks associated with radiographic overexposure can result from frequent x-ray procedures. Personnel in the room with the patient should wear a protective lead apron, stand behind a shield, or leave the area while the examination is being done. Personnel working in the area where the examination is being done should wear badges that reveal their level of exposure to radiation.

Nursing Implications and Procedure · · · · · · · · · · ·

Pretest:

➤ Inform the patient that the procedure assesses the abdomen.

➤ Inform the patient that the procedure is performed in a radiology department by a technologist and a physician and takes approximately 30 to 60 minutes.

➤ Obtain a history of allergies or sensitivities to x-ray contrast medium or shellfish.

➤ Obtain a list of medications the patient is taking.

➤ Obtain a history of the patient's abdominal system and organs, as well as results of previously performed tests and procedures. For related tests, refer to the GI, hepatobiliary, or genitourinary and renal system tables.

➤ Determine previous laboratory abnormalities, especially blood urea nitrogen (BUN) and creatinine, if contrast medium is to be used.

➤ Determine date of last menstrual period and the possibility of pregnancy in perimenopausal women.

➤ Ensure that results of blood tests are obtained and recorded before the procedure.

➤ Inform the patient that iodinated

contrast medium may be injected after the first series of x-rays, which will be followed by a second series of scans.

➤ Patients receiving metformin (Glucophage) for non–insulin-dependent (type 2) diabetes should discontinue the drug on the day of the test and continue to withhold it for 48 hours after the test. Failure to do so may result in lactic acidosis.

➤ Inform the patient that he or she may experience nausea, a feeling of warmth, a salty or metallic taste, or a transient headache after injection of contrast medium, if given. Instruct the patient to take slow, deep breaths if this occurs.

➤ Ensure barium studies have been performed more than 4 days before the scan.

➤ The patient may be requested to drink approximately 450 mL of a dilute barium solution (approximately 1% barium) beginning 1 hour before the examination. This is administered to distinguish GI organs from the other abdominal organs.

➤ Restrict food and fluids for 6 to 8 hours, if contrast medium is to be given.

Intratest: ∎

➤ Administer sedative to a child or to an uncooperative adult, as ordered.

➤ Administer antianxiety agent, as ordered, if the patient is experiencing claustrophobia. Administer an antihistamine or steroid, as ordered by a physician, for patients with a known significant allergic reaction to the IV contrast medium.

➤ Administer an enema to remove barium from the GI tract, as ordered.

➤ Place the patient in a supine position on a flat table with foam wedges that help maintain position and immobilization. Ask the patient to lie still during the procedure because movement produces unclear images. Make sure jewelry, watches, chains, belts, and any other metallic objects have been removed.

➤ Move table into the scanner, and instruct the patient to remain still. The scanner makes noises as it rotates around the body. The patient may be asked to take deep breaths to facilitate visualization. A number of images are taken. A computer reconstructs these images so they can be reviewed.

➤ Administer contrast medium, if ordered. A second series of images is obtained.

Post-test: ∎

➤ Instruct the patient to resume normal activity, diet, and previous medication use, unless otherwise indicated. Renal function should be assessed before metformin is restarted.

➤ Instruct the patient to increase fluid intake to help eliminate the contrast medium, if used.

➤ Inform the patient that diarrhea may occur after ingestion of oral contrast medium.

➤ Instruct the patient or caregiver to note change in urinary output after iodinated contrast medium administration in patients with impaired renal function.

➤ Observe for delayed allergic reactions, such as urticaria (hives), headache, nausea, or vomiting, if contrast medium was administered.

➤ A physician specializing in this branch of medicine sends a written report to the ordering provider, who discusses the results with the patient.

➤ Evaluate test results in relation to the patient's symptoms and other tests performed. Related diagnostic tests include angiogram and magnetic resonance imaging of the abdomen; and kidney, ureter, and bladder (KUB) film.

COMPUTED TOMOGRAPHY, ANGIOGRAPHY

SYNONYM/ACRONYM: Computed axial tomography (CAT) angiography, CTA.

AREA OF APPLICATION: Vessels.

CONTRAST: Iodinated contrast medium.

DESCRIPTION: Computed tomography angiography (CTA) is a noninvasive procedure that enhances certain anatomic views of vascular structures. This procedure complements traditional angiography and allows reconstruction of the images in different planes and removal of surrounding structures, leaving only the vessels to be studied. While lying on a table, the patient moves in and out of a doughnut-like device called a *gantry*, which houses the x-ray tube and associated electronics. The scanner uses multiple x-ray beams and a series of detectors that rotate around the patient to produce cross-sectional views in a three-dimensional fashion by detecting and recording differences in tissue density after having an x-ray beam passed through the tissues. CTA uses spiral CT technology and collects large amounts of data with each scan. Retrospectively, the data can be manipulated to produce the desired image without exposure to additional radiation or contrast medium. Multiplanar reconstruction images are reviewed by the physician at a computerized workstation. These images are helpful when there are heavily calcified vessels. The axial images give the most precise information regarding the true percentage of stenosis, and they can also evaluate intracerebral aneurysms. Small ulcerations and plaque irregularity are readily seen with CTA; the degree of stenosis can be estimated better with CTA because of the increased number of imaging planes. Density measurements are sent to a computer that produces a digital image of the anatomy, enabling a physician to look at slices or thin sections of certain anatomic views of the vessels. Iodinated contrast medium is given intravenously for vascular evaluation. Images can be recorded on photographic or x-ray film or stored in digital format as digitized computer data. ∎

INDICATIONS:

• Detect vascular disease

• Differentiate between vascular and nonvascular tumors

• Detect stenosis

- Detect aneurysms

- Differentiate aortic aneurysms from tumors near the aorta

- Evaluate atherosclerosis

- Detect embolism or other occlusions

- Detect fistula

- Evaluate hemorrhage or trauma

- Monitor and evaluate the effectiveness of medical or surgical therapies

RESULT

Normal Findings:

- Normal size, position, and shape of vascular structures

Abnormal Findings:

- Aortic aneurysm

- Cysts or abscesses

- Emboli

- Hemorrhage

- Neoplasm

- Occlusion

- Shunting

- Stenosis

CRITICAL VALUES: N/A

INTERFERING FACTORS:

This procedure is contraindicated for:

- Patients with allergies to shellfish or ⚠ iodinated dye. The contrast medium used may cause a life-threatening allergic reaction. Patients with a known hypersensitivity to the medium may benefit from premedication with corticosteroids or the use of nonionic contrast medium.

- Patients who are claustrophobic.

- Patients who are pregnant or suspected of being pregnant, unless the potential benefits of the procedure far outweigh the risks to the fetus and mother.

- Elderly and other patients who are ⚠ chronically dehydrated before the test, because of their risk of contrast-induced renal failure.

- ⚠ Patients who are in renal failure.

- Young patients (17 years old and younger), unless the benefits of the x-ray diagnosis outweigh the risks of exposure to high levels of radiation.

Factors that may impair clear imaging:

- Inability of the patient to cooperate or remain still during the procedure because of age, significant pain, or mental status

- Patients with extreme claustrophobia unless sedation is given before the study

- Improper adjustment of the radiographic equipment to accommodate obese or thin patients, which can cause overexposure or underexposure and a poor-quality study

- Patients who are very obese, who may exceed the weight limit for the equipment

- Incorrect positioning of the patient, which may produce poor visualization of the area to be examined

- Gas or feces in the gastrointestinal tract, resulting from inadequate cleansing or failure to restrict food intake before the study

- Metallic objects within the examination field (e.g., jewelry or body rings), which may inhibit organ visualization and can produce unclear images

Other considerations:

- Consultation with a physician should occur before the procedure for radiation safety concerns regarding infants of patients who are lactating.

• Risks associated with radiographic overexposure can result from frequent x-ray procedures. Personnel in the room with the patient should wear a protective lead apron, stand behind a shield, or leave the area while the examination is being done. Personnel working in the area where the examination is being done should wear badges that reveal their level of exposure to radiation.

Nursing Implications and Procedure • • • • • • • • • •

Pretest:

➤ Inform the patient that the procedure assesses the vessels.

➤ Inform the patient that the procedure is performed in a radiology department by a technologist and a physician and takes approximately 30 to 60 minutes.

➤ Obtain a history of allergies or sensitivities to contrast medium or shellfish.

➤ Obtain a list of medications the patient is taking.

➤ Determine previous laboratory abnormalities, especially blood urea nitrogen and creatinine, if contrast medium is to be used.

➤ Ensure that results of blood tests are obtained and recorded before the procedure.

➤ Obtain a history of patient's cardiovascular system and results from previously performed tests and procedures. For related tests, refer to the cardiovascular system table.

➤ Inform the patient that intravenous iodinated contrast medium will be used.

➤ Patients receiving metformin (Glucophage) for non–insulin-dependent (type 2) diabetes should discontinue the drug on the day of the test and continue to withhold it for 48 hours after the test. Failure to do so may result in lactic acidosis.

➤ Inform the patient that he or she may experience nausea, a feeling of warmth, a salty or metallic taste, or a transient headache after injection of contrast medium, if given. Instruct the patient to take slow, deep breaths if this occurs.

➤ Restrict food and fluids for 6 to 8 hours.

Intratest:

➤ Administer sedative to a child or to an uncooperative adult, as ordered.

➤ Administer antianxiety agent, as ordered, if the patient is experiencing claustrophobia.

➤ Administer an antihistamine or steroid, as ordered by a physician, for patients with a known significant allergic reaction to the IV contrast medium.

➤ Place the patient in a supine position on a flat table with foam wedges to help maintain position and immobilization. Ask the patient to lie still during the procedure because movement produces unclear images. Make sure jewelry, watches, chains, belts, and any other metallic objects have been removed.

➤ Instruct the patient to remain still while the table moves into the scanner. The scanner will make noises as it rotates around the body. The patient may be asked to take deep breaths to facilitate visualization. A number of images are taken. A computer reconstructs these images so they can be reviewed.

➤ Contrast medium is administered.

Post-test:

➤ Instruct the patient to resume normal activity and diet, unless otherwise indicated. Renal function should be assessed before metformin is restarted.

➤ Instruct the patient to increase fluid intake to help eliminate the contrast medium.

➤ Instruct the patient or caregiver to note change in urinary output after iodinated contrast medium administration in patients with impaired renal function.

➤ Observe for delayed allergic reactions, such as urticaria (hives), headache, nausea, or vomiting.

➤ A physician specializing in this branch of medicine sends a written report to the ordering provider, who discusses the results with the patient.

➤ Evaluate test results in relation to the patient's symptoms and other tests performed. Related diagnostic tests include Doppler ultrasound, angiography, and magnetic resonance angiography.

COMPUTED TOMOGRAPHY, BILIARY TRACT AND LIVER

• •

SYNONYMS/ACRONYMS: Computed axial tomography (CAT), computed transaxial tomography (CTT), abdominal CT.

AREA OF APPLICATION: Liver, biliary tract, and adjacent structures.

CONTRAST: Can be done with or without iodinated contrast medium.

DESCRIPTION: Computed tomography (CT) of the liver and biliary tract is a noninvasive procedure that enhances certain anatomic views of these structures, but it becomes invasive with the use of contrast medium. The patient lies on a table that moves in and out of a doughnut-like device called a *gantry*, which houses the x-ray tube and associated electronics. The scanner uses multiple x-ray beams and a series of detectors that rotate around the patient to produce cross-sectional views in a three-dimensional fashion by detecting and recording differences in tissue density after having an x-ray beam passed through the tissues. These density measurements are sent to a computer that produces a digital image of the anatomy, enabling a physician to look at slices or thin sections of certain anatomic views of the liver, biliary tract, and vascular system. Differentiations can be made among solid, cystic, inflammatory, or vascular lesions, and suspected hematomas and aneurysms can be identified. Iodinated contrast medium is given intravenously for blood vessel and vascular evaluation. Images can be recorded on photographic or x-ray film or stored in digital format as digitized computer data. Cine scanning produces a series of moving images of the area scanned. The CT scan can be used to guide biopsy needles into areas of suspected tumors to obtain tissue for laboratory analysis and placement of catheters for drainage of abscesses. Tumors, before and after therapy, may be monitored with CT scanning. ∎

INDICATIONS:

• Assist in differentiating between benign and malignant tumors

• Detect dilation or obstruction of the biliary ducts with or without calcification or gallstone

• Detect tumor extension of masses and metastasis into the hepatic area

• Distinguish between obstructive and nonobstructive jaundice

• Differentiate aortic aneurysms from tumors near the aorta

• Differentiate infectious from inflammatory processes

• Evaluate hepatic cysts, masses, abscesses, hematomas, or hepatic trauma

• Detect liver abnormalities, such as cirrhosis with ascites and fatty liver

• Monitor and evaluate effectiveness of medical, radiation, or surgical therapies

RESULT

Normal Findings:

• Normal size, position, and contour of the liver and biliary ducts

Abnormal Findings:

• Dilation of the common hepatic duct, common bile duct, or gallbladder

• Hepatic cysts or abscesses

• Hematomas

• Gallstones

• Jaundice (obstructive or nonobstructive)

• Primary and metastatic neoplasms

CRITICAL VALUES: N/A

INTERFERING FACTORS:

This procedure is contraindicated for:

• Patients with allergies to shellfish or ⚠ iodinated dye. The contrast medium used may cause a life-threatening allergic reaction. Patients with a known hypersensitivity to the medium may benefit from premedication with corticosteroids or the use of nonionic contrast medium.

• Patients who are claustrophobic.

• Patients who are pregnant or suspected of being pregnant, unless the potential benefits of the procedure far outweigh the risks to the fetus and mother.

• Elderly and other patients who are ⚠ chronically dehydrated before the test, because of their risk of contrast-induced renal failure.

• ⚠ Patients who are in renal failure.

• Young patients (17 years old and younger), unless the benefits of the x-ray diagnosis outweigh the risks of exposure to high levels of radiation.

Factors that may impair clear imaging:

• Inability of the patient to cooperate or remain still during the procedure because of age, significant pain, or mental status

• Patients with extreme cases of claustrophobia unless sedation is given before the study

• Improper adjustment of the radiographic equipment to accommodate obese or thin patients, which can cause overexposure or underexposure and a poor-quality study

• Patients who are very obese, who may exceed the weight limit for the equipment

- Incorrect positioning of the patient, which may produce poor visualization of the area to be examined

- Gas or feces in the gastrointestinal tract resulting from inadequate cleansing or failure to restrict food intake before the study

- Retained barium from a previous radiologic procedure

- Metallic objects within the examination field (e.g., jewelry or body rings), which may inhibit organ visualization and can produce unclear images

Other considerations:

- Consultation with a physician should occur before the procedure for radiation safety concerns regarding infants of patients who are lactating.

- Risks associated with radiographic overexposure can result from frequent x-ray procedures. Personnel in the room with the patient should wear a protective lead apron, stand behind a shield, or leave the area while the examination is being done. Personnel working in the area where the examination is being done should wear badges that reveal their level of exposure to radiation.

Nursing Implications and Procedure • • • • • • • • • • •

Pretest:

➤ Inform the patient that the procedure assesses the liver and bile ducts.

➤ Inform the patient that the procedure is performed in a radiology department by a technologist and a physician and takes approximately 30 minutes.

➤ Obtain a history of allergies or sensitivities to contrast medium or shellfish.

➤ Obtain a list of medications the patient is taking.

➤ Obtain a history of the patient's

hepatobiliary and gastrointestinal systems, as well as results of previously performed tests and procedures. For related tests, refer to the hepatobiliary and gastrointestinal system tables.

➤ Determine previous laboratory abnormalities, especially blood urea nitrogen (BUN) and creatinine, if contrast medium is to be used.

➤ Ensure that the results of blood tests are obtained and recorded before the procedure.

➤ Determine date of last menstrual period and the possibility of pregnancy in perimenopausal women.

➤ Inform the patient that iodinated contrast medium may be injected after the first series of x-rays, which will be followed by a second series of scans.

➤ Patients receiving metformin (Glucophage) for non–insulin-dependent (type 2) diabetes should discontinue the drug on the day of the test and continue to withhold it for 48 hours after the test. Failure to do so may result in lactic acidosis.

➤ Inform the patient that he or she may experience nausea, a feeling of warmth, a salty or metallic taste, or a transient headache after injection of contrast medium, if given. Instruct the patient to take slow, deep breaths if this occurs.

➤ Question the patient to ensure that barium studies were performed more than 4 days before the scan.

➤ Restrict food and fluids for 6 to 8 hours, if contrast medium is to be given.

Intratest:

➤ Administer sedative to a child or to an uncooperative adult, as ordered.

➤ Administer antianxiety agent, as ordered, if the patient is experiencing claustrophobia.

➤ Administer an antihistamine or steroid, as ordered by a physician, for patients with a known significant allergic reaction to the IV contrast medium.

➤ Administer an enema to remove barium from the gastrointestinal tract, as ordered.

➤ Place the patient in a supine position on a flat table with foam wedges to help maintain position and immobilization. Ask the patient to lie still during the procedure because movement produces unclear images. Make sure jewelry, watches, chains, belts, and any other metallic objects have been removed.

➤ As the table moves into the scanner, instruct the patient to remain still. The scanner makes noises as it rotates around the body. The patient may be asked to take deep breaths to facilitate visualization. A number of images are taken. A computer reconstructs these images so they can be reviewed.

➤ Administer contrast medium, if ordered. A second series of images is obtained.

Post-test:

➤ Instruct the patient to resume normal activity, diet, and previous medication use, unless otherwise indicated. Renal function should be assessed before metformin is restarted.

➤ Instruct the patient to increase fluid intake to help eliminate the contrast medium, if used.

➤ Instruct the patient or caregiver to note changes in urinary output after iodinated contrast medium administration in patients with impaired renal function.

➤ Observe for delayed allergic reactions, such as urticaria (hives), headache, nausea, or vomiting, if contrast medium was used.

➤ A physician specializing in this branch of medicine sends a written report to the ordering provider, who discusses the results with the patient.

➤ Evaluate test results in relation to the patient's symptoms and other tests performed. Related diagnostic tests include hepatobiliary scan; ultrasound of the liver; kidney, ureter, and bladder (KUB) film; and magnetic resonance imaging of the abdomen.

COMPUTED TOMOGRAPHY, BRAIN

SYNONYMS/ACRONYMS: Computed axial tomography (CAT) of the head, computed transaxial tomography (CTT) of the head, brain CT.

AREA OF APPLICATION: Brain.

CONTRAST: Can be done with or without iodinated contrast medium.

DESCRIPTION: Computed tomography (CT) of the brain is a noninvasive procedure used to assist in diagnosing abnormalities of the head, brain tissue, cerebrospinal fluid, and blood circulation. Brain CT becomes invasive if contrast medium is used for image enhancement when pathology causing destruction of the blood-brain barrier is suspected. CT is useful for evaluating suspected brain tumors, infarction, intracranial hemorrhage, hematomas, arteriovenous malformations, ventricular abnormalities, aneurysms, and other vascular abnormalities. The patient lies on a table and is moved in and out of a doughnut-like device called a *gantry,* which houses the x-ray tube and associated electronics. The scanner uses multiple x-ray beams and a series of detectors that rotate around the patient to produce cross-sectional views in a three-dimensional fashion by detecting and recording differences in tissue density after having an x-ray beam passed through the tissues. Low-density tissue appears black on the images, medium-density tissue appears in shades of gray, and high-density tissue appears nearly white. These density measurements are sent to a computer that produces a digital image of the anatomy, enabling a physician to look at slices or thin sections of certain anatomic views of the pituitary and associated vascular system. Differentiations can be made among solid, cystic, inflammatory, or vascular lesions, and suspected hematomas or aneurysms can be identified. The procedure may be repeated after iodinated contrast medium is given intravenously for blood vessel and vascular evaluation. Images can be recorded on photographic or x-ray film or stored in digital format as digitized computer data. Cine scanning is used to produce a series of moving images of the area scanned. Tumor progression, before and after therapy, and effectiveness of medical interventions may be monitored by CT scanning. ∎

INDICATIONS:

- Determine the presence of multiple sclerosis, as evidenced by sclerotic plaques 3 to 4 mm in diameter

- Determine cause of increased intracranial pressure

- Determine benign and cancerous intracranial tumors and cyst formation, as evidenced by changes in tissue densities (white indicating increased density, darker areas indicating decreased density)

- Determine size and location of a lesion causing a stroke, such as an infarct or hemorrhage

- Detect ventricular enlargement or displacement by increased cerebrospinal fluid

- Determine the presence and type of hemorrhage in infants and children experiencing signs and symptoms of intracranial trauma, or of congenital conditions such as hydrocephalus and arteriovenous malformations

- Differentiate between cerebral infarction and hemorrhage

- Detect the presence of a brain infection or inflammatory condition, such as abscess or necrosis, as evidenced by decreased density on the image

- Differentiate among hematoma locations after trauma (e.g., subdural, epidural, cerebral), and determine the extent of edema resulting from injury, as evidenced by higher blood densities compared with normal tissue

- Evaluate abnormalities of the middle ear ossicles, auditory nerve, and optic nerve

- Monitor and evaluate the effectiveness of medical, radiation, or surgical therapies

RESULT

Normal Findings:

- Normal size, position, and shape of intracranial contents and vascular system

Abnormal Findings:

- Abscess
- Aneurysm
- Arteriovenous malformations
- Cerebral atrophy
- Cerebral edema
- Cerebral infarction
- Congenital abnormalities
- Craniopharyngioma
- Cysts
- Hematomas (e.g., epidural, subdural, intracerebral)
- Hemorrhage
- Hydrocephaly
- Increased intracranial pressure or trauma
- Infection
- Sclerotic plaques suggesting multiple sclerosis
- Tumor
- Ventricular or tissue displacement or enlargement

CRITICAL VALUES: N/A

INTERFERING FACTORS:

This procedure is contraindicated for:

- Patients with allergies to shellfish or iodinated dye. The contrast medium used may cause a life-threatening allergic reaction. Patients with a known hypersensitivity to the medium may benefit from premedication with corticosteroids or the use of nonionic contrast medium.

- Patients who are claustrophobic.

- Patients who are pregnant or suspected of being pregnant, unless the potential benefits of the procedure far outweigh the risks to the fetus and mother.

- Elderly and other patients who are chronically dehydrated before the test, because of their risk of contrast-induced renal failure.

- Patients who are in renal failure.

- Young patients (17 years old and younger), unless the benefits of the x-ray diagnosis outweigh the risks of exposure to high levels of radiation.

Factors that may impair clear imaging:

- Inability of the patient to cooperate or remain still during the procedure because of age, significant pain, or mental status

- Patients with extreme claustrophobia unless sedation is given before the study

- Improper adjustment of the radiographic equipment to accommodate obese or thin patients, which can cause overexposure or underexposure and a poor-quality study

- Patients who are very obese, who may exceed the weight limit for the equipment

- Incorrect positioning of the patient, which may produce poor visualization of the area to be examined

- Retained barium from a previous radiologic procedure

- Metallic objects within the examination field (e.g., jewelry, body rings), which may inhibit organ visualization and can produce unclear images

Other considerations:

- Consultation with a physician should occur before the procedure for radiation safety concerns regarding infants of patients who are lactating.

• Risks associated with radiographic overexposure can result from frequent x-ray procedures. Personnel in the room with the patient should wear a protective lead apron, stand behind a shield, or leave the area while the examination is being done. Personnel working in the area where the examination is being done should wear badges that reveal their level of exposure to radiation.

Nursing Implications and Procedure • • • • • • • • • • •

Pretest: ■

➤ Inform the patient that the procedure assesses the brain.

➤ Inform the patient that the procedure is done in a radiology department or imaging center by a technologist and a physician and takes approximately 15 to 30 minutes.

➤ Obtain a history of allergies or sensitivities to contrast medium or shellfish.

➤ Obtain a list of medications the patient is taking.

➤ Obtain a history of the patient's neurological system and results of previously performed tests, procedures, treatments, and surgeries on the brain and cerebrovascular system. For related tests, refer to the musculoskeletal and cardiovascular system tables.

➤ Determine previous laboratory abnormalities, especially blood urea nitrogen (BUN) and creatinine, if contrast medium is to be used.

➤ Determine date of last menstrual period and the possibility of pregnancy in perimenopausal women.

➤ Ensure that results of blood tests are obtained and recorded before the procedure.

➤ Patients receiving metformin

(Glucophage) for non–insulin-dependent (type 2) diabetes should discontinue the drug on the day of the test and continue to withhold it for 48 hours after the test. Failure to do so may result in lactic acidosis.

➤ Inform the patient that he or she may experience nausea, a feeling of warmth, a salty or metallic taste, or a transient headache after injection of contrast medium, if given. Instruct the patient to take slow, deep breaths if this occurs.

➤ Do not restrict food and fluids before this procedure.

Intratest: ■

➤ Administer sedative to a child or to an uncooperative adult, as ordered.

➤ Administer antianxiety agent, as ordered, if the patient is experiencing claustrophobia.

➤ Administer an antihistamine or steroid, as ordered by a physician, for patients with a known significant allergic reaction to the IV contrast medium.

➤ Place the patient in a supine position on a flat table with foam wedges, which help maintain position and immobilization. Ask the patient to lie still during the procedure because movement produces unclear images. Make sure jewelry, watches, chains, belts, and any other metallic objects have been removed.

➤ As the table moves into the scanner, instruct the patient to remain still. The scanner makes noises as it rotates around the body. The patient may be asked to take deep breaths to facilitate visualization. A number of images are taken. A computer reconstructs these images so they can be reviewed.

➤ Administer contrast medium if ordered, and obtain a second series of images.

Post-test: ■

➤ Instruct the patient to increase fluid intake to help eliminate the contrast medium, if used.

➤ Instruct the patient or caregiver to note change in urinary output after iodinated contrast medium administration in patients with impaired renal function. Renal function should be assessed before metformin is restarted.

➤ Observe for delayed allergic reactions, such as urticaria (hives), headache, nausea, or vomiting, if contrast medium was used.

➤ A physician specializing in this branch of medicine sends a written report to the ordering provider, who discusses the results with the patient.

➤ Evaluate test results in relation to the patient's symptoms and other tests performed. A related test is magnetic resonance imaging of the brain.

COMPUTED TOMOGRAPHY, CARDIAC SCORING

SYNONYMS/ACRONYMS: Computed axial tomography (CAT), computed transaxial tomography (CTT), heart vessel calcium CT, cardiac plaque CT.

AREA OF APPLICATION: Heart.

CONTRAST: Done without iodinated contrast medium.

DESCRIPTION: Cardiac scoring is a noninvasive test for quantifying coronary artery calcium content. Coronary artery disease (CAD) occurs when the arteries that carry blood and oxygen to the heart muscle become clogged or built up with plaque. Plaque buildup slows the flow of blood to the heart muscle, causing ischemia and increasing the risk of heart failure. The procedure begins with a computed tomography (CT) scan of the heart. The patient lies on a table and is moved in and out of a doughnut-like device called a *gantry*, which houses the x-ray tube and associated electronics. The scanner uses multiple x-ray beams and a series of detectors that rotate around the patient to produce cross-sectional views in a three-dimensional fashion by detecting and recording differences in plaque density after having an x-ray beam passed through the tissues. The scanner takes an image of the beating heart while the patient holds his or her breath for approximately 20 seconds. The procedure requires no contrast medium injections. These density measurements are sent to a computer that produces a digital analysis of the anatomy, enabling a physician to look at the quantified amount of calcium (cardiac plaque score) in the coronary arteries. The data can be recorded on photographic or x-ray film or stored in digital format as digitized computer data. ■

INDICATIONS:

- Detect and quantify coronary artery calcium content

  CAD is the leading cause of death in most industrialized nations

  Cardiac scoring is a more powerful predictor of CAD than cholesterol screening

  Of all myocardial infarctions (MIs), 45 percent occur in people younger than age 65

  Of women who have had MIs, 44 percent will die within 1 year after the attack

  Women are more likely to die of heart disease than of breast cancer

- Screening for coronary artery calcium in patients with:

  High blood pressure

  Diabetes

  High cholesterol

  Family history of heart disease

  Personal history of smoking

  Sedentary lifestyle

  Overweight by 20 percent or more

  High-stress lifestyle

- Screening for coronary artery plaque in patients with chest pain of unknown cause

RESULT

Normal Findings:

- If the score is 100 or less, the probability of having significant CAD is minimal or is unlikely to be causing a narrowing at the time of the examination.

Abnormal Findings:

- If the score is between 101 and 400, a significant amount of calcified plaque was found in the coronary arteries. There is an increased risk of a future

MI, and a medical assessment of cardiac risk factors needs to be done. Additional testing may be needed.

- If the score is greater than 400, the procedure has detected extensive calcified plaque in the coronary arteries, which may have caused a critical narrowing of the vessels. A full medical assessment is needed as soon as possible. Further testing may be needed, and treatment may be needed to reduce the risk of MI.

CRITICAL VALUES: N/A

INTERFERING FACTORS:

This procedure is contraindicated for:

- Patients who are claustrophobic

- Patients who are pregnant or suspected of being pregnant, unless the potential benefits of the procedure far outweigh the risks to the fetus and mother

- Young patients, unless the benefits of the x-ray diagnosis outweigh the risks of exposure to high levels of radiation

Factors that may impair clear imaging:

- Inability of the patient to cooperate or remain still during the procedure because of age, significant pain, or mental status

- Patients with extreme claustrophobia unless sedation is given before the study

- Improper adjustment of the radiographic equipment to accommodate obese or thin patients, which can cause overexposure or underexposure and a poor-quality study

- Patients who are very obese, who may exceed the weight limit for the equipment

- Incorrect positioning of the patient,

which may produce poor visualization of the area to be examined

• Patients with metal stents in their coronary arteries or metal overlying the chest area

• Metallic objects within the examination field (e.g., jewelry or body rings), which can produce unclear images

Other considerations:

• Risks associated with radiographic overexposure can result from frequent x-ray procedures. Personnel in the room with the patient should wear a protective lead apron, stand behind a shield, or leave the area while the examination is being done. Personnel working in the area where the examination is being done should wear badges that reveal their level of exposure to radiation.

Nursing Implications and Procedure • • • • • • • • • • • •

Pretest: ■

➤ Inform the patient that the procedure assesses the coronary arteries.

➤ Inform the patient that the procedure is performed in a CT scanner by a technologist and takes approximately 5 minutes.

➤ Obtain a list of medications the patient is taking.

➤ Obtain a history of the patient's respiratory and cardiac systems, as well as results of previously performed tests and procedures. For related tests, refer to the respi-

ratory and cardiovascular system tables.

➤ Do not restrict food and fluids.

Intratest: ■

➤ Administer sedative to a child or to an uncooperative adult, as ordered.

➤ Administer antianxiety agent, as ordered, if the patient is experiencing claustrophobia.

➤ Place the patient in a supine position on a flat table with foam wedges, which help maintain position and immobilization. Ask the patient to lie still during the procedure because movement produces unclear images. Make sure jewelry, watches, chains, belts, and any other metallic objects have been removed.

➤ The table is moved into the scanner, and the patient is instructed to remain still. The scanner makes noises as it rotates around the body. The patient may be asked to take deep breaths to facilitate visualization. A number of images are taken. A computer reconstructs these images so they can be reviewed.

Post-test: ■

➤ A physician specializing in this branch of medicine sends a written report to the ordering provider, who discusses the results with the patient.

➤ Evaluate test results in relation to the patient's symptoms and other tests performed. Related diagnostic tests include chest x-ray, coronary angiogram, echocardiogram, electrocardiogram, CT scan and magnetic resonance imaging of the chest, and lung scan.

COMPUTED TOMOGRAPHY, COLONOSCOPY

SYNONYMS/ACRONYMS: Computed axial tomography (CAT), computed transaxial tomography (CTT), CT virtual colonoscopy, CT colonography.

AREA OF APPLICATION: Colon.

CONTRAST: Screening examinations are done without intravenous (IV) iodinated contrast medium. Examinations done to clarify questionable or abnormal areas may require IV iodinated contrast medium.

DESCRIPTION: Computed tomography (CT) colonoscopy is a noninvasive technique that involves examining the colon by taking multiple CT scans of the patient's colon and rectum and using computer software to create three-dimensional images. The procedure is used to detect polyps, which are growths of tissue in the colon or rectum. Some types of polyps increase the risk of colon cancer, especially if they are large or if a patient has several polyps. Compared to conventional colonoscopy, CT colonoscopy is less effective in detecting polyps smaller than 5 mm, more effective when the polyps are between 5 and 9.9 mm, and most effective when the polyps are 10 mm or larger. This test may be valuable for patients who have diseases rendering them unable to undergo conventional colonoscopy (e.g., bleeding disorders, lung or heart disease) and for patients who are unable to undergo the sedation required for traditional colonoscopy. The procedure is less invasive than

conventional colonoscopy with little risk of complications and no recovery time. CT colonoscopy can be done as an outpatient procedure, and the patient may return to work or usual activities the same day.

CT colonoscopy and conventional colonoscopy require the bowel to be cleansed before the examination. The patient lies on a table and is moved in and out of a doughnut-like device called a *gantry,* which houses the x-ray tube and associated electronics. The scanner uses multiple x-ray beams and a series of detectors that rotate around the patient to produce cross-sectional views in a three-dimensional fashion by detecting and recording differences in densities in the colon after having an x-ray beam passed through it. The scanner takes an image of the colon while the patient holds his or her breath for approximately 10 to 30 seconds. The screening procedure requires no contrast medium injections, but if a suspicious area or abnormality is detected, a repeat series of images may be completed after IV contrast medium is given. These density measurements are sent to a computer that produces a digital analysis of the anatomy. The data can be recorded on photographic or x-ray film or stored in digital format as digitized computer data. A drawback of CT colonoscopy is that polyp removal and biopsies of tissue in the colon must be done using conventional colonoscopy. Therefore, if polyps are discovered during CT colonoscopy and biopsy becomes necessary, the patient must undergo bowel preparation a second time. ▪

INDICATIONS:

- Detect polyps in the colon
- Investigate cause of positive occult blood test
- Investigate further when flexible sigmoidoscopy is positive for polyps
- Investigate further after an abnormal barium enema
- Examine the colon in patients with heart or lung disease, patients unable to be sedated, and patients unable to undergo colonoscopy
- Failure to visualize the entire colon during conventional colonoscopy
- Evaluate the site of resection for local recurrence of lesions
- Evaluate the colon for metachronous lesions
- Identify metastases
- Evaluate polyposis syndromes
- Evaluate the colon in patients with obstructing rectosigmoid disease

RESULT

Normal Findings:

- Normal colon and rectum, with no evidence of polyps or growths

Abnormal Findings:

- Polyps or growths in colon or rectum
- Abnormal endoluminal wall of the colon
- Extraluminal extension of primary cancer
- Mesenteric and retroperitoneal lymphadenopathy
- Metachronous lesions
- Metastases of cancer
- Tumor recurrence after surgery

CRITICAL VALUES: N/A

INTERFERING FACTORS:

This procedure is contraindicated for:

- Patients who are claustrophobic
- Patients who are pregnant or suspected of being pregnant, unless the potential benefits of the procedure far outweigh the risks to the fetus and mother
- Young patients (17 years old and younger), unless the benefits of the x-ray diagnosis outweigh the risks of exposure to high levels of radiation

Factors that may impair clear imaging:

- Inability of the patient to cooperate or remain still during the procedure because of age, significant pain, or mental status
- Patients with extreme claustrophobia unless sedation is given before the study
- Poor patient preparation or inability to retain air in the colon
- Inability of the patient to hold his or her breath, which may cause artifacts on the scan
- Improper adjustment of the radio-

graphic equipment to accommodate obese or thin patients, which can cause overexposure or underexposure and a poor-quality study

• Patients who are very obese, who may exceed the weight limit for the equipment

• Incorrect positioning of the patient, which may produce poor visualization of the area to be examined

• Gas or feces in the gastrointestinal tract resulting from inadequate cleansing or failure to restrict food intake before the study

• Retained barium from a previous radiologic procedure

• Metallic objects within the examination field (e.g., jewelry or body rings), which can produce unclear images

Other considerations:

• Failure to follow dietary restrictions before the procedure may cause the procedure to be canceled or repeated.

• Risks associated with radiographic overexposure can result from frequent x-ray procedures. Personnel in the room with the patient should wear a protective lead apron, stand behind a shield, or leave the area while the examination is being done. Personnel working in the area where the examination is being done should wear badges that reveal their level of exposure to radiation.

Nursing Implications and Procedure • • • • • • • • • • •

Pretest:

➤ Inform the patient that the procedure assesses the rectum and colon.

➤ Inform the patient that the procedure is performed in a CT scanner by a technologist and takes approximately 5 to 10 minutes.

➤ Obtain a list of medications the patient is taking.

➤ Obtain a history of the patient's gastrointestinal system and results of previously performed tests and procedures. For related tests, refer to the gastrointestinal system tables.

➤ Restrict diet to clear liquids for 48 hours before beginning oral bowel preparation.

➤ Ensure that ordered laxative has been administered late in the afternoon the day before the procedure.

Intratest:

➤ Administer sedative to a child or to an uncooperative adult, as ordered.

➤ Administer antianxiety agent, as ordered, if the patient is experiencing claustrophobia.

➤ The colon is distended with room air or carbon dioxide by means of a rectal tube and balloon retention device. Maximal colonic distention is guided by patient tolerance.

➤ Place the patient in a supine position on a flat table with foam wedges, which help maintain position and immobilization. Ask the patient to lie still during the procedure because movement produces unclear images. Make sure jewelry, watches, chains, belts, and any other metallic objects have been removed.

➤ The table is moved into the scanner, and the patient is instructed to remain still. The scanner makes noises as it rotates around the body. The patient may be asked to take a deep breath and hold it to facilitate visualization. A number of images are taken. A computer reconstructs these images so they can be reviewed.

➤ The sequence of images is repeated in the prone position.

Post-test:

➤ Instruct the patient to resume normal activity and diet, unless otherwise indicated.

➤ A physician specializing in this branch of medicine sends a written report to the ordering provider, who discusses the results with the patient.

➤ Evaluate test results in relation to the patient's symptoms and other

tests performed. Related diagnostic tests include colonoscopy; CT and magnetic resonance imaging of the abdomen; kidney, ureter, and bladder (KUB) film; barium enema; and proctosigmoidoscopy.

COMPUTED TOMOGRAPHY, PANCREAS

SYNONYMS/ACRONYMS: Computed axial tomography (CAT), computed transaxial tomography (CTT).

AREA OF APPLICATION: Pancreas.

CONTRAST: Can be done with or without oral or intravenous iodinated contrast medium.

DESCRIPTION: Computed tomography (CT) is a noninvasive procedure used to enhance certain anatomic views of the abdominal structures, but it becomes an invasive procedure when contrast medium is used. CT of the pancreas aids in the diagnosis or evaluation of pancreatic cysts, pseudocysts, inflammation, tumors, masses, metastases, abscesses, and trauma. In all but the thinnest or most emaciated patients, the pancreas is surrounded by fat that clearly defines its margins. While lying on a table, the patient is moved in and out of a doughnut-like device called a *gantry*, which houses the x-ray tube and associated electronics. The scanner uses multiple x-ray beams and a series of detectors that rotate around

the patient to produce cross-sectional views in a three-dimensional fashion by detecting and recording differences in tissue density, surrounding organs, and vessels after having an x-ray beam passed through them. These density measurements are sent to a computer that produces a digital image of the anatomy, enabling the radiologist to look at slices or thin sections of certain anatomic views of the pancreas and associated vascular system. Differentiations can be made among solid, cystic, inflammatory, or vascular lesions. CT scanning can detect the swelling that accompanies acute inflammation of the gland and, in chronic cases, the calcium deposits missed on other examinations. Intravenous iodinated contrast medium is given for blood vessel and vascular evaluation, and oral contrast medium is given for bowel and adjacent structure evaluation. Images can be recorded on photographic or x-ray film or stored in digital format as digitized computer data. Cine scanning produces a series of moving images of the scanned area. The CT scan can be used to guide biopsy needles into areas of pancreatic masses to obtain tissue for laboratory analysis and for placement of needles to aspirate cysts or abscesses. CT scanning can monitor mass, cyst, or tumor growth and post-therapy response. ■

INDICATIONS:

• Evaluate benign or cancerous tumors or metastasis to the pancreas

• Evaluate pancreatic abnormalities (e.g., bleeding, pancreatitis, pseudocyst, abscesses)

• Detect dilation or obstruction of the pancreatic ducts

• Monitor and evaluate effectiveness of medical or surgical therapies

• Differentiate between pancreatic disorders and disorders of the retroperitoneum

• Evaluate unexplained weight loss, jaundice, and epigastric pain

RESULT

Normal Findings:

• Normal size, position, and contour of the pancreas, which lies obliquely in the upper abdomen

Abnormal Findings:

• Acute or chronic pancreatitis
• Obstruction of the pancreatic ducts
• Pancreatic abscesses
• Pancreatic carcinoma

• Pancreatic pseudocyst
• Pancreatic tumor

CRITICAL VALUES: N/A

INTERFERING FACTORS:

This procedure is contraindicated for:

• Patients with allergies to shellfish or ⚠ iodinated dye. The contrast medium used may cause a life-threatening allergic reaction. Patients with a known hypersensitivity to the medium may benefit from premedication with corticosteroids or the use of nonionic contrast medium.

• Patients who are claustrophobic.

• Patients who are pregnant or suspected of being pregnant, unless the potential benefits of the procedure far outweigh the risks to the fetus and mother.

• Elderly and other patients who are ⚠ chronically dehydrated before the test, because of their risk of contrast-induced renal failure.

• ⚠ Patients who are in renal failure.

• Young patients (17 years old and younger), unless the benefits of the x-ray diagnosis outweigh the risks of exposure to high levels of radiation.

Factors that may impair clear imaging:

• Inability of the patient to cooperate or remain still during the procedure because of age, significant pain, or mental status

• Patients with extreme claustrophobia unless sedation is given before the study

• Improper adjustment of the radiographic equipment to accommodate obese or thin patients, which can cause overexposure or underexposure and a poor-quality study

- Patients who are very obese, who may exceed the weight limit for the equipment

- Incorrect positioning of the patient, which may produce poor visualization of the area to be examined

- Gas or feces in the gastrointestinal tract resulting from inadequate cleansing or failure to restrict food intake before the study

- Retained barium from a previous radiologic procedure

- Metallic objects within the examination field (e.g., jewelry or body rings), which may inhibit organ visualization and can produce unclear images

Other considerations:

- Failure to follow dietary restrictions before the procedure may cause the procedure to be canceled or repeated.

- Consultation with a physician should occur before the procedure for radiation safety concerns regarding infants of patients who are lactating.

- Risks associated with radiographic overexposure can result from frequent x-ray procedures. Personnel in the room with the patient should wear a protective lead apron, stand behind a shield, or leave the area while the examination is being done. Personnel working in the area where the examination is being done should wear badges that reveal their level of exposure to radiation.

Nursing Implications and Procedure • • • • • • • • • •

Pretest: █

➤ Inform the patient that the procedure assesses the pancreas.

➤ Inform the patient that the proce-

dure is performed in a radiology department by a technologist and a physician and takes approximately 30 minutes.

➤ Obtain a history of allergies or sensitivities to contrast medium or shellfish.

➤ Obtain a list of medications the patient is taking.

➤ Obtain a history of the patient's abdominal system and organs, as well as results of previously performed tests, trauma, treatments, surgeries, therapies, and procedures. For related tests, refer to the hepatobiliary, endocrine, and gastrointestinal system tables.

➤ Determine previous laboratory abnormalities, especially blood urea nitrogen (BUN) and creatinine, if contrast medium is to be used.

➤ Determine date of last menstrual period and the possibility of pregnancy in perimenopausal women.

➤ Ensure that results of blood tests are obtained and recorded before the procedure.

➤ Patients receiving metformin (Glucophage) for non–insulin-dependent (type 2) diabetes should discontinue the drug on the day of the test and continue to withhold it for 48 hours after the test. Failure to do so may result in lactic acidosis.

➤ Inform the patient that he or she may experience nausea, a feeling of warmth, a salty or metallic taste, or a transient headache after injection. Instruct the patient to take slow, deep breaths if this occurs.

➤ Ensure that barium studies have been performed more than 2 days before the scan.

➤ The patient may be asked to drink approximately 450 mL of a dilute barium solution (approximately 1% barium) beginning 1 hour before the examination. This is done to distinguish gastrointestinal organs from the pancreas.

➤ Restrict food and fluids for 6 to 8 hours, if contrast medium is to be given.

Intratest: ■

➤ Administer sedative to a child or to an uncooperative adult, as ordered.

➤ Administer antianxiety agent, as ordered, if the patient is experiencing claustrophobia.

➤ Administer an antihistamine or steroid, as ordered by a physician, for patients with a known significant allergic reaction to the IV contrast medium.

➤ Place the patient in a supine position on a flat table with foam wedges to help maintain position and immobilization. Ask the patient to lie still during the procedure because movement produces unclear images. Make sure jewelry, watches, chains, belts, and any other metallic objects have been removed.

➤ As the table moves into the scanner, instruct the patient to remain still. The scanner makes noises as it rotates around the body. The patient may be asked to take deep breaths to facilitate visualization. A number of images are taken. A computer reconstructs these images so they can be reviewed.

➤ Administer contrast medium, if ordered, and obtain a second series of images.

Post-test: ■

➤ Instruct the patient to resume normal activity, diet, and previous medications, unless otherwise indicated. Renal function should be assessed before metformin is restarted.

➤ Instruct the patient to increase fluid intake to help eliminate the contrast medium if used.

➤ Inform the patient that diarrhea may occur after ingesting oral contrast medium.

➤ Instruct the patient or caregiver to note change in urinary output after iodinated contrast medium administration in patients with impaired renal function.

➤ Observe for delayed allergic reactions, such as urticaria (hives), headache, nausea, or vomiting, if contrast medium was used.

➤ A physician specializing in this branch of medicine sends a written report to the ordering provider, who discusses the results with the patient.

➤ Evaluate test results in relation to the patient's symptoms and other tests performed. Related diagnostic tests include angiogram and magnetic resonance imaging of the abdomen and ultrasound of the pancreas.

COMPUTED TOMOGRAPHY, PELVIS

SYNONYMS/ACRONYMS: Computed axial tomography (CAT), computed transaxial tomography (CTT), pelvic CT.

AREA OF APPLICATION: Pelvis.

CONTRAST: Can be done with or without iodinated contrast medium.

DESCRIPTION: Computed tomography (CT) of the pelvis is a noninvasive procedure used to enhance certain anatomic views of the pelvic structures, but it becomes an invasive procedure when intravenous contrast medium is used. The patient lies on a table and moves in and out of a doughnut-like device called a *gantry*, which houses the x-ray tube and associated electronics. The scanner uses multiple x-ray beams and a series of detectors that rotate around the patient to produce cross-sectional views in a three-dimensional fashion by detecting and recording differences in tissue density after having an x-ray beam pass through them. These density measurements are sent to a computer that produces a digital image of the anatomy, enabling a physician to look at slices or thin sections of certain anatomic views, as appropriate depending on gender, of the ovaries, uterus, fallopian tubes, bladder, rectum, sigmoid colon, prostate, seminal vesicles, cervix, and associated vascular system and to determine the presence and extent of malignancy. Differentiations can be made among solid, cystic, inflammatory, or vascular lesions, and suspected hematomas or aneurysms can be identified. Iodinated contrast medium is given intravenously for blood vessel and vascular evaluation or orally for bowel and adjacent structure evaluation. Images can be recorded on photographic or x-ray film or stored in digital format as digitized computer data. Cine scanning produces a series of moving images of the scanned area. The CT scan can be used to guide biopsy needles into areas of suspected tumor to obtain tissue for laboratory analysis and to place catheters for drainage of abscesses. Tumor size, progression, and changes before and after therapy may be monitored with CT scanning. In rare cases, CT pelvimetry may be performed on a pregnant woman whose fetus is in a breech position. CT measurements are accurate, and less radiation exposure occurs to the mother and the fetus than with radiographic pelvimetry. ∎

INDICATIONS:

• Assist in differentiating between benign and malignant tumors

• Evaluate pelvic lymph nodes

• Detect tumor extension of masses and metastasis into the pelvic area

• Differentiate infectious from inflammatory processes

• Evaluate cysts, masses, abscesses, ureteral and bladder calculi, gastrointestinal bleeding and obstruction, and trauma

• Monitor and evaluate effectiveness of medical, radiation, or surgical therapies

RESULT

Normal Findings:

• Normal size, position, and shape of pelvic organs and vascular system

Abnormal Findings:

• Bladder calculi

• Ectopic pregnancy

• Fibroid tumors

• Hydrosalpinx

• Ovarian cyst or abscess

• Primary and metastatic neoplasms

CRITICAL VALUES: N/A

INTERFERING FACTORS:

This procedure is contraindicated for:

- Patients with allergies to shellfish or ⚠ iodinated dye. The contrast medium used may cause a life-threatening allergic reaction. Patients with a known hypersensitivity to the medium may benefit from premedication with corticosteroids or the use of a nonionic contrast medium.

- Patients who are claustrophobic.

- Patients who are pregnant or suspected of being pregnant, unless the potential benefits of the procedure far outweigh the risks to the fetus and mother.

- Elderly and other patients who are ⚠ chronically dehydrated before the test, because of their risk of contrast-induced renal failure.

- ⚠ Patients who are in renal failure.

- Young patients (17 years old and younger), unless the benefits of the x-ray diagnosis outweigh the risks of exposure to high levels of radiation.

Factors that may impair clear imaging:

- Inability of the patient to cooperate or remain still during the procedure because of age, significant pain, or mental status

- Patients with extreme claustrophobia unless sedation is given before the study

- Improper adjustment of the radiographic equipment to accommodate obese or thin patients, which can cause overexposure or underexposure and a poor-quality study

- Patients who are very obese, who may exceed the weight limit for the equipment

- Incorrect positioning of the patient, which may produce poor visualization of the area to be examined

- Gas or feces in the gastrointestinal tract resulting from inadequate cleansing or failure to restrict food intake before the study

- Retained barium from a previous radiologic procedure

- Metallic objects within the examination field (e.g., jewelry or body rings), which may inhibit organ visualization and can produce unclear images

Other considerations:

- Consultation with a physician should occur before the procedure for radiation safety concerns regarding infants of patients who are lactating.

- Risks associated with radiographic overexposure can result from frequent x-ray procedures. Personnel in the room with the patient should wear a protective lead apron, stand behind a shield, or leave the area while the examination is being done. Personnel working in the area where the examination is being done should wear badges that reveal their level of exposure to radiation.

Nursing Implications and Procedure • • • • • • • • • •

Pretest:

➤ Inform the patient that the procedure assesses the pelvis.

➤ Inform the patient that the procedure is done in a radiology department by a technologist and a physician and takes approximately 30 to 60 minutes.

➤ Obtain a history of allergies or sensitivities to contrast medium or shellfish.

➤ Obtain a list of medications the patient is taking.

➤ Obtain a history of the patient's pelvic system and organs, as well as results of previously performed tests, procedures, surgeries, and therapies. For related tests, refer to the reproductive, genitourinary/renal and gastrointestinal system tables.

➤ Determine previous laboratory abnormalities, especially blood urea nitrogen (BUN) and creatinine, if contrast medium is to be used.

➤ Determine date of last menstrual period and the possibility of pregnancy in perimenopausal women.

➤ Ensure that results of blood tests are obtained and recorded before the procedure.

➤ Patients receiving metformin (Glucophage) for non–insulin-dependent (type 2) diabetes should discontinue the drug on the day of the test and continue to withhold it for 48 hours after the test. Failure to do so may result in lactic acidosis.

➤ Inform the patient that he or she may experience nausea, a feeling of warmth, a salty or metallic taste, or a transient headache after injection of contrast medium, if used. Instruct the patient to take slow, deep breaths if this occurs.

➤ Ensure that any barium studies have been performed more than 4 days before the scan.

➤ The patient may be requested to drink approximately 450 mL of a dilute barium solution (approximately 1% barium) beginning 1 hour before the examination. This is done to distinguish gastrointestinal organs from the other abdominal organs.

➤ Restrict food and fluids for 6 to 8 hours, if contrast medium is to be given.

Intratest: ■

➤ Administer sedative to a child or to an uncooperative adult, as ordered.

➤ Administer antianxiety agent, as ordered, if patient is experiencing claustrophobia.

➤ Administer an antihistamine or steroid, as ordered by a physician, for patients with a known significant allergic reaction to the IV contrast medium.

➤ If the patient has had a previous barium procedure and some barium is still retained, administer an enema to remove barium from the gastrointestinal tract.

➤ Place the patient in a supine position on a flat table with foam wedges to help maintain position and immobilization. Ask the patient to lie still during the procedure because movement produces unclear images. Make sure jewelry, watches, chains, belts, and any other metallic objects have been removed.

➤ Instruct the patient to remain still when the table moves into the scanner. The scanner makes noises as it rotates around the body. The patient may be asked to take deep breaths to facilitate visualization. A number of images are taken. A computer reconstructs these images so they can be reviewed.

➤ Administer contrast medium, if ordered. A second series of images is obtained.

Post-test: ■

➤ Instruct the patient to resume normal activity, diet, and previous medication use, unless otherwise indicated. Renal function should be assessed before metformin is restarted.

➤ Instruct the patient to increase fluid intake to help eliminate the contrast medium, if used.

➤ Inform the patient that diarrhea may occur after ingesting oral contrast medium.

➤ Instruct the patient or caregiver to note change in urinary output after iodinated contrast medium administration in patients with impaired renal function.

➤ If contrast enhancement was used, observe for delayed allergic reactions, such as urticaria (hives), itching, headache, nausea, or vomiting.

➤ A physician specializing in this branch of medicine sends a written report to the ordering provider, who discusses the results with the patient.

➤ Evaluate test results in relation to the patient's symptoms and other tests performed. Related diagnostic tests include angiogram; ultrasound; kidney, ureter, and bladder (KUB) film; and magnetic resonance imaging of the abdomen.

COMPUTED TOMOGRAPHY, PITUITARY

SYNONYMS/ACRONYMS: Computed axial tomography (CAT), computed transaxial tomography (CTT), pituitary CT.

AREA OF APPLICATION: Pituitary/brain.

CONTRAST: Can be done with or without iodinated contrast medium.

DESCRIPTION: Computed tomography (CT) of the pituitary is a noninvasive procedure that enhances certain anatomic views of the pituitary gland and perisellar region, but it becomes an invasive procedure when a contrast medium is used. CT scanning is a safe and rapid method for pituitary gland evaluation. This procedure aids in the evaluation of pituitary adenoma, craniopharyngioma, meningioma, aneurysm, metastatic disease, exophthalmos, and cysts. It provides unique cross-sectional anatomic information; it is also unsurpassed in evaluating lesions containing calcium. Visualization of bony septa in the sphenoid sinus and evaluation for nonpneumatization of the sphenoid sinus are best performed with this procedure. The patient lies on a table and moves in and out of a doughnut-like device called a *gantry*, which houses the x-ray tube and associated electronics. The scanner uses multiple x-ray beams and a series of detectors that rotate around the patient to produce cross-sectional views in a three-dimensional fashion by detecting and recording differences in tissue density after having an x-ray beam passed through tissue and bone. These density measurements are sent to a computer that produces a digital image of the anatomy, enabling a physician to look at slices or thin sections of certain anatomic views of the pituitary and associated vascular system. Differentiations can be made among solid, cystic, inflammatory, or vascular lesions, and suspected hematomas and aneurysms can be identified. The procedure may be repeated after iodinated contrast medium is given intravenously for blood vessel and vascular evaluation. Images can be recorded on photographic or x-ray film or stored in digital format as digitized computer data. Cine scanning produces a series of moving images of the scanned area. Tumors, before and after therapy, may be monitored by CT scanning. ▪

INDICATIONS:

- Assist in differentiating between benign and malignant tumors

- Detect congenital anomalies, such as partially empty sella

- Detect tumor extension of masses and metastasis

- Detect aneurysms and vascular abnormalities

- Determine pituitary size and location in relation to surrounding structures

- Evaluate cysts, masses, abscesses, and trauma

- Monitor and evaluate effectiveness of medical, radiation, or surgical therapies

RESULT

Normal Findings:

- Normal size, position, and shape of the pituitary fossa, cavernous sinuses, and vascular system

Abnormal Findings:

- Abscess
- Adenoma
- Aneurysm
- Chordoma
- Craniopharyngioma
- Cyst
- Meningioma
- Metastasis
- Pituitary hemorrhage

CRITICAL VALUES: N/A

INTERFERING FACTORS:

This procedure is contraindicated for:

- Patients with allergies to shellfish or iodinated dye. The contrast medium used may cause a life-threatening allergic reaction. Patients with a known hypersensitivity to the contrast medium may benefit from premedication with corticosteroids or the use of nonionic contrast medium.

- Patients who are claustrophobic.

- Patients who are pregnant or suspected of being pregnant, unless the potential benefits of the procedure far outweigh the risks to the fetus and mother.

- Elderly and other patients who are chronically dehydrated before the test, because of their risk of contrast-induced renal failure.

- Patients who are in renal failure.

- Young patients (17 years old and younger), unless the benefits of the x-ray diagnosis outweigh the risks of exposure to high levels of radiation.

Factors that may impair clear imaging:

- Inability of the patient to cooperate or remain still during the procedure because of age, significant pain, or mental status

- Patients with extreme cases of claustrophobia, unless sedation is given before the study

- Improper adjustment of the radiographic equipment to accommodate obese or thin patients, which can cause overexposure or underexposure and a poor-quality study

- Patients who are very obese, who may exceed the weight limit for the equipment

- Incorrect positioning of the patient, which may produce poor visualization of the area to be examined

- Inability of the patient to hyperextend the neck to obtain proper images

- Metallic objects within the examination field (e.g., jewelry or body rings), which may inhibit organ visualization and can produce unclear images

Other considerations:

- Consultation with a physician should occur before the procedure for radiation safety concerns regarding infants of patients who are lactating.

- Risks associated with radiographic overexposure can result from frequent x-ray procedures. Personnel in the room with the patient should wear a protective lead apron, stand behind a shield, or leave the area while the examination is being done. Personnel working in the area where the examination is being done should wear badges that reveal their level of exposure to radiation.

Nursing Implications and Procedure • • • • • • • • • •

Pretest:

➤ Inform the patient that the procedure assesses the pituitary gland.

➤ Inform the patient that the procedure is performed in a radiology department by a technologist and a physician and takes approximately 30 to 60 minutes.

➤ Obtain a history of allergies or sensitivities to contrast medium or shellfish.

➤ Obtain a list of medications the patient is taking.

➤ Obtain a history of the patient's endocrine system as well as results of previously performed tests, procedures, treatments, and surgeries. For related tests, refer to the musculoskeletal, endocrine, and cardiovascular system tables.

➤ Determine previous laboratory abnormalities, especially blood urea nitrogen (BUN) and creatinine, if contrast medium is to be used.

➤ Determine date of last menstrual period and the possibility of pregnancy in perimenopausal women.

➤ Ensure that the results of blood tests are obtained and recorded before the procedure.

➤ Patients receiving metformin (Glucophage) for non–insulin-dependent (type 2) diabetes should discontinue the drug on the day of the test and continue to withhold it for 48 hours after the test. Failure to do so may result in lactic acidosis.

➤ Inform the patient that he or she may experience nausea, a feeling of warmth, a salty or metallic taste, or a transient headache after injection of contrast medium, if given. Instruct the patient to take slow, deep breaths if this occurs.

➤ Do not restrict food and fluids for this procedure; however, if contrast medium is given, restrict food and fluids for 6 to 8 hours.

Intratest:

➤ Administer sedative to a child or to an uncooperative adult, as ordered.

➤ Administer antianxiety agent, as ordered, if the patient is experiencing claustrophobia.

➤ Administer an antihistamine or steroid, as ordered by a physician, for patients with a known significant allergic reaction to the IV contrast medium.

➤ Place the patient in a supine position on a flat table with foam wedges to help maintain position and immobilization. Ask the patient to lie still during the procedure because movement produces unclear images. Make sure jewelry and any other metallic objects have been removed.

➤ As the table moves into the scanner,

instruct the patient to remain still. The scanner makes noises as it rotates around the body. The patient may be asked to take deep breaths to facilitate visualization. A number of images are taken. A computer reconstructs these images so they can be reviewed.

➤ Administer contrast medium, if ordered. A second series of images is obtained.

Post-test:

➤ Instruct the patient to resume normal activity, diet, and previous medication use, unless otherwise indicated. Renal function should be assessed before metformin is restarted.

➤ Instruct the patient to increase fluid intake to help eliminate the contrast medium, if used.

➤ Instruct the patient or caregiver to note any changes in urinary output after iodinated contrast medium administration in patients with impaired renal function.

➤ Observe for delayed allergic reactions, such as urticaria (hives), headache, nausea, or vomiting, if using contrast medium.

➤ A physician specializing in this branch of medicine sends a written report to the ordering provider, who discusses the results with the patient.

➤ Evaluate test results in relation to the patient's symptoms and other tests performed. Related diagnostic tests include CT, positron emission tomography, and magnetic resonance imaging of the brain; and CT angiography and magnetic resonance angiography.

COMPUTED TOMOGRAPHY, RENAL

· ·

SYNONYMS/ACRONYM: Computed axial tomography (CAT), computed transaxial tomography (CTT), kidney CT.

AREA OF APPLICATION: Kidney.

CONTRAST: Can be done with or without iodinated contrast medium.

DESCRIPTION: Renal computed tomography (CT) is a noninvasive procedure used to enhance certain anatomic views of the renal structures, but it becomes an invasive procedure when a contrast medium is used. CT scanning is a safe and rapid method for renal evaluation that is independent of renal function. It provides unique cross-sectional anatomic information and is unsur- passed in evaluating lesions contain- ing fat or calcium. The patient lies on a table and is moved in and out of a doughnut-like device called a *gantry*, which houses the x-ray tube and asso- ciated electronics. The scanner uses multiple x-ray beams and a series of detectors that rotate around the patient to produce cross-sectional views in a three-dimensional fashion by detecting and recording differences in tissue density after having an x-ray beam passed through the tissues. These density measurements are sent to a computer that produces a digital image of the anatomy, enabling a physician to look at slices or thin sections of certain anatomic views of the kidneys and associated vascular system. Differentiations can be made among solid, cystic, inflammatory, or vascular lesions, and suspected hematomas and aneurysms can be identified. The procedure is repeated after iodinated contrast medium is given intravenously for blood vessel and vascular evaluation or orally for bowel and adjacent structure evaluation. Images can be recorded on photographic or x-ray film or stored in digital format as digitized computer data. Cine scanning produces a series of moving images of the area scanned. The CT scan can be used to guide biopsy needles into areas of suspected tumors to obtain tissue for laboratory analysis and to guide placement of catheters for drainage of renal abscesses. Tumors, before and after therapy, may be monitored with CT scanning. ■

INDICATIONS:

• Assist in differentiating between benign and malignant tumors

• Evaluate abnormal fluid accumulation around the kidney

• Aid in the diagnosis of congenital anomalies, such as polycystic kidney disease, horseshoe kidney, absence of one kidney, or kidney displacement

• Detect tumor extension of masses and metastasis into the renal area

• Detect aneurysms and vascular abnormalities

• Determine kidney size and location in

relation to the bladder in post-transplant patients

• Detect bleeding or hyperplasia of the adrenal glands

• Determine presence and type of adrenal tumor, such as benign adenoma, cancer, or pheochromocytoma

• Evaluate spread of a tumor or invasion of nearby retroperitoneal organs

• Aid in the diagnosis of perirenal hematomas and abscesses and assist in localizing for drainage

• Assist in differentiating between an infectious and an inflammatory process

• Evaluate cysts, masses, abscesses, renal calculi, obstruction, and trauma

• Monitor and evaluate effectiveness of medical, radiation, or surgical therapies

RESULT

Normal Findings:

• Normal size, position, and shape of kidneys and vascular system

Abnormal Findings:

• Adrenal tumor or hyperplasia

• Congenital anomalies, such as polycystic kidney disease, horseshoe kidney, absence of one kidney, or kidney displacement

• Dilation of the common hepatic duct, common bile duct, or gallbladder

• Renal artery aneurysm

• Primary and metastatic neoplasms

• Renal cysts or abscesses

• Renal cell carcinoma

• Renal laceration, fracture, tumor, and trauma

• Renal calculi, ureteral obstruction

• Perirenal abscesses and hematomas

CRITICAL VALUES: N/A

INTERFERING FACTORS:

This procedure is contraindicated for:

- Patients with allergies to shellfish ⚠ or iodinated dye. The contrast medium used may cause a life-threatening allergic reaction. Patients with a known hypersensitivity to the contrast medium may benefit from premedication with corticosteroids or the use of nonionic contrast medium.

- Patients who are claustrophobic.

- Elderly and other patients who are ⚠ chronically dehydrated before the test, because of their risk of contrast-induced renal failure.

- ⚠ Patients who are in renal failure.

- Young patients (17 years old and younger), unless the benefits of the x-ray diagnosis outweigh the risks of exposure to high levels of radiation.

Factors that may impair clear imaging:

- Inability of the patient to cooperate or remain still during the procedure because of age, significant pain, or mental status

- Patients with extreme cases of claustrophobia, unless sedation is given before the study

- Improper adjustment of the radiographic equipment to accommodate obese or thin patients, which can cause overexposure or underexposure and a poor-quality study

- Patients who are very obese, who may exceed the weight limit for the equipment

- Incorrect positioning of the patient, which may produce poor visualization of the area to be examined

- Gas or feces in the gastrointestinal tract resulting from inadequate cleansing or failure to restrict food intake before the study

- Retained barium from a previous radiologic procedure

- Metallic objects within the examination field (e.g., jewelry or body rings), which may inhibit organ visualization and can produce unclear images

Other considerations:

- Failure to follow dietary restrictions before the procedure may cause the procedure to be canceled or repeated.

- Consultation with a physician should occur before the procedure for radiation safety concerns regarding infants of patients who are lactating.

- Risks associated with radiographic overexposure can result from frequent x-ray procedures. Personnel in the room with the patient should wear a protective lead apron, stand behind a shield, or leave the area while the examination is being done. Personnel working in the area where the examination is being done should wear badges that reveal their level of exposure to radiation.

Nursing Implications and Procedure • • • • • • • • • • •

Pretest: ■

➤ Inform the patient that the procedure assesses the kidneys.

➤ Inform the patient that the procedure is performed in a radiology department by a technologist and a physician and takes approximately 30 to 60 minutes.

➤ Obtain a history of allergies or sensitivities to contrast medium or shellfish.

➤ Obtain a list of medications the patient is taking.

➤ Obtain a history of the patient's renal system as well as results of previously performed tests, treatments, surgeries, and procedures. For related tests, refer to the genitourinary/renal system table.

➤ Determine previous laboratory abnormalities, especially blood urea nitrogen (BUN) and creatinine, if contrast medium is to be used.

➤ Determine date of last menstrual period and the possibility of pregnancy in perimenopausal women.

➤ Ensure that the results of blood tests are obtained and recorded before the procedure.

➤ Patients receiving metformin (Glucophage) for non–insulin-dependent (type 2) diabetes should discontinue the drug on the day of the test and continue to withhold it for 48 hours after the test. Failure to do so may result in lactic acidosis.

➤ Inform the patient that he or she may experience nausea, a feeling of warmth, a salty or metallic taste, or a transient headache after injection of contrast medium, if given. Instruct the patient to take slow, deep breaths if this occurs.

➤ Question the patient to ensure that barium studies were performed more than 4 days before the scan.

➤ The patient may be requested to drink approximately 450 mL of a dilute barium solution (approximately 1% barium) beginning 1 hour before the examination. A barium study is done to distinguish gastrointestinal organs from the kidneys.

➤ Restrict food and fluids for 6 to 8 hours if contrast medium is to be given.

Intratest: ■

➤ Administer sedative to a child or to an uncooperative adult, as ordered.

➤ Administer antianxiety agent, as ordered, if the patient is experiencing claustrophobia.

➤ Administer an antihistamine or steroid, as ordered by a physician, for patients with a known significant allergic reaction to the IV contrast medium.

➤ Administer an enema to remove barium from the gastrointestinal tract, as ordered.

➤ Place the patient in a supine position on a flat table with foam wedges that help maintain position and immobilization. Ask the patient to lie still during the procedure because movement produces unclear images. Make sure jewelry, watches, chains, belts, and any other metallic objects have been removed.

➤ As the table is moved into the scanner, instruct the patient to remain still. The scanner makes noises as it rotates around the body. The patient may be asked to take deep breaths to facilitate visualization. A number of images are taken. A computer reconstructs these images so they can be reviewed.

➤ Administer a contrast medium, if ordered. A second series of images is obtained.

Post-test: ■

➤ Instruct the patient to resume normal activity, diet, and previous medication use, unless otherwise indicated. Renal function should be assessed before metformin is restarted.

➤ Instruct the patient to increase fluid intake to help eliminate the contrast medium, if used.

➤ Inform the patient that diarrhea may occur after ingesting oral contrast medium.

➤ Instruct the patient or caregiver to note change in urinary output after iodinated contrast medium administration in patients with impaired renal function.

➤ Observe for delayed allergic reactions, such as urticaria (hives), headache, nausea, or vomiting, if contrast enhancement was used.

➤ A physician specializing in this branch of medicine sends a written report to the ordering provider, who discusses the results with the patient.

➤ Evaluate test results in relation to

the patient's symptoms and other tests performed. Related diagnostic tests include intravenous pyelogra- phy; magnetic resonance imaging and CT of the abdomen; and kidney, ureter, and bladder (KUB) film.

COMPUTED TOMOGRAPHY, SPINE

SYNONYMS/ACRONYMS: Computed axial tomography (CAT), computed transaxial tomography (CTT), spine CT, CT myelogram.

AREA OF APPLICATION: Spine.

CONTRAST: Can be done with or without iodinated contrast medium.

DESCRIPTION: Computed tomography (CT) of the spine is a noninvasive procedure that enhances certain anatomic views of the spinal structures, but it becomes an invasive procedure when intravenous contrast medium is used. CT scanning is more versatile than conventional radiography and can easily detect and identify tumors and their types. The patient lies on a table and is moved in and out of a doughnut-like device called a *gantry*, which houses the x-ray tube and associated electronics. The scanner uses multiple x-ray beams and a series of detectors that rotate around the patient to produce cross-sectional views in a three-dimensional fashion by detecting and recording differences in tissue density after having an x-ray beam passed through the tissues. These density measurements are sent to a computer that produces a digital image of the anatomy, enabling a physician to look at slices or thin sections of certain anatomic views of the spine and associated vascular system and to determine the extent of malignancy. Differentiations can be made among solid, cystic, inflammatory, or vascular lesions, and suspected hematomas and aneurysms can be identified. Iodinated contrast medium is given intravenously for blood vessel and vascular evaluation or orally for bowel and adjacent structure evaluation. Images can be recorded on photographic or x-ray film or stored in digital format as digitized computer data. Cine scanning produces a series of moving images of the scanned area. CT scanning can be used to guide biopsy needles into areas of suspected tumor to obtain tissue for laboratory analysis and to guide placement of catheters for drainage of abscesses. Tumor size, progression, and pretherapy and post-therapy changes may be monitored with CT scanning. ■

INDICATIONS:

• Assist in differentiating between benign and malignant tumors

• Detect paraspinal cysts

• Detect vascular malformations

• Detect congenital spinal anomalies, such as spina bifida, meningocele, and myelocele

• Detect herniated intervertebral disks

• Monitor and evaluate effectiveness of medical, radiation, or surgical therapies

RESULT

Normal Findings:

• Normal density, size, position, and shape of spinal structures

Abnormal Findings:

• Congenital spinal malformations, such as meningocele, myelocele, or spina bifida

• Herniated intervertebral disks

• Paraspinal cysts

• Spinal tumors

• Spondylosis (cervical or lumbar)

• Vascular malformations

CRITICAL VALUES: N/A

INTERFERING FACTORS:

This procedure is contraindicated for:

• Patients with allergies to shellfish or iodinated dye. The contrast medium used may cause a life-threatening allergic reaction. Patients with a known hypersensitivity to the contrast medium may benefit from premedication with corticosteroids or the use of nonionic contrast medium.

• Patients who are claustrophobic.

• Patients who are pregnant or suspected of being pregnant, unless the potential benefits of the procedure far outweigh the risks to the fetus and mother.

• Elderly and other patients who are chronically dehydrated before the test, because of their risk of contrast-induced renal failure.

• Patients who are in renal failure.

• Young patients (17 years old and younger), unless the benefits of the x-ray diagnosis outweigh the risks of exposure to high levels of radiation.

Factors that may impair clear imaging:

• Inability of the patient to cooperate or remain still during the procedure because of age, significant pain, or mental status

• Patients with extreme cases of claustrophobia, unless sedation is given before the study

• Improper adjustment of the radiographic equipment to accommodate obese or thin patients, which can cause overexposure or underexposure and a poor-quality study

• Patients who are very obese, who may exceed the weight limit for the equipment

• Incorrect positioning of the patient, which may produce poor visualization of the area to be examined

• Gas or feces in the gastrointestinal tract resulting from inadequate cleansing or failure to restrict food intake before the study

• Retained barium from a previous radiologic procedure

• Metallic objects within the examination field (e.g., jewelry or body rings), which may inhibit organ visualization and can produce unclear images

Other considerations:

- Consultation with a physician should occur before the procedure for radiation safety concerns regarding infants of patients who are lactating.

- Risks associated with radiographic overexposure can result from frequent x-ray procedures. Personnel in the room with the patient should wear a protective lead apron, stand behind a shield, or leave the area while the examination is being done. Personnel working in the area where the examination is being done should wear badges that reveal their level of exposure to radiation.

Nursing Implications and Procedure • • • • • • • • • •

Pretest:

➤ Inform the patient that the procedure assesses the spine.

➤ Inform the patient that the procedure is performed in a radiology department by a technologist and a physician and takes approximately 30 to 60 minutes.

➤ Obtain a history of allergies or sensitivities to contrast medium or shellfish.

➤ Obtain a list of medications the patient is taking.

➤ Obtain a history of the patient's spine as well as results of previously performed tests, procedures, trauma, surgeries, and therapies. For related tests, refer to the musculoskeletal system table.

➤ Determine previous laboratory abnormalities, especially blood urea nitrogen (BUN) and creatinine, if contrast medium is to be used.

➤ Determine date of last menstrual period and the possibility of pregnancy in perimenopausal women.

➤ Ensure that the results of blood tests are obtained and recorded before the procedure.

➤ Patients receiving metformin (Glucophage) for non–insulin-dependent (type 2) diabetes should discontinue the drug on the day of the test and continue to withhold it for 48 hours after the test. Failure to do so may result in lactic acidosis.

➤ Inform the patient that he or she may experience nausea, a feeling of warmth, a salty or metallic taste, or a transient headache after injection of contrast medium, if given. Instruct the patient to take slow, deep breaths if this occurs.

➤ Question the patient to ensure that barium studies were performed more than 4 days before the scan.

➤ Restrict food and fluids for 6 to 8 hours, if contrast medium is to be given.

Intratest:

➤ Administer sedative to a child or to an uncooperative adult, as ordered.

➤ Administer antianxiety agent, as ordered, if the patient is experiencing claustrophobia.

➤ Administer an antihistamine or steroid, as ordered by a physician, for patients with a known significant allergic reaction to the IV contrast medium.

➤ Place the patient in a supine position on a flat table with foam wedges to help maintain position and immobilization. Ask the patient to lie still during the procedure because movement produces unclear images. Make sure jewelry, watches, chains, belts, and any other metallic objects have been removed.

➤ As the table moves into the scanner, instruct the patient to remain still. The scanner makes noises as it rotates around the body. The patient may be asked to take deep breaths to facilitate visualization. A number of images are taken. A computer reconstructs these images so they can be reviewed.

➤ Administer contrast medium, if ordered. A second series of images is obtained.

➤ If a CT myelogram is requested, the patient is removed from the scanner, and a lumbar puncture is performed. A small amount of cerebrospinal fluid is removed and replaced with contrast medium. The patient is placed back into the scanner, and another series of images is obtained.

Post-test:

➤ Instruct the patient to resume normal activity, diet, and previous medication use, unless otherwise indicated. Renal function should be assessed before metformin is restarted.

➤ Instruct the patient to increase fluid intake to help eliminate the contrast medium, if used.

➤ Inform the patient that diarrhea may occur after ingesting oral contrast medium.

➤ Instruct the patient or caregiver to note any change in urinary output after iodinated contrast medium administration in patients with impaired renal function.

➤ Observe for delayed allergic reactions, such as urticaria (hives), headache, nausea, or vomiting, if contrast enhancement was used.

➤ If a CT myelogram was performed, instruct the patient to remain prone for 8 hours.

➤ A physician specializing in this branch of medicine sends a written report to the ordering provider, who discusses the results with the patient.

➤ Evaluate test results in relation to the patient's symptoms and other tests performed. Related diagnostic tests include musculoskeletal magnetic resonance imaging and bone x-rays.

COMPUTED TOMOGRAPHY, SPLEEN

· ·

SYNONYMS/ACRONYMS: Computed axial tomography (CAT), computed transaxial tomography (CTT), splenic CT.

AREA OF APPLICATION: Abdomen/spleen.

CONTRAST: Can be done with or without iodinated contrast medium.

DESCRIPTION: Computed tomography (CT) of the spleen is a noninvasive procedure that enhances certain anatomic views of the splenic structures, but it becomes an invasive procedure with the use of contrast medium. The spleen is not often the organ of interest when abdominal CT scans are obtained. However, a wide variety of splenic variations and abnormalities may be detected on abdominal scans designed to evaluate the liver, pancreas, or retroperitoneum. The patient lies on a table and is moved in and out of a doughnut-like device called a *gantry,* which houses the x-ray tube and associated electronics. The scanner uses multiple x-ray beams and a series of detectors that rotate around the patient to produce cross-sectional views in a three-dimensional fashion by detecting and recording differences in tissue density after having an x-ray beam passed through the tissues. These density measurements are sent to a computer that produces a digital image of the anatomy, enabling a physician to look at slices or thin sections of certain anatomic views of the spleen and vascular system. Differentiations can be made among solid, cystic, inflammatory, or vascular lesions, and suspected hematomas and aneurysms can be identified. CT is the first choice in the evaluation of abdominal trauma because of its diagnostic accuracy. Iodinated contrast medium is given intravenously for blood vessel and vascular evaluation or orally for bowel and adjacent structure evaluation. Images can be recorded on photographic or x-ray film or stored in digital format as digitized computer data. Cine scanning produces a series of moving images of the scanned area. CT scanning can be used to guide biopsy needles into areas of tumor to obtain tissue for laboratory analysis and to guide placement of catheters for drainage of abscesses. Tumors, before and after medical or surgical therapy, may be monitored with CT scanning. ■

INDICATIONS:

- Assist in differentiating between benign and malignant tumors

- Detect tumor extension of masses and metastasis

- Differentiate infectious from inflammatory processes

- Evaluate cysts, masses, abscesses, and trauma

- Monitor and evaluate effectiveness of medical, radiation, or surgical therapies

- Evaluate splenic vein thrombosis

- Evaluate the presence of an accessory spleen, polysplenia, or asplenia

RESULT

Normal Findings:

- Normal size, position, and shape of the spleen and associated vascular system

Abnormal Findings:

- Abdominal aortic aneurysm

- Hematomas

- Hemoperitoneum

- Primary and metastatic neoplasms

- Splenic cysts or abscesses

- Splenic laceration, tumor, infiltration, and trauma

CRITICAL VALUES: N/A

INTERFERING FACTORS:

This procedure is contraindicated for:

- Patients with allergies to shellfish or ⚠ iodinated dye. The contrast medium used may cause a life-threatening allergic reaction. Patients with a known hypersensitivity to the contrast medium may benefit from premedication with corticosteroids or the use of nonionic contrast medium.

- Patients who are claustrophobic.

- Patients who are pregnant or suspected of being pregnant, unless the potential benefits of the procedure far outweigh the risks to the fetus and mother.

- Elderly and other patients who are ⚠ chronically dehydrated before the test, because of their risk of contrast-induced renal failure.

• Patients who are in renal failure.

• Young patients (17 years old and younger), unless the benefits of the x-ray diagnosis outweigh the risks of exposure to high levels of radiation.

Factors that may impair clear imaging include:

• Inability of the patient to cooperate or remain still during the procedure because of age, significant pain, or mental status

• Patients with extreme cases of claustrophobia, unless sedation is given before the study

• Improper adjustment of the radiographic equipment to accommodate obese or thin patients, which can cause overexposure or underexposure and a poor-quality study

• Patients who are very obese, who may exceed the weight limit for the equipment

• Incorrect positioning of the patient, which may produce poor visualization of the area to be examined

• Gas or feces in the gastrointestinal tract, resulting from inadequate cleansing or failure to restrict food intake before the study

• Metallic objects within the examination field (e.g., jewelry or body rings), which may inhibit organ visualization and can produce unclear images

Other considerations:

• Failure to follow dietary restrictions before the procedure may cause the procedure to be canceled or repeated.

• Consultation with a physician should occur before the procedure for radiation safety concerns regarding infants of patients who are lactating.

• Risks associated with radiographic overexposure can result from frequent x-ray procedures. Personnel in the room with the patient should wear a protective lead apron, stand behind a shield, or leave the area while the examination is being done. Personnel working in the area where the examination is being done should wear badges that reveal their level of exposure to radiation.

Nursing Implications and Procedure • • • • • • • • • • •

Pretest: ■

➤ Inform the patient that the procedure assesses the spleen.

➤ Inform the patient that the procedure is performed in a radiology department by a technologist and a physician and takes approximately 30 to 60 minutes.

➤ Obtain a history of allergies or sensitivities to contrast medium or shellfish.

➤ Obtain a list of medications the patient is taking.

➤ Obtain a history of the patient's abdominal systems and organs, as well as results of previously performed tests and procedures. For related tests, refer to the gastrointestinal system table.

➤ Determine previous laboratory abnormalities, especially blood urea nitrogen (BUN) and creatinine, if contrast medium is to be used.

➤ Determine date of last menstrual period and the possibility of pregnancy in perimenopausal women.

➤ Ensure that the results of blood tests are obtained and recorded before the procedure.

➤ Patients receiving metformin (Glucophage) for non–insulin-dependent (type 2) diabetes should discontinue the drug on the day of the test and continue to withhold it for 48 hours after the test. Failure to do so may result in lactic acidosis.

➤ Inform the patient that he or she

may experience nausea, a feeling of warmth, a salty or metallic taste, or a transient headache after injection of contrast medium, if given. Instruct the patient to take slow, deep breaths if this occurs.

➤ Question the patient to ensure that barium studies were performed more than 4 days before the scan.

➤ The patient may be requested to drink approximately 900 mL of a dilute barium solution (approximately 1% barium) beginning 1 hour before the examination. This barium study helps to distinguish the spleen from the other abdominal organs.

➤ Restrict food and fluids for 6 to 8 hours, if contrast medium is to be given.

Intratest:

➤ Administer sedative to a child or to an uncooperative adult, as ordered.

➤ Administer antianxiety agent, as ordered, if the patient is experiencing claustrophobia.

➤ Administer an antihistamine or steroid, as ordered by a physician, for patients with a known significant allergic reaction to the IV contrast medium.

➤ Administer an enema to remove barium from the gastrointestinal tract, as ordered.

➤ Place the patient in a supine position on a flat table with foam wedges to help maintain position and immobilization. Ask the patient to lie still during the procedure because movement produces unclear images. Make sure jewelry, watches, chains, belts, and any other metallic objects have been removed.

➤ As the table moves into the scanner, instruct the patient to remain still.

The scanner makes noises as it rotates around the body. The patient may be asked to take deep breaths to facilitate visualization. A number of images are taken. A computer reconstructs these images so they can be reviewed.

➤ Administer contrast medium, if ordered. A second series of images is obtained.

Post-test:

➤ Instruct the patient to resume normal activity, diet, and previous medication use, unless otherwise indicated. Renal function should be assessed before metformin is restarted.

➤ Instruct the patient to increase fluid intake to help eliminate contrast medium, if used.

➤ Inform the patient that diarrhea may occur after ingesting oral contrast medium.

➤ Instruct the patient or caregiver to note any change in urinary output after iodinated contrast medium administration in patients with impaired renal function.

➤ Observe for delayed allergic reactions, such as urticaria (hives), headache, nausea, or vomiting, if contrast medium was used.

➤ A physician specializing in this branch of medicine sends a written report to the ordering provider, who discusses the results with the patient.

➤ Evaluate test results in relation to the patient's symptoms and other tests performed. Related diagnostic tests include ultrasound of the spleen and CT and magnetic resonance imaging of the abdomen.

COMPUTED TOMOGRAPHY, THORACIC

SYNONYMS/ACRONYMS: Computed axial tomography (CAT), computed transaxial tomography (CTT), chest CT.

AREA OF APPLICATION: Thorax.

CONTRAST: Can be done with or without iodinated contrast medium.

DESCRIPTION: Computed tomography (CT) of the thorax is more detailed than a chest x-ray. It is a noninvasive procedure used to enhance certain anatomic views of the lungs, heart, and mediastinal structures. The patient lies on a table and is moved in and out of a doughnut-like device called a *gantry*, which houses the x-ray tube and associated electronics. The scanner uses multiple x-ray beams and a series of detectors that rotate around the patient to produce cross-sectional views in a three-dimensional fashion by detecting and recording differences in tissue density after having an x-ray beam passed through the tissues. These density measurements are sent to a computer that produces a digital image of the anatomy, enabling a physician to look at slices or thin sections of certain anatomic views of the spine, spinal cord, and lung areas. Iodinated contrast medium is given intravenously for blood vessel and vascular evaluation or orally for esophageal evaluation. Images can be recorded on photographic or x-ray film or stored in digital format as digitized computer data. Cine scanning is used to produce moving images of the heart. ■

INDICATIONS:

• Detect primary and metastatic pulmonary, esophageal, or mediastinal tumors

• Differentiate between benign tumors (granulomas) and malignancies

• Detect mediastinal and hilar lymphadenopathy

• Detect lymphomas, especially Hodgkin's disease

• Detect tumor extension of neck mass to thoracic area

• Differentiate tumor from tuberculosis (which appears as coin-sized, calcified lesions)

• Detect bronchial abnormalities, such as stenosis, dilation, or tumor

• Detect aortic aneurysms

• Differentiate aortic aneurysms from tumors near the aorta

• Differentiate infectious from inflammatory processes (abscess, nodules, or pneumonitis)

- Determine blood, fluid, or fat accumulation in tissues, pleuritic space, or vessels

- Evaluate cardiac chambers and pulmonary vessels

- Evaluate the presence of plaque in cardiac vessels

- Monitor and evaluate effectiveness of medical or surgical therapeutic regimen

RESULT

Normal Findings:

- Normal size, position, and shape of chest organs, tissues, and structures

Abnormal Findings:

- Aortic aneurysm

- Chest lesions (benign lesions, neoplastic tumors, or metastatic mediastinal lesions to ribs or spine)

- Cysts or abscesses

- Enlarged lymph nodes

- Esophageal pathology including tumors

- Hodgkin's disease

- Pleural effusion

- Pneumonitis

CRITICAL VALUES: N/A

INTERFERING FACTORS:

This procedure is contraindicated for:

- Patients with allergies to shellfish or iodinated dye. The contrast medium used may cause a life-threatening allergic reaction. Patients with a known hypersensitivity to the contrast medium may benefit from premedication with corticosteroids or the use of nonionic contrast medium.

- Patients who are claustrophobic.

- Patients who are pregnant or suspected of being pregnant, unless the potential benefits of the procedure far outweigh the risks to the fetus and mother.

- Elderly and other patients who are chronically dehydrated before the test, because of their risk of contrast-induced renal failure.

- Patients who are in renal failure.

- Young patients (17 years old and younger), unless the benefits of the x-ray diagnosis outweigh the risks of exposure to high levels of radiation.

Factors that may impair clear imaging include:

- Inability of the patient to cooperate or remain still during the procedure because of age, significant pain, or mental status

- Patients with extreme cases of claustrophobia, unless sedation is given before the study

- Improper adjustment of the radiographic equipment to accommodate obese or thin patients, which can cause overexposure or underexposure and a poor-quality study

- Patients who are very obese, who may exceed the weight limit for the equipment

- Incorrect positioning of the patient, which may produce poor visualization of the area to be examined

- Metallic objects within the examination field (e.g., jewelry or body rings), which may inhibit organ visualization and can produce unclear images

Other considerations:

- A consultation with a physician should occur before the procedure for radiation safety concerns regarding infants of patients who are lactating.

• Risks associated with radiographic overexposure can result from frequent x-ray procedures. Personnel in the room with the patient should wear a protective lead apron, stand behind a shield, or leave the area while the examination is being done. Personnel working in the area where the examination is being done should wear badges that reveal their level of exposure to radiation.

Nursing Implications and Procedure · · · · · · · · · · · ·

Pretest:

➤ Inform the patient that the procedure assesses the chest.

➤ Inform the patient that the procedure is performed in a radiology department by a technologist and a physician and takes approximately 30 to 60 minutes.

➤ Obtain a history of allergies or sensitivities to contrast medium or shellfish.

➤ Obtain a list of medications the patient is taking.

➤ Obtain a history of the patient's respiratory and cardiac systems, as well as results of previously performed tests and procedures. For related tests, refer to the respiratory and cardiovascular system tables.

➤ Determine previous laboratory abnormalities, especially blood urea nitrogen (BUN) and creatinine, if contrast medium is to be used.

➤ Ensure that the results of blood tests are obtained and recorded before the procedure.

➤ Patients receiving metformin (Glucophage) for non–insulin-dependent (type 2) diabetes should discontinue the drug on the day of the test and continue to withhold it for 48 hours after the test. Failure to do so may result in lactic acidosis.

➤ Inform the patient that he or she may experience nausea, a feeling of

warmth, a salty or metallic taste, or a transient headache after injection of contrast medium, if given. Instruct the patient to take slow, deep breaths if this occurs.

➤ Restrict food and fluids for 6 to 8 hours, if contrast medium is to be given.

Intratest:

➤ Administer sedative to a child or to an uncooperative adult, as ordered.

➤ Administer antianxiety agent, as ordered, if the patient is experiencing claustrophobia.

➤ Administer an antihistamine or steroid, as ordered by a physician, for patients with a known significant allergic reaction to the IV contrast medium.

➤ Place the patient in a supine position on a flat table with foam wedges that help maintain position and immobilization. Ask the patient to lie still during the procedure because movement produces unclear images. Make sure jewelry, watches, chains, belts, and any other metallic objects have been removed.

➤ As the table moves into the scanner, instruct the patient to remain still. The scanner makes noises as it rotates around the body. The patient may be asked to take deep breaths to facilitate visualization. A number of images are taken. A computer reconstructs these images so they can be reviewed.

➤ Administer a contrast medium, if ordered. A second series of images is obtained.

Post-test:

➤ Instruct the patient to resume normal activity, diet, and previous medication use, unless otherwise indicated. Renal function should be assessed before metformin is restarted.

➤ Instruct the patient to increase fluid intake to help eliminate contrast medium, if used.

> Instruct the patient or caregiver to note change in urinary output after iodinated contrast medium administration in patients with impaired renal function.

> Observe for delayed allergic reactions, such as urticaria (hives), headache, nausea, or vomiting, if contrast enhancement was used.

> A physician specializing in this

branch of medicine sends a written report to the ordering provider, who discusses the results with the patient.

> Evaluate test results in relation to the patient's symptoms and other tests performed. Related diagnostic tests include chest x-ray, magnetic resonance imaging of the chest, and lung scan.

COOMBS' ANTIGLOBULIN, DIRECT

SYNONYM/ACRONYM: Direct antiglobulin testing (DAT).

SPECIMEN: Serum (1 mL) collected in a red-top tube. Whole blood (1 mL) collected in lavender-top (ethylenediaminetetra-acetic acid [EDTA]) tube.

REFERENCE VALUE: (Method: Agglutination) Negative (no agglutination).

DESCRIPTION: Direct antiglobulin testing (DAT) detects in *vivo* antibody sensitization of red blood cells (RBCs). Immunoglobulin G (IgG) produced in certain disease states or in response to certain drugs can coat the surface of RBCs, resulting in cellular damage and hemolysis. When DAT is performed, RBCs are taken from the patient's blood sample, washed with saline to remove residual globulins, and mixed with antihuman globulin reagent. If the antihuman globulin reagent causes agglutination of the patient's RBCs, specific antiglobulin reagents can be used to determine whether the patient's RBCs are coated with IgG, comple-

ment, or both. (See monograph titled "Blood Groups and Antibodies" for more information regarding transfusion reactions.) ∎

INDICATIONS:

• Detect autoimmune hemolytic anemia or hemolytic disease of the newborn

• Evaluate suspected drug-induced hemolytic anemia

• Evaluate transfusion reaction

RESULT

Positive in:

• Anemia (autoimmune hemolytic, drug-induced)

- Hemolytic disease of the newborn

- Infectious mononucleosis

- Systemic lupus erythematosus and other connective tissue immune disorders

- Lymphomas

- Mycoplasma pneumonia

- Paroxysmal cold hemoglobinuria (idiopathic or disease related)

- Passively acquired antibodies from plasma products

- Post–cardiac vascular surgery

- Transfusion reactions (blood incompatibility)

Negative in:

- Samples in which sensitization of erythrocytes has not occurred

CRITICAL VALUES: N/A

INTERFERING FACTORS:

- Drugs and substances that may cause a positive DAT include acetaminophen, aminosalicylic acid, aminopyrine, ampicillin, antihistamines, aztreonam, cephalosporins, chlorinated hydrocarbon insecticides, chlorpromazine, chlorpropamide, cisplatin, clonidine, dipyrone, ethosuximide, fenfluramine, hydralazine, hydrochlorothiazide, ibuprofen, insulin, isoniazid, levodopa, mefenamic acid, melphalan, methadone, methicillin, methyldopa, moxalactam, penicillin, phenytoin, probenecid, procainamide, quinidine, quinine, rifampin, streptomycin, stibophen, sulfonamides, and tetracycline.

- Wharton's jelly may cause a false-positive DAT.

- Cold agglutinins and large amounts of paraproteins in the specimen may cause false-positive results.

- Newborns' cells may give negative results in ABO hemolytic disease.

Nursing Implications and Procedure

Pretest:

➤ Obtain a history of the patient's complaints, including a list of known allergens.

➤ Obtain a history of the patient's hematopoietic system as well as results of previously performed tests and procedures. For related tests, refer to the hematopoietic system table.

➤ Obtain a list of all medications the patient is taking, including herbs, nutritional supplements, and nutraceuticals. The requesting health care practitioner and laboratory should be advised if the patient is regularly using these products so that their effects can be taken into consideration when reviewing results.

➤ There are no food, fluid, or medication restrictions unless by medical direction.

➤ Review the procedure with the patient. If a cord sample is to be taken from a newborn, inform parents that the sample will be obtained at the time of delivery and will not result in blood loss to the infant.

➤ Inform the patient that specimen collection takes approximately 5 to 10 minutes.

Intratest:

➤ Direct the patient to breathe normally and to avoid unnecessary movement.

➤ Observe standard precautions and follow the general guidelines in Appendix A. Perform a venipuncture, and collect the specimen in a 5-mL red-top (serum) and lavender-top (whole blood) tube. Cord specimens are obtained by inserting a needle attached to a syringe into the umbilical vein. The specimen is drawn into the syringe and gently expressed into the appropriate collection container.

➤ Label the specimen, and promptly transport it to the laboratory.

Post-test:

➤ Observe venipuncture site for bleeding or hematoma formation. Apply pressure bandage.

➤ Note positive test results in cord blood of neonate; also assess newborn's bilirubin and hematocrit levels. Results may indicate the need for immediate exchange transfusion of fresh whole blood that has been typed and crossmatched with mother's serum.

➤ Inform the postpartum patient of the implications of positive test results in cord blood. Prepare the newborn for exchange transfusion, on medical direction.

➤ Evaluate test results in relation to the patient's symptoms and other tests performed. Related laboratory tests include blood group and type, bilirubin, Coombs' indirect antiglobulin (IAT), Ham's test, haptoglobin, hematocrit, and hemoglobin.

COOMBS' ANTIGLOBULIN, INDIRECT

SYNONYMS/ACRONYM: Indirect antiglobulin test (IAT), antibody screen.

SPECIMEN: Serum (1 mL) collected in a red-top tube.

REFERENCE VALUE: (Method: Agglutination) Negative (no agglutination).

DESCRIPTION: The indirect antiglobulin test (IAT) detects and identifies unexpected circulating complement molecules or antibodies in the patient's serum. The first use of this test was for the detection and identification of anti-D using an indirect method. The test is now commonly used to screen a patient's serum for the presence of antibodies that may react against transfused red blood cells (RBCs). During testing, the patient's serum is allowed to incubate with reagent RBCs. The reagent RBCs used are from group O donors and have most of the clinically significant antigens present (D, C, E c, e, K, M, N, S, s, Fy^a, Fy^b, Jk^a, and Jk^b). Antibodies present in the patient's serum coat antigenic sites on the RBC membrane. The reagent cells are washed with saline to remove any unbound antibody. Antihuman globulin is added in the final step of the test. If the patient's serum contained antibodies, the antihuman globulin would cause the antibody-coated RBCs to stick together or agglutinate. (See monograph titled "Blood Groups and Antibodies" for more information regarding transfusion reactions.) ∎

INDICATIONS:

• Detect other antibodies in maternal blood that can be potentially harmful to the fetus

• Determine antibody titers in Rh-negative women sensitized by an Rh-positive fetus

• Screen for antibodies before blood transfusions

• Test for the weak Rh-variant antigen D^u.

RESULT

Positive in:

• Hemolytic anemia (drug-induced or autoimmune)

• Hemolytic disease of the newborn

• Incompatible crossmatch

• Maternal-fetal Rh incompatibility

Negative in:

• Samples in which sensitization of erythrocytes has not occurred (complete absence of antibodies)

• Samples in which reagent erythrocyte antigens are unable to detect low-prevalence antibodies

• Samples in which the patient's antibodies exhibit dosage effects (i.e., stronger reaction with homozygous than with heterozygous expression of an antigen) and reagent erythrocyte antigens contain single-dose expressions of the corresponding antigen (heterozygous)

CRITICAL VALUES: N/A

INTERFERING FACTORS:

• Drugs that may cause a positive IAT include penicillin, phenacetin, quinidine, and rifampin.

• Recent administration of dextran, whole blood or fractions, or intravenous contrast media can result in a false-positive reaction.

Nursing Implications and Procedure • • • • • • • • • • • •

Pretest:

➤ Obtain a history of the patient's complaints, including a list of known allergens.

➤ Obtain a history of the patient's hematopoietic system as well as results of previously performed tests and procedures. For related tests, refer to the hematopoietic system table.

➤ Obtain a list of all the medications the patient is taking, including herbs, nutritional supplements, and nutraceuticals. The requesting health care practitioner and laboratory should be advised if the patient regularly uses these products so that their effects can be taken into consideration when reviewing results.

➤ Note any recent procedures that can interfere with test results.

➤ There are no food, fluid, or medication restrictions unless by medical direction.

➤ Review the procedure with the patient.

➤ Inform the patient that specimen collection takes approximately 5 to 10 minutes.

Intratest:

➤ Direct the patient to breathe normally and to avoid unnecessary movement.

➤ Observe standard precautions and follow the general guidelines in

Appendix A. Perform a venipuncture, and collect the specimen in a 5-mL red-top tube.

➤ Label the specimen, and promptly transport it to the laboratory.

Post-test:

➤ Observe venipuncture site for bleeding or hematoma formation. Apply pressure bandage.

➤ Inform pregnant women that negative tests during the first 12 weeks' gestation should be repeated at 28 weeks to rule out the presence of an antibody.

➤ Positive test results in pregnant women after 28 weeks' gestation indicate the need for antibody identification testing.

➤ Evaluate test results in relation to the patient's symptoms and other tests performed. Related laboratory tests include blood group and type, bilirubin, Coombs' direct antiglobulin (DAT), haptoglobin, hematocrit, and hemoglobin.

COPPER

. . . .

SYNONYM/ACRONYM: Cu.

SPECIMEN: Serum (1 mL) collected in a royal blue–top, trace element–free tube.

REFERENCE VALUE: (Method: Atomic absorption spectrophotometry)

Age	Conventional Units	SI Units (Conversion Factor ×0.157)
Newborn–5 d	9–46 μg/dL	1.4–7.2 μmol/L
1–5 y	80–150 μg/dL	12.6–23.6 μmol/L
6–9 y	84–136 μg/dL	13.2–21.4 μmol/L
10–14 y	80–121 μg/dL	12.6–19.0 μmol/L
15–19 y	80–171 μg/dL	10.1–18.4 μmol/L
Adult		
Men	70–140 μg/dL	11.0–22.0 μmol/L
Women	80–155 μg/dL	12.6–24.3 μmol/L
Pregnant women	118–302 μg/dL	18.5–47.4 μmol/L

Values for African-Americans are 8% to 12% higher.

DESCRIPTION: Copper is an important cofactor for the enzymes that participate in the formation of hemoglobin and collagen. Copper is also a component of coagulation factor V, assists in the oxidation of glucose, is required for melanin pigment formation, is used to synthesize ceruloplasmin, and is necessary for maintenance of myelin sheaths. Copper levels vary with intake. This mineral is absorbed in the stomach and duodenum, stored in the liver, and excreted in urine and in feces with bile salts. Copper deficiency results in neutropenia and a hypochromic, microcytic anemia that is not responsive to iron therapy. Other signs and symptoms of copper deficiency include osteoporosis, depigmentation of skin and hair, impaired immune system response, and possible neurologic and cardiac abnormalities. ■

INDICATIONS:

- Assist in establishing a diagnosis of Menkes' disease

- Assist in establishing a diagnosis of Wilson's disease

- Monitor patients receiving long-term parenteral nutrition therapy

RESULT

Increased in:

- Anemias
- Ankylosing spondylitis
- Biliary cirrhosis
- Collagen diseases
- Complications of renal dialysis
- Hodgkin's disease
- Infections
- Inflammation
- Leukemia
- Malignant neoplasms
- Myocardial infarction
- Pellagra
- Poisoning from copper-contaminated solutions or insecticides

- Pregnancy
- Pulmonary tuberculosis
- Rheumatic fever
- Rheumatoid arthritis
- Systemic lupus erythematosus
- Thalassemias
- Trauma
- Thyroid disease (hypothyroid or hyperthyroid)
- Typhoid fever
- Use of copper intrauterine device

Decreased in:

- Burns
- Chronic ischemic heart disease
- Cystic fibrosis
- Dysproteinemia
- Infants (especially premature infants) receiving milk deficient in copper
- Iron-deficiency anemias (some)
- Long-term total parenteral nutrition
- Malnutrition
- Menkes' disease
- Malabsorption disorders (celiac disease, tropical sprue)
- Nephrotic syndrome
- Wilson's disease

CRITICAL VALUES: N/A

INTERFERING FACTORS:

- Drugs that may increase copper levels include anticonvulsants and oral contraceptives.

- Drugs that may decrease copper levels include citrates, penicillamine, and valproic acid.

- Excessive therapeutic intake of zinc may interfere with intestinal absorption of copper.

Nursing Implications and Procedure ....

Pretest: ■

➤ Obtain a history of the patient's complaints, including a list of known allergens.

➤ Obtain a history of the patient's hematopoietic, hepatobiliary, and immune systems, as well as results of previously performed tests and procedures. For related tests, refer to the hematopoietic, hepatobiliary, and immune system tables.

➤ Obtain a list of medications the patient is taking, including herbs, nutritional supplements, and nutraceuticals. The requesting health care practitioner and laboratory should be advised if the patient regularly uses these products so that their effects can be taken into consideration when reviewing results.

➤ There are no food, fluid, or medication restrictions unless by medical direction.

➤ Review the procedure with the patient.

➤ Inform the patient that specimen collection takes approximately 5 to 10 minutes.

Intratest: ■

➤ Direct the patient to breathe normally and to avoid unnecessary movement.

➤ Observe standard precautions and follow the general guidelines in Appendix A. Perform a venipuncture, and collect the specimen in a 5-mL royal blue–top, trace element–free tube.

➤ Label the specimen, and promptly transport it to the laboratory.

Post-test: ■

➤ Observe venipuncture site for bleeding or hematoma formation. Apply pressure bandage.

➤ Instruct the patient to avoid or increase intake of foods rich in copper, as appropriate. Organ meats, shellfish, nuts, and legumes are good sources of dietary copper. High intake of zinc, iron, calcium, and manganese interferes with copper absorption. Copper deficiency does not normally occur in adults, but patients receiving long-term total parenteral nutrition should be evaluated if signs and symptoms of copper deficiency appear.

➤ Evaluate test results in relation to the patient's symptoms and other tests performed. Related laboratory tests include ceruloplasmin, complete blood count, liver biopsy, and zinc.

CORTISOL AND CHALLENGE TESTS

· ·

SYNONYMS/ACRONYM: Hydrocortisone, compound F.

SPECIMEN: Serum (1 mL) collected in a red- or tiger-top tube. Plasma (1 mL) collected in green-top (heparin) tube is also acceptable. Care must be taken to use the same type of collection container if serial measurements are to be taken.

Procedure	Medication Administered	Recommended Collection Times
ACTH stimulation	Synthetic ACTH (cosyntropin) IM or IV bolus	3 cortisol levels—baseline immediately before bolus, 30 min after bolus, and 60 min after bolus
CRH stimulation	CRH 1 μg/kg IV 9 a.m.	3 cortisol and ACTH levels—baseline before injection, 30 min after injection, and 60 min after injection
Dexamethasone suppression (overnight)	Oral dose dexamethasone at 11 p.m.	8 a.m. after morning collection of cortisol
Metyrapone stimulation (overnight)	Oral dose of metyrapone at midnight	8 a.m. after morning collection of cortisol and ACTH

ACTH = adrenocorticotropic hormone; CRH = corticotropin-releasing hormone; IM = intramuscular; IV = intravenous.

REFERENCE VALUE: (Method: Immunoassay)

	Conventional Units	SI Units
Cortisol		
		(Conversion Factor ×27.6)
8 a.m.	5–25 μg/dL	138–690 nmol/L
4 p.m.	3–16 μg/dL	83–442 nmol/L
ACTH Challenge Tests		
CRH stimulation	2–4 fold increase over baseline ACTH or cortisol level	2–4 fold increase over baseline values
Dexamethasone Suppressed		
		(Conversion Factor ×27.6)
	Cortisol less than 3 μg/dL next day	Less than 83 nmol/L
ACTH (Cosyntropin) Stimulated		
		(Conversion Factor ×27.6)
	Cortisol greater than 20 μg/dL	Greater than 552 nmol/L

Conventional Units	SI Units
Metyrapone Stimulated	
	(Conversion Factor ×0.22)
ACTH greater than 150 pg/mL	Greater than 33 pmol/L
	(Conversion Factor ×27.6)
Cortisol less than 3 µg/dL next day	Less than 83 nmol/L

ACTH = adrenocorticotropic hormone; CRH = corticotropin-releasing hormone.

DESCRIPTION: Cortisol (hydrocortisone) is the predominant glucocorticoid secreted in response to stimulation by the hypothalamus and pituitary adrenocorticotropic hormone (ACTH). Cortisol stimulates gluconeogenesis, mobilizes fats and proteins, antagonizes insulin, and suppresses inflammation. Measuring levels of cortisol in blood is the best indicator of adrenal function. Cortisol secretion varies diurnally, with highest levels occurring on awakening and lowest levels occurring late in the day. Bursts of cortisol excretion can occur at night. Cortisol and ACTH test results are evaluated together because they each control the other's concentrations (i.e., any change in one causes a change in the other). ACTH levels exhibit a diurnal variation, peaking between 6 and 8 a.m. and reaching the lowest point between 6 and 11 p.m. Evening levels are generally one-half to two-thirds lower than morning levels. (See monograph titled "Adrenocorticotropic Hormone [and Challenge Tests].") ■

INDICATIONS:

• Detect adrenal hyperfunction (Cushing's syndrome)

• Detect adrenal hypofunction (Addison's disease)

RESULT: The dexamethasone suppression test is useful in differentiating the causes for increased cortisol levels. Dexamethasone is a synthetic steroid that suppresses secretion of ACTH. With this test, a baseline morning cortisol level is collected, and the patient is given a 1-mg dose of dexamethasone at bedtime. A second specimen is collected the following morning. If cortisol levels have not been suppressed, adrenal adenoma may be suspected. The dexamethasone suppression test also produces abnormal results in patients with psychiatric illnesses.

The corticotropin-releasing hormone (CRH) stimulation test works as well as the dexamethasone suppression test in distinguishing Cushing's disease from conditions in which ACTH is secreted ectopically. In this test, cortisol levels are measured after an injection of CRH. A fourfold increase in cortisol levels above baseline is seen in Cushing's disease. No increase in cortisol is seen if ectopic ACTH secretion is the cause.

The cosyntropin test is used when adrenal insufficiency is suspected. Cosyntropin is a synthetic form of ACTH. A baseline cortisol level is collected before the injection of cosyntropin. Specimens are subsequently collected at 30- and 60-minute intervals.

If the adrenal glands are functioning normally, cortisol levels rise significantly after administration of cosyntropin.

The metyrapone stimulation test is used to distinguish corticotropin-dependent (pituitary Cushing's disease and ectopic Cushing's disease) from corticotropin-independent (carcinoma of the lung or thyroid) causes of increased cortisol levels. Metyrapone inhibits the conversion of 11-deoxycortisol to cortisol. Cortisol levels should decrease to less than 3 μg/dL if normal pituitary stimulation by ACTH occurs after an oral dose of metyrapone. Specimen collection and administration of the medication are performed as with the overnight dexamethasone test.

Increased in:

- Adrenal adenoma
- Cushing's syndrome
- Ectopic ACTH production
- Hyperglycemia
- Pregnancy
- Stress

Decreased in:

- Addison's disease
- Adrenogenital syndrome
- Hypopituitarism

CRITICAL VALUES: N/A

INTERFERING FACTORS:

- Drugs and substances that may increase cortisol levels include amphetamines, anticonvulsants, clomipramine, corticotropin, CRH, cortisone, cyclic AMP, ether, fenfluramine, hydrocortisone, insulin, lithium, methadone, metoclopramide, naloxone, opiates, oral contraceptives, prednisolone, ranitidine, spironolactone, tetracosactrin, and vasopressin.

- Drugs and substances that may decrease cortisol levels include barbiturates, beclomethasone, betamethasone, clonidine, danazol, desoximetasone, desoxycorticosterone, dexamethasone, ephedrine, etomidate, fluocinolone, ketoconazole, levodopa, lithium, methylprednisolone, metyrapone, midazolam, morphine, nitrous oxide, oxazepam, phenytoin, ranitidine, and trimipramine.

- Test results are affected by the time this test is done because cortisol levels vary diurnally.

- Stress and excessive physical activity can produce elevated levels.

- Normal values can be obtained in the presence of partial pituitary deficiency.

- ⚠ The metyrapone stimulation test is contraindicated in patients with suspected adrenal insufficiency.

- ⚠ Metyrapone may cause gastrointestinal distress and/or confusion.

Nursing Implications and Procedure • • • • • • • • • • •

Pretest: ■

➤ Obtain a history of the patient's complaints, including a list of known allergens.

➤ Obtain a history of the patient's endocrine system as well as results of previously performed tests and procedures. For related tests, refer to the endocrine system table.

➤ Obtain a list of medications the patient is taking, including herbs, nutritional supplements, and nutraceuticals. The requesting health care practitioner and laboratory should be advised if the patient regularly uses these products so that their effects can be taken into consideration when reviewing results.

➤ There are no food, fluid, or medication restrictions unless by medical direction.

> Review the procedure with the patient. Inform the patient that multiple specimens may be required.

> Instruct the patient to minimize stress to avoid raising cortisol levels.

> Inform the patient that specimen collection takes approximately 5 to 10 minutes.

Intratest:

> Direct the patient to breathe normally and to avoid unnecessary movement.

> Collect specimen between 6 and 8 a.m., when cortisol levels are highest.

> Observe standard precautions and follow the general guidelines in Appendix A. Perform a venipuncture, and collect the specimen in a 5-mL red- or tiger-top tube.

> Label the specimen, noting collection time on the label, and promptly transport it to the laboratory.

Post-test:

> Observe venipuncture site for bleeding or hematoma formation. Apply pressure bandage.

> Evaluate test results in relation to the patient's symptoms and other tests performed. Related laboratory tests include ACTH, glucose, and glucose tolerance test.

CREATINE KINASE AND ISOENZYMES

SYNONYM/ACRONYM: CK and isos.

SPECIMEN: Serum (1 mL) collected in a red- or tiger-top tube. Serial specimens are highly recommended. Care must be taken to use the same type of collection container if serial measurements are to be taken.

REFERENCE VALUE: (Method: Enzymatic for CK, electrophoresis for isoenzymes; enzyme immunoassay techniques are in common use for CK-MB)

	Conventional Units	SI Units (Conversion Factor ×0.017)
Total CK		
Newborn	3× adult values	3× adult values
Children and men	38–174 U/L	0.65–2.96 µKat/L
Children and women	26–140 U/L	0.46–2.38 µKat/L

(Continued on the following page)

	SI Units
	Conventional Units (Conversion Factor ×0.017)
CK isoenzymes by electrophoresis	
CK-BB	Absent
CK-MB	Less than 4–6%
CK-MM	94–96%
CK-MB by immunoassay	Less than 10 ng/mL

CK = creatine kinase; CK-BB = CK isoenzyme in brain; CK-MB = CK isoenzyme in heart; CK-MM = CK isoenzyme in skeletal muscle.

DESCRIPTION: Creatine kinase (CK) is an enzyme that exists almost exclusively in skeletal muscle, heart muscle, and, in smaller amounts, in the brain. This enzyme is important in intracellular storage and energy release. Three isoenzymes, based on primary location, have been identified by electrophoresis: brain CK-BB, cardiac CK-MB, and skeletal muscle CK-MM. When injury to these tissues occurs, the enzymes are released into the bloodstream. Levels increase and decrease in a predictable time frame. Measuring the serum levels can help determine the extent and timing of the damage. Noting the presence of the specific isoenzyme helps determine the location of the tissue damage.

Acute myocardial infarction (MI) releases CK into the serum within the first 48 hours; values return to normal in about 3 days. The isoenzyme CK-MB appears in the first 6 to 24 hours and is usually gone in 72 hours. Recurrent elevation of CK suggests reinfarction or extension of ischemic damage. Significant elevations of CK are expected in early phases of muscular dystrophy, even before the clinical signs and symptoms appear. CK elevation diminishes as the disease progresses and muscle mass decreases.

Differences in total CK with age and gender relate to the fact that the predominant isoenzyme is muscle in origin. Body builders have higher values, whereas older individuals have lower values because of deterioration of muscle mass.

The use of the mass assay for CK-MB with cardiac troponin I, in the assessment of MI has largely replaced the use of CK isoenzymes by electrophoresis. CK-MB mass assays are more sensitive and rapid than electrophoresis. The evaluation of serial samples for CK-MB is highly recommended. ■

INDICATIONS:

• Assist in the diagnosis of acute MI and evaluate cardiac ischemia (CK-MB)

• Detect musculoskeletal disorders that do not have a neurological basis, such as dermatomyosis or Duchenne's muscular dystrophy (CK-MM)

• Determine the success of coronary artery reperfusion after streptokinase infusion or percutaneous transluminal angioplasty, as evidenced by a decrease in CK-MB

RESULT

Increased in:

• Alcoholism

- Brain infarction (extensive)
- Congestive heart failure
- Delirium tremens
- Dermatomyositis
- Head injury
- Hypothyroidism
- Hypoxic shock
- Infectious diseases
- Gastrointestinal (GI) tract infarction
- Loss of blood supply to any muscle
- Malignant hyperpyrexia
- Muscular dystrophies
- MI
- Myocarditis
- Neoplasms of the prostate, bladder, and GI tract
- Polymyositis
- Pregnancy
- Prolonged hypothermia
- Pulmonary edema
- Pulmonary embolism
- Reye's syndrome
- Rhabdomyolysis
- Surgery
- Tachycardia
- Tetanus
- Trauma

Decreased in:

- Small stature
- Sedentary lifestyle

CRITICAL VALUES: N/A

INTERFERING FACTORS:

- Drugs that may increase total CK levels include any intramuscularly injected preparations because of tissue trauma caused by injection.
- Drugs that may decrease total CK levels include dantrolene and dobesilate.

Nursing Implications and Procedure • • • • • • • • • •

Pretest:

➤ Obtain a history of the patient's complaints, including a list of known allergens.

➤ Obtain a history of the patient's cardiovascular and musculoskeletal systems, as well as results of previously performed tests and procedures. For related tests, refer to the cardiovascular and musculoskeletal system tables.

➤ Obtain a list of the medications the patient is taking, including herbs, nutritional supplements, and nutraceuticals. The requesting health care practitioner and laboratory should be advised if the patient is regularly using these products so that their effects can be taken into consideration when reviewing results.

➤ There are no food, fluid, or medication restrictions unless by medical direction.

➤ Review the procedure with the patient. Inform the patient that a series of samples will be required. (Samples at time of admission, 2 to 4 hours, 6 to 8 hours, and 12 hours after admission are the minimal recommendations. Additional samples may be requested.)

➤ Inform the patient that specimen collection takes approximately 5 to 10 minutes.

Intratest:

➤ Direct the patient to breathe normally and to avoid unnecessary movement.

➤ Observe standard precautions and

follow the general guidelines in Appendix A. Perform a venipuncture, and collect the specimen in a 5-mL red- or tiger-top tube.

➤ Label the specimen, and promptly transport it to the laboratory.

Post-test:

➤ Observe venipuncture site for bleeding or hematoma formation. Apply pressure bandage.

➤ Increased CK levels may be associated with coronary artery disease (CAD). Nutritional therapy is recommended for individuals identified to be at high risk for developing CAD. If overweight, the patient should be encouraged to achieve a normal weight. The American Heart Association Step 1 and Step 2 diets

may be helpful in achieving a goal of lowering total cholesterol and triglyceride levels. The Step 1 diet emphasizes a reduction in foods high in saturated fats and cholesterol. Red meats, eggs, and dairy products are the major sources of saturated fats and cholesterol. If triglycerides are also elevated, the patient should be advised to eliminate or reduce alcohol and simple carbohydrates from the diet. The Step 2 diet recommends stricter reductions.

➤ Evaluate test results in relation to the patient's symptoms and other tests performed. Related laboratory tests include aspartate aminotransferase, C-reactive protein, calcium, ionized calcium, electrolytes, homocysteine, lactate dehydrogenase and isoenzymes, magnesium, myoglobin, and troponin.

CREATININE, SERUM

SYNONYM/ACRONYM: N/A.

SPECIMEN: Serum (1 mL) collected in a red- or tiger-top tube. Plasma (1 mL) collected in green-top (heparin) tube is also acceptable.

REFERENCE VALUE: (Method: Spectrophotometry)

Age	Conventional Units	SI Units (Conversion Factor ×88.4)
1–5 y	0.3–0.5 mg/dL	27–44 μmol/L
6–10 y	0.5–0.8 mg/dL	44–71 μmol/L
Adult male	0.6–1.2 mg/dL	53–106 μmol/L
Adult female	0.5–1.1 mg/dL	44–97 μmol/L

DESCRIPTION: Creatinine is the end product of creatine metabolism. Creatine resides almost exclusively in skeletal muscle, where it participates

in energy-requiring metabolic reactions. In these processes, a small amount of creatine is irreversibly converted to creatinine, which then circulates to the kidneys and is excreted. The amount of creatinine generated in an individual is proportional to the mass of skeletal muscle present and remains fairly constant, unless there is massive muscle damage resulting from crushing injury or degenerative muscle disease. Creatinine values also decrease with age owing to diminishing muscle mass. Blood urea nitrogen (BUN) is often ordered with creatinine for comparison. The BUN/creatinine ratio is also a useful indicator of disease. The ratio should be between 10:1 and 20:1. Creatinine is the ideal substance for determining renal clearance because a fairly constant quantity is produced within the body. The creatinine clearance test measures a blood sample and a urine sample to determine the rate at which the kidneys are clearing creatinine from the blood; this accurately reflects the glomerular filtration rate. (See monograph titled "Creatinine, Urine, and Creatinine Clearance, Urine" for additional information.) ▪

INDICATIONS:

• Assess a known or suspected disorder involving muscles in the absence of renal disease

• Evaluate known or suspected impairment of renal function

RESULT

Increased in:

• Acromegaly

• Congestive heart failure

• Dehydration

• Gigantism

• Hyperthyroidism

• Poliomyelitis

• Renal disease, acute and chronic renal failure

• Rhabdomyolysis

• Shock

Decreased in:

• Decreased muscle mass owing to debilitating disease or increasing age

• Inadequate protein intake

• Liver disease (severe)

• Muscular dystrophy

• Pregnancy

• Small stature

CRITICAL VALUES: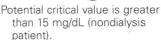

Potential critical value is greater than 15 mg/dL (nondialysis patient).

Possible interventions may include renal or peritoneal dialysis and organ transplant, but early discovery of the cause of elevated creatinine levels might avoid such drastic interventions.

INTERFERING FACTORS:

• Drugs and substances that may increase creatinine levels include acebutolol, acetaminophen (overdose), aldatense, amikacin, amiodarone, amphotericin B, arginine, arsenicals, ascorbic acid, asparaginase, acetylsalicylic acid, barbiturates, capreomycin, captopril, carbutamide, carvedilol, cephalothin, chlorthalidone, cimetidine, cisplatin, clofibrate, colistin, corn oil (Lipomul), cyclosporine, dextran, doxycycline, enalapril, ethylene glycol, gentamicin, indomethacin, ipodate, kanamycin, levodopa, mannitol, methicillin, methoxyflurane, mitomycin, neomycin, netilmycin, nitrofurantoin, nonsteroidal anti-inflammatory drugs, oxyphenbutazone, paromomycin, penicillin, pentamidine, phosphorus, plicamycin, radiographic agents, semustine, streptokinase, streptozocin, tetracycline, thiazides, tobramycin, triamterene, vancomycin, vasopressin, viomycin, and vitamin D.

• Drugs that may decrease creatinine levels include citrates, dopamine, ibuprofen, and lisinopril.

• Bilirubin and glucose can cause false decreases in creatinine.

• A diet high in meat can cause increased creatinine levels.

• Ketosis can cause a significant increase in creatinine.

Nursing Implications and Procedure · · · · · · · · · · ·

Pretest:

➤ Obtain a history of the patient's complaints, including a list of known allergens.

➤ Obtain a history of the patient's genitourinary and musculoskeletal systems, as well as results of previously performed tests and procedures. For related tests, refer to the genitourinary and musculoskeletal system tables.

➤ Obtain a list of medications the patient is taking, including herbs, nutritional supplements, and nutraceuticals. The requesting health care practitioner and laboratory should be advised if the patient is regularly using these products so that their effects can be taken into consideration when reviewing results.

➤ There are no food, fluid, or medication restrictions unless by medical direction.

➤ Instruct the patient to refrain from

excessive exercise for 8 hours before the test.

➤ Review the procedure with the patient.

➤ Inform the patient that specimen collection takes approximately 5 to 10 minutes.

Intratest:

➤ Direct the patient to breathe normally and to avoid unnecessary movement.

➤ Observe standard precautions and follow the general guidelines in Appendix A. Perform a venipuncture, and collect the specimen in a 5-mL red- or tiger-top tube.

➤ Label the specimen, and promptly transport it to the laboratory.

Post-test:

➤ Observe venipuncture site for bleeding or hematoma formation. Apply pressure bandage.

➤ Increased creatinine levels may be associated with kidney disease. The nutritional needs of patients with kidney disease vary widely and are in constant flux. Anorexia, nausea, and vomiting commonly occur, prompting the need for continuous nutritional monitoring for malnutrition, especially among patients receiving long-term hemodialysis therapy.

➤ Evaluate test results in relation to the patient's symptoms and other tests performed. Related laboratory tests include anion gap, urine creatinine, creatinine clearance, serum and urine electrolytes, gentamicin, kidney stone analysis, microalbumin, serum and urine osmolality, tobramycin, serum and urine uric acid, blood and urine urea nitrogen, BUN/creatinine ratio, and vancomycin.

CREATININE, URINE, AND CREATININE CLEARANCE, URINE

SYNONYM/ACRONYM: N/A.

SPECIMEN: Urine (5 mL) from an unpreserved random or timed specimen collected in a clean plastic collection container.

REFERENCE VALUE: (Method: Spectrophotometry)

Age	Conventional Units	SI Units
Urine Creatinine (Conversion Factor × 8.84)		
2–3 y	6–22 mg/kg/24 h	53–194 μmol/kg/24 h
4–18 y	12–30 mg/kg/24 h	106–265 μmol/kg/24 h
Adult male	14–26 mg/kg/24 h	124–230 μmol/kg/24 h
Adult female	11–20 mg/kg/24 h	97–177 μmol/kg/24 h
Creatinine Clearance (Conversion Factor × 0.0167)		
Children	70–140 mL/min/1.73 m^2	1.17–2.33 mL/s/1.73 m^2
Adult male	85–125 mL/min/1.73 m^2	1.42–2.08 mL/s/1.73 m^2
Adult female	75–115 mL/min/1.73 m^2	1.25–1.92 mL/s/1.73 m^2
For each decade after 40 y	Decrease of 6–7 mL/min/1.73 m^2	Decrease of 0.06–0.07 mL/s/1.73 m^2

DESCRIPTION: Creatinine is the end product of creatine metabolism. Creatine resides almost exclusively in skeletal muscle, where it participates in energy-requiring metabolic reactions. In these processes, a small amount of creatine is irreversibly converted to creatinine, which then circulates to the kidneys and is excreted. The amount of creatinine generated in an individual is proportional to the mass of skeletal muscle present and remains fairly constant, unless there is massive muscle damage resulting from crushing injury or degenerative muscle disease. Creatinine values decrease with advancing age owing to diminishing muscle mass. Although the measurement of urine creatinine is an effective indicator of renal function, the creatinine clearance test is more precise. The creatinine clearance test measures a blood sample and a urine sample to determine the rate at which the kidneys are clearing creatinine from the blood; this accurately reflects the glomerular filtration rate and is based on an estimate of body surface. ■

INDICATIONS:

• Determine the extent of nephron damage in known renal disease (at least

50 percent of functioning nephrons must be lost before values are decreased)

• Determine renal function before administering nephrotoxic drugs

• Evaluate accuracy of a 24-hour urine collection, based on the constant level of creatinine excretion

• Evaluate glomerular function

• Monitor effectiveness of treatment in renal disease

RESULT

Increased in:

• Acromegaly

• Acute tubular necrosis

• Carnivorous diets

• Congestive heart failure

• Dehydration

• Diabetes

• Exercise

• Exposure to nephrotoxic drugs and chemicals

• Gigantism

• Glomerulonephritis

• Hypothyroidism

• Infections

• Neoplasms (bilateral renal)

• Nephrosclerosis

• Polycystic kidney disease

• Pyelonephritis

• Renal artery atherosclerosis

• Renal artery obstruction

• Renal disease

• Renal vein thrombosis

• Shock and hypovolemia

• Tuberculosis

Decreased in:

• Acute or chronic glomerulonephritis

• Anemia

• Chronic bilateral pyelonephritis

• Hyperthyroidism

• Leukemia

• Muscle wasting diseases

• Paralysis

• Polycystic kidney disease

• Shock

• Urinary tract obstruction (e.g., from calculi)

• Vegetarian diets

CRITICAL VALUES

Degree of impairment:

Borderline: 62.5–80 mL/min/ 1.73 m^2

Slight: 52–62.5 mL/min/1.73 m^2

Mild: 42–52 mL/min/1.73 m^2

Moderate: 28–42 mL/min/1.73 m^2

Marked: Less than 28 mL/min/ 1.73 m^2

INTERFERING FACTORS:

• Drugs that may increase urine creatinine levels include ascorbic acid, cefoxitin, cephalothin, corticosteroids, fluoxymesterone, levodopa, methandrostenolone, methotrexate, methyldopa, nitrofurans (including nitrofurazone), oxymetholone, phenolphthalein, and prednisone.

• Drugs that may increase urine creatinine clearance include enalapril, oral contraceptives, prednisone, and ramipril.

• Drugs that may decrease urine creatinine levels include anabolic steroids, androgens, captopril, and thiazides.

• Drugs that may decrease the urine

creatinine clearance include amphotericin B, acetylsalicylic acid, carbenoxolone, chlorthalidone, cimetidine, cisplatin, cyclosporine, guancidine, ibuprofen, indomethacin, mitomycin, oxyphenbutazone, paromycin, probenecid (coadministered with digoxin), and thiazides.

• Excessive ketones in urine may cause falsely decreased values.

• Failure to follow proper technique in collecting 24-hour specimen may invalidate test results.

• Failure to refrigerate specimen throughout urine collection period allows decomposition of creatinine, causing falsely decreased values.

• Consumption of large amounts of meat, excessive exercise, and stress should be avoided for 24 hours before the test.

Nursing Implications and Procedure • • • • • • • • • • •

Pretest:

➤ Obtain a history of the patient's complaints, including a list of known allergens.

➤ Obtain a history of the patient's genitourinary system as well as results of previously performed tests and procedures. For related tests, refer to the genitourinary system table.

➤ Obtain a list of medications the patient is taking, including herbs, nutritional supplements, and nutraceuticals. The requesting health care practitioner and laboratory should be advised if the patient regularly uses these products so that their effects can be taken into consideration when reviewing results.

➤ There are no fluid or medication restrictions unless by medical direction.

➤ Instruct the patient to refrain from eating meat during the test.

➤ Review the procedure with the patient. Provide a nonmetallic urinal, bedpan, or toilet-mounted collection device.

➤ Usually a 24-hour time frame for urine collection is ordered. Inform the patient that all urine must be saved during that 24-hour period. Instruct the patient not to void directly into the laboratory collection container. Instruct the patient to avoid defecating in the collection device and to keep toilet tissue out of the collection device to prevent contamination of the specimen. Place a sign in the bathroom to remind the patient to save all urine.

➤ Instruct the patient to void all urine into the collection device and then to pour the urine into the laboratory collection container. Alternatively the specimen can be left in the collection device for a health care staff member to add to the laboratory collection container.

Intratest:

➤ Ensure that the patient has complied with dietary preparations and other pretesting restrictions.

➤ Observe standard precautions and follow the general guidelines in Appendix A.

Random specimen (collect in early morning)

Clean-catch specimen:

➤ Instruct the male patient to (1) thoroughly wash his hands, (2) cleanse the meatus, (3) void a small amount into the toilet, and (4) void directly into the specimen container.

➤ Instruct the female patient to (1) thoroughly wash her hands; (2) cleanse the labia from front to back; (3) while keeping the labia separated, void a small amount into the toilet; and (4) without interrupting the urine stream, void directly into the specimen container.

Pediatric urine collector:

➤ Put on gloves. Appropriately cleanse the genital area and allow the area to dry. Remove the covering over the adhesive strips on the collector bag and apply over the genital area. Diaper the child. When specimen is obtained, place the entire collection bag in a sterile urine container.

Indwelling catheter:

➤ Put on gloves. Empty drainage tube of urine. It may be necessary to clamp off the catheter for 15 to 30 minutes before specimen collection. Cleanse specimen port with antiseptic swab, and then aspirate 5 mL of urine with a 21- to 25-gauge needle and syringe. Transfer urine to a sterile container.

Urinary catheterization:

➤ Place female patient in lithotomy position or male patient in supine position. Using sterile technique, open the straight urinary catheterization kit and perform urinary catheterization. Place the retained urine in a sterile specimen container.

Suprapubic aspiration:

➤ Place the patient in a supine position. Cleanse the area with antiseptic and drape with sterile drapes. Using sterile technique, insert needle and remove sterile sample. Place the returned sample in a sterile specimen container. Place a dry sterile dressing over the site.

➤ Do not collect urine from the pouch from the patient with a urinary diversion (e.g., ilieal conduit). Instead perform catheterization through the stoma.

Timed specimen:

➤ Obtain a clean 3-L urine specimen container, toilet-mounted collection device, and plastic bag (for transport of the specimen container). The specimen must be refrigerated or kept on ice throughout the entire collection period. If an indwelling urinary catheter is in place, the drainage bag must be kept on ice.

➤ Begin the test between 6 and 8 a.m., if possible. Collect first voiding and discard. Record the time the specimen was discarded as the beginning of the timed collection period. The next morning, ask the patient to void at the same time the collection was started and add this last voiding to the container.

➤ If an indwelling catheter is in place, replace the tubing and container system at the start of the collection time. Keep the container system on ice during the collection period, or empty the urine into a larger container periodically during the collection period; monitor to ensure continued drainage, and conclude the test the next morning at the same hour the collection was begun.

➤ At the conclusion of the test, compare the quantity of urine with the urinary output record for the collection; if the specimen contains less than what was recorded as output, some urine may have been discarded, invalidating the test.

➤ Label the specimen, and promptly transport it to the laboratory. Include on the label the amount of urine, test start and stop times, and ingestion of any foods or medications that can affect test results.

Post-test:

➤ Evaluate test results in relation to the patient's symptoms and other tests performed. Related laboratory tests include anion gap, creatinine, serum and urine electrolytes, gentamicin, kidney stone analysis, microalbumin, serum and urine osmolality, tobramycin, serum and urine uric acid, blood and urine urea nitrogen, blood urea nitrogen (BUN)/creatinine ratio, and vancomycin.

CRYOGLOBULIN

SYNONYM/ACRONYM: Cryo.

SPECIMEN: Serum (1 mL) collected in a red-top tube.

REFERENCE VALUE: (Method: Visual observation for changes in appearance)
Negative.

DESCRIPTION: Cryoglobulins are abnormal serum proteins that cannot be detected by protein electrophoresis. Cryoglobulins cause vascular problems because they can precipitate in the blood vessels of the fingers when exposed to cold, causing Raynaud's phenomenon. They are usually associated with immunologic disease. The laboratory procedure to detect cryoglobulins is a two-step process. The serum sample is observed for cold precipitation after 72 hours of storage at 4°C. True cryoglobulins disappear on warming to room temperature, so in the second step of the procedure, the sample is rewarmed to confirm reversibility of the reaction. ∎

INDICATIONS:

• Assist in diagnosis of neoplastic diseases, acute and chronic infections, and collagen diseases

• Detect cryoglobulinemia in patients with symptoms indicating or mimicking Raynaud's disease

• Monitor course of collagen and rheumatic disorders

RESULT

Increased in:

• Type I cryoglobulin (monoclonal)
Chronic lymphocytic leukemia
Lymphoma
Multiple myeloma

• Type II cryoglobulin (mixtures of monoclonal immunoglobulin M [IgM] and polyclonal IgG)
Autoimmune hepatitis
Rheumatoid arthritis
Sjögren's syndrome
Waldenström's macroglobulinemia

• Type III cryoglobulin (mixtures of polyclonal IgM and IgG)
Acute poststreptococcal glomerulonephritis
Chronic infection (especially hepatitis C)
Cirrhosis
Endocarditis
Infectious mononucleosis
Polymyalgia rheumatica
Rheumatoid arthritis
Sarcoidosis
Systemic lupus erythematosus

Decreased in: N/A

CRITICAL VALUES: N/A

INTERFERING FACTORS:

• Testing the sample prematurely (before total precipitation) may yield incorrect results.

• Failure to maintain sample at normal body temperature before centrifugation can affect results.

• A recent fatty meal can increase turbidity of the blood, decreasing visibility.

Nursing Implications and Procedure

Pretest:

➤ Obtain a history of the patient's complaints, including a list of known allergens.

➤ Obtain a history of the patient's immune system as well as results of previously performed tests and procedures. For related tests, refer to the immune system table.

➤ Obtain a list of the medications the patient is taking, including herbs, nutritional supplements, and nutraceuticals. The requesting health care practitioner and laboratory should be advised if the patient regularly uses these products so that their effects can be taken into consideration when reviewing results.

➤ There are no food, fluid, or medication restrictions unless by medical direction.

➤ Review the procedure with the patient.

➤ Inform the patient that specimen collection takes approximately 5 to 10 minutes.

Intratest:

➤ Direct the patient to breathe normally and to avoid unnecessary movement.

➤ Observe standard precautions and follow the general guidelines in Appendix A. Perform a venipuncture, and collect the specimen in a 5-mL red-top tube.

➤ Label the specimen, and promptly transport it to the laboratory.

Post-test:

➤ Observe venipuncture site for bleeding or hematoma formation. Apply pressure bandage.

➤ Evaluate test results in relation to the patient's symptoms and other tests performed. Related laboratory tests include antinuclear antibody, hepatitis C antibody, immunofixation electrophoresis, IgA, IgG, IgM, protein, protein electrophoresis, and rheumatoid factor.

CULTURE AND SMEAR, MYCOBACTERIA

SYNONYMS/ACRONYMS: Acid-fast bacilli (AFB) culture and smear, tuberculosis (TB) culture and smear, *Mycobacterium* culture and smear.

SPECIMEN: Sputum (5 to 10 mL), bronchopulmonary lavage, tissue, material from fine-needle aspiration, bone marrow, cerebrospinal fluid (CSF), gastric aspiration, urine, and stool.

REFERENCE VALUE: (Method: Culture on selected media, microscopic examination of sputum by acid-fast or auramine-rhodamine fluorochrome stain) Rapid methods include: chemiluminescent-labeled DNA probes that target ribosomal RNA of the *Mycobacterium,* radiometric carbon dioxide detection from ^{14}C-labeled media, polymerase chain reaction/amplification techniques.
Culture: No growth
Smear: Negative for AFB

DESCRIPTION: A culture and smear test is used primarily to detect *Mycobacterium tuberculosis,* which is a tubercular bacillus. The cell wall of this mycobacterium contains complex lipids and waxes that do not take up ordinary stains. Cells that resist decolorization by acid alcohol are termed *acid fast.* There are only a few groups of acid-fast bacilli (AFB); this characteristic is helpful in rapid identification so that therapy can be initiated in a timely manner. Smears may be negative 50 percent of the time even though the culture develops positive growth 3 to 8 weeks later. AFB cultures are used to confirm positive and negative AFB smears. *M. tuberculosis* grows in culture slowly. Automated liquid culture systems, such as the Bactec and MGIT (Becton Dickinson and Company, 1 Becton Drive, Franklin Lakes, NJ, 07417), have a turnaround time of approximately 10 days. Results of tests by polymerase chain reaction culture methods are available in 36 to 48 hours.

M. tuberculosis is transmitted via the airborne route to the lungs. It causes areas of granulomatous inflammation, cough, fever, and hemoptysis. It can remain dormant in the lungs for long periods. The incidence of tuberculosis has increased since the late 1980s in depressed inner-city areas, among prison populations, and among human immunodeficiency virus (HIV)–positive patients. Of great concern is the increase in antibiotic-resistant strains of *M. tuberculosis.* HIV-positive patients often become ill from concomitant infections caused by *M. tuberculosis* and *Mycobacterium avium intracellulare.* *M. avium intracellulare* is acquired via the gastrointestinal tract through ingestion of contaminated food or water. The organism's waxy cell wall protects it from acids in the human digestive tract. Isolation of mycobacteria in the stool does not mean the patient has tuberculosis of the intestines because mycobacteria in stool are most often present in sputum that has been swallowed. ■

INDICATIONS:

- Assist in the diagnosis of mycobacteriosis

- Assist in the diagnosis of suspected pulmonary tuberculosis secondary to acquired immunodeficiency syndrome (AIDS)

• Assist in the differentiation of tuberculosis from carcinoma or bronchiectasis

• Investigate suspected pulmonary tuberculosis

• Monitor the response to treatment for pulmonary tuberculosis

RESULT

Identified Organism	Primary Specimen Source	Condition
Mycobacterium avium intracellulare	Sputum, urine, CSF, semen, lymph nodes	Opportunistic pulmonary infection
M. fortuitum	Surgical wound, sputum, joint, bone, tissue	Opportunistic infection (usually pulmonary)
M. leprae	Skin scrapings, CSF, lymph nodes	Hansen's disease (leprosy)
M. kansasii	Skin, joint, sputum, lymph nodes	Pulmonary tuberculosis
M. marinum	Joint	Granulomatous skin lesions
M. tuberculosis	Sputum, urine, CSF, gastric washing	Pulmonary tuberculosis
M. xenopi	Sputum	Pulmonary tuberculosis

CSF = cerebrospinal fluid.

CRITICAL VALUES:

Smear: Positive for AFB

Culture: Growth of pathogenic bacteria

INTERFERING FACTORS:

• Specimen collection after initiation of treatment with antituberculosis drug therapy may result in inhibited or no growth of organisms.

• Contamination of the sterile container with organisms from an exogenous source may produce misleading results.

• Specimens received on a dry swab should be rejected: A dry swab indicates that the sample is unlikely to have been collected properly or unlikely to contain a representative quantity of

significant organisms for proper evaluation.

• Inadequate or improper (e.g., saliva) samples should be rejected.

Nursing Implications and Procedure

Pretest:

➤ Obtain a history of the patient's complaints and exposure to TB. Obtain a list of known allergens.

➤ Obtain a history of the patient's immune and respiratory systems, as well as results of previously performed tests and procedures. For related tests, refer to the immune and respiratory system tables.

➤ Obtain a list of medications the patient is taking, including herbs, nutritional supplements, and nutraceuticals. The requesting health care practitioner and laboratory should be advised if the patient is regularly using these products so that their effects can be taken into consideration when reviewing results.

➤ Note any recent procedures that can interfere with test results.

Culture after bronchoscopy:

➤ The patient should fast and refrain from drinking liquids from midnight the night before the procedure.

➤ Other than antimicrobial drugs, there are no medication restrictions, unless by medical direction.

➤ Assess if the patient has an allergy to local anesthetics, and inform the health care practitioner accordingly.

➤ *Obtain written and informed consent before bronchoscopy is performed.*

Expectorated specimen:

➤ There are no food or fluid restrictions.

➤ Other than antimicrobial drugs, there are no medication restrictions, unless by medical direction.

➤ Additional liquids the night before may assist in liquefying secretions during expectoration the following morning.

➤ Assist patient with oral cleaning before sample collection to reduce the amount of sample contamination by organisms that normally inhabit the mouth.

General:

➤ Review the procedure with the patient. Inform the patient that the culture results will not be reported for 3 to 8 weeks.

➤ The time it takes to collect a proper specimen varies according to the level of cooperation of the patient and the specimen collection site.

Intratest:

➤ Ensure that the patient has complied with dietary preparations and other pretesting restrictions before bronchoscopy.

➤ If the patient is to undergo bronchoscopy, record baseline vital signs.

➤ Instructions regarding the appropriate transport for bone marrow, body fluids, tissue, urine, and stool should be obtained from the laboratory.

➤ Observe standard precautions and follow the general guidelines in Appendix A.

Bronchoscopy:

➤ Record baseline vital signs. The patient is positioned in relation to the type of anesthesia being used. If local anesthesia is used, the patient is seated and the tongue and oropharynx are sprayed and swabbed with anesthetic before the bronchoscope is inserted. For general anesthesia, the patient is placed in a supine position with the neck hyperextended. The patient is helped to a supine or side-lying position and the bronchoscope is inserted. After inspection, the tissue samples are collected from suspicious sites by bronchial brush or biopsy forceps.

Expectorated specimen:

➤ Ask the patient to sit upright, with assistance and support (e.g., with an overbed table) as needed.

➤ Ask the patient to take two or three deep breaths and cough deeply. Any sputum raised should be expectorated directly into a sterile sputum collection container.

➤ If the patient is unable to produce the desired amount of sputum, several strategies may be attempted. One approach is to have the patient drink two glasses of water, and then assume the position for postural drainage of the upper and middle lung segments. Effective coughing may be assisted by placing either the hands or a pillow over the diaphragmatic area and applying slight pressure. Another approach is to place a vaporizer or other humidifying device at the bedside.

➤ After sufficient exposure to adequate humidification, postural drainage of the upper and middle lung segments may be repeated before attempting to obtain the specimen. Other methods may include obtaining an order for an expectorant to be administered with additional water approximately 2 hours before attempting to obtain the specimen. Chest percussion and postural drainage of all lung segments may also be employed. If the patient is still unable to raise sputum, the use of an ultrasonic nebulizer ("induced sputum") may be necessary; this is usually done by a respiratory therapist.

Tracheal suctioning:

➤ Obtain the necessary equipment, including a suction device, suction kit, and Lukens tube or in-line trap.

➤ Position the patient with head elevated as high as tolerated.

➤ Put on sterile gloves. Maintain the dominant hand as sterile and the nondominant hand as clean.

➤ Using the sterile hand, attach the suction catheter to the rubber tubing of the Lukens tube or in-line trap. Then attach the suction tubing to the male adapter of the trap with the clean hand. Lubricate the suction catheter with sterile saline.

➤ Tell nonintubated patients to protrude the tongue and to take a deep breath as the suction catheter is passed through the nostril. When the catheter enters the trachea, a reflex cough is stimulated; immediately advance the catheter into the trachea and apply suction. Maintain suction for approximately 10 seconds, but never longer than 15 seconds. Withdraw the catheter without applying suction. Separate the suction catheter and suction tubing from the trap, and place the rubber tubing over the male adapter to seal the unit.

➤ For intubated patients or patients with a tracheostomy, the previous procedure is followed except that the suction catheter is passed through the existing endotracheal or tracheostomy tube rather than through the nostril. The patient should be hyperoxygenated before and after the procedure in accordance with standard protocols for suctioning these patients.

➤ Generally, a series of three to five early morning sputum samples are collected in sterile containers. If leprosy is suspected, obtain a smear from nasal scrapings or a biopsy specimen from lesions in a sterile container. Label the specimen, and promptly transport it to the laboratory. It is advisable to note antimicrobial therapy on the collection container.

Post-test: ■

➤ Instruct the patient to resume usual diet and medication as directed by the health care practitioner.

➤ Instruct the patient to perform mouth care after the specimen has been obtained. A cool beverage may aid in relieving throat irritation caused by coughing or suctioning.

➤ If a bronchoscopy was performed, inform the patient to drink liquids or eat food only after the gag reflex returns. Monitor vital signs and compare with baseline values. The patient may be placed in isolation pending results of the smear if tuberculosis is suspected.

➤ Instruct the patient to notify someone immediately if he or she begins to have difficulty breathing or if bleeding occurs.

➤ Note the color, consistency, and volume of the specimen collected.

➤ Observe the patient's color and respiratory rate. Administer oxygen, as necessary.

➤ Inform the patient of smoking cessation programs, as appropriate.

➤ Recognize anxiety related to test results and provide support. Provide teaching and information regarding the clinical implications of the test results, as appropriate. Inform the patient of the importance of medical follow-up and suggest ongoing support resources to assist in coping with chronic illness and possible early death.

➤ Evaluate test results in relation to the patient's symptoms and other tests performed. Related laboratory tests include arterial/alveolar oxygen ratio, blood gases, complete blood count, and relevant cultures.

CULTURE, FUNGAL

· ·

SYNONYM/ACRONYM: N/A.

SPECIMEN: Hair, skin, nail, pus, sterile fluids, blood, bone marrow, stool, bronchial washings, sputum, or tissue samples collected in a sterile plastic, tightly capped container.

REFERENCE VALUE: (Method: Culture on selective media; macroscopic and microscopic examination) No presence of fungi.

DESCRIPTION: Fungi, organisms that normally live in soil, can be introduced into humans through the accidental inhalation of spores or inoculation of spores into tissue through trauma. Individuals most susceptible to fungal infection usually are debilitated by chronic disease, are receiving prolonged antibiotic therapy, or have impaired immune systems. Fungal diseases may be classified according to the involved tissue type: dermatophytoses involve superficial and cutaneous tissue; there are also subcutaneous and systemic mycoses. ■

INDICATIONS:

• Determine antimicrobial sensitivity of the organism

• Isolate and identify organisms responsible for nail infections or abnormalities

• Isolate and identify organisms responsible for skin eruptions, drainage, or other evidence of infection

RESULT

Positive findings in:

• Blood

Candida albicans
Histoplasma capsulatum
- Cerebrospinal fluid
Coccidioides immitis
Cryptococcus neoformans
Members of the order Mucorales
Paracoccidioides brasiliensis
Sporothrix schenckii
- Hair
Epidermophyton
Microsporum
Trichophyton
- Nails
Candida albicans
Cephalosporium
Epidermophyton
Trichophyton
- Skin
Actinomyces israelii
Candida albicans
Coccidioides immitis
Epidermophyton
Microsporum
Trichophyton
- Tissue
A. israelii
Aspergillus
Candida albicans
Nocardia
P. brasiliensis

CRITICAL VALUES: N/A

INTERFERING FACTORS: Prompt and proper specimen processing, storage, and analysis are important to achieve accurate results.

Nursing Implications and Procedure • • • • • • • • • • •

Pretest: ■

➤ Obtain a history of the patient's complaints, including a list of known allergens.

➤ Obtain a history of the patient's immune system as well as results of previously performed tests and procedures. For related tests, refer to the immune system table.

➤ Obtain a list of medications the patient is taking, including herbs, nutritional supplements, and nutraceuticals. The requesting health care practitioner and laboratory should be advised that the patient regularly uses these products so that their effects can be taken into consideration when reviewing results.

➤ There are no food, fluid, or medication restrictions unless by medical direction.

➤ Review the procedure with the patient.

➤ Inform the patient that specimen collection may vary depending on collection site but usually takes approximately 5 to 10 minutes.

Intratest: ■

➤ Direct the patient to breathe normally and to avoid unnecessary movement.

➤ Observe standard precautions and follow the general guidelines in Appendix A. Instructions regarding the appropriate transport materials for blood, bone marrow, bronchial washings, sputum, sterile fluids, stool, and tissue samples should be obtained from the laboratory.

Skin:

➤ Clean the collection site with 70% alcohol. Scrape the peripheral margin of the collection site with a sterile scalpel or wooden spatula. Place the scrapings in a sterile collection container.

Hair:

➤ Fungi usually grow at the base of the hair shaft. Infected hairs can be identified by using a Wood's lamp in a darkened room. A Wood's lamp provides rays of ultraviolet light at a wavelength of 366 nm, or 3660 Å. Infected hairs fluoresce a bright yellow-green when exposed to light from the Wood's lamp. Using tweezers, pluck hair from skin.

Nails:

➤ Ideally, softened material from the nail bed is sampled from beneath the nail plate. Alternatively, shavings from the deeper portions of the nail itself can be collected.

➤ The potassium hydroxide (KOH) test is used to indicate the presence of mycelium, mycelial fragments, spores, or budding yeast cells. A portion of the specimen is mixed with 15% KOH on a glass slide, and then the slide is covered and gently heated briefly. The slide is examined under a microscope for the presence of fungal elements.

➤ Label the specimen, and promptly transport it to the laboratory.

Post-test:

➤ Evaluate test results in relation to the patient's symptoms and other tests performed. Related tests include relevant bacterial cultures, tissue biopsies, and body fluid analysis.

CULTURE, VIRAL

SYNONYM/ACRONYM: N/A.

SPECIMEN: Urine, semen, blood, body fluid, stool, tissue, or swabs from the affected site.

REFERENCE VALUE: (Method: Culture in special media, enzyme-linked immunoassays, direct fluorescent antibody techniques, latex agglutination, immunoperoxidase techniques) No virus isolated.

DESCRIPTION: Viruses, the most common cause of human infection, are submicroscopic organisms that invade living cells. They can be classified as either RNA- or DNA-type viruses. Viral titers are highest in the early stages of disease before the host has begun to manufacture significant antibodies against the invader. Specimens need to be collected as early on in the disease process as possible. ∎

INDICATIONS: Assist in the identification of viral infection

RESULT

Positive findings in:

• Acquired immunodeficiency syndrome
  Human immunodeficiency virus (HIV)

• Acute respiratory failure
  Hantavirus

- Anorectal infections
  Herpes simplex virus (HSV)
  Human papillomavirus
- Bronchitis
  Parainfluenza virus
  Respiratory syncytial virus (RSV)
- Condylomata
  Human papilloma DNA virus
- Conjunctivitis/keratitis
  Adenovirus
  Epstein-Barr virus
  HSV
  Measles virus
  Parvovirus
  Rubella virus
  Varicella zoster virus
- Croup
  Parainfluenza virus
  RSV
- Cutaneous infection with rash
  Enteroviruses
  HSV
  Varicella zoster virus
- Encephalitis
  Enteroviruses
  Flaviviruses
  HSV
  HIV
  Measles virus
  Rabies virus
  Togaviruses
- Febrile illness with rash
  Coxsackieviruses
  Echovirus
- Gastroenteritis
  Norwalk virus
  Rotavirus
- Genital herpes
  HSV-1
  HSV-2
- Hemorrhagic cystitis
  Adenovirus

- Hemorrhagic fever
  Ebola virus
  Hantavirus
  Lassa virus
  Marburg virus
- Herpangina
  Coxsackievirus (group A)
- Infectious mononucleosis
  Cytomegalovirus
  Epstein-Barr virus
- Meningitis
  Coxsackieviruses
  Echovirus
  HSV-2
  Lymphocytic choriomeningitis virus
- Myocarditis/pericarditis
  Coxsackievirus
  Echovirus
- Parotitis
  Mumps virus
  Parainfluenza virus
- Pharyngitis
  Adenovirus
  Coxsackievirus (group A)
  Epstein-Barr virus
  HSV
  Influenza virus
  Parainfluenza virus
  Rhinovirus
- Pleurodynia
  Coxsackievirus (group B)
- Pneumonia
  Adenovirus
  Influenza virus
  Parainfluenza virus
  RSV
- Upper respiratory tract infection
  Adenovirus
  Corona virus
  Influenza virus
  Parainfluenza virus
  RSV
  Rhinovirus

CRITICAL VALUES: ⚠ Positive RSV culture should be reported immediately to the requesting health care practitioner.

INTERFERING FACTORS: Viral specimens are unstable. Prompt and proper specimen processing, storage, and analysis are important to achieve accurate results.

Nursing Implications and Procedure • • • • • • • • • • •

Pretest:

➤ Obtain a history of the patient's complaints, including a list of known allergens.

➤ Obtain a history of the patient's gastrointestinal, genitourinary, immune, reproductive, and respiratory systems, as well as results of previously performed tests and procedures. For related tests, refer to the gastrointestinal, genitourinary, immune, reproductive, and respiratory system tables.

➤ Obtain a list of the medications the patient is taking, including herbs, nutritional supplements, and nutraceuticals. The requesting health care practitioner and laboratory should be advised if the patient regularly uses these products so that their effects can be taken into consideration when reviewing results.

➤ There are no food, fluid, or medication restrictions unless by medical direction.

➤ Review the procedure with the patient.

➤ Inform the patient that specimen collection takes approximately 5 to 10 minutes.

Intratest:

➤ Direct the patient to breathe normally and to avoid unnecessary movement.

➤ Observe standard precautions and follow the general guidelines in Appendix A. Instructions regarding the appropriate transport materials for blood, bronchial washings, sputum, sterile fluids, stool, and tissue samples should be obtained from the laboratory. The type of applicator used to obtain swabs should be verified by consultation with the testing laboratory personnel.

➤ The appropriate viral transport material should be obtained from the laboratory. Nasopharyngeal washings for RSV testing should be immediately placed in cold viral transport media.

➤ Label the specimen with the exact site, date, and time of collection; contact person for notification of results; and other pertinent information (e.g., patient immunocompromised owing to organ transplant, radiation, or chemotherapy). Promptly transport the specimen to the laboratory.

Post-test:

➤ Evaluate test results in relation to the patient's symptoms and other tests performed. Related tests include relevant tissue biopsy, bacterial cultures, and viral serology tests.

CYSTOMETRY

• •

SYNONYM/ACRONYM: Urodynamic testing of bladder function, CMG.

AREA OF APPLICATION: Bladder, urethra.

CONTRAST: None.

DESCRIPTION: Cystometry evaluates the motor and sensory function of the bladder when incontinence is present or neurological bladder dysfunction is suspected and monitors the effects of treatment for the abnormalities. This noninvasive manometric study measures the bladder pressure volume characteristics in centimeters of water (cm H$_2$O) during the filling and emptying phases. The test provides information about bladder structure and function that can lead to uninhibited bladder contractions, sensations of bladder fullness and need to void, and ability to inhibit voiding. These abnormalities cause incontinence and other impaired patterns of micturition. Cystometry can be performed with cystoscopy and sphincter electromyography. ∎

INDICATIONS:

• Determine cause of bladder dysfunction and pathology

• Evaluate signs and symptoms of urinary elimination pattern dysfunction

• Determine the type of incontinence: *functional* (involuntary and unpredictable), *reflex* (involuntary when a specific volume is reached), *stress* (weak pelvic muscles), *total* (continuous and unpredictable), *urge* (involuntary when urgency is sensed), and *psychological* (e.g., dementia, confusion affecting awareness)

• Determine type of neurogenic bladder (motor or sensory)

• Evaluate the management of neurological bladder before surgical intervention

• Evaluate the usefulness of drug therapy on detrusor muscle function and tonicity and on internal and external sphincter function

• Determine cause of urinary retention

• Detect congenital urinary abnormalities

• Determine the cause of recurrent urinary tract infections (UTIs)

• Evaluate postprostatectomy incontinence

• Evaluate voiding disorders associated with spinal cord injury

• Evaluate urinary obstruction in male patients experiencing urinary retention

RESULT

Normal Findings:

• Normal sensory perception of bladder fullness, desire to void and ability to inhibit urination, and appropriate response to temperature (hot and cold)

• Normal bladder capacity: 350 to 750 mL for men and 250 to 550 mL for women

• Normal functioning bladder pressure: 8 to 15 cm H_2O

• Normal sensation of fullness: 40 to 100 cm H_2O or 300 to 500 mL

• Normal bladder pressure during voiding: 30 to 40 cm H_2O

• Normal detrusor pressure: less than 10 cm H_2O

• Normal urge to void: 150 to 450 mL

• Urethral pressure that is higher than bladder pressure, ensuring continence

• Normal filling pattern

• Absence of residual urine (0 mL)

Abnormal Findings:

• Flaccid bladder that fills without contracting

• Inability to perceive bladder fullness

• Inability to initiate or maintain urination without applying external pressure

• Sensory or motor paralysis of bladder

• Total loss of conscious sensation and vesical control or uncontrollable micturition (incontinence)

CRITICAL VALUES: N/A

INTERFERING FACTORS:

This procedure is contraindicated for:

• Patients with acute UTIs because the study can cause infection to spread to the kidneys

• Patients who are pregnant or suspected of being pregnant, unless the potential benefits of the procedure far outweigh the risks to the fetus and mother

• Patients with urethral obstruction

• Patients with cervical cord lesions because patients may exhibit autonomic dysreflexia, as seen by bradycardia, flushing, hypertension, diaphoresis, and headache

• Inability to catheterize the patient

Factors that may impair examination results:

• Inability of the patient to cooperate or remain still during the procedure because of age, significant pain, or mental status

• Inability to void in a supine position or straining to void during the study

• A high level of patient anxiety or embarrassment, which may interfere with the study, making it difficult to distinguish whether the results are due to stress or organic pathology

• Administration of drugs that affect bladder function, such as muscle relaxants or antihistamines

Other considerations:

• Failure to follow dietary restrictions before the procedure may cause the procedure to be canceled or repeated.

Nursing Implications and Procedure • • • • • • • • • • •

Pretest:

➤ Inform the patient that the procedure is performed in a special urology room or in a clinic setting by the physician.

➤ Obtain a history of the patient's complaints and medication usage (e.g., antihistamines and muscle relaxants).

➤ Obtain a history of the patient's genitourinary system as well as results of previously performed medical and surgical therapeutic interventions. For related tests, refer to the genitourinary and renal system tables.

➤ Determine date of last menstrual period and the possibility of pregnancy in perimenopausal women.

➤ Determine the patient's allergies or sensitivities to anesthetics, analgesics, antibiotics, and latex.

➤ Assess hematologic status, blood-clotting ability, and urinalysis findings for abnormalities.

➤ Inform the patient that the only discomfort he or she will experience is the insertion of the urethral catheter, and that there may be some sensation of pressure and/or having to void.

➤ *Obtain a written, informed consent for the procedure from the patient.*

➤ Instruct the patient to report pain, sweating, nausea, headache, and the urge to void during the study.

➤ Explain that patient cooperation with positioning and activity before and during the test is crucial for achieving accurate results.

➤ There are no food, fluid, or medication restrictions unless by medical direction.

➤ Review the procedure with the patient.

➤ Inform the patient that the procedure takes approximately 30 to 45 minutes.

Intratest:

➤ Give the patient a gown and robe to wear; ensure that the patient is draped during the procedure to avoid unnecessary exposure.

➤ Position the patient in a supine or lithotomy position on the examining table. If spinal cord injury is present, the patient can remain on a stretcher in a supine position and be draped appropriately.

➤ Ask the patient to void and lie still during the procedure. During voiding, note characteristics such as start time; force and continuity of the stream; volume voided; presence of dribbling, straining, or hesitancy; and stop time.

➤ A urinary catheter is inserted into the bladder under sterile conditions, and residual urine is measured and recorded. A test for sensory response to temperature is done by instilling 30 mL of room-temperature sterile water followed by 30 mL of warm sterile water. Sensations are assessed and recorded.

➤ Fluid is removed from the bladder, and the catheter is connected to a cystometer that measures the pressure. Sterile normal saline or distilled water or carbon dioxide gas is instilled in controlled amounts into the bladder. When the client indicates the urge to void, the bladder is considered full; urination amounts as well as start and stop times are then recorded.

➤ Pressure and volume readings are recorded and graphed for response to heat, full bladder, urge to void, and ability to inhibit voiding. The patient is requested to void without straining, and pressures are taken and recorded during this activity.

➤ After completion of voiding, the bladder is emptied of any other fluid, and the catheter is withdrawn, unless further testing is planned.

➤ If further testing is done to determine if abnormal bladder function is being caused by muscle incompetence or interruption in innervation, anticholinergic medication (e.g., atropine) or cholinergic medication (e.g., bethanechol [Urecholine]) can be injected and the study repeated in 20 or 30 minutes.

Post-test:

➤ Inform the patient that further examinations may be necessary.

➤ Monitor fluid intake and urinary output for 24 hours after the procedure.

➤ Monitor vital signs after the procedure every 15 minutes for 2 hours or as directed. Elevated temperature may indicate infection.

➤ Inform the patient that he or she may experience burning or discomfort on urination for a few voidings after the procedure.

➤ Emphasize that persistent flank or suprapubic pain, fever, chills, blood in urine, difficulty urinating, or change in urinary pattern must be reported to the physician immediately.

➤ Determine if the patient or family members have any further questions or concerns.

➤ A physician specializing in this branch of medicine sends a written report to the ordering provider, who discusses the results with the patient.

➤ Evaluate test results in relation to the patient's symptoms and other tests performed. Related diagnostic tests include pelvic ultrasound, intravenous pyelography, and computed tomography and magnetic resonance imaging of the pelvis.

CYSTOSCOPY

SYNONYMS/ACRONYM: Cystoureterography, cystourethrography, prostatography.

AREA OF APPLICATION: Bladder, urethra, ureteral orifices.

CONTRAST: None.

DESCRIPTION: Cystoscopy provides direct visualization of the urethra, urinary bladder, and ureteral orifices—areas not usually visible with x-ray procedures. This procedure is also used to obtain specimens and treat pathology associated with the aforementioned structures. Cystoscopy is accomplished by transurethral insertion of a cystoscope into the bladder. Rigid cystoscopes contain an obturator and a telescope with a lens and light system; there are also flexible cystoscopes, which use fiberoptic technology. The procedure may be performed during or after ultrasonography or radiography, or during urethroscopy or retrograde pyelography. ■

INDICATIONS:

• Differentiate, through tissue biopsy, between benign and cancerous lesions involving the bladder

• Evaluate the function of each kidney by obtaining urine samples via ureteral catheters

• Evaluate changes in urinary elimination patterns

• Determine the source of hematuria of unknown cause

• Determine the possible source of persistent urinary tract infections

- Evaluate the extent of prostatic hyperplasia and degree of obstruction

- Identify congenital anomalies, such as duplicate ureters, ureteroceles, urethral or ureteral strictures, diverticula, and areas of inflammation or ulceration

- Remove renal calculi from the bladder or ureters

- Place ureteral catheters to drain urine from the renal pelvis or for retrograde pyelography

- Identify and remove polyps and small tumors (including fulguration) from the bladder

- Evacuate blood clots and perform fulguration of bleeding sites within the lower urinary tract

- Implant radioactive seeds

- Evaluate urinary tract abnormalities such as dysuria, frequency, retention, inadequate stream, urgency, and incontinence

- Resect small tumors

- Dilate the urethra and ureters

- Coagulate bleeding areas

- Place ureteral stents and resect prostate gland tissue (transurethral resection of the prostate)

RESULT

Normal Findings:

- Normal ureters, bladder, and urethra structure

Abnormal Findings:

- Diverticulum of the bladder, fistula, stones, and strictures

- Inflammation or infection

- Obstruction

- Polyps

- Prostatic hypertrophy or hyperplasia

- Renal calculi

- Tumors

- Ureteral or urethral stricture

- Urinary tract malformation and congenital anomalies

CRITICAL VALUES: N/A

INTERFERING FACTORS:

This procedure is contraindicated for:

- Patients who are pregnant or suspected of being pregnant, unless the potential benefits of the procedure far outweigh the risks to the fetus and mother

- Patients with bleeding disorders because instrumentation may lead to excessive bleeding from the lower urinary tract

- Patients with acute cystitis or urethritis because instrumentation could allow bacteria to enter the bloodstream, resulting in septicemia

Factors that may impair examination results:

- Inability of the patient to cooperate or remain still during the procedure because of age, significant pain, or mental status

Other considerations:

- Failure to follow dietary restrictions before the procedure may cause the procedure to be canceled or repeated.

Nursing Implications and Procedure

Pretest:

➤ Inform the patient that the procedure is generally performed under general, spinal, or local anesthesia.

➤ Inform the patient that the procedure is performed by a physician in a special cystoscopy suite near or in the operating room (or in a physician's office) and takes approximately 30 to 60 minutes.

➤ Obtain a history of the patient's complaints.

➤ Obtain a history of the patient's genitourinary system as well as results of previously performed tests and procedures for bleeding disorders. For related tests, refer to the genitourinary and renal system tables.

➤ Determine date of last menstrual period and the possibility of pregnancy in perimenopausal women.

➤ Determine the patient's allergies or sensitivities to anesthetics, analgesics, or antibiotics.

➤ Assess hematologic status and blood-clotting ability and urinalysis findings for abnormalities.

➤ *Obtain a written, informed consent for the procedure from the patient.*

➤ Restrict food and fluids for 8 hours if the patient is having general or spinal anesthesia. For local anesthesia, allow only clear liquids 8 hours before the procedure.

➤ Inform the patient that he or she may feel some sensation of pressure and/or having to void.

➤ Obtain and record the patient's vital signs.

➤ Review the procedure with the patient.

Intratest:

➤ Administer ordered preoperative sedation.

➤ Give the patient a gown and robe to wear; ensure that the patient is draped during the procedure to avoid unnecessary exposure.

➤ Position patient on the examination table draped and with legs in stirrups. If general or spinal anesthesia is to be used, it is administered before positioning the patient on the table.

➤ Cleanse external genitalia with antiseptic solution. If local anesthetic is used, it is instilled into the urethra and retained for 5 to 10 minutes. A penile clamp may be used for male patients to aid in retention of anesthetic.

➤ The physician inserts a cystoscope or a urethroscope to examine the urethra before cystoscopy. The urethroscope has a sheath that may be left in place, and the cystoscope is inserted through it, avoiding multiple instrumentations.

➤ After insertion of the cystoscope, a sample of residual urine may be obtained for culture or other analysis.

➤ The bladder is irrigated via an irrigation system attached to the scope. The irrigant is usually sterile water, unless an isotonic solution, such as mannitol, is used during transurethral resection procedures. The irrigation fluid aids in bladder visualization.

➤ If a prostatic tumor is found, a biopsy specimen may be obtained by means of a cytology brush or biopsy forceps inserted through the scope. If the tumor is small and localized, it can be excised and fulgurated. This procedure is termed *transurethral resection of the bladder.* Polyps can also be identified and excised.

➤ Ulcers or bleeding sites can be fulgurated using electrocautery.

➤ Renal calculi can be crushed and removed from the ureters and bladder.

➤ Ureteral catheters can be inserted via the scope to obtain urine samples from each kidney for comparative analysis and radiographic studies.

➤ Ureteral and urethral strictures can also be dilated during this procedure.

➤ Upon completion of the examination and related procedures, the cystoscope is withdrawn.

➤ Place obtained specimens in proper containers, label them properly, and immediately transport them to the laboratory.

Post-test:

➤ Monitor vital and neurological signs until they return to preprocedure levels.

➤ Inform the patient that further examinations may be necessary to evaluate progression of the disease process or to determine the need for a change in therapy.

➤ Instruct the patient to resume his or her usual diet and medications, as directed by the health care provider.

➤ Encourage the patient to drink increased amounts of fluids (125 mL/h for 24 hours) after the procedure.

➤ Monitor fluid intake and urinary output for 24 hours after the procedure. Decreased urine output may indicate bladder edema or perforation caused by forceful advancement of instrumentation.

➤ Inform the patient that burning or discomfort on urination can be experienced for a few voidings after the procedure and that the urine may be blood-tinged for the first and second voidings after the procedure.

➤ Emphasize that persistent flank or suprapubic pain, fever, chills, blood in urine, difficulty urinating, or change in urinary pattern must be reported immediately to the physician.

➤ Determine if the patient or family members have any further questions or concerns.

➤ A physician specializing in this branch of medicine sends a written report to the ordering provider, who discusses the results with the patient.

➤ Evaluate test results in relation to the patient's symptoms and other tests performed. Related diagnostic tests include pelvic ultrasound, intravenous pyelography, and computed tomography and magnetic resonance imaging of the pelvis.

CYSTOURETHROGRAPHY, VOIDING

SYNONYM/ACRONYM: Voiding cystography.

AREA OF APPLICATION: Bladder, urethra.

CONTRAST: Radiopaque iodine–based contrast medium.

DESCRIPTION: Voiding cystourethrography involves visualization of the bladder filled with contrast medium instilled through a catheter by use of a syringe or gravity, and after the catheter is removed, the excretion of the contrast medium. Excretion or micturition is recorded electronically or on videotape for confirmation or exclusion of ureteral reflux and evaluation of the urethra. Fluoroscopic films or plain radiographs may also be taken to record bladder filling and emptying. This procedure is often used to evaluate chronic urinary tract infections (UTIs). ∎

INDICATIONS:

* Evaluate possible cause of frequent UTIs

* Confirm the diagnosis of congenital lower urinary tract anomaly

* Evaluate abnormal bladder emptying and incontinence

* Assess hypertrophy of the prostate lobes

* Assess ureteral stricture

* Evaluate the effects of bladder trauma

* Assess the degree of compromise of a stenotic prostatic urethra

* Evaluate the presence and extent of ureteral reflux

* Evaluate the urethra for obstruction and strictures

RESULT

Normal Findings:

* Normal bladder and urethra structure and function

Abnormal Findings:

* Bladder trauma
* Bladder tumors
* Hematomas
* Neurogenic bladder
* Pelvic tumors
* Prostatic enlargement
* Ureteral stricture
* Ureterocele
* Urethral diverticula
* Vesicoureteral reflux

CRITICAL VALUES: N/A

INTERFERING FACTORS:

This procedure is contraindicated for:

* Patients with allergies to shellfish or iodinated dye. The contrast medium used may cause a life-threatening allergic reaction. Patients with a known hypersensitivity to the contrast medium may benefit from premedication with corticosteroids or the use of nonionic contrast medium.

* Patients with bleeding disorders.

* Patients who are pregnant or suspected of being pregnant, unless the potential benefits of the procedure far outweigh the risks to the fetus and mother.

* Patients with UTI, obstruction, or injury.

* Elderly and other patients who are chronically dehydrated before the test, because of their risk of contrast-induced renal failure.

* Patients who are in renal failure.

Factors that may impair clear imaging:

* Inability of the patient to cooperate or remain still during the procedure because of age, significant pain, or mental status

* Improper adjustment of the radiographic equipment to accommodate obese or thin patients, which can cause overexposure or underexposure and a poor-quality study

* Patients who are very obese, who may exceed the weight limit for the equipment

* Incorrect positioning of the patient, which may produce poor visualization of the area to be examined

* Gas or feces in the gastrointestinal tract

resulting from inadequate cleansing or failure to restrict food intake before the study

• Retained barium from a previous radiologic procedure

• Metallic objects within the examination field (e.g., jewelry or body rings), which may inhibit organ visualization and can produce unclear images

Other considerations:

• Consultation with a physician should occur before the procedure for radiation safety concerns regarding infants of patients who are lactating.

• Risks associated with radiographic overexposure can result from frequent x-ray procedures. Personnel in the room with the patient should wear a protective lead apron, stand behind a shield, or leave the area while the examination is being done. Personnel working in the area where the examination is being done should wear badges that reveal their level of exposure to radiation.

Nursing Implications and Procedure · · · · · · · · · · ·

Pretest:

➤ Inform the patient about the purpose of the procedure, the need to remain still, and the need to hold his or her breath for short periods.

➤ Obtain a history of known or suspected hypersensitivity to radiographic contrast medium or shellfish.

➤ Obtain a history of the patient's complaints.

➤ Obtain a history of the patient's genitourinary and abdominal systems as well as results of previously performed tests and procedures. For related tests, refer to the genitourinary system table.

➤ Determine date of last menstrual period and possibility of pregnancy in perimenopausal women.

➤ *Obtain a written, informed consent for the procedure from the patient.*

➤ Instruct the patient to increase fluid intake the day before the test, but to have only clear fluids 8 hours before the test.

➤ Inform the patient that he or she may feel some pressure when the catheter is inserted and when the contrast medium is instilled through the catheter.

➤ Inform the patient that he or she may receive a laxative the night before the test or an enema or a cathartic the morning of the test, as ordered.

➤ Schedule gastrointestinal or any barium studies after this study.

➤ Inform the patient that the procedure is done by a radiologist and support staff.

➤ Insert a Foley catheter before the procedure, if ordered.

➤ Review the procedure with the patient.

➤ Inform the patient that the procedure takes approximately 30 minutes.

Intratest:

➤ Remove patient's clothing and metallic objects from the lower abdominal area.

➤ Give the patient a gown and robe to wear; ensure that the patient is draped during the procedure to avoid unnecessary exposure.

➤ Have the patient void before the procedure.

➤ Administer an antihistamine or steroid, as ordered by a physician, for patients with a known significant allergic reaction to the IV contrast medium.

➤ Place the patient on the table in a supine or lithotomy position.

➤ A kidney, ureter, and bladder (KUB) film or plain radiograph is taken to ensure that no barium or stool obscures visualization of the urinary system.

➤ A catheter is filled with contrast medium to eliminate air pockets and is inserted until the balloon reaches the meatus. The patient is placed in the right posterior oblique position with the thigh drawn up to a 90° angle and, in men, the penis placed along its axis.

➤ When three-fourths of the contrast medium has been injected, another radiographic exposure is made while the remainder of the contrast medium is injected.

➤ Left lateral and oblique views may be necessary to visualize the area in question.

➤ If the patient is able to void, the catheter is removed and the patient is asked to urinate while films are taken or radiographic images of the bladder and urethra are recorded.

➤ The procedure may be done on women using a double balloon to occlude the bladder neck from above and below the external meatus.

Post-test:

➤ Monitor vital and neurological signs until they return to preprocedure levels.

➤ Inform the patient that further examinations may be necessary to evalu-

ate progression of the disease process or to determine the need for a change in therapy.

➤ Instruct the patient to resume his or her usual diet and medications, as directed by the health care provider.

➤ Maintain the patient on adequate hydration after the procedure Encourage the patient to drink increased amounts of fluids (125 mL/h for 24 hours) after the procedure to prevent stasis and bacterial buildup.

➤ Monitor fluid intake and urinary output for 24 hours after the procedure. Decreased urinary output may indicate impending renal failure or edema caused by instrumentation.

➤ Monitor for signs of sepsis—fever, chills, and severe pelvic pain.

➤ Determine if the patient or family members have any further questions or concerns.

➤ A physician specializing in this branch of medicine sends a written report to the ordering provider, who discusses the results with the patient.

➤ Evaluate test results in relation to the patient's symptoms and other tests performed. Related diagnostic tests include pelvic ultrasound, intravenous pyelography, and computed tomography and magnetic resonance imaging of the pelvis.

CYTOLOGY, SPUTUM

· ·

SYNONYM/ACRONYM: N/A.

SPECIMEN: Sputum (10 to 15 mL) collected on 3 to 5 consecutive first-morning, deep-cough expectorations.

REFERENCE VALUE: (Method: Macroscopic and microscopic examination) Negative for abnormal cells, fungi, ova, and parasites.

DESCRIPTION: Cytology is the study of the origin, structure, function, and pathology of cells. In clinical practice, cytologic examinations are generally performed to detect cell changes resulting from neoplastic or inflammatory conditions. Sputum specimens for cytologic examinations may be collected by expectoration alone, by suctioning, by lung biopsy, during bronchoscopy, or by expectoration after bronchoscopy. A description of the method of specimen collection by bronchoscopy and biopsy is found in the monograph titled "Biopsy, Lung." ∎

INDICATIONS:

• Assist in the diagnosis of lung cancer

• Assist in the diagnosis of *Pneumocystis carinii* in persons with acquired immunodeficiency syndrome (AIDS)

• Detect known or suspected fungal or parasitic infection involving the lung

• Detect known or suspected viral disease involving the lung

• Screen cigarette smokers for neoplastic (nonmalignant) cellular changes

• Screen patients with history of acute or chronic inflammatory or infectious lung disorders, which may lead to benign atypical or metaplastic changes

RESULT: (Method: Microscopic examination) The method of reporting results of cytology examinations varies according to the laboratory performing the test. Terms used to report results may include *negative* (no abnormal cells seen), *inflammatory, benign atypical, suspect for neoplasm,* and *positive for neoplasm.*

Positive findings in:

• Infections caused by fungi, ova, or parasites

• Lipoid or aspiration pneumonia, as seen by lipid droplets contained in macrophages

• Neoplasms

• Viral infections and lung disease

CRITICAL VALUES:

If the patient becomes hypoxic or cyanotic, remove catheter immediately and administer oxygen.

If patient has asthma or chronic bronchitis, watch for aggravated bronchospasms with use of normal saline or acetylcysteine in an aerosol.

INTERFERING FACTORS:

• Improper specimen fixation may be cause for specimen rejection.

• Improper technique used to obtain bronchial washing may be cause for specimen rejection.

Nursing Implications and Procedure

Pretest: ∎

➤ Obtain a history of the patient's complaints, including a list of known allergens.

➤ Obtain a history of the patient's immune and respiratory systems, as well as results of previously performed tests and procedures. For related tests, refer to the immune and respiratory system tables.

➤ Obtain a list of the medications the patient is taking, including herbs, nutritional supplements, and nutraceuticals. The requesting health care practitioner and laboratory should be advised if the patient is regularly using these products so that their effects can be taken into consideration when reviewing results.

➤ For specimens collected by suctioning or expectoration without bronchoscopy, there are no food, fluid, or medication restrictions unless by medical direction.

➤ Instruct the patient to fast and refrain from taking liquids from midnight the night before if bronchoscopy or biopsy is to be performed.

➤ Address concerns about pain related to the procedure. Explain that a sedative and/or anesthetic is administered before the procedure to promote relaxation and reduce discomfort during the procedure, and that general anesthesia is administered for open biopsy. Atropine is usually given before bronchoscopy examinations to reduce bronchial secretions and to prevent vagally induced bradycardia. Meperidine (Demerol) or morphine may be given as a sedative. Lidocaine is sprayed in the patient's throat to reduce discomfort caused by the presence of the tube.

➤ Assess if the patient has an allergy to local anesthetics, and inform the health care practitioner accordingly.

➤ Ensure that nonallergy to anesthesia is confirmed before bronchoscopy or biopsy procedure is performed under general anesthesia.

➤ *Obtain written and informed consent before bronchoscopy or biopsy is performed.*

➤ Inform the patient that the test helps identify cellular changes associated with neoplasms or organisms that result in respiratory tract infections. When the actual infectious organisms are identified by cytology, tell the patient that the findings will be confirmed by culture. Emphasize that sputum and saliva are not the same.

➤ Reassure the patient that he or she will be able to breathe during the procedure if specimen collected is accomplished via suction method. Ensure that oxygen has been administered 20 to 30 minutes before the procedure if the specimen is to be obtained by tracheal suctioning.

➤ Assist in providing extra fluids, unless contraindicated, and proper humidification to decrease tenacious secretions. Inform the patient that increasing fluid intake before retiring on the night before the test aids in liquefying secretions and may make it easier to expectorate in the morning. Also explain that humidifying inspired air also helps to liquefy secretions.

➤ Assist with mouth care (brushing teeth or rinsing mouth with water), if needed, before collection so as not to contaminate the specimen by oral secretions.

➤ Instruct the patient not to touch the edge or inside of the specimen container with the hands or mouth.

➤ Review the procedure with the patient. If the laboratory has provided a container with fixative, instruct the patient that the fixative contents of the specimen collection container should not be ingested or otherwise removed.

➤ Inform the patient that three samples may be required, on three separate mornings, either by passing a small tube (tracheal catheter) and adding suction or by expectoration.

➤ The time it takes to collect a proper specimen varies according to the level of cooperation of the patient and the specimen collection procedure.

Intratest: ■

➤ Ensure that the patient has complied with dietary restrictions before bronchoscopy or biopsy.

➤ Observe standard precautions and follow the general guidelines in Appendix A.

➤ Administer ordered premedication 30 to 60 minutes before the procedure.

Bronchoscopy:

➤ Record baseline vital signs. The

patient is positioned in relation to the type of anesthesia being used. If local anesthesia is used, the patient is seated, and the tongue and oropharynx are sprayed and swabbed with anesthetic before the bronchoscope is inserted. For general anesthesia, the patient is placed in a supine position with the neck hyperextended. The patient is helped to a supine or side-lying position, and the bronchoscope is inserted. After inspection, the tissue samples are collected from suspicious sites by bronchial brush or biopsy forceps.

Expectorated specimen:

➤ Ask the patient to sit upright, with assistance and support (e.g., with an overbed table) as needed.

➤ Ask the patient to take two or three deep breaths and cough deeply. Any sputum raised should be expectorated directly into a sterile sputum collection container.

➤ If the patient is unable to produce the desired amount of sputum, several strategies may be attempted. One approach is to have the patient drink two glasses of water, and then assume the position for postural drainage of the upper and middle lung segments. Effective coughing may be assisted by placing either the hands or a pillow over the diaphragmatic area and applying slight pressure. Another approach is to place a vaporizer or other humidifying device at the bedside.

➤ After sufficient exposure to adequate humidification, postural drainage of the upper and middle lung segments may be repeated before attempting to obtain the specimen. Other methods may include obtaining an order for an expectorant to be administered with additional water approximately 2 hours before attempting to obtain the specimen. Chest percussion and postural drainage of all lung segments may also be employed. If the patient is still unable to raise sputum, the use of an ultrasonic nebulizer ("induced sputum") may be necessary; this is usually done by a respiratory therapist.

Tracheal suctioning:

➤ Obtain the necessary equipment, including a suction device, suction kit, and Lukens tube or in-line trap.

➤ Position the patient with head elevated as high as tolerated.

➤ Put on sterile gloves. Maintain the dominant hand as sterile and the nondominant hand as clean.

➤ Using the sterile hand, attach the suction catheter to the rubber tubing of the Lukens tube or in-line trap. Then attach the suction tubing to the male adapter of the trap with the clean hand. Lubricate the suction catheter with sterile saline.

➤ Tell nonintubated patients to protrude the tongue and to take a deep breath as the suction catheter is passed through the nostril. When the catheter enters the trachea, a reflex cough is stimulated; immediately advance the catheter into the trachea and apply suction. Maintain suction for approximately 10 seconds, but never longer than 15 seconds. Withdraw the catheter without applying suction. Separate the suction catheter and suction tubing from the trap, and place the rubber tubing over the male adapter to seal the unit.

➤ For intubated patients or patients with a tracheostomy, the previous procedure is followed except that the suction catheter is passed through the existing endotracheal or tracheostomy tube rather than through the nostril. The patient should be hyperoxygenated before and after the procedure in accordance with standard protocols for suctioning these patients.

General:

➤ Label the specimen, and promptly transport it to the laboratory. Note antimicrobial therapy on the collection container. Cytology specimens may also be expressed onto a glass slide and sprayed with a fixative or 95% alcohol.

Post-test:

➤ After general anesthesia, monitor vital signs every 15 minutes for an hour, and then every 2 hours for 4 hours, and as ordered. Take temperature every 4 hours for 24 hours.

➤ After local anesthesia, monitor vital signs and compare with baseline values.

➤ To avoid accidental aspiration, instruct the patient not to eat or drink until the effects of the anesthesia have worn off and the gag reflex has returned.

➤ Instruct the patient to resume usual diet as directed by the health care practitioner.

➤ Note the color, consistency, and volume of the specimen collected.

➤ Instruct the patient to perform mouth care after the specimen has been obtained.

➤ Provide comfort measures and treatment as needed, such as antiseptic gargles, inhalants, and warm moist applications. A cool beverage may aid in relieving throat irritation caused by coughing or suctioning.

➤ Instruct the patient to notify someone immediately if he or she begins to have difficulty breathing or if bleeding occurs.

➤ Observe the patient's color and respiratory rate. Administer oxygen, as necessary.

➤ Inform the patient of smoking cessation programs, as appropriate.

➤ Recognize anxiety related to test results and offer support. Provide teaching and information regarding the clinical implications of the test results, as appropriate. Inform the patient with abnormal findings of the importance of medical follow-up, and suggest ongoing support resources to assist in coping with chronic illness and possible early death.

➤ Evaluate test results in relation to the patient's symptoms and other tests performed. Related laboratory tests include arterial/alveolar oxygen ratio, blood gases, complete blood count, Gram stain, and relevant cultures.

CYTOLOGY, URINE

● ●

SYNONYM/ACRONYM: N/A.

SPECIMEN: Urine (180 mL for an adult or at least 10 mL for a child) collected in a clean wide-mouth plastic container.

REFERENCE VALUE: (Method: Microscopic examination) No abnormal cells or inclusions seen.

DESCRIPTION: Cells from the epithelial lining of the urinary tract can be found in the urine. Examination of these cells for abnormalities is useful with suspected infection, inflammatory conditions, or malignancy. ■

INDICATIONS: Assist in the diagnosis of urinary tract diseases, such as cancer, cytomegalovirus infection, and other inflammatory conditions

RESULT

Positive findings in:

• Cancer of the urinary tract

• Cytomegalic inclusion disease

• Inflammatory disease of the urinary tract

Negative findings in: N/A

CRITICAL VALUES: N/A

INTERFERING FACTORS: N/A

Nursing Implications and Procedure • • • • • • • • • • •

Pretest: ■

➤ Obtain a history of the patient's complaints, including a list of known allergens.

➤ Obtain a history of the patient's genitourinary and immune systems, as well as results of previously performed tests and procedures. For related tests, refer to the genitourinary and immune system tables.

➤ Obtain a list of medications the patient is taking, including herbs, nutritional supplements, and nutraceuticals. The requesting health care practitioner and laboratory should be advised if the patient regularly uses these products so that their effects can be taken

into consideration when reviewing results.

➤ There are no food, fluid, or medication restrictions unless by medical direction.

➤ Review the procedure with the patient. If a catheterized specimen is to be collected, explain this procedure to the patient and obtain a catheterization tray.

➤ Inform the patient that specimen collection takes approximately 5 to 10 minutes.

Intratest: ■

➤ Observe standard precautions and follow the general guidelines in Appendix A.

➤ Instruct the patient to obtain a urine specimen.

Clean-catch specimen:

➤ Instruct the male patient to (1) thoroughly wash his hands, (2) cleanse the meatus, (3) void a small amount into the toilet, and (4) void directly into the specimen container.

➤ Instruct the female patient to (1) thoroughly wash her hands; (2) cleanse the labia from front to back; (3) while keeping the labia separated, void a small amount into the toilet; and (4) without interrupting the urine stream, void directly into the specimen container.

Pediatric urine collector:

➤ Put on gloves. Appropriately cleanse the genital area and allow the area to dry. Remove the covering over the adhesive strips on the collector bag and apply over the genital area. Diaper the child. After obtaining the specimen, place the entire collection bag in a sterile urine container.

Indwelling catheter:

➤ Put on gloves. Empty drainage tube of urine. It may be necessary to clamp off the catheter for 15 to 30 minutes before specimen collection. Cleanse specimen port with antiseptic swab, and then aspirate 5 mL of urine with a 21- to 25-gauge needle and syringe. Transfer urine to a sterile container.

Urinary catheterization:

➤ Place female patient in lithotomy position or male patient in supine position. Using sterile technique, open the straight urinary catheterization kit and perform urinary catheterization. Place the retained urine in a sterile specimen container.

Suprapubic aspiration:

➤ Place the patient in a supine position. Cleanse the area with antiseptic and drape with sterile drapes. Using sterile technique, insert needle and remove sterile sample. Place the returned sample in a ster-

ile specimen container. Place a dry sterile dressing over the site. Do not collect urine from the pouch from the patient with a urinary diversion (e.g., ileal conduit). Instead perform catheterization through the stoma.

General:

➤ Label the specimen, and promptly transport it to the laboratory. If a delay in transport is expected, add an equal volume of 50% alcohol to the specimen as a preservative.

Post-test:

➤ Evaluate test results in relation to the patient's symptoms and other tests performed. Related laboratory tests include bladder cancer markers, kidney biopsy, and Papanicolaou smear.

CYTOMEGALOVIRUS, IMMUNOGLOBULIN G AND IMMUNOGLOBULIN M

· ·

SYNONYM/ACRONYM: CMV.

SPECIMEN: Serum (1 mL) collected in a plain red top tube.

REFERENCE VALUE: (Method: Indirect fluorescent antibody) Negative or less than a fourfold increase in titer.

DESCRIPTION: Cytomegalovirus (CMV) is a double-stranded DNA herpesvirus. The incubation period for primary infection is 4 to 8 weeks. Transmission may occur by direct contact with oral, respiratory, or venereal secretions and excretions. CMV infection is of primary concern in pregnant or immunocompromised patients or patients who have recently received an organ transplant. Blood units are sometimes tested for the presence of CMV if patients in these high-risk categories are the transfusion recipients. CMV serology is part of the TORCH (*t*oxoplasmosis, *o*ther [congenital syphilis and viruses], *r*ubella, *C*MV, and *h*erpesvirus type 2) panel used to test pregnant women. CMV, as well as these other infectious agents, can cross the placenta and result in congenital malformations, abortion, or stillbirth. The presence of immunoglobulin M (IgM) antibodies indicates acute infection. The presence of IgG antibodies indicates current or past infection. ∎

INDICATIONS:

• Assist in the diagnosis of congenital CMV infection in newborns

• Determine susceptibility, particularly in pregnant women, immunocompromised patients, and patients who recently have received an organ transplant

• Screen blood for high-risk-category transfusion recipients

RESULT

Positive findings in: CMV infection

Negative findings in: N/A

CRITICAL VALUES: N/A

INTERFERING FACTORS:

• False-positive results may occur in the presence of rheumatoid factor.

• False-negative results may occur if treatment was begun before antibodies developed or if the test was done less than 6 days after exposure to the virus.

Nursing Implications and Procedure • • • • • • • • • • •

Pretest: ▣

➤ Obtain a history of the patient's complaints and history of exposure. Obtain a list of known allergens.

➤ Obtain a history of the patient's

immune and reproductive systems, as well as results of previously performed tests and procedures. For related tests, refer to the immune and reproductive system tables.

➤ Obtain a list of the medications the patient is taking, including herbs, nutritional supplements, and nutraceuticals. The requesting health care practitioner and laboratory should be advised if the patient is regularly using these products so that their effects can be taken into consideration when reviewing results.

➤ There are no food, fluid, or medication restrictions unless by medical direction.

➤ Review the procedure with the patient.

➤ Inform the patient that multiple specimens may be required. Any individual positive result should be repeated in 7 to 14 days to monitor a change in titer.

➤ Inform the patient that each specimen collection takes approximately 5 to 10 minutes.

Intratest: ▣

➤ Direct the patient to breathe normally and to avoid unnecessary movement.

➤ Observe standard precautions and follow the general guidelines in Appendix A. Perform a venipuncture, and collect the specimen in a 5-mL red-top tube.

➤ Label the specimen, and promptly transport it to the laboratory.

Post-test: ▣

➤ Observe venipuncture site for bleeding or hematoma formation. Apply pressure bandage.

➤ Instruct the patient in isolation precautions during time of communicability or contagion.

➤ Emphasize the need to return to have a convalescent blood sample taken in 7 to 14 days.

➤ Warn the patient that there is a

possibility of false-negative or false-positive results.

➤ Recognize anxiety related to test results if the patient is pregnant and offer support. Provide teaching and information regarding the clinical implications of the test results, as appropriate. Educate the patient

regarding access to counseling services.

➤ Evaluate test results in relation to the patient's symptoms and other tests performed. Related laboratory tests include herpesvirus, rubella antibody, and *Toxoplasma* antibody.

D-DIMER

SYNONYMS/ACRONYM: Dimer, fibrin degradation fragment.

SPECIMEN: Plasma (1 mL) collected in a completely filled blue-top (sodium citrate) tube.

REFERENCE VALUE: (Method: Latex semiquantitative screen or quantitative enzyme-linked immunosorbent assay [ELISA])
Semiquantitative: No fragments detected
Quantitative: Less than 250 ng/mL

DESCRIPTION: The D-dimer is an asymmetric carbon compound formed by a crosslink between two identical fibrin molecules. The test is specific for secondary fibrinolysis because the crosslinkage occurs with fibrin and not fibrinogen. A positive test is presumptive evidence of disseminated intravascular coagulation (DIC). ∎

INDICATIONS:
• Assist in the detection of DIC and deep venous thrombosis (DVT)

• Assist in the evaluation of myocardial infarction and unstable angina

• Assist in the evaluation of possible veno-occlusive disease associated with sequelae of bone marrow transplant

• Assist in the evaluation of pulmonary embolism

RESULT: The sensitivity and specificity of the assay varies among test kits and between test methods (e.g., latex vs. ELISA).

Increased in:
• Arterial or venous thrombosis

• DVT

• DIC

• Neoplastic disease

• Pre-eclampsia

• Pregnancy (late and postpartum)

• Pulmonary embolism

• Recent surgery (within 2 days)

- Secondary fibrinolysis

Decreased in: N/A

CRITICAL VALUES: N/A

INTERFERING FACTORS:
- High rheumatoid factor titers can cause a false-positive result.

- Increased CA 125 levels can cause a false-positive result.

- Drugs that may cause an increase in plasma D-dimer include those administered for antiplatelet therapy.

- Drugs that may cause a decrease in plasma D-dimer include pravastatin and warfarin.

- Placement of tourniquet for longer than 1 minute can result in venous stasis and changes in the concentration of plasma proteins to be measured. Platelet activation may also occur under these conditions, causing erroneous results.

- Vascular injury during phlebotomy can activate platelets and coagulation factors, causing erroneous results.

- Hemolyzed specimens must be rejected because hemolysis is an indication of platelet and coagulation factor activation.

- Incompletely filled tubes contaminated with heparin or clotted specimens must be rejected.

- Icteric or lipemic specimens interfere with optical testing methods, producing erroneous results.

Nursing Implications and Procedure

Pretest: ■

➤ Obtain a history of the patient's complaints, including a list of known allergens.

➤ Obtain a history of hematologic diseases and recent surgery.

➤ Obtain a history of the patient's cardiovascular, hematopoietic, and respiratory systems, as well as results of previously performed tests and procedures. For related tests, refer to the cardiovascular, hematopoietic, and respiratory system tables.

➤ Obtain a list of the medications the patient is taking, including herbs, nutritional supplements, and nutraceuticals. The requesting health care practitioner and laboratory should be advised if the patient is regularly using these products so that their effects can be taken into consideration when reviewing results.

➤ There are no food, fluid, or medication restrictions unless by medical direction.

➤ Review the procedure with the patient.

➤ Inform the patient that specimen collection takes approximately 5 to 10 minutes.

Intratest: ■

➤ Direct the patient to breathe normally and to avoid unnecessary movement.

➤ Observe standard precautions and follow the general guidelines in Appendix A. Perform a venipuncture, and collect the specimen in a 5-mL blue-top tube. Fill the tube completely. *Important note*: Two different concentrations of sodium citrate preservative are currently added to blue-top tubes for coagulation studies: 3.2% and 3.8%. The National Committee for Clinical Laboratory Standards (NCCLS) guideline for sodium citrate is 3.2% Laboratories establish reference ranges for coagulation testing based on numerous factors, including sodium citrate concentration, test equipment, and test reagents. It is important to inquire from the laboratory which concentration it recommends, because each concentration will have its own specific reference range.

➤ When multiple specimens are drawn, the blue-top tube should be collected after sterile (i.e., blood culture) and red-top tubes. When coagulation testing is the only work to be done, an extra red-top tube should be collected before the blue-top tube to avoid contaminating the specimen with tissue thromboplastin, which can falsely decrease values.

➤ Label the specimen, and promptly transport it to the laboratory. The NCCLS recommendation for processed and unprocessed samples stored in unopened tubes is that testing should be completed within 1 to 4 hours.

Post-test:

➤ Observe venipuncture site for bleeding or hematoma formation. Apply pressure bandage.

➤ Evaluate test results in relation to the patient's symptoms and other tests performed. Related laboratory tests include fibrin split products, fibrinogen, activated partial thromboplastin time, platelet count, and prothrombin time.

D-XYLOSE TOLERANCE TEST

• •

SYNONYM/ACRONYM: N/A.

SPECIMEN: Plasma (1 mL) collected in gray-top (fluoride/oxalate) tube and urine (10 mL from a 5-hour collection) from a timed collection in a clean amber plastic container.

REFERENCE VALUE: (Method: Spectrophotometry)

Dose by Age	Conventional Units	SI Units
	Plasma	*(Conversion Factor ×0.0666)*
Adult dose		
25 g	Greater than 25 mg/dL	Greater than 1.7 mmol/L
5 g	Greater than 20 mg/dL	Greater than 1.3 mmol/L
Pediatric dose		
0.5 g/kg	Greater than 30 mg/dL	Greater than 2.0 mmol/L
(max. 25 g)		

(Continued on the following page)

Dose by Age	Conventional Units	SI Units
	Urine	*(Conversion Factor × 6.66)*
Adult dose		
25 g	Greater than 4 g/5 h collection	Greater than 26.6 mmol/5 h
5 g	Greater than 1.2 g/5 h collection	Greater than 8 mmol/5 h
Pediatric dose		
0.5 g/kg	Greater than 16–33%	Greater than 16–33%
(max. 25 g)	of dose	of dose

DESCRIPTION: The D-xylose tolerance test is used to screen for intestinal malabsorption of carbohydrates. D-xylose is a pentose sugar not normally present in the blood in significant amounts. It is partially absorbed when ingested and normally passes unmetabolized in the urine. ▪

INDICATIONS: Assist in the diagnosis of malabsorption syndromes

RESULT

Increased in: N/A

Decreased in:
- Postoperative period after massive resection of the intestine
- Amyloidosis
- Bacterial overgrowth
- Eosinophilic gastroenteritis
- Lymphoma
- Nontropical sprue (celiac disease, gluten-induced enteropathy)
- Parasitic infestations (*Giardia*, schistosomiasis, hookworm)
- Radiation enteritis

- Scleroderma
- Small bowel ischemia
- Tropical sprue
- Whipple's disease
- Zollinger-Ellison disease

CRITICAL VALUES: N/A

INTERFERING FACTORS:
- Drugs that may increase urine D-xylose levels include phenazopyridine.
- Drugs and substances that may decrease urine D-xylose levels include acetylsalicylic acid, aminosalicylic acid, arsenicals, colchicine, digitalis, ethionamide, gold, indomethacin, isocarboxazid, kanamycin, monoamine oxidase (MAO) inhibitors, neomycin, and phenelzine.
- Poor renal function or vomiting may cause low urine values.

Nursing Implications and Procedure

Pretest:

➤ Obtain a history of the patient's complaints, including a list of known allergens.

➤ Obtain a history of the patient's gastrointestinal system, as well as results of previously performed tests and procedures. For related tests, refer to the gastrointestinal system table.

➤ Obtain a list of the medications the patient is taking, including herbs, nutritional supplements, and nutraceuticals. The requesting health care practitioner and laboratory should be advised if the patient regularly uses these products so that their effects can be taken into consideration when reviewing results.

➤ The patient should fast for at least 12 hours before the test. In addition, the patient should refrain from eating foods containing pentose sugars such as fruits, jams, jellies, and pastries.

➤ Numerous medications (e.g., acetylsalicylic acid, indomethacin, neomycin) interfere with the test and should be withheld, by medical direction, for 24 hours before testing.

➤ There are no fluid restrictions unless by medical direction.

➤ Review the procedure with the patient. Inform the patient that activity will be restricted during the test. Obtain the pediatric patient's weight to calculate dose of D-xylose to be administered.

➤ Inform the patient that all urine for a 5-hour period must be saved. Provide a nonmetallic urinal, bedpan, or toilet-mounted collection device.

➤ Instruct the patient not to void directly into the laboratory collection container. Instruct the patient to avoid defecating in the collection device and to keep toilet tissue out of the collection device to prevent contamination of the specimen. Place a sign in the bathroom to remind the patient to save all urine.

➤ Instruct the patient to void all urine into the collection device and then to pour the urine into the laboratory collection container. Alternatively the specimen can be left in the collection device for a health care staff member to add to the laboratory collection container.

➤ Inform the patient that blood specimen collection takes approximately 5 to 10 minutes.

Intratest: ■

➤ Ensure that the patient has complied with dietary preparations and other pretesting restrictions.

➤ Observe standard precautions and follow the general guidelines in Appendix A.

Timed specimen:

➤ Obtain a clean 3-L urine specimen container, toilet-mounted collection device, and plastic bag (for transport of the specimen container). The specimen must be refrigerated or kept on ice throughout the entire collection period. If an indwelling urinary catheter is in place, the drainage bag must be kept on ice.

➤ Begin the test between 6 a.m. and 8 a.m., if possible. Remind the patient to remain supine and at rest throughout the duration of the test. Instruct the patient to collect all urine for a 5-hour period after administration of the D-xylose.

➤ Adults are given a 25-g dose of D-xylose dissolved in 250 mL of water to take orally. The dose for pediatric patient is calculated by weight up to a maximum of 25 g. The patient should drink an additional 250 mL of water as soon as the D-xylose solution has been taken. Some adult patients with severe symptoms may be given a 5-g dose, but the test results are less sensitive at the lower dose.

➤ If an indwelling catheter is in place, replace the tubing and container system at the start of the collection time. Keep the container system on ice during the collection period or empty the urine into a larger container periodically during the collection period; monitor to ensure continued drainage.

➤ Blood samples are collected 1 hour postdose for pediatric patients and 2 hours postdose for adults.

➤ Direct the patient to breathe normally and to avoid unnecessary movement. Perform a venipuncture, and collect the specimen in a 5-mL gray-top tube.

➤ At the conclusion of the test, compare the quantity of urine with the urinary output record for the collection; if the specimen contains less than what was recorded as output, some urine may have been discarded, thus invalidating the test.

➤ Label the specimen, and promptly transport it to the laboratory. Include on the label the amount of urine, test start and stop times, and ingestion of any foods or medications that could affect test results.

Post-test:

➤ Observe venipuncture site for bleeding or hematoma formation. Apply pressure bandage.

➤ Recognize anxiety related to test results and offer support to help the patient and/or caregiver cope with the long-term implications of a chronic disorder and related lifestyle changes. Provide teaching and information regarding the clinical implications of the test results, as appropriate. Educate the patient regarding access to counseling services, as appropriate.

➤ Decreased D-xylose levels may be associated with gastrointestinal disease. Nutritional therapy may be indicated in the presence of malabsorption disorders. Encourage the patient, as appropriate, to consult with a qualified nutrition specialist to plan a lactose- and gluten-free diet. This dietary planning is complex because patients are often malnourished and have related nutritional problems.

➤ Evaluate test results in relation to the patient's symptoms and other tests performed. Related laboratory tests include sweat chloride, fecal analysis, fecal fat, intestinal biopsy, and lactose tolerance.

DEHYDROEPIANDROSTERONE SULFATE

• •

SYNONYM/ACRONYM: DHEAS.

SPECIMEN: Serum (1 mL) collected in a red- or tiger-top tube. Plasma (1 mL) collected in lavender-top (ethylenediaminetetra-acetic [EDTA]) tube is also acceptable.

REFERENCE VALUE: (Method: Radioimmunoassay)

Age	Conventional Units	SI Units (Conversion Factor ×0.027)
Newborn		
Male	108–406 μg/dL	2.9–10.9 μmol/L
Female	10–248 μg/dL	0.3–6.7 μmol/L
6–9 y	25–145 μg/dL	0.07–3.9 μmol/L
10–11 y		
Male	15–115 μg/dL	0.4–3.1 μmol/L
Female	15–260 μg/dL	0.4–7.0 μmol/L
12–17 y		
Male	20–555 μg/dL	0.5–15.0 μmol/L
Female	20–535 μg/dL	0.5–14.4 μmol/L
19–30 y		
Male	125–619 μg/dL	3.4–16.7 μmol/L
Female	29–781 μg/dL	0.8–21.1 μmol/L
31–50 y		
Male	59–452 μg/dL	1.6–12.2 μmol/L
Female	12–379 μg/dL	0.8–10.2 μmol/L
51–60 y		
Male	20–413 μg/dL	0.5–11.1 μmol/L
61–83 y		
Male	10–285 μg/dL	0.3–7.7 μmol/L
Postmenopausal woman	30–260 mg/dL	0.8–7.0 mmol/L

DESCRIPTION: Dehydroepiandrosterone sulfate (DHEAS) is the major precursor of 17-ketosteroids. DHEAS is a metabolite of DHEA, the principal adrenal androgen. DHEAS is primarily synthesized in the adrenal gland with a small amount secreted by the ovaries. It is secreted in concert with cortisol, under the control of adrenocorticotropic hormone (ACTH) and prolactin. Excessive production causes masculinization in women and children. DHEAS has replaced measurement of urinary 17-ketosteroids in the estimation of adrenal androgen production. ■

INDICATIONS:
- Assist in the evaluation of androgen excess, including congenital adrenal hyperplasia, adrenal tumor, and Stein-Leventhal syndrome
- Evaluate women with infertility, amenorrhea, or hirsutism

RESULT

Increased in:
- Anovulation
- Cushing's syndrome
- Ectopic ACTH-producing tumors
- Hirsutism
- Hyperprolactinemia
- Polycystic ovary
- Stein-Leventhal syndrome
- Virilizing adrenal tumors

Decreased in:
- Addison's disease

- Adrenal insufficiency (primary or secondary)

- Aging adults

- Hyperlipidemia

- Pregnancy

- Psoriasis

- Psychosis

CRITICAL VALUES: N/A

INTERFERING FACTORS:

- Drugs that may increase DHEAS levels include clomiphene, corticotropin, danazol, DHEA, mifepristone, and nitrendipine.

- Drugs that may decrease DHEAS levels include carbamazepine, dexamethasone, ketoconazole, oral contraceptives, and phenytoin.

- Recent radioactive scans or radiation within 1 week before the test can interfere with test results when radioimmunoassay is the test method.

Nursing Implications and Procedure • • • • • • • • • • •

Pretest:

➤ Obtain a history of the patient's complaints, including a list of known allergens.

➤ Obtain a history of the patient's endocrine system, as well as results of previously performed tests and procedures. For related tests, refer to the endocrine system table.

➤ Obtain a list of the medications the patient is taking, including herbs, nutritional supplements, and nutraceuticals. The requesting health care practitioner and laboratory should be advised if the patient regularly uses these products so that their effects can be taken into consideration when reviewing results.

➤ Note any recent procedures that can interfere with test results.

➤ There are no food, fluid, or medication restrictions unless by medical direction.

➤ Review the procedure with the patient.

➤ Inform the patient that specimen collection takes approximately 5 to 10 minutes.

Intratest:

➤ Direct the patient to breathe normally and to avoid unnecessary movement.

➤ Observe standard precautions and follow the general guidelines in Appendix A. Perform a venipuncture, and collect the specimen in a 5-mL red- or tiger-top tube.

➤ Label the specimen, and promptly transport it to the laboratory.

Post-test:

➤ Observe venipuncture site for bleeding or hematoma formation. Apply pressure bandage.

➤ Evaluate test results in relation to the patient's symptoms and other tests performed. Related laboratory tests include ACTH, cortisol, prolactin, and testosterone.

DRUGS OF ABUSE

Amphetamines
Barbiturates
Benzodiazepines
Cannabinoids
Cocaine

Ethanol
Opiates
Phencyclidine
Tricyclic Antidepressants

SYNONYMS/ACRONYMS: Amphetamines, barbiturates, benzodiazepines (tranquilizers), cannabinoids (THC), cocaine, ethanol (alcohol, ethyl alcohol, EtOH), phencyclidine (PCP), opiates (heroin), tricyclic antidepressants (TCA)

SPECIMEN: For ethanol, serum (1 mL) collected in a red-top tube or plasma (1 mL) collected in gray-top (sodium fluoride/potassium oxalate) tube is also acceptable. For drug screen, urine (15 mL) collected in a clean plastic container. Gastric contents (20 mL) may also be submitted for testing.

Workplace drug-screening programs, because of the potential medicolegal consequences associated with them, require collection of urine and blood specimens using a *chain of custody protocol*. The protocol provides securing the sample in a sealed transport device in the presence of the donor and a representative of the donor's employer, such that tampering would be obvious. The protocol also provides a written document of specimen transfer from donor to specimen collection personnel, to storage, to analyst, and to disposal.

REFERENCE VALUE: (Method: Spectrophotometry for ethanol; immunoassay for drugs of abuse)

Ethanol: None detected
Drug screen: None detected

DESCRIPTION: Drug abuse continues to be one of the most significant social and economic problems in the United States. The National Institute for Drug Abuse (NIDA) has identified opiates, cocaine, cannabinoids, amphetamines, and phencyclidines (PCPs) as the most commonly abused illicit drugs. Ethanol is the most commonly encountered legal substance of abuse. Chronic alcohol abuse can lead to liver disease, high blood pressure, cardiac disease, and birth defects. ■

INDICATIONS:
• Differentiate alcohol intoxication from diabetic coma, cerebral trauma, or drug overdose

• Investigate suspected drug abuse

• Investigate suspected drug overdose

• Investigate suspected noncompliance with drug or alcohol treatment program

• Monitor ethanol levels when administered to treat methanol intoxication

• Routine workplace screening

Cutoff Concentrations for Drugs of Abuse Recommended by NIDA	
Amphetamines	1000 ng/mL
Barbiturates	300 ng/mL
Benzodiazepines	300 ng/mL
Cannabinoids	50 ng/mL
Cocaine	300 ng/mL
Opiates	300 ng/mL
Phencyclidine	25 ng/mL
Tricyclic antidepressants	1000 ng/mL

RESULT: A urine screen merely identifies the presence of these substances in urine: it does not indicate time of exposure, amount used, quality of the source used, or level of impairment. Positive screens should be considered presumptive. Drug-specific confirmatory methods should be used to investigate questionable results of a positive urine screen.

CRITICAL VALUES: ⚠ The legal limit for ethanol intoxication varies from state to state, but in most states greater than 100 mg/dL is considered impaired for driving. Levels greater than 300 mg/dL are associated with amnesia, vomiting, double vision, and hypothermia. Levels 400 to 700 mg/dL are associated with coma and may be fatal. Possible interventions for ethanol toxicity include administration of tap water or 3% sodium bicarbonate lavage, breathing support, and hemodialysis (usually indicated only if levels exceed 300 mg/dL).

Barbiturate and benzodiazepine intoxication causes central nervous system (CNS) depression, which may progress to respiratory failure, hypotension, coma, and death. Do not induce emesis because of the risk of aspiration. Possible interventions include airway protection, administration of oxygen, gastric lavage with water or saline (up to 24 hours after ingestion), administration of activated charcoal, and monitoring CNS depression.

PCP intoxication causes a variety of symptoms depending on the stage of intoxication. Stage I includes psychiatric signs, muscle spasms, fever, tachycardia, flushing, small pupils, salivation, nausea, and vomiting. Stage II includes stupor, convulsions, hallucinations, increased heart rate, and increased blood pressure. Stage III includes further increases of heart rate and blood pressure that may culminate in cardiac and respiratory failure. Possible interventions may include providing respiratory support, administration of activated charcoal with a cathartic such as sorbitol, gastric lavage and suction, administration of intravenous nutrition and electrolytes, and acidification of the urine to promote PCP excretion.

Cocaine intoxication causes short-term symptoms of CNS stimulation, hypertension, tachypnea, mydriasis, and tachycardia. Possible interventions include emesis (if orally ingested and if the patient has a gag reflex and normal CNS function), gastric lavage (if orally ingested), whole bowel irrigation (if packs of the drug were ingested), airway protection, cardiac support, and administration of diazepam or phenobarbital for convulsions. The use of beta blockers is contraindicated.

Amphetamine intoxication causes psychoses, tremors, convulsions, insomnia, tachycardia, dysrhythmias, impotence, cerebrovascular accident, and respiratory failure. Possible interventions include emesis (if orally ingested and if the patient has a gag reflex and normal CNS function), administration of activated charcoal followed by magnesium citrate cathartic, acidification of the urine to promote excretion, and administration of liquids to promote urinary output.

Heroin is an opiate that at toxic levels causes bradycardia, flushing, itching, hypotension, hypothermia, and respiratory depression. Possible interventions include airway protection and the administration of naloxone (Narcan).

Tricyclic antidepressant intoxication causes confusion, agitation, hallucinations, seizures, dysrhythmias, hyperthermia, dilation of the pupils, and coma. Possible interventions may include administration of activated charcoal, gastric lavage with saline, intravenous administration of physostigmine (to counteract coma, hypertension, respiratory depression, and seizures), administration of bicarbonate (to control dysrhythmia), administration of propranolol, lidocaine or phenytoin to control convulsions, and monitoring cardiac function.

INTERFERING FACTORS:
- Codeine-containing cough medicines and antidiarrheal preparations, as well as ingestion of large amounts of poppy seeds, may produce a false-positive opiate result.
- Adulterants such as bleach or other strong oxidizers can produce erroneous urine drug screen results.
- Ethanol is a volatile substance, and specimens should be stored in a tightly stoppered container to avoid falsely decreased values.

Nursing Implications and Procedure

Pretest:
➤ Obtain a history of the patient's complaints, including a list of known allergens.
➤ For related tests, refer to the therapeutic/toxicology table.
➤ Obtain a list of the medications the patient is taking, including herbs, nutritional supplements, and nutraceuticals. The requesting health care practitioner and laboratory should be advised if the patient regularly uses these products so that their effects can be taken into consideration when reviewing results.
➤ There are no food, fluid, or medication restrictions.
➤ Review the entire procedure with the patient, especially if the circumstances require collection of urine and blood specimens using a chain of custody protocol.
➤ *Obtain a written and informed consent, as appropriate.*
➤ Inform the patient that specimen collection takes approximately 5 to 10 minutes but may vary depending on the level of patient cooperation.

Intratest:
➤ Direct the patient to breathe normally and to avoid unnecessary movement.
➤ Observe standard precautions and follow the general guidelines in Appendix A. For ethanol, use a non–alcohol-containing solution to cleanse the venipuncture site before specimen collection.

➤ Perform a venipuncture, and collect the specimen in a 5-mL red-top tube. Cadaver blood is taken from the aorta.

➤ For a drug screen, instruct the patient to obtain clean-catch urine specimen.

Clean-catch specimen:

➤ Instruct the male patient to (1) thoroughly wash his hands, (2) cleanse the meatus, (3) void a small amount into the toilet, and (4) void directly into the specimen container.

➤ Instruct the female patient to (1) thoroughly wash her hands; (2) cleanse the labia from front to back; (3) while keeping the labia separated, void a small amount into the toilet; and (4) without interrupting the urine stream, void directly into the specimen container.

➤ Follow the chain of custody protocol,

if required. Monitor specimen collection, labeling, and packaging to prevent tampering. This protocol may vary by institution.

➤ Label the specimen, and promptly transport it to the laboratory.

Post-test:

➤ Observe venipuncture site for bleeding or hematoma formation. Apply pressure bandage.

➤ Ensure that results are communicated to the proper individual, as indicated in the chain of custody protocol.

➤ Provide support and information regarding detoxification programs, as appropriate.

➤ Evaluate test results in relation to the patient's symptoms and other tests performed.

ECHOCARDIOGRAPHY

SYNONYMS/ACRONYM: Doppler echo, Doppler ultrasound of the heart, echo.

AREA OF APPLICATION: Chest/thorax.

CONTRAST: Can be done with or without noniodinated contrast medium (microspheres).

DESCRIPTION: Echocardiography, a noninvasive ultrasound procedure, uses high-frequency sound waves of various intensities to assist in diagnosing cardiovascular disorders. The procedure records the echoes created by the deflection of an ultrasonic beam off the cardiac structures and allows visualization of the size, shape, position, thickness, and movement of all four valves, atria, ventricular and atria septa, papillary muscles, chordae tendineae, and ventricles. This study can also determine blood-flow velocity, direction, and the presence of pericardial effusion during the movement of the transducer over areas of the chest. Electrocardiography and phonocardiography can be done simultaneously to correlate the findings with the cardiac cycle. These procedures can be done at the bedside or in a specialized department, physician office, or clinic.

Included in the study are the M-mode method, which produces a linear tracing of timed motions of the heart, its structures, and associated measurements over time; and the two-dimensional method, using real-time Doppler color-flow imaging with pulsed and continuous wave Doppler spectral tracings, which produces a cross-section of the structures of the heart and their relationship to one another, changes in the coronary vasculature, velocity and direction of blood flow, and areas of eccentric blood flow. Doppler color-flow imaging may also be helpful in depicting the function of biological and prosthetic valves.

Cardiac contrast medium is used to aid in the diagnosis of intracardiac shunt and tricuspid valve regurgitation. The contrast agent is injected intravenously and outlines the chambers of the heart. ▪

INDICATIONS:

- Determine the severity of valvular abnormalities such as stenosis, prolapse, and regurgitation

- Measure the size of the heart's chambers and determine if hypertrophic cardiomyopathy or congestive heart failure is present

- Evaluate congenital heart disorders

- Detect atrial tumors (myxomas)

- Determine the presence of pericardial effusion, tamponade, and pericarditis

- Detect ventricular or atrial mural thrombi and evaluate cardiac wall motion after myocardial infarction

- Detect subaortic stenosis as evidenced either by displacement of the anterior atrial leaflet or by a reduction in aortic valve flow, depending on the obstruction

- Evaluate unexplained chest pain, electrocardiographic changes, and abnormal chest x-ray (e.g., enlarged cardiac silhouette)

- Evaluate or monitor prosthetic valve function

- Evaluate endocarditis

- Evaluate ventricular aneurysms and/or thrombus

- Establish the presence of shunt flow and continuity of the aorta and pulmonary artery

RESULT

Normal Findings:
- Normal appearance in the size, position, structure, and movements of the heart valves visualized and recorded in a combination of ultrasound modes; and normal heart muscle walls of both ventricles and left atrium, with adequate blood filling. Established values for the measurement of heart activities obtained by the study may vary by physician and institution.

Abnormal Findings:
- Aortic valve abnormalities

- Cardiac neoplasm

- Cardiomyopathy

- Congenital heart defect

- Congestive heart failure

- Coronary artery disease

- Endocarditis

- Mitral valve abnormalities

- Myxoma

- Pericardial effusion, tamponade, and pericarditis

- Pulmonary hypertension

- Pulmonary valve abnormalities

- Septal defects

- Ventricular or atrial mural thrombi

- Ventricular hypertrophy

CRITICAL VALUES: N/A

INTERFERING FACTORS:

Factors that may impair clear imaging:

- Inability of the patient to cooperate or remain still during the procedure because of age, significant pain, or mental status

- Incorrect placement and movement of the transducer over the desired sites or lack of skill in performing the procedure

- Patient obesity, chest thickness, deformity, or other abnormality or trauma, which can affect the transmission of waves to and from the chest because of increased space between the heart and transducer

- The presence of chronic obstructive pulmonary disease or use of mechanical ventilation, which increases the air between the heart and chest wall (hyperinflation) and can attenuate the ultrasound waves

- The presence of arrhythmias

- Metallic objects within the examination field (e.g., jewelry or body rings), which may inhibit organ visualization and can produce unclear image

- The presence of pleural effusion, pericardial fat pad, tumors around the heart, clotted blood, or loculated effusions

Nursing Implications and Procedure

Pretest:

➤ Inform the patient that the procedure assesses heart function.

➤ Inform the patient that the procedure is performed in a special department by a technologist and takes approximately 30 to 60 minutes, and that there is no risk of radiation from the study.

➤ Obtain a list of medications the patient is taking.

➤ Obtain pertinent history of previously performed cardiac tests and procedures, current cardiac conditions or abnormalities, and therapy received for cardiac condition. For related tests, refer to the cardiovascular system table.

➤ Do not restrict food and fluids.

Intratest:

➤ Place the patient in a supine position on a flat table with foam wedges to help maintain position and immobilization. Ask the patient to lie very still during the procedure because movement will produce unclear images.

➤ Patient movement during the procedure will affect the results and make interpretation difficult.

➤ Expose the chest, and attach the electrocardiogram leads for simultaneous tracings, if desired.

➤ Apply conductive gel to the chest slightly to the left of the sternum. Place the transducer on the chest surface along the left sternal border, the subxiphoid area, suprasternal notch, and supraclavicular areas to obtain views and tracings of the portions of the heart. Scan the areas by systematically moving the probe in a perpendicular position to direct the ultrasound waves to each part of the heart. These can be viewed immediately and recorded on moving graph paper (M mode) or videotape (two-dimensional).

> To obtain different views or information about heart function, position the patient on the left side and/or sitting up, or request that the patient breathe slowly or hold breath during the procedure. To evaluate heart function changes, the patient may be asked to inhale amyl nitrate (vasodilator).

> Administer contrast medium, if ordered. A second series of images is obtained.

Post-test:

> Cleanse the patient's skin of remaining gel or mineral oil.

> Instruct the patient to resume normal activity and diet, unless otherwise indicated.

> A physician specializing in this branch of medicine sends a written report to the ordering provider, who discusses the results with the patient.

> Evaluate test results in relation to the patient's symptoms and other tests performed. Related diagnostic tests include positron emission tomography and nuclear thallium scanning of the heart.

ECHOCARDIOGRAPHY, TRANSESOPHAGEAL

· ·

SYNONYM/ACRONYM: Echo, TEE.

AREA OF APPLICATION: Chest/thorax.

CONTRAST: Can be done with or without noniodinated contrast medium (microspheres).

DESCRIPTION: Transesophageal echocardiography (TEE) is performed to assist in the diagnosis of cardiovascular disorders when noninvasive echocardiography is contraindicated or does not reveal enough information to confirm a diagnosis. Noninvasive echocardiography may be an inadequate procedure for patients who are obese, have chest wall structure abnormalities, or have chronic obstructive pulmonary disease (COPD). TEE provides a better view of the posterior aspect of the heart, including the atrium and aorta. It is done with a transducer attached to a gastroscope that is inserted into the esophagus. The transducer and the ultrasound instrument allow the beam to be directed to the back of the heart. The echoes are amplified and recorded on a screen for visualization and recorded on graph paper or videotape. The depth of the endoscope and movement of the transducer is controlled to obtain various images of the heart structures. TEE is usually performed during surgery; it is also used on patients who are in the intensive care unit, in whom the transmission of waves to and from the chest has been compromised and more definitive information is needed. The images obtained by TEE have better resolution than those obtained by routine transthoracic echocardiography because TEE uses higher frequency sound waves and offers closer proximity of the transducer to the cardiac structures. Cardiac contrast medium is used to improve the visualization of viable myocardial tissue within the heart. ■

INDICATIONS:

• Confirm diagnosis if conventional echocardiography does not correlate with other findings

• Monitor cardiac function during open heart surgery

• Detect or determine the severity of valvular abnormalities and regurgitation

• Measure the size of the heart's chambers and determine if hypertrophic cardiomyopathy or congestive heart failure is present

• Detect and evaluate congenital heart disorders

• Detect atrial tumors (myxomas)

• Determine the presence of pericardial effusion

• Detect ventricular or atrial mural thrombi and evaluate cardiac wall motion after myocardial infarction

• Detect subaortic stenosis as evidenced by displacement of the anterior atrial leaflet and reduction in aortic valve flow, depending on the obstruction

• Detect thoracic aortic dissection and coronary artery disease (CAD)

• Evaluate or monitor biological and prosthetic valve function

• Monitor cardiac function during open heart surgery (most sensitive method for monitoring ischemia)

• Reevaluate after inadequate visualization with conventional echocardiography as a result of obesity, trauma to or deformity of the chest wall, or lung hyperinflation associated with COPD

• Evaluate septal defects

• Evaluate aneurysms and ventricular thrombus

RESULT

Normal Findings:

• Normal appearance of the size, position, structure, movements of the heart valves and heart muscle walls, and chamber blood filling; and no evidence of valvular stenosis or insufficiency, cardiac tumor, foreign bodies, or CAD. The established values for the measurement of heart activities obtained by the study may vary by physician and institution.

Abnormal Findings:

• Aneurysm

• Aortic valve abnormalities

• Cardiomyopathy

• CAD

• Congenital heart defects

• Congestive heart failure

• Mitral valve abnormalities

• Myocardial infarction

• Myxoma

• Pericardial effusion

• Pulmonary hypertension

• Pulmonary valve abnormalities

• Septal defects

• Shunting of blood flow

• Thrombus

- Ventricular or atrial mural thrombi

- Ventricular hypertrophy

CRITICAL VALUES: N/A

INTERFERING FACTORS:

This procedure is contraindicated for:
- Patients with significant esophageal pathology (procedure may cause bleeding)

Factors that may impair clear imaging:
- Inability of the patient to cooperate or remain still during the procedure because of age, significant pain, or mental status

- Patients who are very obese, who may exceed the weight limit for the equipment

- Incorrect positioning of the patient, which may produce poor visualization of the area to be examined

- Incorrect placement of the transducer over the desired test site

- Laryngospasm, dysrhythmias, or esophageal bleeding

- Known upper esophageal pathology

- Conditions such as esophageal dysphagia and irradiation of the mediastinum

Other considerations:
- Failure to follow dietary restrictions before the procedure may cause the procedure to be canceled or repeated.

Nursing Implications and Procedure • • • • • • • • •

Pretest:

➤ Inform the patient that the procedure assesses the heart.

➤ Inform the patient that the proce-dure is performed in a special department by a technologist and takes approximately 30 to 60 minutes, and that there is no risk of radiation from the study.

➤ Obtain a list of medications the patient is taking.

➤ Obtain pertinent patient history of cardiac tests and procedures, pres-ent cardiac conditions or abnormali-ties, and therapy received for cardiac condition. For related tests, refer to the cardiovascular system table.

➤ *Obtain a written, informed consent for the procedure from the patient.*

➤ Obtain baseline vital signs.

➤ Establish an intravenous access line for the administration of medications and contrast medium.

➤ Remove dentures from the patient's mouth.

➤ Monitor pulse oximetry to deter-mine oxygen saturation in sedated patients.

➤ Restrict food and fluids 8 to 12 hours before the procedure.

➤ Explain that some discomfort will be experienced during insertion of the scope.

Intratest:

➤ Spray or swab the patient's throat with a local anesthetic, and place the oral bridge device in the mouth to prevent biting of the endoscope.

➤ Place the patient in a left side-lying position on a flat table with foam wedges that will help maintain position and immobilization. Ask the patient to lie very still during the procedure because movement will produce unclear images. The pharyn-geal area is anesthetized and the endoscope with the ultrasound device attached to its tip is inserted 30 to 50 cm to the posterior area of the heart, as in any esophagoscopy procedure.

➤ Ask the patient to swallow as the scope is inserted. When the trans-ducer is in place, the scope is manipulated by controls on the handle to obtain scanning that provides real-time images of the heart motion and recordings of the images for viewing. Actual scanning is usually limited to 15 minutes or until the desired number of image planes is obtained at different depths of the scope.

➤ The images can be viewed immediately and recorded on film, electronic media, or videotape.

➤ Administer a contrast medium, if ordered. A second series of images is obtained.

Post-test:

➤ Instruct the patient to resume normal activity and diet 4 to 6 hours after the test, unless otherwise indicated.

➤ Instruct patient to treat throat discomfort with lozenges and warm gargles when the gag reflex returns.

➤ A physician specializing in this branch of medicine sends a written report to the ordering provider, who discusses the results with the patient.

➤ Evaluate test results in relation to the patient's symptoms and other test performed. Related diagnostic tests include chest or cardiac computed tomography, chest or cardiac magnetic resonance imaging, and nuclear medicine cardiac perfusion study.

ELECTROCARDIOGRAM

SYNONYMS/ACRONYMS: ECG, VCG, ECG.

AREA OF APPLICATION: Heart.

CONTRAST: None.

DESCRIPTION: The cardiac muscle consists of three layers of cells—the inner layer called the *endocardium,* the middle layer called the *myocardium,* and the outer layer called the *epicardium.* The systolic phase reflects the contraction of the myocardium, whereas the diastolic phase takes place when the heart relaxes to allow blood to rush in. All muscle cells have a characteristic rate of contraction called *depolarization.* Therefore, the heart will maintain a predetermined heart rate unless other stimuli are received.

The electrocardiogram (ECG), a noninvasive study, measures the electrical currents or impulses that the heart generates during a cardiac cycle (see figure of a normal ECG). The monitoring of pulse and blood pressure evaluates the mechanical activity of the heart. The ECG is a graphic display of the electrical activity of the heart, which is analyzed by time intervals and segments. Continuous tracing of the cardiac cycle activities is captured as heart cells are electrically stimulated, causing depolarization and movement of the activity through the cells of the myocardium. The ECG study is completed by using 12 electrodes attached to the skin surface to obtain the total electrical activity of the heart. Each lead records the electrical potential between the limbs or between the heart and limbs. The ECG machine records and marks the 12 leads on the strip of paper in the machine in proper sequence, usually 6 inches of the strip for each lead. The ECG pattern, called a *heart rhythm*, is recorded by a machine as a series of waves, intervals, and segments, each of which pertains to a specific occurrence during the contraction of the heart. The ECG tracings are recorded on graph paper with vertical and horizontal lines for analysis and calculations of time measured by the vertical lines (1 mm apart and 0.04 seconds per line) and of voltage measured by the horizontal lines (1 mm apart and 0.5 mV per 5 squares). A pulse rate can be calculated from the ECG strip to obtain the beats per minute. The P wave represents the depolarization of the atrial myocardium; the QRS wave represents the depolarization of the ventricular myocardium; the P-R interval represents the beginning of the excitation of the atrium to the beginning of the ventricular excitation; and the S-T segment has no deflection from baseline, but in an abnormal state may be elevated or depressed. An abnormal rhythm is called an *arrhythmia*. Electrical impulses travel through a conduction system beginning with the SA node to the AV node via internodal pathways. From the AV node, the impulses travel to the bundle of His and onward to the right and left bundle branches. These bundles are located within the right and left ventricles. The impulses continue to the cardiac muscle cells by terminal fibers called *Purkinje fibers.* ■

INDICATIONS:

- Detect arrhythmias, as evidenced by abnormal wave deflections

- Monitor ECG changes during an exercise test

- Monitor rhythm changes during the recovery phase after a myocardial infarction (MI)

- Assess global cardiac function

- Assess the extent of MI or ischemia, as indicated by abnormal S-T wave, interval times, and amplitudes

- Detect pericarditis, shown by S-T segment changes or shortened P-R interval

- Assess the function of heart valves

- Assess the extent of congenital heart disease

- Determine electrolyte imbalances, as evidenced by short or prolonged Q-T interval

- Evaluate and monitor the effect of drugs, such as digitalis antiarrhythmic, or vasodilating agents

- Evaluate and monitor cardiac pacemaker function

- Determine hypertrophy of the chamber of the heart or heart hypertrophy, as evidenced by P or R wave deflections

RESULT

Normal Findings:

- Normal heart rate according to age: range of 60 to 100 beats/min in adults.

- Normal, regular rhythm and wave deflections with normal measurement of ranges of cycle components and height, depth, and duration of complexes as follows:

  P wave: 0.12 seconds or 3 small blocks with amplitude of 2.5 mm

  Q wave: less than 0.04 mm

  R wave: 5 to 27 mm amplitude, depending on lead

  T wave: 1 to 13 mm amplitude, depending on lead

  QRS complex: 0.12 seconds or 3 small blocks

  S-T segment: 1 mm

Abnormal Findings:

- Atrial or ventricular hypertrophy.

- Bundle branch block.

- Arrhythmias.

- MI or ischemia.

- Pericarditis.

- Pulmonary infarction.

- Electrolyte imbalances.

- P wave: An enlarged P wave deflection could indicate atrial enlargement. An absent or altered P wave could suggest that the electrical impulse did not come from the SA node.

- P-R interval: An increased interval could imply a conduction delay in the AV node.

- QRS complex: An enlarged Q wave may indicate an old infarction; an enlarged deflection could indicate ventricular hypertrophy. Increased time duration may indicate a bundle branch block.

- S-T segment: A depressed S-T segment indicates myocardial ischemia. An elevated S-T segment may indicate an acute MI or pericarditis. A prolonged S-T segment may indicate hypocalcemia or hypokalemia (short segment).

- T wave: A flat or inverted T wave may indicate myocardial ischemia, infarction, or hypokalemia. A tall T wave may indicate hyperkalemia.

CRITICAL VALUES: N/A

INTERFERING FACTORS:

Factors that may impair the results of the examination:

- Improper placement of electrodes or inadequate contact between skin and electrodes by insufficient conductive gel or poor placement, which can cause ECG tracing problems

- ECG machine malfunction or interference from electromagnetic waves in the vicinity

- Inability of the patient to remain still during the procedure, because movement, muscle tremor, or twitching can affect accurate test recording

- Strenuous exercise before the procedure

- Anatomic variation of the heart (i.e., the heart may be rotated in both the horizontal and frontal planes)

- Increased patient anxiety, causing hyperventilation or deep respirations

- Distortion of cardiac cycles due to age, sex, weight, or a medical condition (e.g., infants, women [may exhibit slight S-T segment depression], obese patients, pregnant patients, patients with ascites)

- Medications such as barbiturates and digitalis

- High intake of carbohydrates or electrolyte imbalances of potassium or calcium

Nursing Implications and Procedure • • • • • • • • • •

Pretest: ■

➤ Obtain a history of the patient's cardiac disease and present cardiovascular status. For related tests, refer to the cardiovascular system table.

➤ Obtain patient's vital signs.

➤ Obtain a list of the medications the patient is taking.

➤ List previous tests and procedures performed.

➤ *Obtain a written, informed consent for the procedure from the patient, if indicated.*

➤ Review the procedure with the patient.

➤ Recognize anxiety related to the test results.

➤ Ask if the patient has had a heart transplant or pacemaker implanted.

➤ No food, fluid, or medication restrictions exist unless by medical direction.

➤ Inform the patient that the procedure takes approximately 15 minutes.

Intratest: ■

➤ Have the patient remove clothing to the waist and any hosiery. Patients may want to wear a gown (open to the front).

➤ Place patient in a supine position. Expose and appropriately drape the chest, arms, and legs.

➤ Prepare the skin surface with alcohol and remove excess hair. Shaving may be necessary. Dry skin sites.

➤ Apply the electrodes in the proper position. When placing the six unipolar chest leads, place V_1 at the fourth intercostal space at the border of the right sternum, V_2 at the fourth intercostal space at the border of the left sternum, V_3 between V_2 and V_4, V_4 at the fifth intercostal space at the midclavicular line, V_5 at the left

anterior axillary line at the level of V_4 horizontally, and V_6 at the level of V_4 horizontally and at the left midaxillary line. The wires are connected to the matched electrodes and the ECG machine. Chest leads (V_1, V_2, V_3, V_4, V_5, and V_6) record data from the horizontal plane of the heart.

➤ Place three limb bipolar leads (two electrodes combined for each) on the arms and legs. Lead I is the combination of two arm electrodes, lead II is the combination of right arm and left leg electrodes, and lead III is the combination of left arm and left leg electrodes.

➤ Limb leads (I, II, III, AVL, AVF, and AVR) record data from the frontal plane of the heart.

➤ If the patient has any chest discomfort or pain during the procedure, mark the ECG strip indicating that occurrence.

➤ Instruct the patient to lie very still in a relaxed position during the study and to refrain from tensing muscles after electrode placement. The machine is set and turned on after the electrodes, grounding, connections, paper supply, computer, and data storage device are checked.

➤ Direct the patient to breathe normally and to avoid touching the bed or couch.

Post-test: ■

➤ When the procedure is complete, remove the electrodes and clean the skin where the electrode pad was applied.

➤ Evaluate the results in relation to previously performed ECGs.

➤ Denote cardiac rhythm abnormalities on the strip.

➤ Instruct the person to immediately notify a physician of chest pain, changes in pulse rate, or shortness of breath.

➤ Instruct the patient or caregiver regarding the correct administration of heart medications and their possible side effects.

➤ A physician specializing in this branch of medicine sends a written report to the ordering provider, who discusses the results with the patient.

➤ Evaluate test results in relation to the patient's symptoms and other tests performed. Related diagnostic tests include echocardiogram, positron emission tomography scan of the heart, and nuclear thallium scan of the heart.

ELECTROENCEPHALOGRAPHY

SYNONYM/ACRONYM: Sonogram (for sleep disturbances), EEG.

AREA OF APPLICATION: Brain.

CONTRAST: None.

DESCRIPTION: Electroencephalography (EEG) is a noninvasive study that measures the brain's electrical activity and records that activity on graph paper. These electrical impulses arise from the brain cells of the cerebral cortex. Electrodes, placed at 8 to 20 sites (or pairs of sites) on the patient's scalp, transmit the different frequencies and amplitudes of the brain's electrical activity to the EEG machine, which records the results in graph form on a moving paper strip. This procedure can evaluate responses to various stimuli, such as flickering light, hyperventilation, auditory signals, or somatosensory signals generated by skin electrodes. The procedure is usually performed in a room designed to eliminate electrical interference and minimize distractions. EEG can be done at bedside, especially to confirm brain death. A physician analyzes the waveforms. The test is used to detect epilepsy, intracranial abscesses, or tumors; to evaluate cerebral involvement as a result of head injury or meningitis; and to monitor for cerebral tissue ischemia during surgery when cerebral vessels must be occluded. EEG is also used to confirm brain death, which can be defined as absence of electrical activity in the brain. To evaluate abnormal EEG waves further, the patient may be connected to an ambulatory EEG system similar to a Holter monitor for the heart. Patients keep a journal of their activities and any symptoms that occur during the monitoring period. ■

INDICATIONS:
- Detect seizure disorders and identify focus of seizure and seizure activity, as evidenced by abnormal spikes and waves recorded on the graph
- Detect intracranial cerebrovascular lesions, such as hemorrhages and infarcts
- Determine the presence of tumors, abscesses, or infection
- Confirm suspicion of increased intracranial pressure caused by trauma or disease
- Identify area of abnormality in dementia
- Evaluate sleeping disorders, such as sleep apnea and narcolepsy
- Evaluate the effect of drug intoxication on the brain
- Detect cerebral ischemia during endarterectomy
- Confirm brain death

RESULT

Normal Findings:
- Normal occurrences of alpha, beta, theta, and delta waves (rhythms varying depending on the patent's age)
- Normal frequency, amplitude, and characteristics of brain waves

Abnormal Findings:
- Abscess
- Brain death
- Cerebral infarct
- Encephalitis
- Glioblastoma and other brain tumors
- Head injury
- Hypocalcemia or hypoglycemia
- Intracranial hemorrhage
- Meningitis
- Migraine headaches

- Narcolepsy

- Seizure disorders (grand mal, focal, temporal lobe, myoclonic, petit mal)

- Sleep apnea

CRITICAL VALUES: N/A

INTERFERING FACTORS:

Factors that may impair the results of the examination:

- Inability of the patient to cooperate or remain still during the procedure because of age, significant pain, or mental status

- Drugs and substances such as sedatives, anticonvulsants, anxiolytics, alcohol, and stimulants such as caffeine and nicotine

- Hypoglycemic or hypothermic states

- Hair that is dirty, oily, or sprayed or treated with hair preparations

---

Nursing Implications and Procedure • • • • • • • • • • •

Pretest:

➤ Review the procedure with the patient. Inform the patient that the procedure is performed in a special laboratory by a technician trained to do the procedure, and that the results are interpreted by a physician.

➤ Inform the patient that the procedure is performed to measure electrical activity of the brain and takes approximately 1 to 2 hours to complete.

➤ Obtain a history and assessment of the patient's neurological system, known or suspected seizure conditions, intracranial abnormalities, traumatic incidents to head, and sleep disorders, as well as the results of previously performed tests, surgeries, treatments, and procedures. For related tests, refer to the musculoskeletal system table.

➤ Ensure that the patient is able to relax; report any extreme anxiety or restlessness.

➤ Ensure that hair is clean and free of hair sprays, creams, or solutions.

➤ Ensure that caffeine-containing beverages were withheld for 8 hours before the procedure, and that a meal was ingested before the study.

➤ Obtain a list of the medications the patient is taking, including herbs, nutritional supplements, and nutraceuticals, and ensure that all substances with the potential to interfere with test results are withheld for 24 to 48 hours before the test.

➤ Instruct the patient to limit sleep to 5 hours for an adult and 7 hours for a child the night before the study. Young infants and children should not be allowed to nap before the study.

➤ Assure the patient that there is no discomfort during the procedure. Encourage relaxation during the procedure. Indicate to the patient that if needle electrodes are used, a slight pinch may be felt.

➤ Explain that electricity flows *from* the patient's body, not *into* the body, during the procedure.

➤ Explain that the procedure reveals brain activity only, not thoughts, feelings, or intelligence.

➤ *Obtain a written, informed consent for the procedure from the patient, if required.*

➤ Inform the patient that he or she may be asked to alter breathing pattern; be asked to follow simple commands such as opening or closing eyes, blinking, or swallowing; be stimulated with bright light; or be given a drug to induce sleep during the study.

➤ The test recordings are stopped about every 5 minutes to allow the patient to move.

Intratest:

➤ Place the patient in the supine position in a bed or semi-Fowler's position on a recliner in a special room protected from any noise or electrical interferences that could affect the tracings.

➤ Remind the patient to relax and not to move any muscles or parts of the face or head. The technician should be able to observe the patient for movements or other interferences through a window into the test room.

➤ The electrodes are prepared and applied to the scalp. Electrodes are placed in as many as 16 locations over the frontal, temporal, parietal, and occipital areas, and amplifier wires are attached. An electrode is also attached to each ear lobe as grounding electrodes. At this time, a baseline recording can be made with the patient at rest.

➤ Recordings are made with the patient at rest and with eyes closed. Recordings are also made during a drowsy and sleep period, depending on the patient's clinical condition and symptoms.

➤ Procedures (e.g., stroboscopic light stimulation, hyperventilation to induce alkalosis, and sleep induction by administration of sedative to detect abnormalities that occur only during sleep) may be done to bring out abnormal electrical activity or other brain abnormalities.

➤ Observations for seizure activity are carried out during the study, and a description and time of activity is noted by the technician.

Post-test:

➤ When the procedure is complete, remove electrodes from the hair and remove paste by cleansing with oil or witch hazel.

➤ If a sedative was given during the test, allow the patient to recover. Bedside rails are put in the raised position for safety.

➤ Inform the patient to resume medications, as directed.

➤ Instruct the patient to report any seizure activity.

➤ A physician specializing in this branch of medicine sends a written report to the ordering provider, who discusses the results with the patient.

➤ Evaluate test results in relation to the patient's symptoms and other tests performed. Related diagnostic tests include computed tomography and magnetic resonance imaging of the brain.

ELECTROMYOGRAPHY

SYNONYMS/ACRONYM: Electrodiagnostic study, neuromuscular junction testing, EMG.

AREA OF APPLICATION: Muscles.

CONTRAST: None.

DESCRIPTION: Electromyography (EMG) measures skeletal muscle activity during rest, voluntary contraction, and electrical stimulation. Percutaneous extracellular needle electrodes containing fine wires are inserted into selected muscle groups to detect neuromuscular abnormalities and measure nerve and electrical conduction properties of skeletal muscles. The electrical potentials are amplified, displayed on a screen in waveforms, and electronically recorded, similar to electrocardiography. Comparison and analysis of the amplitude, duration, number, and configuration of the muscle activity provide diagnostic information about the extent of nerve and muscle involvement in the detection of primary muscle diseases including lower motor neuron, anterior horn cell, or neuromuscular junction diseases; defective transmission at the neuromuscular junction; and peripheral nerve damage or disease. Responses of a relaxed muscle are electrically silent, but spontaneous muscle movement such as fibrillation and fasciculation can be detected in a relaxed, denervated muscle. Muscle action potentials are detected with minimal or maximal muscle contractions. The differences in the size and numbers of activity potentials during voluntary contractions determine whether the muscle weakness is a disease of the striated muscle fibers or cell membranes (myogenic), or a disease of the lower motor neuron (neurogenic). Nerve conduction studies (electroneurography) are commonly done in conjunction with electromyelography; the combination of the procedures is known as elec-tromyoneurography. The examination's major use lies in differentiating among the following disease classes: primary myopathy, peripheral motor neuron disease, and disease of the neuromuscular junction. ∎

INDICATIONS:

• Assess primary muscle diseases affecting striated muscle fibers or cell membrane, such as muscular dystrophy or myasthenia gravis

• Differentiate secondary muscle disorders caused by polymyositis, sarcoidosis, hypocalcemia, thyroid toxicity, tetanus, and other disorders

• Detect neuromuscular disorders, such as peripheral neuropathy caused by diabetes or alcoholism, and locate the site of the abnormality

• Detect muscle disorders caused by diseases of the lower motor neuron involving the motor neuron on the anterior horn of the spinal cord, such as anterior poliomyelitis, amyotrophic lateral sclerosis, amyotonia, and spinal tumors

• Detect muscle disorders caused by diseases of the lower motor neuron involving the nerve root, such as Guillain-Barré syndrome, herniated disc, or spinal stenosis

• Differentiate between primary and secondary muscle disorders or between neuropathy and myopathy

• Determine if a muscle abnormality is caused by the toxic effects of drugs (e.g., antibiotics, chemotherapy) or toxins (e.g., *Clostridium botulinum*, snake venom, heavy metals)

• Monitor and evaluate progression of myopathies or neuropathies, including confirmation of diagnosis of carpal tunnel syndrome

RESULT

Normal Findings:
- Normal muscle electrical activity during rest and contraction states

Abnormal Findings and possible meanings:
- Evidence of neuromuscular disorders or primary muscle disease (*note:* findings must be correlated with the patient's history, clinical features, and results of other neurodiagnostic tests):
  Amyotrophic lateral sclerosis
  Bell's palsy
  Beriberi
  Carpal tunnel syndrome
  Dermatomyositis
  Diabetic peripheral neuropathy
  Eaton-Lambert syndrome
  Guillain-Barré syndrome
  Multiple sclerosis
  Muscular dystrophy
  Myasthenia gravis
  Myopathy
  Polymyositis
  Radiculopathy
  Traumatic injury

CRITICAL VALUES: N/A

INTERFERING FACTORS:

This procedure is contraindicated for:
- Patients with extensive skin infection
- Patients receiving anticoagulant therapy
- Patients with an infection at the sites of electrode placement

Factors that may impair the results of the examination:
- Inability of the patient to cooperate or remain still during the procedure because of age, significant pain, or mental status

- Age-related decreases in electrical activity
- Medications such as muscle relaxants, cholinergics, and anticholinergics
- Improper placement of surface or needle electrodes

Nursing Implications and Procedure • • • • • • • • • • •

Pretest:

➤ Review the procedure with the patient, indicating that the procedure is performed in a special laboratory by a physician and is done to evaluate electrical activity of muscles. This test takes 1 hour to complete, but can take up to 3 hours depending on the patient's condition.

➤ Obtain a list of the medications the patient is taking.

➤ Obtain a history and assessment of neuromuscular and neurosensory status, disease, or conditions that affect muscle function, level of muscular function and range of motion, traumatic events, and the results of previously performed tests, surgeries, and procedures. For related tests, refer to the musculoskeletal system table.

➤ Ensure that the patient has refrained from smoking and caffeine-containing beverages for 3 hours before the procedure.

➤ Inform the patient that as many as 10 electrodes may be inserted at various locations on the body. Warn the patient that the procedure may be uncomfortable, but that an analgesic or sedative will be administered.

➤ Ask the patient to remain very still and relaxed and to cooperate with instructions given to contract muscles during the procedure.

➤ Ensure that medications such as

muscle relaxants, cholinergics, and anticholinergics have been withheld, as ordered.

➤ Assess for compliance with directions given for exercising during the test.

➤ Appropriate hematologic studies should be ordered to assess coagulopathy.

➤ *Obtain a written, informed consent for the procedure from the patient, if necessary.*

Intratest:

➤ Have patient remove clothing and any hosiery. Patients may want to wear a gown and void.

➤ Administer mild analgesic (adult) or sedative (children), as ordered, to promote a restful state before the procedure.

➤ Place the patient in a supine or sitting position depending on the location of the muscle to be tested. Ensure that the area or room is protected from noise or metallic interference that may affect the test results.

➤ Cleanse the skin thoroughly with alcohol pads, as necessary.

➤ An electrode is applied to the skin to ground the patient, and then 24-gauge needles containing a fine-wire electrode are inserted into the muscle. The electrical potentials of the muscle are amplified, displayed

on a screen, and electronically recorded.

➤ During the test, muscle activity is tested while the patient is at rest, during incremental needle insertion, and during varying degrees of muscle contraction.

➤ Ask the patient to alternate between a relaxed and a contracted muscle state, or to perform progressive muscle contractions while the potentials are being measured.

Post-test:

➤ When the procedure is complete, remove the electrodes and clean the skin where the electrode was applied.

➤ Monitor electrode sites for hematoma or inflammation.

➤ If residual pain is noted after the procedure, instruct the patient to apply warm compresses and to take analgesics, as ordered.

➤ Instruct the patient to resume normal activity, diet, and previous medication use, unless otherwise indicated.

➤ A physician specializing in this branch of medicine sends a written report to the ordering provider, who discusses the results with the patient.

➤ Evaluate test results in relation to the patient's symptoms and any related tests performed.

ELECTROMYOGRAPHY, PELVIC FLOOR SPHINCTER

SYNONYMS/ACRONYM: Electrodiagnostic study, rectal electromyography.

AREA OF APPLICATION: Sphincter muscles.

CONTRAST: None.

DESCRIPTION: Pelvic floor sphincter electromyography, also known as rectal electromyography, is performed to measure electrical activity of the external urinary sphincter. This procedure, often done in conjunction with cystometry and voiding urethrography as part of a full urodynamic study, helps to diagnose neuromuscular dysfunction and incontinence. ■

INDICATIONS: Evaluate neuromuscular dysfunction and incontinence

CRITICAL VALUES: N/A

INTERFERING FACTORS:

This procedure is contraindicated for: Patients who are pregnant or suspected of being pregnant, unless the potential benefits of the procedure far outweigh the risks to the fetus and mother

Other considerations: Failure to follow dietary restrictions before the procedure may cause the procedure to be canceled or repeated.

Nursing Implications and Procedure • • • • • • • • • • •

Pretest: ■

➤ Inform the patient that the procedure is performed in a special room and takes about 30 minutes to complete.

➤ Obtain a history of previously performed tests, procedures, treatments, and surgeries. For related tests, refer to the genitourinary and musculoskeletal systems tables.

➤ Assure the patient that the pain is minimal during the catheter insertion.

Intratest: ■

➤ Ask the patient to void immediately before the test.

➤ Place the patient in a supine position on the examining table and place a drape over the patient, exposing the perineal area.

➤ Two skin electrodes are positioned slightly to the left and right of the perianal area and a grounding electrode is placed on the thigh.

➤ If needle electrodes are used, they are inserted into the muscle surrounding the urethra.

➤ Muscle activity signals are recorded as waves, which are interpreted for number and configurations in diagnosing urinary abnormalities.

➤ An indwelling urinary catheter is inserted, and the bulbocavernosus reflex is tested; the patient is instructed to cough while the catheter is gently pulled.

➤ Voluntary control is tested by requesting the patient to contract and relax the muscle. Electrical activity is recorded during this period of relaxation with the bladder empty.

➤ The bladder is filled with sterile water at a rate of 100 mL/min while the electrical activity during filling is recorded.

➤ The catheter is removed; the patient is then placed in a position to void and is asked to urinate and empty the full bladder. This voluntary urination is then recorded until completed. The complete procedure includes recordings of electrical signals before, during, and at the end of urination.

Post-test:

➤ Advise the patient to take a warm sitz bath.

➤ Encourage fluids unless contraindicated.

➤ If tested with needle electrodes, warn female patients to expect hematuria after the first voiding.

➤ Advise the patient to report symptoms of urethral irritation, such as dysuria, persistent or prolonged hematuria, and urinary frequency.

➤ A physician specializing in this branch of medicine sends a written report to the ordering provider, who discusses the results with the patient.

➤ Evaluate test results in relation to the patient's symptoms and any related tests performed.

ELECTRONEUROGRAPHY

SYNONYMS/ACRONYM: Electrodiagnostic study, nerve conduction study, ENG.

AREA OF APPLICATION: Muscles.

CONTRAST: None.

DESCRIPTION: Electroneurography (ENG) is performed to identify peripheral nerve injury, to differentiate primary peripheral nerve pathology from muscular injury, and to monitor response of the nerve injury to treatment. A stimulus is applied through a surface electrode over a nerve. After a nerve is electrically stimulated proximally, the time for the impulse to travel to a second or distal site is measured. Because the conduction study of a nerve can vary from nerve to nerve, it is important to compare the results of the affected side to those of the contralateral side. The results of the stimulation are shown on a monitor, but the actual velocity must be calculated by dividing the distance in meters between the stimulation point and the response point, by the time between the stimulus and response. Traumatic nerve transection, contusion, or neuropathy will usually cause maximal slowing of conduction velocity in the affected side compared with that in the normal side. A velocity greater than normal does not indicate a pathologic condition. This test is usually performed in conjunction with electromyography in a combined test called *electromyoneurography*. ∎

INDICATIONS: Confirm diagnosis of peripheral nerve damage or trauma

RESULT

Normal Findings:

- No evidence of peripheral nerve injury or disease. Variable readings depend on the nerve being tested. For patients aged 3 years and older, the maximum conduction velocity is 40 to 80 milliseconds; for infants and the elderly, the values are divided by 2.

Abnormal Findings:

- Carpal tunnel syndrome

- Diabetic neuropathy

- Guillain-Barré syndrome

- Herniated disc disease

- Muscular dystrophy

- Myasthenia gravis

- Poliomyelitis

- Tarsal tunnel syndrome

- Thoracic outlet syndrome

CRITICAL VALUES: N/A

INTERFERING FACTORS:

Factors that may impair the results of the examination:

- Inability of the patient to cooperate or remain still during the procedure because of age, significant pain, or mental status

- Age-related decreases in electrical activity

- Poor electrode conduction or failure to obtain contralateral value for comparison

---

Nursing Implications and Procedure

Pretest:

➤ Review the procedure with the patient, indicating that the procedure is performed in a special laboratory by a physiatrist or neurologist and is done to evaluate electrical activity of muscles. Inform the patient that the procedure may be uncomfortable because of a mild electrical shock, but that the electrical shock is brief and is not harmful.

➤ Obtain a list of the medications the patient is taking, including herbs, nutritional supplements, and nutraceuticals.

➤ Obtain a history and assessment of neuromuscular and neurosensory status, disease, or conditions that affect the peripheral neurological system, as well as results of previously performed tests, surgeries, and procedures. For related tests, refer to the musculoskeletal system table.

➤ Obtain a written, informed consent for the procedure from the patient.

➤ Inform the patient that the procedure takes approximately 15 minutes to complete, but can take longer depending on the patient's condition.

Intratest:

➤ Place the patient in a supine or sitting position, depending on the location of the muscle to be tested.

➤ Shave the extremity in the area to be stimulated, and cleanse the skin thoroughly with alcohol pads.

➤ Apply electrode gel and place a recording electrode at a known distance from the stimulation point. Measure the distance between the stimulation point and the site of the recording electrode in centimeters.

➤ Place a reference electrode nearby on the skin surface.

➤ The nerve is electrically stimulated by a shock-emitter device; the time between nerve impulse and electrical contraction, measured in milliseconds (distal latency), is shown on a monitor.

➤ The nerve is also electrically stimulated at a location proximal to the area of suspected injury or disease.

➤ The time required for the impulse to travel from the stimulation site to the muscle contraction (total latency) is recorded in milliseconds.

➤ Calculate the conduction velocity. The conduction velocity is converted to meters per second and computed using the following equation:

$$\text{Conduction velocity (in meters per second)} = \frac{[\text{distance (in meters)}]}{[\text{total latency} - \text{distal latency}]}$$

Post-test:

➤ When the procedure is complete, remove the electrodes and clean the skin where the electrodes were applied.

➤ Monitor electrode sites for hematoma or inflammation.

➤ If residual pain is noted after the procedure, instruct the patient to apply warm compresses and to take analgesics, as ordered.

➤ Instruct the patient to resume normal activity, diet, and previous medication use, unless otherwise indicated.

➤ A physician specializing in this branch of medicine sends a written report to the ordering provider, who discusses the results with the patient.

➤ Evaluate test results in relation to the patient's symptoms and any related tests performed.

EOSINOPHIL COUNT

SYNONYMS/ACRONYM: Eos count, total eosinophil count.

SPECIMEN: Whole blood (1 mL) collected in a lavender-top (ethylenedi-aminetetra-acetic acid [EDTA]) tube.

REFERENCE VALUE: (Method: Manual count using eosinophil stain and hemocytometer or automated analyzer)
Absolute count: 50 to 350/mm^3
Relative percentage: 1 to 4 percent

DESCRIPTION: Eosinophils are white blood cells whose function is phagocytosis of antigen-antibody complexes and response to allergy-inducing substances and parasites. Eosinophils have granules that contain histamine used to kill foreign cells in the body. Eosinophils also contain proteolytic substances that damage parasitic worms. The binding of histamine to receptor sites on cells results in smooth muscle contraction in the bronchioles and upper respiratory tract, constriction of pulmonary vessels, increased mucus production, and secretion of acid by the cells that line the stomach. Eosinophil counts can increase to greater than 30 percent of normal in parasitic infections; however, a significant percentage of children with visceral larva migrans infestations have normal eosinophil counts. ▪

INDICATIONS: Assist in the diagnosis of conditions such as allergies, parasitic infections, drug reactions, collagen diseases, Hodgkin's disease, and myeloproliferative disorders

RESULT

Increased in:
- Addison's disease
- Allergy
- Asthma
- Cancer
- Dermatitis
- Drug reactions
- Eczema
- Hay fever
- Hodgkin's disease
- Hypereosinophilic syndrome
- Löffler's syndrome
- Myeloproliferative disorders
- Parasitic infection (visceral larva migrans)
- Pernicious anemia
- Polycythemia vera
- Rheumatoid arthritis
- Rhinitis
- Sarcoidosis
- Splenectomy
- Tuberculosis

Decreased in:
- Aplastic anemia
- Eclampsia
- Infections (shift to the left)
- Stress

CRITICAL VALUES: N/A

INTERFERING FACTORS:
- Numerous drugs and substances can cause an increase in eosinophil levels as a result of an allergic response or hypersensitivity reaction. These include acetophenazine, allopurinol, aminosalicylic acid, ampicillin, butaperazine, capreomycin, carisoprodol, cephaloglycin, cephaloridine, cephalosporins, cephapirin, cephradine, chloramphenicol, clindamycin, cloxacillin, dapsone, epicillin, erythromycin, fluorides, gold, imipramine, iodides, kanamycin, mefenamic acid, methicillin, methyldopa, minocycline, nalidixic acid, niridazole, nitrofurans (including nitrofurantoin), nonsteroidal anti-inflammatory drugs, nystatin, oxamniquine, penicillin, penicillin G, procainamide, ristocetin, streptokinase, streptomycin, tetracycline, triamterene, tryptophan, and viomycin.

- Drugs that can cause a decrease in eosinophil levels include amphotericin B, acetylsalicylic acid, corticotropin, desipramine, glucocorticoids, hydrocortisone, interferon, niacin, prednisone, and procainamide.

- Clotted specimens should be rejected for analysis.

- Specimens more than 4 hours old should be rejected for analysis.

- There is a diurnal variation in eosinophil counts. The count is lowest in the morning and continues to rise throughout the day until midnight. Therefore, serial measurements should be performed at the same time of day for the purposes of continuity.

Nursing Implications and Procedure • • • • • • • • • • •

Pretest: ■

➤ Obtain a history of the patient's complaints, including a list of known allergens.

➤ Obtain a history of the patient's hematopoietic, immune, and respiratory systems, as well as results of previously performed tests and procedures. For related tests, refer to the hematopoietic, immune, and respiratory system tables.

➤ Obtain a list of the medications the patient is taking, including herbs, nutritional supplements, and nutraceuticals. The requesting health care practitioner and laboratory should be advised if the patient regularly uses these products so that their effects can be taken into consideration when reviewing results.

➤ There are no food, fluid, or medication restrictions unless by medical direction.

➤ Review the procedure with the patient.

➤ Inform the patient that specimen collection takes approximately 5 to 10 minutes.

Intratest: ■

➤ Direct the patient to breathe normally and to avoid unnecessary movement.

➤ Observe standard precautions and follow the general guidelines in Appendix A. Perform a venipuncture, collect the specimen in a 5-mL lavender-top (EDTA) tube.

➤ Label the specimen, and promptly transport it to the laboratory.

Post-test: ■

➤ Observe venipuncture site for bleeding or hematoma formation. Apply pressure bandage.

➤ Consideration should be given to diet if food allergies are present.

➤ Instruct the patient with an elevated eosinophil count to report any signs or symptoms of infection, such as fever.

➤ Instruct the patient with an elevated count to rest and take medications as prescribed, to increase fluid intake as appropriate, and to monitor temperature.

➤ Evaluate test results in relation to the patient's symptoms and other tests performed. Related laboratory tests include allergen-specific immunoglobulin E (IgE), IgE, complete blood count, hypersensitivity pneumonitis screen, fecal analysis, ova and parasites, and stool culture.

ERYTHROCYTE PROTOPORPHYRIN, FREE

• •

SYNONYM/ACRONYM: Free erythrocyte protoporphyrin (FEP).

SPECIMEN: Whole blood (1 mL) collected in lavender-top (ethylenedi-aminetetra-acetic acid [EDTA]) or green-top (heparin) tube.

REFERENCE VALUE: (Method: Fluorometry)

Conventional Units	SI Units (Conversion Factor ×0.0178)
17–77 µg/dL of packed cells	0.3–1.37 µmol/L of packed cells

DESCRIPTION: The free erythrocyte protoporphyrin test measures the concentration of protoporphyrin in red blood cells. Protoporphyrin comprises the predominant porphyrin in red blood cells, which combines with iron to form the heme portion of hemoglobin. Protoporphyrin converts to bilirubin, combines with albumin, and remains unconjugated in the circulation after hemoglobin breakdown. Increased amounts of protoporphyrin can be detected in erythrocytes, urine, and stool in conditions interfering with heme synthesis. Protoporphyria is an autosomal-dominant disorder in which increased amounts of protoporphyrin are secreted and excreted; the disorder is thought to be the result of an enzyme deficiency. Protoporphyria causes photosensitivity and may lead to cirrhosis of the liver and cholelithiasis as a result of protoporphyrin deposits. ∎

INDICATIONS:
- Assist in the diagnosis of erythropoietic protoporphyrias
- Assist in the differential diagnosis of iron deficiency in pediatric patients
- Evaluate lead poisoning

RESULT

Increased in:
- Anemia of chronic disease
- Iron-deficiency anemias
- Some sideroblastic anemias
- Conditions with marked erythropoiesis (e.g., hemolytic anemias)
- Erythropoietic protoporphyria
- Lead poisoning

Decreased in: N/A

CRITICAL VALUES: N/A

INTERFERING FACTORS:
- Drugs that may increase erythrocyte protoporphyrin levels include barbiturates, chlorpropamide, oral contraceptives, sulfomethane, and tolbutamide.
- The test is unreliable in infants less than 6 months of age.

Nursing Implications and Procedure ∙ ∙ ∙ ∙ ∙ ∙ ∙ ∙ ∙ ∙ ∙

Pretest: ∎

➤ Obtain a history of the patient's complaints, including a list of known allergens.

➤ Obtain a history of the patient's hematopoietic system, as well as results of previously performed tests and procedures. For related tests, refer to the hematopoietic system table.

➤ Obtain a list of the medications the patient is taking, including herbs, nutritional supplements, and nutraceuticals. The requesting health care practitioner and laboratory should be advised if the patient regularly uses these products so that their effects can be taken into consideration when reviewing results.

➤ There are no food, fluid, or medication restrictions unless by medical direction.

➤ Review the procedure with the patient.

➤ Inform the patient that specimen collection takes approximately 5 to 10 minutes.

Intratest:

➤ Direct the patient to breathe normally and to avoid unnecessary movement.

➤ Observe standard precautions and follow the general guidelines in Appendix A. Perform a venipuncture, and collect the specimen in a 5-mL lavender-top tube. Specimens should be protected from light.

➤ Label the specimen, and promptly transport it to the laboratory.

Post-test:

➤ Observe venipuncture site for bleeding or hematoma formation. Apply pressure bandage.

➤ Evaluate test results in relation to the patient's symptoms and other tests performed. Related laboratory tests include hematocrit, hemoglobin, iron/total iron-binding capacity, lead, and urine porphyrins.

ERYTHROCYTE SEDIMENTATION RATE

• •

SYNONYM/ACRONYM: Sed rate, ESR.

SPECIMEN: Whole blood (5 mL) collected in a lavender-top (ethylenedi-aminetetra-acetic acid [EDTA]) tube for the modified Westergren method or gray-top (3.8% sodium citrate) tube for the original Westergren method.

REFERENCE VALUE: (Method: Westergren)

Age	Male	Female
Newborn	0–2 mm/h	0–2 mm/h
Less than 50 y	0–15 mm/h	0–25 mm/h
50 y and older	0–20 mm/h	0–30 mm/h

DESCRIPTION: The erythrocyte sedimentation rate (ESR) is a measure of the rate of sedimentation of red blood cells (RBCs) in an anticoagulated whole blood sample over a specified period of time. The basis of the ESR test is the alteration of blood proteins by inflammatory and necrotic processes that cause the RBCs to stick together, become heavier, and rapidly settle at the bottom of a vertically held, calibrated tube over time. In general, relatively little settling occurs in normal blood because normal RBCs do not form rouleaux and would not stack together increasing their mass and rate of sedimentation. The sedimentation rate is proportional to the size or mass of the falling RBCs and is inversely proportional to plasma viscosity. The test is a nonspecific indicator of disease but is fairly sensitive and is frequently the earliest indicator of widespread inflammatory reaction due to infection or autoimmune disorders. Prolonged elevations are also present in malignant disease. The ESR can also be used to monitor the course of a disease and the effectiveness of therapy. The two most commonly used methods to measure the ESR are the Westergren (or modified Westergren) method and the Wintrobe hematocrit method. ■

INDICATIONS:

- Assist in the diagnosis of acute infection, such as tuberculosis or tissue necrosis
- Assist in the diagnosis of acute inflammatory processes
- Assist in the diagnosis of chronic infections
- Assist in the diagnosis of rheumatoid or autoimmune disorders
- Assist in the diagnosis of temporal arthritis and polymyalgia rheumatica
- Monitor inflammatory and malignant disease

RESULT

Increased in:
- Acute myocardial infarction (MI)
- Anemia
- Cat scratch fever

- Carcinoma
- Collagen diseases including systemic lupus erythematosus (SLE)
- Crohn's disease
- Endocarditis
- Heavy metal poisoning
- Increased plasma protein level
- Infections (e.g., pneumonia, syphilis)
- Inflammatory diseases
- Lymphoma
- Lymphosarcoma
- Multiple myeloma
- Nephritis
- Pregnancy
- Pulmonary embolism
- Rheumatic fever
- Rheumatoid arthritis
- Subacute bacterial endocarditis
- Temporal arteritis
- Toxemia
- Tuberculosis
- Waldenström's macroglobulinemia

Normal in:
- Congestive heart failure
- Glucose-6-phosphate dehydrogenase deficiency
- Hemoglobin C disease
- Hypofibrinogenemia
- Polycythemia
- Sickle cell anemia
- Spherocytosis

Decreased in:
- Conditions resulting in high hemoglobin and RBC count
- Elevated blood glucose

CRITICAL VALUES: N/A

INTERFERING FACTORS:

• Some drugs cause an SLE-like syndrome that results in a physiologic increase in ESR. These include anticonvulsants, hydrazine derivatives, nitrofurantoin, procainamide, and quinidine. Other drugs that may cause an increased ESR include acetylsalicylic acid, cephalothin, cephapirin, cyclosporine A, dextran, and oral contraceptives.

• Drugs that may cause a decrease in ESR include aurothiomalate, corticotropin, cortisone, and quinine.

• Menstruation may cause falsely increased test results.

• Prolonged tourniquet constriction around the arm may cause hemoconcentration and falsely low values.

• The Westergren and modified Westergren method are affected by heparin, which causes a false elevation in values.

• Bubbles in the Westergren tube or pipette, or tilting the measurement column more than 3° from vertical will falsely increase the values.

• Movement or vibration of the surface on which the test is being conducted will affect the results.

• Inaccurate timing will invalidate test results.

• Specimens that are clotted, hemolyzed, or insufficient in volume should be rejected for analysis.

• The test should be performed within 4 hours of collection when the specimen has been stored at room temperature; delays in testing may result in decreased values. If a delay in testing is anticipated, refrigerate the sample at 2°C to 4°C; stability at refrigerated temperature is reported to be extended up to 12 hours. Refrigerated specimens should be brought to room temperature before testing.

Nursing Implications and Procedure

Pretest:

➤ Obtain a history of the patient's complaints, including a list of known allergens.

➤ Obtain a history of infectious, autoimmune, or neoplastic diseases.

➤ Obtain a history of the patient's hematopoietic, immune, and respiratory systems, as well as results of previously performed tests and procedures. For related tests, refer to the hematopoietic, immune, and respiratory system tables.

➤ Obtain a list of the medications the patient is taking, including herbs, nutritional supplements, and nutraceuticals. The requesting health care practitioner and laboratory should be advised if the patient regularly uses these products so that their effects can be taken into consideration when reviewing results.

➤ There are no food, fluid, or medication restrictions unless by medical direction.

➤ Review the procedure with the patient.

➤ Inform the patient that specimen collection takes approximately 5 to 10 minutes.

Intratest:

➤ Direct the patient to breathe normally and to avoid unnecessary movement.

➤ Observe standard precautions and follow the general guidelines in Appendix A. Perform a venipuncture and collect the specimen in a 5-mL gray-top (sodium citrate) tube if the Westergren method will be used. Collect the specimen in a 5-mL purple-top (EDTA) tube if the modified Westergren method will be used.

➤ Label the specimen, and promptly transport it to the laboratory.

Post-test: ■

➤ Observe venipuncture site for bleeding or hematoma formation. Apply pressure bandage.

➤ Evaluate test results in relation to the patient's symptoms and other tests performed. Related laboratory tests include complete blood count, C-reactive protein, rheumatoid factor, microorganism-specific serologies, and related cultures.

ERYTHROPOIETIN

. . . .

SYNONYM/ACRONYM: EPO.

SPECIMEN: Serum (2 mL) collected in a red- or tiger-top tube.

REFERENCE VALUE: (Method: Radioimmunoassay)

Conventional Units	SI Units (Conversion Factor ×1)
5–36 mU/mL	5–36 U/L

DESCRIPTION: Erythropoietin (EPO) is a glycoprotein produced mainly by the kidney. Its function is to stimulate the bone marrow to make red blood cells. EPO levels fall after removal of the kidney but do not disappear completely. It is thought that small amounts of EPO may be produced by the liver. Erythropoiesis is regulated by EPO and tissue pO_2. When pO_2 is normal, EPO levels decrease; when pO_2 falls, EPO secretion occurs and EPO levels increase. ■

INDICATIONS:

• Assist in assessment of anemia of end-stage renal disease

• Assist in the diagnosis of EPO-producing tumors

• Evaluate the presence of rare anemias

• Monitor patients receiving EPO therapy

RESULT

Increased in:

• Anemias

• After moderate bleeding in an otherwise healthy patient

• Hepatoma

• Kidney transplant rejection

• Nephroblastoma

• Pheochromocytoma

• Secondary polycythemia (high-altitude hypoxia, chronic obstructive pulmonary disease [COPD], pulmonary fibrosis)

• Polycystic kidney disease

• Pregnancy

Decreased in:

• Chemotherapy

• Primary polycythemia

• Renal failure

CRITICAL VALUES: N/A

INTERFERING FACTORS:

• Drugs that may increase EPO levels include anabolic steroids.

• Drugs that may decrease EPO levels include amphotericin B, cisplatin, enalapril, estrogens, and theophylline.

• Blood transfusions may also decrease EPO levels.

• Recent radioactive scans or radiation within 1 week before the test can interfere with test results when radioimmunoassay is the test method.

Nursing Implications and Procedure • • • • • • • • • • •

Pretest: ■

➤ Obtain a history of the patient's complaints, including a list of known allergens.

➤ Obtain a history of the patient's hematopoietic and genitourinary systems, as well as results of previously performed tests and procedures. For related tests, refer to the hematopoietic and genitourinary system tables.

➤ Obtain a list of the medications the patient is taking, including herbs, nutritional supplements, and nutraceuticals. The requesting health care practitioner and laboratory should be advised if the patient regularly uses these products so that their effects can be taken into consideration when reviewing results.

➤ Note any recent procedures that can interfere with test results.

➤ There are no food, fluid, or medication restrictions unless by medical direction.

➤ Review the procedure with the patient.

➤ Inform the patient that specimen collection takes approximately 5 to 10 minutes.

Intratest: ■

➤ Direct the patient to breathe normally and to avoid unnecessary movement.

➤ Observe standard precautions and follow the general guidelines in Appendix A. Perform a venipuncture, and collect the specimen in a 5-mL red- or tiger-top tube.

➤ Label the specimen, and promptly transport it to the laboratory.

Post-test: ■

➤ Observe venipuncture site for bleeding or hematoma formation. Apply pressure bandage.

➤ Evaluate test results in relation to the patient's symptoms and other tests performed. Related laboratory tests include complete blood count, ferritin, iron/total iron-binding capacity, and vitamin B_{12}.

ESOPHAGEAL MANOMETRY

• •

SYNONYMS/ACRONYM: Esophageal function study, esophageal acid study (Tuttle test), acid reflux test, Bernstein test (aid perfusion), esophageal motility study.

AREA OF APPLICATION: Esophagus.

CONTRAST: Done with or without noniodinated contrast medium.

DESCRIPTION: Esophageal manometry (EM) consists of a group of invasive studies performed to assist in diagnosing abnormalities of esophageal muscle function and esophageal structure. These studies measure esophageal pressure, the effects of gastric acid in the esophagus, lower esophageal sphincter pressure, and motility patterns that result during swallowing. EM can be used to document and quantify gastroesophageal reflux (GER). It is indicated when a patient is experiencing difficulty swallowing, heartburn, regurgitation, or vomiting; or has chest pain for which no diagnosis has been found. Tests performed in combination with EM include the acid reflux, acid clearing, and acid perfusion (Bernstein) tests. ■

INDICATIONS:
• Evaluate pyrosis and dysphagia to determine if the cause is GER or esophagitis

• Aid in the diagnosis of GER, evidenced by low pressure in EM, decreased pH in acidity test, and pain in acid reflux and perfusion tests

• Aid in the diagnosis of esophagitis, evidenced by decreased motility

• Aid in the diagnosis of achalasia, evidenced by increased pressure in EM

• Aid in the diagnosis of chalasia in children, evidenced by decreased pressure in EM

• Aid in the diagnosis of esophageal scleroderma, evidenced by decreased pressure in EM

• Differentiate between esophagitis or cardiac condition as the cause of epigastric pain

RESULT

Normal Findings:
• Esophageal sphincter pressure: 10 to 20 mm Hg

• Esophageal secretions: pH 5 to 6

• Acid reflux: no regurgitation into the esophagus

• Acid perfusion: no GER

• Acid clearing: fewer than 10 swallows

• Bernstein test: negative

Abnormal Findings:
• Achalasia (sphincter pressure of 50 mm Hg)

- Chalasia

- Esophageal scleroderma

- Esophagitis

- GER (sphincter pressure of 0 to 5 mm Hg, pH of 1 to 3)

- Hiatal hernia

- Progressive systemic sclerosis (scleroderma)

- Spasms

CRITICAL VALUES: N/A

INTERFERING FACTORS:

This procedure is contraindicated for:

- Patients with unstable cardiopulmonary status, blood coagulation defects, recent gastrointestinal (GI) surgery, esophageal varices, or bleeding should not have this test performed.

Factors that may impair the results of the examination:

- Inability of the patient to cooperate or remain still during the procedure because of age, significant pain, or mental status

- Administration of medications (e.g., sedatives, antacids, anticholinergics, cholinergics, corticosteroids) that can change pH or relax the sphincter muscle, causing inaccurate results

Other considerations:

- Failure to follow dietary restrictions before the procedure may cause the procedure to be canceled or repeated.

Nursing Implications and Procedure · · · · · · · · · · ·

Pretest:

➤ Explain that the procedure is generally performed in an endoscopy suite by a physician with support staff and

usually takes 30 to 60 minutes to complete.

➤ Explain to the patient the purpose of the study and how the procedure is performed.

➤ *Obtain a written, informed consent for the procedure from the patient.*

➤ Obtain a history of upper GI distress or disorders, hiatal hernia, and related symptoms.

➤ Obtain the results of previously performed tests, treatments, surgeries, and procedures done to diagnose or treat disorders of the upper GI system. For related tests, refer to the gastrointestinal system table.

➤ Determine date of last menstrual period and possibility of pregnancy in perimenopausal women.

➤ Inform the patient that there will be some discomfort and gagging when the tube is inserted, but there are no complications resulting from the procedure and the throat will be anesthetized with a spray or swab.

➤ Inform the patient that dentures and eyewear will be removed before the test.

➤ Inform the patient that he or she will not be able to speak during the procedure, but that breathing will not be affected.

➤ Restrict food, fluids, and smoking for 8 hours before the procedure.

➤ Ensure that medications are withheld for 24 hours before the study; special arrangements may be necessary for diabetic patients.

➤ Resuscitation and suctioning equipment should be readily available.

➤ Obtain and record baseline vital signs.

Intratest:

➤ During the procedure, monitor the patient to prevent aspiration of stomach contents into the lungs. Note any change in respirations (dyspnea, tachypnea, adventitious sounds).

➤ Suction mouth, pharynx, and trachea, and administer oxygen as ordered.

➤ Have the patient put on a hospital gown and void.

➤ Place the patient on the examining table, and spray the throat with local anesthetic.

➤ Wear gloves throughout the procedure.

Esophageal manometry:

➤ One or more small tubes are inserted through the nose into the esophagus and stomach.

➤ A small transducer is attached to the ends of the tubes; pressures are measured at the lower esophageal sphincter, and intraluminal pressures as well as regularity and duration of peristaltic contractions are measured.

➤ The patient is asked to swallow small amounts of water or flavored gelatin.

➤ Pressures are taken and recorded, and a motility pattern is recorded on a graph.

Esophageal acid and clearing (Tuttle test):

➤ With the tube in place, a pH electrode probe is inserted into the esophagus with Valsalva maneuvers performed to stimulate reflux of stomach contents into the esophagus.

➤ If acid reflux is absent, 100 mL of 0.1% hydrochloric acid is instilled into the stomach during a 3-minute period, and then the pH measurement is repeated.

➤ To determine acid clearing, hydrochloric acid is instilled into the esophagus and the patient is asked to swallow while the probe measures the pH.

Acid perfusion (Bernstein test):

➤ A catheter is inserted through the nose into the esophagus and the patient is asked to inform the technician when pain is experienced.

➤ Normal saline solution is allowed to

drip into the catheter at about 10 mL/min. Then hydrochloric acid is allowed to drip into the catheter.

➤ Pain experienced when the hydrochloric acid is instilled determines the presence of an esophageal abnormality. If no pain is experienced, symptoms are the result of some other condition.

Post-test:

➤ Tell the patient to expect some throat soreness and possible hoarseness. Advise the patient to use warm gargles, lozenges, or ice packs to the neck; or to drink cool fluids to alleviate throat discomfort.

➤ Monitor the patient for signs of respiratory depression (less than 15 respirations per minute). Resuscitation equipment should be available.

➤ Observe the patient for indications of perforation: painful swallowing with neck movement, substernal pain with respiration, shoulder pain, dyspnea, abdominal or back pain, cyanosis, and fever.

➤ Emphasize that any severe pain, fever, difficulty breathing, or expectoration of blood must be reported to the physician immediately.

➤ Do not allow the patient to eat or drink until the gag reflex returns; then allow the patient to eat lightly for 12 to 24 hours.

➤ Instruct the patient to resume normal activity, medication, and diet 24 hours after the examination or as tolerated, unless otherwise indicated.

➤ A physician specializing in this branch of medicine sends a written report to the ordering provider, who discusses the results with the patient.

➤ Inform the patient that an abnormal examination may indicate the need for further studies.

➤ Evaluate test results in relation to the patient's symptoms and any related tests performed.

ESOPHAGOGASTRODUODENOSCOPY

SYNONYMS/ACRONYMS: Esophagoscopy, gastroscopy, upper GI endoscopy, EGD.

AREA OF APPLICATION: Esophagus, stomach, and upper duodenum.

CONTRAST: Done without contrast.

DESCRIPTION: Esophagogastroduodenoscopy (EGD) allows direct visualization of the upper gastrointestinal (GI) tract mucosa, which includes the esophagus, stomach, and upper portion of the duodenum, by means of a flexible endoscope. The standard flexible fiberoptic endoscope contains three channels that allow passage of the instruments needed to perform therapeutic or diagnostic procedures, such as biopsies or cytology washings. The endoscope, a multichannel instrument, allows visualization of the GI tract linings, insufflation of air, aspiration of fluid, removal of foreign bodies by suction or by snare or forceps, and passage of a laser beam for obliteration of abnormal tissue or control of bleeding. Direct visualization yields greater diagnostic data than is possible through radiologic procedures, and therefore EGD is rapidly replacing upper GI as the diagnostic procedure of choice. ■

INDICATIONS:
- Assist in differentiating between benign and neoplastic tumors
- Detect upper GI inflammatory disease

- Evaluate the extent of esophageal injury after ingestion of chemicals
- Detect gastric or duodenal ulcers
- Evaluate stomach or duodenum after surgical procedures
- Determine the presence and location of acute upper GI bleeding
- Evaluate suspected gastric outlet obstruction
- Identify tissue abnormalities and obtain biopsy specimens
- Investigate the cause of dysphagia, dyspepsia, and epigastric pain

RESULT

Normal Findings:
- Esophageal mucosa is normally yellow-pink. At about 9 inches from the incisor teeth, a pulsation indicates the location of the aortic arch. The gastric mucosa is orange-red and contains rugae. The proximal duodenum is reddish and contains a few longitudinal folds, whereas the distal duodenum has circular folds lined with villi. No abnormal structures or functions are observed in the esophagus, stomach, or duodenum.

Abnormal Findings:

- Acute and chronic gastric and duodenal ulcers

- Diverticular disease

- Duodenitis

- Esophagitis or strictures

- Esophageal varices

- Esophageal or pyloric stenosis

- Gastritis

- Hiatal hernia

- Mallory-Weiss syndrome

- Tumors (benign or malignant)

CRITICAL VALUES: N/A

INTERFERING FACTORS:

This procedure is contraindicated for:

- Patients who have had surgery involving the stomach or duodenum, which can make locating the duodenal papilla difficult

- Patients with a bleeding disorder

- Patients with unstable cardiopulmonary status, blood coagulation defects, or cholangitis, unless the patient received prophylactic antibiotic therapy before the test (otherwise the examination must be rescheduled)

- Patients with unstable cardiopulmonary status, blood coagulation defects, known aortic arch aneurysm, large esophageal Zenker's diverticulum, recent GI surgery, esophageal varices, or known esophageal perforation

Factors that may impair clear imaging:

- Inability of the patient to cooperate or remain still during the procedure because of age, significant pain, or mental status

- Gas or feces in the GI tract resulting from inadequate cleansing or failure to restrict food intake before the study

- Retained barium from a previous radiologic procedure

- Patients who are very obese, who may exceed the weight limit for the equipment

- Incorrect positioning of the patient, which may produce poor visualization of the area to be examined

- Barium swallow or upper GI series within the preceding 48 hours, which can hinder adequate visualization

- Severe upper GI bleeding or the presence of blood or clots

Other considerations:

- Failure to follow dietary restrictions before the procedure may cause the procedure to be canceled or repeated.

- Consultation with a physician should occur before the procedure for radiation safety concerns regarding infants of patients who are lactating.

- Risks associated with radiographic overexposure can result from frequent x-ray procedures. Personnel in the room with the patient should wear a protective lead apron, stand behind a shield, or leave the area while the examination is being done. Personnel working in the area where the examination is being done should wear badges that reveal their level of exposure to radiation.

Nursing Implications and Procedure • • • • • • • • • • •

Pretest:

➤ Explain to the patient the purpose of the study and how the procedure is performed.

➤ Explain that the procedure usually takes 30 to 60 minutes to complete and is generally performed in an endoscopy suite by a physician and support staff.

➤ *Obtain a written, informed consent for the procedure from the patient.*

➤ Obtain a history of GI disorders and related symptoms.

➤ Obtain the results of previously performed tests, treatments, surgeries, and procedures done to diagnose or treat disorders of the upper GI system. For related tests, refer to the gastrointestinal system table.

➤ Determine date of last menstrual period and possibility of pregnancy in perimenopausal women.

➤ Inform the patient that the procedure is not painful and that the throat will be anesthetized with a spray or swab.

➤ Inform the patient that dentures and eyewear will be removed before the test.

➤ Inform the patient that he or she will not be able to speak during the procedure, but that breathing will not be affected.

➤ Restrict food and fluids for 8 hours before the procedure.

➤ Note recent administration of barium because it can obscure the area to be examined.

➤ Make resuscitation and suctioning equipment readily available.

➤ Obtain and record baseline vital signs.

Intratest:

➤ Have the patient put on a hospital gown and void.

➤ Wear gloves throughout the procedure.

➤ An intravenous (IV) line may be started to allow for the infusion of a sedative or IV fluids.

➤ Administer ordered sedation.

➤ Spray or swab the oropharynx with a topical local anesthetic.

➤ Provide an emesis basin for the increased saliva and encourage the patient to spit out the saliva

because the gag reflex may be impaired.

➤ Place the patient on an examination table in the left lateral decubitus position with the neck slightly flexed forward.

➤ The endoscope is passed through the mouth with a dental suction device in place to drain secretions. A side-viewing flexible, fiberoptic endoscope is advanced and visualization of the GI tract is started.

➤ Air is insufflated to distend the upper GI tract, as needed. Biopsy specimens are obtained and/or endoscopic surgery is performed.

➤ Label the specimens, and promptly transport them to the laboratory.

➤ At the end of the procedure, excess air and secretions are aspirated through the scope and the endoscope is removed.

Post-test:

➤ Do not allow the patient to eat or drink until the gag reflex returns; then allow the patient to eat lightly for 12 to 24 hours. Instruct the patient to resume normal activity, medication, and diet in 24 hours or as tolerated after the examination, unless otherwise indicated.

➤ Inform the patient that he or she may experience some throat soreness and hoarseness. Instruct patient to treat throat discomfort with lozenges and warm gargles when the gag reflex returns.

➤ Monitor the patient for signs of respiratory depression (less than 15 respirations per minute).

➤ Observe the patient until the effects of the sedation have worn off.

➤ Observe the patient for indications of esophageal perforation (i.e., painful swallowing with neck movement, substernal pain with respiration, shoulder pain or dyspnea, and abdominal or back pain, cyanosis, fever).

➤ Inform the patient that any belching,

bloating, or flatulence is the result of air insufflation and is temporary.

➤ Emphasize that any severe pain, fever, difficulty breathing, or expectoration of blood must be immediately reported to the physician.

➤ A physician specializing in this branch of medicine sends a written report to the ordering provider, who discusses the results with the patient.

➤ Inform the patient that an abnormal examination may indicate the need for further studies.

➤ Evaluate test results in relation to the patient's symptoms and any related tests performed.

ESTRADIOL

SYNONYM/ACRONYM: E2.

SPECIMEN: Serum (1 mL) collected in a red- or tiger-top tube. Plasma (1 mL) collected in green-top (heparin) tube is also acceptable.

REFERENCE VALUE: (Method: Immunoassay)

Age	Conventional Units	SI Units (Conversion Factor ×3.67)
6 m–10 y	Less than 15 pg/mL	Less than 55 pmol/L
11–15 y		
Male	Less than 40 pg/mL	Less than 147 pmol/L
Female	10–300 pg/mL	37–1100 pmol/L
Adult male	10–50 pg/mL	37–184 pmol/L
Adult female		
Early follicular phase	20–150 pg/mL	73–551 pmol/L
Late follicular phase	40–350 pg/mL	147–1285 pmol/L
Midcycle peak	150–750 pg/mL	551–2753 pmol/L
Luteal phase	30–450 pg/mL	110–1652 pmol/L
Postmenopause	Less than 20 pg/mL	Less than 73 pmol/L

DESCRIPTION: Estrogens are hormones secreted in large amounts by the ovaries and during pregnancy by the placenta. Estradiol is also secreted in minute amounts by the adrenal cortex and the testes. Only three types of estrogen are present in the blood in measurable amounts: estrone, estradiol, and estriol. Estradiol is the most active of the estrogens. Estrone (E_1) is the immediate precursor of estradiol (E_2). Estriol (E_3) is secreted in large amounts from the placenta during pregnancy from precursors produced by the fetal liver. ■

INDICATIONS:

- Assist in determining the presence of gonadal dysfunction

- Evaluate menstrual abnormalities, fertility problems, and estrogen-producing tumors in women, and testicular or adrenal tumors and feminization disorders in men

- Monitor menotropin (Pergonal) therapy. Menotropin is a preparation of follicle-stimulating hormone (FSH) and luteinizing hormone (LH) used to induce ovulation and increase the chance of pregnancy

RESULT

Increased in:
- Adrenal tumors
- Estrogen-producing tumors
- Feminization in children
- Gynecomastia
- Hepatic cirrhosis
- Hyperthyroidism

Decreased in:
- Ovarian failure
- Primary and secondary hypogonadism
- Turner's syndrome

CRITICAL VALUES: N/A

INTERFERING FACTORS:

- Drugs that may increase estradiol levels include cimetidine, clomiphene, dehydroepiandrosterone, diazepam, estrogen/progestin therapy, ketoconazole, mifepristone (some patients with meningiomas and not receiving any other drugs), nafarelin, nilutamide, phenytoin, tamoxifen, and troleandomycin.

- Drugs that may decrease estradiol levels include aminoglutethimide, chemotherapy drugs, cimetidine, danazol, fadrozole, formestane, goserelin, leuprolide, megestrol, mepartricin, mifepristone (pregnant women with expulsion of fetus), nafarelin (women being treated for endometriosis), and oral contraceptives.

- Estradiol is secreted in a biphasic pattern during normal menstruation. Knowledge of the phase of the menstrual cycle may assist interpretation of estradiol levels.

Nursing Implications and Procedure • • • • • • • • • • •

Pretest: ■

➤ Obtain a history of the patient's complaints, including a list of known allergens.

➤ Obtain a history of the patient's endocrine and reproductive systems, as well as phase of menstrual cycle and results of previously performed tests and procedures. For related tests, refer to the endocrine and reproductive system tables.

➤ Obtain a list of the medications the patient is taking, including herbs, nutritional supplements, and nutraceuticals. The requesting health care practitioner and laboratory should be advised if the patient regularly uses these products so that their effects can be taken into consideration when reviewing results.

➤ There are no food, fluid, or medication restrictions unless by medical direction.

➤ Review the procedure with the patient.

➤ Inform the patient that specimen collection takes approximately 5 to 10 minutes.

ESTROGEN AND PROGESTERONE RECEPTOR ASSAYS

SYNONYMS/ACRONYMS: Estrogen receptor protein (ERP), progesterone receptor protein (PRP).

SPECIMEN: Breast tissue.

REFERENCE VALUE: (Method: Cytochemical or immunocytochemical) Interpretation of results is subjective depending on the intensity of staining and the number of cells classified as positive. More recently, immunoperoxidase methods employing monoclonal antibodies have been introduced. These antibodies have greater specificity and are not subject to interference by exogenous hormones.

Cytochemical Findings	Values
Favorable findings	Greater than 20% of cell nuclei are stained
Borderline findings	11–20% of cell nuclei are stained
Unfavorable findings	Less than 10% of cell nuclei are stained

DESCRIPTION: Estrogen and progesterone receptor assays are used to identify patients with a type of breast cancer that may be more responsive than other types of tumors to estrogen-deprivation (antiestrogen) therapy or removal of the ovaries. Patients with these types of tumors generally have a better prognosis. DNA ploidy testing by flow cytometry may also be performed on suspicious tissue. Cancer cells contain abnormal amounts of DNA. The higher the grade of tumor cells, the more likely abnormal DNA will be detected. The ploidy or number of chromosome sets in the nucleus is an indication of the speed of cell replication and tumor growth. ■

INDICATIONS:
• Identify patients with breast or other types of cancer that may respond to hormone or antihormone therapy

• Monitor responsiveness to hormone or antihormone therapy

RESULT

Positive findings in:
• Hormonal therapy

• Receptor-positive tumors

Negative findings in:
• Receptor-negative tumors

CRITICAL VALUES: N/A

INTERFERING FACTORS:
• Antiestrogen preparations (e.g., tamoxifen) ingested 2 months before tissue sampling will affect test results.

• Tissue specimens contaminated with formalin or failure to freeze the specimen adequately using liquid nitrogen or dry ice will falsely decrease results.

• Massive tumor necrosis or tumors with low cellular composition falsely decrease results.

• Failure to transport specimen to the laboratory immediately can result in degradation of receptor sites. Prompt and proper specimen processing, storage, and analysis are important to achieve accurate results.

Nursing Implications and Procedure • • • • • • • • • • •

Pretest: ■

➤ Obtain a history of the patient's complaints, including a list of known allergens.

➤ Obtain a history of the patient's endocrine, immune, and reproductive systems, as well as results of previously performed tests and procedures. For related tests, refer to the endocrine, immune, and reproductive system tables.

➤ Obtain a list of the medications the patient is taking, including herbs, nutritional supplements, and nutraceuticals. The requesting health care practitioner and laboratory should be advised if the patient regularly uses these products so that their effects can be taken into consideration when reviewing results.

➤ Ensure that the patient has not received antiestrogen therapy within 2 months of the test.

➤ Inform the patient that the excision is considered a surgical procedure and that fasting for 8 hours before the procedure is required.

➤ Review the procedure with the patient.

➤ Assess if the patient has an allergy to local anesthetics, and inform the health care practitioner accordingly.

➤ Ensure that nonallergy to anesthesia is confirmed before open biopsy procedure is performed under general anesthesia.

➤ *Obtain a written and informed consent before administering any medications prior to the procedure.*

➤ Inform the patient that specimen collection takes approximately 15 to 20 minutes.

Intratest: ■

➤ Ensure that the patient has complied with dietary preparation and other pretesting restrictions.

➤ Record baseline vital signs.

➤ Administer preoperative sedation, as ordered.

➤ Assemble supplies and prepare the patient for surgical biopsy or resection. Supplies should include a waxed cardboard specimen container without preservatives.

➤ Observe standard precautions and follow the general guidelines in Appendix A.

➤ Using needle biopsy or resection, the health care practitioner obtains a tissue specimen weighing at least 200 mg. Place the specimen in a labeled formalin-free container. Label the specimen indicating location (e.g., left or right), and promptly transport it to the laboratory.

Post-test:

➤ Instruct the patient to resume usual diet and medication as directed by the health care practitioner.

➤ After open biopsy, monitor vital signs every 15 minutes for 1 hour, and then every 2 hours for 4 hours, and as ordered. Take temperature every 4 hours for 24 hours.

➤ After local anesthesia, monitor vital signs and compare with baseline values.

➤ Instruct the patient in proper cleansing of the site and of the importance of a follow-up appointment for suture removal, as appropriate.

➤ Instruct the patient to report excessive bleeding, redness, edema, or pain at the biopsy site.

➤ Administer analgesics and antibiotics as ordered, and instruct the patient in the importance of completing the entire course of antibiotic therapy even if no symptoms are present.

➤ Teach the patient how to perform a monthly breast self-examination, and instruct her to have a mammogram performed annually.

➤ Recognize anxiety related to test results and offer support. Provide teaching and information regarding the clinical implications of the test results, as appropriate. Educate the patient regarding access to counseling services.

➤ Inform the patient about hormone therapy, as appropriate based on test results.

➤ Evaluate test results in relation to the patient's symptoms and other tests performed. Related laboratory tests include breast biopsy, CA 15-3, HER-2/neu oncoprotein, and carcinoembryonic antigen.

EVOKED BRAIN POTENTIALS

· ·

SYNONYMS/ACRONYMS: EP studies, brain stem auditory evoked potentials (BAEP), brain stem auditory evoked responses (BAER).

AREA OF APPLICATION: Brain.

CONTRAST: None.

DESCRIPTION: Evoked brain potentials, also known as evoked potential (EP) responses, are electrophysiologic studies performed to measure the brain's electrical responses to various visual, auditory, and somatosensory stimuli. EP studies help diagnose lesions of the nervous system by evaluating the integrity of the visual, somatosensory, and auditory nerve pathways. Three response types are measured: visual evoked response (VER), auditory brain stem response (ABR), and somatosensory evoked response (SER). The stimuli activate the nerve tracts that connect the stimulated (receptor) area with the cortical (visual and somatosensory) or midbrain (auditory) sensory area. A number of stimuli are given and then electronically displayed in waveforms, recorded, and computer analyzed. Abnormalities are determined by a delay in time, measured in milliseconds, between the stimulus and the response. This is known as *increased latency.* VER provides information about visual pathway function to identify lesions of the optic nerves, optic tracts, and demyelinating diseases such as multiple sclerosis. ABR provides information about auditory pathways to identify hearing loss and lesions of the brain stem. SER provides information about the somatosensory pathways to identify lesions at various levels of the central nervous system (spinal cord and brain) and peripheral nerve disease. EP studies are especially useful in patients with problems and those unable to speak or respond to instructions during the test, because they do not require voluntary cooperation or participation in the activity. This allows objective diagnostic information about visual or auditory disorders affecting infants and children, and allows differentiation between organic brain and psychological disorders in adults. EP studies are also used to monitor the progression of or the effectiveness of treatment for deteriorating neurological diseases such as multiple sclerosis. ■

INDICATIONS

VER (potentials):
- Detect neurological disorders such as multiple sclerosis, Parkinson's disease, and Huntington's chorea
- Detect cryptic or past retrobulbar neuritis
- Evaluate optic pathway lesions and visual cortex defects
- Detect lesions of the eye or optic nerves
- Evaluate binocularity in infants

ABR (potentials):
- Detect abnormalities or lesions in the brain stem or auditory nerve areas
- Screen or evaluate neonates, infants, children, and adults for auditory problems (EP studies may be indicated when a child falls below growth chart norms)
- Early detection of brain stem tumors and acoustic neuromas

SER (potentials):
- Evaluate spinal cord and brain injury and function
- Detect sensorimotor neuropathies and cervical pathology
- Detect multiple sclerosis and Guillain-Barré syndrome
- Monitor sensory potentials to deter-

mine spinal cord function during a surgical procedure or medical regimen

ERP (potentials):

- Differentiate between organic brain disorder and cognitive function abnormality

- Detect suspected psychosis or dementia

RESULT

Normal Findings:

VER and ABR: Normal latency in recorded cortical and brain stem waveforms depending on age, sex, and stature

ERP: Normal recognition and attention span

SER: No loss of consciousness or presence of weakness

Abnormal Findings:

- VER (potentials):
  P100 latencies (extended) confined to one eye suggest a lesion anterior to the optic chiasm.
  Bilateral abnormal P100 latencies indicate multiple sclerosis, optic neuritis, retinopathies, spinocerebellar degeneration, sarcoidosis, Parkinson's disease, adrenoleukodystrophy, Huntington's chorea, and amblyopias.

- ABR (potentials):
  Normal response at high intensities; wave V may occur slightly later. Earlier wave distortions suggest cochlear lesion.
  Absent or late waves at high intensities; increased amplitude of wave V suggests retrocochlear lesion.

- SER (potentials):
  Abnormal upper-limb latencies suggest cervical spondylosis or intracerebral lesions.

Abnormal lower limb latencies suggest peripheral nerve root disease such as Guillain-Barré syndrome, multiple sclerosis, transverse myelitis, or traumatic spinal cord injuries.

CRITICAL VALUES: N/A

INTERFERING FACTORS

Factors that may impair the results of the examination:

- Inability of the patient to cooperate or remain still during the procedure because of age, significant pain, or mental status (*note*: significant behavioral problems may limit the ability to complete the test)

- Improper placement of electrodes

- Patient stress, which can affect brain chemistry thus making it difficult to distinguish whether the results are due to the patient's emotional reaction or to organic pathology

- Extremely poor visual acuity, which can hinder accurate determination of VER

- Severe hearing loss, which can interfere with accurate determination of ABR

Nursing Implications and Procedure

Pretest:

➤ Inform the patient that this procedure measures electrical activity in the nervous system.

➤ Inform the patient that the procedure is performed in a special laboratory by a technologist and takes approximately 30 minutes to 2 hours, depending on the test.

➤ Obtain a history and assessment of the neurological system, known or suspected neurological conditions, and trauma to the head or spinal cord, as well as the results of previously performed tests, surgeries, treatments, and procedures. For related tests, refer to the musculoskeletal system table.

➤ *Obtain a written, informed consent for the procedure from the patient.*

➤ Ensure that the patient is able to relax; report any extreme anxiety or restlessness.

➤ Ensure that hair is clean and free of hair sprays, creams, or solutions.

➤ Obtain a list of the medications the patient is taking including herbs, nutritional supplements, and nutraceuticals. The requesting health care practitioner and laboratory should be advised if the patient regularly uses these products so that their effects can be taken into consideration when reviewing results.

➤ Remove any jewelry or metallic objects above the neck.

➤ Assure the patient that there is no discomfort during the procedure, and encourage relaxation.

Intratest:

Visual evoked potentials:

➤ Place the patient in a comfortable position about 1 m from the stimulation source. Attach electrodes to the occipital and vertex lobe areas and a reference electrode to the ear. A light-emitting stimulation or a checkerboard pattern is projected on a screen at a regulated speed. This procedure is done for each eye (with the opposite eye covered) as the patient looks at a dot on the screen without any change in the gaze while the stimuli are delivered. A computer interprets the brain's responses to the stimuli and records them in waveforms.

Auditory evoked potentials:

➤ Place the patient in a comfortable position, and place the electrodes on the scalp at the vertex lobe area and on each earlobe. Earphones are placed on the patient's ears, and a clicking noise stimulus is delivered into one ear while a continuous tone is delivered to the opposite ear. Responses to the stimuli are recorded as waveforms for analysis.

Somatosensory evoked potentials:

➤ Place the patient in a comfortable position, and place the electrodes at the nerve sites of the wrist, knee, and ankle and on the scalp at the sensory cortex of the hemisphere on the opposite side (the electrode that picks up the response and delivers it to the recorder). Additional electrodes can be positioned at the cervical or lumbar vertebrae for upper or lower limb stimulation. The rate at which the electric shock stimulus is delivered to the nerve electrodes and travels to the brain is measured, computer analyzed, and recorded in waveforms for analysis. Both sides of the area being examined can be tested by switching the electrodes and repeating the procedure.

Event-related potentials:

➤ Place the patient in a sitting position in a chair in a quiet room. Earphones are placed on the patient's ears and auditory cues administered. The patient is asked to push a button when the tones are recognized. Flashes of light are also used as visual cues, with the client pushing a button when cues are noted. Results are compared to normal EP waveforms for correct, incorrect, or absent responses.

Post-test:

➤ When the procedure is complete, remove the electrodes and clean the skin where the electrodes were applied.

➤ A physician specializing in this branch of medicine sends a written report to the ordering provider, who discusses the results with the patient.

> Evaluate test results in relation to the patient's symptoms and other tests performed. Related diagnostic tests include electroencephalogra-phy as well as magnetic resonance imaging and computed tomography of the brain.

EXERCISE STRESS TEST

• •

SYNONYMS/ACRONYMS: Exercise electrocardiogram (ECG, EKG), graded exercise tolerance test, stress testing, treadmill test.

AREA OF APPLICATION: Heart.

CONTRAST: None.

DESCRIPTION: The exercise stress test is a noninvasive study to measure cardiac function during physical stress. Exercise electrocardiography is primarily useful in determining the extent of coronary artery occlusion by the heart's ability to meet the need for additional oxygen in response to the stress of exercising in a safe environment. The patient exercises on a treadmill or pedals a stationary bicycle to increase the heart rate to 80 to 90 percent of maximal heart rate determined by age and sex, known as the *target heart rate*. Every 2 to 3 minutes the speed and/or grade of the treadmill is increased to yield an increment of stress. The patient's electrocardiogram (ECG) and blood pressure are monitored during the test. The test proceeds until the patient reaches the target heart rate or experiences chest pain or fatigue. The risks involved in the procedure are possible myocardial infarction (1 in 500) and death (1 in 10,000) in those experiencing frequent angina episodes before the test. Although useful, this procedure is not as accurate as cardiac nuclear scans for diagnosing coronary artery disease (CAD).

For patients unable to complete the test, pharmacologic stress testing can be done. Medications used to increase the patient's heart include vasodilators such as dipyridamole and beta-agonists such as dobutamine. ■

INDICATIONS:
• Evaluate suspected CAD in the presence of chest pain and other symptoms

• Screen for CAD in the absence of pain and other symptoms in patients at risk

• Detect dysrhythmias during exercising, as evidenced by ECG changes

• Evaluate cardiac function after myocardial infarction or cardiac surgery to determine safe exercise levels for cardiac rehabilitation as well as work limitations

- Determine exercise-induced hypertension

- Detect peripheral arterial occlusive disease (intermittent claudication), as evidenced by leg pain or cramping during exercising

- Evaluate effectiveness of medication regimens, such as antianginals or antiarrhythmics

RESULT

Normal Findings:

- Normal heart rate during physical exercise. Heart rate and systolic blood pressure rise in direct proportion to workload and metabolic oxygen demand, which is based on age and exercise protocol. Maximal heart rate for adults is normally 150 to 200 beats/min.

Abnormal Findings:

- Activity intolerance related to oxygen supply and demand imbalance

- Bradycardia

- Chest pain related to ischemia or inflammation

- CAD

- Decreased cardiac output

- Dysrhythmias

- Hypertension

- Peripheral arterial occlusive disease

- S-T segment depression of 1 mm (considered a positive test), indicating myocardial ischemia

- Tachycardia

CRITICAL VALUES: N/A

INTERFERING FACTORS: The following factors may impair interpretation of examination results because they create an artificial state that makes it difficult to determine true physiologic function:

- Improper electrode placement

- High food intake or smoking before testing

- Drugs such as beta blockers, cardiac glycosides, calcium channel blockers, coronary vasodilators, and barbiturates

- Potassium or calcium imbalance

- Hypertension, hypoxia, left bundle branch block, and ventricular hypertrophy

- Wolff-Parkinson-White syndrome (anomalous atrioventricular excitation)

- Anxiety or panic attack

Nursing Implications and Procedure · · · · · · · · · · ·

Pretest: ■

➤ Inform the patient that the test assesses the heart's ability to respond to an increasing workload.

➤ Advise the patient to wear comfortable shoes and clothing for the exercise.

➤ Inform the patient that the procedure is performed in a special department by a technician and takes approximately 30 to 60 minutes.

➤ Assure the patient that the test has very few risks and that exercising can be terminated if extreme symptoms occur.

➤ Obtain a list of medications the patient is taking including herbs, nutritional supplements, and nutraceuticals. The requesting health care practitioner and laboratory should be advised if the patient regularly uses these products so that their effects can be taken into consideration when reviewing results.

➤ Obtain a pertinent history of the results of previously performed cardiac tests and procedures, present cardiac conditions or abnormalities, and therapies received for the cardiac conditions. For related tests, refer to the cardiovascular system table.

➤ *Obtain a written, informed consent for the procedure from the patient.*

➤ Ask the patient if he or she has had any chest pain within the prior 48 hours, or has a history of anginal attacks several times a day; if either of these is the case, inform the physician immediately because the stress test may be too risky and should be rescheduled in 4 to 6 weeks.

➤ Record a baseline 12-lead ECG and vital signs, if these recordings were not already obtained or are not available.

➤ Ensure that the patient has abstained from food, fluids, and smoking for at least 4 hours before the test and that the patient has discontinued specific medications that can interfere with test results, as ordered.

Intratest:

➤ Ask the patient to remove clothing from the waist up (give women a hospital gown that opens in the front).

➤ Electrodes are placed in appropriate positions on the patient, a blood pressure cuff connected to a monitoring device is applied, and if the patient's oxygen consumption is continuously monitored, the patient is connected to a machine via a mouthpiece or to a pulse oximeter via a finger lead.

➤ The patient is asked to walk on a treadmill (most commonly used) or to peddle a bicycle. As the stress is increased, the patient is asked to report any symptoms, such as chest or leg pain, dyspnea, or fatigue.

➤ An intravenous access may be established for emergency use.

➤ Instruct the patient to report symptoms such as dizziness, sweating, breathlessness, or nausea, which can be normal as speed increases. The test is terminated if pain or

fatigue is severe; maximum heart rate under stress is attained; signs of ischemia are present; maximum effort has been achieved; or dyspnea, hypertension (systolic blood pressure greater than 250 mm Hg), tachycardia (greater than 200 beats/minute minus person's age), new dysrhythmias, chest pain that begins or worsens, faintness, extreme dizziness, or confusion develop.

➤ The patient is asked to step onto the treadmill and is instructed to use the handrails to maintain balance.

➤ The treadmill is turned on to a slow speed, but is increased in speed and elevation to increase the patient's heart rate. Stress is increased until the patient's predicted target heart rate is reached.

➤ After the exercise period, a 3- to 15-minute rest period is given with the patient in a sitting position. During this period the ECG, blood pressure, and heart rate monitoring is continued.

Post-test:

➤ Remove the electrodes and cleanse the skin of any remaining gel or ECG electrode adhesive.

➤ Instruct the patient to call the physician to report any anginal pain or other discomforts experienced after the test.

➤ Instruct the patient regarding special dietary intake and medication regimen, as needed.

➤ Instruct the patient to resume activities discontinued before the test.

➤ A physician specializing in this branch of medicine sends a written report to the ordering provider, who discusses the results with the patient.

➤ Evaluate test results in relation to the patient's symptoms and other tests performed. Related diagnostic tests include ECG, as well as positron emission tomography scanning and nuclear thallium scanning of the heart.

FECAL ANALYSIS

SYNONYM/ACRONYM: N/A.

SPECIMEN: Stool.

REFERENCE VALUE: (Method: Macroscopic examination, for appearance and color; microscopic examination, for cell count and presence of meat fibers; leukocyte esterase, for leukocytes; Clinitest [Bayer Corporation, Pittsburgh, Pennsylvania] for reducing substances; guaiac, for occult blood; x-ray paper, for trypsin)

Characteristic	Normal Result
Appearance	Solid and formed
Color	Brown
Epithelial cells	Few to moderate
Fecal fat	See fecal fat monograph
Leukocytes (WBCs)	Negative
Meat fibers	Negative
Occult blood	Negative
Reducing substances	Negative
Trypsin	2+ to 4+

DESCRIPTION: Feces consist mainly of cellulose and other undigested foodstuffs, bacteria, and water. Other substances normally found in feces include epithelial cells shed from the gastrointestinal (GI) tract, small amounts of fats, bile pigments in the form of urobilinogen, GI and pancreatic secretions, electrolytes, and trypsin. Trypsin is a proteolytic enzyme produced in the pancreas. The average adult excretes 100 to 300 g of fecal material per day, the residue of approximately 10 L of liquid material that enters the tract each day. The laboratory analysis of feces includes macroscopic examination (volume, odor, shape, color, consistency, presence of mucus), microscopic examination (leukocytes, epithelial cells, meat fibers), and chemical tests for specific substances (occult blood, trypsin, estimation of carbohydrate). ∎

INDICATIONS:

• Assist in diagnosing disorders associated with GI bleeding or drug therapy that leads to bleeding

• Assist in the diagnosis of pseudomembranous enterocolitis after use of broad-spectrum antibiotic therapy

• Assist in the diagnosis of suspected inflammatory bowel disorder

- Detect altered protein digestion

- Detect intestinal parasitic infestation, as indicated by diarrhea of unknown cause

- Investigate diarrhea of unknown cause

- Monitor effectiveness of therapy for intestinal malabsorption or pancreatic insufficiency

- Screen for cystic fibrosis

RESULT

Unusual Appearance:
- Bloody: Excessive intestinal wall irritation or malignancy

- Bulky or frothy: Malabsorption

- Mucous: Inflammation of intestinal walls

- Slender or ribbonlike: Obstruction

Unusual Color:
- Black: Bismuth (antacid) or charcoal ingestion, iron therapy, upper GI bleed

- Grayish white: Barium ingestion, bile duct obstruction

- Green: Antibiotics, biliverdin, green vegetables

- Red: Beets and food coloring, lower GI bleed, phenazopyridine hydrochloride compounds, rifampin

- Yellow: Rhubarb

Increased:
- Carbohydrates/reducing substances: Malabsorption syndromes

- Epithelial cells: Inflammatory bowel disorders

- Leukocytes: Bacterial infections of the intestinal wall, salmonellosis, shigellosis, and ulcerative colitis

- Meat fibers: Altered protein digestion

- Occult blood: Anal fissure, diverticular disease, esophageal varices, esophagitis, gastritis, hemorrhoids, infectious diarrheas, inflammatory bowel disease, Mallory-Weiss tears, polyps, tumors, ulcers

Decreased:
- Leukocytes: Amebic colitis, cholera, disorders resulting from toxins, parasites, viral diarrhea

- Trypsin: Cystic fibrosis, malabsorption syndromes, pancreatic deficiency

CRITICAL VALUES: N/A

INTERFERING FACTORS:
- Drugs that can cause positive results for occult blood include acetylsalicylic acid, anticoagulants, colchicine, corticosteroids, iron preparations, and phenylbutazone.

- Ingestion of a diet high in red meat, certain vegetables, and bananas can cause false-positive results for occult blood.

- Large doses of vitamin C can cause false-negative occult blood.

- Constipated stools may not indicate any trypsin activity owing to extended exposure to intestinal bacteria.

Nursing Implications and Procedure • • • • • • • • • • • •

Pretest:

➤ Obtain a history of the patient's complaints, including a list of known allergens.

➤ Obtain a history of the patient's GI system as well as results of previously performed tests and procedures. For related tests, refer to the gastrointestinal system table.

➤ Obtain a list of medications the patient is taking, including herbs, nutritional supplements, and nutraceuticals. The requesting health care practitioner and laboratory should be advised if the patient regularly uses these products so that their effects can be taken into consideration when reviewing results.

➤ Instruct the patient to follow a normal diet for several days before the test.

➤ Inform the patient of the procedure for collecting a stool sample, including the importance of good hand-washing techniques. The patient should place the sample in a tightly covered container.

➤ Instruct the patient not to use laxatives, enemas, or suppositories for 3 days before the test.

➤ Instruct the patient not to contaminate the specimen with urine, water, or toilet tissue.

➤ There are no food, fluid, or medication restrictions unless by medical direction.

➤ Review the procedure with the patient.

Intratest:

➤ Ensure that the patient has complied with dietary preparations and other pretesting restrictions.

➤ Observe standard precautions and follow the general guidelines in Appendix A.

➤ Collect a stool specimen in a half-pint waterproof container with a tight-fitting lid; if the patient is not ambulatory, collect it in a clean, dry bedpan. Use a tongue blade to transfer the specimen to the container, and include any mucoid and bloody portions. Collect specimen from the first, middle, and last portion of the stool. The specimen should be refrigerated if it will not be transported to the laboratory within 4 hours after collection.

➤ To collect specimen by rectal swab, insert the swab past the anal sphincter, rotate gently, and withdraw. Place the swab in the appropriate container.

➤ Label the specimen, place it in a leak-proof bag, and promptly transport it to the laboratory. Make sure the label includes the date and time of collection and suspected cause of enteritis, noting any current or recent antibiotic therapy.

Post-test:

➤ Evaluate test results in relation to the patient's symptoms and other tests performed. Related laboratory tests include α_1-antitrypsin/phenotyping, intestinal biopsy, sweat chloride, stool culture, D-xylose tolerance, fecal fat, gliadin antibody, lactose tolerance, and ova and parasites.

FECAL FAT

• •

SYNONYMS/ACRONYM: Stool fat, fecal fat stain.

SPECIMEN: Stool (80 mL) aliquot from an unpreserved and homogenized 24- to 72-hour timed collection. Random specimens may also be submitted.

REFERENCE VALUE: (Method: Stain with Sudan black or oil red O. Treatment with ethanol identifies neutral fats; treatment with acetic acid identifies fatty acids.)

Method

Random, Semiquantitative	
Neutral fat	Less than 50 fat globules/hpf
Fatty acids	Less than 100 fat globules/hpf

Age (diet)	72-hour, Quantitative
Infant (breast milk)	Less than 1 g/24 h
0–6 y	Less than 2 g/24 h
Adult	2–7 g/24 h; less than 20% of total solids
Adult (fat-free)	Less than 4 g/24 h

hpf = high-power field.

DESCRIPTION: Fecal fat primarily consists of triglycerides (neutral fats), fatty acids, and fatty acid salts. Through microscopic examination, the number and size of fat droplets can be determined as well as the type of fat present. Excretion of greater than 7 g of fecal fat in a 24-hour period is abnormal but nonspecific for disease. Increases in excretion of neutral fats are associated with pancreatic exocrine insufficiency, whereas decreases are related to small bowel disease. An increase in triglycerides indicates that insufficient pancreatic enzymes are available to convert the triglycerides into fatty acids. Patients with malabsorption conditions have normal amounts of triglycerides but an increase in total fecal fat because the fats are not absorbed through the intestine. Malabsorption disorders (e.g., cystic fibrosis) cause blockage of the pancreatic ducts by mucus, which prevents the enzymes from reaching the duodenum and results in lack of fat digestion. Without digestion, the fats cannot be absorbed, and steatorrhea results. The appearance and odor of stool from patients with steatorrhea is typically foamy, greasy, soft, and foul-smelling. The semiquantitative test is used to screen for the presence of fecal fat. The quantitative method, which requires a 72-hour stool collection, measures the amount of fat present in grams. ■

INDICATIONS:

• Assist in the diagnosis of malabsorption or pancreatic insufficiency, as indicated by elevated fat levels

• Monitor the effectiveness of therapy

RESULT

Increased in:

• A-β-lipoprotein deficiency

• Addison's disease

• Amyloidosis

• Bile salt deficiency

• Carcinoid syndrome

• Celiac disease

• Crohn's disease

• Cystic fibrosis

• Diabetes

• Enteritis

• Malnutrition

• Multiple sclerosis

• Pancreatic insufficiency or obstruction

• Peptic ulcer disease

• Pernicious anemia

• Progressive systemic sclerosis

- Tropical sprue
- Thyrotoxicosis
- Viral hepatitis
- Whipple's disease
- Zollinger-Ellison syndrome

Decreased in: N/A

CRITICAL VALUES: N/A

INTERFERING FACTORS:

- Cimetidine has been associated with decreased fecal fat in some patients with cystic fibrosis who are also receiving pancreatic enzyme therapy.

- Some drugs cause steatorrhea as a result of mucosal damage. These include colchicine, kanamycin, lincomycin, methotrexate, and neomycin. Other drugs that can cause an increase in fecal fat include aminosalicylic acid, bisacodyl and phenolphthalein (observed in laxative abusers), and cholestyramine (in high doses).

- Use of suppositories, oily lubricants, or mineral oil in the perianal area for 3 days before the test can falsely increase neutral fats.

- Use of herbals with laxative effects, including cascara, psyllium, and senna, for 3 days before the test can falsely increase neutral fats.

- Barium interferes with test results.

- Failure to collect all stools may reflect falsely decreased results.

- Ingestion of a diet too high or low in fats may alter the results.

Nursing Implications and Procedure

Pretest:

➤ Obtain a history of the patient's complaints that indicate a gastrointestinal (GI) disorder—diarrhea related to GI dysfunction, pain related to tissue inflammation or irritation, alteration in diet resulting from an inability to digest certain foods, or fluid volume deficit related to active loss.

➤ Obtain a list of known allergens.

➤ Obtain a history of the patient's GI and respiratory systems, as well as results of previously performed tests and procedures. For related tests, refer to the gastrointestinal and respiratory system tables.

➤ Obtain a list of the medications the patient is taking, including herbs, nutritional supplements, and nutraceuticals. The requesting health care practitioner and laboratory should be advised if the patient regularly uses these products so that their effects can be taken into consideration when reviewing results.

➤ Note any recent procedures that can interfere with test results.

➤ Instruct the patient not to use laxatives, enemas, or suppositories for 3 days before the test.

➤ There are no fluid restrictions unless by medical direction.

➤ Stress the importance of collecting all stools for the quantitative test, including diarrhea, over the timed specimen-collection period.

➤ Inform the patient not to urinate in the stool-collection container and not to put toilet paper in the container.

➤ Review the procedure with the patient. Instruct the patient to ingest a diet containing 50 to 150 g of fat for at least 3 days before beginning specimen collection. This approach does not work well with children; instruct the caregiver to record the child's dietary intake to provide a basis from which an estimate of fat intake can be made.

Intratest:

➤ Ensure that the patient has complied with dietary preparations and other pretesting restrictions.

➤ Observe standard precautions and

follow the general guidelines in Appendix A.

➤ Obtain the appropriate-sized specimen container, toilet-mounted collection container to aid in specimen collection, and plastic bag for specimen transport. A large, clean, preweighed container should be used for the timed test. A smaller, clean container can be used for the collection of the random sample.

➤ For the quantitative procedure, instruct the patient to collect each stool and place it in the 500-mL container during the timed collection period. Keep the container refrigerated in the plastic bag throughout the entire collection period.

➤ Label the specimen, and promptly transport it to the laboratory. Make sure the label includes the date of collection and the start and stop times.

Post-test:

➤ Instruct the patient with abnormal values on the importance of fluid intake and proper diet specific to his or her condition.

➤ Instruct the patient to resume his or her usual diet and medication as directed by the health care practitioner.

➤ Evaluate test results in relation to the patient's symptoms and other tests performed. Related laboratory tests include α_1-antitrypsin/phenotyping, complete blood count, D-xylose tolerance test, and sweat chloride.

FERRITIN

SYNONYM/ACRONYM: N/A.

SPECIMEN: Serum (1 mL) collected in a red- or tiger-top tube.

REFERENCE VALUE: (Method: Immunoassay)

Age	Conventional Units	SI Units (Conversion Factor ×1)
Newborn	25–200 ng/mL	25–200 μg/L
1 mo	200–600 ng/mL	200–600 μg/L
2–5 mo	50–200 ng/mL	50–200 μg/L
6 mo–15 y	7–140 ng/mL	7–140 μg/L
Adult		
Men	20–250 ng/mL	20–250 μg/L
Women younger than 40 y	10–120 ng/mL	10–120 μg/L
Women 40 y and older	12–263 ng/mL	12–263 μg/L

DESCRIPTION: Ferritin, a protein manufactured in the liver, spleen, and bone marrow, consists of a protein shell, apoferritin, and an iron core. The amount of ferritin in the circulation is usually proportional to the amount of stored iron (ferritin and hemosiderin) in body tissues. Levels vary according to age and gender, but they are not affected by exogenous iron intake or subject to diurnal variations. Compared to iron and total iron-binding capacity, ferritin is a more sensitive and specific test for diagnosing iron-deficiency anemia. Iron-deficiency anemia in adults is indicated at ferritin levels less than 10 ng/mL; hemochromatosis or hemosiderosis is indicated at levels greater than 400 ng/mL. ■

INDICATIONS:
• Assist in the diagnosis of iron-deficiency anemia

• Assist in the differential diagnosis of microcytic, hypochromic anemias

• Monitor hematologic responses during pregnancy, when serum iron is usually decreased and ferritin may be decreased

• Support diagnosis of hemochromatosis or other disorders of iron metabolism and storage

RESULT

Increased in:
• Alcoholism (active abusers)

• Breast cancer

• Fasting

• Hemochromatosis

• Hemolytic anemia

• Hemosiderosis

• Hepatocellular disease (acute or chronic)

• Hodgkin's disease

• Hyperthyroidism

• Infection (acute or chronic)

• Inflammatory diseases

• Leukemias

• Oral or parenteral administration of iron

• Thalassemia

Decreased in:
• Hemodialysis

• Iron-deficiency anemia

CRITICAL VALUES: N/A

INTERFERING FACTORS:
• Drugs that may increase ferritin levels include ethanol, ferric polymaltose, iron, and oral contraceptives.

• Drugs that may decrease ferritin levels include erythropoietin, methimazole, propylthiouracil, and thiamazole.

• Recent transfusion can elevate serum ferritin.

Nursing Implications and Procedure • • • • • • • • • • •

Pretest: ■

➤ Obtain a history of the patient's complaints, including a list of known allergens.

➤ Obtain a history of the patient's hematopoietic system as well as results of previously performed tests and procedures. For related tests, refer to the hematopoietic system table.

➤ Obtain a list of the medications the patient is taking, including herbs, nutritional supplements, and nutraceuticals. The requesting health care practitioner and laboratory should be advised if the patient regularly uses these products so that their effects can be taken into consideration when reviewing results.

➤ Note any recent procedures that can interfere with test results.

➤ There are no food, fluid, or medication restrictions unless by medical direction.

➤ Review the procedure with the patient.

➤ Inform the patient that specimen collection takes approximately 5 to 10 minutes.

Intratest:

➤ Direct the patient to breathe normally and to avoid unnecessary movement.

➤ Observe standard precautions and follow the general guidelines in Appendix A. Perform a venipuncture,

and collect the specimen in a 5-mL red- or tiger-top tube.

➤ Label the specimen, and promptly transport it to the laboratory.

Post-test:

➤ Observe venipuncture site for bleeding or hematoma formation. Apply pressure bandage.

➤ Nutritional therapy may be indicated for patients with decreased ferritin values because this may indicate corresponding iron deficiency. Instruct these patients in the dietary inclusion of iron-rich foods and in the administration of iron supplements, including side effects, as appropriate.

➤ Evaluate test results in relation to the patient's symptoms and other tests performed. Related laboratory tests include bone marrow biopsy, complete blood count, erythropoietin, iron/total iron-binding capacity, and liver biopsy.

FETAL FIBRONECTIN

• •

SYNONYM/ACRONYM: fFN.

SPECIMEN: Swab of vaginal secretions.

REFERENCE VALUE: (Method: Immunoassay) Negative.

DESCRIPTION: Fibronectin is a protein found in the vaginal secretions of pregnant women. It is first secreted early in pregnancy and is believed to help implantation of the fertilized egg to the uterus. Fibronectin is not detectable again until 22 to 34 weeks of gestation; if it is detected in vaginal secretions at this gestational age, delivery may happen prematurely. The test is a useful marker for impending membrane rupture within 7 to 14 days if the level rises to greater than 0.05 μg/mL. ■

INDICATIONS: Investigate signs of premature labor

RESULT

Positive in: Premature labor

Negative in: N/A

CRITICAL VALUES: N/A

INTERFERING FACTORS: If signs and symptoms persist in light of negative test results, repeat testing may be necessary.

Nursing Implications and Procedure • • • • • • • • • • •

Pretest: ▪

➤ Obtain a history of the patient's complaints, including a list of known allergens. Ensure that the patient knows the symptoms of premature labor, which include uterine contractions (with or without pain) lasting 20 seconds or longer or increasing in frequency, menstrual-like cramping (intermittent or continuous), pelvic pressure, lower back pain that does not dissipate with a change in position, persistent diarrhea, intestinal cramps, changes in vaginal discharge, or a feeling that something is wrong.

➤ The health care practitioner should be informed if contractions occur more frequently than 4 times per hour.

➤ Obtain a history of the patient's reproductive system as well as results of previously performed tests and procedures. For related tests, refer to the reproductive system table.

➤ Obtain a list of the medications the patient is taking, including herbs, nutritional supplements, and nutraceuticals. The requesting health care practitioner and laboratory should be advised if the patient regularly uses these products so that their effects can be taken into consideration when reviewing results.

➤ There are no food, fluid, or medication restrictions unless by medical direction.

➤ Review the procedure with the patient. Sensitivity to cultural and social issues, as well as concern for modesty, is important in providing psychological support.

➤ Inform the patient that specimen collection takes approximately 5 to 10 minutes.

Intratest: ▪

➤ Direct the patient to breathe normally and to avoid unnecessary movement.

➤ Position the patient on the gynecologic examination table with the feet up in stirrups. Drape the patient's legs to provide privacy and to reduce chilling.

➤ Observe standard precautions and follow the general guidelines in Appendix A. Collect a small amount of vaginal secretion using a special swab from a fetal fibronectin kit.

➤ Label the specimen, and promptly transport it to the laboratory.

Post-test: ▪

➤ Reinforce education on signs and symptoms of labor, as appropriate. Inform the patient that hospitalization or more frequent prenatal checks may be ordered. Other therapies may also be administered, such as antibiotics, corticosteroids, and intravenous tocolytics. Instruct the patient in the importance of completing the entire course of antibiotic therapy, if ordered, even if no symptoms are present.

➤ Explain the possible causes and increased risks associated with premature labor and delivery.

➤ Recognize anxiety related to test results and provide support. Provide teaching and information regarding the clinical implications of the test results, as appropriate.

> ➤ Evaluate test results in relation to the patient's symptoms and other tests performed. Related laboratory

| tests include amniotic fluid analysis, chorionic villus biopsy, and lecithin/ sphingomyelin ratio.

α₁-FETOPROTEIN

SYNONYM/ACRONYM: AFP.

SPECIMEN: Serum (1 mL for tumor marker in men and nonpregnant women; 3 mL for maternal triple-marker testing), collected in a red- or tiger-top tube. For maternal triple-marker testing, include human chorionic gonadotropin and free estriol measurement.

REFERENCE VALUE: (Method: Immunoassay for tumor marker, radioimmunoassay for maternal triple-marker testing)

Tumor Marker, Men and Women

AFP	
Fetus, first-trimester peak	200–400 mg/dL
Cord blood	Less than 5 mg/dL

AFP in Maternal Serum	White AFP (Median)	Black AFP (Median)	Hispanic AFP (Median)	Asian AFP (Median)
Low risk	Less than 2 MoM	Less than 2 MoM	Less than 2 MoM	Less than 2 MoM
Gestational Age (wk)				
14	19.9 ng/mL	23.2 ng/mL	18.3 ng/mL	22.4 ng/mL
15	23.2 ng/mL	26.9 ng/mL	22.6 ng/mL	28.3 ng/mL
16	27.0 ng/mL	31.1 ng/mL	27.3 ng/mL	32.7 ng/mL
17	31.5 ng/mL	35.9 ng/mL	32.3 ng/mL	37.9 ng/mL
18	36.7 ng/mL	41.6 ng/mL	38.1 ng/mL	44.8 ng/mL
19	42.7 ng/mL	48.0 ng/mL	45.0 ng/mL	52.0 ng/mL
20	49.8 ng/mL	55.6 ng/mL	52.2 ng/mL	62.2 ng/mL
21	58.1 ng/mL	64.2 ng/mL	61.9 ng/mL	79.5 ng/mL
22	67.8 ng/mL	74.2 ng/mL	64.3 ng/mL	78.2 ng/mL

MoM = multiples of the median.

HCG and Estriol in Maternal Serum	HCG (Second Trimester)	Free Estriol (Second Trimester)
Gestational Age (wk)	Median Value	Median Value
14	41.5 IU/mL	0.5 ng/mL
15	36.0 IU/mL	0.7 ng/mL
16	31.0 IU/mL	0.9 ng/mL
17	27.0 IU/mL	1.1 ng/mL
18	24.0 IU/mL	1.4 ng/mL
19	21.0 IU/mL	1.8 ng/mL
20	18.0 IU/mL	2.3 ng/mL
21	16.0 IU/mL	2.8 ng/mL
22	14.0 IU/mL	3.6 ng/mL

Results vary widely from laboratory to laboratory and method to method.
HCG = human chorionic gonadotropin.

DESCRIPTION: α_1-Fetoprotein (AFP) is a glycoprotein produced in the fetal liver, gastrointestinal tract, and yolk sac. AFP is the major serum protein produced for 10 weeks in early fetal life. (See amniotic fluid analysis monograph for measurement of AFP levels in amniotic fluid.) After 10 weeks of gestation, levels of fetal AFP can be detected in maternal blood, with peak levels occurring at 16 to 18 weeks. Elevated maternal levels of AFP on two tests taken 1 week apart suggest further investigation into fetal well-being by ultrasound or amniocentesis. Human chorionic gonadotropin (HCG), a hormone secreted by the placenta, stimulates secretion of progesterone by the corpus luteum. (The use of HCG as a triple marker is also discussed in the monograph titled "Human Chorionic Gonadotropin.") During intrauterine development, the normal fetus and placenta produce estriol, a portion of which passes into maternal circulation. Decreased estriol levels are an independent indicator of neural tube defects. The incidence of neural tube defects is about 1 in 1000 births.

The presence of AFP in excessive amounts is abnormal in adults. AFP measurements are used as a tumor marker to assist in the diagnosis of cancer. ■

INDICATIONS:

• Assist in the diagnosis of primary hepatocellular carcinoma or metastatic lesions involving the liver, as indicated by highly elevated levels (30 to 50 percent of Americans with liver cancer do not have elevated AFP levels)

• Investigate suspected hepatitis or cirrhosis, indicated by slightly to moderately elevated levels

• Monitor response to treatment for hepatic carcinoma, with successful treatment indicated by an immediate decrease in levels

• Monitor for recurrence of hepatic carcinoma, with elevated levels occurring 1 to 6 months before the patient becomes symptomatic

• Support diagnosis of embryonal gonadal teratoblastoma, hepatoblastoma, and testicular or ovarian carcinomas

• Routine prenatal screening at 13 to 16 weeks of pregnancy for fetal neural tube defects and other disorders, as indicated by elevated levels in maternal serum and amniotic fluid

- Investigate suspected intrauterine fetal death, as indicated by elevated levels

RESULT: Maternal serum AFP test results report actual values and multiples of the median (MoM) by gestational age (in weeks). MoM are calculated by dividing the patient's AFP by the midpoint (or median) of values expected for a large population of unaffected women at the same gestational age in weeks. MoM should be corrected for maternal weight. The MoM should also be corrected for maternal insulin requirement (achieved by dividing MoM by 1.1 for diabetic African-American patients and by 0.8 for diabetic patients of other races) and multiple fetuses (multiply by 2.13 for twins). Some laboratories also provide additional statistical information regarding Down's syndrome risk.

Increased in:
- Pregnant women:
  Congenital nephrosis
  Fetal abdominal wall defects
  Fetal distress
  Fetal neural tube defects (e.g., anencephaly, spina bifida, myelomeningocele)
  Low birth weight
  Multiple pregnancy
  Polycystic kidneys
  Underestimation of gestational age

- Men or nonpregnant women:
  Cirrhosis
  Hepatic carcinoma
  Hepatitis
  Metastatic lesions involving the liver

Decreased in:
- Pregnant women:
  Down's syndrome (trisomy 21)
  Edwards's syndrome (trisomy 18)
  Fetal demise (undetected over a lengthy period of time)
  Hydatidiform moles

Overestimation of gestational age
Pseudopregnancy
Spontaneous abortion

CRITICAL VALUES: N/A

INTERFERING FACTORS:
- Drugs that may decrease AFP levels in pregnant women include acetaminophen, acetylsalicylic acid, and phenacetin.

- Recent radioactive scans or radiation within 1 week before the test can interfere with test results when radioimmunoassay is the test method.

- Multiple fetuses can cause increased levels.

- Gestational age must be between 15 and 22 weeks for initial and follow-up testing. The most common cause of an abnormal MoM is inaccurate estimation of gestational age (defined as weeks from the first day of the last menstrual period).

- Maternal AFP levels vary by race.

Nursing Implications and Procedure ● ● ● ● ● ● ● ● ● ● ●

Pretest: ■

➤ Obtain a history of the patient's complaints and known or suspected malignancy. Obtain a list of known allergens.

➤ Obtain a history of the patient's immune and reproductive systems, gestational age, and results of previously performed tests and procedures. For related tests, refer to the immune and reproductive system tables.

➤ Provide required information to laboratory for triple-marker testing, including maternal birth date, weight, age, race, calculated gestational age, gestational age by ultrasound, gestational date by physical examination, first day of last menstrual period, estimated date of delivery, and whether the patient has insulin-dependent (type 1) diabetes.

➤ Obtain a list of the medications the patient is taking, including herbs, nutritional supplements, and nutraceuticals. The requesting health care practitioner and laboratory should be advised if the patient is regularly using these products so that their effects can be taken into consideration when reviewing results.

➤ Note any recent procedures that can interfere with test results.

➤ There are no food, fluid, or medication restrictions unless by medical direction.

➤ Review the procedure with the patient.

➤ Inform the patient that specimen collection takes approximately 5 to 10 minutes.

➤ *Obtain written and informed consent before specimen collection.*

Intratest:

➤ Direct the patient to breathe normally and to avoid unnecessary movement.

➤ Observe standard precautions and follow the general guidelines in Appendix A. Perform a venipuncture, and collect the specimen in a 5-mL red-top tube.

➤ The sample may be collected directly from the cord using a syringe and transferred to a red-top tube.

➤ Label the specimen, and promptly transport it to the laboratory.

Post-test:

➤ Observe venipuncture site for bleeding or hematoma formation. Apply pressure bandage.

➤ Hyperhomocysteinemia resulting from folate deficiency in pregnant women is believed to increase the risk of neural tube defects. Elevated levels of homocysteine are thought to chemically damage the exposed neural tissue of the developing fetus. As appropriate, instruct pregnant women to eat foods rich in folate, such as liver, salmon, eggs, asparagus, green leafy vegetables, broccoli, sweet potatoes, beans, and whole wheat.

➤ Inform the pregnant patient that an ultrasound may be performed and AFP levels in amniotic fluid may be analyzed if maternal blood levels are elevated in two samples obtained 1 week apart.

➤ Recognize anxiety related to test results, and encourage the family to seek counseling if concerned with pregnancy termination or to seek genetic counseling if a chromosomal abnormality is determined. Provide teaching and information regarding the clinical implications of the test results, as appropriate. Decisions regarding elective abortion should take place in the presence of both parents. Provide a nonjudgmental, nonthreatening atmosphere for discussing the risks and difficulties of delivering and raising an abnormal infant, as well as exploring other options (termination of pregnancy or adoption). It is also important to discuss feelings the mother and father may experience (e.g., guilt, depression, anger) if fetal abnormalities are detected.

➤ In patients with carcinoma, recognize anxiety related to test results and offer support. Provide teaching and information regarding the clinical implications of the test results, as appropriate. Educate the patient regarding access to counseling services, as appropriate.

➤ Evaluate test results in relation to the patient's symptoms and other tests performed. Related laboratory tests include amniotic fluid analysis, carcinoembryonic antigen, folic acid, and homocysteine.

FIBRIN DEGRADATION PRODUCTS

SYNONYMS/ACRONYMS: Fibrin split products, fibrin breakdown products, FDP, FSP, FBP.

SPECIMEN: Plasma (1mL) collected in special blue-top tube containing thrombin and a protease inhibitor.

REFERENCE VALUE: (Method: Latex agglutination)

Conventional Units	SI Units (Conversion Factor ×1)
Less than 10 μg/mL	Less than 10 mg/dL

DESCRIPTION: This coagulation test evaluates fibrin split products or fibrin/fibrinogen degradation products that interfere with normal coagulation and formation of the hemostatic platelet plug. After a fibrin clot has formed, the fibrinolytic system prevents excessive clotting. In the fibrinolytic system, plasmin digests fibrin. Fibrinogen also can be degraded if there is a disproportion among plasmin, fibrin, and fibrinogen. Seven substances labeled *A, B, C, D, E, X,* and *Y* result from this degradation, which can indicate abnormal coagulation. Under normal conditions, the liver and reticuloendothelial system remove fibrin split products from the circulation. ∎

INDICATIONS:

- Assist in the diagnosis of suspected disseminated intravascular coagulation (DIC)

- Evaluate response to therapy with fibrinolytic drugs

- Monitor the effects on hemostasis of

trauma, extensive surgery, obstetric complications, and disorders such as liver or renal disease

RESULT

Increased in:

- DIC

- Excessive bleeding

- Liver disease

- Myocardial infarct

- Obstetric complications, such as preeclampsia, abruptio placentae, intrauterine fetal death

- Post–cardiothoracic surgery period

- Pulmonary embolism

- Renal disease

- Renal transplant rejection

CRITICAL VALUES: Greater than 40 μg/mL.

INTERFERING FACTORS:
- Traumatic venipunctures and excessive agitation of the sample can alter test results.

- Drugs that may increase fibrin degradation product levels include heparin and fibrinolytic drugs such as streptokinase and urokinase.

- The presence of rheumatoid factor may falsely elevate results with some test kits.

- The test should not be ordered on patients receiving heparin therapy.

Nursing Implications and Procedure

Pretest:

➤ Obtain a history of the patient's complaints, including a list of known allergens.

➤ Obtain a history of the patient's cardiovascular and hematopoietic systems, any bleeding disorders, and results of previously performed tests and procedures, especially bleeding time, clotting time, complete blood count, partial thromboplastin time, platelets, and prothrombin time. For related tests, refer to the cardiovascular and hematopoietic system tables.

➤ Obtain a list of medications the patient takes, including anticoagulant therapy, acetylsalicylic acid, herbals, and nutraceuticals known to affect coagulation. It is recommended that use of these products be discontinued 14 days before dental or surgical procedures. The requesting health care practitioner and laboratory should be advised if the patient regularly uses these products so that their effects can be taken into consideration when reviewing results.

➤ Note any recent procedures that can interfere with test results.

➤ There are no food, fluid, or medication restrictions unless by medical direction.

➤ Review the procedure with the patient.

➤ Inform the patient that specimen collection takes approximately 5 to 10 minutes.

Intratest:

➤ Direct the patient to breathe normally and to avoid unnecessary movement.

➤ Observe standard precautions and follow the general guidelines in Appendix A. Perform a venipuncture, and collect the specimen in a special blue-top tube.

➤ Label the specimen, and promptly transport it to the laboratory.

Post-test:

➤ Observe venipuncture site for bleeding or hematoma formation. Apply pressure bandage.

➤ Tell the patient to report bleeding from skin or mucous membranes.

➤ Inform the patient with increased levels of fibrin degradation products of the importance of taking precautions against bruising and bleeding, including the use of a soft bristle toothbrush, use of an electric razor, avoidance of constipation, avoidance of acetylsalicylic acid and similar products, and avoidance of intramuscular injections.

➤ Evaluate test results in relation to the patient's symptoms and other tests performed. Related laboratory tests include D-dimer, fibrinogen, activated partial thromboplastin time, plasminogen, and platelet count.

FIBRINOGEN

. . . .

SYNONYM/ACRONYM: Factor I.

SPECIMEN: Plasma (1 mL) collected in blue top (sodium citrate) tube.

REFERENCE VALUE: (Method: Photo optical clot detection)

Age	Conventional Units	SI Units (Conversion Factor ×0.01)
Newborn	125–300 mg/dL	1.25–3.00 g/L
Adult	200–400 mg/dL	2.00–4.00 g/L

DESCRIPTION: Fibrinogen (factor I) is synthesized in the liver. In the common final pathway of the coagulation sequence, thrombin converts fibrinogen to fibrin, which then clots blood as it combines with platelets. In normal, healthy individuals, the serum should contain no residual fibrinogen after clotting has occurred. ∎

INDICATIONS:
• Assist in the diagnosis of suspected disseminated intravascular coagulation (DIC), as indicated by decreased fibrinogen levels
• Evaluate congenital or acquired dysfibrinogenemias
• Monitor hemostasis in disorders associated with low fibrinogen levels or elevated levels that can predispose patients to excessive thrombosis

RESULT

Increased in:
• Acute myocardial infarction

• Cancer
• Eclampsia
• Hodgkin's disease
• Inflammation
• Multiple myeloma
• Nephrotic syndrome
• Pregnancy
• Tissue necrosis

Decreased in:
• Congenital fibrinogen deficiency (rare)
• DIC
• Dysfibrinogenemia
• Liver disease (severe)
• Primary fibrinolysis

CRITICAL VALUE: ⚠ Less than 100 mg/dL. Signs and symptoms of microvascular thrombosis include acral cyanosis, ischemic tissue necrosis, hemorrhagic necrosis, tachypnea, dyspnea, pulmonary emboli, venous distention, abdominal pain, and oliguria. Possible interventions include identification and treatment of the underlying cause, support through administration of required blood products (platelets, cryoprecipitate, or fresh frozen plasma), and administration of heparin.

INTERFERING FACTORS:

• Drugs that may increase fibrinogen levels include acetylsalicylic acid, norethandrolone, oral contraceptives, oxandrolone, and oxymetholone.

• Drugs that may decrease fibrinogen levels include anabolic steroids, asparaginase, bezafibrate, danazol, dextran, fenofibrate, fish oils, gemfibrozil, lovastatin, pentoxifylline, phosphorus, and ticlopidine.

• Transfusions of whole blood, plasma, or fractions within 4 weeks of the test invalidate results.

• Placement of tourniquet for longer than 1 minute can result in venous stasis and changes in the concentration of plasma proteins to be measured. Platelet activation may also occur under these conditions, causing erroneous results.

• Vascular injury during phlebotomy can activate platelets and coagulation factors, causing erroneous results.

• Hemolyzed specimens must be rejected because hemolysis is an indication of platelet and coagulation factor activation.

• Incompletely filled tubes contaminated with heparin or clotted specimens must be rejected.

• Icteric or lipemic specimens interfere with optical testing methods, producing erroneous results.

• Traumatic venipuncture and excessive agitation of the sample can alter test results.

Nursing Implications and Procedure • • • • • • • • • • •

Pretest: ■

➤ Obtain a history of the patient's complaints, including a list of known allergens.

➤ Obtain a history of the patient's hematopoietic and hepatobiliary systems, as well as results of previously performed tests and procedures. For related tests, refer to the hematopoietic and hepatobiliary system tables.

➤ Obtain a list of medications the patient is taking, including herbs, nutritional supplements, and nutraceuticals. The requesting health care practitioner and laboratory should be advised if the patient regularly takes these products so that their effects can be taken into consideration when reviewing results.

➤ Note any recent procedures that can interfere with test results.

➤ There are no food, fluid, or medication restrictions unless by medical direction.

➤ Review the procedure with the patient.

➤ Inform the patient that specimen collection takes approximately 5 to 10 minutes.

Intratest: ■

➤ Direct the patient to breathe normally and to avoid unnecessary movement.

➤ Observe standard precautions and follow the general guidelines in Appendix A. Perform a venipuncture, and collect the specimen in a 5-mL blue-top tube. Fill the tube completely. *Important note:* Two different concentrations of sodium citrate preservative are currently added to blue-top tubes for coagulation studies: 3.2% and 3.8%. The National Committee for Clinical Laboratory Standards (NCCLS) guideline for sodium citrate is 3.2%. Laboratories establish reference ranges for coagulation testing based on numerous factors, including sodium citrate concentration, test equipment, and test reagents. It is important to inquire from the laboratory which concentration it recommends, because each concentration will have its own specific reference range.

➤ When multiple specimens are drawn, the blue-top tube should be collected after sterile (i.e., blood culture) and red-top tubes. When coagulation testing is the only work to be done, an extra red-top tube should be collected before the blue-top tube to avoid contaminating the specimen with tissue thromboplastin, which can falsely decrease values.

➤ Label the specimen, and promptly transport it to the laboratory. The NCCLS recommendation for processed and unprocessed specimens stored in unopened tubes is that testing should be completed within 1 to 4 hours of collection.

Post-test:

➤ Observe venipuncture site for bleeding or hematoma formation. Apply pressure bandage.

➤ Tell the patient to report bruising, petechiae, and bleeding from mucous membranes.

➤ Inform the patient with a decreased fibrinogen level of the importance of taking precautions against bruising and bleeding, including the use of a soft bristle toothbrush, use of an electric razor, avoidance of constipation, avoidance of acetylsalicylic acid and similar products, and avoidance of intramuscular injections.

➤ Evaluate test results in relation to the patient's symptoms and other tests performed. Related laboratory tests include activated partial thromboplastin time, alanine aminotransferase, albumin, alkaline phosphatase, aspartate aminotransferase, bilirubin, liver biopsy, clot retraction, D-dimer, erythrocyte sedimentation rate, fibrin degradation products, γ-glutamyl transpeptidase, plasminogen, and prothrombin time.

FOLATE

SYNONYM/ACRONYM: Folic acid.

SPECIMEN: Serum (1 mL) collected in a red- or tiger-top tube.

REFERENCE VALUE: (Method: Radioimmunoassay)

Age	Conventional Units	SI Units (Conversion Factor ×2.265)
Newborn–1 y	5–21 ng/mL	11–48 nmol/L
Adult	Greater than 2.5 ng/mL	Greater than 5.7 nmol/L

DESCRIPTION: Folate, a water-soluble vitamin, is produced by bacteria in the intestines and stored in small amounts in the liver. Dietary folate is absorbed through the intestinal mucosa and stored in the liver. Folate is necessary for normal red blood cell and white blood cell function, DNA replication, and cell division. Folate levels are often measured in association with serum vitamin B_{12} determinations. Hyperhomocysteinemia resulting from folate deficiency in pregnant women is believed to increase the risk of neural tube defects. Elevated levels of homocysteine are thought to cause chemical damage to the exposed neural tissue of the developing fetus. ▪

INDICATIONS:
• Assist in the diagnosis of megaloblastic anemia resulting from deficient folate intake or increased folate requirements, such as in pregnancy and hemolytic anemia

• Monitor the effects of prolonged parenteral nutrition

• Monitor response to disorders that may lead to folate deficiency or decreased absorption and storage

RESULT

Increased in:
• Vitamin B_{12} deficiency

• Blind loop syndrome

• Distal small bowel disease

• Excessive dietary intake of folate or folate supplements

• Pernicious anemia

Decreased in:
• Chronic alcoholism

• Crohn's disease

• Exfoliative dermatitis

• Hemolytic anemias

• Infantile hyperthyroidism

• Liver disease

• Malnutrition

• Megaloblastic anemia

• Myelofibrosis

• Neoplasms

• Pregnancy

• Regional enteritis

• Scurvy

• Sideroblastic anemias

• Sprue

• Ulcerative colitis

• Whipple's disease

CRITICAL VALUES: N/A

INTERFERING FACTORS:
• Drugs that may decrease folate levels include aminopterin, ampicillin, antacids, anticonvulsants, barbiturates, chloramphenicol, chloroguanide, ethanol, erythromycin, glutethimide, lincomycin, metformin, methotrexate, nitrofurans, oral contraceptives, penicillin, pentamidine, phenytoin, pyrimethamine, tetracycline, and triamterene.

• Recent radioactive scans or radiation within 1 week before the test can interfere with test results when radioimmunoassay is the test method.

Nursing Implications and Procedure • • • • • • • • • • •

Pretest: ▪

➤ Obtain a history of the patient's complaints, including a list of known allergens.

➤ Obtain a history of the patient's gastrointestinal and hematopoietic systems, as well as results of previously performed tests and procedures. For related tests, refer to the gastrointestinal and hematopoietic system tables.

➤ Obtain a list of medications the patient is taking, including herbs, nutritional supplements, and nutraceuticals. The requesting health care practitioner and laboratory should be advised if the patient regularly uses these products so that their effects can be taken into consideration when reviewing results.

➤ Note any recent procedures that can interfere with test results.

➤ There are no food, fluid, or medication restrictions unless by medical direction.

➤ Review the procedure with the patient.

➤ Inform the patient that specimen collection takes approximately 5 to 10 minutes.

Intratest: ■

➤ Direct the patient to breathe normally and to avoid unnecessary movement.

➤ Observe standard precautions and follow the general guidelines in Appendix A. Perform a venipuncture, and collect the specimen in a 5-mL red- or tiger-top tube. Protect the specimen from light.

➤ Label the specimen, and promptly transport it to the laboratory.

Post-test: ■

➤ Observe venipuncture site for bleeding or hematoma formation. Apply pressure bandage.

➤ Instruct the folate-deficient patient (especially pregnant women), as appropriate, to eat foods rich in folate, such as liver, salmon, eggs, asparagus, green leafy vegetables, broccoli, sweet potatoes, beans, and whole wheat.

➤ Evaluate test results in relation to the patient's symptoms and other tests performed. Related laboratory tests include complete blood count, homocysteine, and vitamin B_{12}.

FOLLICLE-STIMULATING HORMONE

· ·

SYNONYM/ACRONYM: Follitropin, FSH.

SPECIMEN: Serum (1 mL) collected in a red- or tiger-top tube.

REFERENCE VALUE: (Method: Immunoassay)

Status	Conventional Units	SI Units (Conversion Factor ×1)
Prepuberty	Less than 10 mIU/mL	Less than 10 IU/L
Men	1.4–15.5 mIU/mL	1.4–15.5 IU/L
Women		
Follicular phase	1.4–9.9 mIU/mL	1.4–9.9 IU/L
Ovulatory peak	6.2–17.2 mIU/mL	6.2–17.2 IU/L
Luteal phase	1.1–9.2 mIU/mL	1.1–9.2 IU/L
Postmenopause	19–100 mIU/mL	19–100 IU/L

DESCRIPTION: Follicle-stimulating hormone (FSH) is produced and stored in the anterior portion of the pituitary gland. In women, FSH promotes maturation of the graafian (germinal) follicle, causing estrogen secretion and allowing the ovum to mature. In men, FSH partially controls spermatogenesis, but the presence of testosterone is also necessary. Gonadotropin-releasing hormone secretion is stimulated by a decrease in estrogen and testosterone levels. Gonadotropin-releasing hormone secretion stimulates FSH secretion. FSH production is inhibited by an increase in estrogen and testosterone levels. FSH production is pulsatile, episodic, cyclic, and is subject to diurnal variation. Serial measurement is often required. ■

INDICATIONS:
- Assist in distinguishing between primary and secondary (pituitary or hypothalamic) gonadal failure
- Define menstrual cycle phases as a part of infertility testing
- Evaluate ambiguous sexual differentiation in infants
- Evaluate early sexual development in girls younger than age 9 or boys younger than age 10 (precocious puberty associated with elevated levels)
- Evaluate failure of sexual maturation in adolescence
- Evaluate testicular dysfunction
- Investigate impotence, gynecomastia, and menstrual disturbances

RESULT

Increased in:
- Alcoholism
- Castration

- Gonadal failure
- Gonadotropin-secreting pituitary tumors
- Klinefelter's syndrome
- Menopause
- Orchitis
- Precocious puberty in children
- Primary hypogonadism
- Reifenstein's syndrome
- Turner's syndrome

Decreased in:
- Anorexia nervosa
- Anterior pituitary hypofunction
- Hemochromatosis
- Hyperprolactinemia
- Hypothalamic disorders
- Polycystic ovary disease
- Pregnancy
- Sickle cell anemia

CRITICAL VALUES: N/A

INTERFERING FACTORS:
- Drugs that may increase FSH levels include cimetidine, clomiphene, digitalis, gonadotropin-releasing hormone, ketoconazole, levodopa, nafarelin, naloxone, nilutamide, oxcarbazepine, and pravastatin.

- Drugs that may decrease FSH levels include anabolic steroids, anticonvulsants, buserelin, estrogens, corticotropin-releasing hormone, goserelin, megestrol, mestranol, oral contraceptives, phenothiazine, pimozide, pravastatin, progesterone, stanozolol, tamoxifen, toremifene, and valproic acid.

- In menstruating women, values vary in relation to the phase of the menstrual cycle. Values are higher in post-menopausal women.

Nursing Implications and Procedure • • • • • • • • • •

Pretest: ■

➤ Obtain a history of the patient's complaints, including a list of known allergens.

➤ Obtain a history of the patient's endocrine and reproductive systems, as well as phase of menstrual cycle and results of previously performed tests and procedures. For related tests, refer to the endocrine and reproductive system tables.

➤ Obtain a list of medications the patient is taking, including herbs, nutritional supplements, and nutraceuticals. The requesting health care practitioner and laboratory should be advised if the patient regularly uses these products so that their effects can be taken into consideration when reviewing results.

➤ There are no food, fluid, or medication restrictions unless by medical direction.

➤ Review the procedure with the patient.

➤ Inform the patient that specimen collection takes approximately 5 to 10 minutes.

Intratest: ■

➤ Direct the patient to breathe normally and to avoid unnecessary movement.

➤ Observe standard precautions and follow the general guidelines in Appendix A. Perform a venipuncture, and collect the specimen in a 5-mL red- or tiger-top tube.

➤ Label the specimen, and promptly transport it to the laboratory.

Post-test: ■

➤ Observe venipuncture site for bleeding or hematoma formation. Apply pressure bandage.

➤ Inform the patient that multiple specimens may be required.

➤ Recognize anxiety related to test results. Provide teaching and information regarding the clinical implications of the test results, as appropriate. Provide a supportive, nonjudgmental environment when assisting a patient through the process of fertility testing. Educate the patient and partner regarding access to counseling services, as appropriate.

➤ Evaluate test results in relation to the patient's symptoms and other tests performed. Related laboratory tests include estradiol, luteinizing hormone, prolactin, and testosterone.

FRUCTOSAMINE
• •

SYNONYM/ACRONYM: Glycated albumin.

SPECIMEN: Serum (1 mL) collected in a red- or tiger-top tube.

REFERENCE VALUE: (Method: Spectrophotometry)

Status	Conventional Units	SI Units (Conversion Factor ×0.01)
Normal	174–286 µmol/L	1.74–2.86 mmol/L
Diabetic		
Controlled	210–421 µmol/L	2.10–4.21 mmol/L
Uncontrolled	268–870 µmol/L	2.68–8.70 mmol/L

DESCRIPTION: Fructosamine is the result of a covalent linkage between glucose and albumin or other proteins. Similar to glycated hemoglobin, fructosamine can be used to monitor long-term control of glucose in diabetics. It has a shorter half-life than glycated hemoglobin and is thought to be more sensitive to short-term fluctuations in glucose concentrations. Some glycated hemoglobin methods are affected by hemoglobin variants. Fructosamine is not subject to this interference. ■

INDICATIONS: Evaluate diabetic control

RESULT

Increased in: Diabetic patients with poor glucose control

Decreased in: Severe hypoproteinemia

CRITICAL VALUES: N/A

INTERFERING FACTORS:
• Drugs that may increase fructosamine levels include bendroflumethiazide and captopril.

• Drugs that may decrease fructosamine levels include ascorbic acid, pyridoxine, and terazosin.

• Decreased albumin levels may result in falsely decreased fructosamine levels.

Nursing Implications and Procedure

Pretest:

➤ Obtain a history of the patient's complaints, especially related to diabetic control. Obtain a list of known allergens.

➤ Obtain a history of the patient's endocrine and gastrointestinal systems, as well as results of previously performed tests and procedures. For related tests, refer to the endocrine and gastrointestinal system tables.

➤ Obtain a list of the medications the patient is taking, including herbs, nutritional supplements, and nutraceuticals. The requesting health care practitioner and laboratory should be advised if the patient regularly uses these products so that their effects can be taken into consideration when reviewing results.

➤ There are no food, fluid, or medication restrictions unless by medical direction.

➤ Review the procedure with the patient.

➤ Inform the patient that specimen collection takes approximately 5 to 10 minutes.

Intratest:

➤ Direct the patient to breathe normally and to avoid unnecessary movement.

➤ Observe standard precautions and follow the general guidelines in Appendix A. Perform a venipuncture, collect the specimen in a 5-mL red- or tiger-top tube.

➤ Label the specimen, and promptly transport it to the laboratory.

Post-test:

➤ Observe venipuncture site for bleeding or hematoma formation. Apply pressure bandage.

➤ Abnormal fructosamine levels may be associated with conditions resulting from poor glucose control. Instruct the diabetic patient, as appropriate, in nutritional management of the disease. Patients who adhere to dietary recommendations report a better general feeling of health, better weight management, greater control of glucose and lipid values, and improved use of insulin. There is no "diabetic diet"; however, many meal-planning approaches with nutritional goals are endorsed by the American Dietetic Association. The nutritional needs of each diabetic patient must be determined individually with the appropriate health care professionals, particularly professionals trained in nutrition.

➤ Instruct the patient and caregiver to report signs and symptoms of hypoglycemia (weakness, confusion, diaphoresis, rapid pulse) or hyperglycemia (thirst, polyuria, hunger, lethargy). Emphasize, as appropriate, that good control of glucose levels delays the onset and slows the progression of diabetic retinopathy, nephropathy, and neuropathy.

➤ Evaluate test results in relation to the patient's symptoms and other tests performed. Related laboratory tests include C-peptide, cortisol, glucose, glycated hemoglobin A_{1C}, glucose tolerance test, insulin, insulin antibodies, ketones, and microalbumin.

GALLIUM SCAN

SYNONYMS/ACRONYM: Gallium scan, tumor; gallium scan, abscess; gallium scan, fever of undetermined origin.

AREA OF APPLICATION: Whole body.

CONTRAST: Intravenous radioactive gallium-67 citrate.

DESCRIPTION: Gallium imaging is a nuclear medicine study that assists in diagnosing neoplasm and inflammation activity. Gallium, which has 90 percent sensitivity for inflammatory disease, is readily distributed throughout plasma and body tissues. Gallium imaging is sensitive in detecting abscesses, pneumonia, pyelonephritis, active sarcoidosis, and active tuberculosis. In immunocompromised patients, such as patients with acquired immunodeficiency syndrome (AIDS), gallium imaging can detect complications such as *Pneumocystis carinii* pneumonitis. Gallium imaging is useful but less commonly performed in the diagnosis and staging of some neoplasms, including Hodgkin's disease, lymphoma, melanoma, and leukemia. Imaging can be performed 6 to 72 hours after gallium injection. A gamma camera detects the radiation emitted from the injected radioactive material, and a representative image of the distribution of the radioactive material is obtained. The nonspecificity of gallium imaging requires correlation with other diagnostic studies, such as computed tomography, magnetic resonance imaging, and ultrasonography. ■

INDICATIONS:
- Aid in the diagnosis of infectious or inflammatory diseases

- Evaluate lymphomas

- Evaluate recurrent lymphomas or tumors after radiation therapy or chemotherapy

- Perform as a screening examination for fever of undetermined origin

RESULT

Normal Findings:
- Normal distribution of gallium. Some localization of the radionuclide within the liver, spleen, bone, nasopharynx, lacrimal glands, breast, and bowel is expected.

Abnormal Findings:
- Abscess

- Infection

- Inflammation

- Lymphoma

- Tumor

CRITICAL VALUES: N/A

INTERFERING FACTORS:

This procedure is contraindicated for:
- Patients who are pregnant or suspected of being pregnant, unless the potential benefits of the procedure far outweigh the risks to the fetus and mother

Factors that may impair clear imaging:
- Inability of the patient to cooperate or remain still during the procedure because of age, significant pain, or mental status

- Improper adjustment of the radiographic equipment to accommodate obese or thin patients, which can cause overexposure or underexposure and a poor-quality study

- Metallic objects within the examination field (e.g., jewelry or body rings), which may inhibit organ visualization and can produce unclear images

- Patients who are very obese, who may exceed the weight limit for the equipment

- Incorrect positioning of the patient, which may produce poor visualization of the area to be examined

- Performance of other nuclear scans within the preceding 24 to 48 hours

- Administration of certain medications (e.g., gastrin, cholecystokinin), which may interfere with gastric emptying

Other considerations:
- Failure to follow dietary restrictions before the procedure may cause the procedure to be canceled or repeated.

- Consultation with a physician should occur before the procedure for radiation safety concerns regarding infants of patients who are lactating.

Nursing Implications and Procedure • • • • • • • • • • • •

Pretest:

➤ Inform the patient that the test detects inflammation, infection, or tumor.

➤ Inform the patient that the procedure is performed in a special nuclear medicine department by a technologist and usually takes approximately 60 to 90 minutes. Delayed images need 72 hours after the initial injection. The patient may leave the department and return later for the imaging procedure.

➤ Obtain a list of known allergens.

➤ Obtain a medical history of the patient's complaints as well as results of previously performed tests, treatments, and surgical procedures. For related tests, refer to the immunologic, respiratory, and gastrointestinal system tables.

➤ Obtain a list of medications the patient is taking.

➤ Determine date of last menstrual period and possibility of pregnancy in perimenopausal women.

➤ Inform the patient that the technologist will inject gallium in an arm vein and ask the patient to return later for the imaging procedure, at which time the patient will be placed in a supine position on a flat table.

➤ Fasting before the scan is not required, unless indicated.

➤ Inform the patient that gallium is excreted by the kidneys and colon in 48 to 72 hours.

Intratest:

➤ Ask the patient to void before the procedure. Have the patient put on a hospital gown.

➤ Administer sedative to a child or to an uncooperative adult, as ordered.

➤ Ask the patient to lie still during the procedure because movement produces unclear images. Make sure jewelry, watches, chains, belts, and any other metallic objects have been removed.

➤ The radionuclide is administered intravenously. Delayed views may be taken at 6, 24, 48, and 72 hours after the injection.

➤ If an abdominal abscess or infection is suspected, laxatives or enemas may be ordered before delayed imaging at 48 or 72 hours after the injection.

➤ Wear gloves during the radionuclide administration and while handling the patient's urine.

Post-test:

➤ Instruct the patient to resume normal activity, medications, and diet after imaging is complete, unless otherwise indicated.

➤ Advise the patient to drink increased amounts of fluids for several days to eliminate the radionuclide from the body, unless contraindicated. Tell the patient the radionuclide is eliminated from the body within 48 to 72 hours.

➤ Inform the patient to flush the toilet immediately after each voiding following the procedure and to wash hands meticulously with soap and water after each voiding for 72 hours after the procedure.

➤ Tell all caregivers to wear gloves when discarding urine for 48 hours after the procedure. Wash gloved hands with soap and water before removing gloves. Then wash ungloved hands after removing the gloves.

➤ A physician specializing in this branch of medicine sends a written report to the ordering provider, who discusses the results with the patient.

➤ Evaluate test results in relation to the patient's symptoms and other tests performed. Related diagnostic tests are listed by the specific body area in the computed tomography and magnetic resonance imaging monographs.

GASTRIC ACID STIMULATION TEST

SYNONYM/ACRONYM: N/A.

SPECIMEN: Gastric fluid collected in eight plastic tubes at 15-minute intervals.

REFERENCE VALUE: (Method: Volume measurement and pH by ion-selective electrode)

Basal acid output (BAO)	*Male:* 0–10.5 mmol/h
	Female: 0–5.6 mmol/h
Peak acid output (PAO)	*Male:* 12–60 mmol/h
	Female: 8–40 mmol/h
Peak response time	*Pentagastrin, intramuscular:* 15–45 min
	Pentagastrin, subcutaneous: 10–30 min
BAO/PAO ratio	Less than 0.20

DESCRIPTION: The gastric acid stimulation test is performed to determine the response to substances administered to induce increased gastric acid production. Pentagastrin is the usual drug of choice to induce gastric secretion because it has no major side effects. The samples obtained from gastric acid stimulation tests are examined for volume, pH, and amount of acid secreted. First, basal acid output (BAO) is determined by averaging the results of gastric samples collected before the administration of a gastric stimulant. Then a gastric stimulant is administered and peak acid output (PAO) is determined by adding together the gastric acid output of the highest two consecutive 15-minute stimulation samples. Finally, BAO and PAO are compared as a ratio, which is normally less than 0.20. ■

INDICATIONS:
- Detect duodenal ulcer
- Detect gastric carcinoma
- Detect pernicious anemia
- Detect Zollinger-Ellison syndrome
- Evaluate effectiveness of vagotomy in the treatment of peptic ulcer disease

RESULT

Increased:
- BAO
  Basophilic leukemia
  Duodenal ulcer
  G-cell hyperplasia
  Recurring peptic ulcer
  Retained antrum syndrome
  Systemic mastocytosis
  Vagal hyperfunction
  Zollinger-Ellison syndrome
- PAO

Duodenal ulcer
Zollinger-Ellison syndrome

Decreased:

* BAO
  Gastric ulcer

* PAO
  Chronic gastritis
  Gastric cancers
  Gastric polyps
  Gastric ulcer
  Myxedema
  Pernicious anemia

CRITICAL VALUES: N/A

INTERFERING FACTORS:

* Drugs that may increase gastric volume include atropine, diazepam, ganglionic blocking agents, and insulin.

* Drugs and substances that may increase gastric pH include caffeine, calcium salts, corticotropin, ethanol, rauwolfia, reserpine, and tolazoline.

* Drugs and substances that may decrease gastric pH include atropine, cimetidine, diazepam, famotidine, ganglionic blocking agents, glucagon, nizatidine, omeprazole, oxmetidine, propranolol, prostaglandin $\alpha2$, ranitidine, and secretin.

* Gastric intubation is contraindicated ⚠ in patients with esophageal varices, diverticula, stenosis, malignant neoplasm of the esophagus, aortic aneurysm, severe gastric hemorrhage, and congenital heart failure.

* The use of histamine diphosphate is ⚠ contraindicated in patients with a history of asthma, paroxysmal hypertension, urticaria, or other allergic conditions.

* Failure to follow dietary restrictions may result in stimulation of gastric secretions.

* Exposure to the sight, smell, or

thought of food immediately before and during the test may result in stimulation of gastric secretions.

Nursing Implications and Procedure • • • • • • • • • • •

Pretest: ▮

➤ Obtain a history of the patient's complaints, including a list of known allergens.

➤ Obtain a history of the patient's gastrointestinal system as well as results of previously performed tests and procedures. For related tests, refer to the gastrointestinal system table.

➤ Obtain a list of the medications the patient is taking, including herbs, nutritional supplements, and nutraceuticals. The requesting health care practitioner and laboratory should be advised if the patient regularly uses these products so that their effects can be taken into consideration when reviewing results.

➤ Instruct the patient to fast from food after the evening meal the night before the test and not to drink water for 1 hour before the test. The patient should be instructed to refrain from chewing gum or smoking for at least 12 hours before the test.

➤ Drugs and substances that may alter gastric secretions (e.g., alcohol, histamine, nicotine, adrenocorticotropic steroids, insulin, parasympathetic agents, belladonna alkaloids, anticholinergic drugs, histamine receptor antagonists) should be restricted by medical direction for 72 hours before the test.

➤ Review the procedure with the patient. Explain that some discomfort is experienced from insertion of the nasogastric tube.

➤ *Obtain a written and informed consent before administering any medications prior to the procedure.*

➤ Inform the patient that specimen collection takes approximately 60 to 120 minutes.

Intratest:

➤ Ensure that the patient has complied with dietary preparations and other pretesting restrictions.

➤ Ensure that the patient does not have a history of asthma, paroxysmal hypertension, urticaria, or other allergic conditions if histamine diphosphate is being considered for use in the test.

➤ Direct the patient to breathe normally and to avoid unnecessary movement.

➤ Record baseline vital signs.

➤ If the patient is wearing dentures, remove them.

➤ Observe standard precautions and follow the general guidelines in Appendix A.

➤ Have the patient sit, or help the patient recline on the left side.

➤ A cold lubricated gastric (Levine) tube is inserted orally. Alternatively, if the patient has a hyperactive gag reflex, the tube can be inserted nasally. The tube must have a radiopaque tip.

➤ Fluoroscopy or x-ray is used to confirm proper position of the tube before the start of the test.

➤ Using a constant but gentle suction, gastric contents are collected. Do not use specimens obtained from the first 15 to 30 minutes of suctioning.

➤ The gastric stimulant is administered, and the peak basal specimens are collected over a 60-minute period as four 15-minute specimens.

➤ Number the specimen tubes in the order in which they were collected. Label the specimen, including time of collection, and promptly transport it to the laboratory.

Post-test:

➤ Instruct the patient to resume usual diet and medication as directed by the health care practitioner.

➤ Monitor vital signs and compare with baseline values.

➤ Monitor for side effects of drugs administered to induce gastric secretion (e.g., flushing, headache, nasal stuffiness, dizziness, faintness, nausea).

➤ Evaluate test results in relation to the patient's symptoms and other tests performed. Related laboratory tests include complete blood count, folate, gastrin, intrinsic factor antibodies, *Helicobacter pylori*, and vitamin B_{12}.

GASTRIC EMPTYING SCAN

SYNONYMS/ACRONYM: Gastric emptying quantitation, gastric emptying scintigraphy.

AREA OF APPLICATION: Esophagus, stomach, small bowel.

CONTRAST: Radioactive technetium-99m sulfur colloid.

DESCRIPTION: A gastric emptying scan quantifies gastric emptying physiology. The procedure is indicated for patients with gastric motility symptoms, including diabetic gastroparesis, anorexia nervosa, gastric outlet obstruction syndromes, post-vagotomy and postgastrectomy syndromes, and assessment of medical and surgical treatments for diseases known to affect gastric motility. A radionuclide is administered, and the clearance of solids and liquids may be evaluated. The images are recorded electronically, showing the gastric emptying function over time. ∎

INDICATIONS:
• Measure gastric emptying rate

• Investigate the cause of rapid or slow rate of gastric emptying

RESULT

Normal Findings:
• No delay in gastric emptying rate

• Mean time emptying of liquid phase: 30 minutes (range, 11 to 49 minutes)

• Mean time emptying of solid phase: 40 minutes (range, 28 to 80 minutes)

Abnormal Findings:
• Decreased rate:
  Dumping syndrome
  Duodenal ulcer
  Malabsorption syndromes
  Zollinger-Ellison syndrome

• Increased rate:
  Amyloidosis
  Anorexia nervosa
  Diabetes
  Gastric ulcer
  Gastroenteritis
  Gastroesophageal reflux

Gastric outlet obstruction
Hypokalemia, hypomagnesemia
Post–gastric surgery period
Postoperative ileus
Post–radiation therapy period
Scleroderma

CRITICAL VALUES: N/A

INTERFERING FACTORS:

This procedure is contraindicated for:
• Patients who are pregnant or suspected of being pregnant, unless the potential benefits of the procedure far outweigh the risks to the fetus and mother

• Patients with esophageal motor disorders or swallowing difficulties

Factors that may impair clear imaging:
• Inability of the patient to cooperate or remain still during the procedure because of age, significant pain, or mental status

• Improper adjustment of the radiographic equipment to accommodate obese or thin patients, which can cause a poor-quality study

• Metallic objects within the examination field (e.g., jewelry or body rings), which may inhibit organ visualization and can produce unclear images

• Patients who are very obese, who may exceed the weight limit for the equipment

• Incorrect positioning of the patient, which may produce poor visualization of the area to be examined

• Performance of other nuclear scans within the preceding 24 to 48 hours

• Administration of certain medications (e.g., gastrin, cholecystokinin), which may interfere with gastric emptying

Other considerations:

• Failure to follow dietary restrictions before the procedure may cause the procedure to be canceled or repeated.

• Consultation with a physician should occur before the procedure for radiation safety concerns regarding infants of patients who are lactating.

Nursing Implications and Procedure • • • • • • • • • • •

Pretest:

➤ Inform the patient that the procedure assesses gastric emptying.

➤ Inform the patient that the procedure is performed in a nuclear medicine department by a technologist and usually takes 30 to 120 minutes to complete.

➤ Obtain a history of the patient's complaints, including a list of known allergens.

➤ Obtain a history of signs and symptoms of gastrointestinal disorders as well as results of previously performed tests, treatments, and surgical procedures. For related tests, refer to the gastrointestinal system table.

➤ Obtain a list of medications the patient is taking.

➤ Determine date of last menstrual period and possibility of pregnancy in perimenopausal women.

➤ Assure the patient that the procedure is painless and easily tolerated.

➤ Inform the patient that the technologist will place him or her in an upright position in front of the gamma camera (scanner).

➤ Reassure the patient that the radionuclide poses no radioactive hazard and rarely produces side effects.

➤ Restrict food and fluids for 6 to 8 hours before the scan.

➤ Obtain and record baseline vital signs.

Intratest:

➤ Ask the patient to void before the procedure. Have the patient put on a hospital gown.

➤ Administer sedative to a child or to an uncooperative adult, as ordered.

➤ Ask the patient to lie still during the procedure because movement produces unclear images. Make sure jewelry, watches, chains, belts, and any other metallic objects have been removed.

➤ Place the patient in an upright position in front of the gamma camera.

➤ Ask the patient to take the radionuclide orally, combined with eggs or as a liquid.

➤ Images are recorded and evaluated with regard to the amount of time it takes the stomach to empty.

➤ Wear gloves during the radionuclide administration and while handling the patient's urine.

Post-test:

➤ Evaluate the patient's vital signs.

➤ Instruct the patient to resume normal activity, medications, and diet, unless otherwise indicated.

➤ Advise the patient to drink increased amounts of fluids for 24 to 48 hours to eliminate the radionuclide from the body, unless contraindicated. Tell the patient that radionuclide is eliminated from the body within 6 to 24 hours.

➤ Inform the patient to flush the toilet immediately after each voiding following the procedure and to wash hands meticulously with soap and water after each voiding for 24 hours after the procedure.

➤ Tell all caregivers to wear gloves when discarding urine for 24 hours after the procedure. Wash gloved hands with soap and water before removing gloves. Then wash hands after removing the gloves.

➤ A physician specializing in this branch of medicine sends a written

report of it to the ordering provider, who discusses the results with the patient.
➤ Evaluate test results in relation to the patient's symptoms and other tests performed. A related diagnostic test is the upper gastrointestinal and small bowel series.

GASTRIN AND GASTRIN STIMULATION TEST

SYNONYM/ACRONYM: N/A.

SPECIMEN: Serum (1 mL) collected in a red- or tiger-top tube.

REFERENCE VALUE: (Method: Radioimmunoassay)

Gastrin Level

Age	Conventional Units	SI Units (Conversion Factor ×1)
Infant	120–183 pg/mL	120–183 ng/L
Child	Less than 10–125 pg/mL	Less than 10–125 ng/L
Adult		
Up to 60 y	25–90 pg/mL	25–90 ng/L
60 y and older	Less than 100 pg/mL	Less than 100 ng/L

Stimulation Tests

Gastrin stimulation test with calcium or secretin	No response or slight increase over baseline

DESCRIPTION: Gastrin is a hormone secreted by the stomach and duodenum in response to vagal stimulation; the presence of food, alcohol, or calcium in the stomach; and the alkalinity of gastric secretions. After its absorption into the circulation, gastrin returns to the stomach and acts as a stimulant for acid, insulin, pepsin, and intrinsic factor secretion. Gastrin stimulation tests can be performed after a test meal or intravenous infusion of calcium or secretin. ■

INDICATIONS:
• Assist in the diagnosis of gastric carcinoma, pernicious anemia, or G-cell hyperplasia

- Assist in the diagnosis of Zollinger-Ellison syndrome

- Assist in the differential diagnosis of ulcers from other gastrointestinal peptic disorders

RESULT

Increased in:

- Chronic gastritis

- Chronic renal failure

- G-cell hyperplasia

- Gastric carcinoma

- Gastric and duodenal ulcers

- Hyperparathyroidism

- Pernicious anemia

- Pyloric obstruction

- Retained antrum

- Zollinger-Ellison syndrome

Decreased in:

- Hypothyroidism

- Vagotomy

CRITICAL VALUES: N/A

INTERFERING FACTORS:

- Drugs and substances that may increase gastrin levels include amino acids, cimetidine, catecholamines, insulin, morphine, omeprazole, pantoprazole, sufotidine, terbutaline, calcium products, and coffee.

- Drugs that may decrease gastrin levels include atropine, enprostil, glucagon, secretin, streptozocin, and tolbutamide.

- In some cases, protein ingestion elevates serum gastrin levels.

- Recent radioactive scans or radiation within 1 week before the test can interfere with test results when radioimmunoassay is the test method.

Nursing Implications and Procedure

Pretest:

➤ Obtain a history of the patient's complaints, including a list of known allergens.

➤ Obtain a history of the patient's endocrine and gastrointestinal systems, as well as results of previously performed tests and procedures. For related tests, refer to the endocrine and gastrointestinal system tables.

➤ Obtain a list of medications the patient is taking, including herbs, nutritional supplements, and nutraceuticals. The requesting health care practitioner and laboratory should be advised if the patient regularly uses these products so that their effects can be taken into consideration when reviewing results.

➤ Note any recent procedures that can interfere with test results.

➤ Instruct the patient to fast for 12 hours before the test.

➤ Withhold medications and alcohol for 12 to 24 hours, as ordered by the health care practitioner.

➤ There are no fluid restrictions unless by medical direction.

➤ Review the procedure with the patient.

➤ Inform the patient that specimen collection takes approximately 5 to 10 minutes.

Intratest:

➤ Ensure that the patient has complied with dietary preparations and other pretesting restrictions.

➤ Direct the patient to breathe normally and to avoid unnecessary movement.

➤ Observe standard precautions and follow the general guidelines in Appendix A. Perform a venipuncture, and collect the specimen in a 5-mL red- or tiger-top tube.

➤ Administer gastrin stimulators as appropriate.

➤ Label the specimen, and promptly transport it to the laboratory.

Post-test:

➤ Observe venipuncture site for bleeding or hematoma formation. Apply pressure bandage.

➤ Instruct the patient to resume usual diet and medication as directed by the health care practitioner. Nutritional support with calcium, iron, and vitamin B_{12} supplementation may be ordered, as appropriate.

➤ Evaluate test results in relation to the patient's symptoms and other tests performed. Related laboratory tests include complete blood count, gastric acid stimulation, and *Helicobacter pylori*.

GASTROESOPHAGEAL REFLUX SCAN

· ·

SYNONYMS/ACRONYM: Aspiration scan, GE reflux scan.

AREA OF APPLICATION: Esophagus and stomach.

CONTRAST: Radioactive technetium-99m sulfur colloid.

DESCRIPTION: The gastroesophageal (GE) reflux scan assesses gastric reflux across the esophageal sphincter. Symptoms of GE reflux include heartburn, regurgitation, vomiting, dysphagia, and a bitter taste in the mouth. This procedure may be used to evaluate the medical or surgical treatment of patients with GE reflux and to detect aspiration of gastric contents into the lungs. A radionuclide such as technetium-99m sulfur colloid is ingested orally in orange juice. Scanning studies are done immediately to assess the amount of liquid that has reached the stomach. An abdominal binder is applied and then tightened gradually to obtain images at increasing degrees of abdominal pressure: 0, 20, 40, 60, 80, and 100 mm Hg. Computer calcula-

tion determines the amount of reflux into the esophagus at each of these abdominal pressures as recorded on the images. For aspiration scans, images are taken over the lungs to detect tracheoesophageal aspiration of the radionuclide.

In infants, the study distinguishes between vomiting and reflux. Reflux occurs predominantly in infants younger than age 2, who are mainly on a milk diet. This procedure is indicated when an infant has symptoms such as failure to thrive, feeding problems, and episodes of wheezing with chest infection. The radionuclide is added to the infant's milk, images are obtained of the gastric and esophageal area, and the images are evaluated visually and by computer. ■

INDICATIONS:

- Aid in the diagnosis of GE reflux in patients with unexplained nausea and vomiting

- Distinguish between vomiting and reflux in infants with failure to thrive, feeding problems, and wheezing combined with chest infection

RESULT

Normal Findings:

- Reflux less than or equal to 4 percent across the esophageal sphincter

Abnormal Findings:

- Reflux of greater than 4 percent at any pressure level

- Pulmonary aspiration

CRITICAL VALUES: N/A

INTERFERING FACTORS:

This procedure is contraindicated for:

- Patients who are pregnant or suspected of being pregnant, unless the potential benefits of the procedure far outweigh the risks to the fetus and mother

- Patients with hiatal hernia, esophageal motor disorders, or swallowing difficulties

Factors that may impair clear imaging:

- Inability of the patient to cooperate or remain still during the procedure because of age, significant pain, or mental status

- Improper adjustment of the radiographic equipment to accommodate obese or thin patients, which can cause overexposure or underexposure and a poor-quality study

- Patients who are very obese, who may exceed the weight limit for the equipment

- Incorrect positioning of the patient, which may produce poor visualization of the area to be examined

- Other nuclear scans done within the previous 24 to 48 hours

- Metallic objects within the examination field (e.g., jewelry or body rings), which may inhibit organ visualization and can produce unclear images

Other considerations:

- Failure to follow dietary restrictions before the procedure may cause the procedure to be canceled or repeated.

- Consultation with a physician should occur before the procedure for radiation safety concerns regarding infants of patients who are lactating.

Nursing Implications and Procedure ● ● ● ● ● ● ● ● ● ●

Pretest: ■

➤ Inform the patient that the procedure evaluates gastric reflux.

➤ Inform the patient that the procedure is performed in a nuclear medicine department by a technologist and usually takes approximately 60 minutes to complete.

➤ Obtain a history of the patient's complaints, including a list of known allergens.

➤ Obtain a history of signs and symptoms of gastrointestinal disorders as well as results of previously performed tests, treatments, and surgical procedures. For related tests, refer to the gastrointestinal system table.

➤ Obtain a list of medications the patient is taking.

➤ Determine date of last menstrual period and possibility of pregnancy in perimenopausal women.

➤ Reassure the patient that the radionuclide poses no radioactive hazard and rarely produces side effects.

➤ Fasting before the scan is not required; the patient may be encouraged to eat a full meal before the procedure.

➤ Obtain and record baseline vital signs.

Intratest: ■

➤ Ask the patient to void before the procedure. Have the patient put on a hospital gown.

➤ Administer sedative to a child or to an uncooperative adult, as ordered.

➤ Ask the patient to lie still during the procedure because movement produces unclear images. Make sure jewelry, watches, chains, belts, and any other metallic objects have been removed.

➤ Ask the patient to drink approximately 300 mL of orange juice that contains the radionuclide.

➤ Place the patient in a supine position on a flat table with foam wedges to help maintain position and immobilization. An image is recorded to confirm swallowing of the liquid and emptying into the stomach.

➤ The abdominal binder is applied, and scans are taken as the binder is tightened at various pressures, as described previously.

➤ If reflux occurs at lower pressures, an additional 30 mL of water may be given to clear the esophagus.

➤ Wear gloves during the radionuclide administration and while handling the patient's urine.

Post-test: ■

➤ Evaluate the patient's vital signs.

➤ Instruct the patient to resume normal activity, medications, and diet, unless otherwise indicated.

➤ Advise the patient to drink increased amounts of fluids for 24 to 48 hours to eliminate the radionuclide from the body, unless contraindicated. Tell the patient that radionuclide is eliminated from the body within 6 to 24 hours.

➤ Inform the patient to flush the toilet immediately after each voiding following the procedure and to wash hands meticulously with soap and water after each voiding for 24 hours after the procedure.

➤ Tell all caregivers to wear gloves when discarding urine for 24 hours after the procedure. Wash gloved hands with soap and water before removing gloves. Then wash hands after the gloves are removed.

➤ A physician specializing in this branch of medicine sends a written report to the ordering provider, who discusses the results with the patient.

➤ Evaluate test results in relation to the patient's symptoms and other tests performed. Related diagnostic tests include upper gastrointestinal series and gastric emptying examinations.

GASTROINTESTINAL BLOOD LOSS SCAN

SYNONYMS/ACRONYM: Gastrointestinal bleed localization study, GI bleed scintigraphy, lower GI blood loss scan, GI scintigram.

AREA OF APPLICATION: Abdomen.

CONTRAST: Intravenous radioactive technetium-99m–labeled red blood cells.

DESCRIPTION: Gastrointestinal (GI) blood loss scan is a nuclear medicine study that assists in detecting and localizing active GI tract bleeding (2 or 3 mL/min) for the purpose of better directing endoscopic or angiographic studies. This procedure can detect bleeding if the rate is greater than 0.5 mL/min, but it is not specific for site localization or cause of bleeding. Endoscopy is the procedure of choice for diagnosing upper GI bleeding. After injection of technetium-99m–labeled red blood cells, immediate and delayed images of various views of the abdomen are obtained. The radionuclide remains in the circulation long enough to extravasate and accumulate within the bowel lumen at the site of active bleeding. This procedure is valuable for the detection and localization of recent non-GI intra-abdominal hemorrhage. Images may be taken over an extended period to show intermittent bleeding. ∎

INDICATIONS: Diagnose unexplained abdominal pain and GI bleeding

RESULT

Normal Findings:
• Normal distribution of radionuclide in the large vessels with no extravascular activity

Abnormal Findings:
• Angiodysplasia
• Aortoduodenal fistula
• Diverticulosis

• Inflammatory bowel disease
• Polyps
• GI bleeding
• Tumor
• Ulcer

CRITICAL VALUES: N/A

INTERFERING FACTORS:

This procedure is contraindicated for:
• Patients who are pregnant or suspected of being pregnant, unless the potential benefits of the procedure far outweigh the risks to the fetus and mother

Factors that may impair clear imaging:
• Inability of the patient to cooperate or remain still during the procedure because of age, significant pain, or mental status

• Retained barium from a previous radiologic procedure

• Metallic objects within the examination field (e.g., jewelry or body rings), which may inhibit organ visualization and can produce unclear images

• Improper adjustment of the radiographic equipment to accommodate obese or thin patients, which can cause overexposure or underexposure and a poor-quality study

• Patients who are very obese, who may exceed the weight limit for the equipment

• Incorrect positioning of the patient, which may produce poor visualization of the area to be examined

- Other nuclear scans done within the previous 24 to 48 hours

- Inaccurate timing of imaging after the radionuclide injection

Other considerations:

- The examination detects only active or intermittent bleeding.

- The procedure is of little value in patients with chronic anemia or slowly decreasing hematocrit.

- The scan is less accurate for localization of bleeding sites in the upper GI tract.

- Improper injection of the radionuclide allows the tracer to seep deep into the muscle tissue, producing erroneous hot spots.

- The test is not specific and does not indicate the exact pathologic condition causing the bleeding and may miss small sites of bleeding (less than 0.5 mL/min) caused by diverticular disease or angiodysplasia.

- Physiologically unstable patients may be unable to be scanned over long periods or may need to go to surgery before the procedure is complete.

- Failure to follow dietary restrictions before the procedure may cause the procedure to be canceled or repeated.

- Consultation with a physician should occur before the procedure for radiation safety concerns regarding infants of patients who are lactating.

- Risks associated with radiographic overexposure can result from frequent x-ray procedures. Personnel in the room with the patient should wear a protective lead apron, stand behind a shield, or leave the area while the examination is being done. Personnel working in the area where the examination is being done should wear badges that reveal their level of exposure to radiation.

Nursing Implications and Procedure · · · · · · · · · · ·

Pretest:

➤ Inform the patient that the procedure evaluates GI bleeding.

➤ Inform the patient that the procedure is performed in a special nuclear medicine department by a technologist and usually takes approximately 60 minutes to complete, with additional images taken periodically over 24 hours.

➤ Obtain a history of the patient's complaints, including a list of known allergens.

➤ Obtain a history of signs and symptoms of GI bleeding, pain, intussusception, volvulus, or diverticulitis as well as results of previously performed tests, treatments, and surgical procedures. For related tests, refer to the GI and cardiovascular system tables.

➤ Obtain a list of medications the patient is taking.

➤ Determine date of last menstrual period and possibility of pregnancy in perimenopausal women.

➤ Fasting before the scan is not needed, unless otherwise indicated.

➤ Obtain and record baseline vital signs.

Intratest:

➤ Ask the patient to void before the procedure. Have the patient put on a hospital gown.

➤ Administer sedative to a child or to an uncooperative adult, as ordered.

➤ Ask the patient to lie still during the procedure because movement produces unclear images. Make sure jewelry, watches, chains, belts, and any other metallic objects have been removed.

➤ Inform the technologist doing the procedure to notify the nurse of all bloody bowel movements that occur during the procedure.

➤ Place the patient in a supine position

on a flat table with foam wedges to help maintain position and immobilization. The radionuclide is administered intravenously, and the abdomen is scanned immediately for 1 minute to screen for vascular lesions that cause bleeding. Images are taken every 5 minutes for the next 60 minutes in the anterior, oblique, and lateral views, and a postvoid anterior view is taken.

➤ If the patient is having major GI bleeding, closely monitor vital signs during the procedure.

➤ Wear gloves during the radionuclide injection and while handling the patient's urine.

Post-test:

➤ Evaluate the patient's vital signs.

➤ Instruct the patient to resume normal activity, medications, and diet, unless otherwise indicated.

➤ Advise the patient to drink increased amounts of fluids for 24 to 48 hours to eliminate the radionuclide from the body, unless contraindicated. Tell the patient that radionuclide is eliminated from the body within 6 to 24 hours.

➤ Inform the patient to flush the toilet immediately after each voiding following the procedure and to wash hands meticulously with soap and water after each voiding for 24 hours after the procedure.

➤ Tell all caregivers to wear gloves when discarding urine for 24 hours after the procedure. Wash gloved hands with soap and water before removing gloves. Then wash hands after the gloves are removed.

➤ A physician specializing in this branch of medicine sends a written report to the ordering provider, who discusses the results with the patient.

➤ Evaluate test results in relation to the patient's symptoms and other tests performed. Related diagnostic tests include angiography, magnetic resonance imaging, and computed tomography of the abdomen.

GLUCAGON

· ·

SYNONYM/ACRONYM: N/A.

SPECIMEN: Plasma (1 mL) collected in chilled, lavender-top (ethylenedi-aminetetra-acetic acid [EDTA]) tube. Specimen should be transported tightly capped and in an ice slurry.

REFERENCE VALUE: (Method: Radioimmunoassay)

Age	Conventional Units	SI Unit (Conversion Factor ×1)
Cord blood	0–215 pg/mL	0–215 ng/L
1–3 d	0–1750 pg/mL	0–1750 ng/L
4–14 y	0–148 pg/mL	0–148 ng/L
Adult	20–100 pg/mL	20–100 ng/L

DESCRIPTION: Glucagon is a hormone secreted by the alpha cells of the islets of Langerhans in the pancreas in response to hypoglycemia. This hormone acts primarily on the liver to promote glucose production and to control glucose storage. The coordinated release of insulin, glucagon, and somatostatin ensures an adequate fuel supply while maintaining stable blood glucose. Patients with glucagonoma have values greater than 500 ng/L. Values greater than 1000 ng/L are diagnostic for this condition. Glucagonoma causes three different syndromes:
1. *Syndrome 1:* A characteristic skin rash, diabetes or impaired glucose tolerance, weight loss, anemia, and venous thrombosis
2. *Syndrome 2:* Severe diabetes
3. *Syndrome 3:* Multiple endocrine neoplasia

A dramatic increase in glucagon occurring soon after renal transplant may indicate organ rejection. In the case of kidney transplant rejection, glucagon levels increase several days before an increase in creatinine levels.

Glucagon deficiency can be confirmed by measuring glucagon levels before and after intravenous infusion of 0.5 g arginine/kg. Glucagon deficiency is confirmed when levels fail to rise 30 to 60 minutes after infusion. Newborn infants of diabetic mothers have impaired glucagon secretion, which may play a role in their hypoglycemia. ■

INDICATIONS:
- Assist in confirming glucagon deficiency
- Assist in the diagnosis of suspected glucagonoma (alpha islet-cell neoplastic tumor)
- Assist in the diagnosis of suspected renal failure or renal transplant rejection

RESULT

Increased in:
- Acromegaly
- Acute pancreatitis
- Burns
- Cirrhosis
- Cushing's syndrome
- Diabetes (uncontrolled)
- Glucagonoma
- Hyperlipoproteinemia types III and IV
- Hypoglycemia
- Infections
- Kidney transplant rejection
- Renal failure
- Stress
- Trauma

Decreased in:
- Chronic pancreatitis
- Cystic fibrosis
- Postpancreatectomy period

CRITICAL VALUES: N/A

INTERFERING FACTORS:
- Drugs that may increase glucagon levels include amino acids (e.g., arginine), cholecystokinin, danazol, gastrin, glucocorticoids, insulin, and nifedipine.
- Drugs that may decrease glucagon levels include atenolol, pindolol, propranolol, secretin, and verapamil.
- Recent radioactive scans or radiation within 1 week before the test can interfere with test results when radioimmunoassay is the test method.

Nursing Implications and Procedure • • • • • • • • • • •

Pretest:

➤ Obtain a history of the patient's complaints, including a list of known allergens.

➤ Obtain a history of the patient's endocrine system as well as results of previously performed tests and procedures. For related tests, refer to the endocrine system table.

➤ Obtain a list of medications the patient is taking, including herbs, nutritional supplements, and nutraceuticals. The requesting health care practitioner and laboratory should be advised if the patient regularly uses these products so that their effects can be taken into consideration when reviewing results.

➤ Note any recent procedures that can interfere with test results.

➤ There are no fluid or medication restrictions unless by medical direction.

➤ Instruct the patient to fast at least 12 hours before specimen collection for baseline values. Diabetic patients should be in good glycemic control before testing.

➤ Review the procedure with the patient.

➤ Inform the patient that specimen collection takes approximately 5 to 10 minutes.

Intratest:

➤ Ensure that the patient has complied with dietary preparations and other pretesting restrictions.

➤ Direct the patient to breathe normally and to avoid unnecessary movement.

➤ Observe standard precautions and follow the general guidelines in Appendix A. Perform a venipuncture, and collect the specimen in a chilled 5-mL lavender-top tube.

➤ Label the specimen, and promptly transport it to the laboratory. The tightly capped sample should be placed in an ice slurry immediately after collection. Information on the specimen label can be protected from water in the ice slurry if the specimen is first placed in a protective plastic bag.

Post-test:

➤ Observe venipuncture site for bleeding or hematoma formation. Apply pressure bandage.

➤ Instruct the patient to resume usual diet as directed by the health care practitioner.

➤ Instruct the diabetic patient, as appropriate, in nutritional management of the disease. Patients who adhere to dietary recommendations report a better general feeling of health, better weight management, greater control of glucose and lipid values, and improved use of insulin. There is no "diabetic diet"; however, many meal-planning approaches with nutritional goals are endorsed by the American Dietetic Association. The nutritional needs of each diabetic patient must be determined individually with the appropriate health care professionals, particularly professionals trained in nutrition.

➤ Increased glucagon levels may be associated with diabetes. Instruct the patient and caregiver to report signs and symptoms of hypoglycemia (weakness, confusion, diaphoresis, rapid pulse) or hyperglycemia (thirst, polyuria, hunger, lethargy).

➤ Emphasize, as appropriate, that good glycemic control delays the onset and slows the progression of diabetic retinopathy, nephropathy, and neuropathy.

➤ Evaluate test results in relation to the patient's symptoms and other tests performed. Related laboratory tests include glucose, glucose tolerance tests, glycated hemoglobin A_{1C}, insulin, insulin antibodies, and microalbumin.

GLUCOSE

● ●

SYNONYMS/ACRONYMS: Blood sugar, fasting blood sugar (FBS), postprandial glucose, 2-hour PC.

SPECIMEN: Serum (1 mL) collected in a red- or tiger-top tube. Plasma (1 mL) collected in gray-top (sodium fluoride) or green-top (heparin) tube is also acceptable.

REFERENCE VALUE: (Method: Spectrophotometry)

Age	Conventional Units	SI Units (Conversion Factor ×0.0555)
Fasting		
Cord blood	45–96 mg/dL	2.5–5.3 mmol/L
Premature infant	20–60 mg/dL	1.1–3.3 mmol/L
Neonate	30–60 mg/dL	1.7–3.3 mmol/L
Newborn 1 d	40–60 mg/dL	2.2–3.3 mmol/L
Newborn 2 d 2 y	50–80 mg/dL	2.8–4.4 mmol/L
Child	60–100 mg/dL	3.3–5.6 mmol/L
Adult	75–110 mg/dL	4.2–6.1 mmol/L
60–90 y	80–115 mg/dL	4.7–6.4 mmol/L
Older than 90 y	75–120 mg/dL	4.2–6.7 mmol/L
2-Hour Postprandial		
2-h Postprandial	Less than 105 mg/dL	Less than 5.8 mmol/L

DESCRIPTION: Glucose, a simple six-carbon sugar (monosaccharide), enters the diet as part of the sugars sucrose, lactose, and maltose and as the major constituent of the complex polysaccharide called dietary starch. The body acquires most of its energy from the oxidative metabolism of glucose. Excess glucose is stored in the liver or in muscle tissue as glycogen.

Diabetes is a group of diseases characterized by hyperglycemia or elevated glucose levels. Hyperglycemia results from a defect in insulin secretion (type 1 diabetes), a defect in insulin action, or a combination of defects in secretion and action (type 2 diabetes). The chronic hyperglycemia of diabetes may result over time in damage, dysfunction, and eventually failure of the eyes, kidneys, nerves, heart, and blood vessels. The American Diabetes Association's 1998 revised criteria for diagnosing diabetes include any combination of the following findings or confirmation of any of the individual findings by repetition on a subsequent day:

- Symptoms of diabetes (e.g., polyuria, polydipsia, unexplained weight loss) in addition to a random glucose level greater than 200 mg/dL
- Fasting blood glucose greater than 126 mg/dL, after a minimum of an 8-hour fast
- Glucose level greater than 200 mg/dL 2 hours after glucose challenge with standardized 75-mg load ■

INDICATIONS:

- Assist in the diagnosis of insulinoma
- Determine insulin requirements
- Evaluate disorders of carbohydrate metabolism
- Identify hypoglycemia
- Screen for diabetes

RESULT

Increased in:

- Acromegaly, gigantism
- Acute stress reaction
- Cerebrovascular accident
- Cushing's syndrome
- Diabetes
- Glucagonoma
- Hemochromatosis
- Liver disease (severe)
- Myocardial infarction
- Pancreatic adenoma
- Pancreatitis (acute and chronic)
- Pancreatitis due to mumps
- Pheochromocytoma

- Renal disease (severe)
- Shock, trauma
- Somatostatinoma
- Strenuous exercise
- Thyrotoxicosis
- Vitamin B_1 deficiency

Decreased in:

- Acute alcohol ingestion
- Addison's disease
- Ectopic insulin production from tumors (adrenal carcinoma, carcinoma of the stomach, fibrosarcoma)
- Excess insulin by injection
- Galactosemia
- Glucagon deficiency
- Glycogen storage diseases
- Hereditary fructose intolerance
- Hypopituitarism
- Hypothyroidism
- Insulinoma
- Malabsorption syndromes
- Maple syrup urine disease
- Poisoning resulting in severe liver disease
- Postgastrectomy
- Starvation
- von Gierke disease

CRITICAL VALUES:

Less than 40 mg/dL

Greater than 400 mg/dL

Symptoms of decreased glucose levels include headache, confusion, hunger, irritability, nervousness, restlessness, sweating, and weakness. Possible interventions include oral or intravenous (IV) administration of glucose, IV or intramuscular injection of glucagon, and continuous glucose monitoring.

Symptoms of elevated glucose levels

include abdominal pain, fatigue, muscle cramps, nausea, vomiting, polyuria, and thirst. Possible interventions include subcutaneous or IV injection of insulin with continuous glucose monitoring.

INTERFERING FACTORS:

* Drugs that may increase glucose levels include acetazolamide, alanine, albuterol, anesthetic agents, antipyrine, atenolol, betamethasone, cefotaxime, chlorpromazine, chlorprothixene, clonidine, clorexolone, corticotropin, cortisone, cyclic AMP, cyclopropane, dexamethasone, dextroamphetamine, diapamide, epinephrine, enflurane, ethacrynic acid, ether, fludrocortisone, fluoxymesterone, furosemide, glucagon, glucocorticoids, homoharringtonine, hydrochlorothiazide, hydroxydione, isoniazid, maltose, meperidine, meprednisone, methyclothiazide, metolazone, niacin, nifedipine, nortriptyline, octreotide, oral contraceptives, oxyphenbutazone, pancreozymin, phenelzine, phenylbutazone, piperacetazine, polythiazide, prednisone, quinethazone, reserpine, rifampin, ritodrine, salbutamol, secretin, somatostatin, thiazides, thyroid hormone, and triamcinolone.

* Drugs that may decrease glucose levels include acarbose, acetylsalicylic acid, acipimox, alanine, allopurinol, antimony compounds, arsenicals, ascorbic acid, benzene, buformin, cannabis, captopril, carbutamide, chloroform, clofibrate, dexfenfluramine, enalapril, enprostil, erythromycin, fenfluramine, gemfibrozil, glibornuride, glyburide, guanethidine, niceritrol, nitrazepam, oral contraceptives, oxandrolone, oxymetholone, phentolamine, phosphorus, promethazine, ramipril, rotenone, sulfonylureas, thiocarlide, tolbutamide, tromethamine, and verapamil.

* Elevated urea levels and uremia can lead to falsely elevated glucose levels.

* Extremely elevated white blood cell counts can lead to falsely decreased glucose values.

* Failure to follow dietary restrictions before the fasting test can lead to falsely elevated glucose values.

* Administration of insulin or oral hypoglycemic agents within 8 hours of a fasting blood glucose can lead to falsely decreased values.

* Specimens should never be collected above an IV line because of the potential for dilution when the specimen and the IV solution combine in the collection container, falsely decreasing the result. There is also the potential of contaminating the sample with the substance of interest, contained in the IV solution, falsely increasing the result.

Nursing Implications and Procedure • • • • • • • • • • •

Pretest:

➤ Obtain a history of the patient's complaints, including a list of known allergens.

➤ Obtain a history of the patient's endocrine system as well as results of previously performed tests and procedures. For related tests, refer to the endocrine system table.

➤ Obtain a list of medications the patient is taking, including herbs, nutritional supplements, nutraceuticals, insulin, and any other substances used to regulate glucose levels. The requesting health care practitioner and laboratory should be advised if the patient regularly uses these products so that their effects can be taken into consideration when reviewing results.

➤ There are no fluid or medication restrictions unless by medical direction.

➤ For the fasting glucose test, the patient should be fasting at least 12 hours before specimen collection.

➤ The patient should follow the instructions given for 2-hour postprandial glucose test. Some health care practitioners may order administration of a standard glucose solution, whereas others may instruct the patient to eat a meal with a known carbohydrate composition.

➤ Review the procedure with the patient.

➤ Inform the patient that specimen collection takes approximately 5 to 10 minutes.

Intratest:

➤ Ensure that the patient has complied with dietary preparations and other pretesting restrictions.

➤ Direct the patient to breathe normally and to avoid unnecessary movement.

➤ Observe standard precautions and follow the general guidelines in Appendix A. Perform a venipuncture, and collect the specimen in a 5-mL gray-top tube.

➤ Label the specimen, and promptly transport it to the laboratory.

Post-test:

➤ Observe venipuncture site for bleeding or hematoma formation. Apply pressure bandage.

➤ Instruct the patient to resume usual diet as directed by the health care practitioner.

➤ Increased glucose levels may be associated with diabetes. Instruct the diabetic patient, as appropriate, in nutritional management of the disease. Patients who adhere to dietary recommendations report a better general feeling of health, better weight management, greater control of glucose and lipid values, and improved use of insulin. There is no "diabetic diet"; however, many meal-planning approaches with nutritional goals are endorsed by the American Dietetic Association. The nutritional needs of each diabetic patient must be determined individually with the appropriate health care professionals, particularly professionals trained in nutrition.

➤ Instruct the patient and caregiver to report signs and symptoms of hypoglycemia (weakness, confusion, diaphoresis, rapid pulse) or hyperglycemia (thirst, polyuria, hunger, lethargy). Emphasize, as appropriate, that good glycemic control delays the onset of and slows the progression of diabetic retinopathy, nephropathy, and neuropathy.

➤ Evaluate test results in relation to the patient's symptoms and other tests performed. Related laboratory tests include C-peptide, creatinine, fructosamine, glucose tolerance tests, glycated hemoglobin A_{1C}, insulin, insulin antibodies, ketones, microalbumin, and blood urea nitrogen (BUN).

GLUCOSE-6-PHOSPHATE DEHYDROGENASE

• •

SYNONYM/ACRONYM: G6PD.

SPECIMEN: Whole blood (1 mL) collected in a lavender-top (ethylenediaminetetra-acetic acid [EDTA]) tube.

REFERENCE VALUE: (Method: Fluorescent) Qualitative assay—enzyme activity detected; quantitative assay—the following table reflects enzyme activity in units per gram of hemoglobin and in units per milliliter of erythrocytes:

Age	Conventional Units	SI Units
		(Conversion Factor × 0.0645)
Newborn	7.8–14.4 U/g hemoglobin	0.5–0.93 MU/mol hemoglobin
Adult	5.5–9.3 U/g hemoglobin	0.35–0.60 MU/mol hemoglobin
		(Conversion Factor × 1)
Newborn	2.65–4.90 U/mL erythrocytes	2.65–4.90 kU/L erythrocytes
Adult	1.87–3.16 U/mL erythrocytes	1.87–3.16 kU/L erythrocytes

DESCRIPTION: Glucose-6-phosphate dehydrogenase (G6PD) is a red blood cell enzyme. It is involved in the hexose monophosphate shunt, and its function is to protect hemoglobin from oxidation. G6PD deficiency is an inherited X-linked abnormality; approximately 20 percent of female carriers are heterozygous. This deficiency results in hemolysis of varying degrees and acuity depending on the severity of the abnormality. There are three G6PD variants of high frequency in different ethnic groups. G6PD A⁻ is more common in African-Americans (10 percent of males). G6PD Mediterranean is especially common in Iraqis, Kurds, Sephardic Jews, and Lebanese and less common in Greeks, Italians, Turks, North Africans, Spaniards, Portuguese, and Ashkenazic Jews. G6PD Mahidol is common in Southeast Asians (22 percent of males). ∎

INDICATIONS:
- Assist in identifying the cause of hemolytic anemia resulting from drug sensitivity, metabolic disorder, or infection
- Assist in identifying the cause of hemolytic anemia resulting from enzyme deficiency

RESULT

Increased in:
- Hepatic coma
- Hyperthyroidism
- Idiopathic thrombocytopenic purpura
- Myocardial infarction
- Pernicious anemia
- Viral hepatitis

Decreased in:
- Congenital nonspherocytic anemia
- G6PD deficiency
- Nonimmunologic hemolytic disease of the newborn

CRITICAL VALUES: N/A

INTERFERING FACTORS:
- Sulfates may decrease G6PD levels.

- G6PD levels are increased in reticulocytes; the test results may be falsely positive when a patient is in a period of acute hemolysis. G6PD levels can also be affected by the presence of large numbers of platelets and white blood cells, which also contain significant amounts of the enzyme.

Nursing Implications and Procedure • • • • • • • • • •

Pretest:

➤ Obtain a history of the patient's complaints, including a list of known allergens.

➤ Obtain a history of the patient's hematopoietic system as well as results of previously performed tests and procedures. For related tests, refer to the hematopoietic system table.

➤ Obtain a list of medications the patient is taking, including herbs, nutritional supplements, and nutraceuticals. The requesting health care practitioner and laboratory should be advised if the patient regularly uses these products so that their effects can be taken into consideration when reviewing results.

➤ There are no food, fluid, or medication restrictions unless by medical direction.

➤ Review the procedure with the patient.

➤ Inform the patient that specimen collection takes approximately 5 to 10 minutes.

Intratest:

➤ Direct the patient to breathe normally and to avoid unnecessary movement.

➤ Observe standard precautions and follow the general guidelines in Appendix A. Perform a venipuncture, and collect the specimen in a 5-mL lavender-top tube.

➤ Label the specimen, and promptly transport it to the laboratory.

Post-test:

➤ Observe venipuncture site for bleeding or hematoma formation. Apply pressure bandage.

➤ Educate the patient with G6PD deficiency, as appropriate, to avoid certain foods, vitamins, and drugs that may precipitate an acute episode of intravascular hemolysis, including fava beans, ascorbic acid (large doses), acetanilid, antimalarials, furazolidone, isobutyl nitrate, methylene blue, nalidixic acid, naphthalene, niridazole, nitrofurantoin, phenazopyridine, phenylhydrazine, primaquine, sulfacetamide, sulfamethoxazole, sulfanilamide, sulfapyridine, thiazolesulfone, toluidine blue, trinitrotoluene, and urate oxidase.

➤ Evaluate test results in relation to the patient's symptoms and other tests performed. Related laboratory tests include complete blood count (including examination of peripheral smear for red blood cell abnormalities and the presence of Heinz bodies), bilirubin, Ham's test, haptoglobin, hemosiderin, osmotic fragility, reticulocyte count, and urinalysis (for hemoglobin and urobilinogen).

GLUCOSE TOLERANCE TESTS

• •

SYNONYMS/ACRONYM: Standard oral tolerance test, standard gestational screen, standard gestational tolerance test, GTT.

SPECIMEN: Plasma (1 mL) collected in gray-top (sodium fluoride) tube. Serum (1 mL) collected in a red- or tiger-top tube. Plasma collected in a green-top (heparin) tube is also acceptable. It is important to use the same type of collection container throughout the entire test.

REFERENCE VALUE: (Method: Spectrophotometry)

	Conventional Units	SI Units (Conversion Factor ×0.0555)
Standard Oral Tolerance		
Fasting sample	Less than 126 mg/dL	Less than 7.0 mmol/L
2-hour sample	Less than 200 mg/dL	Less than 11.1 mmol/L
Standard Gestational Screen	Less than 141 mg/dL	Less than 7.8 mmol/L
Standard Gestational Tolerance		
Fasting sample	75–104 mg/dL	4.2–5.8 mmol/L
1-hour sample	75–180 mg/dL	4.2–10.0 mmol/L
2-hour sample	75–164 mg/dL	4.2–9.1 mmol/L
3-hour sample	75–144 mg/dL	4.2–8.0 mmol/L

Plasma glucose values are reported to be 10–20% higher than serum values.

DESCRIPTION: The glucose tolerance test (GTT) measures glucose levels after administration of an oral or intravenous carbohydrate challenge. Patients with diabetes are unable to metabolize glucose at a normal rate. The oral GTT is used for individuals who are able to eat and who are not known to have problems with gastrointestinal malabsorption. The intravenous GTT is used for individuals who are unable to tolerate oral glucose.

Diabetes is a group of diseases characterized by hyperglycemia or elevated glucose levels. Hyperglycemia results from a defect in insulin secretion (type 1 diabetes), a defect in insulin action, or a combination of dysfunction secretion and action (type 2 diabetes). The chronic hyperglycemia of diabetes over time results in damage, dysfunction, and eventually failure of the eyes, kidneys, nerves, heart, and blood vessels. The American Diabetes Association's 1998 revised criteria for diagnosing diabetes include any combination of the following findings or confirmation of any of the individual findings by repetition on a subsequent day:

• Symptoms of diabetes (e.g., polyuria, polydipsia, and unexplained weight loss) in addition to a random glucose level greater than 200 mg/dL

• Fasting blood glucose greater than 126 mg/dL, after a minimum of an 8-hour fast

• Glucose level greater than 200 mg/dL 2 hours after glucose challenge with standardized 75-mg load ■

INDICATIONS:

- Evaluate abnormal fasting or postprandial blood glucose levels that do not clearly indicate diabetes

- Evaluate glucose metabolism in women of childbearing age, especially women who are pregnant and have (1) a history of previous fetal loss or birth of infants weighing 9 pounds or more, and/or (2) a family history of diabetes

- Identify abnormal renal tubular function if glycosuria occurs without hyperglycemia

- Identify impaired glucose metabolism without overt diabetes

- Support the diagnosis of hyperthyroidism and alcoholic liver disease, which are characterized by a sharp rise in blood glucose followed by a decline to subnormal levels

RESULT

Tolerance increased in:

- Decreased absorption of glucose:
  Adrenal insufficiency (Addison's disease, hypopituitarism)
  Hypothyroidism
  Intestinal diseases, such as celiac disease and tropical sprue
  Whipple's disease

- Increased insulin secretion:
  Pancreatic islet cell tumor

Tolerance impaired in:

- Increased absorption of glucose:
  Excessive intake of glucose
  Gastrectomy
  Gastroenterostomy
  Hyperthyroidism
  Vagotomy

- Decreased usage of glucose:
  Central nervous system lesions
  Cushing's syndrome
  Diabetes

Hemochromatosis
Hyperlipidemia

- Decreased glycogenesis:
  Hyperthyroidism
  Infections
  Liver disease (severe)
  Stress
  Pheochromocytoma
  Pregnancy
  von Gierke disease

CRITICAL VALUES: N/A

INTERFERING FACTORS:

- Drugs and substances that may increase GTT values include acetylsalicylic acid, atenolol, bendroflumethiazide, clofibrate, fenfluramine, fluoxymesterone, glyburide, guanethidine, lisinopril, methandrostenolone, metoprolol, nandrolone, niceritrol, nifedipine, nitrendipine, norethisterone, phenformin, phenobarbital, prazosin, terazosin, and caffeine.

- Drugs and substances that may decrease GTT values include acebutolol, beclomethasone, bendroflumethiazide, betamethasone, calcitonin, catecholamines, chlorothiazide, chlorpromazine, chlorthalidone, cimetidine, corticotropin, cortisone, danazol, deflazacort, dexamethasone, diapamide, diethylstilbestrol, ethacrynic acid, fludrocortisone, furosemide, glucagon, glucocorticosteroids, heroin, hydrochlorothiazide, mephenytoin, mestranol, methadone, methandrostenolone, methylprednisolone, muzolimine, niacin, nifedipine, norethindrone, norethynodrel, oral contraceptives, paramethasone, perphenazine, phenolphthalein, phenothiazine, phenytoin, pindolol, prednisolone, prednisone, propranolol, quinethazone, thiazides, triamcinolone, triamterene, and verapamil.

- The test should be performed on

ambulatory patients. Impaired physical activity affects test results.

- Failure of the patient to ingest a diet with sufficient carbohydrate content (e.g., 150 g/day) for at least 3 days before the test can result in falsely decreased values.

- Impaired physical activity can lead to falsely increased values.

- Excessive physical activity before or during the test can lead to falsely decreased values.

- Smoking before or during the test can lead to falsely increased values.

- The patient should not be under recent or current physiologic stress during the test. If the patient has had recent surgery (less than 2 weeks previously), an infectious disease, or a major illness (e.g., myocardial infarction), the test should be delayed or rescheduled.

Nursing Implications and Procedure • • • • • • • • • • •

Pretest: ■

➤ Obtain a history of the patient's complaints, including a list of known allergens.

➤ Obtain a history of the patient's endocrine system as well as results of previously performed tests and procedures. For related tests, refer to the endocrine system table.

➤ Obtain a list of medications the patient is taking, including herbs, nutritional supplements, and nutraceuticals. The requesting health care practitioner and laboratory should be advised if the patient regularly uses these products so that their effects can be taken into consideration when reviewing results.

➤ There are no fluid or medication restrictions unless by medical direction.

➤ The patient should fast for at least 8 to 12 hours before the standard oral and standard gestational GTTs.

➤ Review the procedure with the patient.

➤ Inform the patient that specimen collection takes approximately 5 to 10 minutes.

Intratest: ■

➤ Ensure that the patient has complied with dietary preparations and other pretesting restrictions.

➤ Direct the patient to breathe normally and to avoid unnecessary movement.

➤ Observe standard precautions and follow the general guidelines in Appendix A. Perform the venipuncture, and collect the specimen in a 5-mL gray-top tube.

Standard oral GTT:

➤ The standard oral GTT takes 2 hours. A fasting blood glucose is determined before administration of an oral glucose load. If the fasting blood glucose is less than 126 mg/dL, the patient is given an oral glucose load.

➤ An oral glucose load should not be administered *before* the value of the fasting specimen has been received. *If the fasting blood glucose is greater than 126 mg/dL, the glucola is not administered and the test is canceled.* The laboratory will follow its protocol as far as notifying the patient of his or her glucose level and the reason why the test was canceled. The requesting health care practitioner will then be issued a report indicating the glucose level and the cancellation of the test. A fasting glucose greater than 126 mg/dL indicates diabetes; therefore the glucola would never be administered before allowing the requesting health care practitioner to evaluate the clinical situation.

➤ Adults receive 75 g and children receive 1.75 g/kg ideal weight, not to exceed 75 g. The glucose load should be consumed within 5 minutes, and time 0 begins as soon as the patient begins to ingest the glucose load. A second specimen is collected at 2 hours, concluding the test. The test is discontinued if the patient vomits before all specimens have been collected.

Standard gestational screen:

➤ The standard gestational screen is performed on pregnant women. If results from the screen are abnormal, a full gestational GTT is performed. The gestational screen does not require a fast. The patient is given a 50-g oral glucose load. The glucose load should be consumed within 5 minutes, and time 0 begins as soon as the patient begins to ingest the glucose load. One hour after ingestion, a specimen is collected. The test is discontinued if the patient vomits before the 1-hour specimen has been collected.

Standard gestational GTT:

➤ The standard gestational GTT takes 3 hours. A fasting blood glucose is determined before administration of a 100-g oral glucose load. If the fasting blood glucose is less than 200 mg/dL, the patient is given an oral glucose load.

➤ An oral glucose load should not be administered *before* the value of the fasting specimen has been received. *If the fasting blood glucose is greater than 126 mg/dL, the glucola is not administered and the test is canceled* (see previous explanation).

➤ The glucose load should be consumed within 5 minutes, and time 0 begins as soon as the patient begins to ingest the glucose load. Subsequent specimens are collected at 1, 2, and 3 hours, concluding the test. The test is discontinued if the patient vomits before all specimens have been collected.

➤ Label the specimen, and promptly transport it to the laboratory. You must note the collection time on the specimen label. Do not wait until all specimens have been collected to transport.

Post-test:

➤ Observe venipuncture site for bleeding or hematoma formation. Apply pressure bandage.

➤ Instruct the patient to resume usual diet as directed by the health care practitioner.

➤ The nutritional needs of each diabetic patient need to be determined individually (especially during pregnancy) with the appropriate health care professionals, particularly professionals trained in nutrition. Patients who adhere to dietary recommendations report a better general feeling of health, better weight management, greater control of glucose and lipid values, and improved use of insulin. There is no "diabetic diet"; however, many meal-planning approaches with nutritional goals are endorsed by the American Dietetic Association. The nutritional needs of each diabetic patient need to be determined individually with the appropriate health care professionals, particularly professionals trained in nutrition.

➤ Impaired glucose tolerance may be associated with diabetes. Instruct the patient and caregiver to report signs and symptoms of hypoglycemia (weakness, confusion, diaphoresis, rapid pulse) or hyperglycemia (thirst, polyuria, hunger, lethargy).

➤ Recognize anxiety related to test results and offer support. Provide teaching and information regarding the clinical implications of the test results, as appropriate. Emphasize, as appropriate, that good glycemic control delays the onset of and slows the progression of diabetic retinopathy, nephropathy, and neuropathy. Educate the patient regarding access to counseling services, as appropriate.

➤ Evaluate test results in relation to the patient's symptoms and other tests performed. Related laboratory tests include C-peptide, creatinine, fructosamine, glucose, glycated hemoglobin A_{1C}, insulin, insulin antibodies, ketones, microalbumin, and blood urea nitrogen (BUN).

γ-GLUTAMYLTRANSFERASE

SYNONYMS/ACRONYMS: Serum γ-glutamyltransferase, γ-glutamyl transpeptidase, GGT, SGGT.

SPECIMEN: Serum (1 mL) collected in a red- or tiger-top tube. Plasma (1 mL) collected in green-top (heparin) tube is also acceptable.

REFERENCE VALUE: (Method: Spectrophotometry)

Sex	Conventional Units	SI Units (Conversion Factor ×0.017)
Male	1–94 U/L	0.02–1.6 μKat/L
Female	1–70 U/L	0.02–1.2 μKat/L

DESCRIPTION: γ-Glutamyltransferase (GGT) assists with the reabsorption of amino acids and peptides from the glomerular filtrate and intestinal lumen. Hepatobiliary, renal tubular, and pancreatic tissue contain large amounts of GGT. Other sources include the prostate gland, brain, and heart. GGT is elevated in all types of liver disease and is more responsive to biliary obstruction, cholangitis, or cholecystitis than any of the other enzymes used as markers for liver disease. ∎

INDICATIONS:
• Assist in the diagnosis of obstructive jaundice in neonates

• Detect the presence of liver disease

• Evaluate and monitor patients with known or suspected alcohol abuse (levels rise after ingestion of small amounts of alcohol)

RESULT

Increased in:
• Cirrhosis
• Diabetes with hypertension
• Hepatitis
• Hepatobiliary tract disorders
• Hepatocellular carcinoma
• Hyperthyroidism
• Obstructive liver disease

- Pancreatitis
- Renal transplantation
- Significant alcohol ingestion

Decreased in:
- Hypothyroidism

CRITICAL VALUES: N/A

INTERFERING FACTORS:
- Drugs that may increase GGT levels include acetaminophen, aminoglutethimide, anticonvulsants, barbiturates, captopril, clotiazepam, disulfiram, methyldopa, oral contraceptives, phenothiazines, rifampin, and streptokinase.
- Drugs that may decrease GGT levels include bezafibrate, cefotaxime, clofibrate, fenofibrate, and ursodiol.

Nursing Implications and Procedure

Pretest:

➤ Obtain a history of the patient's complaints, including a list of known allergens.

➤ Obtain a history of the patient's hepatobiliary system as well as results of previously performed tests and procedures. For related tests, refer to the hepatobiliary system table.

➤ Obtain a list of the medications the patient is taking, including herbs, nutritional supplements, and nutraceuticals. The requesting health care practitioner and laboratory should be advised if the patient regularly uses these products so that their effects can be taken into consideration when reviewing results.

➤ There are no food, fluid, or medication restrictions unless by medical direction.

➤ Review the procedure with the patient.

➤ Inform the patient that specimen collection takes approximately 5 to 10 minutes.

Intratest:

➤ Direct the patient to breathe normally and to avoid unnecessary movement.

➤ Observe standard precautions and follow the general guidelines in Appendix A. Perform a venipuncture, collect the specimen in a 5-mL red- or tiger-top tube.

➤ Label the specimen, and promptly transport it to the laboratory.

Post-test:

➤ Observe venipuncture site for bleeding or hematoma formation. Apply pressure bandage.

➤ Increased GGT levels may be associated with liver disease. Dietary recommendations may be indicated and vary depending on the condition and its severity. Currently, there are no specific medications that can be given to cure hepatitis, but elimination of alcohol ingestion and a diet optimized for convalescence are commonly included in the treatment plan. A high-calorie, high-protein, moderate-fat diet with a high fluid intake is often recommended for patients with hepatitis. Treatment of cirrhosis is different because a low-protein diet may be in order if the patient's liver has lost the ability to process the end products of protein metabolism. A diet of soft foods also may be required if esophageal varices have developed. Ammonia levels may be used to determine whether protein should be added to or reduced from the diet. The patient should be encouraged to eat simple carbohydrates and emulsified fats (as in homogenized milk or eggs) as opposed to complex carbohydrates (e.g., starch, fiber, and glycogen [animal carbohydrates]) and complex fats, which would require additional bile to emulsify it so that it could be used. The cirrhotic patient should also be carefully observed for the development of ascites, in which case fluid and electrolyte balance requires strict attention. The alcoholic patient should be encouraged to avoid alcohol and to seek appropriate counseling for substance abuse.

➤ Evaluate test results in relation to the patient's symptoms and other tests performed. Related laboratory tests include alanine aminotransferase, alkaline phosphatase and isoenzymes, ammonia, aspartate aminotransferase, bilirubin, and electrolytes.

GLYCATED HEMOGLOBIN A$_{1C}$

SYNONYMS/ACRONYM: Hemoglobin A$_{1C}$, A$_{1C}$.

SPECIMEN: Whole blood (1 mL) collected in a lavender-top (ethylenediaminetetra-acetic acid [EDTA]) tube.

REFERENCE VALUE: (Method: Chromatography)

Total A$_1$	4.0–7.0%
A$_{1C}$	4.0–5.5%

Values vary widely by method.

DESCRIPTION: *Glycosylated* or *glycated hemoglobin* is a term used to describe the combination of glucose and hemoglobin into a ketamine; the rate at which this occurs is proportional to glucose concentration. The average life span of a red blood cell is approximately 120 days; measurement of glycated hemoglobin is a way to monitor long-term diabetic management.

Diabetes is a group of diseases characterized by hyperglycemia or elevated glucose levels. Hyperglycemia results from a defect in insulin secretion (type 1 diabetes), a defect in insulin action, or a combination of dysfunction secretion and action (type 2 diabetes). The chronic hyperglycemia of diabetes over time results in damage, dysfunction, and eventually failure of the eyes, kidneys, nerves, heart, and blood vessels. Hemoglobin A$_{1C}$ levels are not age dependent and are not affected by exercise, diabetic medications, or nonfasting state before specimen collection. ■

INDICATIONS: Assess long-term glucose control in diabetics

RESULT

Increased in:
• Diabetes (poorly controlled or uncontrolled)

Decreased in:
• Chronic blood loss

• Chronic renal failure

- Conditions that decrease red blood cell life span

- Hemolytic anemia

- Pregnancy

CRITICAL VALUES: N/A

INTERFERING FACTORS:

- Drugs that may increase glycated hemoglobin A_{1C} values include hydrochlorothiazide, indapamide, insulin, morphine, propranolol, and sulfonylureas.

- Drugs that may decrease glycated hemoglobin A_{1C} values include carbamate, galactose, metformin, and salicylate.

- Conditions involving abnormal hemoglobins (hemoglobinopathies) affect the reliability of glycated hemoglobin A_{1C} values, causing (1) falsely increased values, (2) falsely decreased values, or (3) discrepancies in either direction depending on the method.

Nursing Implications and Procedure • • • • • • • • • • •

Pretest: ▪

➤ Obtain a history of the patient's complaints, including a list of known allergens.

➤ Obtain a history of the patient's endocrine system as well as results of previously performed tests and procedures. For related tests, refer to the endocrine system table.

➤ Obtain a list of medications the patient is taking, including herbs, nutritional supplements, and nutraceuticals. The requesting health care practitioner and laboratory should be advised if the patient regularly uses these products so that their effects can be taken into consideration when reviewing results.

➤ There are no food, fluid, or medication restrictions unless by medical direction.

➤ Review the procedure with the patient.

➤ Inform the patient that specimen collection takes approximately 5 to 10 minutes.

Intratest: ▪

➤ Direct the patient to breathe normally and to avoid unnecessary movement.

➤ Observe standard precautions and follow the general guidelines in Appendix A. Perform a venipuncture, and collect the specimen in a 5-mL lavender-top tube.

➤ Label the specimen, and promptly transport it to the laboratory.

Post-test: ▪

➤ Observe venipuncture site for bleeding or hematoma formation. Apply pressure bandage.

➤ Increased glycated hemoglobin A_{1C} levels may be associated with diabetes. Instruct the diabetic patient, as appropriate, in nutritional management of the disease. Patients who adhere to dietary recommendations report a better general feeling of health, better weight management, greater control of glucose and lipid values, and improved use of insulin. There is no "diabetic diet"; however, many meal-planning approaches with nutritional goals are endorsed by the American Dietetic Association. The nutritional needs of each diabetic patient must be determined individually with the appropriate health care professionals, particularly professionals trained in nutrition.

➤ Instruct the patient and caregiver to report signs and symptoms of hypoglycemia (weakness, confusion, diaphoresis, rapid pulse) or hyperglycemia (thirst, polyuria, hunger, lethargy).

➤ Emphasize, as appropriate, that good glycemic control delays the onset of and slows the progression of diabetic retinopathy, nephropathy, and neuropathy.

➤ Evaluate test results in relation to the patient's symptoms and other tests performed. Related laboratory tests include C-peptide, fructosamine, glucose, glucose tolerance tests, insulin, insulin antibodies, ketones, and microalbumin.

GRAM STAIN

SYNONYM/ACRONYM: N/A.

SPECIMEN: Blood, biopsy specimen, or body fluid as collected for culture.

REFERENCE VALUE: N/A.

DESCRIPTION: Gram stain is a technique commonly used to identify bacterial organisms based on their specific staining characteristics. The method involves smearing a small amount of specimen on a slide, and then exposing it to gentian or crystal violet, iodine, alcohol, and safranin O. Gram-positive bacteria retain the gentian or crystal violet and iodine stain complex after a decolorization step and appear purple-blue in color. Gram-negative bacteria do not retain the stain after decolorization but can pick up the pink color of the safranin O counterstain. Gram stain results should be correlated with culture results to interpret the significance of isolated organisms. A sputum Gram stain showing greater than 25 squamous epithelial cells per low-power field, regardless of the number of polymorphonuclear white blood cells, indicates contamination of the specimen with saliva and should be rejected for subsequent culture. The occasional presence of bacteria in an unspun urine Gram stain suggests a correlating colony count of 10,000 bacteria/mL. The presence of bacteria in most fields is clinically significant and suggests greater than 100,000 bacteria/mL of urine. ■

INDICATIONS:

• Provide a rapid determination of the acceptability of the specimen for further analysis

• Provide rapid, presumptive information about the type of potential pathogen present in the specimen (i.e., gram-positive bacteria, gram-negative bacteria, or yeast)

RESULT

Gram Positive	Gram Negative			Acid Fast or Partial Acid Fast
Actinomadura	Acinetobacter	Helicobacter	Xanthomonas	Nocardia
Actinomyces	Aeromonas	Klebsiella	Yersinia	Mycobacterium
Bacillus	Alcaligenes	Legionella		
Clostridium	Bacteroides	Leptospira		
Corynebacterium	Bordetella	Moraxella		
Enterococcus	Borrelia	Neisseria		
Erysipelothrix	Brucella	Pasteurella		
Lactobacillus	Campylobacter	Plesiomonas		
Listeria	Citrobacter	Porphyromonas		
Micrococcus	Chlamydia	Prevotella		
Mycobacterium	Enterobacter	Proteus		
(gram variable)	Escherichia	Pseudomonas		
Peptostreptococcus	Flavobacter	Rickettsia		
Propionibacterium	Francisella	Salmonella		
Rhodococcus	Fusobacterium	Serratia		
Staphylococcus	Gardnerella	Shigella		
Streptococcus	Haemophilus	Vibrio		

Note: *Treponema* species are classified as gram-negative spirochetes, but they are most often visualized using dark-field or silver staining techniques.

CRITICAL VALUES: ⚠ Organisms detected in cerebrospinal fluid or in specimens obtained by aseptic technique should be reported immediately.

INTERFERING FACTORS: Very young, very old, or dead cultures may react atypically to the Gram stain technique.

Nursing Implications and Procedure • • • • • • • • • • •

Pretest: ■

➤ Obtain a history of the patient's complaints, including a list of known allergens.

➤ Obtain a history of the patient's gastrointestinal, genitourinary, immune, reproductive, and respiratory systems, as well as results of previously performed tests and procedures. For related tests, refer to the gastrointestinal, genitourinary, immune, reproductive, and respiratory system tables.

➤ Obtain a list of medications the patient is taking, including herbs, nutritional supplements, and nutraceuticals. The requesting health care practitioner and laboratory should be advised if the patient regularly uses these products so that their effects can be taken into consideration when reviewing results.

➤ There are no food, fluid, or medication restrictions unless by medical direction.

➤ Inform the patient that the test helps identify organisms that cause infections.

➤ Review the procedure with the patient.

➤ The time it takes to collect a proper specimen varies according to the patient's level of cooperation as well as the specimen collection site.

Intratest: ■	**Post-test:** ■
➤ Specific collection instructions are found in the associated culture monograph. ➤ Label the specimen, and promptly transport it to the laboratory.	➤ Evaluate test results in relation to the patient's symptoms and other tests performed. Related laboratory tests include bacterial and viral cultures.

GROUP A STREPTOCOCCAL SCREEN

• •

SYNONYMS/ACRONYM: Strep screen, rapid strep screen, direct strep screen.

SPECIMEN: Throat swab (two swabs should be submitted so that a culture can be performed if the screen is negative).

REFERENCE VALUE: (Method: Enzyme immunoassay or latex agglutination) Negative.

DESCRIPTION: Rheumatic fever is a possible sequela to an untreated streptococcal infection. Early diagnosis and treatment appear to lessen the seriousness of symptoms during the acute phase and overall duration of the infection and sequelae. The onset of strep throat is sudden and includes symptoms such as chills, headache, sore throat, malaise, and exudative gray-white patches on the tonsils or pharynx. The group A streptococcal screen should not be ordered unless the results would be available within 1 to 2 hours of specimen collection to make rapid, effective therapeutic decisions. A positive result can be a reliable basis for the initiation of therapy. A negative result is presumptive for infection and should be backed up by culture results. In general, specimens showing growth of less than 10 colonies on culture yield negative results by the rapid screening method. Evidence of group A streptococci disappears rapidly after the initiation of antibiotic therapy. A nucleic acid probe method has also been developed for rapid detection of group A streptococci. ■

INDICATIONS: Assist in the rapid determination of the presence of group A streptococci

RESULT

Positive findings in:
• Rheumatic fever

• Scarlet fever

• Streptococcal glomerulonephritis

• Strep throat

• Tonsillitis

CRITICAL VALUES: N/A

INTERFERING FACTORS:
• Polyester swabs are favored over cotton for best chance of detection.

• Sensitivity of the method varies from manufacturer to manufacturer.

• Adequate specimen collection in children may be difficult to achieve, which explains the higher percentage of false-negative results in this age group.

Nursing Implications and Procedure • • • • • • • • • • •

Pretest:

➤ Obtain a history of the patient's complaints, including a list of known allergens.

➤ Obtain a history of the patient's immune and respiratory systems, as well as results of previously performed tests and procedures. For related tests, refer to the immune and respiratory system tables.

➤ Obtain a history of prior antibiotic therapy.

➤ Obtain a list of medications the patient is taking, including herbs, nutritional supplements, and nutraceuticals. The requesting health care practitioner and laboratory should be advised if the patient regularly uses these products so that their effects

can be taken into consideration when reviewing results.

➤ There are no food, fluid, or medication restrictions unless by medical direction.

➤ Before specimen collection, verify with the laboratory whether wet or dry swabs are preferred for collection.

➤ Review the procedure with the patient.

➤ Inform the patient that specimen collection takes approximately 5 minutes.

Intratest:

➤ Observe standard precautions and follow the general guidelines in Appendix A. Vigorous swabbing of both tonsillar pillars and the posterior throat enhances the probability of streptococcal antigen detection.

➤ Label the specimen, and promptly transport it to the laboratory.

Post-test:

➤ Administer antibiotics as ordered, and emphasize to the patient the importance of completing the entire course of antibiotic therapy even if no symptoms are present.

➤ Evaluate test results in relation to the patient's symptoms and other tests performed. Related laboratory tests include complete blood count, Gram stain, and relevant cultures.

GROWTH HORMONE, STIMULATION AND SUPPRESSION TESTS

• •

SYNONYMS/ACRONYMS: Somatotropic hormone, somatotropin, GH, hGH.

SPECIMEN: Serum (1 mL) collected in a red- or tiger-top tube.

REFERENCE VALUE: (Method: Radioimmunoassay)

Growth Hormone

Age	Conventional Units	SI Units (Conversion Factor ×1)
Cord blood	8–40 ng/mL	8–40 μg/L
1 d	5–50 ng/mL	5–50 μg/L
1 wk	5–25 ng/mL	5–25 μg/L
Child	2–10 ng/mL	2–10 μg/L
Adult		
Male	0–5 ng/mL	0–5 μg/L
Female	0–10 ng/mL	0–10 μg/L
Male older than 60 y	0–10 ng/mL	0–10 μg/L
Female older than 60 y	0–14 ng/mL	0–14 μg/L
Stimulation Tests		
Rise above baseline	Greater than 5 ng/mL	Greater than 5 μg/L
Peak response	Greater than 10 ng/mL	Greater than 10 μg/L
Suppression Tests		
	0–2 ng/mL	0–2 μg/L

DESCRIPTION: Human growth hormone (GH) is secreted in episodic bursts by the anterior pituitary gland; the highest level is usually secreted during deep sleep. GH plays an integral role in growth from birth to puberty. GH promotes skeletal growth by stimulating hepatic production of proteins; it also affects lipid and glucose metabolism. Random levels are rarely useful because secretion of GH is episodic and pulsatile. Stimulation tests with arginine, glucagon, insulin, or L-dopa, as well as suppression tests with glucose, provide useful information. ■

INDICATIONS:

- Assist in the diagnosis of acromegaly in adults

- Assist in establishing a diagnosis of dwarfism or growth retardation in children with decreased GH levels, indicative of a pituitary cause

- Monitor response to treatment of growth retardation

- Detect suspected disorder associated with decreased GH

- Assist in establishing a diagnosis of gigantism in children with GH increased levels, indicative of a pituitary cause

RESULT

Increased in:

- Acromegaly

- Anorexia nervosa

- Cirrhosis

- Diabetes (uncontrolled)

- Ectopic GH secretion (neoplasms of stomach, lung)

- Exercise

- Gigantism (pituitary)

- Hyperpituitarism

- Laron dwarfism
- Malnutrition
- Renal failure
- Stress

Decreased in:

- Adrenocortical hyperfunction
- Dwarfism (pituitary)
- Hypopituitarism

CRITICAL VALUES: N/A

INTERFERING FACTORS:

- Drugs that may increase GH levels include alanine, anabolic steroids, angiotensin II, apomorphine, arginine, clonidine, corticotropin, cyclic AMP, desipramine dexamethasone, dopamine, fenfluramine, galanin, glucagon, GH-releasing hormone, levodopa, methamphetamine, methyldopa hydrazine, metoclopramide, midazolam, niacin, oral contraceptives, phenytoin, propranolol, and vasopressin.

- Drugs that may decrease GH levels include corticosteroids, corticotropin, hydrocortisone, octreotide, and pirenzepine.

- Recent radioactive scans or radiation within 1 week before the test can interfere with test results when radioimmunoassay is the test method.

Nursing Implications and Procedure • • • • • • • • • • •

Pretest: ▮

➤ Obtain a history of the patient's complaints, including a list of known allergens.

➤ Obtain a history of the patient's endocrine system as well as results of previously performed tests and procedures. For related tests, refer to the endocrine system table.

➤ Obtain a list of medications the patient is taking, including herbs, nutritional supplements, and nutraceuticals. The requesting health care practitioner and laboratory should be advised if the patient regularly uses these products that so their effects can be taken into consideration when reviewing results.

➤ Note any recent procedures that can interfere with test results.

➤ There are no fluid or medication restrictions unless by medical direction.

➤ The patient should fast and avoid strenuous exercise for 12 hours before specimen collection.

➤ The patient should have bed rest for 1 hour before each sample is obtained.

➤ Record pertinent information related to diet, sleep pattern, and activity at the time of the test.

➤ Review the procedure with the patient. Inform the patient that multiple specimens may be required.

➤ Inform the patient that each specimen collection takes approximately 5 to 10 minutes.

Intratest: ▮

➤ Ensure that the patient has complied with dietary preparations and other pretesting restrictions.

➤ Direct the patient to breathe normally and to avoid unnecessary movement.

➤ Observe standard precautions and follow the general guidelines in Appendix A. Perform a venipuncture, and collect the specimen in a 5-mL red- or tiger-top tube.

➤ Test samples may be requested at baseline and 10-, 20-, 30-, 45-, and 60-minute intervals after stimulation and at baseline and 30-, 60-, 90-, and 120-minute intervals after suppression.

➤ Label the specimen, and promptly transport it to the laboratory.

Post-test:

➤ Observe venipuncture site for bleeding or hematoma formation. Apply pressure bandage.

➤ Instruct the patient to resume normal diet as directed by the health care practitioner.

➤ Evaluate test results in relation to the patient's symptoms and other tests performed. A related laboratory test is adrenocorticotropic hormone.

HAM'S TEST FOR PAROXYSMAL NOCTURNAL HEMOGLOBINURIA

SYNONYM/ACRONYM: Acid hemolysis test for PNH.

SPECIMEN: Whole blood (5 mL) collected in lavender-top (ethylenediaminetetra-acetic acid [EDTA]) top tube and serum (3 mL) collected in red-top tube.

REFERENCE VALUE: (Method: Acidified hemolysis) No hemolysis seen.

DESCRIPTION: Paroxysmal nocturnal hemoglobinuria (PNH) is a condition in which the patient experiences nocturnal hemoglobinuria, chronic hemolytic anemia, diminished or absent generation of new red blood cells (RBCs), and a tendency to thrombose. It is caused by an acquired defect in hematopoietic stem cells. In patients with PNH, erythrocytes have an increased sensitivity to complement and will lyse when mixed with acidified serum containing complement. The patient's RBCs are also mixed with fresh normal serum that is ABO compatible with the patient's cells. Some of the control serum is acidified, and some is heated to inactivate the complement. The result is posi-

tive if 10 to 50 percent cell lysis occurs in the samples mixed with patient and control acidified serum. No hemolysis should occur in the heated control serum. The sugar water test can also be performed to investigate the presence of PNH. Platelet and granulocyte membranes are affected as well, but RBC hemolysis in a positive test is clear evidence of PNH. ■

INDICATIONS:

• Evaluate hemolytic anemia, especially with hemosiderinuria

• Evaluate suspected congenital dyserythropoietic anemia, type II (also known as HEMPAS [*h*ereditary *e*rythroblastic *m*ultinuclearity with *p*ositive *a*cidified *s*erum test])

• Evaluate suspected PNH

RESULT

Increased in:

• Paroxysmal nocturnal hemoglobinuria

• Congenital dyserythropoietic anemia, type II

Decreased in: N/A

CRITICAL VALUES: N/A

INTERFERING FACTORS:

• False-positives may occur in the presence of other disorders, such as aplastic anemia, HEMPAS, hereditary or acquired spherocytosis, leukemia, and myeloproliferative syndromes. False-positives may also occur with aged RBCs. The sugar water test is negative in HEMPAS.

• False-negatives can occur if the patient's serum sample contains a low level of complement.

Nursing Implications and Procedure • • • • • • • • • • •

Pretest:

➤ Obtain a history of the patient's complaints, including a list of known allergens.

➤ Obtain a history of the patient's hematopoietic system, as well as results of previously performed tests and procedures. For related tests refer to the hematopoietic system table.

➤ Obtain a list of the medications the patient is taking, including herbs, nutritional supplements, and nutraceuticals. The requesting health care practitioner and laboratory should be advised if the patient regularly uses these products so that their effects can be taken into consideration when reviewing results.

➤ There are no food, fluid, or medication restrictions unless by medical direction.

➤ Review the procedure with the patient.

➤ Inform the patient that specimen collection takes approximately 5 to 10 minutes.

Intratest:

➤ Direct the patient to breathe normally and to avoid unnecessary movement.

➤ Observe standard precautions and follow the general guidelines in Appendix A. Perform a venipuncture, collect the specimen in a 5-mL lavender-top and 5-mL red-top tube.

➤ Label the specimen, and promptly transport it to the laboratory.

Post-test:

➤ Observe venipuncture site for bleeding or hematoma formation. Apply pressure bandage.

➤ Evaluate test results in relation to the patient's symptoms and other tests performed. Related laboratory tests include bone marrow biopsy, complete blood count, direct Coombs' test, glucose-6-phosphate dehydrogenase, hemosiderin, and osmotic fragility.

HAPTOGLOBIN

. . . .

SYNONYMS/ACRONYMS: Hapto, HP, Hp.

SPECIMEN: Serum (1 mL) collected in a red- or tiger-top tube.

REFERENCE VALUE: (Method: Nephelometry)

Age	Conventional Units	SI Units (Conversion Factor ×0.01)
Newborn	5–48 mg/dL	0.05–0.48 g/L
6 mo–16 y	25–138 mg/dL	0.25–1.38 g/L
Adult	15–200 mg/dL	0.15–2.00 g/L

DESCRIPTION: Haptoglobin is an α_2-globulin produced in the liver. It binds with the free hemoglobin released when red blood cells (RBCs) are lysed. If left unchecked, free hemoglobin in the plasma can cause renal damage; haptoglobin prevents it from accumulating. In conditions such as hemolytic anemia, so many hemolyzed RBCs are available for binding that the liver cannot compensate by producing additional haptoglobin fast enough, resulting in low serum levels. ■

INDICATIONS:

• Assist in the investigation of suspected transfusion reaction

• Evaluate known or suspected chronic liver disease, as indicated by decreased levels

• Evaluate known or suspected disorders characterized by excessive RBC hemolysis, as indicated by decreased levels

• Evaluate known or suspected disorders involving a diffuse inflammatory process or tissue destruction, as indicated by elevated levels

RESULT

Increased in:

• Biliary obstruction

• Disorders involving tissue destruction, such as cancers, burns, and acute myocardial infarction

• Infection or inflammatory diseases, such as ulcerative colitis, arthritis, and pyelonephritis

• Neoplasms

• Steroid therapy

Decreased in:

• Autoimmune hemolysis

• Hemolysis due to mechanical destruction (e.g., artificial heart valves, contact sports, subacute bacterial endocarditis)

• Hemolysis due to drug reaction

• Hemolysis due to RBC membrane or metabolic defects

• Hemolysis due to transfusion reaction

- Hypersplenism

- Ineffective hematopoiesis due to conditions such as folate deficiency or hemoglobinopathies

- Liver disease

CRITICAL VALUES: N/A

INTERFERING FACTORS:

- Drugs that may increase haptoglobin levels include anabolic steroids, danazol, ethylestrenol, fluoxymesterone, methandrostenolone, norethandrolone, oxandrolone, oxymetholone, and stanozolol.

- Drugs that may decrease haptoglobin levels include acetanilid, aminosalicylic acid, chlorpromazine, dapsone, dextran, diphenhydramine, furadaltone, furazolidone, isoniazid, nitrofurantoin, norethindrone, oral contraceptives, quinidine, resorcinol, stibophen, tamoxifen, thiazolsulfone, and tripelennamine.

Nursing Implications and Procedure • • • • • • • • • • •

Pretest: ■

➤ Obtain a history of the patient's complaints, including a list of known allergens.

➤ Obtain a history of the patient's hematopoietic, hepatobiliary, and immune systems, as well as results of previously performed tests and procedures. For related tests, refer to the hematopoietic and immune system tables.

➤ Obtain a list of the medications the patient is taking, including herbs, nutritional supplements, and nutraceuticals. The requesting health care practitioner and laboratory should be advised if the patient regularly uses these products so that their effects can be taken into consideration when reviewing results.

➤ There are no food, fluid, or medication restrictions unless by medical direction.

➤ Review the procedure with the patient.

➤ Inform the patient that specimen collection takes approximately 5 to 10 minutes.

Intratest: ■

➤ Direct the patient to breathe normally and to avoid unnecessary movement.

➤ Observe standard precautions and follow the general guidelines in Appendix A. Perform a venipuncture, and collect the specimen in a 5-mL red-top tube.

➤ Label the specimen, and promptly transport it to the laboratory.

Post-test: ■

➤ Observe venipuncture site for bleeding or hematoma formation. Apply pressure bandage.

➤ Instruct the patient to immediately report symptoms of hemolysis, including chills, fever, flushing, back pain, and fast heartbeat.

➤ Evaluate test results in relation to the patient's symptoms and other tests performed. Related laboratory tests include direct antiglobulin test, indirect antiglobulin test, bilirubin, and blood group and type.

HELICOBACTER PYLORI ANTIBODY

SYNONYM/ACRONYM: *H. pylori.*

SPECIMEN: Serum (1 mL) collected in a plain red-top tube.

REFERENCE VALUE: (Method: Enzyme-linked immunosorbent assay [ELISA]) Negative.

DESCRIPTION: There is a strong association between *Helicobacter pylori* infection and gastric cancer, duodenal and gastric ulcer, and chronic gastritis. Immunoglobulin G (IgG) antibodies can be detected for up to 1 year after treatment. The presence of *H. pylori* can also be demonstrated by a positive urea breath test, positive stool culture, or positive endoscopic biopsy. Patients with symptoms and evidence of *H. pylori* infection are considered to be *infected* with the organism; patients who demonstrate evidence of *H. pylori* but are without symptoms are said to be *colonized.* ■

INDICATIONS:
- Assist in differentiating between *H. pylori* infection and nonsteroidal anti-inflammatory drug (NSAID) use as the cause of gastritis or peptic or duodenal ulcer
- Assist in establishing a diagnosis of gastritis, gastric carcinoma, or peptic or duodenal ulcer

RESULT

Positive findings in:
- *H. pylori* infection
- *H. pylori* colonization

Negative findings in: N/A

CRITICAL VALUES: N/A

INTERFERING FACTORS: N/A

Nursing Implications and Procedure

Pretest:
- Obtain a history of the patient's complaints, including a list of known allergens.
- Obtain a history of the patient's gastrointestinal and immune systems, as well as results of previously performed tests and procedures. For related tests, refer to the gastrointestinal and immune system tables.
- Obtain a list of the medications the patient is taking, including herbs, nutritional supplements, and nutraceuticals. The requesting health care practitioner and laboratory should be advised if the patient regularly uses these products so that their effects can be taken into consideration when reviewing results.
- There are no food, fluid, or medication restrictions unless by medical direction.
- Inform the patient that each specimen collection takes approximately 5 to 10 minutes.

Intratest: ■

➤ Direct the patient to breathe normally and to avoid unnecessary movement.

➤ Observe standard precautions and follow the general guidelines in Appendix A. Perform a venipuncture, and collect the specimen in a 5-mL red-top tube.

➤ Label the specimen, and promptly transport it to the laboratory.

Post-test: ■

➤ Observe venipuncture site for bleeding or hematoma formation. Apply pressure bandage.

➤ Inform the patient that a positive test result constitutes an independent risk factor for gastric cancer.

➤ Evaluate test results in relation to the patient's symptoms and other tests performed. Related laboratory tests include gastrin and gastric acid stimulation.

HEMATOCRIT

· ·

SYNONYMS/ACRONYMS: Packed cell volume (PCV), Hct.

SPECIMEN: Whole blood from one full lavender-top (ethylenediaminetetraacetic acid [EDTA]) tube, Microtainer, or capillary. Whole blood from a green-top (lithium or sodium heparin) tube may also be submitted.

REFERENCE VALUE: (Method: Automated, computerized, multichannel analyzers)

Hematocrit

Age	Conventional Units (%)	SI Unit (Volume Fraction, Conversion Factor ×0.01)
Cord blood	47–57	0.47–0.57
1 d	51–65	0.51–0.65
2 wk	47–57	0.47–0.57
1 mo	38–52	0.38–0.52
6 mo	35–41	0.35–0.41
1 y	37–41	0.37–0.41
10 y	36–42	0.36–0.42
Adult		
Male	43–49	0.43–0.49
Female	38–44	0.38–0.44

DESCRIPTION: Blood consists of a fluid portion (plasma) and a solid portion that includes red blood cells (RBCs), white blood cells, and platelets. The hematocrit, or packed cell volume, is the percentage of RBCs in a volume of whole blood. For example, a hematocrit (Hct) of 45 percent means that a 100-mL sample of blood contains 45 mL of packed RBCs. Although Hct depends primarily on the number of RBCs, the average size of the RBCs plays a role. Conditions that cause the RBCs to swell, such as when the serum sodium concentration is elevated, may increase the Hct level.

Hct level is included in the complete blood count (CBC) and is generally tested together with hemoglobin (Hgb). These levels parallel each other and are the best determinant of the degree of anemia or polycythemia. *Polycythemia* is a term used in conjunction with conditions resulting from an abnormal increase in Hgb, Hct, and RBC count. *Anemia* is a term associated with conditions resulting from an abnormal decrease in Hgb, Hct, and RBC count. Results of the Hgb, Hct, and RBC count should be evaluated simultaneously because the same underlying conditions affect this triad of tests similarly. The RBC count multiplied by three should approximate the Hgb concentration. The Hct should be within three times the Hgb if the RBC population is normal in size and shape. The Hct plus six should approximate the first two figures of the RBC count within three (e.g., Hct is 40 percent; therefore 40 + 6 = 46, and the RBC count should be 4.3–4.9). There are some cultural variations in Hgb and Hct (H&H) values. After the first decade of life, the mean Hgb in African-Americans is 0.5 to 1.0 g lower than in Caucasians. Mexican-Americans and Asian-Americans have higher H&H values than Caucasians. ■

INDICATIONS:

- Detect hematologic disorder, neoplasm, or immunological abnormality

- Determine the presence of hereditary hematologic abnormality

- Evaluate known or suspected anemia and related treatment, in combination with Hgb

- Monitor blood loss and response to blood replacement, in combination with Hgb

- Monitor the effects of physical or emotional stress

- Monitor fluid imbalances or their treatment

- Monitor hematologic status during pregnancy, in combination with Hgb

- Monitor the progression of nonhematologic disorders such as chronic obstructive pulmonary disease, malabsorption syndromes, cancer, and renal disease

- Monitor response to drugs or chemotherapy, and evaluate undesired reactions to drugs that may cause blood dyscrasias

- Provide screening as part of a CBC count in a general physical examination, especially upon admission to a health care facility or before surgery

RESULT

Increased in:

- Erythrocytosis

- Hemoconcentration

- Polycythemia

- Shock

Decreased in:

- Anemia

- Blood loss (acute and chronic)

- Bone marrow hyperplasia

- Burns (severe)

- Chronic disease

- Hemolytic reactions

CRITICAL VALUES:

Less than 18 percent
Greater than 54 percent
Note and report to the health care practitioner any critically increased or decreased values and symptoms:

- Severe hemodilution can lead to cardiac failure and death. Symptoms of hemodilution include rales, anxiety, restlessness, edema, hypertension, jugular venous distention, and shortness of breath. Possible interventions include diuretics, restriction of fluids and sodium, and careful monitoring of input and output. Symptoms of blood loss include bleeding, hypotension, and hypoxia. Once the cause of blood loss has been identified, possible interventions include blood transfusion and administration of vasopressin, omeprazole, or isotonic fluids.

- Severe hemoconcentration can lead to spontaneous blood clotting. Symptoms of hemoconcentration include decreased pulse pressure and volume, loss of skin turgor, dry mucous membranes, low central venous pressure, orthostatic hypotension, tachycardia, thirst, and weakness. Possible interventions include intravenous fluids and discontinuance of diuretics if they are believed to be contributing to critically elevated Hct. Symptoms of polycythemic overload crisis include signs of thrombosis, pain and redness in extremities, facial flushing, and irritability. Possible interventions include therapeutic phlebotomy and intravenous fluids.

INTERFERING FACTORS:

- Drugs and substances that may cause a decrease in Hct include those that induce hemolysis due to drug sensitivity or enzyme deficiency, such as aminopyrine, aminosalicylic acid, amphetamine, anticonvulsants, antimalarials, antipyretics, cephalothin, chloroquine, chlorothiazide, chlorpromazine, colchicine, corticosteroids, dapsone, dimercaprol, diphenhydramine, dipyrone, glucosulfone, glycerin, gold, mephytoin, methyldopa, nalidixic acid, neomycin, niridazole, nitrobenzene, nitrofurantoin, novobiocin, penicillin, phenacemide, pipobroman (intended effect for polycythemia), primaquine, probenecid, propranolol, pyrazolones, quinines, streptomycin, sulfamethizole, sulfamethoxypyridazine, sulfisoxazole, suramin, tolbutamide, trimethadione, and tripelennamine.

- Some drugs may also affect Hct values by increasing or decreasing the RBC count (see monograph titled "Red Blood Cell Count").

- The results of RBC counts may vary depending on the patient's position: Hct can decrease when the patient is recumbent as a result of hemodilution and can increase when the patient rises as a result of hemoconcentration.

- Leaving the tourniquet in place for longer than 60 seconds can falsely increase levels by 2 to 5 percent.

- Traumatic venipuncture and hemolysis may result in falsely decreased values.

- Failure to fill the tube sufficiently (i.e., tube less than three-quarters full) may yield inadequate sample volume for automated analyzers and may be reason for specimen rejection.

- Clotted specimens must be rejected for analysis.

- Care should be taken in evaluating the Hct during the first few hours after transfusion or acute blood loss because the value may appear to be normal and may not be a reliable indicator of anemia.

- Abnormalities in the RBC size (macrocytes, microcytes) or shape (spherocytes, sickle cells) may alter values, as in diseases and conditions including sickle cell anemia, hereditary spherocytosis, and iron deficiency

- Elevated blood glucose or serum sodium levels may produce elevated levels because of swelling of the erythrocytes.

Nursing Implications and Procedure • • • • • • • • • • •

Pretest: ■

➤ Obtain a history of the patient's complaints, including a list of known allergens.

➤ Obtain a history of the patient's cardiovascular, gastrointestinal, hematopoietic, hepatobiliary, immune, musculoskeletal, and respiratory systems, as well as results of previously performed tests and procedures. For related tests, refer to the cardiovascular, gastrointestinal, hematopoietic, hepatobiliary, immune, musculoskeletal, and respiratory system tables.

➤ Obtain a list of the medications the patient is taking, including herbs, nutritional supplements, and nutraceuticals. The requesting health care practitioner and laboratory should be advised if the patient regularly uses these products so their that effects can be taken into consideration when reviewing results.

➤ Note any recent procedures that can interfere with test results.

➤ There are no food, fluid, or medication restrictions unless by medical direction.

➤ Review the procedure with the patient.

➤ Inform the patient that specimen collection takes approximately 5 to 10 minutes.

Intratest: ■

➤ Direct the patient to breathe normally and to avoid unnecessary movement.

➤ Observe standard precautions and follow the general guidelines in Appendix A. Perform a venipuncture, and collect the specimen in a 5-mL lavender-top (EDTA) tube. An EDTA Microtainer sample may be obtained from infants, children, and adults for whom venipuncture may not be feasible. The specimen should be mixed gently by inverting the tube 10 times. It is stable when stored for up to 6 hours at room temperature or 24 hours if stored refrigerated. In addition, if it is anticipated that the specimen will not be analyzed within 4 to 6 hours, two blood smears should be made immediately after the venipuncture and submitted with the blood sample.

➤ Label the specimen, and promptly transport it to the laboratory.

Post-test: ■

➤ Observe venipuncture site for bleeding or hematoma formation. Apply pressure bandage.

➤ Nutritional therapy may be indicated for patients with decreased Hct. Iron deficiency is the most common nutrient deficiency in the United States. Patients at risk (e.g., children, pregnant women and women of childbearing age, low-income populations) should be instructed to include foods that are high in iron in their diet, such as meats (especially liver), eggs, grains, vegetables, and multivitamins with iron. Iron absorption is affected by numerous factors (see monograph titled "Iron").

➤ Evaluate test results in relation to the patient's symptoms and other tests performed. Related laboratory tests include CBC count, erythropoietin, ferritin, iron/total iron-binding capacity, peripheral blood smear, and reticulocyte count.

HEMOGLOBIN

· ·

SYNONYM/ACRONYM: Hgb.

SPECIMEN: Whole blood from one full lavender-top (ethylenediaminetetraacetic acid [EDTA]) tube, Microtainer, or capillary. Whole blood from a green-top (lithium or sodium heparin) tube may also be submitted.

REFERENCE VALUE: (Method: Spectrophotometry)

Age	Conventional Units	SI Units (Conversion Factor ×10)
Cord blood	13.5–20.5 g/dL	135–205 mmol/L
2 wk	13.4–19.8 g/dL	134–198 mmol/L
1 mo	10.7–17.1 g/dL	107–171 mmol/L
6 mo	11.1–14.4 g/dL	111–144 mmol/L
1 y	11.3–14.1 g/dL	113–141 mmol/L
9–14 y	12.0–14.4 g/dL	120–144 mmol/L
Adult		
Male	13.2–17.3 g/dL	132–173 mmol/L
Female	11.7–15.5 g/dL	117–155 mmol/L
Older adult (65–74 y)		
Male	12.6–17.4 g/dL	126–174 mmol/L
Female	11.7–16.1 g/dL	117–161 mmol/L

DESCRIPTION: Hemoglobin (Hgb) is the main intracellular protein of erythrocytes. It carries oxygen (O_2) to and removes carbon dioxide (CO_2) from red blood cells (RBCs). It also serves as a buffer to maintain acid-base balance in the extracellular fluid. Each Hgb molecule consists of heme and globulin. Copper is a cofactor necessary for the enzymatic incorporation of iron molecules into heme. Heme contains iron and porphyrin molecules that have a high affinity for O_2. The affinity of Hgb molecules for O_2 is influenced by 2,3-diphosphoglycerate (2,3-DPG), a substance produced by anaerobic glycolysis to generate energy for the RBCs. When Hgb binds with 2,3-DPG, O_2 affinity decreases. The ability of Hgb to bind and release O_2 can be graphically represented by an oxyhemoglobin dissociation curve. The term *shift to the left* is used to describe an increase in the affinity of Hgb for O_2. Conditions that can cause this leftward shift include decreased body temperature, decreased 2,3-DPG, decreased CO_2 concentration, or increased pH. Conversely, a *shift to* *the right* represents a decrease in the affinity of Hgb for O_2. Conditions that can cause a rightward shift include increased body temperature, increased 2,3-DPG levels, increased CO_2 concentration, or decreased pH.

Hgb levels are a direct reflection of the O_2-combining capacity of the blood. It is the combination of heme and O_2 that gives blood its characteristic red color. RBC counts parallel the O_2-combining capacity of Hgb, but because some RBCs contain more Hgb than other cells, the relationship is not directly proportional. As CO_2 diffuses into RBCs, an enzyme called carbonic anhydrase converts the CO_2 into bicarbonate and hydrogen ions. Hgb that is not bound to O_2 combines with the free hydrogen ions, increasing pH. As this binding is occurring, bicarbonate is leaving the RBC in exchange for chloride ions. (For additional information about the relationship between the respiratory and renal components of this buffer system, see monograph titled "Blood Gases.")

Hgb is included in the complete blood count (CBC) and generally performed with a hematocrit (Hct). These levels parallel each other and are frequently used to evaluate anemia. *Polycythemia* is a term used in conjunction with conditions resulting from an abnormal increase in Hgb, Hct, and RBC count. *Anemia* is a term associated with conditions resulting from an abnormal decrease in Hgb, Hct, and RBC count. Results of the Hgb, Hct, and RBC count should be evaluated simultaneously because the same underlying conditions affect this triad of tests similarly. The RBC count multiplied by three should approximate the Hgb concentration. The Hct should be within three times the Hgb if the RBC population is normal in size and shape. The Hct plus six should approximate the first two figures of the RBC count within three (e.g., Hct is 40 percent; therefore $40 + 6 = 46$, and the RBC count should be 4.6 or in the range of 4.3–4.9). There are some cultural variations in Hgb and Hct (H&H) values. After the first decade of life, the mean Hgb in African-Americans is 0.5 to 1.0 g lower than in Caucasians. Mexican-Americans and Asian-Americans have higher Hgb and H&H values than Caucasians. ∎

INDICATIONS:

- Detect hematologic disorder, neoplasm, or immunologic abnormality

- Determine the presence of hereditary hematologic abnormality

- Evaluate known or suspected anemia and related treatment, in combination with Hct

- Monitor blood loss and response to blood replacement, in combination with Hct

- Monitor the effects of physical or emotional stress on the patient

- Monitor hematologic status during pregnancy, in combination with Hct

- Monitor the progression of nonhematologic disorders, such as chronic obstructive pulmonary disease (COPD), malabsorption syndromes, cancer, and renal disease

- Monitor response to drugs or chemotherapy, and evaluate undesired reactions to drugs that may cause blood dyscrasias

- Provide screening as part of a CBC in a general physical examination, especially upon admission to a health care facility or before surgery

RESULT

Increased in:

• Burns

• COPD

• Congestive heart failure

• Dehydration

• Erythrocytosis

• Hemoconcentration

• High altitudes

• Polycythemia vera

Decreased in:

• Anemias

• Carcinoma

• Fluid retention

• Hemolytic disorders

• Hemoglobinopathies

• Hemorrhage (acute and chronic)

• Hodgkin's disease

• Incompatible blood transfusion

• Intravenous overload

• Leukemia

• Lymphomas

• Nutritional deficit

• Pregnancy

• Splenomegaly

CRITICAL VALUES:

Less than 6.0 g/dL

Greater than 18.0 g/dL

Note and report critically increased or decreased values and symptoms to the health care practitioner:

• Severe hemodilution can lead to cardiac failure and death. Symptoms of hemodilution include rales, anxiety, restlessness, edema, hypertension, jugular venous distention, and short-

ness of breath. Possible interventions include diuretics, restriction of fluids and sodium, and careful monitoring of input and output. Symptoms of blood loss include bleeding, hypotension, and hypoxia. Once the cause of blood loss has been identified, possible interventions include blood transfusion and administration of vasopressin, omeprazole, or isotonic fluids.

• Severe hemoconcentration can lead to spontaneous blood clotting. Symptoms of hemoconcentration include decreased pulse pressure and volume, loss of skin turgor, dry mucous membranes, low central venous pressure, orthostatic hypotension, tachycardia, thirst, and weakness. Possible interventions include intravenous fluids and discontinuance of diuretics if they are believed to be contributing to critically elevated Hct. Symptoms of polycythemic overload crisis include signs of thrombosis, pain and redness in extremities, facial flushing, and irritability. Possible interventions include therapeutic phlebotomy and intravenous fluids.

INTERFERING FACTORS:

• Drugs and substances that may cause a decrease in Hgb levels include those that induce hemolysis due to drug sensitivity or enzyme deficiency, such as acetaminophen, aminopyrine, aminosalicylic acid, amphetamine, antipyrine, arsenicals, benzene, busulfan, anticonvulsants, carbenicillin, cephalothin, chemotherapy, chlorate, chloroquine, chlorothiazide, chlorpromazine, colchicine, diphenhydramine, dipyrone, glucosulfone, gold, hydroflumethiazide, indomethacin, mephenytoin, nalidixic acid, neomycin, nitrofurantoin, penicillin, phenacemide, phenazopyridine, phenothiazines; and those that result in anemia, such as miconazole and penicillamine, phenylhydrazine, primaquine, probenecid, pyrazolones, pyrimethamine, quinines, streptomycin, sulfamethizole, sulfamethoxypyridazine, sulfisoxazole, suramin, thioridazine, tolbutamide, trimethadione, and tripelennamine.

- Some drugs may also affect Hgb values by increasing or decreasing the RBC count (see monograph titled "Red Blood Cell Count").

- The results of RBC counts may vary depending on the patient's position: Hct can decrease when the patient is recumbent as a result of hemodilution and can increase when the patient rises as a result of hemoconcentration.

- Use of the neutraceutical liver extract is strongly contraindicated in iron-storage disorders, such as hemochromatosis, because it is rich in heme (the iron-containing pigment in Hgb).

- A severe copper deficiency may result in decreased Hgb levels.

- Cold agglutinins may falsely increase the mean corpuscular Hgb concentration (MCHC) and decrease the RBC count, affecting Hgb values. This can be corrected by warming the blood or replacing the plasma with warmed saline and repeating the analysis.

- Leaving the tourniquet in place for longer than 60 seconds can falsely increase levels by 2 to 5 percent.

- Failure to fill the tube sufficiently (i.e., tube less than three-quarters full) may yield inadequate sample volume for automated analyzers and may be reason for specimen rejection.

- Clotted specimens must be rejected for analysis.

- Care should be taken in evaluating the Hct during the first few hours after transfusion or acute blood loss because the value may appear to be normal.

- Lipemia will falsely increase the Hgb measurement, also affecting the mean corpuscular volume (MCV) and mean corpuscular Hgb (MCH). This can be corrected by replacing the plasma with saline, repeating the measurement, and manually correcting the Hgb, MCH, and MCHC using specific mathematical formulas.

Nursing Implications and Procedure

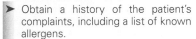

Pretest:

➤ Obtain a history of the patient's complaints, including a list of known allergens.

➤ Obtain a history of the patient's cardiovascular, gastrointestinal, hematopoietic, hepatobiliary, immune, musculoskeletal, and respiratory systems, as well as results of previously performed tests and procedures. For related tests, refer to the cardiovascular, gastrointestinal, hematopoietic, hepatobiliary, immune, musculoskeletal, and respiratory system tables.

➤ Obtain a list of the medications the patient is taking, including herbs, nutritional supplements, and nutraceuticals. The requesting health care practitioner and laboratory should be advised if the patient regularly uses these products so that their effects can be taken into consideration when reviewing results.

➤ Note any recent procedures that can interfere with test results.

➤ There are no food, fluid, or medication restrictions unless by medical direction.

➤ Review the procedure with the patient.

➤ Inform the patient that specimen collection takes approximately 5 to 10 minutes.

Intratest:

➤ Direct the patient to breathe normally and to avoid unnecessary movement.

➤ Observe standard precautions and

follow the general guidelines in Appendix A. Perform a venipuncture, and collect the specimen in a 5-mL lavender-top (EDTA) tube. An EDTA Microtainer sample may be obtained from infants, children, and adults for whom venipuncture may not be feasible. The specimen should be mixed gently by inverting the tube 10 times. It is stable when stored for up to 6 hours at room temperature or 24 hours if stored refrigerated. In addition, if it is anticipated that the specimen will not be analyzed within 4 to 6 hours, two blood smears should be made immediately after the venipuncture and submitted with the blood sample.

➤ Label the specimen, and promptly transport it to the laboratory.

Post-test:

➤ Observe venipuncture site for bleed-ing or hematoma formation. Apply pressure bandage.

➤ Nutritional therapy may be indicated for patients with decreased Hct. Iron deficiency is the most common nutrient deficiency in the United States. Patients at risk (e.g., children, pregnant women and women of childbearing age, low-income populations) should be instructed to include foods that are high in iron in their diet, such as meats (especially liver), eggs, grains, vegetables, and multivitamins with iron. Iron absorption is affected by numerous factors (see monograph titled "Iron").

➤ Evaluate test results in relation to the patient's symptoms and other tests performed. Related laboratory tests include CBC, erythropoietin, ferritin, iron/total iron-binding capacity, peripheral blood smear, and reticulocyte count.

HEMOGLOBIN ELECTROPHORESIS

• •

SYNONYM/ACRONYM: N/A

SPECIMEN: Whole blood (1 mL) collected in a lavender-top (ethylenedi-aminetetra-acetic acid [EDTA]) tube.

REFERENCE VALUE: (Method: Electrophoresis)

Hgb A	
Adult	Greater than 95%

Hgb A₂	
Adult	1.5–3.7%

(Continued on the following page)

Hgb F	
Newborns and infants	
1 d–3 wk	70–77%
6–9 wk	42–64%
3–4 mo	7–39%
6 mo	3–7%
8–11 mo	0.6–2.6%
Adult	Less than 2%

DESCRIPTION: Hemoglobin (Hgb) electrophoresis is a separation process used to identify normal and abnormal forms of Hgb. Hgb A is the main form of Hgb in the normal adult. Hgb F is the main form of Hgb in the fetus, the remainder being composed of Hgb A_1 and A_2. Small amounts of Hgb F are normal in the adult. Hgb D, E, H, S, and C result from abnormal amino acid substitutions during the formation of Hgb and are inherited hemoglobinopathies. ■

INDICATIONS:

• Assist in the diagnosis of Hgb C disease

• Assist in the diagnosis of thalassemia, especially in patients with a family history positive for the disorder

• Differentiate among thalassemia types

• Evaluate hemolytic anemia of unknown cause

• Evaluate a positive sickle cell screening test to differentiate sickle cell trait from sickle cell disease

RESULT

Increased:

• Hgb A_2:
  Megaloblastic anemia
  Thalassemias

• Hgb F:
  Acquired aplastic anemia
  Hereditary persistence of fetal Hgb

Hyperthyroidism
Leakage of fetal blood into maternal circulation
Leukemia (acute or chronic)
Myeloproliferative disorders
Sickle cell disease
Thalassemias

• β-Chain substitutions:

Hgb C (second most common variant in the United States, it has a higher prevalence among African-Americans):
  • Hgb C disease

Hgb D (rare hemoglobinopathy that may also be found in combination with Hgb S or thalassemia):
  • Splenomegaly without other significant clinical implications

Hgb E (second most common hemoglobinopathy in the world, occurs with the highest frequency in Southeast Asians and African-Americans):
  • Thalassemia-like condition

Hgb S (most common variant in the United States, occurs with a frequency of about 8 percent among African-Americans):
  • Sickle cell trait or disease

• α-Chain substitutions:
Hgb H:
  • α Thalassemias
Bart's Hgb:
  • α Thalassemias
  • Hgb Bart's hydrops fetalis syndrome

Decreased:

- Hgb A$_2$:
  Erythroleukemia:
  - Hgb H disease
  - Iron-deficiency anemia (untreated)
  - Sideroblastic anemia

CRITICAL VALUES: N/A

INTERFERING FACTORS:
- High altitude and dehydration may increase values.

- Iron deficiency may decrease Hgb A$_2$, C, and S.

- In patients less than 3 months of age, false-negative results for Hgb S occur in coincidental polycythemia.

- Red blood cell transfusion within 4 months of test can mask abnormal Hgb levels.

Nursing Implications and Procedure • • • • • • • • • •

Pretest:

➤ Obtain a history of the patient's complaints, including a list of known allergens.

➤ Obtain a history of the patient's hematopoietic system, as well as results of previously performed tests and procedures. For related tests, refer to the hematopoietic system table.

➤ Obtain a list of the medications the patient is taking, including herbs, nutritional supplements, and nutraceuticals. The requesting health care practitioner and laboratory should be advised if the patient is regularly using these products so that their effects can be taken into consideration when reviewing results.

➤ Note any recent procedures that can interfere with test results.

➤ There are no food, fluid, or medication restrictions unless by medical direction.

➤ Review the procedure with the patient. Sensitivity to cultural and social issues is important in providing psychological support.

➤ Inform the patient that specimen collection takes approximately 5 to 10 minutes.

Intratest:

➤ Direct the patient to breathe normally and to avoid unnecessary movement.

➤ Observe standard precautions and follow the general guidelines in Appendix A. Perform a venipuncture, and collect the specimen in a 5-mL lavender-top tube.

➤ Label the specimen, and promptly transport it to the laboratory.

Post-test:

➤ Observe venipuncture site for bleeding or hematoma formation. Apply pressure bandage.

➤ Evaluate test results in relation to the patient's symptoms and other tests performed. Related laboratory tests include blood gases, complete blood count (including evaluation of blood smear for RBC morphology), methemoglobin, and sickle cell screen.

HEMOSIDERIN

SYNONYMS/ACRONYM: Hemosiderin stain, Pappenheimer body stain, iron stain.

SPECIMEN: Urine (5 mL) from a random first morning sample, collected in a clean, plastic collection container.

REFERENCE VALUE: (Method: Microscopic examination of Prussian blue–stained specimen) None seen.

DESCRIPTION: Hemosiderin stain is used to indicate the presence of iron storage granules called *hemosiderin* by microscopic examination of urine sediment. Granules of hemosiderin stain blue when potassium ferrocyanide is added to the sample. Hemosiderin is normally found in the liver, spleen, and bone marrow, but not in the urine. Under normal conditions, hemosiderin is absorbed by the renal tubules; however, in extensive hemolysis, renal tubule damage, or an iron metabolism disorder, hemosiderin filters its way into the urine. The Prussian blue stain may also be used to identify siderocytes (iron-containing red blood cells [RBCs]) in peripheral blood. The presence of siderocytes in circulating RBCs is abnormal. ■

INDICATIONS:
• Assist in the diagnosis of hemochromatosis (tissue damage caused by iron toxicity)
• Detect excessive RBC hemolysis within the systemic circulation
• Evaluate renal tubule dysfunction

RESULT

Increased in:
• Burns
• Cold hemagglutinin disease
• Hemochromatosis
• Hemolytic transfusion reactions
• Mechanical trauma to RBCs
• Megaloblastic anemia
• Microangiopathic hemolytic anemia
• Paroxysmal nocturnal hemoglobinuria
• Pernicious anemia
• Sickle cell anemia
• Thalassemia major

Decreased in: N/A

CRITICAL VALUES: N/A

INTERFERING FACTORS: N/A

Nursing Implications and Procedure

Pretest: ■

➤ Obtain a history of the patient's

complaints, including a list of known allergens.

➤ Obtain a history of the patient's hematopoietic system, especially a history of hemolytic anemia, as well as results of previously performed tests and procedures. For related tests, refer to the hematopoietic system table.

➤ Obtain a list of the medications the patient is taking, including herbs, nutritional supplements, and nutraceuticals. The requesting health care practitioner and laboratory should be advised if the patient regularly uses these products so that their effects can be taken into consideration when reviewing results.

➤ There are no food, fluid, or medication restrictions unless by medical direction.

➤ Review the procedure with the patient.

➤ Inform the patient that specimen collection takes approximately 5 to 10 minutes.

Intratest:

➤ Observe standard precautions and follow the general guidelines in Appendix A.

Clean-catch specimen:

➤ Instruct the male patient to (1) thor-oughly wash his hands, (2) cleanse the meatus, (3) void a small amount into the toilet, and (4) void directly into the specimen container.

➤ Instruct the female patient to (1) thoroughly wash her hands; (2) cleanse the labia from front to back; (3) while keeping the labia separated, void a small amount into the toilet; and (4) without interrupting the urine stream, void directly into the specimen container.

Indwelling catheter:

➤ Put on gloves. Empty drainage tube of urine. It may be necessary to clamp off the catheter for 15 to 30 minutes before specimen collection. Cleanse specimen port with antiseptic swab, and then aspirate 5 mL of urine with a 21- to 25-gauge needle and syringe. Transfer urine to a collection container.

➤ Label the specimen, and promptly transport it to the laboratory.

Post-test:

➤ Evaluate test results in relation to the patient's symptoms and other tests performed. Related laboratory tests include bone marrow studies, complete blood count (CBC), iron/total iron-binding capacity, ferritin, kidney biopsy, lead, and RBC morphology.

HEPATITIS A ANTIBODY

• •

SYNONYM/ACRONYM: HAV serology.

SPECIMEN: Serum (1 mL) collected in a red- or tiger-top tube.

REFERENCE VALUE: (Method: Enzyme immunoassay) Negative.

DESCRIPTION: The hepatitis A virus is classified as a picornavirus. Its primary mode of transmission is by the fecal-oral route under conditions of poor personal hygiene or inadequate sanitation. The incubation period is about 28 days, with a range of 15 to 50 days. Onset is usually abrupt, with the acute disease lasting about 1 week. Therapy is supportive and there is no development of chronic or carrier states. Assays for total (immunoglobulin G [IgG] and IgM) hepatitis A antibody and IgM-specific hepatitis A antibody assist in differentiating recent infection from prior exposure. If results from the IgM-specific or from both assays are positive, recent infection is suspected. If the IgM-specific test results are negative and the total antibody test results are positive, past infection is indicated. The clinically significant assay—IgM-specific antibody—is often the only test requested. Jaundice occurs in 70 to 80 percent of adult cases of HAV infection and in 70 percent of pediatric cases. ∎

INDICATIONS:

• Screen individuals at high risk of exposure, such as those in institutions or correctional facilities

• Screen individuals with suspected HAV infection

RESULT

Positive findings in:

• Individuals with current hepatitis A infection

• Individuals with past hepatitis A infection

CRITICAL VALUES: N/A

INTERFERING FACTORS: N/A

Nursing Implications and Procedure

Pretest:

➤ Obtain a history of the patient's complaints, including a list of known allergens.

➤ Obtain a history of the patient's hepatobiliary and immune systems, as well as results of previously performed tests and procedures. For related tests, refer to the hepatobiliary and immune system tables.

➤ Obtain a list of the medications the patient is taking, including herbs, nutritional supplements, and nutraceuticals. The requesting health care practitioner and laboratory should be advised if the patient regularly uses these products so that their effects can be taken into consideration when reviewing results.

➤ There are no food, fluid, or medication restrictions unless by medical direction.

➤ Review the procedure with the patient.

➤ Inform the patient that specimen collection takes approximately 5 to 10 minutes.

Intratest:

➤ Direct the patient to breathe normally and to avoid unnecessary movement.

➤ Observe standard precautions and follow the general guidelines in Appendix A. Perform a venipuncture, and collect the specimen in a 5-mL red- or tiger-top tube.

➤ Label the specimen, and promptly transport it to the laboratory.

Post-test:

➤ Observe venipuncture site for bleeding or hematoma formation. Apply pressure bandage.

➤ Dietary recommendations may be indicated and will vary depending on the type and severity of the condition. Elimination of alcohol ingestion and a diet optimized for convalescence are commonly included in the treatment plan.

➤ Recognize anxiety related to test results and offer support. Provide teaching and information regarding the clinical implications of the test results, as appropriate.

➤ Counsel the patient, as appropriate, regarding risk of transmission and proper prophylaxis. Immune globulin can be given before exposure (in the case of individuals who may be traveling to a location where the disease is endemic) or after exposure, during the incubation period. Prophylaxis is most effective when administered 2 weeks after exposure.

➤ Evaluate test results in relation to the patient's symptoms and other tests performed. Related laboratory tests include alanine aminotransferase, alkaline phosphatase, aspartate aminotransferase, bilirubin, γ-glutamyl transpeptidase, and hepatitis B and C antigens and antibodies.

HEPATITIS B, ANTIGEN AND ANTIBODY

SYNONYMS/ACRONYMS: HBeAg, HBeAb, HBcAb, HBsAb, HBsAg.

SPECIMEN: Serum (1 mL) collected in a red- or tiger-top tube.

REFERENCE VALUE: (Method: Enzyme immunoassay) Negative.

DESCRIPTION: The hepatitis B virus (HBV) is classified as a double-stranded DNA retrovirus of the Hepadnaviridae family. Its primary modes of transmission are parenteral, perinatal, and sexual contact. Serological profiles vary with different scenarios (i.e., asymptomatic infection, acute/resolved infection, coinfection, and chronic carrier state). The formation and detectability of markers is also dose dependent. The following description refers to HBV infection that becomes resolved. The incubation period is generally 6 to 16 weeks. The hepatitis B surface antigen (HBsAg) is the first marker to appear after infection. It is detectable 8 to 12 weeks after exposure and often precedes symptoms. At about the time liver enzymes fall back to normal levels, the HBsAg titer has fallen to nondetectable levels. If the HBsAg remains detectable after 6 months, the patient will likely become a chronic carrier who can transmit the virus. Hepatitis Be antigen (HBeAg) appears in the serum 10 to 12 weeks after exposure. HBeAg can be found in the serum of patients with acute or chronic HBV infection and is a sign of active viral replication and infectivity. Levels of hepatitis Be antibody (HBeAb) appear about 14 weeks after exposure, suggesting resolution of the infection and reduction of the patient's ability to transmit the disease. The more quickly HBeAg disappears, the shorter the acute phase of the infection. IgM-specific hepatitis B core antibody (HBcAb) appears 6 to 14 weeks after exposure to HBsAg and continues to be detectable either until the infection is resolved or over the life span in patients who are in a chronic carrier state. In some cases HBcAb may be the only detectable marker; hence its lone appearance has sometimes been referred to as the *core window.* HBcAb is not an indicator of recovery or immunity; however, it does indicate current or previous infection. Hepatitis B surface antibody (HBsAb) appears 2 to 16 weeks after HBsAg disappears. Appearance of HBsAb represents clinical recovery and immunity to the virus. Onset of HBV infection is usually insidious. Most children and half of infected adults are asymptomatic. During the acute phase of infection, symptoms range from mild to severe. Chronicity decreases with age. HBsAg and HBcAb tests are used to screen donated blood before transfusion. HBsAg testing is often part of the routine prenatal screen. ■

INDICATIONS:

• Detect exposure to HBV

• Detect possible carrier status

• Screen donated blood before transfusion

• Screen for individuals at high risk of exposure, such as hemodialysis patients, persons with multiple sex partners, persons with a history of other sexually transmitted diseases, intravenous drug abusers, infants born to infected mothers, individuals residing in institutions or correctional facilities, recipients of blood- or plasma-derived products, allied health care workers, and public service employees who come in contact with blood and blood products.

RESULT

Positive findings in:

• Patients currently infected with HBV

• Patients with a past HBV infection

CRITICAL VALUES: N/A

INTERFERING FACTORS: Drugs that may decrease HBeAb and HBsAb include interferon.

Nursing Implications and Procedure • • • • • • • • • •

Pretest:

➤ Obtain a history of the patient's complaints, including a list of known allergens.

➤ Obtain a history of the patient's hepatobiliary and immune systems, as well as results of previously performed tests and procedures. For related tests, refer to the hepatobiliary and immune system tables.

➤ Obtain a history of intravenous drug use, high-risk sexual activity, or occupational exposure.

➤ Obtain a list of the medications the patient is taking, including herbs, nutritional supplements, and nutraceuticals. The requesting health care practitioner and laboratory should be advised if the patient is regularly using these products so that their effects can be taken into consideration when reviewing results.

➤ There are no food, fluid, or medication restrictions unless by medical direction.

➤ Review the procedure with the patient.

➤ Inform the patient that specimen collection takes approximately 5 to 10 minutes.

Intratest:

➤ Direct the patient to breathe normally and to avoid unnecessary movement.

➤ Observe standard precautions and follow the general guidelines in Appendix A. Perform a venipuncture, and collect the specimen in a 5-mL red- or tiger-top tube.

➤ Label the specimen, and promptly transport it to the laboratory.

Post-test:

➤ Observe venipuncture site for bleeding or hematoma formation. Apply pressure bandage.

➤ Dietary recommendations may be indicated and will vary depending on the type and severity of the condition. Elimination of alcohol ingestion and a diet optimized for convalescence are commonly included in the treatment plan. A high-calorie, high-protein, moderate-fat diet with a high fluid intake is often recommended for patients with hepatitis.

➤ Recognize patient anxiety related to test results and offer support. Provide teaching and information regarding the clinical implications of the test results, as appropriate. Counsel the patient, as appropriate, regarding risk of transmission and proper prophylaxis. Hepatitis B immune globulin (HBIG) vaccination should be given immediately after situations in which there is a potential for HBV exposure (e.g. accidental

needle stick, perinatal period, sexual contact) for temporary, passive protection. Some studies have indicated that alpha interferon may be useful in the treatment of chronic hepatitis.

➤ Counsel the patient and significant contacts, as appropriate, that HBIG immunization is available and has in fact become a requirement in many places as part of childhood immunization and employee health programs. Parents may choose to sign a waiver preventing their newborns from receiving the vaccine; they may choose not to vaccinate on the basis of philosophical, religious, or medical reasons. Vaccination regulations vary from state to state.

➤ Inform the patient that positive findings must be reported to local health department officials, who will question him or her regarding sexual partners.

➤ Offer support, as appropriate, to patients who may be the victims of rape or other forms of sexual assault including children and elderly individuals. Educate the patient regarding access to counseling services. Provide a nonjudgmental, nonthreatening atmosphere for a discussion during which the risks of sexually transmitted diseases are explained. It is also important to discuss the problems that the patient may experience (e.g., guilt, depression, anger) if test results indicate the presence of hepatitis B antigen.

➤ Evaluate test results in relation to the patient's symptoms and other tests performed. Related laboratory tests include alanine aminotransferase, alkaline phosphatase, aspartate aminotransferase, bilirubin, liver biopsy, γ-glutamyl transpeptidase, human immunodeficiency virus (HIV) serology, and hepatitis C serology.

HEPATITIS C ANTIBODY

SYNONYMS/ACRONYMS: HCV serology, hepatitis non-A/non-B.

SPECIMEN: Serum (1 mL) collected in a red- or tiger-top tube.

REFERENCE VALUE: (Method: Enzyme immunoassay, branch DNA [bDNA], polymerase chain reaction [PCR], recombinant immunoblot assay [RIBA]) Negative.

DESCRIPTION: The hepatitis C virus (HCV) causes the majority of blood-borne non-A, non-B hepatitis. Its primary modes of transmission are parenteral, perinatal, and sexual contact. The virus is thought to be a flavivirus and contains a single-stranded RNA core. The incubation period varies widely, from 2 to 52 weeks. Onset is insidious, and the risk of chronic liver disease after infection is high. On average, antibodies to hepatitis C are detectable in approximately 45 percent of infected individuals within 6 weeks of infection. The remaining 55 percent produce antibodies within the next 6 to 12 months. Once infected with HCV, 50 percent of patients will become chronic carriers. Infected individuals and carriers have a high frequency of chronic liver diseases such as cirrhosis and chronic active hepatitis, and they have a higher risk of developing hepatocellular cancer. The transmission of hepatitis C by blood transfusion has decreased dramatically since it became part of the routine screening panel for blood donors. The possibil-ity of prenatal transmission exists, especially in the presence of human immunodeficiency virus (HIV) coinfection. Therefore, this test is often included in prenatal testing packages. ∎

INDICATIONS:

• Assist in the diagnosis of non-A, non-B viral hepatitis infection

• Monitor patients suspected of HCV infection but who have not yet produced antibody

• Screen donated blood before transfusion

RESULT

Positive findings in:

• Patients currently infected with HCV

• Patients with a past HCV infection

Negative findings in: N/A

CRITICAL VALUES: N/A

INTERFERING FACTORS: Drugs that may decrease hepatitis C antibody levels include interferon.

Nursing Implications and Procedure • • • • • • • • • • •

➤ Obtain a history of the patient's complaints, including a list of known allergens.

➤ Obtain a history of the patient's hepatobiliary and immune systems, as well as results of previously performed tests and procedures. For related tests, refer to the hepatobiliary and immune system tables.

➤ Obtain a history of intravenous drug use, high-risk sexual activity, or occupational exposure.

➤ Obtain a list of the medications the patient is taking, including herbs, nutritional supplements, and nutraceuticals. The requesting health care practitioner and laboratory should be advised if the patient is regularly using these products so that their effects can be taken into consideration when reviewing results.

➤ There are no food, fluid, or medication restrictions unless by medical direction.

➤ Review the procedure with the patient.

➤ Inform the patient that specimen collection takes approximately 5 to 10 minutes.

Intratest:

➤ Direct the patient to breathe normally and to avoid unnecessary movement.

➤ Observe standard precautions and follow the general guidelines in Appendix A. Perform a venipuncture, and collect the specimen in a 5-mL red- or tiger-top tube.

➤ Label the specimen, and promptly transport it to the laboratory.

Post-test:

➤ Observe venipuncture site for bleeding or hematoma formation. Apply pressure bandage.

➤ Dietary recommendations may be indicated and will vary depending on the type and severity of the condition. Currently, for example, there are no specific medications that can be given to cure hepatitis; however, bed rest, elimination of alcohol ingestion, and a diet optimized for convalescence are commonly included in the treatment plan. A high-calorie, high-protein, moderate-fat diet with a high fluid intake is often recommended for patients with hepatitis.

➤ Recognize patient anxiety related to test results and offer support. Provide teaching and information regarding the clinical implications of the test results, as appropriate. Counsel the patient, as appropriate, regarding the risk of transmission and proper prophylaxis. Alpha interferon was approved in 1991 by the U.S. Food and Drug Administration (FDA) for use as a therapeutic agent in the treatment of chronic HCV infection.

➤ Inform the patient that positive findings must be reported to local health department officials, who will question him or her regarding sexual partners.

➤ Offer support, as appropriate, to patients who may be the victims of rape or other forms of sexual assault including children and elderly individuals. Educate the patient regarding access to counseling services. Provide a nonjudgmental, nonthreatening atmosphere for a discussion during which risks of sexually transmitted diseases are explained. It is also important to discuss problems the patient may experience (e.g., guilt, depression, anger) if test results indicate the presence of hepatitis C antibodies.

➤ Evaluate test results in relation to the patient's symptoms and other tests performed. Related laboratory tests include alanine aminotransferase, alkaline phosphatase, aspartate aminotransferase, bilirubin, liver biopsy, γ-glutamyl transpeptidase, HIV serology, and hepatitis B serology.

HEPATITIS D ANTIBODY

SYNONYM/ACRONYM: Delta hepatitis.

SPECIMEN: Serum (1 mL) collected in a red- or tiger-top tube.

REFERENCE VALUE: (Method: Enzyme immunoassay, EIA) Negative.

DESCRIPTION: Symptoms of hepatitis D virus (HDV) infection are similar but often more severe than those of hepatitis B virus (HBV) infection. As with HBV, the primary modes of HDV transmission are parenteral, perinatal, and sexual contact. The virus contains a single-stranded RNA core. In order to replicate, it requires the presence of the hepatitis B outer coat. Therefore, HDV infection can only occur with hepatitis B coinfection or superinfection. Onset is abrupt, after an incubation period of 3 to 13 weeks. Because of its dependence on HBV, prevention can be accomplished by using the same preexposure and postexposure protective measures used for HBV (see monograph titled "Hepatitis B, Antigen and Antibody.") ■

INDICATIONS: Establish the presence of coinfection or superinfection in patients with HBV (clinical course of superinfection is more severe)

RESULT

Positive findings in:
• Individuals currently infected with HDV

• Individuals with a past HDV infection

CRITICAL VALUES: N/A

INTERFERING FACTORS: Drugs that may decrease hepatitis D antibody levels include interferon.

Nursing Implications and Procedure

Pretest:

➤ Obtain a history of the patient's complaints, including a list of known allergens.

➤ Obtain a history of the patient's hepatobiliary and immune systems, as well as results of previously performed tests and procedures. For related tests, refer to the hepatobiliary and immune system tables.

➤ Obtain a history of intravenous drug use, high-risk sexual activity, or occupational exposure.

➤ Obtain a list of the medications the patient is taking, including herbs, nutritional supplements, and nutraceuticals. The requesting health care practitioner and laboratory should be advised if the patient is regularly using these products so that their effects can be taken into consideration when reviewing results.

> There are no food, fluid, or medication restrictions unless by medical direction.

> Review the procedure with the patient.

> Inform the patient that specimen collection takes approximately 5 to 10 minutes.

Intratest:

> Direct the patient to breathe normally and to avoid unnecessary movement.

> Observe standard precautions and follow the general guidelines in Appendix A. Perform a venipuncture, and collect the specimen in a 5-mL red- or tiger-top tube.

> Label the specimen, and promptly transport it to the laboratory.

Post-test:

> Observe venipuncture site for bleeding or hematoma formation. Apply pressure bandage.

> Dietary recommendations may be indicated and will vary depending on the type and severity of the condition. Elimination of alcohol ingestion and a diet optimized for convalescence are commonly included in the treatment plan. A high-calorie, high-protein, moderate-fat diet with a high fluid intake is often recommended for patients with hepatitis.

> Recognize patient anxiety related to test results and offer support. Provide teaching and information regarding the clinical implications of the test results, as appropriate. Counsel the patient, as appropriate, regarding the risk of transmission and proper prophylaxis. Hepatitis B immune globulin (HBIG) vaccination should be given immediately after situations in which there is a potential for HBV exposure (e.g., accidental needle stick, perinatal period, sexual contact) for temporary, passive protection. Counsel the patient and significant contacts, as appropriate, that HBIG immunization is available and has in fact become a requirement in many places as part of childhood immunization and employee health programs. Parents may choose to sign a waiver preventing their newborns from receiving the vaccine; they may choose not to vaccinate on the basis of philosophical, religious, or medical reasons. Vaccination regulations vary from state to state.

> Evaluate test results in relation to the patient's symptoms and other tests performed. Related laboratory tests include hepatitis B serology.

HEPATOBILIARY SCAN

SYNONYM/ACRONYM: Hepatobiliary imaging, biliary tract radionuclide scan, hepatobiliary scintigraphy, gallbladder scan, cholescintigraphy, HIDA (a technetium-99m disopropyl analogue) scan.

AREA OF APPLICATION: Bile ducts.

CONTRAST: Intravenous contrast medium (aminodiacetic acid compounds), usually combined with technetium-99m.

DESCRIPTION: The hepatobiliary scan is a nuclear medicine study of the hepatobiliary excretion system. It is primarily used to determine the patency of the cystic and common bile ducts, but it can also be used to determine overall hepatic function, gallbladder function, presence of gallstones (indirectly), and sphincter of Oddi dysfunction. Technetium (Tc-99m) HIDA (tribromoethyl, an aminodiacetic acid) is injected intravenously (IV) and excreted into the bile duct system. A gamma camera detects the radiation emitted from the injected contrast medium, and a representative image of the duct system is obtained. The results are correlated with other diagnostic studies, such as IV cholangiography, computed tomography (CT) scan of the gallbladder, and ultrasonography. Gallbladder emptying or ejection fraction can be determined by administering a fatty meal or cholecystokinin to the patient. This procedure can be used before and after surgery to determine the extent of bile reflux. ■

INDICATIONS:
- Aid in the diagnosis of suspected gallbladder disorders, such as inflammation, perforation, or calculi
- Aid in the diagnosis of acute and chronic cholecystitis
- Determine common duct obstruction caused by tumors or choledocholithiasis
- Evaluate biliary enteric bypass patency
- Assess obstructive jaundice when done in combination with radiography or ultrasonography
- Assess enterogastric reflux

- Postoperatively evaluate gastric surgical procedures and abdominal trauma

RESULT

Normal Findings:
- Normal shape, size, and function of the gallbladder with patent cystic and common bile ducts

Abnormal Findings:
- Acalculous cholecystitis
- Acute cholecystitis
- Chronic cholecystitis
- Common bile duct obstruction secondary to gallstones, tumor, or stricture
- Congenital biliary atresia or choledochal cyst
- Postoperative biliary leak, fistula, or obstruction
- Trauma-induced bile leak or cyst

CRITICAL VALUES: N/A

INTERFERING FACTORS:

This procedure is contraindicated for:
- Patients who are pregnant or suspected of being pregnant, unless the potential benefits of the procedure far outweigh the risks to the fetus and mother

Factors that may impair clear imaging:
- Inability of the patient to cooperate or remain still during the procedure because of age, significant pain, or mental status
- Improper adjustment of the radiographic equipment to accommodate obese or thin patients, which can cause overexposure or underexposure and poor-quality study

- Patients who are very obese, who may exceed the weight limit for the equipment

- Incorrect positioning of the patient, which may produce poor visualization of the area to be examined

- Retained barium from a previous radiologic procedure

- Metallic objects within the examination field (e.g., jewelry or body rings), which may inhibit organ visualization and can produce unclear images

- Bilirubin levels greater than or equal to 30 mg/dL, depending on the radionuclide used, which may decrease hepatic uptake

- Other nuclear scans done within the previous 24 to 48 hours

- Fasting for more than 24 hours before the procedure, total parenteral nutrition, and alcoholism

- Ingestion of food or liquids within 2 to 4 hours before the scan

Other considerations:

- Failure to follow dietary restrictions before the procedure may cause the procedure to be canceled or repeated.

- Improper injection of the radionuclide that allows the tracer to seep deep into the muscle tissue can produce erroneous hot spots.

- Inaccurate timing of imaging after the radionuclide injection can affect the results.

- Consultation with a physician should occur before the procedure for radiation safety concerns regarding infants of patients who are lactating.

- Risks associated with radiographic overexposure can result from frequent x-ray procedures. Personnel in the room with the patient should wear a protective lead apron, stand behind a shield, or leave the area while the examination is being done. Personnel working in the area where the examination is being done should wear badges that reveal their level of exposure to radiation.

Nursing Implications and Procedure

Pretest:

➤ Inform the patient that the procedure detects inflammation or obstruction of the gallbladder or bile duct system.

➤ Inform the patient that the procedure is performed in a special nuclear medicine department by a technologist and usually takes approximately 60 to 90 minutes, and that delayed images are needed up to 24 hours after the initial injection. The patient may leave the department and return later to undergo delayed imaging.

➤ Obtain a history of the patient's complaints, including a list of known allergens.

➤ Obtain a history of the patient's gallbladder and hepatobiliary systems, as well as results of previously performed tests, treatments, surgeries, and procedures. For related tests, refer to the hepatobiliary system table.

➤ Obtain a list of the medications the patient is taking.

➤ Determine date of last menstrual period and possibility of pregnancy in perimenopausal women.

➤ Inform the patient that the technologist will place him or her in a supine position on a flat table for the injection.

➤ Ask the patient to lie very still during the procedure because movement will produce unclear images.

➤ Ensure that the patient fasted for 4 to 6 hours before the scan, unless otherwise indicated.

Intratest:

➤ Ask the patient to void before the procedure. Have the patient put on a hospital gown.

➤ Administer sedative to a child or to an uncooperative adult, as ordered.

➤ Ask the patient to lie still during the procedure because movement produces unclear images. Make sure jewelry, watches, chains, belts, and any other metallic objects have been removed.

➤ Place the patient in a supine position on a flat table with foam wedges to help maintain position and immobilization.

➤ IV radionuclide is administered, and the upper-right quadrant of the abdomen is scanned immediately with images taken every 5 minutes for the first 30 minutes and every 10 minutes for the next 30 minutes. Delayed views are taken in 2, 4, and 24 hours if the gallbladder cannot be visualized, in order to differentiate acute from chronic cholecystitis or to detect the degree of obstruction.

➤ IV morphine may be administered during the study to initiate spasms of the sphincter of Oddi, forcing the radionuclide into the gallbladder if the organ is not visualized within 1 hour of injection of the radionuclide. Imaging is then done 20 to 50 minutes later to determine delayed visualization or nonvisualization of the gallbladder.

➤ If gallbladder function or bile reflux is being assessed, the patient will be given a fatty meal or cholecystokinin 60 minutes after the injection.

➤ Wear gloves during the radionuclide administration and while handling the patient's urine.

Post-test:

➤ Instruct the patient to resume normal activity, medications, and diet, unless otherwise indicated.

➤ Advise patient to drink increased amounts of fluids for 24 to 48 hours to eliminate the radionuclide from the body, unless contraindicated. Tell the patient that radionuclide is eliminated from the body within 6 to 24 hours.

➤ Inform the patient to immediately flush the toilet after each voiding after the procedure and to meticulously wash hands with soap and water after each voiding for 24 hours after the procedure.

➤ Tell all caregivers to wear gloves when discarding urine for 24 hours after the procedure. Wash gloved hands with soap and water before removing gloves. Then wash ungloved hands after the gloves are removed.

➤ A physician specializing in this branch of medicine sends a written report to the ordering health care provider, who discusses the results with the patient.

➤ Evaluate test results in relation to the patient's symptoms and other tests performed. Related diagnostic tests include ultrasound of the liver and bile ducts, and CT and magnetic resonance imaging of the abdomen.

HER-2/NEU ONCOPROTEIN

• •

SYNONYM/ACRONYM: c-erb-B2.

SPECIMEN: Breast tissue or cells.

REFERENCE VALUE: (Method: Immunocytochemical) Negative.

DESCRIPTION: Breast cancer is the most common newly diagnosed cancer in American women. It is the second leading cause of cancer-related death. The presence of abnormal amounts of a protein called human epidermal growth factor receptor 2 (HER-2/neu oncoprotein) is helpful in establishing histologic evidence of metastatic breast cancer. Overexpression of this protein results from an acquired genetic mutation and occurs in 25 to 30 percent of patients with metastatic breast cancer. Metastatic breast cancer patients with high levels of HER-2/neu oncoprotein have a poor prognosis: They have rapid tumor progression, increased rate of recurrence, poor response to standard therapies, and a lower survival rate.

The specimen is collected by fine-needle or open biopsy. The tissue sample is treated with a material that binds to HER-2/neu oncoprotein. A dye is added to the tissue sample; areas of tissue that have large amounts of HER-2/neu oncoprotein are indicated by high-intensity color on the tissue sample. ■

INDICATIONS: Evidence of breast lesion by palpation, mammography, or ultrasound

RESULT

Positive findings in: Breast cancer

CRITICAL VALUES: N/A

INTERFERING FACTORS: N/A

Nursing Implications and Procedure • • • • • • • • • • •

Pretest:

➤ Obtain a history of the patient's complaints, including a list of known allergens.

➤ Obtain a history of the patient's immune and reproductive systems, as well as results of previously performed tests and procedures. For related tests, refer to the immune and reproductive system tables.

➤ Obtain a list of the medications the patient is taking, including herbs, nutritional supplements, and nutraceuticals. The requesting health care practitioner and laboratory should be advised if the patient regularly uses these products so that their effects can be taken into consideration when reviewing results.

➤ There are no food, fluid, or medication restrictions before fine-needle biopsy unless by medical direction; however, food and fluids are restricted for at least 12 hours before an open biopsy.

➤ Review the procedure with the patient. Sensitivity to cultural and social issues, as well as concern for modesty, is important in providing psychological support.

➤ Address concerns about pain related to the procedure, and explain that a sedative may be administered to promote relaxation during the procedure.

➤ Assess whether the patient has an allergy to local anesthetics, and inform the health care practitioner accordingly.

➤ Ensure that nonallergy to anesthesia is confirmed before open biopsy procedure is performed under general anesthesia.

➤ *Obtain written and informed consent before administering any medications prior to the procedure.*

➤ Prophylactic antibiotics may be administered before or after the procedure in certain cases.

➤ Inform the patient that specimen collection takes approximately 20 to 30 minutes.

Intratest:

➤ Observe standard precautions and follow the general guidelines in Appendix A.

Open biopsy:

➤ Record baseline vital signs. Ensure that the patient is in compliance with pretesting dietary restrictions before open biopsy. The specimen is obtained by surgical excision.

Needle biopsy:

➤ Assist the patient into a supine position and cleanse the area undergoing biopsy with an antiseptic. The local anesthetic is injected, and the biopsy site is protected with sterile drapes. Direct the patient to breathe normally and to avoid unnecessary movement. A needle is inserted into the mass, and tissue and fluid are aspirated.

General:

➤ Apply a sterile dressing to the site.

➤ Place the specimen in the appropriate containers.

➤ Label the specimen, indicating location (especially left or right), and promptly transport it to the laboratory.

Post-test:

➤ If the patient has undergone open biopsy, monitor vital signs and compare to baseline values.

➤ Instruct the patient to resume usual diet and medication, if withheld, as directed by the health care practitioner.

➤ Instruct the patient in proper cleansing of the site and of the importance of a follow-up appointment for suture removal, as appropriate.

➤ Instruct the patient to report excessive bleeding, redness, edema, or pain at the biopsy site.

➤ Administer analgesics and antibiotics as ordered, and instruct the patient in the importance of completing the entire course of antibiotic therapy, if prescribed, even if no symptoms are present.

➤ Instruct and educate the patient regarding monthly breast self-examination, and emphasize, as appropriate, the importance of having a mammogram performed annually.

➤ Recognize anxiety related to test results and offer support. Provide teaching and information regarding the clinical implications of the test results, as appropriate. Educate the patient regarding access to counseling services.

➤ Evaluate test results in relation to the patient's symptoms and other tests performed. Related laboratory tests include breast biopsy, CA 15-3, carcinoembryonic antigen, and estrogen and progesterone receptors.

HEXOSAMINIDASE A AND B

SYNONYM/ACRONYM: N/A.

SPECIMEN: Serum (3 mL) collected in a red-top tube. After the specimen is collected it *must* be brought immediately to the laboratory. The specimen must be allowed to clot for 1 to 1.5 hours in the refrigerator. The serum should be removed and frozen immediately.

REFERENCE VALUE: (Method: Fluorometry)

Total Hexosaminidase	Conventional Units	SI Units (Conversion Factor ×0.0167)
Noncarrier	589–955 nmol/h/mL	9.83–15.95 U/L
Heterozygote	465–675 nmol/h/mL	3.30–5.39 U/L
Tay-Sachs homozygote	Greater than 1027 nmol/h/mL	Greater than 17.15 U/L

Hexosaminidase A	Conventional Units	SI Units (Conversion Factor ×0.0167)
Noncarrier	456–592 nmol/h/mL	7.2–9.88 U/L
Heterozygote	197–323 nmol/h/mL	3.3–5.39 U/L
Tay-Sachs homozygote	0 nmol/h/mL	0 U/L

Hexosaminidase B	Conventional Units	SI Units (Conversion Factor ×0.0167)
Noncarrier	12–32 nmol/h/mL	0.2–0.54 U/L
Heterozygote	21–81 nmol/h/mL	0.35–1.35 U/L
Tay-Sachs homozygote	Greater than 305 nmol/h/mL	Greater than 5.09 U/L

DESCRIPTION: Hexosaminidase is a lysosomal enzyme. There are three predominant isoenzymes: hexosaminidase A, B, and S. Deficiency results in the accumulation of complex sphingolipids and gangliosides in the brain. There are more than 70 lysozymal enzyme disorders. Testing for hexosaminidase A is done to determine the presence of Tay-Sachs disease, a genetic autosomal-recessive condition characterized by early and progressive retardation of physical and mental development. This enzyme deficiency is most common among Ashkenazic Jews. Patients who are homozygous for this trait have no hexosaminidase A and have greatly elevated levels of hexosaminidase B; signs and symptoms include red spot in the retina, blindness, and muscular weakness. Tay-Sachs disease results in early death, usually by age 3 or 4 years. ■

INDICATIONS:

• Assist in the diagnosis of Tay-Sachs disease

• Identify carriers with hexosaminidase deficiency

RESULT

Increased in:

• Total

Gastric cancer
Hepatic disease
Myeloma
Myocardial infarct
Pregnancy
Symptomatic porphyria
Vascular complications of diabetes

• Hexosaminidase A
Diabetes
Pregnancy

• Hexosaminidase B
Tay-Sachs disease

Decreased in:
• Total
Sandhoff's disease

• Hexosaminidase A
Tay-Sachs disease

• Hexosaminidase B
Sandhoff's disease

CRITICAL VALUES: N/A

INTERFERING FACTORS: Drugs that may increase hexosaminidase levels include ethanol, isoniazid, oral contraceptives, and rifampin.

Nursing Implications and Procedure

Pretest:

➤ Obtain a history of the patient's complaints, including a list of known allergens.

➤ Obtain a history of the patient's reproductive system and results of previously performed tests and procedures. For related tests, refer to the reproductive system table.

➤ Obtain a list of the medications the patient is taking, including herbs,

nutritional supplements, and nutraceuticals. The requesting health care practitioner and laboratory should be advised if the patient regularly uses these products so that their effects can be taken into consideration when reviewing results.

➤ There are no food, fluid, or medication restrictions unless by medical direction.

➤ Review the procedure with the patient. Sensitivity to cultural and social issues is important in providing psychological support.

➤ Inform the patient that specimen collection takes approximately 5 to 10 minutes.

Intratest:

➤ Direct the patient to breathe normally and to avoid unnecessary movement.

➤ Observe standard precautions and follow the general guidelines in Appendix A. Perform a venipuncture, and collect the specimen in a 5-mL red-top tube.

➤ Label the specimen, and promptly transport it to the laboratory.

Post-test:

➤ Observe venipuncture site for bleeding or hematoma formation. Apply pressure bandage.

➤ Recognize anxiety related to test results and offer support. Provide teaching and information regarding the clinical implications of the test results, as appropriate. Encourage the family to seek genetic counseling if results are abnormal. It is also important to discuss feelings the mother and father may experience (e.g., guilt, depression, anger) if abnormalities are detected.

➤ Evaluate test results in relation to the patient's symptoms and other tests performed. A related laboratory test is chromosomal analysis.

HOLTER MONITOR

SYNONYMS/ACRONYM: Holter electrocardiography, ambulatory monitoring, ambulatory electrocardiography, event recorder.

AREA OF APPLICATION: Heart.

CONTRAST: None.

DESCRIPTION: The Holter monitor records electrical cardiac activity on a continuous basis for 24 to 48 hours. This noninvasive study includes the use of a portable device worn around the waist or over the shoulder that records cardiac electrical impulses on a magnetic tape. The recorder has a clock that allows accurate time markings on the tape. The patient is asked to keep a log or diary of daily activities and to record any occurrence of cardiac symptoms. When the client pushes a button indicating that symptoms (e.g., pain, palpitations, dyspnea, syncope) have occurred, an event marker is placed on the tape for later comparison with the cardiac activity recordings and the daily activity log. Some recorders allow the data to be transferred to the physician's office by telephone, where the tape is interpreted by a computer to detect any significantly abnormal variations in the recorded waveform patterns. ■

INDICATIONS:

- Detect arrhythmias that occur during normal daily activities, and correlate them with symptoms experienced by the patient
- Evaluate the effectiveness of antiar-

rhythmic medications for dosage adjustment, if needed

- Monitor for ischemia and arrhythmias after myocardial infarction or cardiac surgery before changing rehabilitation and other therapy regimens
- Evaluate pacemaker function
- Evaluate chest pain, dizziness, syncope, and palpitations
- Evaluate activity intolerance related to oxygen supply and demand imbalance

RESULT

Normal Findings:
- Normal sinus rhythm

Abnormal Findings:
- Cardiomyopathy
- Arrhythmias such as premature ventricular contractions, bradyarrhythmias, tachyarrhythmias, conduction defects, bradycardia
- Hypoxic or ischemic changes
- Mitral valve abnormality
- Palpitations

CRITICAL VALUES: N/A

INTERFERING FACTORS:

Factors that may impair the results of the examination:

- Improper placement of the electrodes or movement of the electrodes

- Failure of the patient to maintain a daily log of symptoms or to push the button to produce a mark on the strip when experiencing a symptom

Nursing Implications and Procedure • • • • • • • • • • •

Pretest:

➤ Inform the patient that the procedure evaluates how the heart responds to normal activity or to a medication regimen.

➤ Explain that no electricity is delivered to the body during this procedure and that no discomfort is experienced during monitoring.

➤ Obtain a history of cardiac disease and present cardiovascular status as well as results of previously performed tests and procedures. For related tests, refer to the cardiovascular system table.

➤ Determine previous abnormalities in laboratory tests and diagnostic procedures.

➤ Obtain a list of the medications the patient is taking, including herbs, nutritional supplements, and nutraceuticals.

➤ Inform the patient that the electrocardiography (ECG) recorder is worn for 24 to 48 hours, at which time the patient is to return to the laboratory with an activity log to have the monitor and strip removed for interpretation.

➤ Advise the patient to avoid contact with electrical devices that can affect the strip tracings (e.g., shavers, toothbrush, massager, blanket) and to avoid showers and tub bathing.

➤ Instruct the patient to perform normal activities, such as walking, sleeping, climbing stairs, sexual activity, bowel or urinary elimination, cigarette smoking, emotional upsets, and medications, and to record them in an activity log.

➤ Instruct the patient to wear loose-fitting clothing over the electrodes and not to disturb or disconnect the electrodes or wires.

➤ Ensure that the skin where electrodes will be placed is cleansed with an alcohol wipe.

➤ Instruct the patient regarding recording and pressing the button upon experiencing pain or discomfort.

➤ Advise the patient to report a light signal on the monitor, which indicates equipment malfunction or that an electrode has come off.

Intratest:

➤ Ask the patient to void before the procedure. Have the patient put on a hospital gown.

➤ Place the patient in a supine position.

➤ Expose the chest; cleanse the skin sites thoroughly with alcohol and rub until red in color.

➤ Shave excessive hair at sites and apply electropaste to the skin sites to provide conduction between the skin and electrodes, or apply disk electrodes that are prelubricated and disposable.

➤ Apply two electrodes on the manubrium (negative electrodes), one in the V_1 position (fourth intercostal space at the border of the right sternum), and one at the V_5 position (level of the fifth intercostal space at the midclavicular line, horizontally and at the left axillary line). A ground electrode is also placed and secured to the skin of the chest or abdomen.

➤ After checking to ensure that the electrodes are secure, attach the electrode cable to the monitor and the lead wires to the electrodes.

➤ Check the monitor for paper supply and battery, insert the tape, and turn on the recorder. Tape all wires to the chest, and place the belt or shoulder strap in the proper position.

Post-test:

➤ Gently remove the tape and other items securing the electrodes to the patient.

➤ Instruct the patient to resume ordered medications that were discontinued before the procedure.

➤ Instruct the patient to resume pretest activities after the procedure, or as ordered, and to resume previous diet.

➤ Advise the patient to immediately report symptoms such as fast heart rate or difficulty breathing.

➤ Compare the activity log and tape recordings for changes during the monitoring period.

➤ A physician specializing in this branch of medicine sends a written report to the ordering provider, who discusses the results with the patient.

➤ Evaluate test results in relation to the patient's symptoms and other tests performed. Related tests include ECG and echocardiogram.

HOMOCYSTEINE AND METHYLMALONIC ACID

SYNONYM/ACRONYM: N/A.

SPECIMEN: Serum (4 mL) collected in a red- or tiger-top tube if methylmalonic acid and homocysteine are to be measured together. Alternatively, plasma collected in a lavender-top (ethylenediaminetetra-acetic acid [EDTA]) tube may be acceptable for the homocysteine measurement. The laboratory should be consulted before specimen collection because specimen type may be method dependent. Care must be taken to use the same type of collection container if serial measurements are to be taken.

REFERENCE VALUE: (Method: Chromatography) Homocysteine 8 to 20 μmol/L; methylmalonic acid 80 to 560 μmol/L.

DESCRIPTION: Homocysteine is an amino acid formed from methionine. Normally homocysteine is rapidly remetabolized in a biochemical pathway that requires vitamin B_{12} and folate, preventing the buildup of homocysteine in the blood. Excess levels damage the endothelial lining of blood vessels; change coagulation factor levels, increasing the risk of blood clot formation; prevent smaller arteries from dilating, increasing the risk of plaque formation; cause platelet aggregation; and cause smooth muscle cells lining the arterial wall to multiply, promoting atherosclerosis.

Approximately one-third of patients with hyperhomocysteinuria have normal fasting levels. Patients with a heterozygous biochemical enzyme defect in cystathionine B synthase or with a nutritional deficiency in vitamin B$_6$ can be identified through the administration of a methionine challenge or loading test. Specimens are collected while fasting and 2 hours later. An increase in homocysteine after 2 hours is indicative of hyperhomocysteinuria. In patients with vitamin B$_{12}$ deficiency, elevated levels of methylmalonic acid and homocysteine develop fairly early in the course of the disease. Unlike vitamin B$_{12}$ levels, homocysteine levels will remain elevated for at least 24 hours after the start of vitamin therapy. This may be useful if vitamin therapy is inadvertently begun before specimen collection. Patients with folate deficiency, for the most part, will only develop elevated homocysteine levels. Hyperhomocysteinemia due to folate deficiency in pregnant women is believed to increase the risk of neural tube defects. Elevated levels of homocysteine are thought to chemically damage the exposed neural tissue of the developing fetus. ■

INDICATIONS:

- Evaluate inherited enzyme deficiencies that result in homocystinuria

- Evaluate the risk for cardiovascular disease

- Evaluate the risk for venous thrombosis

RESULT

Increased in:
- Chronic renal failure
- Folic acid deficiency
- Homocystinuria
- Vitamin B$_{12}$ deficiency
- Coronary artery disease

Decreased in: N/A

CRITICAL VALUES: N/A

INTERFERING FACTORS:

- Drugs that may increase plasma homocysteine levels include anticonvulsants, cycloserine, hydralazine, isoniazid, methotrexate, theophylline, penicillamine, and phenelzine.

- Specimens should be kept at a refrigerated temperature and delivered immediately to the laboratory for processing.

Nursing Implications and Procedure • • • • • • • • • • •

Pretest:

➤ Obtain a history of the patient's complaints, including a list of known allergens.

➤ Obtain a history of the patient's cardiovascular and hematopoietic systems, as well as results of previously performed tests and procedures. For related tests, refer to the cardiovascular and hematopoietic system tables.

➤ Obtain a list of the medications the patient is taking, including herbs, nutritional supplements, and nutraceuticals. The requesting health care practitioner and laboratory should be advised if the patient regularly uses these products so that their effects can be taken into consideration when reviewing results.

➤ There are no food, fluid, or medication restrictions unless by medical direction.

➤ Review the procedure with the patient.

➤ Inform the patient that specimen collection takes approximately 5 to 10 minutes.

Intratest:

➤ Direct the patient to breathe normally and to avoid unnecessary movement.

➤ Observe standard precautions and follow the general guidelines in Appendix A. Perform a venipuncture, and collect the specimen for combined methylmalonic acid and homocysteine studies in two 5-mL red-, tiger-, or lavender-top tubes. If only homocysteine is to be measured, a 5-mL red-, tiger-, or lavender-top tube is acceptable.

➤ Label the specimen, and promptly transport it to the laboratory.

Post-test:

➤ Observe venipuncture site for bleeding or hematoma formation. Apply pressure bandage.

➤ Increased homocysteine levels may be associated with atherosclerosis and coronary artery disease. Nutritional therapy is recommended for individuals identified to be at high risk for developing coronary artery

disease. If overweight, these patients should be encouraged to achieve a normal weight. The American Heart Association has Step 1 and Step 2 diets that may be helpful in achieving a goal of lowering total cholesterol and triglyceride levels. The Step 1 diet emphasizes a reduction in foods high in saturated fats and cholesterol. Red meats, eggs, and dairy products are the major sources of saturated fats and cholesterol. If triglycerides are also elevated, patients should be advised to eliminate or reduce alcohol and simple carbohydrates from their diet. The Step 2 diet recommends stricter reductions.

➤ Diets rich in fruits, grains, and cereals, in addition to a multivitamin containing B_{12} and folate, may be recommended for patients with elevated homocysteine levels. Processed and refined foods should be kept to a minimum.

➤ Evaluate test results in relation to the patient's symptoms and other tests performed. Related laboratory tests include C-reactive protein, complete blood count, creatine kinase and isoenzymes, folate, lactate dehydrogenase and isoenzymes, myoglobin, troponin, and vitamin B_{12}.

HOMOVANILLIC ACID

SYNONYM/ACRONYM: HVA.

SPECIMEN: Urine (10 mL) from a timed specimen collected in a clean plastic collection container with 6N HCl as a preservative.

REFERENCE VALUE: (Method: Chromatography)

Age	Conventional Units	SI Units
	Homovanillic acid	
		(Conversion Factor ×5.49)
3–6 y	1.4–4.3 mg/24 h	8–24 μmol/24 h
7–10 y	2.1–4.7 mg/24 h	12–26 μmol/24 h
11–16 y	2.4–8.7 mg/24 h	13–48 μmol/24 h
Adult	1.4–8.8 mg/24 h	8–48 μmol/24 h
	Vanillylmandelic Acid	
		(Conversion Factor ×5.05)
3–6 y	1.0–2.6 mg/24 h	5–13 μmol/24 h
7–10 y	2.0–3.2 mg/24 h	10–16 μmol/24 h
11–16 y	2.3–5.2 mg/24 h	12–26 μmol/24 h
Adult	1.4–6.5 mg/24 h	7–33 μmol/24 h

DESCRIPTION: Homovanillic acid (HVA) is the main terminal metabolite of dopamine. Vanillylmandelic acid (VMA) is a major metabolite of epinephrine and norepinephrine. Both of these tests should be evaluated together for the diagnosis of neuroblastoma. Excretion may be intermittent; therefore, a 24-hour specimen is preferred. Creatinine is usually measured simultaneously to ensure adequate collection and to calculate an excretion ratio of metabolite to creatinine. ∎

INDICATIONS:
• Assist in the diagnosis of pheochromocytoma, neuroblastoma, and ganglioblastoma

• Monitor the course of therapy

RESULT

Increased in:
• Ganglioblastoma

• Neuroblastoma

• Pheochromocytoma

• Riley-Day syndrome

Decreased in:
• Schizotypal personality disorders

CRITICAL VALUES: N/A

INTERFERING FACTORS:
• Drugs that may increase HVA levels include acetylsalicylic acid, disulfiram, levodopa, pyridoxine, and reserpine.

• Drugs that may decrease HVA levels include moclobemide.

• All urine voided for the timed collection period must be included in the collection or else falsely decreased values may be obtained. Compare output records with volume collected to verify that all voids were included in the collection.

Nursing Implications and Procedure . . . .

Pretest: ∎

➤ Obtain a history of the patient's complaints, including a list of known allergens.

➤ Obtain a history of the patient's endocrine system and results of previously performed tests and procedures. For related tests, refer to the endocrine system table.

➤ Obtain a list of the medications the patient is taking, including herbs, nutritional supplements, and nutraceuticals. The requesting health care

practitioner and laboratory should be advised if the patient regularly uses these products so that their effects can be taken into consideration when reviewing results.

➤ If possible, and with medical direction, patients should withhold acetylsalicylic acid, disulfiram, pyridoxine, and reserpine for 2 days before specimen collection. Levodopa should be withheld for 2 weeks before specimen collection.

➤ There are no food or fluid restrictions unless by medical direction.

➤ Review the procedure with the patient. Provide a nonmetallic urinal, bedpan, or toilet-mounted collection device.

➤ Usually a 24-hour time frame for urine collection is ordered. Inform the patient that all urine must be saved during that 24-hour period. Instruct the patient not to void directly into the laboratory collection container. Instruct the patient to avoid defecating in the collection device and to keep toilet tissue out of the collection device to prevent contamination of the specimen. Place a sign in the bathroom to remind the patient to save all urine.

➤ Instruct the patient to void all urine into the collection device and then to pour the urine into the laboratory collection container. Alternatively the specimen can be left in the collection device for a health care staff member to add to the laboratory collection container.

refrigerated or kept on ice throughout the entire collection period. If an indwelling urinary catheter is in place, the drainage bag must be kept on ice.

➤ Begin the test between 6 and 8 a.m., if possible. Collect first voiding and discard. Record the time the specimen was discarded as the beginning of the timed collection period. The next morning, ask the patient to void at the same time the collection was started and add this last voiding to the container.

➤ If an indwelling catheter is in place, replace the tubing and container system at the start of the collection time. Keep the container system on ice during the collection period, or empty the urine into a larger container periodically during the collection period; monitor to ensure continued drainage, and conclude the test the next morning at the same hour the collection was begun.

➤ At the conclusion of the test, compare the quantity of urine with the urinary output record for the collection; if the specimen contains less than what was recorded as output, some urine may have been discarded, invalidating the test.

➤ Label the specimen, and promptly transport it to the laboratory. Include on the label the amount of urine, test start and stop times, and ingestion of any foods or medications that can affect test results.

Intratest: ■

➤ Ensure that the patient has complied with dietary preparations and other pretesting restrictions.

➤ Observe standard precautions and follow the general guidelines in Appendix A. Obtain a clean 3-L urine specimen container, toilet-mounted collection device, and plastic bag (for transport of the specimen container). The specimen must be

Post-test: ■

➤ Instruct the patient to resume usual medication as directed by the health care practitioner.

➤ Evaluate test results in relation to the patient's symptoms and other tests performed. Related laboratory tests include carcinoembryonic antigen, catecholamines, urine catecholamines, metanephrines, and vanillylmandelic acid.

HUMAN CHORIONIC GONADOTROPIN
· ·

SYNONYMS/ACRONYMS: Chorionic gonadotropin, pregnancy test, HCG, hCG, β-HCG, β-subunit HCG.

SPECIMEN: Serum (1 mL) collected in a red- or tiger-top tube. Plasma (1 mL) collected in green-top (heparin) tube is also acceptable.

REFERENCE VALUE: (Method: Immunoassay)

	Conventional Units	SI Units (Conversion Factor ×1)
Males and nonpregnant females	Less than 5 mIU/mL	Less than 5 IU/L
Pregnant females by week of gestation:		
Less than 1 wk	5–50 mIU/mL	5–50 IU/L
2 wk	50–500 mIU/mL	50–500 IU/L
3 wk	100–10,000 mIU/mL	100–10,000 IU/L
4 wk	1,000–30,000 mIU/mL	1,000–30,000 IU/L
5 wk	3,500–115,000 mIU/mL	3,500–115,000 IU/L
6–8 wk	12,000–270,000 mIU/mL	12,000–270,000 IU/L
12 wk	15,000–220,000 mIU/mL	15,000–220,000 IU/L

DESCRIPTION: Human chorionic gonadotropin (HCG) is a hormone secreted by the placenta beginning 8 to 10 days after conception, which coincides with implantation of the fertilized ovum. It stimulates secretion of progesterone by the corpus luteum. HCG levels peak at 8 to 12 weeks of gestation and then fall to less than 10 percent of first trimester levels by the end of pregnancy. By postpartum week 2, levels are undetectable. HCG levels increase at a slower rate in ectopic pregnancy and spontaneous abortion than in normal pregnancy; a low rate of change between serial specimens is predictive of a nonviable fetus. As assays improve in sensitivity over time, ectopic pregnancies are increasingly being identified before rupture. HCG is used along with estriol and α₁-fetoprotein in prenatal screening for neural tube defects. These prenatal measurements are also known as *triple markers.* Serial measurements are needed for an accurate estimate of gestational stage and determination of fetal viability. Triple marker testing has also been used to screen for neural tube defects and trisomy 21 (Down syndrome). (To compare HCG to other tests in the triple marker screening procedure, see monograph titled "α_1-Fetoprotein.") HCG is also produced by some germ cell tumors. Most assays measure both the intact and free β-HCG subunit, but if HCG is to be used as a tumor marker, the assay must be capable of detecting both intact and free β-HCG. ■

INDICATIONS:

• Assist in the diagnosis of suspected HCG-producing tumors, such as choriocarcinoma, germ cell tumors of the ovary and testes, or hydatidiform moles

• Confirm pregnancy, assist in the diagnosis of suspected ectopic pregnancy, or determine threatened or incomplete abortion

• Determine adequacy of hormonal levels to maintain pregnancy

• Monitor effects of surgery or chemotherapy

• Monitor ovulation induction treatment

• Prenatally detect neural tube defects and trisomy 21 (Down's syndrome)

RESULT

Increased in:

• Choriocarcinoma

• Ectopic HCG-producing tumors (stomach, lung, colon, pancreas, liver, breast)

• Erythroblastosis fetalis

• Germ cell tumors (ovary and testes)

• Hydatidiform mole

• Islet cell tumors

• Multiple gestation pregnancy

• Pregnancy

Decreased in:

• Ectopic pregnancy

• Incomplete abortion

• Intrauterine fetal demise

• Spontaneous abortion

• Threatened abortion

CRITICAL VALUES: N/A

INTERFERING FACTORS:

• Drugs that may decrease HCG levels include epostane and mifepristone.

• Results may vary widely depending on the sensitivity and specificity of the assay. Performance of test too early in pregnancy may cause false-negative results. HCG is composed of an alpha and a beta subunit. The structure of the alpha subunit is essentially identical to the alpha subunit of follicle-stimulating hormone, luteinizing hormone, and thyroid-stimulating hormone. The structure of the beta subunit differentiates HCG from the other hormones. False-positive results can therefore be obtained if the HCG assay does not detect beta subunit.

Nursing Implications and Procedure • • • • • • • • • •

Pretest: ■

➤ Obtain a history of the patient's complaints, including a list of known allergens.

➤ Obtain a history of the patient's endocrine, immune, and reproductive systems, as well as results of previously performed tests and procedures. For related tests, refer to the endocrine, immune, and reproductive system tables.

➤ Obtain a list of the medications the patient is taking, including herbs, nutritional supplements, and nutraceuticals. The requesting health care practitioner and laboratory should be advised if the patient regularly uses these products so that their effects can be taken into consideration when reviewing results.

➤ There are no food, fluid, or medication restrictions unless by medical direction.

➤ Review the procedure with the patient.

➤ Inform the patient that specimen collection takes approximately 5 to 10 minutes.

Intratest:

➤ Direct the patient to breathe normally and to avoid unnecessary movement.

➤ Observe standard precautions and follow the general guidelines in Appendix A. Perform a venipuncture, and collect the specimen in a 5-mL red- or tiger-top tube.

➤ Label the specimen, and promptly transport it to the laboratory.

Post-test:

➤ Observe venipuncture site for bleeding or hematoma formation. Apply pressure bandage.

➤ Recognize anxiety related to test results, and encourage the family to seek counseling if concerned with pregnancy termination or to seek genetic counseling if a chromosomal abnormality is determined. Provide teaching and information regarding the clinical implications of the test results, as appropriate. Decisions

regarding elective abortion should take place in the presence of both parents. Provide a nonjudgmental, nonthreatening atmosphere for discussing the risks and difficulties of delivering and raising an abnormal infant, as well as exploring other options (termination of pregnancy or adoption). It is also important to discuss feelings the mother and father may experience (e.g., guilt, depression, anger) if fetal abnormalities are detected.

➤ Offer support, as appropriate, to patients who may be the victims of rape or sexual assault. Educate the patient regarding access to counseling services. Provide a nonjudgmental, nonthreatening atmosphere for a discussion during which risks of sexually transmitted diseases are explained. It is also important to discuss problems the patient may experience (e.g., guilt, depression, anger) if test results indicate the presence of organisms responsible for causing syphilis or if faced with the possibility of pregnancy.

➤ In patients with carcinoma, recognize anxiety related to test results and offer support. Provide teaching and information regarding the clinical implications of the test results, as appropriate. Educate the patient regarding access to counseling services, as appropriate.

➤ Evaluate test results in relation to the patient's symptoms and other tests performed. Related laboratory tests include α_1-fetoprotein and progesterone.

HUMAN IMMUNODEFICIENCY VIRUS TYPE 1 AND TYPE 2 ANTIBODIES

SYNONYM/ACRONYM: HIV-1/HIV-2.

SPECIMEN: Serum (1 mL) collected in a red-top tube.

REFERENCE VALUE: (Method: Enzyme immunoassay) Negative.

DESCRIPTION: Human immunodeficiency virus (HIV) is the etiologic agent of acquired immunodeficiency syndrome (AIDS) and is transmitted through bodily secretions, especially by blood or sexual contact. The virus preferentially binds to the T4 helper lymphocytes and replicates within the cells. Current assays detect several viral proteins. Positive results should be confirmed by Western Blot assay. This test is routinely recommended as part of a prenatal workup and is required for evaluating donated blood units before release for transfusion. ■

INDICATIONS:

• Evaluate donated blood units before transfusion

• Perform as part of prenatal screening

• Screen organ transplant donors

• Test individuals who have documented and significant exposure to other infected individuals

• Test exposed high-risk individuals for detection of antibody (e.g., persons with multiple sex partners, persons with a history of other sexually transmitted diseases, intravenous drug users, infants born to infected mothers, allied health care workers, public service employees who have contact with blood and blood products)

RESULT

Positive findings in: HIV-1 or HIV-2 infection

CRITICAL VALUES: N/A

INTERFERING FACTORS:

• Drugs that may decrease HIV antibody levels include didanosine, dideoxycytidine, zalcitabine, and zidovudine.

• Nonreactive HIV test results occur during the acute stage of the disease, when the virus is present but antibodies have not sufficiently developed to be detected. It may take up to 6 months for the test to become positive. During this stage, the test for HIV antigen may not confirm an HIV infection.

• Test kits for HIV are very sensitive. As a result, nonspecific reactions may occur, resulting in a false-positive result.

Nursing Implications and Procedure • • • • • • • • • •

Pretest: ■

➤ Obtain a history of the patient's complaints, including a list of known allergens.

➤ Obtain a history of the patient's immune and reproductive systems, a history of high-risk behaviors, and results of previously performed tests and procedures. For related tests, refer to the immune and reproductive system tables.

➤ Obtain a list of the medications the patient is taking, including herbs, nutritional supplements, and nutraceuticals. The requesting health care practitioner and laboratory should be advised if the patient regularly uses these products so that their effects can be taken into consideration when reviewing results.

➤ There are no food, fluid, or medication restrictions unless by medical direction.

➤ Review the procedure with the patient.

➤ *Obtain written and informed consent before the procedure is initiated.*

➤ Inform the patient that specimen collection takes approximately 5 to 10 minutes.

Intratest:

➤ Direct the patient to breathe normally and to avoid unnecessary movement.

➤ Observe standard precautions and follow the general guidelines in Appendix A. Perform a venipuncture, and collect the specimen in a 5-mL red-top tube.

➤ Label the specimen, and promptly transport it to the laboratory.

Post-test:

➤ Observe venipuncture site for bleeding or hematoma formation. Apply pressure bandage.

➤ Warn the patient that false-positive results occur and that the absence of antibody does not guarantee absence of infection, because the virus may be latent or may not have produced detectable antibody at the time of testing.

➤ Recognize anxiety related to test results and offer support. Provide teaching and information regarding the clinical implications of the test results, as appropriate. Educate the patient regarding access to counseling services.

➤ Counsel the patient, as appropriate, regarding risk of transmission and proper prophylaxis, and reinforce the importance of strict adherence to the treatment regimen.

➤ Inform patients that positive findings must be reported to local health department officials, who will question him or her regarding sexual partners.

➤ Offer support, as appropriate, to patients who may be the victims of rape or sexual assault. Educate the patient regarding access to counseling services. Provide a nonjudgmental, nonthreatening atmosphere for a discussion during which risks of sexually transmitted diseases are explained. It is also important to discuss problems the patient may experience (e.g., guilt, depression, anger) if test results indicate the presence of HIV.

➤ Inform the patient that retesting may be necessary.

➤ Evaluate test results in relation to the patient's symptoms and other tests performed. Related laboratory tests include β_2-microglobulin, complete blood count, CD4/ CD8 enumeration, skin culture, cytomegalovirus, and human T-cell lymphotropic virus types I and II.

HUMAN LEUKOCYTE ANTIGEN B27

• •

SYNONYM/ACRONYM: HLA-B27.

SPECIMEN: Whole blood (5 mL) collected in green-top (heparin) or yellow-top (acid-citrate-dextrose [ACD]) tube.

REFERENCE VALUE: (Method: Flow cytometry) Negative (indicating absence of the antigen).

DESCRIPTION: The human leukocyte antigens (HLAs) are gene products of the major histocompatibility complex, derived from their respective loci on the short arm of chromosome six. There are more than 27 identified HLAs. HLA-B27 is an allele (one of two or more genes for an inheritable trait that occupy the same location on each chromosome, paternal and maternal) of the HLA-B locus. The presence of HLA-B27 is associated with several specific conditions listed below, but HLA-B27 should not be used as a screening test for these conditions. ■

INDICATIONS: Assist in diagnosing ankylosing spondylitis and Reiter's syndrome

RESULT

Positive findings in:
• Ankylosing spondylitis
• Juvenile rheumatoid arthritis
• Psoriatic arthritis
• Reiter's syndrome

CRITICAL VALUES: N/A

INTERFERING FACTORS:
• The specimen should be stored at room temperature and should be received by the laboratory performing the assay within 24 hours of collection. It is highly recommended that the laboratory be contacted before specimen collection to avoid specimen rejection.

Nursing Implications and Procedure ● ● ● ● ● ● ● ● ● ● ●

Pretest: ■

➤ Obtain a history of the patient's complaints, including a list of known allergens.

➤ Obtain a history of the patient's immune and musculoskeletal systems as well as results of previously performed tests and procedures. For related tests, refer to the immune and musculoskeletal system tables.

➤ Obtain a list of the medications the patient is taking, including herbs, nutritional supplements, and nutraceuticals. The requesting health care practitioner and laboratory should be advised if the patient regularly uses these products so that their effects can be taken into consideration when reviewing results.

➤ There are no food, fluid, or medication restrictions unless by medical direction.

➤ Review the procedure with the patient.

➤ Inform the patient that specimen collection takes approximately 5 to 10 minutes.

Intratest: ■

➤ Direct the patient to breathe normally and to avoid unnecessary movement.

➤ Observe standard precautions and follow the general guidelines in Appendix A. Perform a venipuncture, and collect the specimen in a 5-mL green- or yellow-top tube.

➤ Label the specimen, and promptly transport it to the laboratory.

Post-test: ■

➤ Observe venipuncture site for bleeding or hematoma formation. Apply pressure bandage.

➤ Recognize patient anxiety related to test results and offer support. These diseases can be moderately to severely debilitating, resulting in significant lifestyle changes. Provide teaching and information regarding

the clinical implications of the test results, as appropriate. Educate the patient regarding access to counseling services.

➤ Inform the patient that false-positive test results occur and that retesting may be required.

➤ Evaluate test results in relation to the patient's symptoms and other tests performed. A related laboratory test is rheumatoid factor.

HUMAN T-LYMPHOTROPIC VIRUS TYPE I AND TYPE II ANTIBODIES

· ·

SYNONYM/ACRONYM: HTLV-I and HTLV-II.

SPECIMEN: Serum (1 mL) collected in a red-top tube.

REFERENCE VALUE: (Method: Enzyme immunoassay) Negative.

DESCRIPTION: Human T-lymphotropic virus type I (HTLV-I) and type II (HTLV-II) are two closely related retroviruses known to remain latent for extended periods before becoming reactive. The viruses are transmitted by sexual contact, contact with blood, placental transfer from mother to fetus, or ingestion of breast milk. As with human immunodeficiency virus type 1 (HIV-1) and type 2 (HIV-2), HTLV targets the T4 lymphocytes. The disease is uncommon in the United States, but retrospective studies conducted by the American Red Cross demonstrated that a small percentage of transfusion recipients became infected by HTLV-positive blood. The results of this study led to

a requirement that all donated blood units be tested for HTLV-I/HTLV-II before release for transfusion. ■

INDICATIONS:

• Distinguish HTLV-I/HTLV-II infection from spastic myelopathy

• Establish HTLV-I as the causative agent in adult lymphoblastic (T-cell) leukemia

• Evaluate donated blood units before transfusion

• Evaluate HTLV-II as a contributing cause of chronic neuromuscular disease

RESULT

Positive findings in: HTLV-I/ HTLV-II infection

CRITICAL VALUES: N/A

INTERFERING FACTORS: N/A

Nursing Implications and Procedure • • • • • • • • • •

Pretest: ■

➤ Obtain a history of the patient's complaints, including a list of known allergens.

➤ Obtain a history of the patient's immune system, a history of high-risk behaviors, and results of previously performed tests and procedures. For related tests, refer to the immune system table.

➤ Obtain a list of the medications the patient is taking, including herbs, nutritional supplements, and nutraceuticals. The requesting health care practitioner and laboratory should be advised if the patient regularly uses these products so that their effects can be taken into consideration when reviewing results.

➤ There are no food, fluid, or medication restrictions unless by medical direction.

➤ Review the procedure with the patient.

➤ Inform the patient that specimen collection takes approximately 5 to 10 minutes.

Intratest: ■

➤ Direct the patient to breathe normally and to avoid unnecessary movement.

➤ Observe standard precautions and follow the general guidelines in Appendix A. Perform a venipuncture, and collect the specimen in a 5-mL red-top tube.

➤ Label the specimen, and promptly transport it to the laboratory.

Post-test: ■

➤ Observe venipuncture site for bleeding or hematoma formation. Apply pressure bandage.

➤ Warn the patient that false-positive results occur and that the absence of antibody does not guarantee absence of infection, because the virus may be latent or not have produced detectable antibody at the time of testing.

➤ Recognize anxiety related to test results and offer support. Provide teaching and information regarding the clinical implications of the test results, as appropriate. Counsel the patient, as appropriate, regarding risk of transmission and proper prophylaxis, and reinforce the importance of strict adherence to the treatment regime.

➤ Inform the patient that the presence of HTLV-I/HTLV-II antibodies precludes blood donation, but it does not mean that leukemia or a neurologic disorder is present or will develop.

➤ Inform the patient that subsequent retesting may be necessary.

➤ Evaluate test results in relation to the patient's symptoms and other tests performed. Related laboratory tests include complete blood count, HIV-1/HIV-2, and hepatitis antigens and antibodies.

5-HYDROXYINDOLEACETIC ACID

SYNONYM/ACRONYM: 5-HIAA.

SPECIMEN: Urine (10 mL) from a timed specimen collected in a clean plastic collection container with boric acid as a preservative.

REFERENCE VALUE: (Method: High-pressure liquid chromatography)

Conventional Units	SI Units (Conversion Factor ×5.23)
2–7 mg/24 h	10.5–36.6 μmol/24 h

DESCRIPTION: Because 5-hydroxyindoleacetic acid (5-HIAA) is a metabolite of serotonin, 5-HIAA levels reflect plasma serotonin concentrations. 5-HIAA is excreted in the urine. Increased urinary excretion occurs in the presence of carcinoid tumors. This test, which replaces serotonin measurement, is most accurate when obtained from a 24-hour urine specimen. ■

INDICATIONS: Detect early, small, or intermittently secreting carcinoid tumors

RESULT

Increased in:
- Celiac and tropical sprue
- Cystic fibrosis
- Foregut and midgut carcinoid tumors
- Oat cell carcinoma of the bronchus
- Ovarian carcinoid tumors
- Whipple's disease

Decreased in:
- Depressive illnesses
- Hartnup disease
- Mastocytosis
- Phenylketonuria
- Renal disease
- Small intestinal resection

CRITICAL VALUES: N/A

INTERFERING FACTORS:
- Drugs that may increase 5-HIAA levels include acetaminophen, cisplatin, ephedrine, fluorouracil, cough syrups containing glyceryl guaiacolate, melphalan, mephenesin, methocarbamol, naproxen, phenacetin, pindolol, and rauwolfia alkaloids.

- Drugs that may decrease 5-HIAA levels include corticotropin, ethanol, imipramine, isoniazid, levodopa, monoamine oxidase inhibitors, methenamine, methyldopa, and phenothiazines.

- Foods containing serotonin, such as

avocados, bananas, chocolate, eggplant, pineapples, plantain, red plums, tomatoes, and walnuts, can falsely elevate levels if ingested within 4 days of specimen collection.

• Severe gastrointestinal disturbance or diarrhea can interfere with test results.

• Failure to collect all the urine and store the specimen properly during the 24-hour test period invalidates the results.

Nursing Implications and Procedure • • • • • • • • • • •

Pretest: ■

➤ Obtain a history of the patient's complaints, including a list of known allergens.

➤ Obtain a history of the patient's endocrine, gastrointestinal, and immune system and results of previously performed tests and procedures. For related tests, refer to the endocrine, gastrointestinal, and immune system tables.

➤ Obtain a list of the medications the patient is taking, including herbs, nutritional supplements, and nutraceuticals. Advise the requesting health care practitioner and laboratory that the patient regularly uses these products so that their effects can be taken into consideration when reviewing results. The requesting health care practitioner and laboratory should be advised if the patient regularly uses these products so that their effects can be taken into consideration when reviewing results.

➤ There are no fluid restrictions unless by medical direction.

➤ Inform the patient that foods and medications (herbs, nutritional supplements, and nutraceuticals) listed under "Interfering Factors" should be restricted by medical direction for at least 4 days before specimen collection.

➤ Review the procedure with the patient. Provide a nonmetallic urinal, bedpan, or toilet-mounted collection device.

➤ Inform the patient that all urine collected over a 24-hour period must be saved; if a preservative has been added to the container, instruct the patient not to discard the preservative. Instruct the patient not to void directly into the container. Instruct the patient to avoid defecating in the collection device and to keep toilet tissue out of the collection device to prevent contamination of the specimen. Place a sign in the bathroom as a reminder to save all urine.

➤ Instruct the patient to void all urine into the collection device, then pour the urine into the laboratory collection container. Alternatively, the specimen can be left in the collection device for a health care staff member to add to the laboratory collection container.

Intratest: ■

➤ Ensure that the patient is in compliance with dietary preparation and other pretesting restrictions.

➤ Observe standard precautions and follow the general guidelines in Appendix A.

Timed specimen:

➤ Obtain a clean 3-L urine specimen container, toilet-mounted collection device, and plastic bag (for transport of the specimen container). The specimen must be refrigerated or kept on ice throughout the entire collection period. If an indwelling urinary catheter is in place, the drainage bag must be kept on ice.

➤ Begin the test between 6 and 8 a.m., if possible. Collect first voiding and discard. Record the time the specimen was discarded as the beginning of the timed collection period. The next morning, ask the patient to void at the same time the collection was started, and add this last voiding to the container.

➤ If an indwelling catheter is in place,

replace the tubing and container system at the start of the collection time. Keep the container system on ice during the collection period, or empty the urine into a larger container periodically during the collection period; monitor to ensure continued drainage. Conclude the test the next morning at the same hour the collection was begun.

➤ At the conclusion of the test, compare the quantity of urine with the urinary output record for the collection; if the specimen contains less than what was recorded as output, some urine may have been discarded, invalidating the test.

➤ Label the specimen, and promptly transport it to the laboratory. Include on the label the amount of urine, test start and stop times, and ingestion of any foods or medications that can affect test results.

Post-test: ■

➤ Instruct the patient to resume usual diet and medication as directed by the requesting health care practitioner. Consideration may be given to niacin supplementation and increased protein, if appropriate, for patients with abnormal findings. In some cases, the tumor may divert dietary tryptophan to serotonin, resulting in pellagra.

➤ Evaluate test results in relation to the patient's symptoms and other tests performed. A related laboratory test is biopsy of the affected tissue.

HYPERSENSITIVITY PNEUMONITIS SEROLOGY

· ·

SYNONYM/ACRONYM: Farmer's lung disease serology, extrinsic allergic alveolitis.

SPECIMEN: Serum (2 mL) collected in a red-top tube.

REFERENCE VALUE: (Method: Immunodiffusion) Negative.

DESCRIPTION: Hypersensitivity pneumonitis is a respiratory disease caused by the inhalation of organisms from an organic source. Affected and symptomatic individuals will demonstrate acute bronchospastic reaction 4 to 6 hours after exposure to the offending antigen. Inhalation of the antigen stimulates the production of immunoglobulin G (IgG) antibodies.

The combination of immune-complexing and cell-mediated immunopathogenesis results in a chronic granulomatous pneumonitis of the interstitial space of the lung. Hypersensitivity pneumonitis serology includes detection of antibodies to *Aspergillus fumigatus, Micropolyspora faeni, Thermoactinomyces vulgaris* and *T. candidus.* A negative test result does not rule out hypersensitivity pneumonitis as a possible diagnosis, nor does a positive test result confirm the diagnosis. Also, individuals with a positive test result may not exhibit the typical symptoms, and patients with severe symptoms may not have detectable levels of antibody while their disease is inactive. To confirm the diagnosis, it is necessary to obtain a sputum culture and chest x-rays. ■

INDICATIONS: Assist in establishing a diagnosis of hypersensitivity pneumonitis in patients experiencing fever, chills, and dyspnea after repeated exposure to moist organic sources

RESULT

Increased in: Hypersensitivity pneumonitis

CRITICAL VALUES: N/A

INTERFERING FACTORS: N/A

Nursing Implications and Procedure • • • • • • • • • • • •

Pretest: ■

➤ Obtain a history of the patient's complaints, including a list of known allergens.

➤ Obtain a history of the patient's immune and respiratory systems, as well as results of previously performed tests and procedures. For related tests, refer to the immune and respiratory system tables.

➤ Obtain a list of the medications the patient is taking, including herbs, nutritional supplements, and nutraceuticals. The requesting health care practitioner and laboratory should be advised if the patient regularly uses these products so that their effects can be taken into consideration when reviewing results.

➤ There are no food, fluid, or medication restrictions unless by medical direction.

➤ Review the procedure with the patient.

➤ Inform the patient that specimen collection takes approximately 5 to 10 minutes.

Intratest: ■

➤ Direct the patient to breathe normally and to avoid unnecessary movement.

➤ Observe standard precautions and follow the general guidelines in Appendix A. Perform a venipuncture and collect the specimen in a 5-mL red-top tube.

➤ Label the specimen, and promptly transport it to the laboratory.

Post-test: ■

➤ Observe venipuncture site for bleeding or hematoma formation. Apply pressure bandage.

➤ Positive test results may be associated with respiratory disease. Malnutrition is commonly seen in patients with severe respiratory disease for reasons including fatigue and lack of appetite. The importance of following the prescribed diet should be stressed to the patient and/or caregiver.

➤ Instruct the patient in preventive measures for protecting his or her lungs (e.g., avoid contact with persons who have respiratory or other infections, avoid use of tobacco, avoid highly polluted areas as well as work environments with hazards such as fumes, dust, and other respiratory pollutants).

➤ Instruct the patient in deep breathing and pursed-lip breathing to enhance breathing patterns, as appropriate.

➤ Inform the patient of smoking cessation programs, as appropriate.

➤ Evaluate test results in relation to the patient's symptoms and other tests performed. Related laboratory tests include allergen-specific IgE, arterial/alveolar oxygen ratio, complete blood count, eosinophil count, lung biopsy, and sputum culture.

HYSTEROSALPINGOGRAPHY

· ·

SYNONYMS/ACRONYM: Uterography, uterosalpingography, hysterogram.

AREA OF APPLICATION: Uterus and fallopian tubes.

CONTRAST: Iodinated contrast medium.

DESCRIPTION: Hysterosalpingography is generally performed as part of an infertility study to identify anatomical abnormalities of the uterus or occlusion of the fallopian tubes. The procedure allows visualization of the uterine cavity, fallopian tubes, and peritubal area after the injection of contrast medium into the cervix. The contrast medium should flow through the uterine cavity, through the fallopian tubes, and into the peritoneal cavity, where it can be absorbed if no obstruction exists. Passage of the contrast medium through the tubes may clear mucous plugs, straighten kinked tubes, or break up adhesions, thus restoring fertility. This procedure is also used to evaluate the fallopian tubes after tubal ligation and to evaluate the results of reconstructive surgery. Risks include uterine perforation, exposure to radiation, infection, allergic reaction to contrast medium, bleeding, and pulmonary embolism. ▪

INDICATIONS:

• Confirm tubal abnormalities such as adhesions and occlusions

• Confirm uterine abnormalities such as congenital malformation, traumatic injuries, or the presence of foreign bodies

• Confirm the presence of fistulas or adhesions

• Detect bicornate uterus

• Evaluate adequacy of surgical tubal ligation and reconstructive surgery

RESULT

Normal Findings:

• Normal position, shape, and size of the uterine cavity

• Contrast medium flowing freely into the fallopian tubes and not leaking from the uterus

Abnormal Findings:

• Bicornate uterus

• Developmental abnormalities

• Extrauterine pregnancy

• Internal scarring

• Kinking of the fallopian tubes due to adhesions

• Partial or complete blockage of fallopian tube(s)

• Tumors

• Uterine cavity anomalies

• Uterine fistulas

• Uterine masses or foreign body

• Uterine fibroid tumors (leiomyomas)

INTERFERING FACTORS:

This procedure is contraindicated for:

• Patients with allergies to shellfish or ⚠ iodinated dye. The contrast medium used may cause a life-threatening allergic reaction. Patients with a known hypersensitivity to the contrast medium may benefit from premedication with corticosteroids or the use of nonionic contrast medium.

• Patients with bleeding disorders.

• Patients who are pregnant or suspected of being pregnant, unless the potential benefits of the procedure far outweigh the risks to the fetus and mother.

• Elderly and other patients who are ⚠ chronically dehydrated before the test, because of their risk of contrast-induced renal failure.

• ⚠ Patients who are in renal failure.

• Patients with menses, undiagnosed vaginal bleeding, or pelvic inflammatory disease.

• Young patients (17 years and younger),

unless the benefits of the x-ray diagnosis outweigh the risks of exposure to high levels of radiation.

Factors that may impair clear imaging:

• Inability of the patient to cooperate or remain still during the procedure because of age, significant pain, or mental status

• Retained barium from a previous radiologic procedure

• Metallic objects within the examination field (e.g., jewelry or body rings), which may inhibit organ visualization and can produce unclear images

• Gas or feces in the gastrointestinal tract resulting from inadequate cleansing or failure to restrict food intake before the study

• Insufficient injection of contrast medium

• Excessive traction during the test or tubal spasm, which may cause the appearance of a stricture in an otherwise normal fallopian tube

Other considerations:

• Excessive traction during the test may displace adhesions, making the fallopian tubes appear normal.

• Consultation with a physician should occur before the procedure for radiation safety concerns regarding infants of patients who are lactating.

• Risks associated with radiographic overexposure can result from frequent x-ray procedures. Personnel in the room with the patient should wear a protective lead apron, stand behind a shield, or leave the area while the examination is being done. Personnel working in the area where the examination is being done should wear badges that reveal their level of exposure to radiation.

Nursing Implications and Procedure • • • • • • • • • • •

➤ Inform the patient that the procedure assesses the uterus and fallopian tubes and takes approximately 30 minutes.

➤ Obtain a history of allergies or sensitivities to contrast medium, shellfish, or latex.

➤ Obtain a list of the medications the patient is taking.

➤ Assess date of last menstrual period and possibility of pregnancy in perimenopausal women.

➤ The procedure should be performed 2 to 5 days after menstruation ends.

➤ Obtain a history of the patient's reproductive system and previously performed laboratory tests (especially blood urea nitrogen and creatinine), surgeries, therapies, and procedures. For related tests, refer to the reproductive system table.

➤ Patients receiving metformin (Glucophage) for non–insulin-dependent (type 2) diabetes should discontinue the drug on the day of the test and continue to withhold it for 48 hours after the test. Failure to do so may result in lactic acidosis.

➤ Instruct the patient to take a laxative or an enema the night before the test, or as ordered.

➤ Restrict food and fluids for 8 hours before the test.

➤ Explain to the patient that she may feel menstrual-like cramping during the procedure and shoulder pain from subphrenic irritation from the contrast medium as it spills into the peritoneal cavity.

➤ *Obtain a written, informed consent for the procedure from the patient.*

➤ Schedule barium and colonoscopy studies after completion of the study, if ordered.

➤ Wear gloves throughout the procedure.

➤ Ask the patient to void before the procedure. Have the patient put on a hospital gown.

➤ Ask the patient to lie still during the procedure because movement produces unclear images. Make sure jewelry, watches, chains, belts, and any other metallic objects have been removed.

➤ Remove any wires connected to electrodes, if allowed.

➤ Administer enemas or suppositories on the morning of the test, as ordered.

➤ Administer sedative, as ordered, before the test.

➤ Place patient in a lithotomy position on the fluoroscopy table.

➤ A kidney, ureter, and bladder (KUB) film is taken to ensure that no stool, gas, or barium will obscure visualization of the uterus and fallopian tubes.

➤ A speculum is inserted into the vagina, and contrast medium is introduced into the uterus through the cervix via a cannula, after which both fluoroscopic and radiographic films are taken.

➤ The patient may experience temporary sensations of nausea, dizziness, bradycardia, or uterine cramping as the contrast medium is instilled. The patient may have shoulder pain caused by subphrenic irritation from the contrast medium as it leaks into the peritoneal cavity.

➤ To take oblique views, the table may be tilted or the patient may be asked to change position during the procedure.

➤ Direct the patient to resume usual diet, activity, and medication, if withheld and as directed by the physician. Renal function should be assessed before metformin is restarted.

➤ Inform the patient of the possible

need for further testing to evaluate her condition and determine the need for a change in therapy.

➤ Monitor the patient's vital and neurological signs per institution policy until stable.

➤ Evaluate the patient for signs of hypersensitivity reaction to contrast medium, such as urticaria, headache, nausea, respiratory distress, hypotension, edema, hives, rash, tachycardia, laryngeal stridor, or vomiting, and alert the patient to be watchful for these symptoms.

➤ Evaluate the patient for signs of infection, such as pain, fever, increased pulse rate, chills, flushing, abdominal pain, tachycardia, or muscle aches.

➤ Inform the patient that a vaginal discharge is common and that it may be bloody, lasting 1 to 2 days after the test.

➤ Inform the patient that dizziness and cramping may follow this procedure.

➤ Inform the patient that analgesia may be given if there is persistent cramping after the procedure.

➤ Inform the patient to contact the physician in the event of severe cramping or profuse bleeding.

➤ Determine if the patient or family members have any further questions or concerns.

➤ A physician specializing in this branch of medicine sends a written report to the ordering provider, who discusses the results with the patient.

➤ Evaluate test results in relation to the patient's symptoms and any related tests performed.

IMMUNOFIXATION ELECTROPHORESIS, SERUM AND URINE

· ·

SYNONYM/ACRONYM: IFE.

SPECIMEN: Serum (1 mL) collected in a red-top tube. Urine (10 mL) from a random collection in a clean plastic container.

REFERENCE VALUE: (Method: Immunoprecipitation combined with electrophoresis) Test results are interpreted by a pathologist. Normal placement and intensity of staining provide information about the immunoglobulin bands.

DESCRIPTION: Immunofixation electrophoresis (IFE) is a qualitative technique that provides a detailed separation of individual immunoglobulins according to their electrical charges. Abnormalities are revealed by changes produced in the individual bands, such as displacement, color, or absence of color. Urine IFE has replaced the Bence Jones screening test for light chains. IFE has replaced immunoelectrophoresis because it is more sensitive and easier to interpret. ■

INDICATIONS:

• Assist in the diagnosis of multiple myeloma and amyloidosis

• Assist in the diagnosis of suspected immunodeficiency

• Assist in the diagnosis of suspected immunoproliferative disorders, such as multiple myeloma and Waldenström's macroglobulinemia

• Identify biclonal or monoclonal gammopathies

• Identify cryoglobulinemia

• Monitor the effectiveness of chemotherapy or radiation therapy

RESULT: See monograph titled "Immunoglobulins A, D, G, and M."

CRITICAL VALUES: N/A

INTERFERING FACTORS:

• Drugs that may increase immunoglobulin levels include asparaginase, cimetidine, and narcotics.

• Drugs that may decrease immunoglobulin levels include dextran, oral contraceptives, phenytoin, and methylprednisolone (high doses).

• Chemotherapy and radiation treatments may alter the width of the bands and make interpretation difficult.

Nursing Implications and Procedure

Pretest:

➤ Obtain a history of the patient's complaints, including a list of known allergens.

➤ Obtain a history of the patient's hematopoietic and immune systems, as well as results of previously performed tests and procedures. Assess whether the patient received any vaccinations or immunizations within the last 6 months or any blood or blood components within the last 6 weeks. For related tests, refer to the hematopoietic and immune system tables.

➤ Obtain a list of medications the patient is taking, including herbs, nutritional supplements, and nutraceuticals. The requesting health care practitioner and laboratory should be advised if the patient regularly uses these products so that their effects can be taken into consideration when reviewing results.

➤ Note any recent procedures that can interfere with test results.

➤ There are no food, fluid, or medication restrictions unless by medical direction.

➤ Review the procedure with the patient. Provide a nonmetallic urinal, bedpan, or toilet-mounted collection device.

➤ Usually a 24-hour time frame for urine collection is ordered. Inform the patient that all urine must be saved during that 24-hour period. Instruct the patient not to void directly into the laboratory collection container. Instruct the patient to avoid defecating in the collection device and to keep toilet tissue out of the collection device to prevent contamination of the specimen. Place a sign in the bathroom to remind the patient to save all urine.

➤ Instruct the patient to void all urine into the collection device and then to pour the urine into the laboratory collection container. Alternatively the specimen can be left in the collection device for a health care staff member to add to the laboratory collection container.

➤ Inform the patient that specimen collection takes approximately 5 to 10 minutes.

Intratest:

➤ Direct the patient to breathe normally and to avoid unnecessary movement. Observe standard precautions and follow the general guidelines in Appendix A.

Blood:

➤ Perform a venipuncture, and collect the specimen in a 5-mL red-top tube.

Urine:

Clean-catch specimen:

➤ Instruct the male patient to (1) thoroughly wash his hands, (2) cleanse the meatus, (3) void a small amount into the toilet, and (4) void directly into the specimen container.

➤ Instruct the female patient to (1) thoroughly wash her hands; (2) cleanse the labia from front to back; (3) while keeping the labia separated, void a small amount into the toilet; and (4) without interrupting the urine stream, void directly into the specimen container.

Blood or urine:

➤ Label the specimen, and promptly transport it to the laboratory.

Post-test:

➤ Observe venipuncture site for bleeding or hematoma formation. Apply pressure bandage.

➤ Evaluate test results in relation to the patient's symptoms and other tests performed. Related laboratory tests include bone marrow biopsy, lymph node biopsy, complete blood count with examination of peripheral smear, quantitative immunoglobulin levels, protein, urine protein, protein electrophoresis, urine protein electrophoresis, and urinalysis.

IMMUNOGLOBULIN E

· ·

SYNONYM/ACRONYM: IgE.

SPECIMEN: Serum (1 mL) collected in a red- or tiger-top tube.

REFERENCE VALUE: (Method: Immunoassay)

Age	Conventional Units	SI Unit (Conversion Factor ×1)
Newborn	Less than 12 IU/mL	Less than 12 kIU/mL
Less than 1 y	Less than 50 IU/mL	Less than 50 kIU/mL
2–4 y	Less than 100 IU/mL	Less than 100 kIU/mL
5 y and older	Less than 300 IU/m	Less than 300 kIU/mL

DESCRIPTION: Immunoglobulin E (IgE) is an antibody whose primary response is to allergic reactions and parasitic infections. Most of the body's IgE is bound to specialized tissue cells; little is available in the circulating blood. IgE binds to the membrane of special granulocytes called *basophils* in the circulating blood and *mast cells* in the tissues. Basophil and mast cell membranes have receptors for IgE. Mast cells are abundant in the skin and the tissues lining the respiratory and alimentary tracts. When IgE antibody becomes cross-linked with antigen/allergen, the release of histamine, heparin, and other chemicals from the granules in the cells is triggered. A sequence of events follows activation of IgE that affects smooth muscle contraction, vascular permeability, and inflammatory reactions. The inflammatory response allows proteins from the bloodstream to enter the tissues. Helminths (worm parasites) are especially susceptible to immunoglobulin-mediated cytotoxic chemicals. The inflammatory reaction proteins attract macrophages from the circulatory system and granulocytes, such as eosinophils, from circulation and bone marrow. Eosinophils also contain enzymes effective against the parasitic invaders. ∎

INDICATIONS: Assist in the evaluation of allergy and parasitic infection

RESULT

Increased in:
• Asthma
• Alcoholism
• Allergy

• Bronchopulmonary aspergillosis
• Dermatitis
• Eczema
• Hay fever
• IgE myeloma
• Parasitic infestation
• Rhinitis
• Sinusitis
• Wiskott-Aldrich syndrome

Decreased in:
• Advanced carcinoma
• Agammaglobulinemia
• Ataxia-telangiectasia
• IgE deficiency

CRITICAL VALUES: N/A

INTERFERING FACTORS:
• Drugs that may cause a decrease in IgE levels include phenytoin and tryptophan.

• Penicillin G has been associated with increased IgE levels in some patients with drug-induced acute interstitial nephritis.

• Normal IgE levels do not eliminate allergic disorders as a possible diagnosis.

Nursing Implications and Procedure • • • • • • • • • •

Pretest: ∎

➤ Obtain a history of the patient's complaints, including a list of known allergens.

➤ Obtain a history of the patient's immune and respiratory systems, as well as results of previously performed tests and procedures. For related tests, refer to the immune and respiratory system tables.

➤ Obtain a list of the medications the patient is taking, including herbs, nutritional supplements, and neutraceuticals. The requesting health care practitioner and laboratory should be advised if the patient regularly uses these products so that their effects can be taken into consideration when reviewing results.

➤ There are no food, fluid, or medication restrictions unless by medical direction.

➤ Review the procedure with the patient.

➤ Inform the patient that specimen collection takes approximately 5 to 10 minutes.

Intratest:

➤ Direct the patient to breathe normally and to avoid unnecessary movement.

➤ Observe standard precautions and follow the general guidelines in Appendix A. Perform a venipuncture, and collect the specimen in a 5-mL red- or tiger-top tube.

➤ Label the specimen, and promptly transport it to the laboratory.

Post-test:

➤ Observe venipuncture site for bleeding or hematoma formation. Apply pressure bandage.

➤ Consideration should be given to diet if the patient has food allergies.

➤ Evaluate test results in relation to the patient's symptoms and other tests performed. Related laboratory tests include allergen-specific IgE, alveolar/arterial gradient and arterial/alveolar oxygen ratio, blood gases, complete blood count, eosinophil count, hypersensitivity pneumonitis, and theophylline.

IMMUNOGLOBULINS A, D, G, AND M
• •

SYNONYMS/ACRONYMS: IgA, IgD, IgG, and IgM.

SPECIMEN: Serum (1 mL) collected in a red-top tube.

REFERENCE VALUE: (Method: Nephelometry)

Age	Conventional Units	SI Units
Immunoglobulin A		
		(Conversion Factor × 10)
Newborn	1–4 mg/dL	10–40 mg/L
1–9 mo	2–80 mg/dL	20–800 mg/L
10–12 mo	15–90 mg/dL	150–900 mg/L
2–3 y	18–150 mg/dL	180–1500 mg/L
4–5 y	25–160 mg/dL	250–1600 mg/L
6–8 y	35–200 mg/dL	350–2000 mg/L
9–12 y	45–250 mg/dL	450–2500 mg/L
Older than 12 y	40–350 mg/dL	400–3500 mg/L

(Continued on the following page)

Immunoglobulin D		
		(Conversion Factor × 10)
Newborn	Greater than 2 mg/dL	Greater than 20 mg/L
Adult	Less than 15 mg/dL	Less than 150 mg/L
Immunoglobulin G		
		(Conversion Factor × 0.01)
Newborn	650–1600 mg/dL	6.5–16 g/L
1–9 mo	250–900 mg/dL	2.5–9 g/L
10–12 mo	290–1070 mg/dL	2.9–10.7 g/L
2–3 y	420–1200 mg/dL	4.2–12 g/L
4–6 y	460–1240 mg/dL	4.6–12.4 g/L
Greater than 6 y	650–1600 mg/dL	6.5–16 g/L
Immunoglobulin M		
		(Conversion Factor × 10)
Newborn	Less than 25 mg/dL	Less than 250 mg/L
1–9 mo	20–125 mg/dL	200–1250 mg/L
10–12 mo	40–150 mg/dL	400–1500 mg/L
2–8 y	45–200 mg/dL	450–2000 mg/L
9–12 y	50–250 mg/dL	500–2500 mg/L
Greater than 12 y	50–300 mg/dL	500–3000 mg/L

DESCRIPTION: Immunoglobulins A, D, E, G, and M are made by plasma cells in response to foreign particles. Immunoglobulins neutralize toxic substances, support phagocytosis, and destroy invading microorganisms. They are made up of heavy and light chains. Immunoglobulins produced by the proliferation of a single plasma cell (clone) are called *monoclonal.* Polyclonal increases result when multiple cell lines produce antibody. IgA is found mainly in secretions such as tears, saliva, and breast milk. It is believed to protect mucous membranes from viruses and bacteria. The function of IgD is not well understood. For details on IgE, see monograph titled "Immunoglobulin E." IgG is the predominant serum immunoglobulin and is important in long-term defense against disease. It is the only antibody that crosses the placenta. IgM is the largest immunoglobulin, and it is the first antibody to react to an antigenic stimulus. IgM also forms natural antibodies, such as ABO blood group antibodies. The presence of IgM in cord blood is an indication of congenital infection. ■

INDICATIONS:
• Assist in the diagnosis of multiple myeloma

• Evaluate humoral immunity status

• Monitor therapy for multiple myeloma

• IgA: Evaluate anaphylaxis associated with the transfusion of blood and blood products (anti-IgA antibodies may develop in patients with low levels of IgA, possibly resulting in anaphylaxis when donated blood is transfused)

RESULT

Increases in:

IgA:
• Polyclonal:

Chronic infections, especially gastrointestinal (GI) and respiratory tracts
Chronic liver disease
Immunodeficiency states, such as Wiskott-Aldrich syndrome
Inflammatory bowel disease
Lower GI cancer
Rheumatoid arthritis

• Monoclonal:
IgA-type multiple myeloma

IgD:
• Polyclonal:
Chronic infections
Certain liver diseases
Connective tissue disorders

• Monoclonal:
IgD-type multiple myeloma

IgG:
• Polyclonal:
Autoimmune diseases, such as systemic lupus erythematosus, rheumatoid arthritis, and Sjögren's syndrome
Chronic liver disease
Chronic or recurrent infections
Intrauterine devices
Sarcoidosis

• Monoclonal:
IgG-type multiple myeloma
Leukemias
Lymphomas

IgM:
• Polyclonal:
Active sarcoidosis
Chronic hepatocellular disease
Collagen vascular disease
Early response to bacterial or parasitic infection
Hyper-IgM dysgammaglobulinemia
Rheumatoid arthritis
Variable in nephrotic syndrome

Viral infection (hepatitis or mononucleosis)

• Monoclonal:
Cold agglutinin hemolysis disease
Malignant lymphoma
Neoplasms (especially GI tract)
Reticulosis
Waldenström's macroglobulinemia

Decreases in:

IgA:
• Ataxia-telangiectasia
• Chronic sinopulmonary disease
• Genetic IgA deficiency

IgD:
• Genetic IgD deficiency
• Malignant melanoma of the skin
• Preeclampsia

IgG:
• Burns
• Genetic IgG deficiency
• Nephrotic syndrome
• Pregnancy

IgM:
• Burns
• Secondary IgM deficiency associated with IgG or IgA gammopathies

CRITICAL VALUES: N/A

INTERFERING FACTORS:
• Drugs that may increase immunoglobulin levels include asparaginase, cimetidine, and narcotics.

• Drugs that may decrease immunoglobulin levels include dextran, oral contraceptives, phenytoin, and methylprednisolone (high doses).

• Chemotherapy, immunosuppressive therapy, and radiation treatments decrease immunoglobulin levels.

- Specimens with macroglobulins, cryoglobulins, or cold agglutinins tested at cold temperatures may give falsely low values.

Nursing Implications and Procedure • • • • • • • • • •

Pretest:

➤ Obtain a history of the patient's complaints, including a list of known allergens.

➤ Obtain a history of the patient's GI, hematopoietic, immune, and musculoskeletal systems, as well as results of previously performed tests and procedures. For related tests, refer to the gastrointestinal, hematopoietic, immune, and musculoskeletal system tables.

➤ Obtain a list of medications the patient is taking, including herbs, nutritional supplements, and nutraceuticals. The requesting health care practitioner and laboratory should be advised if the patient regularly uses these products so that their effects can be taken into consideration when reviewing results.

➤ Note any recent procedures that can interfere with test results.

➤ There are no food, fluid, or medication restrictions unless by medical direction.

➤ Review the procedure with the patient.

➤ Inform the patient that specimen collection takes approximately 5 to 10 minutes.

Intratest:

➤ Direct the patient to breathe normally and to avoid unnecessary movement.

➤ Observe standard precautions and follow the general guidelines in Appendix A. Perform a venipuncture, and collect the specimen in a 5-mL red-top tube.

➤ Label the specimen, and promptly transport it to the laboratory.

Post-test:

➤ Observe venipuncture site for bleeding or hematoma formation. Apply pressure bandage.

➤ Evaluate test results in relation to the patient's symptoms and other tests performed. Related laboratory tests include bone marrow biopsy, complete blood count with evaluation of peripheral smear, immunofixation electrophoresis, urine immunofixation electrophoresis, protein, urine protein, protein electrophoresis, and urinalysis.

IMMUNOSUPPRESSANTS: CYCLOSPORINE, METHOTREXATE

• •

SYNONYMS/ACRONYM: Cyclosporine (Sandimmune), methotrexate (MTX, amethopterin, Folex, Rheumatrex), methotrexate sodium (Mexate).

SPECIMEN: Whole blood (1 mL) collected in lavender-top tube for cyclosporine. Serum (1 mL) collected in a red-top tube for methotrexate.

Immunosuppressant	Route of Administration	Recommended Collection Time
Cyclosporine	Oral	12 hours after dose
Methotrexate	Oral	Varies according to dosing protocol
	Intramuscular	Varies according to dosing protocol

REFERENCE VALUE: (Method: Immunoassay)

	Therapeutic Dose		Half-Life	Volume of Distribution	Protein Binding	Excretion
	Conventional Units	*SI Units (Conversion Factor ×0.832)*				
Cyclosporine	100–400 ng/mL Renal transplant	83–333 nmol/L	8–24 h	4–6 L/kg	90%	Renal
	100–300 ng/mL Cardiac transplant	83–250 nmol/L	8–24 h	4–6 L/kg	90%	Renal
	100–250 ng/mL Bone marrow transplant	83–208 nmol/L	8–24 h	4–6 L/kg	90%	Renal
Methotrexate	Dependent on therapeutic approach		8–15 h	0.4–1.0 L/kg	50–70%	Renal

DESCRIPTION: Cyclosporine is an immunosuppressive drug used in the management of organ rejection, especially rejection of the heart, liver, and kidney. Its most serious side effect is renal impairment or renal failure. Methotrexate is a highly toxic drug that causes cell death by disrupting DNA synthesis.

Many factors must be considered in effective dosing and monitoring of therapeutic drugs, including patient age, weight, interacting medications, electrolyte balance, protein levels, water balance, and conditions that affect absorption and excretion; as well as foods, herbals, vitamins, and minerals that can either potentiate or inhibit the intended target concentration. Collection times should be documented carefully in relation to the time of medication administration. It is essential that this information be communicated clearly and accurately to avoid misunderstanding of the dose time in relation to the collection time. Miscommunication between the individual administering the medication and the individual collecting the specimen is the most frequent cause of subtherapeutic levels, toxic levels, and misleading information used in calculation of future doses. ■

INDICATIONS

Cyclosporine:
• Assist in the management of treatments to prevent organ rejection

• Monitor for toxicity

Methotrexate:
• Monitor effectiveness of treatment of cancer and some autoimmune disorders

• Monitor for toxicity

RESULT

Normal levels	Therapeutic effect
Toxic levels	Adjust dose as indicated
Cyclosporine	Renal impairment
Methotrexate	Renal impairment

CRITICAL VALUES: ⚠ It is important to note the adverse effects of subtherapeutic levels. Care should be taken to investigate signs and symptoms of too little and too much medication.

Cyclosporine: Greater than 400 ng/mL

Signs and symptoms of cyclosporine toxicity include increased severity of expected side effects, which include nausea, stomatitis, vomiting, anorexia, hypertension, infection, fluid retention, hypercalcemic metabolic acidosis, tremor, seizures, headache, and flushing. Possible interventions include close monitoring of blood levels to make dosing adjustments, inducing emesis (if orally ingested), performing gastric lavage (if orally ingested), withholding the drug, and initiating alternative therapy for a short time until the patient is stabilized.

Methotrexate: Low-dose therapy, greater than 9.1 ng/mL; high-dose therapy, greater than 454 ng/mL

Signs and symptoms of methotrexate toxicity include increased severity of expected side effects, which include nausea, stomatitis, vomiting, anorexia, bleeding, infection, bone marrow depression, and over a prolonged period of use, hepatotoxicity. The effect of methotrexate on normal cells can be reversed by administration of 5-formyltetrahydrofolate (citrovorum or leucovorin). 5-Formyltetrahydrofolate allows higher doses of methotrexate to be given.

INTERFERING FACTORS:
• Numerous drugs interact with and either increase cyclosporine levels or increase the risk of toxicity. These drugs include acyclovir, aminoglycosides, amiodarone, amphotericin B, anabolic steroids, cephalosporins, cimetidine, danazol, erythromycin, furosemide, ketoconazole, melphalan, methylprednisolone, miconazole, nonsteroidal anti-inflammatory drugs (NSAIDs), oral contraceptives, and trimethoprim-sulfamethoxazole.

• Drugs that may decrease cyclosporine levels include carbamazepine, ethotoin, mephenytoin, phenobarbital, phenytoin, primidone, and rifampin.

• Drugs that may increase methotrexate levels or increase the risk of toxicity include NSAIDs, probenecid, salicylate, and sulfonamides.

• Antibiotics may decrease the absorption of methotrexate.

Nursing Implications and Procedure • • • • • • • • • •

Pretest:

➤ Obtain a history of the patient's complaints, including a list of known allergens.

➤ Obtain a history of the patient's genitourinary system as well as results of previously performed tests and procedures. For related tests, refer to the genitourinary system and therapeutic/toxicology table.

➤ Obtain a list of the medications the patient is taking, including herbs, nutritional supplements, and nutraceuticals. The requesting health care practitioner and laboratory should be advised if the patient regularly uses these products so that their effects can be taken into consideration when reviewing results. For related tests, refer to the therapeutic/toxicology table.

➤ There are no food, fluid, or medication restrictions unless by medical direction.

➤ Review the procedure with the patient.

➤ Inform the patient that specimen collection takes approximately 5 to 10 minutes.

Intratest:

➤ Direct the patient to breathe normally and to avoid unnecessary movement.

➤ Observe standard precautions and follow the general guidelines in Appendix A. Consider recommended collection time around dosing schedule. Perform a venipuncture, and collect the specimen in a lavender-top tube for cyclosporine and a red-top tube for methotrexate.

➤ Label the specimen, and promptly transport it to the laboratory.

Post-test:

➤ Observe venipuncture site for bleeding or hematoma formation. Apply pressure bandage.

➤ Explain to the patient the importance of following the medication regimen and instructions regarding food and drug interactions.

➤ Instruct the patient to be prepared to list to the pharmacist the other medications he or she already is taking in the event that the requesting health care practitioner prescribes a medication.

➤ Recognize anxiety related to test results and offer support. Patients receiving these drugs usually have conditions that can be intermittently moderate to severely debilitating and resulting in significant lifestyle changes. Educate the patient regarding access to counseling services, as appropriate.

➤ Evaluate test results in relation to the patient's symptoms and other tests performed. Related laboratory tests include creatinine and blood urea nitrogen (BUN).

INFECTIOUS MONONUCLEOSIS SCREEN

• •

SYNONYMS/ACRONYM: Monospot, heterophil antibody test, IM serology.

SPECIMEN: Serum (1 mL) collected in a red-top tube.

REFERENCE VALUE: (Method: Agglutination) Negative.

DESCRIPTION: Infectious mononucleosis is caused by the Epstein-Barr virus (EBV). The incubation period is 10 to 50 days, and the symptoms last 1 to 4 weeks after the infection has fully developed. The hallmark of EBV infection is the presence of heterophil antibodies, also called *Paul-Bunnell-Davidsohn antibodies*, which are immunoglobulin M (IgM) antibodies that agglutinate sheep or horse red blood cells. The disease induces formation of abnormal lymphocytes in the lymph nodes; stimulates increased formation of heterophil antibodies; and is characterized by fever, cervical lymphadenopathy, tonsillopharyngitis, and hepatosplenomegaly. EBV is also thought to play a role in Burkitt's lymphoma, nasopharyngeal carcinoma, and chronic fatigue syndrome. If the results of the heterophil antibody screening test are negative and infectious mononucleosis is highly suspected, EBV-specific serology should be requested. ■

INDICATIONS: Assist in confirming infectious mononucleosis

RESULT

Positive findings in: Infectious mononucleosis

CRITICAL VALUES: N/A

INTERFERING FACTORS:
• False-positive results may occur in the presence of narcotic addiction, serum sickness, lymphomas, hepatitis, leukemia, cancer of the pancreas, and phenytoin therapy.

• A false-negative result may occur if treatment was begun before antibodies developed or if the test was done less than 6 days after exposure to the virus.

Nursing Implications and Procedure

Pretest:

➤ Obtain a history of the patient's complaints, including a list of known allergens. Obtain a history of exposure.

➤ Obtain a history of the patient's hepatobiliary and immune systems, as well as results of previously performed tests and procedures. For related tests, refer to the hepatobiliary and immune system tables.

➤ Obtain a list of medications the patient is taking, including herbs, nutritional supplements, and nutraceuticals. The requesting health care practitioner and laboratory should be advised if the patient regularly uses these products so that their effects can be taken into consideration when reviewing results.

➤ Note any recent therapies that can interfere with test results.

➤ There are no food, fluid, or medication restrictions unless by medical direction.

➤ Review the procedure with the patient. Inform the patient that specimen collection takes approximately 5 to 10 minutes.

Intratest:

➤ Direct the patient to breathe normally and to avoid unnecessary movement.

➤ Observe standard precautions and follow the general guidelines in Appendix A. Perform a venipuncture, and collect the specimen in a 5-mL red-top tube.

➤ Label the specimen, and promptly transport it to the laboratory.

Post-test:

➤ Observe venipuncture site for bleeding or hematoma formation. Apply pressure bandage.

➤ Advise the patient to refrain from direct contact with others because the disease is transmitted through saliva.

➤ Inform the patient that approximately 10 percent of all results are false-negative or false-positive. Inform the patient that signs and symptoms of infection include fever, chills, sore throat, enlarged lymph nodes and fatigue. Self-care while the disease runs its course includes adequate fluid and nutritional intake along with sufficient rest. Activities that cause fatigue or stress should be avoided.

➤ Evaluate test results in relation to the patient's symptoms and other tests performed. Related laboratory tests include complete blood count with peripheral blood smear evaluation.

INSULIN AND INSULIN RESPONSE TO GLUCOSE

SYNONYM/ACRONYM: N/A.

SPECIMEN: Serum (1 mL) collected in a red-top tube.

REFERENCE VALUE: (Method: Radioimmunoassay)

	Insulin	Insulin ×6.945 = SI Units	Glucose (Tolerance for Hypoglycemia)
Fasting	Less than 25 mIU/L	Less than 174 pmol/L	65–115 mg/dL
30 min	30–230 mIU/L	208–1597 pmol/L	N/A
1 h	18–276 mIU/L	125–1917 pmol/L	Less than 200 mg/dL
2 h	16–166 mIU/L	111–1153 pmol/L	Less than 140 mg/dL
3 h	Less than 25 mIU/L	Less than 174 pmol/L	65–120 mg/dL
4 h	Less than 25 mIU/L	Less than 174 pmol/L	65–120 mg/dL
5 h	Less than 25 mIU/L	Less than 174 pmol/L	65–115 mg/dL

DESCRIPTION: Insulin is secreted in response to elevated blood glucose, and its overall effect is to promote glucose use and energy storage. The insulin response test measures the rate of insulin secreted by the beta cells of the islets of Langerhans in the pancreas; it may be performed simultaneously with a 5-hour glucose tolerance test for hypoglycemia. ■

INDICATIONS:

- Assist in the diagnosis of early or developing non–insulin-dependent (type 2) diabetes, as indicated by excessive production of insulin in relation to blood glucose levels (best shown with glucose tolerance tests or 2-hour postprandial tests)

- Assist in the diagnosis of insulinoma, as indicated by sustained high levels of insulin and absence of blood glucose–related variations

- Confirm functional hypoglycemia, as indicated by circulating insulin levels appropriate to changing blood glucose levels

- Differentiate between insulin-resistant diabetes, in which insulin levels are high, and non–insulin-resistant diabetes, in which insulin levels are low

- Evaluate fasting hypoglycemia of unknown cause

- Evaluate postprandial hypoglycemia of unknown cause

- Evaluate uncontrolled insulin-dependent (type 1) diabetes

RESULT

Increased in:

- Acromegaly

- Alcohol use

- Cushing's syndrome

- Diabetes

- Excessive administration of insulin

- Insulin- and proinsulin-secreting tumors (insulinomas)

- Obesity

- Reactive hypoglycemia in developing diabetes

- Severe liver disease

Decreased in:

- Beta cell failure

CRITICAL VALUES:
Greater than 35 mIU/L
Symptoms of elevated insulin levels include dizziness, diaphoresis, faintness, pallor, weakness, stupor, and seizures. Possible interventions include administering 50% dextrose in water (D$_5$W) solution, administering glucagon, and monitoring blood glucose level hourly.

INTERFERING FACTORS:

- Drugs and substances that may increase insulin levels include acetohexamide, alanine, albuterol, amino acids, beclomethasone, betamethasone, broxaterol, calcium gluconate, cannabis, chlorpropamide, cyclic AMP, glibornuride, glipizide, glisoxepide, glucagon, glyburide, ibopamine, insulin, insulin-like growth factor–I, oral contraceptives, pancreozymin, prednisolone, prednisone, rifampin, salbutamol, terbutaline, tolazamide, tolbutamide, trichlormethiazide, and verapamil.

- Drugs that may decrease insulin levels include acarbose, asparaginase, calcitonin, cimetidine, clofibrate, dexfenfluramine, diltiazem, doxazosin, enalapril, enprostil, ether, hydroxypropyl methylcellulose, insulin-like growth factor–I, metformin, niacin, nifedipine, nitrendipine, octreotide, phenytoin, propranolol, and psyllium.

- Administration of insulin or oral hypoglycemic agents within 8 hours of the test can lead to falsely elevated levels.

- Hemodialysis destroys insulin and affects test results.

- Recent radioactive scans or radiation can interfere with test results when radioimmunoassay is the test method.

Nursing Implications and Procedure • • • • • • • • • • •

Pretest:

➤ Obtain a history of the patient's complaints, including a list of known allergens.

➤ Obtain a history of the patient's endocrine system and results of previously performed tests and procedures. For related tests, refer to the endocrine system table.

➤ Obtain a list of the medications the patient is taking, including herbs, nutritional supplements and nutraceuticals. The requesting health care practitioner and laboratory should be advised if the patient regularly uses these products so their effects can be taken into consideration when reviewing results.

➤ Note any recent procedures that can interfere with test results.

➤ There are no fluid restrictions unless by medical direction.

➤ If a single sample is to be collected, the patient should have fasted and refrained, with medical direction, from taking insulin or other oral hypoglycemic agents for at least 8 hours before specimen collection.

➤ Hypoglycemia: Serial specimens for insulin levels are collected in conjunction with glucose levels after administration of a 100-g dose of glucola. The patient should be prepared as for a standard oral glucose tolerance test over a 5-hour period.

➤ Review the procedure with the patient. Inform the patient that multiple specimens may be required.

➤ Inform the patient that specimen collection takes approximately 5 to 10 minutes.

Intratest:

➤ Ensure that the patient has complied with dietary preparations and other pretesting restrictions.

➤ Direct the patient to breathe normally and to avoid unnecessary movement.

➤ Observe standard precautions and follow the general guidelines in Appendix A. Perform a venipuncture, and collect the specimen in a 5-mL red-top tube.

➤ Label the specimen, and promptly transport it to the laboratory.

Post-test:

➤ Observe venipuncture site for bleeding or hematoma formation. Apply pressure bandage.

➤ Instruct the patient to resume usual diet and medication as directed by the requesting health care practitioner.

➤ Increased insulin levels may be associated with diabetes. Instruct the diabetic patient, as appropriate, in nutritional management of the disease. Patients who adhere to dietary recommendations report a better general feeling of health, better weight management, greater control of glucose and lipid values, and improved use of insulin. There is no "diabetic" diet; however, there are many meal-planning approaches with nutritional goals endorsed by the American Dietetic Association. The nutritional needs of each diabetic patient must be determined individually with the appropriate health care professionals, particularly professionals trained in nutrition.

➤ Instruct the patient and caregiver to report signs and symptoms of hypoglycemia (weakness, confusion, diaphoresis, rapid pulse) or hyperglycemia (thirst, polyuria, hunger, and lethargy).

➤ Recognize anxiety related to test results and provide support. Provide teaching and information regarding the clinical implications of the test results, as appropriate.

➤ Emphasize, as appropriate, that good glycemic control delays the onset and slows the progression of diabetic retinopathy, nephropathy, and neuropathy.

➤ Evaluate test results in relation to the patient's symptoms and other tests performed. Related laboratory tests include C-peptide, fructosamine, glucose, glycated hemoglobin, insulin antibodies, and microalbumin.

INSULIN ANTIBODIES

SYNONYM/ACRONYM: N/A.

SPECIMEN: Serum (1 mL) collected in a red-top tube.

REFERENCE VALUE: (Method: Radioimmunoassay) Less than 3 percent; includes binding of human, beef, and pork insulin to antibodies in patient's serum.

DESCRIPTION: The most common anti-insulin antibody is immunoglobulin G (IgG), but IgA, IgM, IgD, and IgE antibodies also have anti-insulin properties. These antibodies usually do not cause clinical problems, but they may complicate insulin assay testing. IgM is thought to participate in insulin resistance and IgE in insulin allergy. Improvements in the purity of animal insulin and increased use of human insulin have resulted in a significant decrease in the incidence of insulin antibody formation. ■

INDICATIONS:
• Assist in confirming insulin resistance
• Assist in determining if hypoglycemia is caused by insulin abuse
• Assist in determining insulin allergy

RESULT

Increased in:
• Insulin allergy or resistance

• Factitious hypoglycemia

• Polyendocrine autoimmune syndromes

• Steroid-induced diabetes (a side effect of treatment for systemic lupus erythematosus)

Decreased in: N/A

CRITICAL VALUES: N/A

INTERFERING FACTORS: Recent radioactive scans or radiation can interfere with test results when radioimmunoassay is the test method.

Nursing Implications and Procedure • • • • • • • • • • •

Pretest:

➤ Obtain a history of the patient's complaints, including a list of known allergens.

➤ Obtain a history of the patient's endocrine and immune systems, as well as results of previously performed tests and procedures. For related tests, refer to the endocrine and immune system tables.

➤ Obtain a list of medications the patient is taking, including herbs, nutritional supplements, and nutraceuticals. The requesting health care practitioner and laboratory should be advised if the patient is regularly using these products so that their effects can be taken into consideration when reviewing results.

➤ Note any recent procedures that can interfere with test results.

➤ There are no food, fluid, or medication restrictions unless by medical direction.

➤ Review the procedure with the patient.

➤ Inform the patient that specimen collection takes approximately 5 to 10 minutes.

Intratest:

➤ Direct the patient to breathe normally and to avoid unnecessary movement.

➤ Observe standard precautions and follow the general guidelines in Appendix A. Perform a venipuncture, and collect the specimen in a 5-mL red-top tube.

➤ Label the specimen, and promptly transport it to the laboratory.

Post-test:

➤ Observe venipuncture site for bleeding or hematoma formation. Apply pressure bandage.

➤ Instruct the patient and caregiver to report signs and symptoms of hypoglycemia (weakness, confusion, diaphoresis, rapid pulse) or hyperglycemia (thirst, polyuria, hunger, and lethargy).

➤ Emphasize, as appropriate, that good glycemic control delays the onset and slows the progression of diabetic retinopathy, nephropathy, and neuropathy.

➤ Evaluate test results in relation to the patient's symptoms and other tests performed. Related laboratory tests include C-peptide, glucose, and insulin.

INTRAVENOUS PYELOGRAPHY
• •

SYNONYMS/ACRONYMS: Excretory urography (EUG), intravenous urography (IVU, IUG), IVP.

AREA OF APPLICATION: Kidneys, ureters, bladder, and renal pelvis.

CONTRAST: Intravenous radiopaque iodine-based contrast medium.

DESCRIPTION: Intravenous pyelography (IVP) is the most commonly performed test to determine urinary tract dysfunction or renal disease. IVP uses IV radiopaque contrast medium to visualize the kidneys, ureters, bladder, and renal pelvis. The contrast medium concentrates in the blood and is filtered out by the glomeruli; it passes out through the renal tubules and is concentrated in the urine. Renal function is reflected by the length of time it takes the contrast medium to appear and to be excreted by each kidney. A series of x-rays is performed during a 30-minute period to view passage of the medium through the kidneys and ureters into the bladder. A final film is taken after the patient empties the bladder (postvoiding film). Computed tomography (CT) may be employed during the examination to permit the examination of an individual layer or plane of the organ that may be obscured by surrounding overlying structures. ■

INDICATIONS:

- Evaluate known or suspected ureteral obstruction

- Evaluate function of the kidneys, ureters, and bladder

- Evaluate the presence of renal, ureter, or bladder calculi

- Evaluate the cause of blood in the urine

- Aid in the diagnosis of renovascular hypertension

- Evaluate space-occupying lesions or congenital anomalies of the urinary system

- Evaluate the effects of urinary system trauma

RESULT

Normal Findings:

- Normal size and shape of kidneys, ureters, and bladder

- Normal bladder and absence of masses or renal calculi, with prompt visualization of contrast medium through the urinary system

Abnormal Findings:

- Absence of a kidney (congenital malformation)

- Benign and malignant kidney tumors

- Bladder tumors

- Congenital renal or urinary tract abnormalities

- Glomerulonephritis

- Hydronephrosis

- Prostatic enlargement

- Pyelonephritis

- Renal cysts

- Renal hematomas

- Renal or ureteral calculi

- Soft-tissue masses

- Tumors of the collecting system

CRITICAL VALUES: N/A

INTERFERING FACTORS:

This procedure is contraindicated for:

- Patients with allergies to shellfish or iodinated dye. The contrast medium used may cause a life-threatening allergic reaction. Patients with a known hypersensitivity to the contrast medium may benefit from premedication with corticosteroids or the use of nonionic contrast medium.

- Patients with bleeding disorders.

- Patients who are pregnant or suspected of being pregnant, unless the potential benefits of the procedure far outweigh the risks to the fetus and mother.

- Elderly and other patients who are ⚠ chronically dehydrated before the test, because of their risk of contrast-induced renal failure.

- ⚠ Patients who are in renal failure.

- Patients with renal insufficiency, indicated by a blood urea nitrogen (BUN) value greater than 40 mg/dL, because contrast medium can complicate kidney function.

- Young patients (17 years old and younger), unless the benefits of the x-ray diagnosis outweigh the risks of exposure to high levels of radiation.

- Patients with multiple myeloma, who may experience decreased kidney function subsequent to administration of contrast medium.

Factors that may impair clear imaging:

- Inability of the patient to cooperate or remain still during the procedure because of age, significant pain, or mental status

- Improper adjustment of the radiographic equipment to accommodate obese or thin patients, which can cause overexposure or underexposure and a poor-quality study

- Patients who are very obese, who may exceed the weight limit for the equipment

- Incorrect positioning of the patient, which may produce poor visualization of the area to be examined, especially for oblique and decubitus views and for films done by portable equipment

- Metallic objects within the examination field (e.g., jewelry or body rings), which may inhibit organ visualization and can produce unclear images

- Retained barium from a previous radiologic procedure

- Gas or feces in the gastrointestinal tract resulting from inadequate cleansing or failure to restrict food intake before the study

- End-stage renal disease, which may produce an examination of poor quality

Other considerations:

- Consultation with a physician should occur before the procedure for radiation safety concerns regarding infants of patients who are lactating.

- Risks associated with radiographic overexposure can result from frequent x-ray procedures. Personnel in the room with the patient should wear a protective lead apron, stand behind a shield, or leave the area while the examination is being done. Personnel working in the area where the examination is being done should wear badges that reveal their level of exposure to radiation.

Nursing Implications and Procedure • • • • • • • • • • •

Pretest: ■

➤ Inform the patient that the procedure assesses the kidneys, ureters, and bladder.

➤ Inform the patient that the procedure is performed in a radiology department by a technologist and a physician and takes approximately 30 minutes.

➤ Ask the patient to lie still during the procedure because movement produces unclear images; the patient may be asked to hold his or her breath for short periods.

➤ Obtain a history of allergies or sensitivities to contrast medium or shellfish.

➤ Obtain a history of the patient's complaints.

➤ Obtain a history of the patient's genitourinary and abdominal systems, as well as results of previously performed tests and procedures. For related tests and procedures. For related tests, refer to the genitourinary system table.

➤ Determine date of last menstrual period and the possibility of pregnancy in perimenopausal women.

➤ Patients receiving metformin (Glucophage) for non–insulin-dependent (type 2) diabetes should discontinue the drug on the day of the test and continue to withhold it for 48 hours after the test. Failure to do so may result in lactic acidosis.

➤ Instruct the patient to increase fluid intake the day before the test but to withhold food and fluids for 8 hours before the test.

➤ Schedule gastrointestinal or any barium studies after this study.

Intratest:

➤ Give the patient a laxative or a cathartic, as ordered, on the evening before the examination.

➤ Give the patient an enema or suppository on the morning of the test, as ordered.

➤ Have the patient put on a hospital gown, but instruct the patient not to void until after the test is performed.

➤ Administer sedative to a child or to an uncooperative adult, as ordered.

➤ Ask the patient to lie still during the procedure because movement produces unclear images. Make sure jewelry, watches, chains, belts, and any other metallic objects have been removed from the abdominal area.

➤ Remove any wires connected to electrodes, if allowed.

➤ Place the patient on the table in the supine position with hands over the head or relaxed at the patient's side.

➤ For male patients, place lead protection over the testicles to prevent their irradiation but remove it for bladder exposures.

➤ A kidney, ureter, and bladder (KUB) or plain film is taken to ensure that no barium or stool obscures visualization of the urinary system.

➤ Insert an IV line, if one is not already in place, and inject the contrast medium.

➤ X-ray exposures are made at 1-, 5-, 10-, 15-, 20-, and 30-minute intervals to follow the course of the contrast medium through the urinary system. Instruct the patient to exhale deeply and to hold his or her breath while the x-ray is taken, and then to breathe after the film is taken.

➤ Ask the patient to void; a postvoiding exposure is done to visualize the empty bladder.

Post-test:

➤ Direct the patient to resume usual diet, activity, and medication, if withheld and as directed by the physician. Renal function should be assessed before metformin is restarted.

➤ Inform the patient that the contrast medium may cause a temporary flushing of the face, a feeling of warmth, or nausea.

➤ Inform the patient that further examinations may be necessary to evaluate progression of the disease process or to determine the need for a change in therapy.

➤ Maintain the patient on adequate hydration after the procedure.

➤ Monitor urinary output after the procedure. Decreased urine output may indicate impending renal failure.

➤ Determine if the patient or family members have any further questions or concerns.

➤ A physician specializing in this branch of medicine sends a written report to the ordering provider, who discusses the results with the patient.

➤ Evaluate test results in relation to the patient's symptoms and other tests performed. Related diagnostic tests include renogram, renal ultrasound, and CT scan of the kidneys.

INTRINSIC FACTOR ANTIBODIES

SYNONYM/ACRONYM: IF antibodies.

SPECIMEN: Serum (1 mL) collected in a red-top tube. Plasma (1 mL) collected in a lavender-top (ethylenediaminetetra-acetic acid) tube is also acceptable.

REFERENCE VALUE: (Method: Radioimmunoassay) None detected.

DESCRIPTION: Intrinsic factor (IF) is produced by the parietal cells of the gastric mucosa and is required for the normal absorption of vitamin B_{12}. In some diseases, antibodies are produced that bind the cobalamin-IF complex, prevent the complex from binding to ileum receptors, and prevent vitamin B_{12} absorption. There are two types of antibodies: type 1, the more commonly present blocking antibody; and type 2, the binding antibody. The blocking antibody inhibits uptake of vitamin B_{12} at the binding site of IF. Binding antibody combines with either free or complexed IF. ∎

INDICATIONS:
• Assist in the diagnosis of pernicious anemia

• Evaluate patients with decreased vitamin B_{12} levels

RESULT

Increased in:
• Megaloblastic anemia

• Pernicious anemia

• Some patients with insulin-dependent (type 1) diabetes

• Some patients with hyperthyroidism

Decreased in: N/A

CRITICAL VALUES: N/A

INTERFERING FACTORS:
• Recent treatment with methotrexate or another folic acid antagonist can interfere with test results.

• Vitamin B_{12} injected or ingested within 48 hours of the test invalidates results.

• Recent radioactive scans or radiation can interfere with test results when radioimmunoassay is the test method.

Nursing Implications and Procedure

Pretest:

➤ Obtain a history of the patient's complaints, including a list of known allergens.

➤ Obtain a history of the patient's hematopoietic and gastrointestinal systems, as well as results of previously performed tests and procedures. For related tests, refer to the hematopoietic and gastrointestinal system tables.

➤ Obtain a list of the medications the patient is taking, including herbs, nutritional supplements, and nutraceuticals. The requesting health care practitioner and laboratory should be advised if the patient is regularly using these products so that their effects can be taken into consideration when reviewing results.

➤ Note any recent procedures that can interfere with test results.

➤ There are no food or fluid restrictions unless by medical direction. Administration of vitamin B$_{12}$ should be withheld within 48 hours before testing.

➤ Review the procedure with the patient.

➤ Inform the patient that specimen collection takes approximately 5 to 10 minutes.

Intratest:

➤ Direct the patient to breathe normally and to avoid unnecessary movement.

➤ Observe standard precautions and follow the general guidelines in Appendix A. Perform a venipuncture, and collect the specimen in a 5-mL red-top tube.

➤ Label the specimen, and promptly transport it to the laboratory.

Post-test:

➤ Observe venipuncture site for bleeding or hematoma formation. Apply pressure bandage.

➤ Evaluate test results in relation to the patient's symptoms and other tests performed. Related laboratory tests include complete blood count, folic acid, and vitamin B$_{12}$.

IRON

• •

SYNONYM/ACRONYM: Fe.

SPECIMEN: Serum (1 mL) collected in a red- or tiger-top tube.

REFERENCE VALUE: (Method: Spectrophotometry)

Age	Conventional Units	SI Units (Conversion Factor ×0.179)
Newborn	100–250 μg/dL	17.9–44.8 μmol/L
Infant–9 y	20–105 μg/dL	3.6–18.8 μmol/L
10–14 y	20–145 μg/dL	3.6–26.0 μmol/L
Adult		
Male	65–175 μg/dL	11.6–31.3 μmol/L
Female	50–170 μg/dL	9–30.4 μmol/L

DESCRIPTION: Iron plays a principal role in erythropoiesis. Iron is necessary for the proliferation and maturation of red blood cells and is required for hemoglobin synthesis. Of the body's normal 4 g of iron, approximately 65 percent of iron resides in hemoglobin and 3 percent in myoglobin. A small amount is also found in cellular enzymes that catalyze the oxidation and reduction of iron. The remainder of iron is stored in the liver, bone marrow, and spleen as ferritin or hemosiderin. Any iron present in the serum is in transit among the alimentary tract, the bone marrow, and available iron storage forms. Iron travels in the bloodstream bound to transferrin, a protein manufactured by the liver. Normally, iron enters the body by oral ingestion; only 10 percent is absorbed, but 20 percent can be absorbed in patients with iron-deficiency anemia. Unbound iron is highly toxic, but there is generally an excess of transferrin available to prevent the buildup of unbound iron in circulation. Iron overload is as clinically significant as iron deficiency, especially in the accidental poisoning of children caused by excessive intake of iron-containing multivitamins. ∎

INDICATIONS:
- Assist in the diagnosis of blood loss, indicated by decreased serum iron
- Assist in the diagnosis of hemochromatosis or other disorders of iron metabolism and storage
- Determine the presence of disorders that involve diminished protein synthesis or defects in iron absorption
- Determine the differential diagnosis of anemia
- Evaluate accidental iron poisoning
- Evaluate iron overload in dialysis patients or patients with transfusion-dependent anemias
- Evaluate thalassemia and sideroblastic anemia
- Monitor hematologic responses during pregnancy, when serum iron is usually decreased
- Monitor response to treatment for anemia

RESULT

Increased in:
- Acute iron poisoning (children)
- Acute leukemia
- Acute liver disease
- Aplastic anemia
- Excessive iron therapy
- Hemochromatosis
- Hemolytic anemias
- Lead toxicity
- Nephritis
- Pernicious anemias
- Sideroblastic anemias
- Thalassemia
- Transfusions (repeated)
- Vitamin B_6 deficiency

Decreased in:
- Acute and chronic infection
- Carcinoma
- Chronic blood loss (gastrointestinal, uterine)
- Hypothyroidism
- Iron-deficiency anemia
- Nephrosis
- Postoperative state

- Protein malnutrition (kwashiorkor)

- Remission of pernicious anemia

CRITICAL VALUES: ⚠ Ingestion of 30 mg/kg of elemental iron by a child may be sufficient to induce toxicity. Greater than 400 μg/dL is indicative of possible toxicity. Intervention may include chelation therapy by administration of deferoxamine mesylate (Desferal).

INTERFERING FACTORS:

- Drugs that may increase iron levels include blood transfusions, chemotherapy, iron (intramuscular), iron dextran, iron-protein-succinylate, methimazole, methotrexate, oral contraceptives, and rifampin.

- Drugs that may decrease iron levels include allopurinol, acetylsalicylic acid, cholestyramine, corticotropin, cortisone, deferoxamine, and metformin.

- Failure to withhold iron-containing medications 24 hours before the test may falsely increase values.

Nursing Implications and Procedure • • • • • • • • • • • •

Pretest: ■

➤ Obtain a history of the patient's complaints, including a list of known allergens.

➤ Obtain a history of the patient's hematopoietic system and results of previously performed tests and procedures. For related tests, refer to the hematopoietic system table.

➤ Obtain a list of medications the patient is taking, including herbs, nutritional supplements, and nutraceuticals. The requesting health care practitioner and laboratory should be advised if the patient regularly uses these products so that their effects can be taken into consideration when reviewing results.

➤ Note any recent therapies that can interfere with test results.

➤ There are no fluid restrictions unless by medical direction.

➤ Instruct the patient to fast for at least 12 hours before testing, and with medical direction, to refrain from taking iron-containing medicines before specimen collection.

➤ Specimen collection should be delayed for several days after blood transfusion.

➤ Gross hemolysis can interfere with test results.

➤ Review the procedure with the patient.

➤ Inform the patient that specimen collection takes approximately 5 to 10 minutes.

Intratest: ■

➤ Ensure that the patient has complied with dietary preparations and other pretesting restrictions.

➤ Direct the patient to breathe normally and to avoid unnecessary movement.

➤ Observe standard precautions and follow the general guidelines in Appendix A. Perform a venipuncture, and collect the specimen in a 5-mL red- or tiger-top tube.

➤ Label the specimen, and promptly transport it to the laboratory.

Post-test: ■

➤ Observe venipuncture site for bleeding or hematoma formation. Apply pressure bandage.

➤ Instruct the patient to resume usual diet as directed by the requesting health care practitioner.

➤ Educate the patient with abnormally elevated iron values, as appropriate, on the importance of reading food labels either to avoid or to ingest foods containing iron. Foods high in iron include meats, eggs, grains, and vegetables. It is also important to explain that iron levels in foods can be increased if foods are cooked in cookware containing iron.

➤ Educate the patient with abnormal iron values that numerous factors affect the absorption of iron, enhancing or decreasing absorption regardless of the original content of the iron-containing dietary source. Consumption of large amounts of alcohol damages the intestine and allows increased absorption of iron. A high intake of calcium and ascorbic acid also increases iron absorption. Iron absorption after a meal is also increased by factors in meat, fish, or poultry. Iron absorption is decreased by the absence (gastric resection) or diminished presence (use of antacids) of gastric acid. Phytic acids from cereals, tannins from tea and coffee, oxalic acid from vegetables, and minerals such as copper, zinc, and manganese interfere with iron absorption.

➤ Evaluate test results in relation to the patient's symptoms and other tests performed. Related laboratory tests include bone marrow biopsy, liver biopsy, complete blood count, erythropoietin, ferritin, hemosiderin, iron/total iron-binding capacity, lead, porphyrins, and transferrin.

IRON-BINDING CAPACITY (TOTAL), TRANSFERRIN, AND IRON SATURATION

SYNONYMS/ACRONYMS: TIBC, Fe Sat.

SPECIMEN: Serum (1 mL) collected in a red- or tiger-top tube.

REFERENCE VALUE: (Method: Spectrophotometry for TIBC and nephelometry for transferrin)

Test	Conventional Units	SI Unit
		(Conversion Factor ×0.179)
TIBC	250–350 μg/dL	45–63 μmol/L
		(Conversion Factor ×0.01)
Transferrin	200–380 mg/dL	2–3.8 g/L
Iron saturation	20–50%	

TIBC = total iron-binding capacity.

DESCRIPTION: Iron plays a principal role in erythropoiesis. It is necessary for proliferation and maturation of red blood cells and for hemoglobin synthesis. Of the body's normal 4 g of iron (less in women), about 65 percent is present in hemoglobin and about 3 percent in myoglobin. A small amount is also found in cellular enzymes that catalyze the oxidation and reduction of iron. The remainder of iron is stored in the liver, bone marrow, and spleen as ferritin or hemosiderin. Any iron present in the serum is in transit among the alimentary tract, the bone marrow, and available iron storage forms. Iron travels in the bloodstream bound to transport proteins. Transferrin is the major iron-transport protein, carrying 60 to 70 percent of the body's iron. For this reason, total iron-binding capacity (TIBC) and transferrin are sometimes referred to interchangeably, even though other proteins carry iron and contribute to the TIBC. Unbound iron is highly toxic, but there is generally an excess of transferrin available to prevent the buildup of unbound iron in circulation. The percentage of iron saturation is calculated by dividing the serum iron value by the TIBC value and multiplying by 100. ■

INDICATIONS:
- Assist in the diagnosis of iron-deficiency anemia
- Differentiate between iron-deficiency anemia and anemia secondary to chronic disease
- Monitor hematologic response to therapy during pregnancy and iron-deficiency anemias
- Provide support for diagnosis of hemochromatosis or diseases of iron metabolism and storage

RESULT

Increased in:
- Acute liver disease
- Hypochromic   (iron-deficiency) anemias
- Late pregnancy

Decreased in:
- Chronic infections
- Cirrhosis
- Hemochromatosis
- Hemolytic anemias
- Protein depletion
- Neoplastic diseases
- Renal disease
- Sideroblastic anemias
- Thalassemia

CRITICAL VALUES: N/A

INTERFERING FACTORS:
- Drugs that may increase TIBC levels include mestranol and oral contraceptives.
- Drugs that may decrease TIBC levels include asparaginase, chloramphenicol, corticotropin, cortisone, and testosterone.

Nursing Implications and Procedure • • • • • • • • • • • •

Pretest:
➤ Obtain a history of the patient's complaints, including a list of known allergens.

➤ Obtain a history of the patient's hematopoietic system and results of previously performed tests and procedures. For related tests, refer to the hematopoietic system table.

➤ Obtain a list of the medications the patient is taking, including herbs, nutritional supplements, and nutraceuticals. The requesting health care practitioner and laboratory should be advised if the patient is regularly using these products so that their effects can be taken into consideration when reviewing results.

➤ There are no food, fluid, or medication restrictions unless by medical direction.

➤ Review the procedure with the patient.

➤ Inform the patient that specimen collection takes approximately 5 to 10 minutes.

Intratest:

➤ Direct the patient to breathe normally and to avoid unnecessary movement.

➤ Observe standard precautions and follow the general guidelines in Appendix A. Perform a venipuncture, and collect the specimen in a 5-mL red- or tiger-top tube.

➤ Label the specimen, and promptly transport it to the laboratory.

Post-test:

➤ Observe venipuncture site for bleeding or hematoma formation. Apply pressure bandage.

➤ Evaluate test results in relation to the patient's symptoms and other tests performed. Related laboratory tests include bone marrow biopsy, complete blood count, erythropoietin, ferritin, iron, hemosiderin, lead, and porphyrins.

KETONES, BLOOD AND URINE

SYNONYMS/ACRONYM: Ketone bodies, acetoacetate, acetone.

SPECIMEN: Serum (1 mL) collected from red- or tiger-top tube. Urine (5 mL), random or timed specimen, collected in a clean plastic collection container.

REFERENCE VALUE: (Method: Colorimetric nitroprusside reaction) Negative.

DESCRIPTION: Ketone bodies refer to the three intermediate products of metabolism: acetone, acetoacetic acid, and β-hydroxybutyrate. Even though β-hydroxybutyrate is not a ketone, it is usually listed with the ketone bodies. In healthy individuals, ketones are produced and completely metabolized by the liver so that measurable amounts are not normally present in serum. Ketones appear in the urine before a significant serum level is detectable. If the patient has

excessive fat metabolism, ketones are found in blood and urine. Excessive fat metabolism may occur if the patient has impaired ability to metabolize carbohydrates, inadequate carbohydrate intake, inadequate insulin levels, excessive carbohydrate loss, or increased carbohydrate demand. A strongly positive acetone result without severe acidosis, accompanied by normal glucose, electrolyte, and bicarbonate levels, is strongly suggestive of isopropyl alcohol poisoning. A low-carbohydrate or low-fat diet may cause a positive acetone test. Ketosis in diabetics is usually accompanied by increased glucose and decreased bicarbonate and pH. Extremely elevated levels of ketone bodies can result in coma. This situation is particularly life-threatening in children younger than 10 years old. ▪

INDICATIONS:
• Assist in the diagnosis of starvation, stress, alcoholism, suspected isopropyl alcohol ingestion, glycogen storage disease, and other metabolic disorders

• Detect and monitor treatment of diabetic ketoacidosis

• Monitor the control for diabetes

• Screen for ketonuria to assist in the assessment of inborn errors of metabolism

• Screen for ketonuria to assist in the diagnosis of suspected isopropyl alcohol poisoning

• Screen for ketonuria due to acute illness or stress in nondiabetic patients

RESULT

Increased in:
• Acidosis

• Branched-chain ketonuria

• Carbohydrate deficiency

• Eclampsia

• Fasting or starvation

• Gestational diabetes

• Glycogen storage diseases

• Hyperglycemia

• High-fat or high-protein diet

• Ketoacidosis of alcoholism and diabetes

• Illnesses with marked vomiting and diarrhea

• Isopropyl alcohol ingestion

• Methylmalonic aciduria

• Postanesthesia period

• Propionyl coenzyme A carboxylase deficiency

Decreased in: N/A

CRITICAL VALUES: ⚠ An elevated level of ketone bodies is evidenced by fruity-smelling breath, acidosis, ketonuria, and decreased level of consciousness. Administration of insulin and frequent blood-glucose measurement may be indicated.

INTERFERING FACTORS:
• Drugs that may cause an increase in serum ketone levels include acetylsalicylic acid (if therapy results in acidosis, especially in children),albuterol, fenfluramine, levodopa, nifedipine, and paraldehyde.

• Drugs that may cause a decrease in serum ketone levels include acetylsalicylic acid and valproic acid. Increases have been shown in hyperthyroid patients receiving propranolol and propylthiouracil.

• Drugs that may increase urine ketone levels include acetylsalicylic acid (if therapy results in acidosis, especially in children), captopril, dimercaprol, ether, ifosfamide, insulin, levodopa, mesna, metformin, methyldopa, N-acetylcysteine, niacin, paraldehyde, penicillamine, phenazopyridine, phenolphthalein, phenolsulfonphthalein, pyrazinamide, streptozocin, sulfobromophthalein, and valproic acid.

• Drugs that may decrease urine ketone levels include acetylsalicylic acid and phenazopyridine.

• Urine should be checked within 60 minutes of collection.

- Bacterial contamination of urine can cause false-negative results.

- Failure to keep reagent strip tightly closed can cause false-negative results. Light and moisture affect the ability of the chemicals in the strip to perform as expected.

- False-negative or weakly false-positive test results can be obtained when β-hydroxybutyrate is the predominating ketone body in cases of lactic acidosis.

Nursing Implications and Procedure • • • • • • • • • • •

Pretest:

➤ Obtain a history of the patient's complaints, including a list of known allergens.

➤ Obtain a history of the patient's endocrine system and results of previously performed tests and procedures. For related tests, refer to the endocrine system table.

➤ Obtain a list of the medications the patient is taking, including herbs, nutritional supplements, and nutraceuticals. The requesting health care practitioner and laboratory should be advised if the patient regularly uses these products so that their effects can be taken into consideration when reviewing results.

➤ There are no food, fluid, or medication restrictions unless by medical direction.

➤ Review the procedure with the patient.

➤ Inform the patient that blood specimen collection takes approximately 5 to 10 minutes. The amount of time required to collect a urine specimen depends on the level of cooperation from the patient.

Intratest:

➤ Observe standard precautions and follow the general guidelines in Appendix A.

Blood:

➤ Direct the patient to breathe normally and to avoid unnecessary movement.

➤ Perform a venipuncture, and collect the specimen in a 5-mL red- or tiger-top tube. Alternatively, a finger- or heel-stick method of specimen collection can be used.

Urine:

➤ Review the procedure with the patient. Explain to the patient how to collect a second-voided midstream specimen: (1) void, then drink a glass of water; and (2) wait 30 minutes, and then try to void again.

➤ Instruct the patient to avoid excessive exercise and stress before specimen collection.

Clean-catch specimen:

➤ Instruct the male patient to (1) thoroughly wash his hands, (2) cleanse the meatus, (3) void a small amount into the toilet, and (4) void directly into the specimen container.

➤ Instruct the female patient to (1) thoroughly wash her hands; (2) cleanse the labia from front to back; (3) while keeping the labia separated, void a small amount into the toilet; and (4) without interrupting the urine stream, void directly into the specimen container.

Blood or urine:

➤ Label the specimen, and promptly transport it to the laboratory.

Post-test:

➤ Observe venipuncture site for bleeding or hematoma formation. Apply pressure bandage.

➤ Increased levels of ketone bodies may be associated with diabetes. Instruct the diabetic patient, as appropriate, in nutritional management of the disease. Patients who adhere to dietary recommendations report a better general feeling of health, better weight management, greater control of glucose and lipid values, and improved use of insulin. There is no "diabetic" diet; however, there are many meal-planning approaches with nutritional goals endorsed by the American Dietetic Association. The nutritional needs of each diabetic patient must be determined individually with the appropriate health care professionals, particularly professionals trained in nutrition.

➤ Instruct the patient and caregiver to report signs and symptoms of hypoglycemia (weakness, confusion, diaphoresis, rapid pulse) or hyper-

glycemia (thirst, polyuria, hunger, and lethargy). Emphasize, as appropriate, that good glycemic control delays the onset and slows the progression of diabetic retinopathy, nephropathy, and neuropathy.

➤ Evaluate test results in relation to the patient's symptoms and other tests performed. Related laboratory tests include anion gap, blood gases, electrolytes, glucose, glycated hemoglobin, urine ketones, lactic acid, osmolality, urine osmolality, phosphorus, and routine urinalysis.

KIDNEY, URETER, AND BLADDER STUDY

SYNONYMS/ACRONYM: Flat plate of the abdomen, plain film of the abdomen, scout film, KUB.

AREA OF APPLICATION: Kidneys, ureters, bladder, and abdomen.

CONTRAST: None.

DESCRIPTION: A kidney, ureter, and bladder (KUB) x-ray examination provides information regarding the structure, size, and position of the abdominal organs; it also indicates whether there is any obstruction or abnormality of the abdomen caused by disease or congenital malformation. Calcifications of the renal calyces or renal pelvis, as well as any radiopaque calculi present in the urinary tract or surrounding organs, may be visualized. Patterns of air and gas appear light and bright on the image. Air normally remains contained within the intestinal tract; perforation of either the stomach or

the intestines causes air to escape into the abdominal cavity. When there is an intestinal obstruction, air and fluid collect above the area of obstruction, distending the lumen of the intestine. KUB x-rays are among the first examinations done to diagnose intra-abdominal diseases such as intestinal obstruction, masses, tumors, ruptured organs, abnormal gas accumulation, and ascites. ■

INDICATIONS:

• Evaluate known or suspected intestinal obstruction

• Evaluate the size, shape, and position of the liver, kidneys, and spleen

- Evaluate the presence of renal, ureter, or other organ calculi

- Determine the cause of acute abdominal pain or palpable mass

- Evaluate suspected abnormal fluid, air, or metallic object or obstruction in the abdomen

- Evaluate the effects of lower abdominal trauma, such as internal hemorrhage

RESULT

Normal Findings:

- Normal size and shape of kidneys

- Normal bladder, absence of masses and renal calculi, and no abnormal accumulation of air or fluid

Abnormal Findings:

- Abnormal accumulation of bowel gas

- Ascites

- Bladder distention

- Congenital renal anomaly

- Hydronephrosis

- Intestinal obstruction

- Organomegaly

- Renal hematomas

- Renal calculi

- Ruptured viscus

- Soft-tissue masses

- Trauma to liver, spleen, kidneys, and bladder

- Vascular calcification

CRITICAL VALUES: N/A

INTERFERING FACTORS:

This procedure is contraindicated for:

- Patients who are pregnant or suspected of being pregnant, unless the potential benefits of the procedure far outweigh the risks to the fetus and mother

Factors that may impair clear imaging:

- Inability of the patient to cooperate or remain still during the procedure because of age, significant pain, or mental status

- Metallic objects within the examination field (e.g., jewelry or body rings), which may inhibit organ visualization and can produce unclear images

- Improper adjustment of the radiographic equipment to accommodate obese or thin patients, which can cause overexposure or underexposure and a poor-quality study

- Patients who are very obese, who may exceed the weight limit for the equipment

- Incorrect positioning of the patient, which may produce poor visualization of the area to be examined, especially for oblique and decubitus views and for films done by portable equipment

- Retained barium from a previous radiologic procedure

- Gas or feces in the gastrointestinal tract resulting from inadequate cleansing or failure to restrict food intake before the study

- Ascites, uterine tumors, and ovarian tumors, which can interfere with the quality of the procedure

Other considerations:

- Consultation with a physician should occur before the procedure for radiation safety concerns regarding infants of patients who are lactating.

- Risks associated with radiographic overexposure can result from frequent x-ray procedures. Personnel in the room with the patient should wear a protective lead apron, stand behind a shield, or leave the area while the examination is being done. Personnel working in the area where the examination is being done should wear badges that reveal their level of exposure to radiation.

Nursing Implications and Procedure ●●●●●●●●●●●

Pretest: ■

➤ Inform the patient about the purpose of the procedure, various positions to assume, and the need to hold his or her breath.

➤ Inform the patient that the procedure is performed in a radiology department by a technologist and takes approximately 10 minutes.

➤ Obtain a history of the patient's complaints.

➤ Obtain a history of the patient's genitourinary and abdominal systems, as well as results of previously performed tests and procedures. For related tests, refer to the genitourinary and gastrointestinal system tables.

➤ Determine date of last menstrual period and possibility of pregnancy in perimenopausal women.

➤ Inform the patient that there are no food or fluid restrictions and that no pain is associated with the study.

➤ Schedule intravenous pyelography (IVP) or gastrointestinal studies after this study.

Intratest: ■

➤ Have the patient put on a hospital gown.

➤ Ask the patient to lie still during the procedure because movement produces unclear images. Make sure jewelry, watches, chains, belts, and any other metallic objects have been removed from the abdominal area.

➤ Remove any wires connected to electrodes, if allowed.

➤ Place the patient on the table in a supine position with hands over the head or relaxed at the side.

➤ For portable examinations, lower the head of the bed such that the patient is lying as flat as he or she can tolerate.

➤ For male patients, place lead protection over the testicles to prevent their irradiation.

➤ Instruct the patient to inhale deeply and to hold his or her breath while the x-ray is taken, and then to exhale after the film is taken.

Post-test: ■

➤ Inform the patient that further examinations may be necessary to evaluate progression of the disease process or to determine the need for a change in therapy.

➤ Determine if the patient or family members have any further questions or concerns.

➤ A physician specializing in this branch of medicine sends a written report to the ordering provider, who discusses the results with the patient.

➤ Evaluate test results in relation to the patient's symptoms and other tests performed. Related diagnostic tests include IVP as well as ultrasound and computed tomography of the abdomen.

KLEIHAUER-BETKE TEST

· ·

SYNONYMS/ACRONYM: Fetal hemoglobin, hemoglobin F, acid elution slide test.

SPECIMEN: Whole blood (1 mL) collected in a lavender-top (ethylenedi-aminetetra-acetic acid [EDTA]) tube. Freshly prepared blood smears are also acceptable. Cord blood may be requested for use as a positive control.

REFERENCE VALUE: (Method: Microscopic examination of treated and stained peripheral blood smear) Less than 1 percent.

DESCRIPTION: The Kleihauer-Betke test is used to determine the degree of fetal-maternal hemorrhage and to help calculate the dosage of RhoGAM to be given in some cases of Rh-negative mothers. The test can also be used to distinguish some forms of thalassemia from the hereditary persistence of fetal hemoglobin, but hemoglobin electrophoresis and flow-cytometry methods are more commonly used for this purpose. ■

INDICATIONS:
• Assist in the diagnosis of certain types of anemia.

• Calculating dosage of RhoGAM

• Screening postpartum maternal blood for the presence of fetal-maternal hemorrhage

RESULT

Positive in:
• Fetal-maternal hemorrhage

• Hereditary persistence of fetal hemo-globin

Negative in: N/A

CRITICAL VALUES: N/A

INTERFERING FACTORS: Specimens must be obtained before transfusion.

Nursing Implications and Procedure · · · · · · · · · · ·

Pretest: ■

➤ Obtain a history of the patient's complaints, including a list of known allergens.

➤ Obtain a history of the patient's hematopoietic and reproductive systems, as well as results of previously performed tests and procedures. For related tests, refer to the hematopoietic and reproductive system tables.

➤ Obtain a list of medications the patient is taking, including herbs, nutritional supplements, and nutraceuticals. The requesting health care practitioner and laboratory should be advised if the patient regularly uses these products so that their effects can be taken into consideration when reviewing results.

➤ Note any recent procedures that can interfere with test results.

➤ There are no food, fluid, or medication restrictions unless by medical direction.

➤ Review the procedure with the patient.

➤ Inform the patient that specimen collection takes approximately 5 to 10 minutes.

Intratest:

➤ Direct the patient to breathe normally and to avoid unnecessary movement.

➤ Observe standard precautions and follow the general guidelines in Appendix A. Perform a venipuncture, and collect the specimen in a 5-mL lavender-top tube.

➤ Label the specimen, and promptly transport it to the laboratory. Sample must be less than 6 hours old.

Post-test:

➤ Observe venipuncture site for bleeding or hematoma formation. Apply pressure bandage.

➤ Evaluate test results in relation to the patient's symptoms and other tests performed. Related laboratory tests include blood group and type.

LACTATE DEHYDROGENASE AND ISOENZYMES

SYNONYMS/ACRONYMS: LDH and isos, LD and isos.

SPECIMEN: Serum (1 mL) collected in a red- or tiger-top tube.

REFERENCE VALUE: (Method: Enzymatic analysis for lactate dehydrogenase, electrophoretic analysis for isoenzymes) Reference ranges are method dependent and may vary from laboratory to laboratory.

Lactate Dehydrogenase

Age	Conventional Units	SI Units (Conversion Factor ×1)
1–3 y	500–920 U/L	500–920 U/L
4–6 y	470–900 U/L	470–900 U/L
7–9 y	420–750 U/L	420–750 U/L
10–13 y	432–750 U/L	432–750 U/L
14–15 y	360–730 U/L	360–730 U/L
16–19 y	340–670 U/L	340–670 U/L
Adult	313–618 U/L	313–618 U/L

LDH Fraction	% of Total	Fraction of Total
LDH$_1$	14–26	0.14–0.26
LDH$_2$	29–39	0.29–0.39
LDH$_3$	20–26	0.20–0.26
LDH$_4$	8–16	0.08–0.16
LDH$_5$	6–16	0.06–0.16

DESCRIPTION: Lactate dehydrogenase (LDH) is an enzyme that catalyzes the reversible conversion of lactate to pyruvate within cells. Because many tissues contain LDH, elevated total LDH is considered a nonspecific indicator of cellular damage unless other clinical data make the tissue origin obvious. Determining tissue origin is aided by electrophoretic analysis of the five isoenzymes specific to certain tissues. The heart and erythrocytes are rich sources of LDH$_1$, LDH$_2$, and LDH$_3$; the kidneys contain large amounts of LDH$_3$ and LDH$_4$; and the liver and skeletal muscles are high in LDH$_4$ and LDH$_5$. Certain glands (e.g., thyroid, adrenal, thymus), the pancreas, spleen, lungs, lymph nodes, and white blood cells contain LDH$_3$, whereas the ilium is an additional source of LDH$_5$. There have been documented reports of a sixth isoenzyme of LDH. It is seen in patients with severe liver disease and is an indicator of a very poor prognosis. LDH is found in every tissue of the body. It is of no use as a specific diagnostic marker. Testing for the presence of LDH and isoenzymes is rarely used anymore to confirm acute myocardial infarction (MI), having been replaced by more sensitive and specific creatine kinase (CK-MB) and troponin assays. ■

INDICATIONS:
• Differentiate acute MI, evidenced by elevated LDH$_1$ and LDH$_2$, from pulmonary infarction and liver problems, which elevate LDH$_4$ and LDH$_5$

• Evaluate the degree of muscle wasting in muscular dystrophy (LDH levels rise early in this disorder and approach normal as muscle mass is reduced by atrophy)

• Evaluate the effectiveness of cancer chemotherapy (LDH levels should fall with successful treatment)

• Evaluate red cell hemolysis or renal infarction, especially as indicated by reversal of the LDH$_1$:LDH$_2$ ratio

• Investigate acute MI or extension thereof, as indicated by elevation (usually) of total LDH, elevation of LDH$_1$ and LDH$_2$, and reversal of the LDH$_1$:LDH$_2$ ratio within 48 hours of the infarction

• Investigate chronicity of liver, lung, and kidney disorders, as evidenced by LDH levels that remain persistently high

RESULT

Total LDH increased in:
• Carcinoma of the liver
• Chronic alcoholism
• Cirrhosis
• Congestive heart failure
• Hemolytic anemias
• Hypoxia
• Leukemias
• MI or pulmonary infarction

- Megaloblastic and pernicious anemia
- Musculoskeletal disease
- Obstructive jaundice
- Pancreatitis
- Renal disease (severe)
- Shock
- Viral hepatitis

Total LDH decreased in: N/A

LDH Isoenzymes:
- LDH$_1$ fraction increased over LDH$_2$ can be seen in acute MI, anemias (pernicious, hemolytic, acute sickle cell, megaloblastic, hemolytic), and acute renal cortical injury due to any cause. The LDH$_1$ fraction in particular is elevated in cases of germ cell tumors.

- Increases in the middle fractions are associated with conditions in which massive platelet destruction has occurred (e.g., pulmonary embolism, post-transfusion period), and in lymphatic system disorders (e.g., infectious mononucleosis, lymphomas, lymphocytic leukemias).

- An increase in LDH$_5$ occurs with musculoskeletal damage and many types of liver damage (e.g., cirrhosis, cancer, hepatitis).

CRITICAL VALUES: N/A

INTERFERING FACTORS:
- Drugs that may increase total LDH levels include amiodarone, etretinate, fluosol-DA, methotrexate, oxacillin, plicamycin, propoxyphene and streptokinase.

- Drugs that may decrease total LDH levels include ascorbic acid, cefotaxime, enalapril, fluorides, naltrexone, and oxalate.

- Hemolysis will cause significant false elevations in total LDH and a false "flip" pattern of the isoenzymes

because LDH$_1$ fraction is of red blood cell origin.

- Some isoenzymes are temperature sensitive; therefore prolonged storage at refrigerated temperatures may cause false decreases.

Nursing Implications and Procedure • • • • • • • • • • •

Pretest:
➤ Obtain a history of the patient's complaints, including a list of known allergens.

➤ Obtain a history of the patient's cardiovascular, hematopoietic, hepatobiliary, and musculoskeletal systems, as well as results of previously performed tests and procedures. For related tests, refer to the cardiovascular, hematopoietic, hepatobiliary, and musculoskeletal system tables.

➤ Obtain a list of the medications the patient is taking, including herbs, nutritional supplements, and nutraceuticals. The requesting health care practitioner and laboratory should be advised if the patient regularly uses these products so that their effects can be taken into consideration when reviewing results.

➤ There are no food, fluid, or medication restrictions unless by medical direction.

➤ Review the procedure with the patient.

➤ Inform the patient that specimen collection takes approximately 5 to 10 minutes.

Intratest:
➤ Direct the patient to breathe normally and to avoid unnecessary movement.

➤ Observe standard precautions and follow the general guidelines in Appendix A. Perform a venipuncture, and collect the specimen in a 5-mL red- or tiger-top tube.

➤ Label the specimen, and promptly transport it to the laboratory.

Post-test:

➤ Observe venipuncture site for bleeding or hematoma formation. Apply pressure bandage.

➤ Evaluate test results in relation to the patient's symptoms and other tests performed. Related laboratory tests include alanine aminotransferase, aspartate aminotransferase, C-reactive protein, complete blood count, creatine kinase and isoenzymes, γ-glutamyl transpeptidase, homocysteine, body fluid LDH, magnesium, myoglobin, and troponin.

LACTIC ACID

· ·

SYNONYM/ACRONYM: Lactate.

SPECIMEN: Plasma (1 mL) collected in a gray-top (sodium fluoride) or green-top (lithium heparin) tube. Specimen should be transported tightly capped and in an ice slurry.

REFERENCE VALUE: (Method: Spectrophotometry/enzymatic analysis)

Conventional Units	SI Units (Conversion Factor ×0.111)
3–23 mg/dL	0.3–2.6 mmol/L

DESCRIPTION: Lactic acid (present in blood as lactate) is a byproduct of carbohydrate metabolism. Normally metabolized in the liver, lactate concentration is based on the rate of production and metabolism. Levels increase during strenuous exercise, which results in insufficient oxygen delivery to the tissues. Pyruvate, the normal end product of glucose metabolism, is converted to lactate in emergency situations when energy is needed but there is insufficient oxygen in the system to favor the aerobic and customary energy cycle. When hypoxia or circulatory collapse increases production of lactate, or when the hepatic system doesn't metabolize lactate sufficiently, lactate levels become elevated. The lactic acid test can be performed in conjunction with pyruvic acid testing to monitor tissue oxygenation. Lactic acidosis can be differentiated from ketoacidosis by the absence of ketosis and grossly elevated glucose levels. ■

INDICATIONS:
• Assess tissue oxygenation

• Evaluate acidosis

RESULT

Increased in:
• Cardiac failure

• Diabetes

- Hemorrhage

- Hepatic coma

- Ingestion of large doses of ethanol or acetaminophen

- Lactic acidosis

- Pulmonary embolism

- Pulmonary failure

- Reye's syndrome

- Shock

- Strenuous exercise

Decreased in: N/A

CRITICAL VALUES:

Greater than or equal to 45 mg/dL

Observe the patient for signs and symptoms of elevated levels, such as Kussmaul's breathing and increased pulse rate. In general, there is an inverse relationship between critically elevated lactate levels and survival.

INTERFERING FACTORS:

- Drugs that may increase lactate levels include albuterol, anticonvulsants (long-term use), epinephrine, intravenous glucose, lactose, oral contraceptives, sodium bicarbonate, and sorbitol.

- Falsely low lactate levels are obtained in samples with elevated levels of the enzyme lactate dehydrogenase (LDH) because this enzyme reacts with the available lactate substrate.

- Using a tourniquet or instructing the patient to clench his or her fist during a venipuncture can cause elevated levels.

- Engaging in strenuous physical activity (i.e., activity in which blood flow and oxygen distribution cannot keep pace with increased energy needs) before specimen collection can cause an elevated result.

- Delay in transport of the specimen to the laboratory must be avoided. Specimens not processed by centrifugation in a tightly stoppered collection container within 15 minutes of collection should be rejected for analysis. It is preferable to transport specimens to the laboratory in an ice slurry to further retard cellular metabolism that might shift lactate levels in the sample before analysis.

Nursing Implications and Procedure

Pretest:

➤ Obtain a history of the patient's complaints, including a list of known allergens.

➤ Obtain a history of the patient's cardiovascular, endocrine, hepatobiliary, musculoskeletal, and respiratory systems, as well as results of previously performed tests and procedures. For related tests, refer to the cardiovascular, endocrine, hepatobiliary, musculoskeletal, and respiratory system tables.

➤ Obtain a list of the medications the patient is taking, including herbs, nutritional supplements, and nutraceuticals. The requesting health care practitioner and laboratory should be advised if the patient regularly uses these products so that their effects can be taken into consideration when reviewing results.

➤ There are no medication restrictions unless by medical direction.

➤ Instruct the patient to fast and to restrict fluids overnight. Instruct the patient not to ingest alcohol for 12 hours before the test.

➤ Instruct the patient to rest for 1 hour before specimen collection.

➤ Review the procedure with the patient.

➤ Inform the patient that specimen

collection takes approximately 5 to 10 minutes.

➤ Prepare an ice slurry in a cup or plastic bag to have on hand for immediate transport of the specimen to the laboratory.

Intratest:

➤ Ensure that the patient has complied with dietary preparations and other pretesting restrictions.

➤ Direct the patient to breathe normally and to avoid unnecessary movement. Instruct the patient *not* to clench and unclench fist immediately before or during specimen collection. Do not use a tourniquet.

➤ Observe standard precautions and follow the general guidelines in Appendix A. Perform a venipuncture, and collect the specimen in a 5-mL

gray-top (sodium fluoride) or green-top (lithium heparin) tube.

➤ Label the specimen, and promptly transport it to the laboratory. The tightly capped sample should be placed in an ice slurry immediately after collection. Information on the specimen label can be protected from water in the ice slurry if the specimen is first placed in a protective plastic bag.

Post-test:

➤ Observe venipuncture site for bleeding or hematoma formation. Apply pressure bandage.

➤ Evaluate test results in relation to the patient's symptoms and other tests performed. Related laboratory tests include arterial/alveolar oxygen ratio, anion gap, blood gases, and electrolytes.

LACTOSE TOLERANCE TEST

· ·

SYNONYM/ACRONYM: LTT.

SPECIMEN: Plasma (1 mL) collected in gray-top (fluoride/oxalate) tube.

REFERENCE VALUE: (Method: Spectrophotometry)

Change in Glucose Value	Conventional Units	SI Units (Conversion Factor ×0.0555)
Normal*	Greater than 30 mg/dL	Greater than 1.7 mmol/L
Inconclusive*	20–30 mg/dL	1.1–1.7 mmol/L
Abnormal*	Less than 20 mg/dL	Less than 1.1 mmol/L

* Compared to fasting sample.

DESCRIPTION: Lactose is a disaccharide found in dairy products. When ingested, lactose is broken down in the intestine, by the sugar-splitting enzyme lactase, into glucose and galactose. When sufficient lactase is not available, intestinal bacteria metabolize the lactose, resulting in abdominal bloating, pain, flatus, and diarrhea. The lactose tolerance test screens for lactose intolerance by monitoring glucose levels after ingestion of a dose of lactose. ■

INDICATIONS: Evaluate patients for suspected lactose intolerance

RESULT

Glucose levels increased in: N/A

Glucose levels decreased in:
Lactose intolerance

CRITICAL VALUES: N/A

INTERFERING FACTORS:

• Numerous medications may alter glucose levels (see monograph titled "Glucose").

• Failure to restrict diet and exercise may alter test results.

• Delayed gastric emptying may decrease glucose levels.

• Smoking may falsely increase glucose levels.

Nursing Implications and Procedure • • • • • • • • • • •

Pretest:

➤ Obtain a history of the patient's complaints, including a list of known allergens.

➤ Obtain a history of the patient's gastrointestinal system and results of previously performed tests and procedures. For related tests, refer to the gastrointestinal system table.

➤ Obtain a list of the medications the patient is taking, including herbs, nutritional supplements, and nutraceuticals. The requesting health care practitioner and laboratory should be advised if the patient regularly uses these products so that their effects can be taken into consideration when reviewing results.

➤ There are no medication restrictions unless by medical direction.

➤ Inform the patient that fasting for at least 12 hours before the test is required and that strenuous activity should also be avoided for at least 12 hours before the test.

➤ Review the procedure with the patient. Inform the patient that the test may produce symptoms such as cramps and diarrhea. Instruct the patient not to smoke cigarettes or chew gum during the test.

➤ Obtain the pediatric patient's weight to calculate dose of lactose to be administered.

➤ Inform the patient that multiple samples over a 90-minute interval will be collected and that each specimen collection takes approximately 5 to 10 minutes.

Intratest:

➤ Ensure that the patient has complied with dietary preparations and other pretesting restrictions.

➤ Administer 50 g of lactose dissolved in a small amount of water to adults over a 5- to 10-minute period. Pediatric dosage is based on weight: 0.6 to 1.3 g lactose per kilogram of body weight for infants less than 12 months old; 1.7 g lactose per kilogram of body weight for children 1 to 12 years old. Record time of ingestion. Encourage the patient to drink one to two glasses of water.

➤ Observe standard precautions and follow the general guidelines in Appendix A. Perform a venipuncture, and collect the specimen in a 5-mL red-top tube or red pediatric Microtainer. Samples should be collected at baseline, 30, 45, 60, and 90 minutes. Record any symptoms the patient reports throughout the course of the test.

➤ Glucose values change rapidly in an unprocessed, unpreserved specimen; therefore, if a Microtainer is used, each sample should be transported immediately after collection. Label the specimen, and promptly transport it to the laboratory.

Post-test:

➤ Observe venipuncture site for bleeding or hematoma formation. Apply pressure bandage.

➤ Provide teaching and information regarding the clinical implications of the test results, as appropriate.

➤ Instruct the patient that resuming his or her usual diet may not be possible if lactose intolerance is identified. Educate patients on the importance of following the dietary advice of a nutritionist to ensure proper nutritional balance. Recognize anxiety caused by a perceived change in lifestyle, and offer support.

➤ Instruct the patient with lactose intolerance to avoid milk products and to carefully read labels on prepared products. Yogurt, which contains inactive lactase enzyme, may be ingested. The lactase in yogurt is activated by the temperature and pH of the duodenum and substitutes for the lack of endogenous lactase. Advise the patient that products such as Lactaid tablets or drops may allow ingestion of milk products without sequelae. Lactose-free milk is also available.

➤ Evaluate test results in relation to the patient's symptoms and other tests performed. Related laboratory tests include D-xylose absorption and fecal analysis.

LAPAROSCOPY, ABDOMINAL

SYNONYM/ACRONYM: Abdominal peritoneoscopy.

AREA OF APPLICATION: Pelvis.

CONTRAST: Carbon dioxide (CO_2).

DESCRIPTION: Abdominal or gastrointestinal laparoscopy provides direct visualization of the liver, gallbladder, spleen, and stomach after insufflation of carbon dioxide (CO_2). In this procedure, a rigid laparoscope is introduced into the body cavity through a 1- to 2-cm abdominal incision. The endoscope has a microscope to allow visualization of the organs, and it can be used to insert instruments for performing certain procedures, such as biopsy and tumor resection. Under general anesthesia, the peritoneal cavity is inflated with 2 to 3 L of CO_2. The gas distends the abdominal wall so that the instruments can be inserted safely. Advantages of this procedure compared to an open laparotomy include reduced pain, reduced length of stay at the hospital or surgical center, and reduced time off from work. ■

INDICATIONS:

• Evaluate abdominal pain or abdominal mass of unknown origin

• Obtain biopsy specimens of benign or cancerous tumors

• Evaluate jaundice of unknown origin

• Evaluate and treat appendicitis

- Assist in performing surgical procedures such as cholecystectomy, appendectomy, hernia repair, hiatal hernia repair, and bowel resection
- Detect cirrhosis of the liver
- Stage neoplastic disorders such as lymphomas, Hodgkin's disease, and hepatic carcinoma
- Detect pancreatic disorders
- Evaluate the extent of splenomegaly due to portal hypertension
- Evaluate abdominal trauma in an emergency

RESULT

Normal Findings:
- Normal appearance of the liver, spleen, gallbladder, pancreas, and other abdominal contents

Abnormal Findings:
- Abdominal adhesions
- Appendicitis
- Ascites
- Cancer of any of the organs
- Cirrhosis of the liver
- Gangrenous gallbladder
- Intra-abdominal bleeding
- Portal hypertension
- Splenomegaly

CRITICAL VALUES: N/A

INTERFERING FACTORS:

This procedure is contraindicated for:
- Patients who are pregnant or suspected of being pregnant, unless the potential benefits of the procedure far outweigh the risk of radiation exposure to the fetus
- Patients with bleeding disorders, especially those associated with uremia and cytotoxic chemotherapy
- Patients with cardiac conditions or dysrhythmias
- Patients with advanced respiratory or cardiovascular disease
- Patients with intestinal obstruction, abdominal mass, abdominal hernia, or suspected intra-abdominal hemorrhage

Factors that may impair clear visualization:
- Inability of the patient to cooperate or remain still during the procedure because of age, significant pain, or mental status
- Patients who are very obese, who may exceed the weight limit for the equipment
- Incorrect positioning of the patient, which may produce poor visualization of the area to be examined
- A history of peritonitis or multiple abdominal operations causing dense adhesions

Other considerations:
- Failure to follow dietary restrictions before the procedure may cause the procedure to be canceled or repeated.
- Patients who are in a hypoxemic or hypercapnic state will require continuous oxygen administration.
- Patients with acute infection or advanced malignancy involving the abdominal wall are at increased risk because organisms may be introduced into the normally sterile peritoneal cavity.

Nursing Implications and Procedure

Pretest:

▶ Inform the patient that the procedure assesses the abdominal organs.

➤ Inform the patient that the procedure is generally performed in an operating room by a physician while the patient is under general anesthesia, but that it may be done under local anesthesia. Inform the patient that the procedure takes approximately 15 to 30 minutes.

➤ Assess whether the patient is allergic to latex.

➤ Determine date of last menstrual period and the possibility of pregnancy in perimenopausal women.

➤ Obtain a history of the patient's reproductive system and previously performed laboratory tests (especially complete blood count, prothrombin time, partial thromboplastin time, clotting and bleeding times), surgeries, therapies, and procedures. For related tests, refer to the gastrointestinal system table.

➤ Obtain a history of the patient's complaints, including a list of known allergens and sensitivities to anesthetics and analgesics.

➤ Obtain a list of the medications the patient is taking.

➤ Restrict food or fluids for at least 8 hours before the procedure.

➤ *Obtain a written, informed consent before administering any medications prior to the procedure.*

➤ Wear gloves and gowns throughout the procedure.

➤ Obtain and record baseline vital signs.

Intratest:

➤ Administer a cleansing enema 4 hours before the procedure.

➤ Ask the patient to void before the procedure. Have the patient put on a hospital gown.

➤ Ask the patient to lie still during the procedure because movement impairs clear visualization. Make sure jewelry, watches, chains, belts, and any other metallic objects have been removed from the abdominal area.

➤ Insert an intravenous line or venous access device at a low "keep open" rate.

➤ Administer medications, as ordered, to reduce discomfort and to promote relaxation and sedation.

➤ Place the patient on the laparoscopy table. General anesthesia is administered. Then place the patient in a modified lithotomy position with the head tilted downward. Cleanse the abdomen with an antiseptic solution, and drape and catheterize the patient, if ordered.

➤ The physician identifies the site for the scope insertion and administers local anesthesia. After deeper layers are anesthetized, a pneumoperitoneum needle is placed between the visceral and parietal peritoneum.

➤ Cleanse the abdomen with antiseptic solution and drape with sterile drapes. CO_2 is insufflated through the pneumoperitoneum needle to separate the abdominal wall from the viscera and to aid in visualization of the abdominal structures. The pneumoperitoneum needle is removed, and the trocar and laparoscope are inserted through the incision.

➤ After the examination, collection of tissue samples, and performance of therapeutic procedures, the scope is withdrawn. All possible CO_2 is evacuated via the trocar, which is then removed. The skin incision is closed with sutures, clips, or sterile strips, and a small dressing or adhesive strip is applied.

Post-test:

➤ Inform the patient to resume usual diet when the vital signs return to baseline levels, usually within 2 hours after the procedure, but instruct the patient to restrict activity for 2 to 7 days after the procedure.

➤ Inform the patient that further examinations may be necessary to evaluate progression of the disease process or to determine the need for a change in therapy.

➤ Inform the patient that shoulder discomfort may be experienced for 1 or 2 days after the procedure as a result abdominal distention caused by insufflation of CO_2 into the abdomen, and that mild analgesics and cold compresses, as ordered, can be used to relieve the discomfort.

➤ Emphasize that any persistent shoulder pain, abdominal pain, vaginal bleeding, fever, redness, or swelling of the incisional area must be reported to the physician immediately.

➤ Determine whether the patient or family members have any further questions or concerns.

➤ A physician specializing in this branch of medicine sends a written report to the ordering provider, who discusses the results with the patient.

➤ Evaluate test results in relation to the patient's symptoms and other tests performed. Related diagnostic tests include abdominal ultrasound and pelvic ultrasound.

LAPAROSCOPY, GYNECOLOGIC

SYNONYMS/ACRONYM: Gynecologic pelviscopy, gynecologic laparoscopy, pelvic endoscopy, peritoneoscopy.

AREA OF APPLICATION: Pelvis.

CONTRAST: Carbon dioxide (CO_2).

DESCRIPTION: Gynecologic laparoscopy provides direct visualization of the internal pelvic contents including the ovaries, fallopian tubes, and uterus after insufflation of carbon dioxide (CO_2). It is done to diagnose and treat pelvic organ disorders, as well as to perform surgical procedures on the organs. In this procedure, a rigid laparoscope is introduced into the body cavity through a 1- to 2-cm periumbilical incision. The endoscope has a microscope to allow visualization of the organs, and it can be used to insert instruments for performing certain procedures, such as biopsy and tumor resection. Under general or local anesthesia, the peritoneal cavity is inflated with 2 to 3 L of CO_2. The gas distends the abdominal wall so that the instruments can be inserted safely. Advantages of this procedure compared to an open laparotomy include reduced pain, reduced length of stay at the hospital or surgical center, and reduced time off from work. ■

INDICATIONS:

• Evaluate amenorrhea and infertility

• Evaluate fallopian tubes and anatomic defects to determine the cause of infertility

• Evaluate reproductive organs after therapy for infertility

- Evaluate pelvic pain or masses of unknown cause
- Evaluate known or suspected endometriosis, salpingitis, and hydrosalpinx
- Detect ectopic pregnancy and determine the need for surgery
- Detect pelvic inflammatory disease or abscess
- Detect uterine fibroids, ovarian cysts, and uterine malformations (ovarian cysts may be aspirated during the procedure)
- Obtain biopsy specimens to confirm suspected pelvic malignancies or metastasis
- Treat endometriosis through electrocautery or laser vaporization
- Remove adhesions or foreign bodies such as intrauterine devices (IUDs)
- Perform vaginal hysterectomy
- Perform tubal sterilization and ovarian biopsy

RESULT

Normal Findings:

- Normal appearance of uterus, ovaries, fallopian tubes, and other pelvic contents

Abnormal Findings:

- Ectopic pregnancy
- Endometriosis
- Ovarian cyst
- Ovarian tumor
- Pelvic adhesions
- Pelvic inflammatory disease
- Pelvic tumor
- Salpingitis
- Uterine fibroids

CRITICAL VALUES: N/A

INTERFERING FACTORS:

This procedure is contraindicated for:

- Patients who are pregnant or suspected of being pregnant, unless the potential benefits of the procedure far outweigh the risks to the fetus and mother
- Patients with bleeding disorders, especially those associated with uremia and cytotoxic chemotherapy
- Patients with cardiac conditions or dysrhythmias
- Patients with advanced respiratory or cardiovascular disease
- Patients with intestinal obstruction, abdominal mass, abdominal hernia, or suspected intra-abdominal hemorrhage

Factors that may impair clear visualization:

- Inability of the patient to cooperate or remain still during the procedure because of age, significant pain, or mental status
- Patients who are very obese, who may exceed the weight limit for the equipment
- Incorrect positioning of the patient, which may produce poor visualization of the area to be examined
- A history of peritonitis or multiple abdominal operations causing dense adhesions

Other considerations:

- Failure to follow dietary restrictions before the procedure may cause the procedure to be canceled or repeated.
- Patients who are in a hypoxemic or hypercapnic state will require continuous oxygen administration.
- Patients with acute infection or advanced malignancy involving the

abdominal wall are at increased risk because organisms may be introduced into the normally sterile peritoneal cavity.

Nursing Implications and Procedure • • • • • • • • • •

Pretest:

➤ Inform the patient that the procedure assesses the pelvic organs.

➤ Inform the patient that the procedure is generally performed in an operating room by a physician while the patient is under general anesthesia, but that it may be done under local anesthesia. Inform the patient that the procedure takes approximately 15 to 30 minutes.

➤ Assess whether the patient is allergic to latex.

➤ Determine the date of last menstrual period and the possibility of pregnancy in perimenopausal women. The procedure should not be done when the patient is menstruating and is best performed 1 week after menses ends.

➤ Obtain a history of the patient's reproductive system and previously performed laboratory tests (especially complete blood count, prothrombin time, partial thromboplastin time, clotting and bleeding times), surgeries, therapies, and procedures. For related tests, refer to the genitourinary and reproductive system tables.

➤ Obtain a history of the patient's complaints, including a list of known allergens and sensitivities to anesthetics and analgesics.

➤ Obtain a list of the medications the patient is taking.

➤ Restrict food or fluids for at least 8 hours before the procedure.

➤ *Obtain a written, informed consent before administering any medications prior to the procedure.*

➤ Wear gloves and gowns throughout the procedure.

➤ Obtain and record baseline vital signs.

Intratest:

➤ Administer a cleansing enema 4 hours before the procedure.

➤ Ask the patient to void before the procedure. Have the patient put on a hospital gown.

➤ Ask the patient to lie still during the procedure because movement impairs clear visualization. Make sure jewelry, watches, chains, belts, and any other metallic objects have been removed.

➤ Insert an intravenous line or venous access device at a low "keep open" rate.

➤ Administer medications, as ordered, to reduce discomfort and to promote relaxation and sedation.

➤ Place the patient on the laparoscopy table. General anesthesia is administered. Then place the patient in a modified lithotomy position with the head tilted downward. Cleanse the abdomen with an antiseptic solution and drape and catheterize the patient, if ordered.

➤ The physician inserts a uterine manipulator through the vagina and cervix and into the uterus so that the uterus, fallopian tubes, and ovaries can be moved to permit better visualization.

➤ Cleanse the abdomen with antiseptic solution and drape with sterile drapes. CO_2 is insufflated through the pneumoperitoneum needle to separate the abdominal wall from the viscera and to aid in visualization of the abdominal structures. The pneumoperitoneum needle is removed, and the trocar and laparoscope are inserted through the incision.

➤ After the examination, collection of tissue samples, and performance of therapeutic procedures (e.g., tubal ligation), the scope is withdrawn. All possible CO_2 is evacuated via the trocar, which is then removed. The skin incision is closed with sutures, clips, or sterile strips, and a small dressing or adhesive strip is applied. After the perineum is cleansed, the uterine manipulator is removed and a sterile pad applied.

Post-test:

➤ Inform the patient to resume usual diet when the vital signs return to baseline levels, usually within 2 hours after the procedure, but instruct the patient to restrict activity for 2 to 7 days after the procedure.

➤ Inform the patient that further examinations may be necessary to evaluate progression of the disease process or to determine the need for a change in therapy.

➤ Inform the patient that shoulder discomfort may be experienced for 1 or 2 days after the procedure as a result of abdominal distention caused by insufflation of CO_2 into the abdomen, and that mild anal-

gesics and cold compresses, as ordered, can be used to relieve the discomfort.

➤ Emphasize that any persistent shoulder pain, abdominal pain, vaginal bleeding, fever, redness, or swelling of the incisional area must be reported to the physician immediately.

➤ Determine whether the patient or family members have any further questions or concerns.

➤ A physician specializing in this branch of medicine sends a written report to the ordering provider, who discusses the results with the patient.

➤ Evaluate test results in relation to the patient's symptoms and other tests performed. Related diagnostic tests include ultrasound or computed tomography of the pelvis as well as ultrasound the abdomen.

LATEX ALLERGY

SYNONYM/ACRONYM: N/A.

SPECIMEN: Serum (1 mL) collected in a red-top tube.

REFERENCE VALUE: (Method: Immunoassay) Negative.

DESCRIPTION: Latex is found in numerous medical supplies, such as gloves, catheters, and bandages. Some individuals who are routinely exposed to latex products, particularly as part of their occupation, have become highly allergic to latex. Health care workers are classified as high risk, especially since the 1987 mandate of standard/universal precautions that resulted in increased use of latex

gloves. It is estimated that 8 to 17 percent of health care workers have become allergic to latex. There are two types of allergic reactions. Type IV allergic contact dermatitis is caused by chemicals used in the process of manufacturing latex. It is a delayed reaction occurring within 6 to 48 hours of direct-skin or mucous-membrane contact with latex products. The type I allergic reaction occurs in response to proteins in the natural latex products by direct-skin or mucous-membrane contact or by inhaling aerosolized powder from a latex glove. Other high-risk individuals include people with spina bifida, spinal cord injury, myelodysplasia, atopic dermatitis, eczema, history of allergies (personal or family), history of chronic illness, or multiple surgeries. ▪

INDICATIONS: Suspected latex allergy

RESULT

Positive findings in: Latex allergy

Negative findings in: N/A

CRITICAL VALUES: N/A

INTERFERING FACTORS: N/A

Nursing Implications and Procedure ․ ․ ․ ․ ․ ․ ․ ․ ․ ․

Pretest: ■

➤ Obtain a history of the patient's complaints, including a list of known allergens.

➤ Obtain a history of the patient's immune system, a history of latex exposure, and results of previously performed tests and procedures. For related tests, refer to the immune system table.

➤ Obtain a list of the medications the patient is taking, including herbs,

nutritional supplements, and nutraceuticals. The requesting health care practitioner and laboratory should be advised if the patient regularly uses these products so that their effects can be taken into consideration when reviewing results.

➤ There are no food, fluid, or medication restrictions unless by medical direction.

➤ Review the procedure with the patient.

➤ Inform the patient that specimen collection takes approximately 5 to 10 minutes.

Intratest: ■

➤ Direct the patient to breathe normally and to avoid unnecessary movement.

➤ Observe standard precautions and follow the general guidelines in Appendix A. Perform a venipuncture, and collect the specimen in a 5-mL red-top tube.

➤ Label the specimen, and promptly transport it to the laboratory.

Post-test: ■

➤ Observe venipuncture site for bleeding or hematoma formation. Apply pressure bandage.

➤ Assist the patient, as appropriate, in identifying sources of exposure in order for the patient to eliminate or reduce the opportunity for continued exposure.

➤ Evaluate test results in relation to the patient's symptoms, history of exposure, and other tests performed. Related laboratory tests include complete blood count and immunoglobulin E.

LEAD

SYNONYM/ACRONYM: Pb.

SPECIMEN: Whole blood (1 mL) collected in a special lead-free royal blue–or tan-top tube. Plasma (1 mL) collected in lavender-top (ethylenedi-aminetetra-acetic acid [EDTA]) tube is also acceptable.

REFERENCE VALUE: (Method: Atomic absorption spectrophotometry)

	Conventional Units	SI Units (Conversion Factor ×0.0483)
Children	0–9.9 μg/dL	0–0.48 μmol/L
Adults	0–25.0 μg/dL	0–1.20 μmol/L
OSHA action limit for occupational exposure	Up to 40 μg/dL	Up to 1.93 μmol/L

OSHA = Occupational Safety and Health Administration.

DESCRIPTION: Lead is a heavy metal and trace element. It is absorbed through the respiratory and gastrointestinal systems. It can also be transported from mother to fetus through the placenta. When there is frequent exposure to lead-containing items (e.g., paint, batteries, gasoline, pottery, bullets, printing materials) or occupations (mining, automobile, printing, and welding industries), many organs of the body are affected. Lead poisoning can cause severe behavioral and neurologic effects. The blood test is considered the best indicator of lead poisoning, and confirmation is made by the lead mobilization test performed on a 24-hour urine specimen. ■

INDICATIONS: Assist in the diagnosis and treatment of lead poisoning

RESULT

Increased in:
• Anemia of lead intoxication
• Lead encephalopathy
• Metal poisoning

Decreased in: N/A

CRITICAL VALUES: N/A

INTERFERING FACTORS: Contamination of the collection site and/or specimen with lead in dust can be avoided by taking special care to have the surfaces surrounding the collection location cleaned. Extra care should also be used to avoid contamination during the actual venipuncture.

Nursing Implications and Procedure • • • • • • • • • • •

Pretest:

➤ Obtain a history of the patient's complaints, including a list of known allergens.

➤ Obtain a history of the patient's hematopoietic system and results of previously performed tests and procedures. For related tests, refer to the hematopoietic system and therapeutic/toxicology tables.

➤ Obtain a history of the patient's exposure to lead.

➤ Obtain a list of the medications the patient is taking, including herbs, nutritional supplements, and nutraceuticals. The requesting health care practitioner and laboratory should be advised if the patient regularly uses these products so that their effects can be taken into consideration when reviewing results.

➤ There are no food, fluid, or medication restrictions unless by medical direction.

➤ Review the procedure with the patient.

➤ Inform the patient that specimen collection takes approximately 5 to 10 minutes.

Intratest:

➤ Direct the patient to breathe normally and to avoid unnecessary movement.

➤ Observe standard precautions and follow the general guidelines in Appendix A. Perform a venipuncture, and collect the specimen in a 5-mL royal blue– or tan-top tube.

➤ Label the specimen, and promptly transport it to the laboratory.

Post-test:

➤ Observe venipuncture site for bleeding or hematoma formation. Apply pressure bandage.

➤ Evaluate test results in relation to the patient's symptoms and other tests performed. Related laboratory tests include complete blood count, δ-aminolevulinic acid, erythrocyte protoporphyrin, and urine porphyrins.

LECITHIN/SPHINGOMYELIN RATIO

• •

SYNONYM/ACRONYM: L/S ratio.

SPECIMEN: Amniotic fluid (10 mL) collected in a sterile, brown glass or plastic tube or bottle protected from light.

REFERENCE VALUE: (Method: Thin-layer chromatography)

Mature (nondiabetic): Greater than 2:1 in the presence of phosphatidyl glycerol

Borderline: 1.5 to 1.9:1

Immature: Less than 1.5:1

DESCRIPTION: Respiratory distress syndrome (RDS) is the most common problem encountered in the care of premature infants. RDS, also called hyaline membrane disease, results from a deficiency of phospholipid lung surfactants. The phospholipids in surfactant are produced by specialized alveolar cells and stored in granular lamellar bodies in the lung. In normally developed lungs, surfactant coats the surface of the alveoli. Surfactant reduces the surface tension of the alveolar wall during breathing. When there is an insufficient quantity of surfactant, the alveoli are unable to expand normally and gas exchange is inhibited. Amniocentesis is a procedure by which fluid is removed from the amniotic sac to assess fetal lung maturity.

Lecithin is the primary surfactant phospholipid, and it is a stabilizing factor for the alveoli. It is produced at a low but constant rate until the 35th week of gestation, after which its production sharply increases. Sphingomyelin, another phospholipid component of surfactant, is also produced at a constant rate after the 26th week of gestation. Before the 35th week, the lecithin/sphingomyelin (L/S) ratio is usually less than 1.6:1. The ratio increases to 2.0 or greater when the rate of lecithin production increases after the 35th week of gestation. Other phospholipids, such as phosphatidyl glycerol (PG) and phosphatidyl inositol (PI), increase over time in amniotic fluid as well. The presence of PG indicates that the fetus is within 2 to 6 weeks of lung maturity (i.e., at full term). Simultaneous measurement of PG with the L/S ratio improves diagnos-

tic accuracy. Production of phospholipid surfactant is delayed in diabetic mothers. Therefore, caution must be used when interpreting the results obtained from a diabetic patient, and a higher ratio is expected to predict maturity. ∎

INDICATIONS:
• Assist in the evaluation of fetal lung maturity

• Determine the optimal time for obstetric intervention in cases of threatened fetal survival caused by stresses related to maternal diabetes, toxemia, hemolytic diseases of the newborn, or postmaturity

• Identify fetuses at risk of developing respiratory distress syndrome (RDS)

RESULT

Increased in:
• Hypertension

• Intrauterine growth retardation

• Malnutrition

• Maternal diabetes

• Placenta previa

• Placental infarction

• Premature rupture of the membranes

Decreased in:
• Immature fetal lungs

• Advanced maternal age

• Polyhydramnios

• Multiple gestation

CRITICAL VALUES: ⚠ An L/S ratio less than 1.5:1 is predictive of RDS at the time of delivery. Infants known to be at risk for RDS can be treated with surfactant by intratracheal administration at birth.

INTERFERING FACTORS:

• Fetal blood falsely elevates L/S ratio.

• Exposing the specimen to light may cause falsely decreased values.

• There is some risk to having an amniocentesis performed, and this should be weighed against the need to obtain the desired diagnostic information. A small percentage (0.5%) of patients have experienced complications including premature rupture of the membranes, premature labor, spontaneous abortion, and stillbirth.

Nursing Implications and Procedure • • • • • • • • • • •

Pretest: ■

➤ Obtain a history of the patient's complaints, including a list of known allergens.

➤ Obtain a history of the patient's reproductive and respiratory system and results of previously performed tests and procedures. For related tests, refer to the reproductive and respiratory system tables.

➤ Obtain a list of the medications the patient is taking, including herbs, nutritional supplements, and nutraceuticals. The requesting health care practitioner and laboratory should be advised if the patient regularly uses these products so that their effects can be taken into consideration when reviewing results.

➤ There are no food, fluid, or medication restrictions unless by medical direction.

➤ If the patient is less than 20 weeks' gestation, instruct her to drink extra fluids 1 hour before the test and to refrain from urination. The full bladder assists in raising the uterus up and out of the way to provide better visualization during the ultrasound procedure. Patients who are at 20 weeks' gestation or beyond do not need to drink extra fluids and should

void before the test, because an empty bladder is less likely to be accidentally punctured during specimen collection.

➤ Review the amniocentesis procedure with the patient.

➤ Assess whether the patient has an allergy to local anesthetics, and inform the health care practitioner accordingly.

➤ *Obtain written and informed consent before administering any medications prior to the procedure.*

➤ Inform the patient that specimen collection usually takes 20 to 30 minutes.

Intratest: ■

➤ Record maternal and fetal baseline vital signs. Monitor for uterine contractions.

➤ Ultrasound is used to locate the fetus, placenta, and amniotic fluid.

➤ Observe standard precautions and follow the general guidelines in Appendix A.

➤ Assemble the necessary equipment, including an amniocentesis tray with solution for skin preparation, local anesthetic, 10- or 20-mL syringe, needles of various sizes (including a 22-gauge, 5-inch spinal needle), sterile drapes, sterile gloves, and foil-covered or amber specimen collection containers.

➤ Ensure that the patient has a full bladder before the procedure if gestation is 20 weeks or less; have patient void before the procedure if gestation is 21 weeks or more.

➤ Assist the patient to a supine position. Raise her head or legs slightly to promote comfort and to relax abdominal muscles. If the uterus is large, place a pillow or rolled blanket under the patient's right side to prevent hypertension caused by great-vessel compression.

➤ Note fetal position and pocket of amniotic fluid as determined by ultrasound and palpation.

➤ Cleanse suprapubic area with an antiseptic solution and protect with sterile drapes. A local anesthetic is injected. Explain that this may cause a stinging sensation.

➤ A 22-gauge, 5-inch spinal needle is inserted through the abdominal and uterine walls. Explain that a sensation of pressure may be experienced when the needle is inserted. Explain to the patient how to use focusing and controlled breathing for relaxation during the procedure.

➤ After the fluid is collected and the needle withdrawn, apply slight pressure to the site. If there is no evidence of bleeding or other drainage, apply a sterile adhesive bandage to the site.

Post-test:

➤ Fetal heart rate and maternal life ⚠ signs (i.e., heart rate, blood pressure, pulse, and respiration) must be compared to baseline values and closely monitored every 15 minutes for 30 to 60 minutes after the amniocentesis procedure.

➤ Observe the patient after the procedure for symptoms of discomfort, such as nausea, faintness, or cramping. Instruct the patient to lie on her right side if symptoms are present.

➤ Instruct the patient to rest until all symptoms have disappeared before resuming normal levels of activity.

➤ Instruct the patient to immediately report any symptoms of itching at the collection site, fever, leakage of fluid, severe abdominal pain, or change in fetal activity (either increased or decreased).

➤ A Kleihauer-Betke test should be performed on maternal blood after amniocentesis of an Rh-negative patient to determine if fetal-maternal hemorrhage has occurred. Administration of Rh immune globulin is recommended if the results are increased. Some protocols may recommend automatically administering Rh immune globulin after amniocentesis of an Rh-negative patient and ignoring Kleihauer-Betke testing.

➤ Recognize anxiety related to test results and offer support. Provide teaching and information regarding the clinical implications of the test results, as appropriate. Encourage the family to seek counseling if concerned with pregnancy termination or to seek genetic counseling if a chromosomal abnormality is determined. Provide teaching and information regarding the clinical implications of the test results, as appropriate. Decisions regarding elective abortion should take place in the presence of both parents. Provide a nonjudgmental, nonthreatening atmosphere for discussing the risks and difficulties of delivering and raising an abnormal infant, as well as exploring other options (termination of pregnancy or adoption). It is also important to discuss feelings the mother and father may experience (e.g., guilt, depression, anger) if fetal abnormalities are detected.

➤ Evaluate test results in relation to the patient's symptoms and other tests performed. Related laboratory tests include α_1-fetoprotein, amniotic fluid analysis, Kleihauer-Betke test, and chromosomal analysis.

LEUKOCYTE ALKALINE PHOSPHATASE

SYNONYMS/ACRONYM: LAP, LAP score, LAP smear.

SPECIMEN: Whole blood (1 mL) collected in a lavender-top (ethylenedi-aminetetra-acetic acid [EDTA]) tube.

REFERENCE VALUE: (Method: Microscopic evaluation of specially stained blood smears) 32 to 182 (score based on 0 to 4+ rating of 100 neutrophils).

DESCRIPTION: Alkaline phosphatase is an enzyme important for intracellular metabolic processes. It is present in the cytoplasm of neutrophilic granulocytes from the metamyelocyte to the segmented stage. Leukocyte alkaline phosphatase (LAP) concentrations may be altered by the presence of infection, stress, chronic inflammatory diseases, Hodgkin's disease, and hematologic disorders. Levels are low in leukemic leukocytes and high in normal white blood cells (WBCs), making this test useful as a supportive test in the differential diagnosis of leukemia. It should be noted that test results must be correlated with the patient's condition because LAP levels increase toward normal in response to therapy. ■

INDICATIONS:
• Differentiate chronic myelocytic leukemia from other disorders that increase the WBC count

• Monitor response of Hodgkin's disease to therapy

RESULT

Increased in:
• Aplastic leukemia

• Chronic inflammation

• Down syndrome

• Hodgkin's disease

• Hairy cell leukemia

• Leukemia (acute and chronic lymphoblastic)

• Myelofibrosis with myeloid metaplasia

• Multiple myeloma

• Polycythemia vera

• Pregnancy

• Stress

• Thrombocytopenia

Decreased in:
• Chronic myelogenous leukemia

• Hereditary hypophosphatemia

• Idiopathic thrombocytopenia purpura

• Nephrotic syndrome

• Paroxysmal nocturnal hemoglobinuria

• Sickle cell anemia

• Sideroblastic anemia

CRITICAL VALUES: N/A

INTERFERING FACTORS: Drugs that may increase the LAP score include steroids.

Nursing Implications and Procedure · · · · · · · · · · ·

Pretest: ■

➤ Obtain a history of the patient's complaints, including a list of known allergens.

➤ Obtain a history of the patient's hematopoietic and immune systems, as well as results of previously performed tests and procedures. For related tests, refer to the hematopoietic and immune system tables.

➤ Obtain a list of the medications the patient is taking, including herbs, nutritional supplements, and nutraceuticals. The requesting health care

practitioner and laboratory should be advised if the patient regularly uses these products so that their effects can be taken into consideration when reviewing results.

➤ There are no food, fluid, or medication restrictions unless by medical direction.

➤ Review the procedure with the patient.

➤ Inform the patient that specimen collection takes approximately 5 to 10 minutes.

Intratest:

➤ Direct the patient to breathe normally and to avoid unnecessary movement.

➤ Observe standard precautions and

follow the general guidelines in Appendix A. Perform a venipuncture, and collect the specimen in a 5-mL lavender-top tube.

➤ Label the specimen, and promptly transport it to the laboratory.

Post-test:

➤ Observe venipuncture site for bleeding or hematoma formation. Apply pressure bandage.

➤ Instruct the patient to avoid exposure to infection if WBC count is decreased.

➤ Evaluate test results in relation to the patient's symptoms and other tests performed. Related laboratory tests include bone marrow biopsy and WBC count.

LIPASE

• •

SYNONYM/ACRONYM: Triacylglycerol acylhydrolase.

SPECIMEN: Serum (1 mL) collected in a red- or tiger-top tube. Plasma (1 mL) collected in green-top (heparin) tube is also acceptable.

REFERENCE VALUE: (Method: Spectrophotometry) Plasma values may be 15 percent lower than serum values.

Conventional Units	SI Units (Conversion Factor ×0.017)
40–375 U/L	0.68–6.38 μKat/L

DESCRIPTION: Lipases are digestive enzymes secreted by the pancreas into the duodenum. Different lipolytic enzymes have specific substrates, but overall activity is collectively described as lipase. Lipase participates in fat digestion by breaking down triglycerides into fatty acids and glycerol. Lipase is released into the blood-

stream when damage occurs to the pancreatic acinar cells. Its presence in the blood indicates pancreatic disease because it is the only organ that secretes this enzyme. ■

INDICATIONS:

• Assist in the diagnosis of acute and chronic pancreatitis

- Assist in the diagnosis of pancreatic carcinoma

RESULT

Increased in:

- Acute cholecystitis

- Obstruction of the pancreatic duct

- Pancreatic cyst or pseudocyst

- Pancreatic carcinoma (early)

- Pancreatic inflammation

- Pancreatitis (acute and chronic)

- Renal failure (early)

Decreased in: N/A

CRITICAL VALUES: N/A

INTERFERING FACTORS:

- Drugs that may increase lipase levels include asparaginase, azathioprine, cholinergics, codeine, deoxycholate, didanosine, glycocholate, indomethacin, methacholine, methylprednisolone, morphine, narcotics, pancreozymin, pentazocine, and taurocholate.

- Drugs that may decrease lipase levels include protamine and saline (intravenous infusions).

- Endoscopic retrograde cholangiopancreatography may increase lipase levels.

- Serum lipase levels increase with hemodialysis. Therefore, predialysis specimens should be collected for lipase analysis.

Nursing Implications and Procedure

Pretest:

➤ Obtain a history of the patient's complaints, including a list of known allergens.

➤ Obtain a history of the patient's gastrointestinal and hepatobiliary systems, as well as results of previously performed tests and procedures. For related tests, refer to the gastrointestinal and hepatobiliary system tables.

➤ Obtain a list of the medications the patient is taking, including herbs, nutritional supplements, and nutraceuticals. The requesting health care practitioner and laboratory should be advised if the patient regularly uses these products so that their effects can be taken into consideration when reviewing results.

➤ Note any recent procedures that can interfere with test results.

➤ There are no food, fluid, or medication restrictions unless by medical direction.

➤ Review the procedure with the patient.

➤ Inform the patient that specimen collection takes approximately 5 to 10 minutes.

Intratest:

➤ Direct the patient to breathe normally and to avoid unnecessary movement.

➤ Observe standard precautions and follow the general guidelines in Appendix A. Perform a venipuncture, and collect the specimen in a 5-mL red- or tiger-top tube.

➤ Label the specimen, and promptly transport it to the laboratory.

Post-test:

➤ Observe venipuncture site for bleeding or hematoma formation. Apply pressure bandage.

➤ Increased lipase levels may be associated with pancreatic disorders.

➤ Instruct the patient to ingest small, frequent meals if he or she has a gastrointestinal disorder; advise the patient to consider other dietary alterations as well. After acute symptoms subside and bowel sounds return, patients are usually prescribed a clear liquid diet, progressing to a low-fat, high-carbohydrate diet.

➤ Administer vitamin B$_{12}$, as ordered, to the patient with decreased lipase levels, especially if his or her disease prevents adequate absorption of the vitamin.

➤ Encourage the alcoholic patient to avoid alcohol and to seek appropriate counseling for substance abuse.

➤ Evaluate test results in relation to the patient's symptoms and other tests performed. Related laboratory tests include alanine aminotransferase, alkaline phosphatase, amylase, fluid amylase, aspartate aminotransferase, bilirubin, CA 19-9, calcium, fecal fat, γ-glutamyl transpeptidase, magnesium, mumps serology, triglycerides, and white blood cell count.

LIPOPROTEIN ELECTROPHORESIS

SYNONYMS/ACRONYMS: Lipid fractionation; lipoprotein phenotyping; α$_1$-lipoprotein cholesterol, high-density lipoprotein (HDL); β-lipoprotein cholesterol, low-density lipoprotein (LDL); pre-β-lipoprotein cholesterol, very-low-density lipoprotein (VLDL).

SPECIMEN: Serum (3 mL) collected in a red- or tiger-top tube.

REFERENCE VALUE: (Method: Electrophoresis and 4°C test for specimen appearance) There is no quantitative interpretation of this test. The specimen appearance and electrophoretic pattern is visually interpreted.

Hyperlipoproteinemia: Fredrickson Type	Specimen Appearance	Electrophoretic Pattern
Type I	Clear with creamy top layer	Heavy chylomicron band
Type IIa	Clear	Heavy β band
Type IIb	Clear or faintly turbid	Heavy β and pre-β band
Type III	Slightly to moderately turbid	Heavy β band
Type IV	Slightly to moderately turbid	Heavy pre-β band
Type V	Slightly to moderately turbid with creamy top layer	Intense chylomicron band and heavy pre-β band

DESCRIPTION: Lipoprotein electrophoresis measures lipoprotein fractions to determine abnormal distribution and concentration of lipoproteins in the serum, an impor-tant risk factor in the development of coronary artery disease (CAD). The lipoprotein fractions in order of increasing density are (1) chylomicrons, (2) very-low-density lipoprotein (VLDL), (3) low-density lipoprotein (LDL), and (4) high-density lipoprotein (HDL). Chylomicrons and VLDL contain the highest levels of triglycerides and lower amounts of cholesterol and protein. LDL and HDL contain the lowest amounts of triglycerides and relatively higher amounts of cholesterol and protein. ∎

INDICATIONS:

• Evaluate known or suspected disorders associated with altered lipoprotein levels

• Evaluate patients with serum cholesterol levels greater than 250 mg/dL, which indicate a high risk for CAD

• Evaluate the response to treatment for high cholesterol, and determine the need for drug therapy

RESULT:

Type I: Hyperlipoproteinemia or increased chylomicrons can be primary, resulting from an inherited deficiency of lipoprotein lipase; or secondary, caused by uncontrolled diabetes, systemic lupus erythematosus, and dysgammaglobulinemia. Total cholesterol is normal to moderately elevated and triglycerides (mostly exogenous chylomicrons) are grossly elevated. If the condition is inherited, symptoms will appear in childhood.

Type IIa: Hyperlipoproteinemia can be primary, resulting from inherited characteristics or secondary, caused by hypothyroidism, nephrotic syndrome, and dysgammaglobulinemia. Total cholesterol is elevated, triglycerides are normal, and LDL cholesterol (LDLC) is elevated. If the condition is inherited, symptoms will appear in childhood.

Type IIb: Hyperlipoproteinemia can

occur for the same reasons as in Type IIa. Total cholesterol, triglycerides, and LDLC are all elevated.

Type III: Hyperlipoproteinemia can be primary, resulting from inherited characteristics; or secondary, caused by hypothyroidism, uncontrolled diabetes, alcoholism, and dysgammaglobulinemia. Total cholesterol and triglycerides are elevated, whereas LDLC is normal.

Type IV: Hyperlipoproteinemia can be primary, resulting from inherited characteristics; or secondary, caused by poorly controlled diabetes, alcoholism, nephrotic syndrome, chronic renal failure, and dysgammaglobulinemia. Total cholesterol is normal to moderately elevated, triglycerides are moderately to grossly elevated, and LDLC is normal.

Type V: Hyperlipoproteinemia can be primary, resulting from inherited characteristics; or secondary, caused by uncontrolled diabetes, alcoholism, nephrotic syndrome, and dysgammaglobulinemia. Total cholesterol is normal to moderately elevated, triglycerides are grossly elevated, and LDLC is normal.

CRITICAL VALUES: N/A

INTERFERING FACTORS:

• Failure to follow usual diet for 2 weeks before the test can yield results that do not accurately reflect patient's cholesterol values.

• Ingestion of alcohol 24 hours before the test, ingestion of food 12 hours before the test, and excessive exercise 12 hours before the test can alter results.

• Numerous drugs can alter results (see

monographs titled "Cholesterol, Total" and "Triglycerides").

Nursing Implications and Procedure • • • • • • • • • • • •

➤ Obtain a history of the patient's complaints, including a list of known allergens.

➤ Obtain a history of the patient's cardiovascular system and risk for heart disease, as well as results of previously performed tests and procedures, particularly the results of lipid tests. For related tests, refer to the cardiovascular system table.

➤ Obtain a list of the medications the patient is taking, including herbs, nutritional supplements, and nutraceuticals. The requesting health care practitioner and laboratory should be advised if the patient regularly uses these products so that their effects can be taken into consideration when reviewing results.

➤ There are no medication restrictions unless by medical direction.

➤ Instruct the patient to follow his or her usual diet for 2 weeks before testing.

➤ Instruct the patient to fast and to avoid excessive exercise for at least 12 hours before testing, and to refrain from alcohol consumption for 24 hours before testing.

➤ Review the procedure with the patient.

➤ Inform the patient that specimen collection takes approximately 5 to 10 minutes.

➤ Ensure that the patient has complied with dietary preparations and other pretesting restrictions.

➤ Direct the patient to breathe normally and to avoid unnecessary movement.

➤ Observe standard precautions and follow the general guidelines in Appendix A. Perform a venipuncture, and collect the specimen in a 5-mL red- or tiger-top tube.

➤ Label the specimen, and promptly transport it to the laboratory.

➤ Observe venipuncture site for bleeding or hematoma formation. Apply pressure bandage.

➤ Instruct the patient to resume usual medication as directed by the requesting health care practitioner.

➤ Abnormal lipoprotein electrophoresis patterns may be associated with cardiovascular disease. Nutritional therapy is recommended for the patient identified to be at high risk for developing CAD. If overweight, the patient should be encouraged to achieve a normal weight. The American Heart Association Step 1 and Step 2 diets may be helpful in achieving a goal of lowering total cholesterol and triglyceride levels. The Step 1 diet emphasizes a reduction in foods high in saturated fats and cholesterol. Red meats, eggs, and dairy products are the major sources of saturated fats and cholesterol. If triglycerides also are elevated, the patient should be advised to eliminate or reduce alcohol and simple carbohydrates from the diet. The Step 2 diet recommends stricter reductions.

➤ Numerous studies point to the prevalence of excess body weight in American children and adolescents. Experts estimate that obesity is present in 25 percent of the population aged 6 to 11 years. The medical, social, and emotional consequences of excess body weight are significant. Special attention should be given to instructing the child and caregiver regarding health risks and weight control education.

➤ Evaluate test results in relation to the patient's symptoms and other tests performed. Related laboratory tests include apolipoprotein A and B, total cholesterol, HDL cholesterol, LDL cholesterol, and triglycerides.

LIVER AND SPLEEN SCAN

• •

SYNONYMS/ACRONYM: Liver and spleen scintigraphy, liver-spleen scan, radionuclide liver scan, spleen scan.

AREA OF APPLICATION: Abdomen.

CONTRAST: Intravenous radioactive technetium-99m sulfur colloid.

DESCRIPTION: The liver and spleen scan is performed to help diagnose abnormalities in the function and structure of the liver and spleen. It is often performed in combination with lung scanning to help diagnose masses or inflammation in the diaphragmatic area. This procedure is useful for evaluating right-upper-quadrant pain, metastatic disease, jaundice, cirrhosis, ascites, traumatic infarction, and radiation-induced organ cellular necrosis. Technetium-99m (Tc-99m) sulfur colloid is injected intravenously and rapidly taken up by the reticuloendothelial cells through phagocytosis, which normally function to remove particulate matter, including radioactive colloids in the liver and spleen. False-negative results may occur in patients with space-occupying lesions (e.g., tumors, cysts, abscesses) smaller than 2 cm. This scan can detect portal hypertension, demonstrated by a greater uptake of the radionuclide in the spleen than in the liver. Single photon emission computed tomography (SPECT) has significantly improved the resolution and accuracy of liver scanning. SPECT enables images to be recorded from multiple angles around the body and reconstructed by a computer to produce images representing the organ at different levels or "slices." For evaluation of a suspected hemangioma, the patient's red blood cells are combined with Tc-99m and images are recorded over the liver. To confirm diagnosis, liver and spleen scans are done in conjunction with CT, magnetic resonance imaging (MRI), ultrasonography, and SPECT scans and interpreted in light of the results of liver function tests. ■

INDICATIONS:

• Detect and differentiate between primary and metastatic tumor focal disease

• Detect diffuse hepatocellular disease, such as hepatitis and cirrhosis

• Detect benign tumors, such as adenoma and cavernous hemangioma

• Detect a bacterial or amebic abscess

• Detect cystic focal disease

• Evaluate the effects of lower abdominal trauma, such as internal hemorrhage

• Assess the condition of the liver and spleen after abdominal trauma

- Detect infiltrative processes that affect the liver, such as sarcoidosis and amyloidosis

- Evaluate palpable abdominal masses

- Differentiate between splenomegaly and hepatomegaly

- Determine superior vena cava obstruction or Budd-Chiari syndrome

- Evaluate liver and spleen damage caused by radiation therapy or toxic drug therapy

- Evaluate jaundice

RESULT

Normal Findings:
- Normal size, contour, position, and function of the liver and spleen

Abnormal Findings:
- Abscesses

- Cirrhosis

- Cysts

- Inflammation of the diaphragmatic area

- Hemangiomas

- Hematoma

- Hepatitis

- Hodgkin's disease

- Infection

- Infarction

- Infiltrate process (amyloidosis and sarcoidosis)

- Metastatic tumors

- Nodular hyperplasia

- Portal hypertension

- Primary benign or malignant tumors

- Traumatic lesions

CRITICAL VALUES: N/A

INTERFERING FACTORS:

This procedure is contraindicated for:
- Patients who are pregnant or suspected of being pregnant, unless the potential benefits of the procedure far outweigh the risks to the fetus and mother

Factors that may impair clear imaging:
- Inability of the patient to cooperate or remain still during the procedure because of age, significant pain, or mental status

- Metallic objects within the examination field (e.g., jewelry or body rings), which may inhibit organ visualization and can produce unclear images

- Patients who are very obese, who may exceed the weight limit for the equipment

- Incorrect positioning of the patient, which may produce poor visualization of the area to be examined, especially for oblique and decubitus views

- Other nuclear scans done within the preceding 24 to 48 hours

Other considerations:
- The scan may fail to detect focal lesions smaller than 2 cm in diameter.

- Improper injection of the radionuclide may allow the tracer to seep deep into the muscle tissue, producing erroneous hot spots.

- Consultation with a physician should occur before the procedure for radiation safety concerns regarding infants of patients who are lactating.

- Risks associated with radiologic overexposure can result from frequent x-ray procedures. Personnel in the room with the patient should wear a protective lead apron, stand behind a shield, or leave the area while the examination is being done. Personnel working in the area where the examination is being done should wear badges that reveal their level of exposure to radiation.

Nursing Implications and Procedure • • • • • • • • • • •

Pretest:

➤ Inform the patient that the procedure assesses liver and spleen function.

➤ Inform the patient that the procedure is performed in a nuclear medicine department by a technologist and usually takes approximately 30 to 60 minutes.

➤ Obtain a history of the patient's complaints, including a list of known allergens.

➤ Obtain a history of the patient's liver and spleen, as well as results of previously performed tests (especially liver function tests) and surgical procedures. For related tests, refer to the hepatobiliary and gastrointestinal systems tables.

➤ Obtain a list of the medications the patient is taking.

➤ Determine date of last menstrual period and possibility of pregnancy in perimenopausal women.

➤ Fasting before the scan is not necessary, unless otherwise indicated.

Intratest:

➤ Ask the patient to void before the procedure. Have the patient put on a hospital gown.

➤ Administer sedative to a child or to an uncooperative adult, as ordered.

➤ Make sure jewelry, watches, chains, belts, and any other metallic objects have been removed from the abdominal area.

➤ Place the patient in a supine position on a flat table with foam wedges, which help maintain position and immobilization. Ask the patient to lie still during the procedure because movement produces unclear images. The radionuclide is administered intravenously and the abdomen is scanned immediately for 1 minute to screen for vascular lesions. Then images are taken in the anterior, oblique, lateral, and posterior oblique positions.

➤ Wear gloves during the radionuclide administration and while handling the patient's urine.

Post-test:

➤ Evaluate the patient's vital signs.

➤ Instruct the patient to resume normal activity, medications, and diet, unless otherwise indicated.

➤ Advise patient to drink increased amounts of fluids for 24 to 48 hours to eliminate the radionuclide from the body, unless contraindicated. Tell the patient that radionuclide is eliminated from the body within 6 to 24 hours.

➤ Inform the patient to flush the toilet immediately after each voiding following the procedure and to wash hands meticulously with soap and water after each voiding for 24 hours after the procedure.

➤ Tell all caregivers to wear gloves when discarding urine for 24 hours after the procedure. Wash gloved hands with soap and water before removing gloves. Then wash hands after the gloves are removed.

➤ A physician specializing in this branch of medicine sends a written report to the ordering provider, who discusses the results with the patient.

➤ Evaluate test results in relation to the patient's symptoms and other tests performed. Related diagnostic tests include hepatobiliary scan, liver and abdominal ultrasound, and CT and MRI of the abdomen.

LUNG PERFUSION SCAN

SYNONYMS/ACRONYM: Radioactive perfusion scan, lung scintiscan, lung perfusion scintigraphy, perfusion-ventilation scan, pulmonary scan, radionuclide perfusion lung scan, V/Q scan.

AREA OF APPLICATION: Chest/thorax.

CONTRAST: Intravenous radioactive material, usually macroaggregated albumin (MAA).

DESCRIPTION: The lung perfusion scan is a nuclear medicine study performed to evaluate a patient for pulmonary embolus (PE) or other pulmonary disorders. Technetium (Tc-99m) is injected intravenously and distributed throughout the pulmonary vasculature because of the gravitational effect on perfusion. The scan, which produces a visual image of pulmonary blood flow, is useful in diagnosing or confirming pulmonary vascular obstruction. The diameter of the intravenously injected macroaggregated albumin (MAA) is larger than that of the pulmonary capillaries; therefore the MAA temporarily becomes lodged in the pulmonary vasculature. A gamma camera detects the radiation emitted from the injected radioactive material, and a representative image of the lung is obtained. This procedure is often done in conjunction with the ventilation scan to obtain clinical information that assists in differentiating among the many possible pathologic conditions revealed by the procedure. The results are correlated with other diagnostic studies, such as pulmonary function, chest x-ray, pulmonary angiography, and arterial blood gases. A recent chest x-ray is essential for accurate interpretation of the lung perfusion scan. An area of nonperfusion seen in the same area as a pulmonary parenchymal abnormality on the chest x-ray indicates that a PE is not present; the defect may represent some other pathologic condition, such as pneumonia. ∎

INDICATIONS:
- Aid in the diagnosis of PE in a patient with a normal chest x-ray
- Differentiate between PE and other pulmonary diseases, such as pneumonia, pulmonary effusion, atelectasis, asthma, bronchitis, emphysema, and tumors
- Evaluate perfusion changes associated with congestive heart failure and pulmonary hypertension
- Detect malignant tumor
- Evaluate pulmonary function preoperatively in a patient with pulmonary disease

RESULT

Normal Findings:
- Diffuse and homogeneous uptake of the radioactive material by the lungs

Abnormal Findings:

• Asthma

• Atelectasis

• Bronchitis

• Chronic obstructive pulmonary disease

• Emphysema

• Left atrial or pulmonary hypertension

• Lung displacement by fluid or chest masses

• Pneumonia

• Pneumonitis

• Pulmonary embolism

• Tuberculosis

CRITICAL VALUES: N/A

INTERFERING FACTORS:

This procedure is contraindicated for:

• Patients who are pregnant or suspected of being pregnant, unless the potential benefits of the procedure far outweigh the risks to the fetus and mother

• Patients with atrial and ventricular septal defects, because the MAA particles will not reach the lungs

• Patients with pulmonary hypertension

Factors that may impair clear imaging:

• Inability of the patient to cooperate or remain still during the procedure because of age, significant pain, or mental status

• Metallic objects within the examination field (e.g., jewelry or body rings), which may inhibit organ visualization and can produce unclear images

• Patients who are very obese, who may exceed the weight limit for the equipment

• Incorrect positioning of the patient, which may produce poor visualization

of the area to be examined, especially for oblique and decubitus views and for films done by portable equipment

• Other nuclear scans done on the same day

Other considerations:

• Improper injection of the radionuclide may allow the tracer to seep deep into the muscle tissue, producing erroneous hot spots.

• Consultation with a physician should occur before the procedure for radiation safety concerns regarding infants of patients who are lactating.

• Risks associated with radiologic overexposure can result from frequent x-ray procedures. Personnel in the room with the patient should wear a protective lead apron, stand behind a shield, or leave the area while the examination is being done. Personnel working in the area where the examination is being done should wear badges that reveal their level of exposure to radiation.

Nursing Implications and Procedure • • • • • • • • • • •

Pretest:

➤ Inform the patient that the procedure assesses blood flow to the lungs.

➤ Inform the patient that the procedure is performed in a special department by a technologist and is usually done in conjunction with a ventilation test; the combined procedures take approximately 60 minutes.

➤ Obtain pertinent history, pulmonary findings, and chest x-ray results on the same day as the ventilation examination. For related tests, refer to the respiratory system table.

➤ Obtain a history of the patient's complaints, including a list of known allergens.

➤ Obtain a list of the medications the patient is taking.

➤ Determine date of last menstrual period and possibility of pregnancy in perimenopausal women.

➤ Do not restrict food and fluids, unless otherwise indicated.

Intratest: ■

➤ Ask the patient to void before the procedure. Have the patient put on a hospital gown.

➤ Administer sedative to a child or to an uncooperative adult, as ordered.

➤ Make sure jewelry, chains, and any other metallic objects have been removed from the chest area.

➤ Place the patient in a supine position on a flat table with foam wedges, which help maintain position and immobilization. Ask the patient to lie still during the procedure because movement produces unclear images. The radionuclide is administered intravenously after the syringe is shaken to resuspend the particles. Images of the lungs are obtained in the anterior, posterior, both lateral, and both oblique views.

➤ Wear gloves during the radionuclide administration and while handling the patient's urine.

Post-test: ■

➤ Evaluate the patient's vital signs. Monitor vital signs every 15 to 30 minutes and compare with baseline readings until the patient is stable.

➤ Instruct the patient to resume normal activity, medications, and diet, unless otherwise indicated.

➤ Advise the patient to drink increased amounts of fluids for 24 to 48 hours to eliminate the radionuclide from the body, unless contraindicated. Tell the patient that radionuclide is eliminated from the body within 6 to 24 hours.

➤ The presence of conditions that affect perfusion or ventilation (e.g., tumors that obstruct the pulmonary artery, vasculitis, pulmonary edema, sickle cell disease, parasitic disease, emphysema, effusion, infection) can simulate a perfusion defect similar to PE.

➤ Observe the patient for up to 60 minutes after the study for a possible anaphylactic reaction to the radionuclide, such as rash, tightening of throat, or difficulty breathing.

➤ Inform the patient to flush the toilet immediately after each voiding following the procedure and to wash hands meticulously with soap and water after each voiding for 24 hours after the procedure.

➤ Tell all caregivers to wear gloves when discarding urine for 24 hours after the procedure. Wash gloved hands with soap and water before removing gloves. Then wash hands after the gloves are removed.

➤ A physician specializing in this branch of medicine sends a written report to the ordering provider, who discusses the results with the patient.

➤ Evaluate test results in relation to the patient's symptoms and other tests performed. Related diagnostic tests include x-ray, computed tomography, and magnetic resonance imaging of the chest.

LUNG VENTILATION SCAN

SYNONYMS/ACRONYM: Radioactive ventilation scan, VQ lung scan, aerosol lung scan, ventilation scan, xenon lung scan.

AREA OF APPLICATION: Chest/thorax.

CONTRAST: Done with inhaled radioactive material (xenon gas or technetium-DTPA).

DESCRIPTION: The lung ventilation scan is a nuclear medicine study performed to evaluate a patient for pulmonary embolus (PE) or other pulmonary disorders. It can evaluate respiratory function (i.e., demonstrating areas of the lung that are patent and capable of ventilation) and dysfunction (e.g., parenchymal abnormalities affecting ventilation, such as pneumonia). The procedure is performed after the patient inhales air mixed with a radioactive gas through a face mask and mouthpiece. The radioactive gas delineates areas of the lung during ventilation. The distribution of the gas throughout the lung is measured in three phases:

Wash-in phase: Phase during buildup of the radioactive gas

Equilibrium phase: Phase after the patient rebreathes from a closed delivery system

Wash-out phase: Phase after the radioactive gas has been removed

This procedure is usually performed along with a lung perfusion scan. When PE is present, ventilation scans display a normal wash-in and wash-out of radioactivity from the lung areas. Parenchymal disease responsible for perfusion abnormalities will produce abnormal wash-in and wash-out phases. This test can be used to quantify regional ventilation in patients with pulmonary disease. ∎

INDICATIONS:

• Aid in the diagnosis of PE

• Differentiate between PE and other pulmonary diseases, such as pneumonia, pulmonary effusion, atelectasis, asthma, bronchitis, emphysema, and tumors

• Evaluate regional respiratory function

• Identify areas of the lung that are capable of ventilation

• Locate hypoventilation (regional), which can result from chronic obstructive pulmonary disease (COPD) or excessive smoking

RESULT

Normal Findings:

• Equal distribution of radioactive gas throughout both lungs and a normal wash-out phase

Abnormal Findings:

• Atelectasis

• Bronchogenic carcinoma

- Bronchitis

- COPD

- Emphysema

- Pneumonia

- PE

- Regional hypoventilation

- Sarcoidosis

- Tuberculosis

- Tumor

INTERFERING FACTORS:

This procedure is contraindicated for:
- Patients who are pregnant or suspected of being pregnant, unless the potential benefits of the procedure far outweigh the risks to the fetus and mother

Factors that may impair clear imaging:
- Inability of the patient to cooperate or remain still during the procedure because of age, significant pain, or mental status

- Metallic objects within the examination field (e.g., jewelry or body rings), which may inhibit organ visualization and can produce unclear images

- Patients who are very obese, who may exceed the weight limit for the equipment

- Incorrect positioning of the patient, which may produce poor visualization of the area to be examined, especially for oblique and decubitus views and for films done by portable equipment

- Other nuclear scans done within the preceding 24 to 48 hours

Other considerations:
- Consultation with a physician should occur before the procedure for radiation safety concerns regarding infants of patients who are lactating.

- Risks associated with radiographic overexposure can result from frequent x-ray procedures. Personnel in the room with the patient should wear a protective lead apron, stand behind a shield, or leave the area while the examination is being done. Personnel working in the area where the examination is being done should wear badges that reveal their level of exposure to radiation.

Nursing Implications and Procedure • • • • • • • • • •

Pretest: ■

➤ Inform the patient that the procedure assesses airflow to the lungs.

➤ Inform the patient that the procedure is performed in a special department by a technologist and usually is done in conjunction with a lung perfusion scan; the combined tests take approximately 60 minutes.

➤ Obtain pertinent history, pulmonary findings, and chest x-ray results on the same day as the ventilation examination. For related tests, refer to the respiratory system table.

➤ Determine date of last menstrual period and possibility of pregnancy in perimenopausal women.

➤ Do not restrict food and fluids, unless otherwise indicated.

Intratest: ■

➤ Ask the patient to void before the procedure. Have the patient put on a hospital gown.

➤ Administer sedative to a child or to an uncooperative adult, as ordered.

➤ Make sure jewelry, chains, and any other metallic objects have been removed from the chest area.

➤ Place the patient in a supine position on a flat table with foam wedges, which help maintain position and immobilization. Ask the patient to lie still during the procedure because movement produces unclear images. The radionuclide is administered through a mask, which is placed over the patient's nose and mouth. The patient is asked to hold his or her breath for a short period of time while the scan is taken. The distribution of the radioactive gas is monitored and measured on a nuclear scanner. The patient's chest is imaged while the gas is in the lungs. Images of the lungs are obtained in the posterior and, when possible, both oblique views.

➤ Wear gloves during the radionuclide administration and while handling the patient's urine.

Post-test:

➤ Evaluate the patient's vital signs. Monitor vital signs every 15 to 30 minutes and compare with baseline readings until the patient is stable.

➤ Advise patient to drink increased amounts of fluids for 24 to 48 hours to eliminate the radionuclide from the body, unless contraindicated. Tell the patient that radionuclide is eliminated from the body within 6 to 24 hours.

➤ The presence of conditions that affect perfusion or ventilation (e.g., tumors that obstruct the pulmonary

artery, vasculitis, pulmonary edema, sickle cell disease, parasitic disease, emphysema, effusion, infection) can simulate a perfusion defect similar to PE.

➤ Observe patient for up to 60 minutes after the study for a possible anaphylactic reaction to the radionuclide, such as rash, tightening of throat, or difficulty breathing.

➤ Inform the patient to flush the toilet immediately after each voiding following the procedure and to wash hands meticulously with soap and water after each voiding for 24 hours after the procedure.

➤ Tell all caregivers to wear gloves when discarding urine for 24 hours after the procedure. Wash gloved hands with soap and water before removing gloves. Then wash hands after the gloves are removed.

➤ A physician specializing in this branch of medicine sends a written report to the ordering provider, who discusses the results with the patient.

➤ Evaluate test results in relation to the patient's symptoms and other tests performed. Related diagnostic tests include lung perfusion scan as well as x-ray and computed tomography of the chest.

LUPUS ANTICOAGULANT ANTIBODIES

• •

SYNONYMS/ACRONYM: Lupus inhibitor phospholipid type, lupus antiphospholipid antibodies.

SPECIMEN: Plasma (1 mL) collected in blue-top (sodium citrate) tube.

REFERENCE VALUE: (Method: Dilute Russell venom viper test time) Negative.

DESCRIPTION: Lupus anticoagulant antibodies are immunoglobulins, usually of the IgG class. They are also referred to as lupus antiphospholipid antibodies because they interfere with phospholipid-dependent coagulation tests such as activated partial thromboplastin time (APTT) by reacting with the phospholipids in the test system. They are not associated with a bleeding disorder unless thrombocytopenia or antiprothrombin antibodies are already present. They are associated with an increased risk of thrombosis. ■

INDICATIONS:

• Evaluate prolonged activated partial thromboplastin times

• Investigate reasons for fetal death

RESULT

Positive in:

• Fetal loss

• Raynaud's syndrome

• Rheumatoid arthritis

• Systemic lupus erythematosus

• Thromboembolism

Negative in: N/A

CRITICAL VALUES: N/A

INTERFERING FACTORS:

• Drugs that may cause a positive lupus anticoagulant test result include chlorpromazine and heparin.

• Placement of tourniquet for longer than 1 minute can result in venous stasis and changes in the concentration of plasma proteins to be measured. Platelet activation may also occur under these conditions, causing erroneous results.

• Vascular injury during phlebotomy can activate platelets and coagulation factors, causing erroneous results.

• Hemolyzed specimens must be rejected because hemolysis is an indication of platelet and coagulation factor activation.

• Incompletely filled tubes contaminated with heparin or clotted specimens must be rejected.

• Icteric or lipemic specimens interfere with optical testing methods, producing erroneous results.

Nursing Implications and Procedure

Pretest: ■

➤ Obtain a history of the patient's complaints, including a list of known allergens.

➤ Obtain a history of the patient's hematopoietic, immune, musculoskeletal, and reproductive systems, as well as results of previously performed tests and procedures. For related tests, refer to the hematopoietic, immune, musculoskeletal, and reproductive system tables.

➤ Obtain a list of the medications the patient is taking, including herbs, nutritional supplements, and nutraceuticals. The requesting health care practitioner and laboratory should be advised if the patient regularly uses these products so that their effects can be taken into consideration when reviewing results.

➤ There are no food or fluid restrictions unless by medical direction.

➤ Heparin therapy should be discontinued 2 days before specimen collection, with medical direction. Coumarin therapy should be discontinued 2 weeks before specimen collection, with medical direction.

➤ Review the procedure with the patient.

➤ Inform the patient that specimen

collection takes approximately 5 to 10 minutes.

Intratest:

➤ Ensure that the patient has complied with pretesting restrictions.

➤ Direct the patient to breathe normally and to avoid unnecessary movement.

➤ Observe standard precautions and follow the general guidelines in Appendix A. Perform a venipuncture, and collect the specimen in a 5-mL blue-top tube. *Important note:* Two different concentrations of sodium citrate preservative are currently added to blue-top tubes for coagulation studies: 3.2% and 3.8%. The National Committee for Clinical Laboratory Standards (NCCLS) guideline for sodium citrate is 3.2%. Laboratories establish reference ranges for coagulation testing based on numerous factors, including sodium citrate concentration, test equipment, and test reagents. It is important to inquire from the laboratory which concentration it recommends, because each concentration will have its own specific reference range.

➤ When multiple specimens are drawn, the blue-top tube should be collected after sterile (i.e., blood culture) and red-top tubes. When coagulation testing is the only test to be done, an extra red-top tube should be collected before the blue-top tube to avoid contaminating the specimen with tissue thromboplastin, which can falsely decrease values.

➤ Label the specimen, and promptly transport it to the laboratory. The NCCLS recommendation for processed and unprocessed samples stored in unopened tubes is that testing should be completed within 1 to 4 hours of collection.

Post-test:

➤ Observe venipuncture site for bleeding or hematoma formation. Apply pressure bandage.

➤ Evaluate test results in relation to the patient's symptoms and other tests performed. Related laboratory tests include anticardiolipin antibody, antinuclear antibody, activated partial thromboplastin time, and protein S.

LUTEINIZING HORMONE

SYNONYMS/ACRONYMS: LH, luteotropin, interstitial cell–stimulating hormone (ICSH).

SPECIMEN: Serum (1 mL) collected in a red- or tiger-top tube. Plasma (1 mL) collected in green-top (heparin) tube is also acceptable.

REFERENCE VALUE: (Method: Immunoassay)

Concentration by Sex and by Phase (in Women)	Conventional Units	SI Units (Conversion Factor ×1)
Male		
Less than 2 y	0.5–1.9 mIU/mL	0.5–1.9 IU/L
2–10 y	Less than 0.5 mIU/mL	Less than 0.5 IU/L
11–20 y	0.5–5.3 mIU/mL	0.5–5.3 IU/L
Adult	1.2–7.8 mIU/mL	1.2–7.8 IU/L
Female		
Less than 2–10 y	Less than 0.5 mIU/mL	Less than 0.5 IU/L
11–20 y	0.5–9.0 mIU/mL	0.5–9.0 IU/L
Phase in Women		
Follicular	1.7–15.0 mIU/mL	1.7–15.0 IU/L
Ovulatory	21.9–56.6 mIU/mL	21.9–56.6 IU/L
Luteal	0.6–16.3 mIU/mL	0.6–16.3 IU/L
Postmenopausal	14.2–52.3 mIU/mL	14.2–52.3 IU/L

DESCRIPTION: Luteinizing hormone (LH) is secreted by the anterior pituitary gland in response to stimulation by gonadotropin-releasing hormone, the same hypothalamic releasing factor that stimulates follicle-stimulating hormone release. LH affects gonadal function in both men and women. In women, a surge of LH normally occurs at the midpoint of the menstrual cycle (ovulatory phase); this surge is believed to be induced by high estrogen levels. LH causes the ovum to be expelled from the ovary and stimulates development of the corpus luteum and progesterone production. As progesterone levels rise, LH production decreases. In males, LH stimulates the interstitial cells of Leydig, located in the testes, to produce testosterone. For this reason, in reference to males, LH is sometimes called interstitial cell stimulating hormone. Secretion of LH is pulsatile and follows a circadian rhythm in response to the normal intermittent secretion of gonadotropin-releasing hormone. ■

INDICATIONS:

- Distinguish between primary and secondary causes of gonadal failure
- Evaluate children with precocious puberty
- Evaluate male and female infertility, as indicated by decreased LH levels
- Evaluate response to therapy to induce ovulation
- Support diagnosis of infertility caused by anovulation, as evidenced by lack of LH surge at the midpoint of the menstrual cycle

RESULT

Increased in:
- Anorchia
- Gonadal failure
- Menopause
- Primary gonadal dysfunction

Decreased in:
- Anorexia nervosa
- Kallmann's syndrome

- Malnutrition

- Pituitary or hypothalamic dysfunction

- Severe stress

CRITICAL VALUES: N/A

INTERFERING FACTORS:

- Drugs and hormones that may increase LH levels include clomiphene, gonadotropin-releasing hormone, goserelin, ketoconazole, mestranol, nafarelin, naloxone, nilutamide, spironolactone, and tamoxifen.

- Drugs and hormones that may decrease LH levels include anabolic steroids, anticonvulsants, conjugated estrogens, danazol, digoxin, D-Trp-6-LHRH, estrogen/progestin therapy, goserelin, megestrol, norethindrone, octreotide, oral contraceptives, phenothiazine, pimozide, pravastatin, progesterone, stanozolol, and tamoxifen.

- In menstruating women, values vary in relation to the phase of the menstrual cycle.

- LH secretion follows a circadian rhythm, higher levels occurring during sleep.

Nursing Implications and Procedure • • • • • • • • • • •

Pretest:

➤ Obtain a history of the patient's complaints, including a list of known allergens.

➤ Obtain a history of the patient's endocrine and reproductive systems, as well as results of previously performed tests and procedures. For related tests, refer to the endocrine and reproductive system tables.

➤ Obtain a list of the medications the patient is taking, including herbs, nutritional supplements, and nutraceuticals. The requesting health care practitioner and laboratory should be advised if the patient regularly uses these products so that their effects can be taken into consideration when reviewing results.

➤ There are no food, fluid, or medication restrictions unless by medical direction.

➤ Review the procedure with the patient.

➤ If the test is being performed to detect ovulation, inform the patient that it may be necessary to obtain a series of samples over a period of several days to detect peak LH levels.

➤ Inform the patient that specimen collection takes approximately 5 to 10 minutes.

Intratest:

➤ Direct the patient to breathe normally and to avoid unnecessary movement.

➤ Observe standard precautions and follow the general guidelines in Appendix A. Perform a venipuncture, and collect the specimen in a 5-mL red- or tiger-top tube.

➤ Label the specimen, and promptly transport it to the laboratory. Provide date of last menstrual period.

Post-test:

➤ Observe venipuncture site for bleeding or hematoma formation. Apply pressure bandage.

➤ Evaluate test results in relation to the patient's symptoms and other tests performed. Related laboratory tests include adrenocorticotropic hormone, antisperm antibody, estradiol, follicle-stimulating hormone, prolactin, and testosterone.

LYME ANTIBODY

. . . .

SYNONYM/ACRONYM: N/A.

SPECIMEN: Serum (1 mL) collected in a red-top tube.

REFERENCE VALUE: (Method: Indirect immunofluorescence) Negative.

DESCRIPTION: *Borrelia burgdorferi*, a deer tick–borne spirochete, is the organism that causes Lyme disease. Lyme disease affects multiple systems and is characterized by fever, arthralgia, and arthritis. The circular, red rash characterizing erythema migrans can appear 3 to 30 days after the tick bite. About one-half of patients in the early stage of Lyme disease (stage 1) and generally all of those in the advanced stage (stage 2)—with cardiac, neurologic, and rheumatoid manifestations—will have a positive test result. Patients in remission will also have a positive test response. The presence of immunoglobulin M (IgM) antibodies indicates acute infection. The presence of IgG antibodies indicates current or past infection. ■

INDICATIONS: Assist in establishing a diagnosis of Lyme disease

RESULT

Positive findings in: Lyme disease

Negative findings in: N/A

CRITICAL VALUES: N/A

INTERFERING FACTORS:
• High rheumatoid-factor titers as well as cross-reactivity with Epstein-Barr virus and other spirochetes (e.g., *Rickettsia, Treponema*) may cause false-positive results.

• Positive test results should be confirmed by the Western Blot method.

Nursing Implications and Procedure

. . . .

Pretest:

➤ Obtain a history of the patient's complaints, including a list of known allergens.

➤ Obtain a history of the patient's immune and musculoskeletal systems, as well as results of previously performed tests and procedures and history of exposure. For related tests, refer to the immune and musculoskeletal system tables.

➤ Obtain a list of the medications the patient is taking, including herbs, nutritional supplements, and nutraceuticals. The requesting health care practitioner and laboratory should be advised if the patient regularly uses these products so that their effects can be taken into consideration when reviewing results.

➤ There are no food, fluid, or medication restrictions unless by medical direction.

➤ Review the procedure with the patient. Inform the patient that several tests may be necessary to confirm diagnosis.

➤ Inform the patient that each specimen collection takes approximately 5 to 10 minutes.

Intratest: ■

➤ Direct the patient to breathe normally and to avoid unnecessary movement.

➤ Observe standard precautions and follow the general guidelines in Appendix A. Perform a venipuncture, and collect the specimen in a 5-mL red-top tube.

➤ Label the specimen, and promptly transport it to the laboratory.

Post-test: ■

➤ Observe venipuncture site for bleed-ing or hematoma formation. Apply pressure bandage.

➤ Warn the patient that false-positive test results can occur and that false-negative test results frequently occur.

➤ Recognize anxiety related to test results and offer support. Provide teaching and information regarding the clinical implications of the test results, as appropriate. Educate the patient regarding access to counseling services if results are positive, because Lyme disease can be debilitating and can result in significant changes in lifestyle.

➤ Advise the patient to wear light-colored clothing that covers extremities when in areas infested by deer ticks, and to check body for ticks after returning from infested area.

➤ Evaluate test results in relation to the patient's symptoms and other tests performed. A related test is synovial fluid analysis.

LYMPHANGIOGRAPHY

• •

SYNONYM/ACRONYM: Lymphangiogram.

AREA OF APPLICATION: Lymphatic system.

CONTRAST: Iodine based.

DESCRIPTION: Lymphangiography involves visualization of the lymphatic system after the injection of an iodinated oil–based contrast medium into a lymphatic vessel in the hand or foot. The lymphatic system consists of lymph vessels and nodes. Assessment of this system is important be-cause cancer (lymphomas and Hodgkin's disease) often spreads via the lymphatic system. When the lymphatic system becomes obstructed, painful edema of the extremities usually results. The procedure is usually performed for cancer staging in patients with an established diagnosis of lymphoma or metastatic tumor. Injection into the hand allows visualization of the axillary and supraclavicular nodes. Injection into the foot allows visualization of the lymphatics of the leg, inguinal and iliac regions, and retroperitoneum up to the thoracic duct. Less commonly, injection into the foot can be used to visualize the cervical region (retroauricular area). This procedure can assess progression of the disease, assist in planning surgery, and monitor the effectiveness of chemotherapy or radiation treatment. ■

INDICATIONS:

* Determine lymphatic cancer staging

* Evaluate effects of chemotherapy or radiation therapy

* Evaluate edema of an extremity without known cause

* Determine the extent of adenopathy

* Distinguish primary from secondary lymphedema

* Plan surgical treatment or evaluate effectiveness of chemotherapy or radiation therapy in controlling malignant tumors

RESULT

Normal Findings:
* Normal lymphatic vessels and nodes that fill completely with contrast medium on the initial films. On the 24-hour films, the lymph nodes are fully opacified and well circumscribed. The lymphatic channels are emptied a few hours after injection of the contrast medium.

Abnormal Findings:
* Abnormal lymphatic vessels

* Hodgkin's disease

* Metastatic tumor involving the lymph glands

* Nodal lymphoma

* Retroperitoneal lymphomas associated with Hodgkin's disease

CRITICAL VALUES: N/A

INTERFERING FACTORS:

This procedure is contraindicated for:
* Patients with pulmonary insufficiencies, cardiac diseases, or severe renal or hepatic disease.

* Patients with allergies to shellfish or iodinated dye. The contrast medium used may cause a life-threatening allergic reaction. Patients with a known hypersensitivity to the contrast medium may benefit from premedication with corticosteroids or the use of nonionic contrast medium.

* Patients who are pregnant or suspected of being pregnant, unless the potential benefits of the procedure far outweigh the risks to the fetus and mother

* Elderly and other patients who are chronically dehydrated before the test, because of their risk of contrast-induced renal failure.

* Patients who are in renal failure.

* Young patients (17 years old and younger), unless the benefits of the x-ray diagnosis outweigh the risks of exposure to high levels of radiation.

Factors that may impair clear imaging:
* Inability of the patient to cooperate or remain still during the procedure because of age, significant pain, or mental status

* Metallic objects within the examination field (e.g., jewelry or body rings), which may inhibit organ visualization and can produce unclear images

* Improper adjustment of the radiographic equipment to accommodate obese or thin patients, which can cause

overexposure or underexposure and a poor-quality study

- Patients who are very obese, who may exceed the weight limit for the equipment

- Incorrect positioning of the patient, which may produce poor visualization of the area to be examined

- Gas or feces in the gastrointestinal tract resulting from inadequate cleansing or failure to restrict food intake before the study

- Retained barium from a previous radiologic procedure

- Inability to cannulate the lymphatic vessels

Other considerations:

- Be aware of risks associated with the ⚠ contrast medium. The oil-based contrast medium may embolize into the lungs and will temporarily diminish pulmonary function. This can produce lipid pneumonia, which is a life-threatening complication.

- Consultation with a physician should occur before the procedure for radiation safety concerns regarding infants of patients who are lactating.

- Risks associated with radiographic overexposure can result from frequent x-ray procedures. Personnel in the room with the patient should wear a protective lead apron, stand behind a shield, or leave the area while the examination is being done. Personnel working in the area where the examination is being done should wear badges that reveal their level of exposure to radiation.

Nursing Implications and Procedure · · · · · · · · · · ·

Pretest:

➤ Inform the patient that the procedure assesses the lymphatic system.

➤ Inform the patient that the procedure is performed by a physician and takes 1 to 2 hours. Inform the patient that he or she may have to return the next day, but that this set of images will take only 30 minutes.

➤ Obtain a history of allergies or sensitivities to contrast medium or shellfish.

➤ Obtain a history of the patient's complaints, including a list of known allergens.

➤ Obtain a history of the patient's lymphatic system and previously performed tests, treatments, and procedures. For related tests, refer to the endocrine and immunologic system tables.

➤ Ascertain recent coagulation times and other laboratory tests, as ordered, especially blood urea nitrogen (BUN) and creatinine.

➤ Inform the patient that the procedure may be painful and that there may be moments of discomfort.

➤ Inform the patient that he or she may feel some discomfort when the contrast medium and anesthesia are injected.

➤ *Obtain a written and informed consent before administering any medications prior to the procedure.*

➤ Instruct the patient on the importance of lying motionless throughout the procedure.

➤ Instruct patient to withhold anticoagulant medication or to reduce dosage before the procedure, as ordered.

➤ Determine date of last menstrual period and possibility of pregnancy in perimenopausal women.

➤ Do not restrict food and fluids, unless otherwise indicated.

➤ Obtain and record baseline vital signs, and assess neurologic status.

Intratest:

➤ Have emergency equipment readily accessible.

➤ Administer an antihistamine or steroid, as ordered by a physician, for patients with a known significant allergic reaction to the IV contrast medium.

➤ Ask the patient to void before the procedure. Have the patient put on a hospital gown.

➤ Administer a mild sedative, as ordered.

➤ Place the patient in a supine position on an x-ray table. Cleanse the selected vein and cover with a sterile drape.

➤ A local anesthetic is injected at the site, and a small incision is made or a needle inserted. The contrast medium is injected intradermally into the area between the toes or fingers. The lymphatic vessels are identified as the contrast medium moves. A local anesthetic is then injected into the dorsum of each foot or hand, and a small incision is made and cannulated for injection of the contrast medium.

➤ The contrast medium is then injected, and the flow of the contrast medium is followed by fluoroscopy. When the contrast medium reaches the upper lumbar level, the infusion of contrast medium is discontinued. X-ray images are taken of the chest, abdomen, and pelvis to determine the extent of filling of the lymphatic vessels.

➤ Twenty-four–hour delayed images may be taken to examine the lymphatic system after a period of time has elapsed and to monitor the progress of delayed flow.

➤ Monitor the patient for complications related to the contrast medium (e.g., allergic reaction, anaphylaxis, bronchospasm).

➤ When the procedure is complete, the cannula is removed and the incision sutured.

Post-test:

➤ Instruct the patient to resume normal activity, diet, and previous medication use, unless otherwise indicated.

➤ Instruct patient to maintain bedrest up to 24 hours to reduce extremity swelling after the procedure, or as ordered.

➤ Advise patient to drink increased amounts of fluids for 24 to 48 hours to eliminate the radionuclide from the body, unless contraindicated. Tell the patient that radionuclide is eliminated from the body within 6 to 24 hours.

➤ Advise the patient to immediately report symptoms such as fast heart rate, difficulty breathing, skin rash, itching, nausea, vomiting, or decreased urinary output.

➤ Observe the cannula insertion site for bleeding, inflammation, or hematoma formation.

➤ Instruct the patient to apply cold compresses to the cannulated site, as needed, to reduce discomfort or edema.

➤ Monitor for signs of infection, such as pain, fever, increased pulse rate, and muscle aches.

➤ Assess neurologic status and vital signs as directed.

➤ Observe for a delayed allergic reaction to contrast medium or pulmonary embolus, which may include shortness of breath, increased heart rate, pleuritic pain, hypotension, low-grade fever, and cyanosis.

➤ A physician specializing in this branch of medicine sends a written report to the ordering provider, who discusses the results with the patient.

➤ Evaluate test results in relation to the patient's symptoms and other tests performed. Related diagnostic tests include computed tomography of the abdomen and pelvis.

MAGNESIUM, SERUM

SYNONYM/ACRONYM: Serum Mg^{++}.

SPECIMEN: Serum (1 mL) collected in a red- or tiger-top tube.

REFERENCE VALUE: (Method: Spectrophotometry)

Age	Conventional Units	Alternative Units (Conversion Factor ×0.8229)	SI Units (Conversion Factor ×0.4114)
Newborn	1.5–2.2 mg/dL	1.23–1.81 mEq/L	0.62–0.91 mmol/L
Child	1.7–2.1 mg/dL	1.40–1.73 mEq/L	0.70–0.86 mmol/L
Adult	1.6–2.6 mg/dL	1.32–2.14 mEq/L	0.66–1.07 mmol/L

DESCRIPTION: Magnesium is required as a cofactor in numerous crucial enzymatic processes, such as protein synthesis, nucleic acid synthesis, and muscle contraction. Magnesium is also required for the use of adenosine diphosphate as a source of energy. It is the fourth most abundant cation and the second most abundant intracellular ion. Magnesium is needed for the transmission of nerve impulses and muscle relaxation. It controls absorption of sodium, potassium, calcium, and phosphorus; utilization of carbohydrate, lipid, and protein; and activation of enzyme systems that enable the B vitamins to function. Magnesium is also essential for oxidative phosphorylation, nucleic acid synthesis, and blood clotting. Urine magnesium levels reflect magnesium deficiency before serum levels. Magnesium deficiency severe enough to cause hypocalcemia and cardiac arrhythmias can exist despite normal serum magnesium levels. ■

INDICATIONS:
- Determine electrolyte balance in renal failure and chronic alcoholism
- Evaluate cardiac arrhythmias (decreased magnesium levels can lead to excessive ventricular irritability)
- Evaluate known or suspected disorders associated with altered magnesium levels
- Monitor the effects of various drugs on magnesium levels

RESULT

Increased in:
- Addison's disease
- Adrenocortical insufficiency
- Dehydration
- Diabetic acidosis (severe)
- Hypothyroidism
- Systemic lupus erythematosus

- Multiple myeloma
- Overuse of antacids
- Renal insufficiency
- Tissue trauma

Decreased in:
- Alcoholism
- Diabetic acidosis
- Glomerulonephritis (chronic)
- Hemodialysis
- Hyperaldosteronism
- Hypercalcemia
- Hypoparathyroidism
- Inadequate intake
- Inappropriate secretion of antidiuretic hormone
- Long-term hyperalimentation
- Malabsorption
- Pancreatitis
- Pregnancy
- Severe loss of body fluids (diarrhea, lactation, sweating, laxative abuse)

CRITICAL VALUES:

Less than 1.2 mg/dL

Greater than 6.1 mg/dL

Symptoms such as tetany, weakness, dizziness, tremors, hyperactivity, nausea, vomiting, and convulsions occur at decreased (less than 1.2 mg/dL) concentrations. Electrocardiographic (ECG) changes (prolonged P-R and Q-T intervals, broad flat T waves, and ventricular tachycardia) may also occur. Treatment may include administration of magnesium salts, monitoring for respiratory depression and areflexia (intravenous [IV] administration of magnesium salts), and monitoring for diarrhea and metabolic alkalosis (oral administration to replace magnesium).

Respiratory paralysis, decreased reflexes, and cardiac arrest occur at grossly elevated (greater than 15 mg/dL) levels. ECG changes, such as prolonged

P-R and Q-T intervals, and bradycardia may be seen. Toxic levels of magnesium may be reversed with the administration of calcium, dialysis treatments, and removal of the source of excessive intake.

INTERFERING FACTORS:
- Drugs that may increase magnesium levels include acetylsalicylic acid and progesterone.
- Drugs that may decrease magnesium levels include albuterol, aminoglycosides, amphotericin B, bendroflumethiazide, chlorthalidone, citrates, cyclosporines, cisplatin, digoxin, gentamicin, glucagon, and oral contraceptives.
- Hemolysis results in a false elevation in values; such specimens should be rejected for analysis.
- Specimens should never be collected above an IV line because of the potential for dilution when the specimen and the IV solution combine in the collection container, falsely decreasing the result. There is also the potential of contaminating the sample with the substance of interest, contained in the IV solution, falsely increasing the result.

Nursing Implications and Procedure ● ● ● ● ● ● ● ● ● ●

Pretest:

➤ Obtain a history of the patient's complaints, including a list of known allergens.

➤ Obtain a history of the patient's cardiovascular, endocrine, gastrointestinal, genitourinary, and reproductive systems, as well as results of previously performed tests and procedures. For related tests, refer to the cardiovascular, endocrine, gastrointestinal, genitourinary, and reproductive system tables.

➤ Obtain a list of medications the patient is taking, including herbs, nutritional supplements, and nutraceuticals. The requesting health care practitioner and laboratory should be advised if the patient regularly uses these products so that their effects can be taken into consideration when reviewing results.

➤ There are no food, fluid, or medication restrictions unless by medical direction.

➤ Review the procedure with the patient.

➤ Inform the patient that specimen collection takes approximately 5 to 10 minutes.

Intratest:

➤ Direct the patient to breathe normally and to avoid unnecessary movement.

➤ Observe standard precautions and follow the general guidelines in Appendix A. Perform a venipuncture, and collect the specimen in a 5-mL red- or tiger-top tube.

➤ Label the specimen, and promptly transport it to the laboratory.

Post-test:

➤ Observe venipuncture site for bleeding or hematoma formation. Apply pressure bandage.

➤ Educate the magnesium-deficient patient regarding good dietary sources of magnesium, such as green vegetables, seeds, legumes, shrimp, and some bran cereals. Advise the patient that high intake of substances such as phosphorus, calcium, fat, and protein interferes with the absorption of magnesium.

➤ Instruct the patient to report any signs or symptoms of electrolyte imbalance, such as dehydration, diarrhea, vomiting, or prolonged anorexia.

➤ Evaluate test results in relation to the patient's symptoms and other tests performed. Related laboratory tests include aspartate aminotransferase, C-reactive protein, calcium, creatine kinase and isoenzymes, lactate dehydrogenase and isoenzymes, kidney stone analysis, urine magnesium, myoglobin, potassium, troponin, and vitamin D.

MAGNESIUM, URINE

SYNONYMS/ACRONYM: Urine Mg^{++}.

SPECIMEN: Urine (5 mL) from a random or timed specimen collected in a clean plastic collection container with 6N hydrochloride as a preservative.

REFERENCE VALUE: (Method: Spectrophotometry)

Conventional Units	Alternative Units (Conversion Factor ×0.8229)	SI Units (Conversion Factor ×0.4114)
7.3–12.2 mg/24 h	6.0–10.0 mEq/24 h	3.0–5.0 mmol/24 h

DESCRIPTION: Magnesium is required as a cofactor in numerous crucial enzymatic processes, such as protein synthesis, nucleic acid synthesis, and muscle contraction. Magnesium is also required for the use of adenosine diphosphate as a source of energy. It is the fourth most abundant cation and the second most abundant intracellular ion. Magnesium is needed for the transmission of nerve impulses and muscle relaxation. It controls absorption of sodium, potassium, calcium, and phosphorus; utilization of carbohydrate, lipid, and protein; and activation of enzyme systems that enable the B vitamins to function. Magnesium is also essential for oxidative phosphorylation, nucleic acid synthesis, and blood clotting. Urine magnesium levels reflect magnesium deficiency before serum levels. Magnesium deficiency severe enough to cause hypocalcemia and cardiac arrhythmias can exist despite normal serum magnesium levels.

Regulating electrolyte balance is one of the major functions of the kidneys. In normally functioning kidneys, urine levels increase when serum levels are high and decrease when serum levels are low to maintain homeostasis. Analyzing these urinary levels can provide important clues as to the functioning of the kidneys and other major organs. Tests for electrolytes, such as magnesium, in urine usually involve timed urine collections over a 12- or 24-hour period. Measurement of random specimens may also be requested. ■

INDICATIONS:
- Determine the potential cause of renal calculi

- Evaluate known or suspected endocrine disorder
- Evaluate known or suspected renal disease
- Evaluate magnesium imbalance
- Evaluate a malabsorption problem

RESULT

Increased in:
- Alcoholism
- Bartter's syndrome
- Transplant recipients on cyclosporine and prednisone
- Use of diuretics
- Use of corticosteroids

Decreased in:
- Abnormal renal function
- Crohn's disease
- Inappropriate secretion of antidiuretic hormone
- Salt-losing conditions

CRITICAL VALUES: N/A

INTERFERING FACTORS:
- Drugs that may increase urine magnesium levels include cisplatin, cyclosporine, ethacrynic acid, furosemide, mercaptomerin, mercurial diuretics, and thiazides.

- Drugs that may decrease urine magnesium levels include amiloride, angiotensin, oral contraceptives, parathyroid extract, phosphates.

- Magnesium levels follow a circadian rhythm, and for this reason 24-hour collections are recommended.

- All urine voided for the timed collection period must be included in the collection, or else falsely decreased values may be obtained. Compare output records with volume collected to verify that all voids were included in the collection.

Nursing Implications and Procedure · · · · · · · · · · ·

Pretest:

➤ Obtain a history of the patient's complaints, including a list of known allergens.

➤ Obtain a history of the patient's endocrine, gastrointestinal, and genitourinary systems, as well as results of previously performed tests and procedures. For related tests, refer to the endocrine, gastrointestinal, and genitourinary system tables.

➤ Obtain a list of medications the patient is taking, including herbs, nutritional supplements, and nutraceuticals. The requesting health care practitioner and laboratory should be advised if the patient regularly uses these products so that their effects can be taken into consideration when reviewing results.

➤ There are no food, fluid, or medication restrictions unless by medical direction.

➤ Instruct the patient to avoid excessive exercise and stress during the 24-hour collection of urine.

➤ Review the procedure with the patient. Provide a nonmetallic urinal, bedpan, or toilet-mounted collection device.

➤ Usually a 24-hour time frame for urine collection is ordered. Inform the patient that all urine must be saved during that 24-hour period. Instruct the patient not to void directly into the laboratory collection container. Instruct the patient to avoid defecating in the collection device and to keep toilet tissue out of the collection device to prevent contamination of the specimen. Place a sign in the bathroom to remind the patient to save all urine.

➤ Instruct the patient to void all urine into the collection device and then to pour the urine into the laboratory collection container. Alternatively the specimen can be left in the collection device for a health care staff member to add to the laboratory collection container.

Intratest:

➤ Observe standard precautions and follow the general guidelines in Appendix A.

Random specimen (collect in early morning):

Clean-catch specimen:

➤ Instruct the male patient to (1) thoroughly wash his hands, (2) cleanse the meatus, (3) void a small amount into the toilet, and (4) void directly into the specimen container.

➤ Instruct the female patient to (1) thoroughly wash her hands; (2) cleanse the labia from front to back; (3) while keeping the labia separated, void a small amount into the toilet; and (4) without interrupting the urine stream, void directly into the specimen container.

Indwelling catheter:

➤ Put on gloves. Empty drainage tube of urine. It may be necessary to clamp off the catheter for 15 to 30 minutes before specimen collection. Cleanse specimen port with antiseptic swab, and then aspirate 5 mL of urine with a 21- to 25-gauge needle and syringe. Transfer urine to a sterile container.

Timed specimen:

➤ Obtain a clean 3-L urine specimen container, toilet-mounted collection device, and plastic bag (for transport of the specimen container). The specimen must be refrigerated or kept on ice throughout the entire collection period. If an indwelling urinary catheter is in place, the drainage bag must be kept on ice.

➤ Begin the test between 6 and 8

a.m., if possible. Collect first voiding and discard. Record the time the specimen was discarded as the beginning of the timed collection period. The next morning, ask the patient to void at the same time the collection was started and add this last voiding to the container.

➤ If an indwelling catheter is in place, replace the tubing and container system at the start of the collection time. Keep the container system on ice during the collection period, or empty the urine into a larger container periodically during the collection period; monitor to ensure continued drainage, and conclude the test the next morning at the same hour the collection was begun.

➤ At the conclusion of the test, compare the quantity of urine with the urinary output record for the collection; if the specimen contains less than what was recorded as output, some urine may have been discarded, invalidating the test.

➤ Label the specimen, and promptly transport it to the laboratory. Include on the label the amount of urine, test start and stop times, and ingestion of any foods or medications that can affect test results.

Post-test:

➤ Educate the magnesium-deficient patient regarding good dietary sources of magnesium, such as green vegetables, seeds, legumes, shrimp, and some bran cereals. Advise the patient that high intake of substances such as phosphorus, calcium, fat, and protein interferes with the absorption of magnesium.

➤ Instruct the patient to report any signs or symptoms of electrolyte imbalance, such as dehydration, diarrhea, vomiting, or prolonged anorexia.

➤ Evaluate test results in relation to the patient's symptoms and other tests performed. Related laboratory tests include calcium, kidney stone analysis, magnesium, phosphorus, potassium, and vitamin D.

MAGNETIC RESONANCE IMAGING, ABDOMEN

SYNONYM/ACRONYM: Abdominal MRI.

AREA OF APPLICATION: Liver/abdominal area.

CONTRAST: Can be done with or without contrast medium (gadolinium).

DESCRIPTION: Magnetic resonance imaging (MRI) uses a magnet and radio waves to produce an energy field that can be displayed as an image. Use of magnetic fields with the aid of radiofrequency energy produces images primarily based on water content of tissue. The magnetic field causes the hydrogen atoms in tissue to line up, and when radio waves are directed toward the magnetic field, the atoms absorb the radio waves and change their position. When the radio waves are turned off, the atoms go back to their original position; this change in the energy field is sensed by the equipment, and an image is generated by the attached computer system. Abdominal MRI produces cross-sectional images of the abdomen in multiple planes without the use of ionizing radiation or the interference of bone.

Abdominal MRI is performed to assist in diagnosing abnormalities of abdominal and hepatic structures. Contrast-enhanced imaging is effective for distinguishing peritoneal metastases from primary tumors of the gastrointestinal tract. Primary tumors of the stomach, pancreas, colon, and appendix often spread by intraperitoneal tumor shedding and subsequent peritoneal carcinomatosis. MRI uses the noniodinated contrast medium gadopentetate dimeglumine (Magnevist), which is administered intravenously to enhance contrast differences between normal and abnormal tissues.

Magnetic resonance angiography (MRA) is an application of MRI that provides images of blood flow and diseased and normal blood vessels. In patients who are allergic to iodinated contrast medium, MRA is used in place of angiography (see monograph titled "Angiography, Magnetic Resonance"). ■

INDICATIONS:

- Detect abdominal aortic diseases
- Detect and stage cancer (primary or metastatic tumors of liver, pancreas, prostate, uterus, and bladder)
- Detect chronic pancreatitis
- Determine vascular complications of

pancreatitis, venous thrombosis, or pseudoaneurysm

- Differentiate liver tumors from liver abnormalities, such as cysts, cavernous hemangiomas, and hepatic amebic abscesses
- Detect renal vein thrombosis
- Evaluate postoperative angioplasty sites and bypass grafts
- Detect soft tissue abnormalities
- Determine and monitor tissue damage in renal transplant patients
- Differentiate aortic aneurysms from tumors near the aorta
- Determine the presence of blood clots, cysts, fluid or fat accumulation in tissues, hemorrhage, and infarctions
- Monitor and evaluate the effectiveness of medical or surgical interventions and the course of the disease

RESULT

Normal Findings:
- Normal anatomic structures, soft tissue density, and biochemical constituents of body tissues, including blood flow

Abnormal Findings:
- Acute tubular necrosis
- Glomerulonephritis
- Hydronephrosis
- Masses, lesions, infections, or inflammations
- Renal vein thrombosis
- Vena cava obstruction

CRITICAL VALUES: N/A

INTERFERING FACTORS:

This procedure is contraindicated for:
- Patients with certain ferrous metal prostheses, valves, aneurysm clips,

inner ear prostheses, or other metallic objects

• Patients with metal in their body, such as shrapnel or ferrous metal in the eye

• Patients with cardiac pacemakers, ⚠ because the pacemaker can be deactivated by MRI

• Patients who are claustrophobic

• Patients who are pregnant or suspected of being pregnant, unless the potential benefits of the procedure far outweigh the risks to the fetus and mother

Factors that may impair clear imaging:

• Inability of the patient to cooperate or remain still during the procedure because of age, significant pain, or mental status

• Patients with extreme cases of claustrophobia, unless sedation is given before the study

• Patients who are very obese, who may exceed the weight limit for the equipment

• Incorrect positioning of the patient, which may produce poor visualization of the area to be examined

• Metallic objects within the examination field (e.g., jewelry, body rings), which may inhibit organ visualization and can produce unclear images

Other considerations:

• If contrast medium is allowed to seep deep into the muscle tissue, vascular visualization will be impossible.

Nursing Implications and Procedure · · · · · · · · · · · ·

Pretest: ▮

➤ Inform the patient that the procedure assesses the abdomen.

➤ Inform the patient that the procedure is performed in a special

department by a technologist and a physician and takes approximately 30 to 60 minutes.

➤ Obtain a history of allergies or sensitivities to contrast medium.

➤ Obtain a list of medications the patient is taking.

➤ Obtain a history of the patient's hepatic and abdominal systems, as well as results of previously performed tests, treatments, surgeries, and procedures. Determine if the patient has ever had any device implanted into the body, including copper intrauterine devices, pacemakers, ear implants, and heart valves.

➤ For related tests, refer to the gastrointestinal system table.

➤ Determine previous laboratory abnormalities, especially blood urea nitrogen (BUN) and creatinine, if contrast medium is to be used.

➤ Ensure that the results of blood tests are obtained and recorded before the procedure.

➤ Obtain occupational history to determine the presence of metal in the body, such as shrapnel or flecks of ferrous metal in the eye (which can cause retinal hemorrhage).

➤ Determine date of last menstrual period and possibility of pregnancy in perimenopausal women.

➤ Ensure that the patient and staff have removed all external metallic objects from the patient before he or she enters the scanning room.

➤ Inform the patient that the technologist will place him or her in a supine position on a flat table in a large, cylindrical scanner.

➤ Tell the patient to expect to hear loud banging from the scanner and possibly to see magnetophosphenes (flickering lights in the visual field); these will stop when the procedure is over.

➤ Instruct the patient to take slow, deep breaths if nausea occurs during the procedure.

➤ Do not restrict food and fluids.

Intratest:

> Ask the patient to remove jewelry, including watches, hairpins, and other metallic objects, and credit cards.

> Ask the patient to void before the procedure.

> Administer a sedative to a child or to an uncooperative adult, as ordered.

> Administer an antianxiety agent, as ordered, if the patient has claustrophobia.

> Place the patient in a supine position on a flat table; use foam wedges to help maintain position and immobilization. Ask the patient to lie still during the procedure because movement produces unclear images, thus affecting the results and making interpretation difficult.

> Supply earplugs to the patient to block out the loud, banging sounds that occur during the test.

> If an electrocardiogram or respiratory gating is to be performed in conjunction with the scan, apply MRI-safe electrodes to the appropriate sites.

> The patient can communicate with the technologist doing the examination via a microphone within the machine.

> The table is moved into the scanner. Instruct the patient to remain still. The scanner makes noises as it acquires images of the body. The patient may be asked to hold his or her breath to facilitate visualization. A number of images are taken. These images are reconstructed by a computer and reviewed.

> Administer the contrast medium, if ordered. A second series of images is obtained.

Post-test:

> Instruct the patient to resume medications, normal activity, and diet, unless otherwise indicated.

> Observe for delayed allergic reactions, such as urticaria, hives, nausea, or vomiting, if contrast medium was used.

> A physician specializing in this branch of medicine sends a written report to the ordering provider, who discusses the results with the patient.

> Evaluate test results in relation to the patient's symptoms and other tests performed. Related diagnostic tests include ultrasound, angiogram, and computed tomography of the abdomen; and kidney, ureter, and bladder (KUB) film.

MAGNETIC RESONANCE IMAGING, BRAIN

SYNONYM/ACRONYM: Brain MRI.

AREA OF APPLICATION: Brain area.

CONTRAST: Can be done with or without contrast medium (gadolinium).

DESCRIPTION: Magnetic resonance imaging (MRI) uses a magnet and radio waves to produce an energy field that can be displayed as an image. Use of magnetic fields with the aid of radiofrequency energy produces images primarily based on water content of tissue. The magnetic field causes the hydrogen atoms in tissue to line up, and when radio waves are directed toward the magnetic field, the atoms absorb the radio waves and change their position. When the radio waves are turned off, the atoms go back to their original position, this change in the energy field is sensed by the equipment, and an image is generated by the attached computer system. MRI produces cross-sectional images of the pathologic lesions in multiple planes without the use of ionizing radiation or the interference of bone or surrounding tissue.

Brain MRI can distinguish solid, cystic, and hemorrhagic components of lesions. This procedure is done to aid in the diagnosis of intracranial abnormalities, including tumors, ischemia, infection, and multiple sclerosis, and assessment of brain maturation in pediatric patients. Rapidly flowing blood on spin-echo MRI appears as an absence of signal or a void in the vessel's lumen. Blood flow can be evaluated in the cavernous and carotid arteries. Aneurysms may be diagnosed without traditional iodine contrast–based angiography, and old clotted blood in the walls of the aneurysms appears white. MRI uses the noniodinated contrast medium gadopentetate dimeglumine (Magnevist), which is administered intravenously to enhance contrast differences between normal and abnormal tissues.

Magnetic resonance angiography (MRA) is an application of MRI that provides images of blood flow and diseased and normal blood vessels. In patients who are allergic to iodinated contrast medium, MRA is used in place of angiography (see monograph titled "Angiography, Magnetic Resonance"). ■

INDICATIONS:
• Detect and locate brain tumors

• Detect cause of cerebrovascular accident, cerebral infarct, or hemorrhage

• Evaluate vascularity of the brain and evaluate vascular integrity

• Evaluate the solid, cystic, and hemorrhagic components of lesions

• Detect cranial bone, face, throat, and neck soft tissue lesions

• Evaluate the potential causes of headache, visual loss, and vomiting

• Evaluate intracranial infections

• Evaluate the cause of seizures, such as intracranial infection, edema, or increased intracranial pressure

• Evaluate demyelinating disorders

• Evaluate cerebral changes associated with dementia

• Evaluate shunt placement and function in patients with hydrocephalus

• Monitor and evaluate the effectiveness of medical or surgical interventions, chemotherapy, and radiation therapy and the course of disease

RESULT

Normal Findings:
• Normal anatomic structures, soft tissue density, blood flow rate, face, nasopharynx, neck, tongue, and brain

Abnormal Findings:
• Abscess

- Acoustic neuroma

- Aneurysm

- Arteriovenous malformation

- Benign meningioma

- Cerebral aneurysm

- Cerebral infarction

- Craniopharyngioma or meningioma

- Granuloma

- Intraparenchymal hematoma or hemorrhage

- Lipoma

- Metastasis

- Multiple sclerosis

- Optic nerve tumor

- Pituitary microadenoma

- Subdural empyema

- Ventriculitis

CRITICAL VALUES: N/A

INTERFERING FACTORS:

This procedure is contraindicated for:

- Patients with certain ferrous metal prostheses, valves, aneurysm clips, inner ear prostheses, or other metallic objects

- Patients with metal in their body, such as shrapnel or ferrous metal in the eye

- Patients with cardiac pacemakers ⚠ because the pacemaker can be deactivated by MRI

- Patients who are claustrophobic

- Patients who are pregnant or suspected of being pregnant, unless the potential benefits of the procedure far outweigh the risks to the fetus and mother

Factors that may impair clear imaging:

- Inability of the patient to cooperate or remain still during the procedure because of age, significant pain, or mental status

- Patients with extreme cases of claustrophobia, unless sedation is given before the study.

- Metallic objects within the examination field (e.g., jewelry or body rings), which may inhibit organ visualization and can produce unclear images

- Patients who are very obese, who may exceed the weight limit for the equipment

- Incorrect positioning of the patient, which may produce poor visualization of the area to be examined

Other considerations:

- If contrast medium is allowed to seep deep into the muscle tissue, vascular visualization will be impossible.

Nursing Implications and Procedure • • • • • • • • • • •

Pretest:

➤ Inform the patient that the procedure assesses the pituitary.

➤ Inform the patient that the procedure is performed in a special department by a technologist and a physician and takes approximately 30 to 60 minutes.

➤ Obtain a history of allergies or sensitivities to contrast medium.

➤ Obtain a list of medications the patient is taking.

➤ Obtain a history of the patient's pituitary, endocrine, and cranial findings, as well as results of previously performed tests, treatments, surgeries, and procedures. Determine if the patient has ever had any device implanted into the body, including copper intrauterine devices, pacemakers, ear implants, and heart valves.

➤ For related tests, refer to the

endocrine and musculoskeletal system tables.

➤ Determine previous laboratory abnormalities, especially blood urea nitrogen (BUN) and creatinine, if contrast medium is to be used.

➤ Ensure that the results of blood tests are obtained and recorded before the procedure.

➤ Obtain occupational history to determine the presence of metal in the body, such as shrapnel or flecks of ferrous metal in the eye (which can cause retinal hemorrhage).

➤ Determine date of last menstrual period and possibility of pregnancy in perimenopausal women.

➤ Ensure that the patient and staff have removed all external metallic objects from the patient before he or she enters the scanning room.

➤ Inform the patient that the technologist will place him or her in a supine position on a flat table in a large, cylindrical scanner.

➤ Tell the patient to expect to hear loud banging from the scanner and possibly to see magneto-phosphenes (flickering lights in the visual field); these will stop when the procedure is over.

➤ Instruct the patient to take slow, deep breaths if nausea occurs during the procedure.

➤ Do not restrict food and fluids.

Intratest:

➤ Ask the patient to remove jewelry, including watches, hairpins, and other metallic objects, and credit cards.

➤ Ask the patient to void before the procedure.

➤ Administer a sedative to a child or to an uncooperative adult, as ordered.

➤ Administer an antianxiety agent, as ordered, if the patient has claustrophobia.

➤ Place the patient in a supine position on a flat table; use foam wedges to help maintain position and immobilization. Ask the patient to lie still during the procedure because movement produces unclear images, thus affecting the results and making interpretation difficult.

➤ Supply earplugs to the patient to block out the loud, banging sounds that occur during the test.

➤ If an electrocardiogram or respiratory gating is to be performed in conjunction with the scan, apply MRI-safe electrodes to the appropriate sites.

➤ The patient can communicate with the technologist doing the examination via a microphone within the machine.

➤ The table is moved into the scanner. Instruct the patient to remain still. The scanner makes noises as it acquires images of the body. The patient may be asked to hold his or her breath to facilitate visualization. A number of images are taken. These images are reconstructed by a computer and reviewed.

➤ Administer the contrast medium, if ordered. A second series of images is obtained.

Post-test:

➤ Instruct the patient to resume medications, normal activity, and diet, unless otherwise indicated.

➤ Observe for delayed allergic reactions, such as urticaria, hives, nausea, or vomiting, if contrast medium was used.

➤ A physician specializing in this branch of medicine sends a written report to the ordering provider, who discusses the results with the patient.

➤ Evaluate test results in relation to the patient's symptoms and other tests performed. Related diagnostic tests include computed tomography of the brain and electroencephalography.

MAGNETIC RESONANCE IMAGING, CHEST

SYNONYM/ACRONYM: Chest MRI.

AREA OF APPLICATION: Chest/thorax.

CONTRAST: Can be done with or without contrast medium (gadolinium).

DESCRIPTION: Magnetic resonance imaging (MRI) uses a magnet and radio waves to produce an energy field that can be displayed as an image. Use of magnetic fields with the aid of radiofrequency energy produces images primarily based on water content of tissue. The magnetic field causes the hydrogen atoms in tissue to line up, and when radio waves are directed toward the magnetic field, the atoms absorb the radio waves and change their position. When the radio waves are turned off, the atoms go back to their original position, this change in the energy field is sensed by the equipment, and an image is generated by the attached computer system. MRI produces cross-sectional images of the pathologic lesions in multiple planes without the use of ionizing radiation or the interference of bone or surrounding tissue.

Chest MRI scanning is performed to assist in diagnosing abnormalities of cardiovascular and pulmonary structures. Two special techniques are available for evaluation of cardiovascular structures. One is the electrocardiograph (ECG)–gated multislice spin-echo sequence, used to diagnose anatomical abnormalities of the heart and aorta, and the other is the ECG-referenced gradient refocused sequence, used to diagnose heart function and analyze blood flow patterns.

Magnetic resonance angiography (MRA) is an application of MRI that provides images of blood flow and diseased and normal blood vessels. In patients who are allergic to iodinated contrast medium, MRA is used in place of angiography (see monograph titled "Angiography, Magnetic Resonance"). ■

INDICATIONS:

• Detect thoracic aortic diseases

• Confirm diagnosis of cardiac and pericardiac masses

• Identify congenital heart diseases

• Determine cardiac ventricular function

• Detect myocardial infarction and cardiac muscle ischemia

• Detect pleural effusion

• Evaluate postoperative angioplasty sites and bypass grafts

• Detect pericardial abnormalities

- Detect aortic aneurysms

- Differentiate aortic aneurysms from tumors near the aorta

- Determine blood, fluid, or fat accumulation in tissues, pleuritic space, or vessels

- Evaluate cardiac chambers and pulmonary vessels

- Monitor and evaluate the effectiveness of medical or surgical therapeutic regimen

RESULT

Normal Findings:

- Normal heart and lung structures, soft tissue, and function, including blood flow rate

Abnormal Findings:

- Aortic dissection

- Congenital heart diseases, including pulmonary atresia, aortic coarctation, agenesis of the pulmonary artery, and transposition of the great vessels

- Constrictive pericarditis

- Intramural and periaortic hematoma

- Myocardial infarction

- Pericardial hematoma or effusion

- Pleural effusion

CRITICAL VALUES: N/A

INTERFERING FACTORS:

This procedure is contraindicated for:

- Patients with certain ferrous metal prostheses, valves, aneurysm clips, inner ear prostheses, or other metallic objects

- Patients with metal in their body, such as shrapnel or ferrous metal in the eye

- Patients with cardiac pacemakers

 because the pacemaker can be deactivated by MRI

- Patients who are claustrophobic

- Patients who are pregnant or suspected of being pregnant, unless the potential benefits of the procedure far outweigh the risks to the fetus and mother

Factors that may impair clear imaging:

- Inability of the patient to cooperate or remain still during the procedure because of age, significant pain, or mental status

- Patients with extreme cases of claustrophobia, unless sedation is given before the study

- Patients who are very obese, who may exceed the weight limit for the equipment

- Incorrect positioning of the patient, which may produce poor visualization of the area to be examined

- Metallic objects within the examination field (e.g., jewelry or body rings), which may inhibit organ visualization and can produce unclear images

Other considerations:

- If contrast medium is allowed to seep deep into the muscle tissue, vascular visualization will be impossible.

Nursing Implications and Procedure · · · · · · · · · · ·

Pretest:

➤ Inform the patient that the procedure assesses the chest.

➤ Inform the patient that the procedure is performed in a special department by a technologist and a physician and takes approximately 30 to 60 minutes.

➤ Obtain a history of allergies or sensitivities to contrast medium.

➤ Obtain a list of medications the patient is taking.

➤ Obtain a history of the patient's cardiac and pulmonary findings, as well as results of previously performed tests, treatments, surgeries, and procedures. Determine if the patient has ever had any device implanted into the body, including copper intrauterine devices, pacemakers, ear implants, and heart valves.

➤ For related tests, refer to the respiratory system table.

➤ Determine previous laboratory abnormalities, especially blood urea nitrogen (BUN) and creatinine, if contrast medium is to be used.

➤ Ensure that the results of blood tests are obtained and recorded before the procedure.

➤ Obtain occupational history to determine the presence of metal in the body, such as shrapnel or flecks of ferrous metal in the eye (which can cause retinal hemorrhage).

➤ Determine date of last menstrual period and possibility of pregnancy in perimenopausal women.

➤ Ensure that the patient and staff have removed all external metallic objects from the patient before he or she enters the scanning room.

➤ Inform the patient that the technologist will place him or her in a supine position on a flat table in a large, cylindrical scanner.

➤ Tell the patient to expect to hear loud banging from the scanner and possibly to see magnetophosphenes (flickering lights in the visual field); these will stop when the procedure is over.

➤ Instruct the patient to take slow, deep breaths if nausea occurs during the procedure.

➤ Do not restrict food and fluids.

Intratest:

➤ Ask the patient to remove jewelry, including watches, hairpins, and other metallic objects, and credit cards.

➤ Ask the patient to void before the procedure.

➤ Administer a sedative to a child or to an uncooperative adult, as ordered.

➤ Administer an antianxiety agent, as ordered, if the patient has claustrophobia.

➤ Place the patient in a supine position on a flat table; use foam wedges to help maintain position and immobilization. Ask the patient to lie still during the procedure because movement produces unclear images, thus affecting the results and making interpretation difficult.

➤ Supply earplugs to the patient to block out the loud, banging sounds that occur during the test.

➤ If an electrocardiogram or respiratory gating is to be performed in conjunction with the scan, apply MRI-safe electrodes to the appropriate sites.

➤ The patient can communicate with the technologist doing the examination via a microphone within the machine.

➤ The table is moved into the scanner. Instruct the patient to remain still. The scanner makes noises as it acquires images of the body. The patient may be asked to hold his or her breath to facilitate visualization. A number of images are taken. These images are reconstructed by a computer and reviewed.

➤ Administer the contrast medium, if ordered. A second series of images is obtained.

Post-test:

➤ Instruct the patient to resume medications, normal activity, and diet, unless otherwise indicated.

➤ Observe for delayed allergic reactions, such as urticaria, hives, nausea, or vomiting, if contrast medium was used.

➤ A physician specializing in this

branch of medicine sends a written report to the ordering provider, who discusses the results with the patient.

➤ Evaluate test results in relation to the patient's symptoms and other tests performed. Related tests include computed tomography and x-ray of the chest, echocardiogram, and myocardial scan.

MAGNETIC RESONANCE IMAGING, MUSCULOSKELETAL

SYNONYM/ACRONYM: Musculoskeletal (knee, shoulder, hand, wrist, foot, elbow, hip) MRI.

AREA OF APPLICATION: Bones, joints, soft tissues.

CONTRAST: Can be done with or without contrast medium (gadolinium).

DESCRIPTION: Magnetic resonance imaging (MRI) uses a magnet and radio waves to produce an energy field that can be displayed as an image. Use of magnetic fields with the aid of radiofrequency energy produces images primarily based on water content of tissue. The magnetic field causes the hydrogen atoms in tissue to line up, and when radio waves are directed toward the magnetic field, the atoms absorb the radio waves and change their position. When the radio waves are turned off, the atoms go back to their original position, this change in the energy field is sensed by the equipment, and an image is generated by the attached computer system. MRI produces cross-sectional images of bones and joints in multiple planes without the use of ionizing radiation or the interference of bone or surrounding tissue.

Musculoskeletal MRI is performed to assist in diagnosing abnormalities of bones and joints and surrounding soft tissue structures, including cartilage, synovium, ligaments, and tendons. MRI eliminates the risks associated with exposure to x-rays and causes no harm to cells. Contrast-enhanced imaging is effective for evaluating scarring from previous surgery, vascular abnormalities, and differentiation of metastases from primary tumors. MRI uses the noniodinated contrast medium gadopentetate dimeglumine (Magnevist), which is administered intravenously to enhance contrast differences between normal and abnormal tissues.

Magnetic resonance angiography (MRA) is an application of MRI that provides images of blood flow and diseased and normal blood vessels. In patients who are allergic to iodinated contrast medium, MRA is used in place of angiography (see monograph titled "Angiography, Magnetic Resonance"). ■

INDICATIONS:

- Detect benign and cancerous tumors and cysts of the bone or soft tissue
- Determine cause of low back pain, including herniated disk and spinal degenerative disease
- Detect avascular necrosis of the femoral head or knee
- Detect bone infarcts in the epiphyseal or diaphyseal sites
- Confirm diagnosis of osteomyelitis
- Differentiate between primary and secondary malignant processes of the bone marrow
- Detect changes in bone marrow
- Detect tears or degeneration of ligaments, tendons, and meniscus resulting from trauma or pathology
- Differentiate between a stress fracture and a tumor
- Evaluate meniscal detachment of the temporomandibular joint

RESULT

Normal Findings:

- Normal bones, joints, and surrounding tissue structures; no articular disease, bone marrow disorders, tumors, infections, or trauma to the bones, joints, or muscles

Abnormal Findings:

- Avascular necrosis of femoral head or knee, as found in Legg-Calvé-Perthes disease
- Bone marrow disease, such as Gaucher's disease, aplastic anemia, sickle cell disease, or polycythemia
- Degenerative spinal disease, such as spondylosis or arthritis

- Fibrosarcoma
- Hemangioma (muscular or osseous)
- Herniated disk
- Infection
- Meniscal tears or degeneration
- Rotator cuff tears
- Osteochondroma
- Osteogenic sarcoma
- Osteomyelitis
- Spinal stenosis
- Stress fracture
- Synovitis
- Tumor

CRITICAL VALUES: N/A

INTERFERING FACTORS:

This procedure is contraindicated for:

- Patients with cardiac pacemakers because the pacemaker can be deactivated by MRI
- Patients with certain ferrous metal prostheses, valves, aneurysm clips, inner ear prostheses, or other metallic objects
- Patients with metal in their body, such as shrapnel or ferrous metal in the eye
- Patients who are claustrophobic
- Patients who are pregnant or suspected of being pregnant, unless the potential benefits of the procedure far outweigh the risks to the fetus and mother

Factors that may impair clear imaging:

- Inability of the patient to cooperate or remain still during the procedure because of age, significant pain, or mental status
- Patients with extreme cases of claustro-

phobia unless sedation is given before the study

• Patients who are very obese, who may exceed the weight limit for the equipment

• Incorrect positioning of the patient, which may produce poor visualization of the area to be examined

• Metallic objects within the examination field (e.g., jewelry or body rings), which may inhibit organ visualization and can produce unclear images

Other considerations:

• If contrast medium is allowed to seep deep into the muscle tissue, vascular visualization will be impossible.

Nursing Implications and Procedure

Pretest:

➤ Inform the patient that the procedure assesses the bones and joints.

➤ Inform the patient that the procedure is performed in a special department by a technologist and a physician and takes approximately 30 to 60 minutes.

➤ Obtain a history of allergies or sensitivities to contrast medium.

➤ Obtain a list of medications the patient is taking.

➤ Obtain a history of the patient's trauma or disease process of the bones and joints, as well as results of previously performed tests, treatments, surgeries, and procedures. Determine if the patient has ever had any device implanted into the body, including copper intrauterine devices, pacemakers, ear implants, and heart valves.

➤ For related tests, refer to the musculoskeletal system table.

➤ Determine previous laboratory abnormalities, especially blood urea nitrogen (BUN) and creatinine, if contrast medium is to be used.

➤ Ensure that the results of blood tests are obtained and recorded before the procedure.

➤ Obtain occupational history to determine the presence of metal in the body, such as shrapnel or flecks of ferrous metal in the eye (which can cause retinal hemorrhage).

➤ Determine date of last menstrual period and possibility of pregnancy in perimenopausal women.

➤ Ensure that the patient and staff have removed all external metallic objects from the patient before he or she enters the scanning room.

➤ Inform the patient that the technologist will place him or her in a supine position on a flat table in a large, cylindrical scanner.

➤ Tell the patient to expect to hear loud banging from the scanner and possibly to see magnetophosphenes (flickering lights in the visual field); these will stop when the procedure is over.

➤ Instruct the patient to take slow, deep breaths if nausea occurs during the procedure.

➤ Do not restrict food and fluids.

Intratest:

➤ Ask the patient to remove jewelry, including watches, hairpins, and other metallic objects, and credit cards.

➤ Ask the patient to void before the procedure.

➤ Administer a sedative to a child or to an uncooperative adult, as ordered.

➤ Administer an antianxiety agent, as ordered, if the patient has claustrophobia.

➤ Place the patient in a supine position on a flat table; use foam wedges to help maintain position and immobilization. Ask the patient to lie still during the procedure because movement produces unclear images, thus affecting the results and making interpretation difficult.

➤ Supply earplugs to the patient to block out the loud, banging sounds that occur during the test.

➤ If an electrocardiogram or respiratory gating is to be performed in conjunction with the scan, apply MRI-safe electrodes to the appropriate sites.

➤ The patient can communicate with the technologist doing the examination via a microphone within the machine.

➤ The table is moved into the scanner. Instruct the patient to remain still. The scanner makes noises as it acquires images of the body. The patient may be asked to hold his or her breath to facilitate visualization. A number of images are taken. These images are reconstructed by a computer and reviewed.

➤ Administer the contrast medium, if ordered. A second series of images is obtained.

Post-test:

➤ Instruct the patient to resume medications, normal activity, and diet, unless otherwise indicated.

➤ Observe for delayed allergic reactions, such as urticaria, hives, nausea, or vomiting, if contrast medium was used.

➤ A physician specializing in this branch of medicine sends a written report to the ordering provider, who discusses the results with the patient.

➤ Evaluate test results in relation to the patient's symptoms and other tests performed. Related diagnostic tests include bone x-rays, arthroscopy, and bone mineral density.

MAGNETIC RESONANCE IMAGING, PANCREAS

· ·

SYNONYM/ACRONYM: Pancreatic MRI.

AREA OF APPLICATION: Pancreatic/upper abdominal area.

CONTRAST: Can be done with or without contrast medium (gadolinium).

DESCRIPTION: Magnetic resonance imaging (MRI) uses a magnet and radio waves to produce an energy field that can be displayed as an image. Use of magnetic fields with the aid of radiofrequency energy produces images primarily based on water content of tissue. The magnetic field causes the hydrogen atoms in tissue to line up, and when radio waves are directed toward the magnetic field, the atoms absorb the radio waves and change their position. When the radio waves are turned off, the atoms go back to their original position, this change in the energy field is sensed by the equipment, and an image is generated by the attached computer system. MRI produces cross-sectional images of the abdominal area in multiple planes without the use of ionizing radiation or the interference of bone or surrounding tissue.

MRI of the pancreas is employed to evaluate small pancreatic adenocarcinomas, islet cell tumors, ductal abnormalities and calculi, or parenchymal abnormalities. A T1-weighted, fat-saturation series of images is probably the best series of images for evaluating the pancreatic parenchyma. This sequence is ideal for showing fat planes between the pancreas and peripancreatic structures and for identifying abnormalities, such as fatty infiltration of the pancreas, hemorrhage, adenopathy, and carcinomas. T2-weighted images are most useful for depicting intrapancreatic or peripancreatic fluid collections, pancreatic neoplasms, and calculi. Imaging sequences can be adjusted to display fluid in the biliary tree and pancreatic ducts.

MRI uses the noniodinated contrast medium gadopentetate dimeglumine (Magnevist), which is administered intravenously to enhance contrast differences between normal and abnormal tissues.

Magnetic resonance angiography (MRA) is an application of MRI that provides images of blood flow and diseased and normal blood vessels that supply the pancreas and peripancreatic organs. In patients who are allergic to iodinated contrast medium, MRA is used in place of angiography (see monograph titled "Angiography, Magnetic Resonance"). When the Food and Drug Administration approves gastrointestinal contrast agents, they may be useful for delineating the exact relationship among the stomach, duodenum, and proximal jejunum and the pancreas. These agents would assist in identifying areas of bowel wall thickening, stricture, and intraluminal abnormalities, such as tumors, sites of perforation, and fistula. ∎

INDICATIONS:

- Detect a pancreatic mass

- Detect primary or metastatic tumors of the pancreas and provide cancer staging

- Detect pancreatitis

- Determine vascular complications of pancreatitis, venous thrombosis, or pseudoaneurysm

- Differentiate tumors from other abnormalities, such as cysts, cavernous hemangiomas, and pancreatic abscesses

- Detect soft tissue abnormalities

- Detect pancreatic fatty infiltration, hemorrhage, and adenopathy

- Monitor and evaluate the effectiveness of medical or surgical interventions and course of disease

RESULT

Normal Findings:
- Normal anatomic structures and soft tissue density and biochemical constituents of the pancreatic parenchyma, including blood flow

Abnormal Findings:
- Islet cell tumor

- Metastasis

- Pancreatic mass

- Pancreatitis

- Pancreatic fatty infiltration, hemorrhage, and adenopathy

- Pancreatic duct obstruction or calculi

CRITICAL VALUES: N/A

INTERFERING FACTORS:

This procedure is contraindicated for:

- Patients with certain ferrous metal prostheses, valves, aneurysm clips, inner ear prostheses, or other metallic objects

- Patients with metal in their body, such as shrapnel or ferrous metal in the eye

- Patients with cardiac pacemakers ⚠ because the pacemaker can be deactivated by MRI

- Patients who are claustrophobic

- Patients who are pregnant or suspected of being pregnant, unless the potential benefits of the procedure far outweigh the risks to the fetus and mother

Factors that may impair clear imaging:

- Inability of the patient to cooperate or remain still during the procedure because of age, significant pain, or mental status

- Patients with extreme cases of claustrophobia, unless sedation is given before the study

- Patients who are very obese, who may exceed the weight limit for the equipment

- Incorrect positioning of the patient, which may produce poor visualization of the area to be examined

- Metallic objects within the examination field (e.g., jewelry or body rings), which may inhibit organ visualization and can produce unclear images

Other considerations:

- If contrast medium is allowed to seep deep into the muscle tissue, vascular visualization will be impossible.

Nursing Implications and Procedure • • • • • • • • • •

Pretest: ■

➤ Inform the patient that the procedure assesses the pancreas.

➤ Inform the patient that the procedure is performed in a special department by a technologist and a physician and takes approximately 30 to 60 minutes.

➤ Obtain a history of allergies or sensitivities to contrast medium.

➤ Obtain a list of medications the patient is taking.

➤ Obtain a history of the patient's hepatic and pancreatic findings, as well as results of previously performed tests, treatments, surgeries, and procedures. Determine if the patient has ever had any device implanted into the body, including copper intrauterine devices, pacemakers, ear implants, and heart valves.

➤ For related tests, refer to the hepatobiliary system table.

➤ Determine previous laboratory abnormalities, especially blood urea nitrogen (BUN) and creatinine, if contrast medium is to be used.

➤ Ensure that the results of blood tests are obtained and recorded before the procedure.

➤ Obtain occupational history to determine the presence of metal in the body, such as shrapnel or flecks of ferrous metal in the eye (which can cause retinal hemorrhage).

➤ Determine date of last menstrual period and possibility of pregnancy in perimenopausal women.

➤ Ensure that the patient and staff have removed all external metallic objects from the patient before he or she enters the scanning room.

➤ Inform the patient that the technologist will place him or her in a supine position on a flat table in a large, cylindrical scanner.

➤ Tell the patient to expect to hear loud banging from the scanner and possibly to see magneto-phosphenes (flickering lights in the visual field); these will stop when the procedure is over.

➤ Instruct the patient to take slow, deep breaths if nausea occurs during the procedure.

➤ Do not restrict food and fluids.

Intratest:

➤ Ask the patient to remove jewelry, including watches, hairpins, and other metallic objects, and credit cards.

➤ Ask the patient to void before the procedure.

➤ Administer a sedative to a child or to an uncooperative adult, as ordered.

➤ Administer an antianxiety agent, as ordered, if the patient has claustrophobia.

➤ Place the patient in a supine position on a flat table; use foam wedges to help maintain position and immobilization. Ask the patient to lie still during the procedure because movement produces unclear images, thus affecting the results and making interpretation difficult.

➤ Supply earplugs to the patient to block out the loud, banging sounds that occur during the test.

➤ If an electrocardiogram or respiratory gating is to be performed in conjunction with the scan, apply MRI-safe electrodes to the appropriate sites.

➤ The patient can communicate with the technologist doing the examination via a microphone within the machine.

➤ The table is moved into the scanner. Instruct the patient to remain still. The scanner makes noises as it acquires images of the body. The patient may be asked to hold his or her breath to facilitate visualization. A number of images are taken. These images are reconstructed by a computer and reviewed.

➤ Administer the contrast medium, if ordered. A second series of images is obtained.

Post-test:

➤ Instruct the patient to resume medications, normal activity, and diet, unless otherwise indicated.

➤ Observe for delayed allergic reactions, such as urticaria, hives, nausea, or vomiting, if contrast medium was used.

➤ A physician specializing in this branch of medicine sends a written report to the ordering provider, who discusses the results with the patient.

➤ Evaluate test results in relation to the patient's symptoms and other tests performed. Related diagnostic tests include computed tomography, ultrasound, and angiogram of the abdomen; hepatobiliary scan; and ultrasound of the biliary ducts.

MAGNETIC RESONANCE IMAGING, PELVIS

SYNONYM/ACRONYM: Pelvic MRI.

AREA OF APPLICATION: Pelvic area.

CONTRAST: Can be done with or without contrast (gadolinium).

DESCRIPTION: Magnetic resonance imaging (MRI) uses a magnet and radio waves to produce an energy field that can be displayed as an image. Use of magnetic fields with the aid of radiofrequency energy produces images primarily based on water content of tissue. The magnetic field causes the hydrogen atoms in tissue to line up, and when radio waves are directed toward the magnetic field, the atoms absorb the radio waves and change their position. When the radio waves are turned off, the atoms go back to their original position, this change in the energy field is sensed by the equipment, and an image is generated by the attached computer system. MRI produces cross-sectional images of the pelvic area in multiple planes without the use of ionizing radiation or the interference of bone or surrounding tissue.

Pelvic MRI is performed to assist in diagnosing abnormalities of the pelvis and associated structures. Contrast-enhanced MRI is effective for evaluating metastases from primary tumors. MRI is highly effective for depicting small-volume peritoneal tumors, carcinomatosis, and peritonitis and for determining the response to surgical and chemical therapies. MRI uses the noniodinated contrast medium gadopentetate dimeglumine (Magnevist), which is administered intravenously to enhance contrast differences between normal and abnormal tissues. Oral and rectal contrast administration may be used to isolate the bowel from adjacent pelvic organs and improve organ visualization.

Magnetic resonance angiography (MRA) is an application of MRI that provides images of blood flow and diseased and normal blood vessels. In patients who are allergic to iodinated contrast medium, MRA is used in place of angiography (see monograph titled "Angiography, Magnetic Resonance"). When the Food and Drug Administration approves gastrointestinal contrast agents, these agents would assist in identifying areas of bowel wall thickening, stricture, and intraluminal abnormalities, such as tumors, sites of perforation, and fistula. ■

INDICATIONS:

• Detect pelvic vascular diseases

• Detect cancer (primary or metastatic tumors of ovary, prostate, uterus, and bladder) and provide cancer staging

• Detect peritonitis

• Differentiate tumors from tissue abnormalities, such as cysts, cavernous hemangiomas, and abscesses

• Detect soft tissue abnormalities

• Determine blood clots, cysts, fluid or fat accumulation in tissues, hemorrhage, and infarctions

• Monitor and evaluate the effectiveness of medical or surgical interventions and course of the disease

RESULT

Normal Findings:
• Normal pelvic structures and soft tissue density and biochemical constituents of pelvic tissues, including blood flow

Abnormal Findings:
• Ascites

- Masses, lesions, infections, or inflammations

- Peritonitis

- Peritoneal tumor or carcinomatosis

- Pseudomyxoma peritonei

CRITICAL VALUES: N/A

INTERFERING FACTORS:

This procedure is contraindicated for:
- Patients with certain ferrous metal prostheses, valves, aneurysm clips, inner ear prostheses, or other metallic objects

- Patients with metal in their body, such as shrapnel or ferrous metal in the eye

- Patients with cardiac pacemakers, ⚠ because the pacemaker can be deactivated by MRI

- Patients who are claustrophobic

- Patients who are pregnant or suspected of being pregnant, unless the potential benefits of the procedure far outweigh the risks to the fetus and mother

Factors that may impair clear imaging:
- Inability of the patient to cooperate or remain still during the procedure because of age, significant pain, or mental status

- Patients with extreme cases of claustrophobia, unless sedation is given before the study

- Patients who are very obese, who may exceed the weight limit for the equipment

- Metallic objects within the examination field (e.g., jewelry or body rings), which may inhibit organ visualization and can produce unclear images

- Incorrect positioning of the patient, which may produce poor visualization of the area to be examined

Other considerations:
- If contrast medium is allowed to seep deep into the muscle tissue, vascular visualization will be impossible.

Nursing Implications and Procedure ● ● ● ● ● ● ● ● ● ● ●

Pretest: ■

➤ Inform the patient that the procedure assesses the pelvis.

➤ Inform the patient that the procedure is performed in a special department by a technologist and a physician and takes approximately 30 to 60 minutes.

➤ Obtain a history of allergies or sensitivities to contrast medium.

➤ Obtain a list of medications the patient is taking.

➤ Obtain a history of the patient's pelvic and reproductive systems, as well as results of previously performed tests, treatments, surgeries, and procedures. Determine if the patient has ever had any device implanted into the body, including copper intrauterine devices, pacemakers, ear implants, and heart valves.

➤ For related tests, refer to the reproductive and gastrointestinal system table.

➤ Determine previous laboratory abnormalities, especially blood urea nitrogen (BUN) and creatinine, if contrast medium is to be used.

➤ Ensure that the results of blood tests are obtained and recorded before the procedure.

➤ Obtain occupational history to determine the presence of metal in the body, such as shrapnel or flecks of ferrous metal in the eye (which can cause retinal hemorrhage).

➤ Determine date of last menstrual period and possibility of pregnancy in perimenopausal women.

➤ Ensure that the patient and staff have removed all external metallic objects from the patient before he or she enters the scanning room.

➤ Inform the patient that the technologist will place him or her in a supine position on a flat table in a large, cylindrical scanner.

➤ Tell the patient to expect to hear loud banging from the scanner and possibly to see magneto-phosphenes (flickering lights in the visual field); these will stop when the procedure is over.

➤ Instruct the patient to take slow, deep breaths if nausea occurs during the procedure.

➤ Do not restrict food and fluids.

Intratest:

➤ By physician direction, the patient is given dilute barium to drink or a tap water enema to distend the bowel before the examination, improving visualization of adjacent organs.

➤ Ask the patient to remove jewelry, including watches, hairpins, and other metallic objects, and credit cards.

➤ Ask the patient to void before the procedure.

➤ Administer a sedative to a child or to an uncooperative adult, as ordered.

➤ Administer an antianxiety agent, as ordered, if the patient has claustrophobia.

➤ Place the patient in a supine position on a flat table; use foam wedges to help maintain position and immobilization. Ask the patient to lie still during the procedure because movement produces unclear images, thus affecting the results and making interpretation difficult.

➤ Supply earplugs to the patient to block out the loud, banging sounds that occur during the test.

➤ If an electrocardiogram or respiratory gating is to be performed in conjunction with the scan, apply MRI-safe electrodes to the appropriate sites.

➤ The patient can communicate with the technologist doing the examination via a microphone within the machine.

➤ The table is moved into the scanner. Instruct the patient to remain still. The scanner makes noises as it acquires images of the body. The patient may be asked to hold his or her breath to facilitate visualization. A number of images are taken. These images are reconstructed by a computer and reviewed.

➤ Administer the contrast medium, if ordered. A second series of images is obtained.

Post-test:

➤ Instruct the patient to resume medications, normal activity, and diet, unless otherwise indicated.

➤ Observe for delayed allergic reactions, such as urticaria, hives, nausea, or vomiting, if contrast medium was used.

➤ A physician specializing in this branch of medicine sends a written report to the ordering provider, who discusses the results with the patient.

➤ Evaluate test results in relation to the patient's symptoms and other tests performed. Related diagnostic tests include ultrasound and computed tomography of the pelvis, as well as a kidney, ureter, and bladder (KUB) film.

MAGNETIC RESONANCE IMAGING, PITUITARY

SYNONYMS/ACRONYM: Pituitary MRI, MRI of the perisellar region.

AREA OF APPLICATION: Brain/pituitary area.

CONTRAST: Can be done with or without contrast medium (gadolinium).

DESCRIPTION: Magnetic resonance imaging (MRI) uses a magnet and radio waves to produce an energy field that can be displayed as an image. Use of magnetic fields with the aid of radiofrequency energy produces images primarily based on water content of tissue. The magnetic field causes the hydrogen atoms in tissue to line up, and when radio waves are directed toward the magnetic field, the atoms absorb the radio waves and change their position. When the radio waves are turned off, the atoms go back to their original position, this change in the energy field is sensed by the equipment, and an image is generated by the attached computer system. MRI produces cross-sectional images of the pituitary and perisellar region in multiple planes without the use of ionizing radiation or the interference of bone or surrounding tissue.

Pituitary MRI shows the relationship of pituitary lesions to the optic chiasm and cavernous sinuses. MRI has the capability of distinguishing the solid, cystic, and hemorrhagic components of lesions. Rapidly flowing blood on spin-echo MRI appears as an absence of signal or a void in the vessel's lumen. Blood flow can be evaluated in the cavernous and carotid arteries. Suprasellar aneurysms may be diagnosed without angiography, and old clotted blood in the walls of the aneurysms appears white. MRI uses the noniodinated contrast medium gadopentetate dimeglumine (Magnevist), which is administered intravenously to enhance contrast differences between normal and abnormal tissues.

Magnetic resonance angiography (MRA) is an application of MRI that provides images of blood flow and diseased and normal blood vessels. In patients who are allergic to iodinated contrast medium, MRA is used in place of angiography (see monograph titled "Angiography, Magnetic Resonance"). ∎

INDICATIONS:
• Detect microadenoma or macroadenoma of the pituitary

• Detect tumors of the pituitary

• Evaluate vascularity of the pituitary

• Evaluate the solid, cystic, and hemorrhagic components of lesions

- Detect perisellar abnormalities

- Evaluate potential cause of headache, visual loss, and vomiting

- Monitor and evaluate the effectiveness of medical or surgical interventions and course of disease

RESULT

Normal Findings:

- Normal anatomic structures, density, and biochemical constituents of the pituitary, including blood flow

Abnormal Findings:

- Abscess

- Aneurysm

- Choristoma

- Craniopharyngioma or meningioma

- Granuloma

- Infarct or hemorrhage

- Empty sella

- Macroadenoma or microadenoma

- Metastasis

- Parasitic infection

CRITICAL VALUES: N/A

INTERFERING FACTORS:

This procedure is contraindicated for:

- Patients with certain ferrous metal prostheses, valves, aneurysm clips, inner ear prostheses, or other metallic objects

- Patients with metal in their body, such as shrapnel or ferrous metal in the eye

- Patients with cardiac pacemakers, ⚠ because the pacemaker can be deactivated by MRI

- Patients who are claustrophobic

- Patients who are pregnant or suspected of being pregnant, unless the potential benefits of the procedure far outweigh the risks to the fetus and mother

Factors that may impair clear imaging:

- Inability of the patient to cooperate or remain still during the procedure because of age, significant pain, or mental status

- Patients with extreme cases of claustrophobia, unless sedation is given before the study

- Patients who are very obese, who may exceed the weight limit for the equipment

- Incorrect positioning of the patient, which may produce poor visualization of the area to be examined

- Metallic objects within the examination field (e.g., jewelry or rings), which may inhibit organ visualization and can produce unclear images

Other considerations:

- If contrast medium is allowed to seep deep into the muscle tissue, vascular visualization will be impossible.

Nursing Implications and Procedure • • • • • • • • • • • •

Pretest: ■

➤ Inform the patient that the procedure assesses the pituitary.

➤ Inform the patient that the procedure is performed in a special department by a technologist and a physician and takes approximately 30 to 60 minutes.

➤ Obtain a history of allergies or sensitivities to contrast medium.

➤ Obtain a list of medications the patient is taking.

➤ Obtain a history of the patient's pituitary, endocrine, and cranial findings, as well as results of previously performed tests, treatments, surgeries, and procedures. Determine if the patient has ever had any device implanted into the body, including copper intrauterine devices, pacemakers, ear implants, and heart valves.

➤ For related tests, refer to the endocrine system table.

➤ Determine previous laboratory abnormalities, especially blood urea nitrogen (BUN) and creatinine, if contrast medium is to be used.

➤ Ensure that the results of blood tests are obtained and recorded before the procedure.

➤ Obtain occupational history to determine the presence of metal in the body, such as shrapnel or flecks of ferrous metal in the eye (which can cause retinal hemorrhage).

➤ Determine date of last menstrual period and possibility of pregnancy in perimenopausal women.

➤ Ensure that the patient and staff have removed all external metallic objects from the patient before he or she enters the scanning room.

➤ Inform the patient that the technologist will place him or her in a supine position on a flat table in a large, cylindrical scanner.

➤ Tell the patient to expect to hear loud banging from the scanner and possibly to see magneto-phosphenes (flickering lights in the visual field); these will stop when the procedure is over.

➤ Instruct the patient to take slow, deep breaths if nausea occurs during the procedure.

➤ Do not restrict food and fluids.

Intratest:

➤ Ask the patient to remove jewelry, including watches, hairpins, and other metallic objects, and credit cards.

➤ Ask the patient to void before the procedure.

➤ Administer a sedative to a child or to an uncooperative adult, as ordered.

➤ Administer an antianxiety agent, as

ordered, if the patient has claustrophobia.

➤ Place the patient in a supine position on a flat table; use foam wedges to help maintain position and immobilization. Ask the patient to lie still during the procedure because movement produces unclear images, thus affecting the results and making interpretation difficult.

➤ Supply earplugs to the patient to block out the loud, banging sounds that occur during the test.

➤ If an electrocardiogram or respiratory gating is to be performed in conjunction with the scan, apply MRI-safe electrodes to the appropriate sites.

➤ The patient can communicate with the technologist doing the examination via a microphone within the machine.

➤ The table is moved into the scanner. Instruct the patient to remain still. The scanner makes noises as it acquires images of the body. The patient may be asked to hold his or her breath to facilitate visualization. A number of images are taken. These images are reconstructed by a computer and reviewed.

➤ Administer the contrast medium, if ordered. A second series of images is obtained.

Post-test:

➤ Instruct the patient to resume medications, normal activity, and diet, unless otherwise indicated.

➤ Observe for delayed allergic reactions, such as urticaria, hives, nausea, or vomiting, if contrast medium was used.

➤ A physician specializing in this branch of medicine sends a written report to the ordering provider, who discusses the results with the patient.

➤ Evaluate test results in relation to the patient's symptoms and other tests performed. Related diagnostic tests include electroencephalography, as well as MRI and computed tomography of the brain.

MAMMOGRAPHY

. . . .

SYNONYMS/ACRONYM: Mammogram, breast x-ray.

AREA OF APPLICATION: Breast.

CONTRAST: None.

DESCRIPTION: Mammography, an x-ray examination of the breast, is most commonly used to detect breast cancer; however, it can also be used to detect and evaluate symptomatic changes associated with other breast diseases, including mastitis, abscess, cystic changes, cysts, benign tumors, masses, and lymph nodes. Mammography is usually performed with traditional x-ray film, but totally electronic image recording is becoming commonplace. This type of radiologic procedure reduces the amount or radiation exposure to the patient and produces detailed images with excellent contrast. Two views of each breast are usually taken. Benign cysts appear as clearly defined, regular, clear spots that are bilateral; cancer appears as irregular, poorly defined, unilateral opaque areas or clusters of calcifications. Mammography can be used to locate a nonpalpable lesion for biopsy. Mammography cannot detect breast cancer with 100 percent accuracy: In approximately 15 percent of breast cancer cases, the cancer is not detected with mammography. To assist in early detection of nonpalpable breast lesions, computer-assisted diagnosis is currently being used. With this technique, a computer performs automated scanning

of the mammogram before the physician interprets the findings.

When a mass is detected, additional studies are performed to help differentiate the nature of the mass, as follows:

Magnification views of the area in question

Focal or "spot" views of the area in question, done with a specialized paddle-style compression device

Ultrasound images of the area in question, which help differentiate between a fluid-filled cystic lesion and a solid lesion indicative of cancer

The American Cancer Society recommends that all women follow a personal breast-care plan according to age:

Women aged 20 to 39: Clinical breast examination performed by a health care professional every 3 years and a monthly breast self-examination

Women aged 40 and older: Annual mammogram, clinical breast examination every year by a health care professional (near time of the mammogram), and monthly breast self-examination. ■

INDICATIONS:

• Evaluate known or suspected breast cancer

- Evaluate size, shape, and position of breast masses
- Evaluate breast pain, skin retraction, nipple erosion, or nipple discharge
- Differentiate between benign and neoplastic breast disease
- Evaluate nonpalpable breast masses
- Monitor postoperative and post–radiation treatment status of the breast
- Evaluate opposite breast after mastectomy

RESULT

Normal Findings:
- Normal breast tissue, with no cysts, tumors, or calcifications

Abnormal Findings:
- Breast cysts or abscesses
- Breast tumors
- Breast calcifications
- Hematoma resulting from trauma
- Mastitis
- Soft-tissue masses
- Vascular calcification

CRITICAL VALUES: N/A

INTERFERING FACTORS:

This procedure is contraindicated for:
- Patients who are pregnant or suspected of being pregnant, unless the potential benefits of the procedure far outweigh the risks to the fetus and mother
- Patients younger than age 25, because the density of the breast tissue is such that diagnostic x-rays are of limited value

Factors that may impair clear imaging:
- Inability of the patient to cooperate or remain still during the procedure because of age, significant pain, or mental status

- Metallic objects within the examination field (e.g., jewelry or body rings), which may inhibit organ visualization and can produce unclear images
- Improper adjustment of the radiographic equipment to accommodate obese or thin patients, which can cause overexposure or underexposure and a poor-quality study
- Incorrect positioning of the patient, which may produce poor visualization of the area to be examined
- Application of substances such as talcum powder or creams to the skin of breasts or underarms, which may alter test results
- Previous breast surgery, breast augmentation, or the presence of breast implants, which may decrease the readability of the examination

Other considerations:
- Consultation with a physician should occur before the procedure for radiation safety concerns regarding infants of patients who are lactating.
- Risks associated with radiographic overexposure can result from frequent x-ray procedures. Personnel in the room with the patient should wear a protective lead apron, stand behind a shield, or leave the area while the examination is being done. Personnel working in the area where the examination is being done should wear badges that reveal their level of exposure to radiation.

Nursing Implications and Procedure · · · · · · · · · · ·

Pretest:

➤ Inform the patient about the purpose of the procedure, various positions to assume, and the need to hold her breath during x-ray exposures.
➤ Obtain a history of the patient's complaints, if any.

➤ Obtain a history of known or suspected breast disease, family history of breast disease, and results of previously performed tests, treatments, therapies, surgeries, biopsies, and other procedures.

➤ For related tests, refer to the reproductive system table.

➤ Inform the patient not to apply deodorant, body creams, or powders on the day of the procedure.

➤ Inform the patient there may be discomfort associated with the study, while the breast is being compressed. The compression allows for better visualization of the breast tissue.

➤ Determine date of last menstrual period and possibility of pregnancy in perimenopausal women.

➤ Inform the patient the best time to schedule the examination is 1 week after menses, when breast tenderness is decreased.

➤ Explain to the patient that the radiation dose will be kept to an absolute minimum.

➤ Do not restrict food and fluids, unless otherwise indicated.

➤ Inform the patient that the procedure lasts 15 to 30 minutes.

Intratest: ■

➤ Ask the patient to void before the procedure. Have the patient put on a hospital gown.

➤ Make sure jewelry, chains, and any other metallic objects have been removed from the chest area.

➤ Assist the patient to a standing or sitting position in front of the x-ray machine, which is adjusted to the level of the breasts. Position the patient's arms out of the range of the area to be filmed.

➤ Place breasts, one at a time, between the compression apparatus. Usually two views or exposures are taken of each breast. Ask the patient to hold her breath during exposures.

Post-test: ■

➤ Inform the patient that further examinations may be necessary to further evaluate questionable areas of the breast, evaluate progression of the disease process, or determine the need for a change in therapy.

➤ Determine if patient or family members have any further questions or concerns.

➤ Educate the patient regarding the techniques for breast self-examination.

➤ A physician specializing in this branch of medicine sends a written report to the ordering provider, who discusses the results with the patient.

➤ Evaluate test results in relation to the patient's symptoms and any related tests performed.

MECKEL'S DIVERTICULUM SCAN

· ·

SYNONYMS/ACRONYM: Meckel's scan, Meckel's scintigraphy, ectopic gastric mucosa scan.

AREA OF APPLICATION: Abdomen.

CONTRAST: Intravenous radioactive technetium-99m pertechnetate.

DESCRIPTION: Meckel's diverticulum scan is a nuclear medicine study performed to assist in diagnosing the cause of abdominal pain or occult gastrointestinal (GI) bleeding, and to assess the presence and size of a congenital anomaly of the GI tract. After intravenous injection of technetium-99m pertechnetate, immediate and delayed imaging is performed, with various views of the abdomen obtained. The radionuclide is taken up and concentrated by parietal cells of the gastric mucosa, whether located in the stomach or in a Meckel's diverticulum. Up to 25 percent of Meckel's diverticulum is lined internally with ectopic gastric mucosal tissue. This tissue is usually located in the ileum and right lower quadrant of the abdomen; it secretes acid that causes ulceration of intestinal tissue, which results in abdominal pain and occult blood in stools. ∎

INDICATIONS:
• Aid in the diagnosis of unexplained abdominal pain and GI bleeding caused by hydrochloric acid and pepsin secreted by ectopic gastric mucosa, which ulcerates nearby mucosa

• Detect sites of ectopic gastric mucosa

RESULT

Normal Findings:
• Normal distribution of radionuclide by gastric mucosa at normal sites

Abnormal Findings:
• Meckel's diverticulum, evidenced by focally increased radioactive uptake in areas other than normal structures

CRITICAL VALUES: N/A

INTERFERING FACTORS:

This procedure is contraindicated for:
• Patients who are pregnant or suspected of being pregnant, unless the potential benefits of the procedure far outweigh the risks to the fetus and mother

Factors that may impair clear imaging:
• Inability of the patient to cooperate or remain still during the procedure because of age, significant pain, or mental status

• Metallic objects within the examination field (e.g., jewelry or body rings), which may inhibit organ visualization and can produce unclear images

• Patients who are very obese, who may exceed the weight limit for the equipment

• Incorrect positioning of the patient, which may produce poor visualization of the area to be examined

• Retained barium from a previous radiologic procedure

• Other nuclear scans done within preceding 24 hours

Other considerations:
• False-positive results may come from nondiverticular bleeding, intussusception, duplication cysts, inflammatory bowel disease, hemangioma of the bowel, and other organ infections.

• Inadequate amount of gastric mucosa within Meckel's diverticulum can affect the ability to visualize abnormalities.

• Inaccurate timing for imaging after the radionuclide injection can affect the results.

• Failure to follow dietary restrictions before the procedure may cause the procedure to be canceled or repeated.

• Improper injection of the radionuclide that allows the tracer to seep deep into the muscle tissue produces erroneous hot spots.

• Consultation with a physician should occur before the procedure for radiation safety concerns regarding infants of patients who are lactating.

• Risks associated with radiographic overexposure can result from frequent x-ray procedures. Personnel in the room with the patient should wear a protective lead apron, stand behind a shield, or leave the area while the examination is being done. Personnel working in the area where the examination is being done should wear badges that reveal their level of exposure to radiation.

Nursing Implications and Procedure • • • • • • • • • •

Pretest:

➤ Inform the patient that the procedure assesses GI bleeding.

➤ Inform the patient that the procedure is performed in a special nuclear medicine department by a technologist and usually takes approximately 60 minutes.

➤ Obtain a history of allergies or sensitivities to contrast medium.

➤ Obtain a list of medications the patient is taking.

➤ Obtain a history of signs and symptoms of Meckel's diverticulum, such as bleeding, pain, intussusception, volvulus, or diverticulitis, as well as results of previously performed tests and surgical procedures. For related tests, refer to the cardiovascular and gastrointestinal system tables.

➤ Determine date of last menstrual period and possibility of pregnancy in perimenopausal women.

➤ Ensure that a histamine blocker is administered, as ordered, 2 days before the study to block GI secretion, as appropriate.

➤ Occasionally, gastrin is given to increase the uptake of the radionuclide by the ectopic gastric mucosa.

➤ Obtain and record baseline vital signs.

➤ Ensure that the patient has fasted for 6 to 8 hours before the scan, unless otherwise indicated.

Intratest:

➤ Ask the patient to void before the procedure. Have the patient put on a hospital gown.

➤ Administer sedative to a child or to an uncooperative adult, as ordered.

➤ Make sure jewelry, watches, chains, belts, and any other metallic objects have been removed from the abdominal area.

➤ Place the patient in a supine position on a flat table with foam wedges, which help maintain position and immobilization. Ask the patient to lie still during the procedure because movement produces unclear images. The radionuclide is administered intravenously, and the abdomen is scanned immediately for 1 minute to screen for vascular lesions that cause bleeding. Then images are taken every 5 minutes for the next 60 minutes in the anterior, oblique, lateral, and postvoid anterior views.

➤ Wear gloves during the radionuclide injection and while handling the patient's urine.

Post-test:

➤ Instruct the patient to resume normal activity, medications, and diet, unless otherwise indicated.

➤ Evaluate the patient's vital signs. Monitor vital signs every 15 to 30 minutes and compare with baseline readings until the patient is stable.

➤ Advise patient to drink increased amounts of fluids for 24 to 48 hours to eliminate the radionuclide from the body, unless contraindicated. Tell the patient that radionuclide is eliminated from the body within 6 to 24 hours.

➤ Instruct the patient to flush the toilet immediately after each voiding following the procedure and to wash hands meticulously with soap and water after each voiding for 24 hours after the procedure.

➤ Tell all caregivers to wear gloves when discarding urine for 24 hours after the procedure. Wash gloved hands with soap and water before removing gloves. Then wash hands after the gloves are removed.

➤ A physician specializing in this branch of medicine sends a written report to the ordering provider, who discusses the results with the patient.

➤ Evaluate test results in relation to the patient's symptoms and other tests performed. Related diagnostic tests include abdominal, computed tomography (CT), and magnetic resonance angiography; and CT and magnetic resonance imaging of the abdomen.

MEDIASTINOSCOPY

. . . .

SYNONYM/ACRONYM: None.

AREA OF APPLICATION: Mediastinum.

CONTRAST: None.

DESCRIPTION: Mediastinoscopy provides direct visualization of the structures that lie beneath the mediastinum, which is the area behind the sternum and between the lungs. The test is performed under general anesthesia by means of a mediastinoscope inserted through a surgical incision at the suprasternal notch. Structures that can be viewed include the trachea, the esophagus, the heart and its major vessels, the thymus gland, and the lymph nodes that receive drainage from the lungs. The procedure is performed primarily to visualize and obtain biopsy specimens of the mediastinal lymph nodes, and to determine the extent of metastasis into the mediastinum for the determination of treatment planning in cancer patients. ■

INDICATIONS:

• Confirm radiologic or cytologic evidence of carcinoma or sarcoidosis

• Confirm radiologic evidence of a thoracic infectious process of an indeterminate nature, coccidioidomycosis, or histoplasmosis

• Detect Hodgkin's disease

• Determine stage of known bronchogenic carcinoma, as indicated by the extent of mediastinal lymph node involvement

• Detect metastasis into the anterior

mediastinum or extrapleurally into the chest

- Evaluate a patient with signs and symptoms of obstruction of mediastinal lymph flow and a history of head or neck cancer to determine recurrence or spread

RESULT

Normal Findings:

- Normal appearance of mediastinal structures

- No abnormal lymph node tissue

Abnormal Findings:

- Bronchogenic carcinoma

- Coccidioidomycosis

- Granulomatous infections

- Histoplasmosis

- Hodgkin's disease

- *Pneumocystis carinii* infection

- Sarcoidosis

- Tuberculosis

Critical values: N/A

INTERFERING FACTORS:

This procedure is contraindicated for:

- Patients who have had a previous mediastinoscopy, because scarring can make insertion of the scope and biopsy of lymph nodes difficult

- Patients who have superior vena cava obstruction, because this condition causes increased venous collateral circulation in the mediastinum

- Patients who are pregnant or suspected of being pregnant, unless the potential benefits of the procedure far outweigh the risks to the fetus and mother

Other considerations:

- Failure to follow dietary restrictions

before the procedure may cause the procedure to be canceled or repeated.

Nursing Implications and Procedure • • • • • • • • • • •

Pretest:

➤ Inform the patient that the procedure is usually performed under general anesthesia in an operating room by a physician and takes approximately 60 minutes.

➤ Obtain a history of complaints; allergies or sensitivities to anesthetics, analgesics, or antibiotics; thoracic or hematologic disorders; and treatment regimen. For related tests, refer to the respiratory and immunologic system tables.

➤ Obtain a list of medications the patient is taking.

➤ Obtain a history of the patient's respiratory problems as well as results of previously performed tests and procedures.

➤ Ensure that the results of blood typing and cross-matching are obtained and recorded before the procedure in the event that an emergency thoracotomy should be required.

➤ *Obtain a written, informed consent before administering any medications prior to the procedure.*

➤ Ensure that the patient has fasted for 6 to 8 hours before the scan, unless otherwise indicated.

➤ Obtain and record baseline vital signs.

Intratest:

➤ Prepare the patient for surgery, and administer sedation, as ordered.

➤ Place the patient in the supine position. General anesthesia is administered via an endotracheal tube.

➤ An incision is made at the suprasternal notch, and a path for the mediastinoscope is made using finger dissection. The lymph nodes can be palpated at this time. The lymph nodes on the right side of the mediastinum are most accessible and safest to biopsy by med astinoscopy; the lymph nodes on the left side are more difficult to explore and biopsy because of their proximity to the aorta. Biopsy specimens of nodes on the left side of the mediastinum may need to be obtained by mediastinotomy, which involves performing a left anterior thoracotomy.

➤ Label the specimens for biopsy or culture, place them in appropriate containers, and promptly send them to the laboratory.

➤ The scope is removed, and the incision is closed.

➤ If the patient is stable and if no further surgery is immediately indicated, the patient is extubated.

Post-test:

➤ Instruct the patient to resume usual diet and medications, if withheld and directed by the physician.

➤ Monitor vital signs according to institution's policy.

➤ Inform the patient that some chest discomfort may be present and that the throat may be slightly sore after the procedure.

➤ Warm gargles or lozenges can be administered for throat discomfort.

➤ Inform the patient and caregiver that food, fluids, and activities are resumed when the patient has recovered from general anesthesia.

➤ Instruct the patient to immediately report to the physician any difficulty breathing, other abnormal sensations or discomforts, or changes in vocal patterns.

➤ Instruct the patient on the symptoms of incisional infection, and inform the patient of the need to promptly report any symptoms to the physician.

➤ A physician specializing in this branch of medicine sends a written report to the ordering provider, who discusses the results with the patient.

➤ Evaluate test results in relation to the patient's symptoms and other tests performed. Related tests include computed tomography and magnetic resonance imaging of the chest.

METANEPHRINES

SYNONYM/ACRONYM: N/A.

SPECIMEN: Urine (25 mL) from a timed specimen collected in a clean amber, plastic collection container with 6N hydrochloride as a preservative.

REFERENCE VALUE: (Method: High-pressure liquid chromatography)

Age	Conventional Units	SI Units
	Normetanephrines	
		(Conversion Factor × 5.46)
0–3 mo	47–156 μg/24 h	257–852 nmol/24 h
4–6 mo	31–111 μg/24 h	171–607 nmol/24 h
7–9 mo	42–109 μg/24 h	230–595 nmol/24 h
10–12 mo	23–103 μg/24 h	127–562 nmol/24 h
1–2 y	32–118 μg/24 h	175–647 nmol/24 h
2–6 y	50–111 μg/24 h	274–604 nmol/24 h
6–10 y	47–176 μg/24 h	255–964 nmol/24 h
10–16 y	53–290 μg/24 h	289–1586 nmol/24 h
Adult	82–500 μg/24 h	448–2730 nmol/24 h
	Metanephrines	
		(Conversion Factor × 5.07)
0–3 mo	5.9–37 μg/24 h	30–188 nmol/24 h
4–6 mo	6.1–42 μg/24 h	31–213 nmol/24 h
7–9 mo	12–41 μg/24 h	61–210 nmol/24 h
10–12 mo	8.5–101 μg/24 h	43–510 nmol/24 h
1–2 y	6.7–52 μg/24 h	34–264 nmol/24 h
2–6 y	11–99 μg/24 h	56–501 nmol/24 h
6–10 y	54–138 μg/24 h	275–701 nmol/24 h
10–16 y	39–243 μg/24 h	200–1231 nmol/24 h
Adult	45–290 μg/24 h	228–1470 nmol/24 h

DESCRIPTION: Metanephrines are the inactive metabolites of epinephrine and norepinephrine. Metanephrines are either excreted or further metabolized into vanillylmandelic acid. Release of metanephrines in the urine is indicative of disorders associated with excessive catecholamine production, particularly pheochromocytoma. Vanillylmandelic acid and catecholamines are normally measured with urinary metanephrines. Creatinine is usually measured simultaneously to ensure adequate collection and to calculate an excretion ratio of metabolite to creatinine. ■

INDICATIONS:
• Assist in the diagnosis of suspected pheochromocytoma

• Assist in identifying the cause of hypertension

• Verify suspected tumors associated with excessive catecholamine secretion

RESULT

Increased in:
• Ganglioneuroma
• Neuroblastoma
• Pheochromocytoma
• Severe stress

Decreased in: N/A

CRITICAL VALUES: N/A

INTERFERING FACTORS:
• Drugs that may increase metanephrine levels include labetalol, monoamine

oxidase inhibitors, oxprenolol, oxytetracycline, and prochlorperazine.

• Methylglucamine in x-ray contrast medium may cause false-negative results.

Nursing Implications and Procedure • • • • • • • • • • •

Pretest: ■

➤ Obtain a history of the patient's complaints, including a list of known allergens.

➤ Obtain a history of the patient's endocrine system and results of previously performed tests and procedures. For related tests, refer to the endocrine system table.

➤ Obtain a list of the medications the patient is taking, including herbs, nutritional supplements, and nutraceuticals. The requesting health care practitioner and laboratory should be advised if the patient regularly uses these products so that their effects can be taken into consideration when reviewing results.

➤ Note any recent procedures that can interfere with test results.

➤ There are no food, fluid, or medication restrictions unless by medical direction.

➤ Instruct the patient to avoid excessive exercise and stress during the 24-hour collection of urine.

➤ Review the procedure with the patient. Provide a nonmetallic urinal, bedpan, or toilet-mounted collection device.

➤ Usually a 24-hour time frame for urine collection is ordered. Inform the patient that all urine must be saved during that 24-hour period. Instruct the patient not to void directly into the laboratory collection container. Instruct the patient to avoid defecating in the collection device and to keep toilet tissue out

of the collection device to prevent contamination of the specimen. Place a sign in the bathroom to remind the patient to save all urine.

➤ Instruct the patient to void all urine into the collection device and then to pour the urine into the laboratory collection container. Alternatively the specimen can be left in the collection device for a health care staff member to add to the laboratory collection container.

Intratest: ■

➤ Observe standard precautions and follow the general guidelines in Appendix A.

Timed specimen:

➤ Obtain a clean 3-L urine specimen container, toilet-mounted collection device, and plastic bag (for transport of the specimen container). The specimen must be refrigerated or kept on ice throughout the entire collection period. If an indwelling urinary catheter is in place, the drainage bag must be kept on ice.

➤ Begin the test between 6 and 8 a.m., if possible. Collect first voiding and discard. Record the time the specimen was discarded as the beginning of the timed collection period. The next morning, ask the patient to void at the same time the collection was started and add this last voiding to the container.

➤ If an indwelling catheter is in place, replace the tubing and container system at the start of the collection time. Keep the container system on ice during the collection period, or empty the urine into a larger container periodically during the collection period; monitor to ensure continued drainage, and conclude the test the next morning at the same hour the collection was begun.

➤ At the conclusion of the test, compare the quantity of urine with the urinary output record for the collection; if the specimen contains less than what was recorded as output, some urine may have been discarded, invalidating the test.

➤ Label the specimen, and promptly transport it to the laboratory. Include on the label the amount of urine and test start and stop times.

➤ Evaluate test results in relation to the patient's symptoms and other tests performed. Related laboratory tests include catecholamines, homovanillic acid, and vanillylmandelic acid.

METHEMOGLOBIN

• •

SYNONYMS/ACRONYM: Hemoglobin, hemoglobin M, MetHb, Hgb M.

SPECIMEN: Whole blood (1 mL) collected in green-top (heparin) tube. Specimen should be transported tightly capped and in an ice slurry.

REFERENCE VALUE: (Method: Spectrophotometry)

Conventional Units	SI Units (Conversion Factor ×155)
0.06–0.24 g/dL*	9.3–37.2 µmol/L*

* Percentage of total hemoglobin = 0.41–1.15 percent.
Note: The conversion factor of ×155 is based on the molecular weight of hemoglobin of 64,500 daltons (d) or 64.5 kd.

DESCRIPTION: Methemoglobin is a structural hemoglobin variant formed when the heme portion of the deoxygenated hemoglobin is oxidized to a ferric state that renders it incapable of combining with and transporting oxygen to tissues. Visible cyanosis can result as levels approach 10 to 15 percent of total hemoglobin. ■

INDICATIONS:

• Assist in the detection of acquired methemoglobinemia caused by the toxic effects of chemicals and drugs

• Assist in the detection of congenital methemoglobinemia, indicated by deficiency of red blood cell nicotinamide

adenine dinucleotide (NADH)-methemoglobin reductase or presence of methemoglobin.

• Evaluate cyanosis in the presence of normal blood gases

RESULT

Increased in:

• Acquired methemoglobinemia (drugs, tobacco smoking, or ionizing radiation)

• Carbon monoxide poisoning

• Hereditary methemoglobinemia (deficiency of NADH-methemoglobin reductase or hemoglobinopathy)

Decreased in: N/A

CRITICAL VALUES: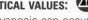

Cyanosis can occur at levels greater than 10 percent.

Dizziness, fatigue, headache, and tachycardia can occur at levels greater than 30 percent.

Signs of central nervous system depression can occur at levels greater than 45 percent.

Death may occur at levels greater than 70 percent.

Possible interventions include airway protection, administration of oxygen, monitoring neurologic status every hour, continuous pulse oximetry, hyperbaric oxygen therapy, and exchange transfusion. Administration of activated charcoal or gastric lavage may be effective if performed soon after the toxic agent is ingested. Emesis should never be induced in patients with no gag reflex because of the risk of aspiration. Methylene blue may be used to reverse the process of methemoglobin formation, but it should be used cautiously when methemoglobin levels are greater than 30 percent. Use of methylene blue is contraindicated in the presence of glucose-6-phosphate dehydrogenase deficiency.

INTERFERING FACTORS:

• Drugs that may increase methemoglobin levels include acetanilid, amyl nitrate, aniline derivatives, benzocaine, chlorates, chloroquine, dapsone, glucosulfone, isoniazid, lidocaine, phenacetin, phenytoin, primaquine, nitroglycerin, resorcinol, sulfonamides, and thiazolsulfone.

• Well water containing nitrate is the most common cause of methemoglobinemia in infants.

• Breastfeeding infants are capable of converting inorganic nitrate from common topical anesthetic applications containing nitrate to the nitrite

ion, causing nitrite toxicity and increased methemoglobin.

• Prompt and proper specimen processing, storage, and analysis are important to achieve accurate results. Methemoglobin is unstable and should be transported on ice within a few hours of collection, or else the specimen should be rejected.

Nursing Implications and Procedure

Pretest:

➤ Obtain a history of the patient's complaints, including a list of known allergens.

➤ Obtain a history of the patient's hematopoietic system and results of previously performed tests and procedures. For related tests, refer to the hematopoietic system table.

➤ Obtain a list of medications the patient is taking, including herbs, nutritional supplements, and nutraceuticals. The requesting health care practitioner and laboratory should be advised if the patient regularly uses these products so that their effects can be taken into consideration when reviewing results.

➤ There are no food, fluid, or medication restrictions unless by medical direction.

➤ Review the procedure with the patient.

➤ Inform the patient that specimen collection takes approximately 5 to 10 minutes.

➤ Prepare an ice slurry in a cup or plastic bag to have on hand for immediate transport of the specimen to the laboratory.

Intratest:

➤ Direct the patient to breathe normally and to avoid unnecessary movement.

➤ Observe standard precautions and follow the general guidelines in

Appendix A. Perform a venipuncture, and collect the specimen in a 5-mL green-top tube.

➤ Label the specimen, and promptly transport it to the laboratory. The tightly stoppered specimen should be placed in an ice slurry immediately after collection. Information on the specimen label can be protected from water in the ice slurry if the specimen is first placed in a protective plastic bag.

Post-test:

➤ Observe venipuncture site for bleeding or hematoma formation. Apply pressure bandage.

➤ Evaluate test results in relation to the patient's symptoms and other tests performed. Related laboratory tests include arterial/alveolar oxygen ratio, blood gases, carboxyhemoglobin, and hemoglobin electrophoresis.

MICROALBUMIN

SYNONYMS/ACRONYM: Albumin, urine.

SPECIMEN: Urine (10 mL) from a random or timed specimen collected in a clean plastic collection container.

REFERENCE VALUE: (Method: Nephelometry immunoassay)

Test	Conventional Units	SI Units (Conversion Factor ×0.001)
Random microalbumin	0–30 µg/mL	0–0.03 g/L
24-h microalbumin	Greater than 40 µg/24 h	Greater than 0.04 g/24 h

Simultaneous measurement of urine creatinine or creatinine clearance may be requested. Normal ratio of microalbumin to creatinine is less than 15.

DESCRIPTION: The term *microalbumin* is used to describe concentrations of albumin in urine that are greater than normal but undetectable by dipstick or traditional spectrophotometry methods. Microalbuminuria precedes the nephropathy associated with diabetes and is often elevated years before creatinine clearance shows abnormal values. Studies have shown that the median duration from onset of microalbuminuria to development of nephropathy is 5 to 7 years. ∎

INDICATIONS:

• Evaluate renal disease

• Screen diabetic patients for early signs of nephropathy

RESULT

Increased in:
- Cardiomyopathy
- Diabetic nephropathy
- Exercise
- Hypertension (uncontrolled)
- Preeclampsia
- Renal disease
- Urinary tract infections

Decreased in: N/A

CRITICAL VALUES: N/A

INTERFERING FACTORS:
- Drugs that may decrease microalbumin levels include captopril, dipyridamole, enalapril, furosemide, indapamide, perindopril, quinapril, ramipril, tolrestat, and triflusal.

- All urine voided for the timed collection period must be included in the collection or else falsely decreased values may be obtained. Compare output records with volume collected to verify that all voids were included in the collection.

Nursing Implications and Procedure • • • • • • • • • • •

Pretest: ■

➤ Obtain a history of the patient's complaints, including a list of known allergens.

➤ Obtain a history of the patient's endocrine and genitourinary systems as well as results of previously performed tests and procedures. For related tests, refer to the endocrine and genitourinary system tables.

➤ Obtain a list of medications the patient is taking, including herbs,

nutritional supplements, and nutraceuticals. The requesting health care practitioner and laboratory should be advised if the patient regularly uses these products so that their effects can be taken into consideration when reviewing results.

➤ There are no food, fluid, or medication restrictions unless by medical direction.

➤ Instruct the patient to avoid excessive exercise and stress during the 24-hour collection of urine.

➤ Review the procedure with the patient. Provide a nonmetallic urinal, bedpan, or toilet-mounted collection device.

➤ Usually a 24-hour time frame for urine collection is ordered. Inform the patient that all urine must be saved during that 24-hour period. Instruct the patient not to void directly into the laboratory collection container. Instruct the patient to avoid defecating in the collection device and to keep toilet tissue out of the collection device to prevent contamination of the specimen. Place a sign in the bathroom to remind the patient to save all urine.

➤ Instruct the patient to void all urine into the collection device and then to pour the urine into the laboratory collection container. Alternatively the specimen can be left in the collection device for a health care staff member to add to the laboratory collection container.

Intratest: ■

➤ Observe standard precautions and follow the general guidelines in Appendix A.

Random specimen (collect in early morning):

Clean-catch specimen:

➤ Instruct the male patient to (1) thoroughly wash his hands, (2) cleanse the meatus, (3) void a small amount into the toilet, and (4) void directly into the specimen container.

> Instruct the female patient to (1) thoroughly wash her hands; (2) cleanse the labia from front to back; (3) while keeping the labia separated, void a small amount into the toilet; and (4) without interrupting the urine stream, void directly into the specimen container.

Indwelling catheter:

> Put on gloves. Empty drainage tube of urine. It may be necessary to clamp off the catheter for 15 to 30 minutes before specimen collection. Cleanse specimen port with antiseptic swab, and then aspirate 5 mL of urine with a 21- to 25-gauge needle and syringe. Transfer urine to a sterile container.

Timed specimen:

> Obtain a clean 3-L urine specimen container, toilet-mounted collection device, and plastic bag (for transport of the specimen container). The specimen must be refrigerated or kept on ice throughout the entire collection period. If an indwelling urinary catheter is in place, the drainage bag must be kept on ice.

> Begin the test between 6 and 8 a.m., if possible. Collect first voiding and discard. Record the time the specimen was discarded as the beginning of the timed collection period. The next morning, ask the patient to void at the same time the collection was started and add this last voiding to the container.

> If an indwelling catheter is in place, replace the tubing and container system at the start of the collection time. Keep the container system on ice during the collection period, or empty the urine into a larger container periodically during the collection period; monitor to ensure continued drainage, and conclude the test the next morning at the same hour the collection was begun.

> At the conclusion of the test, compare the quantity of urine with the urinary output record for the collection; if the specimen contains less than what was recorded as output, some urine may have been discarded, invalidating the test.

> Label the specimen, and promptly transport it to the laboratory. Include on the label the amount of urine and test start and stop times.

Post-test:

> Instruct the patient, as appropriate, in nutritional management of diabetes. Patients who adhere to dietary recommendations report a better general feeling of health, better weight management, greater control of glucose and lipid values, and improved use of insulin. There is no "diabetic diet"; however, there are many meal-planning approaches with nutritional goals endorsed by the American Dietetic Association. The nutritional needs of each diabetic patient need to be determined individually with the appropriate health care professionals, particularly professionals trained in nutrition.

> Instruct the patient and caregiver to report signs and symptoms of hypoglycemia or hyperglycemia.

> Recognize anxiety related to test results and offer support. Provide teaching and information regarding the clinical implications of the test results, as appropriate. Emphasize, if indicated, that good glycemic control delays the onset and slows the progression of diabetic retinopathy, nephropathy, and neuropathy. Educate the patient regarding access to counseling services, as appropriate.

> Evaluate test results in relation to the patient's symptoms and other tests performed. Related laboratory tests include cortisol, urine creatinine, creatinine clearance, glucose, glycated hemoglobin, glucose tolerance test, insulin, insulin antibodies, urine protein and fractions, and urinalysis.

β₂-MICROGLOBULIN

SYNONYM/ACRONYM: β₂-M.

SPECIMEN: Serum (1 mL) collected in a red-top tube or 5 mL urine from a timed collection in a clean, plastic container with 1N NaOH as a preservative.

REFERENCE VALUE: (Method: Immunoassay for serum sample, radioimmunoassay for urine sample)

Sample	Conventional Units	SI Units (Conversion Factor ×10)
Serum		
Newborn	Less than 0.3 mg/dL	Less than 3 mg/L
Adult	Less than 0.2 mg/dL	Less than 2 mg/L
Urine	0.03–0.37 mg/24 h	

DESCRIPTION: β₂-Microglobulin is an amino acid peptide component of human leukocyte antigen (HLA) complexes. β₂-Microglobulin increases in inflammatory conditions and when lymphocyte turnover increases, such as in lymphocytic leukemia or when T-lymphocyte helper (OKT4) cells are attacked by human immunodeficiency virus (HIV). Serum β₂-microglobulin becomes elevated with malfunctioning glomeruli, but decreases with malfunctioning tubules because it is metabolized by the renal tubules. Conversely, urine β₂-microglobulin decreases with malfunctioning glomeruli, but becomes elevated with malfunctioning tubules. ■

INDICATIONS:
- Detect aminoglycoside toxicity (becomes elevated before creatinine)
- Detect chronic lymphocytic leukemia, multiple myeloma, lung cancer, hepatoma, or breast cancer
- Detect HIV infection (*note:* levels do not correlate with stages of infection)
- Evaluate renal disease to differentiate glomerular from tubular dysfunction
- Monitor antiretroviral therapy

RESULT

Increased in:
- Acquired immune deficiency syndrome (AIDS)
- Aminoglycoside toxicity
- Amyloidosis
- Autoimmune disorders
- Breast cancer
- Crohn's disease
- Felty's syndrome

- Hepatitis
- Hepatoma
- Hyperthyroidism
- Inflammation of all types
- Leukemia (chronic lymphocytic)
- Lung cancer
- Lymphoma
- Multiple myeloma
- Poisoning with heavy metals, such as mercury or cadmium
- Renal dialysis
- Renal disease (glomerular): serum only
- Renal disease (tubular): urine only
- Sarcoidosis
- Systemic lupus erythematosus
- Vasculitis
- Viral infections (e.g., cytomegalovirus)

Decreased in:

- Renal disease (glomerular): urine only
- Renal disease (tubular): serum only
- Response to zidovudine (AZT)

CRITICAL VALUES: N/A

INTERFERING FACTORS:

- Drugs and proteins that may increase serum β$_2$-microglobulin levels include cefuroxime, cyclosporine A, gentamicin, interferon-α, pentoxifylline, and tumor necrosis factor.

- Drugs that may decrease serum β$_2$-microglobulin levels include zidovudine.

- Drugs that may increase urine β$_2$-microglobulin levels include azathioprine, cisplatin, cyclosporine A, furosemide, gentamicin, mannitol, nifedipine, sisomicin, and tobramycin.

- Drugs that may decrease urine β$_2$-microglobulin levels include cilostazol.

- Urinary β$_2$-microglobulin is unstable at pH less than 5.5.

- Recent radioactive scans or radiation within 1 week before the test can interfere with test results when radioimmunoassay is the test method.

Nursing Implications and Procedure • • • • • • • • • •

Pretest: ▮

➤ Obtain a history of the patient's complaints, including a list of known allergens.

➤ Obtain a history of the patient's genitourinary and immune system, as well as results of previously performed tests and procedures. For related tests, refer to the genitourinary and immune system tables.

➤ Obtain a list of the medications the patient takes including herbs, nutritional supplements, and nutraceuticals. The requesting health care practitioner and laboratory should be advised if the patient regularly uses these products so their effects can be taken into consideration when reviewing results.

➤ Note any recent procedures that can interfere with test results.

➤ There are no food, fluid, or medication restrictions unless by medical direction.

➤ Review the procedure with the patient.

Blood:

➤ Inform the patient that blood specimen collection takes approximately 5 to 10 minutes.

Urine:

➤ Review the procedure with the patient. Provide a nonmetallic urinal, bedpan, or toilet-mounted collection device.

➤ Usually a 24-hour urine collection is ordered. Inform the patient that all urine over a 24-hour period must be saved; instruct the patient to avoid defecating in the collection device and to keep toilet tissue out of the collection device to prevent contamination of the specimen. Place a sign in the bathroom as a reminder to save all urine.

➤ Instruct the patient to void all urine into the collection device and then pour the urine into the laboratory collection container. Alternatively, the specimen can be left in the collection device for a health care staff member to add to the laboratory collection container.

Intratest:

Blood:

➤ Direct the patient to breathe normally and to avoid unnecessary movement.

➤ Observe standard precautions and follow the general guidelines in Appendix A. Perform a venipuncture, and collect the specimen in a 5-mL red-top tube.

Urine:

➤ Obtain a clean 3-L urine specimen container, toilet-mounted collection device, and plastic bag (for transport of the specimen container). The specimen must be refrigerated or kept on ice throughout the entire collection period. If an indwelling urinary catheter is in place, the drainage bag must be kept on ice.

➤ If possible, begin the test between 6 and 8 a.m. Collect first voiding and discard. Record the time the specimen was discarded as the beginning of the timed collection period. At the same time the next morning, ask the patient to void and add this last voiding to the container.

➤ If an indwelling catheter is in place, replace the tubing and container system at the start of the collection time. Keep the container system on ice during the collection period, or empty the urine into a larger container periodically during the collection period; monitor to ensure

continued drainage, and conclude the test the next morning at the same hour the collection started.

➤ At the conclusion of the test, compare the quantity of urine with the urinary output record for the collection. If the specimen contains less than what was recorded as output, some urine may have been discarded, thus invalidating the test.

➤ Observe standard precautions and follow the general guidelines in Appendix A. Label the specimen, and promptly transport it to the laboratory. Include on the label the amount of urine and ingestion of any medications that can affect test results.

Post-test:

➤ Observe venipuncture site for bleeding or hematoma formation. Apply pressure bandage.

➤ Educate the patient regarding the risk of infection related to immunosuppressed inflammatory response and fatigue related to decreased energy production.

➤ Stress the importance of good nutrition, and suggest that the patient meet with a nutritional specialist. Also, stress the importance of following the care plan for medications and follow-up visits.

➤ Recognize anxiety related to test results and offer support. Provide teaching and disease information, as appropriate. Educate the patient regarding access to counseling services.

➤ Evaluate test results in relation to the patient's symptoms and other tests performed. Related laboratory tests include biopsy of the suspect tissue; CD4/CD8 enumeration; complete blood count; creatinine; erythrocyte sedimentation rate; gentamicin; hepatitis serology; HIV-1/HIV-2 serology; immunofixation electrophoresis; immunoglobulins A, G, and M; protein electrophoresis; total protein; tobramycin; and urinalysis.

MUMPS SEROLOGY

● ●

SYNONYMS/ACRONYM: N/A.

SPECIMEN: Serum (1 mL) collected in a red-top tube.

REFERENCE VALUE: (Method: Indirect immunofluorescence) Negative or less than a fourfold increase in titer.

DESCRIPTION: Mumps serology is done to determine the presence of mumps antibody, indicating exposure to or active presence of mumps. Mumps, also known as *parotitis,* is an infectious viral disease of the parotid glands caused by a myxovirus that is transmitted by direct contact with or droplets spread from the saliva of an infected person. The incubation period averages 3 weeks. Virus can be shed in saliva for 2 weeks after infection and in urine for 2 weeks after the onset of symptoms. Complications of infection include aseptic meningitis, encephalitis, and inflammation of the testes, ovaries, and pancreas. The presence of immunoglobulin M (IgM) antibodies indicates acute infection. The presence of IgG antibodies indicates current or past infection. ■

INDICATIONS:
- Determine resistance to or protection against the mumps virus by a positive reaction, or susceptibility to mumps by a negative reaction
- Document immunity
- Evaluate mumpslike diseases and differentiate between these and actual mumps

RESULT

> **Positive findings in:** Past or current mumps infection.

CRITICAL VALUES: N/A

INTERFERING FACTORS: N/A

Nursing Implications and Procedure ● ● ● ● ● ● ● ● ● ● ●

Pretest: ■

➤ Obtain a history of the patient's complaints, including a list of known allergens. Obtain a history of exposure.

➤ Obtain a history of the patient's immune system as well as results of previously performed tests and procedures. For related tests, refer to the immune system table.

➤ Obtain a list of medications the patient is taking, including herbs, nutritional supplements, and nutraceuticals. The requesting health care practitioner and laboratory should be advised if the patient regularly uses these products so that their effects can be taken into consideration when reviewing results.

➤ There are no food, fluid, or medication restrictions unless by medical direction.

➤ Review the procedure with the patient.

➤ Inform the patient that several tests may be necessary to confirm diagnosis. Any individual positive result should be repeated in 7 to 14 days to monitor a change in titer.

➤ Inform the patient that each specimen collection takes approximately 5 to 10 minutes.

Intratest:

➤ Direct the patient to breathe normally and to avoid unnecessary movement.

➤ Observe standard precautions and follow the general guidelines in Appendix A. Perform a venipuncture, and collect the specimen in a 5-mL red-top tube.

➤ Label the specimen, and promptly transport it to the laboratory.

Post-test:

➤ Observe venipuncture site for bleeding or hematoma formation. Apply pressure bandage.

➤ Instruct the patient in isolation precautions during the time of communicability or contagion.

➤ Emphasize that the patient must return to have a convalescent blood sample taken in 7 to 14 days.

➤ Inform the patient that the presence of mumps antibodies ensures lifetime immunity.

➤ Evaluate test results in relation to the patient's symptoms and other tests performed.

MYOCARDIAL INFARCT SCAN

SYNONYMS/ACRONYM: PYP cardiac scan, infarct scan, pyrophosphate cardiac scan, acute myocardial infarction scan.

AREA OF APPLICATION: Heart, chest/thorax.

CONTRAST: Intravenous contrast medium.

DESCRIPTION: Technetium-99m stannous pyrophosphate (PYP) scanning, also known as *myocardial infarct imaging,* reveals the presence of myocardial perfusion and the extent of myocardial infarction (MI). This procedure can distinguish new from old infarct when a patient has had abnormal electrocardiograms (ECGs) and cardiac enzymes have returned to normal. PYP uptake by acutely infarcted tissue may be related to the influx of calcium through damaged cell membranes, which accompanies myocardial necrosis; that is, the radionuclide may be binding to calcium phosphates or to hydroxyapatite. The PYP in these damaged cells can be viewed as spots of increased radionuclide uptake that appear in 12 hours at the earliest.

PYP uptake usually takes place 24 to 72 hours after MI, and the radionuclide remains detectable for approximately 10 to 14 days after the MI. PYP uptake is proportional to the blood flow to the affected area; with large areas of necrosis, PYP uptake may be maximal around the periphery of a necrotic area, with little uptake being detectable in the poorly perfused center. Most of the PYP is concentrated in regions that have 20 to 40 percent of the normal blood flow.

Single-photon emission computed tomography (SPECT) can be used to visualize the heart from multiple angles and planes, enabling areas of MI to be viewed with greater accuracy and resolution. This technique removes overlying structures that may confuse interpretation of the results. With the availability of assays of troponins, myocardial infarct imaging has become less important in the diagnosis of acute MI. ▪

INDICATIONS:
- Aid in the diagnosis of (or confirm and locate) acute MI when ECG and enzyme testing do not provide a diagnosis

- Evaluate possible reinfarction or extension of the infarct

- Obtain baseline information about infarction before cardiac surgery

- Aid in the diagnosis of perioperative MI

- Differentiate between a new and old infarction

RESULT

Normal Findings:
- Normal coronary blood flow and tissue perfusion, with no PYP localization in the myocardium

- No uptake above background activity in the myocardium (*note:* when PYP

uptake is present, it is graded in relation to adjacent rib activity)

Abnormal Findings:
- MI, indicated by increased PYP uptake in the myocardium

CRITICAL VALUES: N/A

INTERFERING FACTORS:

This procedure is contraindicated for:
- Patients who are pregnant or suspected of being pregnant, unless the potential benefits of the procedure far outweigh the risk of radiation exposure to the fetus

- Patients with hypersensitivity to the radionuclide.

Factors that may impair clear imaging:
- Inability of the patient to cooperate or remain still during the procedure because of age, significant pain, or mental status

- Conditions such as chest wall trauma, cardiac trauma, or recent cardioversion procedure

- Myocarditis

- Pericarditis

- Left ventricular aneurysm

- Metastasis

- Valvular and coronary artery calcifications

- Cardiac neoplasms

- Aneurysms

Nursing Implications and Procedure • • • • • • • • • • •

Pretest: ▇

➤ Inform the patient that the procedure assesses blood flow to the heart.

➤ Inform the patient that the procedure is performed in a special department by a technologist and takes approximately 30 to 60 minutes for each set of images; the patient may be imaged several times, hours apart.

➤ Obtain a history of allergies or sensitivities to contrast medium.

➤ Obtain a list of medications the patient is taking.

➤ Obtain a history of cardiac tests, other diagnostic procedure results, laboratory test results, present cardiac conditions or abnormalities, and therapy received for cardiac conditions. For related tests, refer to the cardiovascular system table.

➤ Determine date of last menstrual period and possibility of pregnancy in perimenopausal women.

➤ Reassure the patient that the radioactive material poses no radioactive hazard and rarely produces side effects.

➤ Restrict food for 4 hours, nicotine for 4 to 6 hours, and medications for 24 hours before the procedure.

Intratest:

➤ Ensure that emergency equipment is readily available during the procedure.

➤ Ask the patient to void before the procedure. Have the patient put on a hospital gown.

➤ Inform the patient that movement during the procedure affects the results and makes interpretation difficult.

➤ Images of the patient's heart begin 2 to 4 hours after injection of the radionuclide.

➤ Images of the heart are taken from a minimum of three angles: anterior, left anterior oblique, and left lateral. In most circumstances, however, SPECT is done so that the heart can be viewed from multiple angles and planes.

Post-test:

➤ Instruct the patient to resume normal activity and diet, unless otherwise indicated.

➤ If the patient must return for additional imaging, advise the patient to rest in the interim and restrict diet to liquids before redistribution studies.

➤ Observe the injection site for redness, swelling, or hematoma.

➤ Advise patient to drink increased amounts of fluids for 24 to 48 hours to eliminate the radionuclide from the body, unless contraindicated. Tell the patient that radionuclide is eliminated from the body within 6 to 24 hours.

➤ Observe patient for up to 60 minutes after the study for a possible anaphylactic reaction to the radionuclide, such as rash, tightening of throat, or difficulty breathing.

➤ Instruct the patient to flush the toilet immediately after each voiding following the procedure and to wash hands meticulously with soap and water after each voiding for 24 hours after the procedure.

➤ Tell all caregivers to wear gloves when discarding urine for 24 hours after the procedure. Wash gloved hands with soap and water before removing gloves. Then wash hands after the gloves are removed.

➤ A physician specializing in this branch of medicine sends a written report to the ordering provider, who discusses the results with the patient.

➤ Evaluate test results in relation to the patient's symptoms and other tests performed. Related diagnostic tests include electrocardiogram, echocardiogram, myocardial perfusion scan, and computed tomography and magnetic resonance imaging of the chest.

MYOCARDIAL PERFUSION HEART SCAN

SYNONYMS/ACRONYM: Thallium scan, sestamibi scan, stress thallium.

AREA OF APPLICATION: Heart, chest/thorax.

CONTRAST: Intravenous contrast medium.

DESCRIPTION: Cardiac scanning is a nuclear medicine study that reveals clinical information about coronary blood flow, ventricular size, and cardiac function. Thallium-201 chloride rest or stress studies are used to evaluate myocardial blood flow to assist in diagnosing or determining the risk for ischemic cardiac disease, coronary artery disease (CAD), and myocardial infarction (MI). This procedure is an alternative to angiography or cardiac catheterization in cases where these procedures may pose a risk to the patient. Thallium-201 is a potassium analogue and is taken up by myocardial cells proportional to blood flow to the cell and cell viability. During stress studies, the radionuclide is injected at peak exercise, after which the patient continues to exercise for several minutes. During exercise, areas of heart muscle supplied by normal arteries increase their blood supply, as well as the supply of thallium-201 delivery to the heart muscle, to a greater extent than regions of the heart muscle supplied by stenosed coronary arteries. This discrepancy in blood flow becomes apparent and quantifiable in subsequent imaging. Comparison of early stress images with 3 to 4 hours' redistribution (delayed images) enables differentiation between normally perfused, healthy myocardium (which is normal at rest but ischemic on stress) and infarcted myocardium.

Technetium-99m agents such as sestamibi (2-methoxyisobutylisonitrile) are delivered similarly to thallium-201 during myocardial perfusion imaging, but they are extracted to a lesser degree on the first pass through the heart and are taken up by the mitochondria. Over a short period, the radionuclide concentrates in the heart to the same degree as thallium-201. The advantage to technetium-99m agents is that immediate imaging is unnecessary because the radionuclide remains fixed to the heart muscle for several hours. The examination requires two separate injections, one for the rest portion and one for the stress portion of the procedure. These injections can take place on the same day or preferably over a 2-day period. Examination quality is improved if the patient is given a light, fatty meal after the radionuclide is injected to facilitate hepatobiliary clearance of the radioactivity. If stress testing cannot be performed by exercising, dipyridamole (Persantine) or adenosine, a vasodilator, can be administered orally or intravenously. A coronary vasodilator is administered before the thallium-201, or other radionuclide, and the scanning procedure is then performed. Vasodilators increase blood flow in normal coronary arteries twofold to threefold without exercise, and they reveal perfusion defects when blood flow is compromised by vessel pathology. Vasodilator-mediated myocardial perfusion scanning is reserved for patients who are unable to participate in treadmill, bicycle, or handgrip exercises for stress testing because of lung disease, neurologic disorders (e.g., multiple sclerosis, spinal cord injury), morbid obesity, and orthopedic disorders (e.g., arthritis, limb amputation). Single photon emission computed tomography (SPECT) can be used to visualize the heart from multiple angles and planes, enabling areas of MI to be viewed with greater accuracy and resolution. This technique removes overlying structures that may confuse interpretation of the results. ∎

INDICATIONS:

- Aid in the diagnosis of or risk for CAD

- Evaluate the extent of CAD and determine cardiac function

- Assess the function of collateral coronary arteries

- Evaluate bypass graft patency and general cardiac status after surgery

- Evaluate the site of an old MI to determine obstruction to cardiac muscle perfusion

- Determine rest defects and reperfusion with delayed imaging in unstable angina

- Evaluate the effectiveness of medication regimen and balloon angioplasty procedure on narrow coronary arteries

RESULT

Normal Findings:

- Normal wall motion, coronary blood flow, tissue perfusion, and ventricular size and function

Abnormal Findings:

- Abnormal stress images with normal resting images, indicating transient ischemia

- Abnormal stress and resting images, indicating previous MI

- Cardiac hypertrophy, indicated by increased radionuclide uptake in the myocardium

- Enlarged left ventricle

- Heart chamber disorder

- Ventricular septal defects

CRITICAL VALUES: N/A

INTERFERING FACTORS:

This procedure is contraindicated for:

- Patients who are pregnant or suspected of being pregnant, unless the potential benefits of the procedure far outweigh the risk of radiation exposure to the fetus

- Patients with hypersensitivity to the radionuclide

- Patients with left ventricular hypertrophy, right and left bundle-branch block, or hypokalemia, and patients receiving cardiotonic therapy

- Patients with anginal pain at rest or patients with severe atherosclerotic coronary vessels, in whom dipyridamole testing cannot be performed

- Patients with asthma, because chemical stress with vasodilators can cause bronchospasms

Factors that may impair clear imaging:

- Inability of the patient to cooperate or

remain still during the procedure because of age, significant pain, or mental status

- Medications such as digitalis and quinidine, which can alter cardiac contractility; and nitrates, which can affect cardiac performance

- Single-vessel disease, which can produce false-negative thallium-201 scanning results

- Conditions such as chest wall or cardiac trauma, angina that is difficult to control, significant cardiac arrhythmias, and recent cardioversion procedure

- Suboptimal cardiac stress or patient exhaustion preventing maximum heart rate testing

- Excessive eating or exercising between initial and redistribution imaging 4 hours later, which produces false-positive results

- Improper adjustment of the radiologic equipment to accommodate obese or thin patients, which can cause overexposure or underexposure and a poor-quality study

- Patients who are very obese, who may exceed the weight limit for the equipment

- Incorrect positioning of the patient, which may produce poor visualization of the area to be examined

- Metallic objects within the examination field (e.g., jewelry or body rings), which may inhibit organ visualization and can produce unclear images

Other considerations:

- Failure to follow dietary restrictions before the procedure may cause the procedure to be canceled or repeated.

- Improper injection of the radionuclide that allows the tracer to seep deep into the muscle tissue produces erroneous hot spots.

- Inaccurate timing for imaging after radionuclide injection can affect the results.

- Consultation with a physician should occur before the procedure for radiation safety concerns regarding infants of patients who are lactating.

- Risks associated with radiographic overexposure can result from frequent x-ray procedures. Personnel in the room with the patient should wear a protective lead apron, stand behind a shield, or leave the area while the examination is being done. Personnel working in the area where the examination is being done should wear badges that reveal their level of exposure to radiation.

Nursing Implications and Procedure · · · · · · · · · ·

Pretest: ■

➤ Inform the patient that the procedure assesses blood flow to the heart.

➤ Inform the patient that the procedure is performed in a special department by a technologist and takes approximately 30 to 60 minutes for each rest and stress part of the examination.

➤ Obtain a history of allergies or sensitivities to contrast medium.

➤ Obtain a list of medications the patient is taking.

➤ Obtain a history of cardiac tests, other diagnostic procedure results, laboratory test results, present cardiac conditions or abnormalities, and therapy received for cardiac conditions. For related tests, refer to the cardiovascular system table.

➤ Determine date of last menstrual period and possibility of pregnancy in perimenopausal women.

➤ Reassure the patient that radioactive material poses no radioactive hazard and rarely produces side effects.

➤ *Obtain a written, informed consent*

before administering any medications prior to the procedure.

➤ Tell the patient to wear walking shoes for treadmill exercise, and emphasize the importance of the patient reporting fatigue, pain, or shortness of breath.

➤ Restrict food for 4 hours, nicotine for 4 to 6 hours, and medications for 24 hours before the test.

➤ Establish an intravenous access before the procedure.

➤ Obtain and record baseline vital signs and electrocardiographic (ECG) tracings.

Intratest:

➤ Ensure that emergency equipment is readily available during the procedure.

➤ Ask the patient to void before the procedure. Have the patient put on a hospital gown.

➤ Make sure jewelry, chains, and any other metallic objects have been removed from the chest area.

➤ Expose the chest, and attach the ECG leads for simultaneous tracings; apply a blood pressure cuff.

➤ Assist the patient onto the treadmill or bicycle ergometer and ask the patient to exercise to a calculated 80 to 85 percent of the maximum heart rate, as determined by the protocol selected.

➤ Thallium-201 is injected 60 to 90 seconds before exercise is terminated, and imaging is done immediately in the supine position and repeated in 4 hours.

➤ Patients who cannot exercise are given dipyridamole 4 minutes before thallium-201 is injected.

➤ Inform the patient that movement during the procedure affects the results and makes interpretation difficult.

Post-test:

➤ Instruct the patient to resume normal activity, medications, and diet, unless otherwise indicated. If the patient must return for further thallium-201 imaging, advise the patient to rest in the interim and to restrict diet to liquids before redistribution studies.

➤ Evaluate the patient's vital signs. Observe the patient for 60 minutes after the procedure for possible reaction to the radionuclide or for complications from the exercise.

➤ Monitor ECG tracings and compare with baseline readings until stable.

➤ Observe the injection site for redness, swelling, or hematoma.

➤ Advise patient to drink increased amounts of fluids for 24 to 48 hours to eliminate the radionuclide from the body, unless contraindicated. Tell the patient that radionuclide is eliminated from the body within 6 to 24 hours.

➤ Instruct the patient to flush the toilet immediately after each voiding following the procedure and to wash hands meticulously with soap and water after each voiding for 24 hours after the procedure.

➤ Tell all caregivers to wear gloves when discarding urine for 24 hours after the procedure. Wash gloved hands with soap and water before removing gloves. Then wash hands after the gloves are removed.

➤ A physician specializing in this branch of medicine sends a written report to the ordering provider, who discusses the results with the patient.

➤ Inform the patient that abnormalities found of the heart scan may indicate the need for further procedures, including cardiac catheterization.

➤ Evaluate test results in relation to the patient's symptoms and other tests performed. Related diagnostic tests include echocardiogram, computed tomography and magnetic resonance imaging of the chest, ECG, and Holter monitoring.

MYOGLOBIN

. . . .

SYNONYM/ACRONYM: MB.

SPECIMEN: Serum (1 mL) collected in a red- or tiger-top tube.

REFERENCE VALUE: (Method: Nephelometry)

Conventional Units	SI Units (Conversion Factor ×1)
5–70 µg/dL	5–70 µg/dL

DESCRIPTION: Myoglobin is an oxygen-binding muscle protein normally found in skeletal and cardiac muscle. It is released into the bloodstream after muscle damage from ischemia, trauma, or inflammation. Although myoglobin testing is more sensitive than creatinine kinase and isoenzymes, it does not indicate the specific site involved. ■

INDICATIONS:
• Assist in predicting a flare-up of polymyositis
• Estimate damage from skeletal muscle injury or myocardial infarction

RESULT

Increased in:
• Cardiac surgery
• Cocaine use
• Exercise
• Malignant hyperthermia
• Myocardial infarction
• Progressive muscular dystrophy
• Renal failure

• Rhabdomyolysis
• Shock
• Thrombolytic therapy

Decreased in:
• Myasthenia gravis
• Presence of antibodies to myoglobin as seen in patients with polymyositis
• Rheumatoid arthritis

CRITICAL VALUES: N/A

INTERFERING FACTORS: N/A

Nursing Implications and Procedure . . . .

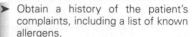

Pretest:

➤ Obtain a history of the patient's complaints, including a list of known allergens.

➤ Obtain a history of the patient's cardiovascular and musculoskeletal system as well as results of previously performed tests and procedures. For related tests, refer to the cardiovascular and musculoskeletal system tables.

➤ Obtain a list of medications the patient is taking, including herbs, nutritional supplements, and nutraceuticals. The requesting health care practitioner and laboratory should be advised if the patient regularly uses these products so that their effects can be taken into consideration when reviewing results.

➤ There are no food, fluid, or medication restrictions unless by medical direction.

➤ Review the procedure with the patient.

➤ Inform the patient that specimen collection takes approximately 5 to 10 minutes.

Intratest:

➤ Direct the patient to breathe normally and to avoid unnecessary movement.

➤ Observe standard precautions and

follow the general guidelines in Appendix A. Perform a venipuncture, and collect the specimen in a 5-mL red- or tiger-top tube.

➤ Label the specimen, and promptly transport it to the laboratory.

Post-test:

➤ Observe venipuncture site for bleeding or hematoma formation. Apply pressure bandage.

➤ Evaluate test results in relation to the patient's symptoms and other tests performed. Related laboratory tests include apolipoprotein A and B; muscle biopsy; C-reactive protein; high-density, low-density, and very-low-density lipoprotein cholesterol; chylomicrons; triglycerides; creatine kinase and isoenzymes; homocysteine, lactate dehydrogenase and isoenzymes; lipoprotein electrophoresis; magnesium; and troponin.

OSMOLALITY, SERUM AND URINE

· ·

SYNONYM/ACRONYM: Osmo.

SPECIMEN: Serum (1 mL) collected in a red- or tiger-top tube; urine (5 mL) from an unpreserved random specimen collected in a clean, plastic collection container.

REFERENCE VALUE: (Method: Freezing point depression)

	Conventional Units	SI Units (Conversion Factor ×1)
Serum	275–295 mOsm/kg	275–295 mmol/kg
Urine		
Newborn	75–300 mOsm/kg	75–300 mmol/kg
Children	250–900 mOsm/kg	250–900 mmol/kg
and adults		

DESCRIPTION: Osmolality refers to the number of particles in solution; it is independent of particle size, shape, and charge. Measurement of osmotic concentration in serum provides clinically useful information about water and dissolved-particle transport across fluid compartment membranes. Osmolality is used to assist in the diagnosis of metabolic, renal, and endocrine disorders. The simultaneous determination of serum and urine osmolality provides the opportunity to compare values between the two fluids. A normal urine-to-serum ratio is approximately 0.2 to 4.7 for random samples and greater than 3.0 for first-morning samples (dehydration normally occurs overnight). The major dissolved particles that contribute to osmolality are sodium, chloride, bicarbonate, urea, and glucose. Some of these substances are used in the following calculated estimate:

$$\text{Serum osmolality} = \{[2\ (Na^+)] + [glucose/18] + [BUN/2.8]\}$$

Measured osmolality is higher than the estimated value. The osmolal gap is the difference between the measured and calculated values and is normally 5 to 10 mOsm/kg. If the difference is greater than 15 mOsm/kg, consider ethylene glycol, isopropanol, methanol, or ethanol toxicity. These substances behave like antifreeze, lowering the freezing point in the blood, and provide misleadingly high results. ■

INDICATIONS

Serum:
- Assist in the evaluation of antidiuretic hormone (ADH) function

- Assist in rapid screening for toxic substances, such as ethylene glycol, ethanol, isopropanol, and methanol
- Evaluate electrolyte and acid-base balance
- Evaluate state of hydration

Urine:
- Evaluate concentrating ability of the kidneys
- Evaluate diabetes insipidus
- Evaluate neonatal patients with protein or glucose in the urine
- Perform workup for renal disease

RESULT

Increased in:
- Serum:
  Azotemia
  Dehydration
  Diabetes insipidus
  Diabetic ketoacidosis
  Hypercalcemia
  Hypernatremia

- Urine:
  Amyloidosis
  Azotemia
  Congestive heart failure
  Dehydration
  Hyponatremia
  Syndrome of inappropriate antidiuretic hormone production (SIADH)

Decreased in:
- Serum:
  Adrenocorticoid insufficiency
  Hyponatremia
  SIADH
  Water intoxication

- Urine:
  Diabetes insipidus
  Hypokalemia

Hypernatremia

Primary polydipsia

CRITICAL VALUES: Serum:

Less than 265 mOsm/kg

Greater than 320 mOsm/kg

Serious clinical conditions may be associated with elevated or decreased serum osmolality. The following conditions are associated with elevated serum osmolality:

Respiratory arrest: 360 mOsm/kg

Stupor of hyperglycemia: 385 mOsm/kg

Grand mal seizures: 420 mOsm/kg

Death: greater than 420mOsm/kg

Symptoms of critically high levels include poor skin turgor, listlessness, acidosis (decreased pH), shock, seizures, coma, and cardiopulmonary arrest. Intervention may include close monitoring of electrolytes, administering intravenous fluids with the appropriate composition to shift water either in or out of the intravascular space as needed, monitoring cardiac signs, continuing neurologic checks, and taking seizure precautions.

INTERFERING FACTORS:

- Drugs that may increase serum osmolality include citrates (as an anticoagulant), corticosteroids, ethylene glycol, glycerin, inulin, ioxithalamic acid, mannitol, and methoxyflurane.

- Drugs that may decrease serum osmolality include bendroflumethiazide, carbamazepine, chlorpromazine, chlorthalidone, cyclophosphamide, cyclothiazide, hydrochlorothiazide, lorcainide, methyclothiazide, and polythiazide.

- Drugs that may increase urine osmolality include anesthetic agents, chlorpropamide, cyclophosphamide, furosemide, mannitol, metolazone, octreotide, phloridzin, and vincristine.

- Drugs that may decrease urine osmolality include captopril, demeclocycline, glyburide, lithium, methoxyflurane, octreotide, tolazamide, and verapamil.

Nursing Implications and Procedure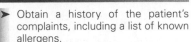

Pretest:

➤ Obtain a history of the patient's complaints, including a list of known allergens.

➤ Obtain a history of the patient's endocrine and genitourinary systems, as well as results of previously performed tests and procedures. For related tests, refer to the endocrine and genitourinary system tables.

➤ Obtain a list of the medications the patient is taking, including herbs, nutritional supplements, and nutraceuticals. The requesting health care practitioner and laboratory should be advised if the patient regularly uses these products so that their effects can be taken into consideration when reviewing results.

➤ There are no food, fluid, or medication restrictions unless by medical direction.

➤ Review the procedure with the patient.

➤ Inform the patient that specimen collection takes approximately 5 to 10 minutes.

Intratest:

➤ Direct the patient to breathe normally and to avoid unnecessary movement. Observe standard precautions and follow the general guidelines in Appendix A.

Blood:

➤ Perform a venipuncture, and collect the specimen in a 5-mL red-top tube.

Urine:

➤ Review the procedure with the

patient. Provide a nonmetallic urinal, bedpan, or toilet-mounted collection device.

➤ Either a random specimen or a timed collection may be requested. For timed specimens, a 12- or 24-hour time frame for urine collection may be ordered. Inform the patient that all urine must be saved during that 24-hour period. Instruct the patient not to void directly into the laboratory collection container. Instruct the patient to avoid defecating in the collection device and to keep toilet tissue out of the collection device to prevent contamination of the specimen. Place a sign in the bathroom to remind the patient to save all urine.

➤ Instruct the patient to void all urine into the collection device and then to pour the urine into the laboratory collection container. Alternatively the specimen can be left in the collection device for a health care staff member to add to the laboratory collection container.

Clean-catch specimen:

➤ Instruct the male patient to (1) thoroughly wash his hands, (2) cleanse the meatus, (3) void a small amount into the toilet, and (4) void directly into the specimen container.

➤ Instruct the female patient to (1) thoroughly wash her hands; (2) cleanse the labia from front to back; (3) while keeping the labia separated, void a small amount into the toilet; and (4) without interrupting the urine stream, void directly into the specimen container.

Indwelling catheter:

➤ Put on gloves. Empty drainage tube of urine. It may be necessary to clamp off the catheter for 15 to 30 minutes before specimen collection. Cleanse specimen port with antiseptic swab, and then aspirate 5 mL of urine with a 21- to 25-gauge needle and syringe. Transfer urine to a sterile container.

Blood or urine:

➤ Label the specimen, and promptly transport it to the laboratory.

Post-test:

➤ Observe venipuncture site for bleeding or hematoma formation. Apply pressure bandage.

➤ Decreased osmolality may be associated with overhydration. Observe the patient for signs and symptoms of fluid-volume excess related to excess electrolyte intake, fluid-volume deficit related to active loss, or risk of injury related to an alteration in body chemistry. (For electrolyte-specific dietary references, see monographs titled "Chloride," "Potassium," and "Sodium.")

➤ Increased osmolality may be associated with dehydration. Evaluate the patient for signs and symptoms of dehydration. Dehydration is a significant and common finding in geriatric and other patients in whom renal function has deteriorated.

➤ Evaluate test results in relation to the patient's symptoms and other tests performed. Related laboratory tests include ADH, ammonia, serum and urine creatinine, serum and urine electrolytes, ethanol, ketones, urine ketones, glucose, blood urea nitrogen (BUN), and urine urea nitrogen.

OSMOTIC FRAGILITY

SYNONYM/ACRONYM: Red blood cell osmotic fragility, OF.

SPECIMEN: Whole blood (1 mL) collected in a green-top (heparin) tube and two peripheral blood smears.

REFERENCE VALUE: (Method: Spectrophotometry) Hemolysis begins at 0.5 w/v sodium chloride (NaCl) solution and is complete at 0.3 w/v NaCl solution. Results are compared to a normal curve.

DESCRIPTION: Osmotic fragility (OF) is an indication of the ability of red blood cells (RBCs) to take on water without lysing. In this test, RBCs are placed in graded dilutions of sodium chloride. Swelling of the cells occurs at lower concentrations of NaCl as they take on water in the hypotonic solution. Thicker cells, such as spherocytes, have an increased OF; thinner cells have a decreased OF. ∎

INDICATIONS: Evaluate hemolytic anemia.

RESULT

Increased in:

• Acquired immune hemolytic anemias

• Hemolytic disease of the newborn

• Hereditary spherocytosis

• Malaria

• Pyruvate kinase deficiency

Decreased in:

• Asplenia

• Hemoglobinopathies

• Iron deficiency anemia

• Liver disease

• Reticulocytosis

• Thalassemias

CRITICAL VALUES: N/A

INTERFERING FACTORS:

• Drugs that may increase osmotic fragility include dapsone.

• Parasitic infestations, such as malaria, may independently cause cell hemolysis.

• Specimens should be submitted for analysis immediately after collection.

Nursing Implications and Procedure

Pretest:

➤ Obtain a history of the patient's complaints, including a list of known allergens.

➤ Obtain a history of the patient's hematopoietic system and results of previously performed tests and procedures. For related tests, refer to the hematopoietic system table.

➤ Obtain a list of the medications the patient is taking, including herbs, nutritional supplements, and nutraceuticals. The requesting health care practitioner and laboratory should be advised if the patient regularly uses these products so that their effects can be taken into consideration when reviewing results.

➤ There are no food, fluid, or medication restrictions unless by medical direction.

➤ Review the procedure with the patient.

➤ Inform the patient that specimen collection takes approximately 5 to 10 minutes.

Intratest:

➤ Direct the patient to breathe normally and to avoid unnecessary movement.

➤ Observe standard precautions and follow the general guidelines in Appendix A. Perform a venipuncture, and collect the specimen in a 5-mL green-top tube.

➤ Label the specimen, and promptly transport it to the laboratory.

Post-test:

➤ Observe venipuncture site for bleeding or hematoma formation. Apply pressure bandage.

➤ Evaluate test results in relation to the patient's symptoms and other tests performed. Related laboratory tests include complete blood count, glucose-6-phosphate dehydrogenase, Ham's test, and pyruvate kinase.

OSTEOCALCIN

SYNONYMS/ACRONYMS: Bone GLA protein, BGP.

SPECIMEN: Serum (1 mL) collected in a red-top tube.

REFERENCE VALUE: (Method: Radioimmunoassay)

Age and Sex	Conventional Units	SI Units (Conversion Factor ×1)
Newborn	20–40 ng/mL	20–40 µg/L
1–17 y	2.8–41 ng/mL	2.8–41 µg/L
Adult		
Male	3–13 ng/mL	3–13 µg/L
Female		
Premenopausal	0.4–8.2 ng/mL	0.4–8.2 µg/L
Postmenopausal	1.5–11 ng/mL	1.5–11 µg/L

DESCRIPTION: Osteocalcin is an important bone cell matrix protein and sensitive marker in bone metabolism. It is produced by osteoblasts during the matrix mineralization phase of bone formation and is the most abundant noncollagenous bone cell protein. Synthesis of osteocalcin is dependent on vitamin K. Osteocalcin levels parallel alkaline phosphatase levels. Osteocalcin levels are affected by a number of factors, including the hormone estrogen. Assessment of osteocalcin levels permits indirect measurement of osteoblast activity and bone formation. Because it is released into the bloodstream during bone resorption, there is some question as to whether osteocalcin might also be considered a marker for bone matrix degradation and turnover. ∎

INDICATIONS:

• Assist in the diagnosis of bone cancer

• Evaluate bone disease

• Evaluate bone metabolism

• Monitor effectiveness of estrogen replacement therapy

RESULT

Increased in:

• Adolescents undergoing a growth spurt

• Chronic renal failure

• Hyperthyroidism (primary and secondary)

• Metastatic skeletal disease

• Paget's disease

• Renal osteodystrophy

• Some patients with osteoporosis

Decreased in:

• Growth hormone deficiency

• Pregnancy

• Primary biliary cirrhosis

CRITICAL VALUES: N/A

INTERFERING FACTORS:

• Drugs that may increase calcitonin

levels include anticonvulsants, calcitriol, and estrogens.

• Drugs that may decrease calcitonin levels include glucocorticoids.

• Recent radioactive scans or radiation within 1 week before the serum osteocalcin test can interfere with test results when radioimmunoassay is the test method.

Nursing Implications and Procedure ∙ ∙ ∙ ∙ ∙ ∙ ∙ ∙ ∙ ∙ ∙

Pretest:

➤ Obtain a history of the patient's complaints, including a list of known allergens.

➤ Obtain a history of the patient's musculoskeletal system and results of previously performed tests and procedures. For related tests, refer to the musculoskeletal system table.

➤ Obtain a list of the medications the patient is taking, including herbs, nutritional supplements, and nutraceuticals. The requesting health care practitioner and laboratory should be advised if the patient regularly uses these products so that their effects can be taken into consideration when reviewing results.

➤ Note any recent procedures that can interfere with test results.

➤ There are no food, fluid, or medication restrictions unless by medical direction.

➤ Review the procedure with the patient.

➤ Inform the patient that specimen collection takes approximately 5 to 10 minutes.

Intratest:

➤ Direct the patient to breathe normally and to avoid unnecessary movement.

➤ Observe standard precautions and follow the general guidelines in Appendix A. Perform a venipuncture, and collect the specimen in a 5-mL red-top tube.

➤ Label the specimen, and promptly transport it to the laboratory.

Post-test:

➤ Observe venipuncture site for bleeding or hematoma formation. Apply pressure bandage.

➤ Increased osteocalcin levels may be associated with skeletal disease. Nutritional therapy is indicated for individuals identified as being at high risk for developing osteoporosis. Educate the patient regarding the National Osteoporosis Foundation's guidelines, which include a regular regimen of weight-bearing exercises, limited alcohol intake, avoidance of tobacco products, and adequate dietary intake of vitamin D (400 to 800 IU/day) and calcium (120 mg/day). Dietary calcium can be obtained from animal or plant sources. Milk and milk products, sardines, clams, oysters, salmon, rhubarb, spinach, beet greens, broc-

coli, kale, tofu, legumes, and fortified orange juice are high in calcium. Milk and milk products also contain vitamin D and lactose, which assist calcium absorption. Cooked vegetables yield more absorbable calcium than raw vegetables. Patients should be informed of the substances that can inhibit calcium absorption by irreversibly binding to some of the calcium, making it unavailable for absorption, such as oxalates, which naturally occur in some vegetables; phytic acid, found in some cereals; and insoluble dietary fiber (in excessive amounts). Excessive protein intake can also negatively affect calcium absorption, especially if it is combined with foods high in phosphorus. Vitamin D is synthesized by the skin and is also available in fortified dairy foods and cod liver oil.

➤ Evaluate test results in relation to the patient's symptoms and other tests performed. Related laboratory tests include alkaline phosphatase, calcium, urine calcium, phosphorus, collagen crosslinked N-telopeptides, parathyroid hormone, phosphorus, and vitamin D.

OVA AND PARASITES, STOOL

· ·

SYNONYM/ACRONYM: O & P.

SPECIMEN: Stool collected in a clean plastic, tightly capped container.

REFERENCE VALUE: (Method: Macroscopic and microscopic examination) No presence of parasites, ova, or larvae.

DESCRIPTION: This test evaluates stool for the presence of intestinal parasites and their eggs. Some para-

sites are nonpathogenic; others, such as protozoa and worms, can cause serious illness. ∎

INDICATIONS: Assist in the diagnosis of parasitic infestation

RESULT

Positive findings in:

- Amebiasis—*Entamoeba histolytica* infection
- Ascariasis—*Ascaris lumbricoides* infection
- Blastocystis—*Blastocystis hominis* infection
- Cryptosporidiosis—*Cryptosporidium parvum* infection
- Enterobiasis—*Enterobius vermicularis* (pinworm) infection
- Giardiasis—*Giardia lamblia* infection
- Hookworm disease—*Ancylostoma duodenale, Necator americanus* infection
- Isospora—*Isospora belli* infection
- Schistosomiasis—*Schistosoma haematobium, Schistosoma japonicum, Schistosoma mansoni* infection
- Strongyloidiasis—*Strongyloides stercoralis* infection
- Tapeworm disease—*Diphyllobothrium, Hymenolepiasis, Taenia saginata, Taenia solium* infection
- Trematode disease—*Clonorchis sinensis, Fasciola hepatica, Fasciolopsis buski* infection
- Trichuriasis—*Trichuris trichiura* infection

CRITICAL VALUES: N/A

INTERFERING FACTORS:
- Failure to test a fresh specimen may yield a false-negative result.
- Antimicrobial or antiamebic therapy within 10 days of test may yield a false-negative result.
- Failure to wait 1 week after a gastrointestinal study using barium or after laxative use can affect test results.

- Medications such as antacids, antibiotics, bismuth, castor oil, antidiarrheal compounds, iron, magnesia, or psyllium fiber (Metamucil) may interfere with analysis.

Nursing Implications and Procedure   • • • • • • • • • •

Pretest: ▮

- ➤ Obtain a history of the patient's complaints, and document any travel to foreign countries. Obtain a list of known allergens.

- ➤ Obtain a history of the patient's gastrointestinal and immune systems, as well as results of previously performed tests and procedures. For related tests, refer to the gastrointestinal and immune system tables.

- ➤ Obtain a list of the medications the patient is taking, including herbs, nutritional supplements, and nutraceuticals. The requesting health care practitioner and laboratory should be advised if the patient regularly uses these products so their effects can be taken into consideration when reviewing results.

- ➤ Instruct the patient to avoid medications that interfere with test results.

- ➤ Note any recent therapies that can interfere with test results.

- ➤ Instruct the patient on handwashing procedures, and inform the patient that the infection may be contagious.

- ➤ There are no food or fluid restrictions unless by medical direction.

- ➤ Review the procedure with the patient. Warn the patient not to contaminate the specimen with urine, toilet paper, or toilet water.

Intratest: ▮

- ➤ Obtain a waterproof specimen container with a tight-fitting lid.

- ➤ Observe standard precautions and follow the general guidelines in Appendix A. Collect a stool specimen directly into the container. If the patient is bedridden, use a clean bedpan and transfer the specimen into the container using a tongue depressor.

➤ Specimens to be examined for the presence of pinworms are collected by the "Scotch tape" method in the morning before bathing or defecation. A small paddle with a piece of cellophane tape (sticky side facing out) is pressed against the perianal area. The tape is placed in a collection container and submitted to determine if ova are present. Sometimes adult worms are observed protruding from the rectum.

➤ Label the specimen, and promptly transport it to the laboratory.

Post-test: ■

➤ Recognize anxiety related to test results and offer support. Educate the patient with positive findings on the transmission of the parasite, as indicated. Provide teaching and information regarding the clinical implications of the test results, as appropriate.

➤ Warn the patient that one negative result does not rule out parasitic infestation and that additional specimens may be required.

➤ Evaluate test results in relation to the patient's symptoms and other tests performed. Related laboratory tests include immunoglobulin E, stool culture, and fecal analysis.

OXALATE, URINE

. . . .

SYNONYM/ACRONYM: N/A.

SPECIMEN: Urine (25 mL) from a timed specimen collected in a clean, plastic collection container with hydrogen chloride (HCl) as a preservative.

REFERENCE VALUE: (Method: Spectrophotometry)

Conventional Units	SI Units (Conversion Factor ×11.4)
0–40 mg/24 h	0–456 μmol/24 h

DESCRIPTION: Oxalate is derived from the metabolism of oxalic acid, glycine, and ascorbic acid. Some individuals with malabsorption disorders absorb and excrete abnormally high amounts of oxalate, resulting in *hyperoxaluria.* Hyperoxaluria may be seen in patients who consume large amounts of animal protein, certain fruits and vegetables, or mega-doses of vitamin C (ascorbic acid). Hyperoxaluria is also associated with ethylene glycol poisoning (oxalic acid is used in cleaning and bleaching agents). Patients who absorb and excrete large amounts of oxalate may form calcium oxalate kidney stones. Simultaneous measurement of serum and urine calcium is often requested. ■

INDICATIONS:

* Assist in the evaluation of patients with ethylene glycol poisoning

* Assist in the evaluation of patients with malabsorption syndromes or patients who have had jejunoileal bypass surgery

* Assist in the evaluation of patients with a history of kidney stones

RESULT

Increased in:

* Bacterial overgrowth

* Biliary tract disease

* Bowel disease

* Celiac disease

* Cirrhosis

* Crohn's disease

* Diabetes

* Ethylene glycol poisoning

* Ileal resection

* Jejunal shunt

* Pancreatic disease

* Primary hereditary hyperoxaluria (rare)

* Pyridoxine (vitamin B_6) deficiency

* Sarcoidosis

Decreased in:

* Hypercalciuria

* Renal failure

CRITICAL VALUES: N/A

INTERFERING FACTORS:

* Drugs and vitamins that may increase oxalate levels include methoxyflurane, ascorbic acid, and calcium.

* Drugs that may decrease oxalate levels include nifedipine and pyridoxine.

Nursing Implications and Procedure

Pretest:

➤ Obtain a history of the patient's complaints, including a list of known allergens.

➤ Obtain a history of the patient's gastrointestinal and genitourinary systems, as well as results of previously performed tests and procedures. For related tests, refer to the gastrointestinal and genitourinary system tables.

➤ Obtain a list of the medications the patient is taking, including herbs, nutritional supplements and nutraceuticals. The requesting health care practitioner and laboratory should be advised if the patient regularly uses these products so that their effects can be taken into consideration when reviewing results.

➤ There are no fluid restrictions unless by medical direction.

➤ Calcium supplements, gelatin, rhubarb, spinach, strawberries, tomatoes, and vitamin C should be restricted for at least 24 hours before the test. High-protein meals should also be avoided 24 hours before specimen collection.

➤ Review the procedure with the patient. Provide a nonmetallic urinal, bedpan, or toilet-mounted collection device.

➤ Usually a 24-hour time frame for urine collection is ordered. Inform the patient that all urine must be saved during that 24-hour period. Instruct the patient not to void directly into the laboratory collection container. Instruct the patient to avoid defecating in the collection device and to keep toilet tissue out of the collection device to prevent contamination of the specimen. Place a sign in the bathroom to remind the patient to save all urine.

➤ Instruct the patient to void all urine into the collection device and then to pour the urine into the laboratory collection container. Alternatively the specimen can be left in the collection device for a health care staff member to add to the laboratory collection container.

➤ Ensure that the patient has complied with dietary preparations and other pretesting restrictions.

➤ Observe standard precautions and follow the general guidelines in Appendix A.

Random specimen (collect in early morning):

Clean-catch specimen:

➤ Instruct the male patient to (1) thoroughly wash his hands, (2) cleanse the meatus, (3) void a small amount into the toilet, and (4) void directly into the specimen container.

➤ Instruct the female patient to (1) thoroughly wash her hands; (2) cleanse the labia from front to back; (3) while keeping the labia separated, void a small amount into the toilet; and (4) without interrupting the urine stream, void directly into the specimen container.

Timed specimen:

➤ Obtain a clean 3-L urine specimen container, toilet-mounted collection device, and plastic bag (for transport of the specimen container). The specimen must be refrigerated or kept on ice throughout the entire collection period. If an indwelling urinary catheter is in place, the drainage bag must be kept on ice.

➤ Begin the test between 6 and 8 a.m., if possible. Collect first voiding and discard. Record the time the specimen was discarded as the beginning of the timed collection period. The next morning, ask the patient to void at the same time the

collection was started and add this last voiding to the container.

➤ If an indwelling catheter is in place, replace the tubing and container system at the start of the collection time. Keep the container system on ice during the collection period, or empty the urine into a larger container periodically during the collection period; monitor to ensure continued drainage, and conclude the test the next morning at the same hour the collection was begun.

➤ At the conclusion of the test, compare the quantity of urine with the urinary output record for the collection; if the specimen contains less than what was recorded as output, some urine may have been discarded, invalidating the test.

➤ Label the specimen, and promptly transport it to the laboratory. Include on the label the amount of urine, test start and stop times, and ingestion of any foods or medications that can affect test results.

➤ Instruct the patient to resume usual diet and medication as directed by the requesting health care practitioner. Consideration may be given to lessen dietary intake of oxalate if urine levels are increased. Encourage patients with abnormal results to seek advice regarding dietary modifications from a trained nutritionist. Magnesium supplementation may be recommended for patients with gastrointestinal disease to prevent the development of calcium oxalate kidney stones.

➤ Evaluate test results in relation to the patient's symptoms and other tests performed. Related laboratory tests include serum and urine calcium, kidney stone analysis, serum and urine magnesium, urine uric acid, urinalysis, and vitamin C.

PAPANICOLAOU SMEAR

- -

SYNONYMS/ACRONYM: Pap smear, cervical smear.

SPECIMEN: Cervical and endocervical cells.

REFERENCE VALUE: (Method: Microscopic examination of fixed and stained smear) Reporting of Pap smear findings may follow one of several formats and may vary from laboratory to laboratory. Simplified content of the two most common formats for interpretation are listed.

Traditional Method	Description
Class I	Normal cells only
Class II	Atypical cells but not malignant or inflammatory
Class III	Atypical cells suspicious of malignancy/mild cervical dysplasia
Class IV	Atypical cells suggestive of malignancy/severe cervical dysplasia
Class V	Cancerous cells conclusive for malignancy

Bethesda System	Description
Adequacy of the specimen	Satisfactory
	Satisfactory but limited by lack of required patient information, contamination, or poor technique, which prevents evaluation of 50–70% of the cells
	Unsatisfactory—should be rejected and recollected
General interpretation	Within normal limits
	Benign cellular changes
	Cellular abnormality
Descriptive diagnoses	
Benign cellular changes	Infection or reactive changes
Epithelial cell abnormalities	Graded squamous and glandular cell description
	Description of other malignant neoplasms
	Hormonal evaluation (vaginal smears only)

DESCRIPTION: The Papanicolaou (Pap) smear is primarily used for the early detection of cervical cancer. The interpretation of Pap smears is as heavily dependent on the collection and fixation technique as it is on the completeness and accuracy of the clinical information provided with the specimen. The patient's age, date of last menstrual period, parity, surgical status, postmenopausal status, hormone therapy (including use of oral contraceptives), history of radiation or chemotherapy, abnormal vaginal bleeding, and history of previous Pap smears are essential for proper interpretation.

Improvements in specimen preparation have added to the increased quality of screening procedures. The Cytyc ThinPrep PapTest (Cytyc Corporation, Boxborough, MA), approved by the U.S. Food and Drug Administration in 1996, is a technique that provides a uniform monolayer of cells free of debris such as blood and mucus. Computerized scanning systems are also being used to reduce the number of smears that require manual review by a cytotechnologist or pathologist. ∎

INDICATIONS:
- Assist in the diagnosis of cervical dysplasia
- Assist in the diagnosis of endometriosis, condyloma, and vaginal adenosis
- Assist in the diagnosis of genital infections (herpes, *Candida* spp., *Trichomonas vaginalis*, cytomegalovirus, *Chlamydia*, lymphogranuloma venereum, human papillomavirus, and *Actinomyces* spp.
- Assist in the diagnosis of primary and metastatic neoplasms
- Evaluate hormonal function

RESULT

Positive findings in: (See table [Bethesda system], listed earlier under "Reference value")

Decreased in: N/A

CRITICAL VALUES: N/A

INTERFERING FACTORS:
- The smear should not be allowed to air dry before fixation.

- Lubricating jelly should not be used on the speculum.

- Improper collection site may result in specimen rejection. Samples for cancer screening are obtained from the posterior vaginal fornix and from the cervix. Samples for hormonal evaluation are obtained from the vagina.

- Contamination with blood from samples collected during the patient's menstrual period may be cause for specimen rejection.

Nursing Implications and Procedure

Pretest:

➤ Obtain a history of the patient's complaints, including a list of known allergens.

➤ Obtain a history of the patient's immune and reproductive systems, as well as results of previously performed tests and procedures. For related tests, refer to the immune and reproductive system table.

➤ Obtain a list of the medications the patient is taking, including herbs, nutritional supplements, and nutraceuticals. The requesting health care practitioner and laboratory should be advised if the patient regularly uses these products so that their effects can be taken into consideration when reviewing results.

➤ There are no food or fluid restrictions unless by medical direction.

➤ If the patient is taking vaginal antibiotic medication, testing should be delayed for 1 month after the treatment has been completed.

➤ Review the procedure with the patient. Sensitivity to cultural and social issues, as well as concern for modesty, is important in providing psychological support.

➤ Instruct the patient to avoid douching or sexual intercourse for 24 hours before specimen collection. Verify that the patient is not menstruating.

➤ Instruct the patient to void before specimen collection.

➤ Inform the patient that specimen collection takes approximately 5 to 10 minutes.

Intratest:

➤ Position the patient on the gynecologic examination table with the feet in stirrups. Drape the patient's legs to provide privacy and reduce chilling.

➤ Direct the patient to breathe normally and to avoid unnecessary movement.

➤ Observe standard precautions and follow the general guidelines in Appendix A.

Conventional collection:

➤ The speculum may be dipped in warm water to aid in comfortable insertion. After the speculum is properly positioned, the specimen is obtained (using a wooden spatula, cotton-tipped applicator, or synthetic fiber brush) and smeared onto slides. The speculum is removed, and the slides are immediately fixed with a liquid or spray containing 95% ethanol. A pelvic and/or rectal examination may be performed, if necessary, after specimen collection.

ThinPrep collection:

➤ The specimen is obtained using a special broomlike device. The central bristles of the device are inserted deep enough into the endocervical canal to allow the bristles to contact the ectocervix. The device is rotated five times in a clockwise direction, and then removed and rinsed in a special solution vial. The device is pushed against the bottom of the solution vial 10 times and then vigorously swirled to detach the cells brushed from the patient's tissue.

General:

➤ Label the specimen, and promptly transport it to the laboratory.

Post-test:

➤ Cleanse or allow the patient to clean secretions or excess lubricant (if a pelvic and/or rectal examination is also performed) from the perineal area. Provide a sanitary pad if cervical bleeding occurs.

➤ Inform the patient, as appropriate, that repeat testing may be requested in the event of specimen rejection or abnormal findings.

➤ Recognize anxiety related to test results and offer support. Provide teaching and information regarding the clinical implications of the test results, as appropriate. Educate the patient regarding access to counseling services.

➤ Inform the patient that women aged 20 to 40 should have a Pap smear *at least* every 3 years; women older than 40 should have a Pap smear annually. Women at risk (e.g., with a positive family history of cervical cancer) may need to have more frequent Pap smears.

➤ Evaluate test results in relation to the patient's symptoms and other tests performed. Related laboratory tests include *Chlamydia*, related cultures, and cervical biopsy.

PARATHYROID HORMONE: INTACT, C-TERMINAL, AND N-TERMINAL

SYNONYM/ACRONYM: Parathormone, PTH.

SPECIMEN: Serum (1 mL) collected in a red- or tiger-top tube is recommended for C-terminal and N-terminal. Plasma (1 mL) collected in lavender-top (EDTA) tube is recommended for intact PTH. Specimen should be transported tightly capped and in an ice slurry.

REFERENCE VALUE: (Method: Immunoassay)

	Conventional Units	SI Units (Conversion Factor ×1)
C-terminal		
1–16 y	51–217 pg/mL	51–217 ng/L
Adults	50–330 pg/mL	50–330 ng/L
N-terminal		
2–13 y	14–21 pg/mL	14–21 ng/L
Adult	8–24 pg/mL	8–24 ng/L
Intact		
Cord blood	Less than 3 pg/mL	Less than 3 ng/L
2–20 y	9–52 pg/mL	9–52 ng/L
Adult	10–65 pg/mL	10–65 ng/L

DESCRIPTION: Parathyroid hormone (PTH) is secreted by the parathyroid glands in response to decreased levels of circulating calcium. PTH assists in the mobilization of calcium from bone into the bloodstream, promoting renal tubular reabsorption of calcium and depression of phosphate reabsorption, thereby reducing calcium excretion and increasing phosphate excretion by the kidneys. PTH also decreases the renal secretion of hydrogen ions, which leads to increased renal excretion of bicarbonate and chloride. PTH enhances renal production of active vitamin D metabolites, causing increased calcium absorption in the small intestine. The net result of PTH action is maintenance of adequate serum calcium levels. In normal individuals, intact PTH has a circulating half-life of about 5 minutes. N-terminal PTH has a circulating half-life of about 2 minutes and is found in very small quantities. Intact and N-terminal PTH are the only biologically active forms of the hormone. Ninety percent of circulating PTH is composed of inactive C-terminal and midregion fragments. PTH is cleared from the body by the kidneys. ∎

INDICATIONS:

- Assist in the diagnosis of hyperparathyroidism

- Assist in the diagnosis of suspected secondary hyperparathyroidism due to chronic renal failure, malignant tumors that produce ectopic PTH, and malabsorption syndromes

- Detect incidental damage or inadvertent removal of the parathyroid glands during thyroid or neck surgery

- Differentiate parathyroid and nonparathyroid causes of hypercalcemia

- Evaluate autoimmune destruction of the parathyroid glands

- Evaluate parathyroid response to altered serum calcium levels, especially those that result from malignant processes, leading to decreased PTH production

- Evaluate source of altered calcium metabolism

RESULT

Increased in:
- Fluorosis

- Primary, secondary, or tertiary hyperparathyroidism

- Pseudogout

- Pseudohypoparathyroidism

- Spinal cord trauma

- Zollinger-Ellison syndrome

Decreased in:
- Autoimmune destruction of the parathyroids

- DiGeorge syndrome

- Hyperthyroidism

- Hypomagnesemia

- Nonparathyroid hypercalcemia (in the absence of renal failure)

- Sarcoidosis

- Secondary hypoparathyroidism due to surgery

CRITICAL VALUES: N/A

INTERFERING FACTORS:

- Drugs that may increase PTH levels include clodronate, dopamine, estrogen/progestin therapy, foscarnet, furosemide, hydrocortisone, isoniazid, lithium, octreotide, pamidronate, phosphates, prednisone, tamoxifen, and verapamil.

- Drugs and vitamins that may decrease PTH levels include alfacalcidol, aluminum hydroxide, calcitriol, cimetidine (C-terminal only), diltiazem, magnesium sulfate, pindolol, prednisone (intact), and vitamin D.

- PTH levels are subject to diurnal variation, with highest levels occurring in the morning.

- PTH levels should always be measured in conjunction with calcium for proper interpretation.

Nursing Implications and Procedure

Pretest:

➤ Obtain a history of the patient's complaints, including a list of known allergens.

➤ Obtain a history of the patient's endocrine system and results of previously performed tests and procedures. For related tests, refer to the endocrine system table.

➤ Obtain a list of the medications the patient is taking, including herbs, nutritional supplements, and nutraceuticals. The requesting health care practitioner and laboratory should be advised if the patient regularly uses these products so that their effects can be taken into consideration when reviewing results.

➤ The patient should fast for 12 hours before specimen collection.

➤ There are no fluid or medication restrictions unless by medical direction.

➤ Early morning specimen collection is recommended because of the diurnal variation in PTH levels.

➤ Review the procedure with the patient.

➤ Inform the patient that specimen collection takes approximately 5 to 10 minutes.

➤ Prepare an ice slurry in a cup or plastic bag to have on hand for immediate transport of the specimen to the laboratory.

Intratest:

➤ Ensure that the patient has complied with dietary preparations and other pretesting restrictions.

➤ Direct the patient to breathe normally and to avoid unnecessary movement.

➤ Observe standard precautions and follow the general guidelines in Appendix A. Perform a venipuncture, and collect the specimen in a 5-mL red- and lavender-top tube.

➤ Label the specimen, and promptly transport it to the laboratory. The tightly capped sample should be placed in an ice slurry immediately after collection. Information on the specimen label can be protected from water in the ice slurry if the specimen is first placed in a protective plastic bag.

Post-test:

➤ Observe venipuncture site for bleeding or hematoma formation. Apply pressure bandage.

➤ Patients with abnormal parathyroid levels are also likely to experience the effects of calcium level imbalances. Instruct the patient to report signs and symptoms of hypocalcemia and hypercalcemia to the requesting health care practitioner. (For critical values, signs and symptoms of calcium imbalance, and nutritional information, see monograph titled "Calcium.")

➤ Evaluate test results in relation to the patient's symptoms and other tests performed. Related laboratory tests include calcium, ionized calcium, serum and urine phosphorus, and vitamin D.

PARATHYROID SCAN

SYNONYM/ACRONYM: Parathyroid scintiscan.

AREA OF APPLICATION: Parathyroid.

CONTRAST: Intravenous technetium-99m (Tc-99m) pertechnetate, Tc-99m sestamibi, oral iodine-123, and thallium.

DESCRIPTION: Parathyroid scanning is performed to assist in the preoperative localization of parathyroid adenomas in clinically proven primary hyperparathyroidism; it is useful for distinguishing between intrinsic and extrinsic parathyroid adenomas. It is also performed after surgery to verify the presence of the parathyroid gland in children, and it is done after thyroidectomy as well.

The radionuclide is administered 10 to 20 minutes before the imaging is performed. The thyroid and surrounding tissues should be carefully palpated.

Fine-needle aspiration biopsy guided by ultrasound is occasionally necessary to differentiate thyroid pathology, as well as pathology of other tissues, from parathyroid neoplasia. ∎

INDICATIONS:
• Aid in the diagnosis of hyperparathyroidism

• Differentiate between extrinsic and intrinsic parathyroid adenoma, but not between benign and malignant conditions

• Evaluate the parathyroid in patients with severe hypercalcemia or in patients before parathyroidectomy

RESULT

Normal Findings:
• No areas of increased perfusion or uptake in the thyroid or parathyroid

Abnormal Findings:
• Intrinsic and extrinsic parathyroid adenomas

CRITICAL VALUES: N/A

INTERFERING FACTORS:

This procedure is contraindicated for:
• Patients who are pregnant or suspected of being pregnant, unless the potential benefits of the procedure far outweigh the risks to the fetus and mother

Factors that may impair clear imaging:
• Inability of the patient to cooperate or remain still during the procedure because of age, significant pain, or mental status

• Ingestion of foods containing iodine (e.g., iodized salt) and medications containing iodine (e.g., cough syrup, potassium iodide, vitamins, Lugol's solution, thyroid replacement medications), which can decrease uptake of the radionuclide

• Recent use of iodinated contrast medium for radiographic studies or recently performed nuclear medicine procedures, which can affect the uptake of the radionuclide

• Patients who are very obese, who may exceed the weight limit for the equipment

• Incorrect positioning of the patient, which may produce poor visualization of the area to be examined

• Metallic objects within the examination field (e.g., jewelry or body rings), which may inhibit organ visualization and can produce unclear images

Other considerations:
• Improper injection of the radionuclide that allows the tracer to seep deep into the muscle tissue produces erroneous hot spots.

• Consultation with a physician should occur before the procedure for radiation safety concerns regarding infants of patients who are lactating.

• Risks associated with radiographic overexposure can result from frequent x-ray procedures. Personnel in the room with the patient should stand behind a shield or leave the area while the examination is being done. Personnel working in the area where the examination is being done should wear badges that reveal their level of exposure to radiation.

Nursing Implications and Procedure • • • • • • • • • • •

Pretest: ■

➤ Inform the patient that the procedure assesses the parathyroid glands.

➤ Inform the patient that the procedure is performed in a special nuclear medicine department by a technologist and takes 30 to 60 minutes.

➤ Obtain a history of the patient's complaints, including a list of known allergens.

➤ Obtain a history of the patient's parathyroid and thyroid, as well as results of previously performed laboratory tests, surgical procedures, other radiology procedures, and parathyroid therapy. For related tests, refer to the endocrine system table.

➤ Obtain a list of the medications the patient is taking.

➤ Determine whether the patient has had any recent intake of iodine.

➤ Make sure all blood tests are obtained before the test is performed.

➤ Determine date of last menstrual period and possibility of pregnancy in perimenopausal women.

➤ Do not restrict food or fluids unless otherwise indicated.

➤ All radiographic procedures done with iodinated contrast medium should be done after this procedure is completed.

➤ Ensure that the patient has not been scheduled for more than one radionuclide scan on the same day. Multiple procedures on the same day may interfere with interpretation of results.

Intratest: ■

➤ Ask the patient to void before the procedure. Have the patient put on a hospital gown.

➤ Make sure jewelry, chains, and any other metallic objects have been removed from the neck area.

➤ Administer technetium-99m (Tc-99m) pertechnetate intravenously before scanning.

➤ To scan the parathyroid gland, the patient is placed in a supine position under a radionuclide gamma camera 15 minutes after the radionuclide injection. Imaging is performed over the anterior neck area.

➤ Ask the patient to lie still during the procedure because movement produces unclear images.

➤ The images are recorded on film or stored electronically for recall and future analysis and interpretation by a physician.

➤ With the patient in the same position, Tc-99m sestamibi is injected, and after 10 minutes a second image is obtained and stored in the computer. The computer subtracts the technetium-visualized thyroid structures from the thallium accumulation in a parathyroid adenoma.

➤ Iodine-123 may be administered orally in place of Tc-99m pertechnetate; the imaging sequence, as described above, is performed 24 hours later.

➤ Wear gloves during the radionuclide injection and while handling the patient's urine.

Post-test: ■

➤ Assess injection site for redness or swelling. Apply warm soaks to promote comfort if a hematoma develops.

➤ Advise patient to drink increased amounts of fluids for 24 to 48 hours to eliminate the radionuclide from the body, unless contraindicated. Tell the patient that radionuclide is eliminated from the body within 6 to 24 hours.

➤ Instruct the patient to flush the toilet immediately after each voiding following the procedure and to wash hands meticulously with soap and water after each voiding for 24 hours after the procedure.

➤ Tell all caregivers to wear gloves when discarding urine for 24 hours after the procedure. Wash gloved hands with soap and water before removing gloves. Then wash hands after the gloves are removed.

➤ A physician specializing in this branch of medicine sends a written report to the ordering provider, who discusses the results with the patient.

➤ Evaluate test results in relation to the patient's symptoms and other tests performed. Related diagnostic tests include computed tomography and magnetic resonance imaging of the chest.

PARTIAL THROMBOPLASTIN TIME, ACTIVATED

· ·

SYNONYM/ACRONYM: APTT.

SPECIMEN: Plasma (1 mL) collected in a completely filled blue-top (sodium citrate) tube.

REFERENCE VALUE: (Method: Clot detection) 25 to 39 seconds, usually compared +10 seconds to a normal control. Reference ranges vary with respect to the equipment and reagents used to perform the assay.

DESCRIPTION: The activated partial thromboplastin time (APTT) coagulation test evaluates the function of the intrinsic (factors XII, XI, IX, and VIII) and common (factors V, X, II, and I) pathways of the coagulation sequence, specifically the intrinsic thromboplastin system. It represents the time required for a firm fibrin clot to form after tissue thromboplastin or phospholipid reagents similar to thromboplastin and calcium are added to the specimen. The APTT is abnormal in 90 percent of patients with coagulation disorders and is useful in monitoring the inactivation of factor II effect of heparin therapy. The test is prolonged when there is a

30 to 40 percent deficiency in one of the factors required, or when factor inhibitors (e.g., antithrombin III, protein C, or protein S) are present. The APTT has additional activators, such as kaolin, Celite, or elegiac acid, that more rapidly activate factor XII, making this test faster and more reliably reproducible than the partial thromboplastin time (PTT). A comparison between the results of APTT and prothrombin time (PT) tests can allow some inferences to be made that a factor deficiency exists. A normal APTT with a prolonged PT can only occur with factor VII deficiency. A prolonged APTT with a normal PT could indicate a defi-

ciency in factors XII, XI, IX, VIII, and VIII:C (von Willebrand factor). Factor deficiencies can also be identified by correction or substitution studies using normal serum. These studies are easy to perform and are accomplished by adding plasma from a normal patient to a sample from a patient suspected to be factor-deficient. When the APTT is repeated and is corrected, or within the reference range, it can be assumed that the prolonged APTT is caused by a factor deficiency. The administration of prophylactic low-dose heparin does not require serial monitoring of APTT. (For more information on factor deficiencies, see monograph titled "Fibrinogen.") ∎

INDICATIONS:

- Detect congenital deficiencies in clotting factors, as seen in diseases such as hemophilia A (factor VIII) and hemophilia B (factor IX)

- Evaluate response to anticoagulant therapy with heparin or coumarin derivatives

- Identify individuals who may be prone to bleeding during surgical, obstetric, dental, or invasive diagnostic procedures

- Identify the possible cause of abnormal bleeding, such as epistaxis, hematoma, gingival bleeding, hematuria, and menorrhagia

- Monitor the hemostatic effects of conditions such as liver disease, protein deficiency, and fat malabsorption

RESULT

Prolonged in:

- Afibrinogenemia

- Circulating products of fibrin and fibrinogen degradation

- Disseminated intravascular coagulation

- Factor deficiencies

- Hemodialysis patients

- Polycythemia

- Severe liver disease

- Vitamin K deficiency

- Von Willebrand's disease

CRITICAL VALUES: ⚠ Greater than 70 seconds. Important signs to note are prolonged bleeding, hematoma at the puncture site, hemorrhage, blood in stool, bleeding gums, and shock. Monitoring vital signs and neurologic changes until values are within normal range is indicated. Administration of protamine sulfate may be requested.

The requesting health care practitioner should also be notified if the APTT is less than 53 seconds in a patient receiving heparin therapy. Low values indicate that the therapy is providing inadequate anticoagulation.

INTERFERING FACTORS:

- Drugs and vitamins such as anistreplase, antihistamines, chlorpromazine, salicylates, and ascorbic acid may cause prolonged APTT.

- Anticoagulant therapy with heparin will prolong the APTT.

- Copper is a component of factor V, and severe copper deficiencies may result in prolonged APTT values.

- Traumatic venipunctures can activate the coagulation sequence by contamination of the sample with tissue thromboplastin and can produce falsely shortened results.

- Failure to fill the tube sufficiently to yield a proper blood-to-anticoagulant ratio invalidates the results and is reason for specimen rejection.

- Excessive agitation that causes sample

hemolysis can falsely shorten the APTT because the hemolyzed cells activate plasma-clotting factors.

• Inadequate mixing of the tube can produce erroneous results.

• Specimens left unprocessed for longer than 4 hours should be rejected for analysis.

• High platelet count or inadequate centrifugation will result in decreased values.

• Hematocrit greater than 55 percent may cause falsely prolonged results because of anticoagulant excess. The excess anticoagulant chelates the calcium reagent in the test system, making it unavailable to react properly with the patient sample.

Nursing Implications and Procedure • • • • • • • • • • • •

Pretest:

➤ Obtain a history of the patient's complaints, including a list of known allergens.

➤ Obtain a history of the patient's hematopoietic and hepatobiliary systems, history of any bleeding disorders, and results of previously performed tests and procedures, especially bleeding time, clotting time, complete blood count, PTT, platelets, and prothrombin time. For related tests, refer to the hematopoietic and hepatobiliary system tables.

➤ Obtain a list of the medications the patient is taking, including anticoagulant therapy, acetylsalicylic acid, herbs, and nutraceuticals known to affect coagulation. It is recommended that use of these products be discontinued 14 days before dental or surgical procedures. The requesting health care practitioner and laboratory should be advised if the patient regularly uses these products so that their effects can be taken into consideration when reviewing results. If the patient is receiving anticoagulant therapy, note the time and amount of the last dose.

➤ There are no food, fluid, or medication restrictions unless by medical direction.

➤ Review the procedure with the patient.

➤ Inform the patient that specimen collection takes approximately 5 to 10 minutes.

Intratest:

➤ Direct the patient to breathe normally and to avoid unnecessary movement.

➤ Observe standard precautions and follow the general guidelines in Appendix A. Perform a venipuncture, and collect the specimen in a 5-mL blue-top tube. Fill the tube completely. *Important note*: Two different concentrations of sodium citrate preservative are currently added to blue-top tubes for coagulation studies: 3.2% and 3.8%. The National Committee for Clinical Laboratory Standards (NCCLS) guideline for sodium citrate is 3.2%. Laboratories establish reference ranges for coagulation testing based on numerous factors, including sodium citrate concentration, test equipment, and test reagents. It is important to inquire from the laboratory which concentration it recommends, because each concentration will have its own specific reference range.

➤ When multiple specimens are drawn, the blue-top tube should be collected after sterile (i.e., blood culture) and red-top tubes. When coagulation testing is the only work to be done, an extra red-top tube should be collected before the blue-top tube to avoid contaminating the specimen with tissue thromboplastin.

➤ Label the specimen, and promptly transport it to the laboratory. The NCCLS recommendation for processed and unprocessed specimens stored in unopened tubes is that testing should be completed within 1 to 4 hours of collection.

Post-test:

➤ Observe venipuncture site for bleeding or hematoma formation. Apply pressure bandage.

➤ Instruct the patient to report severe bruising or bleeding from any areas of the skin or mucous membranes.

➤ Inform the patient with prolonged APTT values of the importance of taking precautions against bruising and bleeding, including the use of a soft bristle toothbrush, use of an electric razor, avoidance of constipation, avoidance of acetylsalicylic acid and similar products, and avoidance of intramuscular injections.

➤ Inform the patient of the importance of periodic laboratory testing while taking an anticoagulant.

➤ Evaluate test results in relation to the patient's symptoms and other tests performed. Related laboratory tests include antithrombin III, specific factor assays, fibrin breakdown products, platelet count, protein C, and protein S.

PARVOVIRUS B19 IMMUNOGLOBULIN G AND IMMUNOGLOBULIN M ANTIBODIES

● ●

SYNONYM/ACRONYM: N/A.

SPECIMEN: Serum (2 mL) collected in a red- or tiger-top tube.

REFERENCE VALUE: (Method: Immunoassay)

Negative	Less than 0.8
Equivocal	0.8–1.2

DESCRIPTION: Parvovirus B19, a single-stranded DNA virus transmitted by respiratory secretions, is the only parvovirus known to infect humans. Its primary site of replication is in red blood cell precursors in the bone marrow. It is capable of causing disease along a wide spectrum ranging from a self-limited erythema (fifth disease) to bone marrow failure or aplastic crisis in patients with sickle cell anemia, spherocytosis, or thalassemia. Fetal hydrops and spontaneous abortion may also occur as a result of infection during pregnancy. The incubation period is approximately 1 week after exposure. B19-specific antibodies appear in the serum approximately 3 days after the onset of symptoms. The presence of immunoglobulin M (IgM) antibodies indicates acute infection. The presence of IgG antibodies indicates past infection and is believed to confer lifelong immunity. Parvovirus can also be detected by DNA hybridization using a polymerase chain reaction. ▪

INDICATIONS: Assist in establishing a diagnosis of parvovirus B19 infection

RESULT

Positive findings in:

• Arthritis

• Erythema infectiosum (fifth disease)

• Erythrocyte aplasia

• Hydrops fetalis

Negative findings in: N/A

CRITICAL VALUES: N/A

INTERFERING FACTORS: Immunocompromised patients may not develop sufficient antibody to be detected.

Nursing Implications and Procedure • • • • • • • • • •

Pretest: ▪

➤ Obtain a history of the patient's complaints, including a list of known allergens.

➤ Obtain a history of the patient's immune system and results of previously performed tests and procedures. For related tests, refer to the immune system table.

➤ Obtain a list of the medications the patient is taking, including herbs, nutritional supplements, and nutraceuticals. The requesting health

care practitioner and laboratory should be advised if the patient regularly uses these products so that their effects can be taken into consideration when reviewing results.

➤ There are no food, fluid, or medication restrictions unless by medical direction.

➤ Review the procedure with the patient. Inform the patient that a subsequent sample will be required in 7 to 14 days.

➤ Inform the patient that specimen collection takes approximately 5 to 10 minutes.

Intratest: ▪

➤ Direct the patient to breathe normally and to avoid unnecessary movement.

➤ Observe standard precautions and follow the general guidelines in Appendix A. Perform a venipuncture, and collect the specimen in a 5-mL red-top tube.

➤ Label the specimen, and promptly transport it to the laboratory.

Post-test: ▪

➤ Observe venipuncture site for bleeding or hematoma formation. Apply pressure bandage.

➤ Emphasize the need for the patient to return to have a convalescent blood sample taken in 7 to 14 days.

➤ Evaluate test results in relation to the patient's symptoms and other tests performed. Related laboratory tests include complete blood count, bone marrow biopsy, hemoglobin electrophoresis, red blood cell morphology, and sickle cell screen.

PERICARDIAL FLUID ANALYSIS

SYNONYM/ACRONYM: N/A.

SPECIMEN: Pericardial fluid (5 mL) collected in a red- or green-top (heparin) tube for glucose, lavender-top (ethylenediaminetetra-acetic acid [EDTA]) tube for cell count, and sterile containers for microbiology specimens. Ensure that there is an equal amount of fluid to fixative in a clear container for cytology.

REFERENCE VALUE: (Method: Spectrophotometry for glucose, automated or manual cell count, macroscopic examination of cultured organisms, and microscopic examination of specimen for microbiology and cytology; microscopic examination of cultured microorganisms)

Pericardial Fluid	Reference Value
Appearance	Clear
Color	Pale yellow
Glucose	Parallel serum values
Red blood cell count	None seen
White blood cell count	Less than 1000/mm^3
Culture	No growth
Gram stain	No organisms seen
Cytology	No abnormal cells seen

DESCRIPTION: The heart is located within a protective membrane called the *pericardium*. The fluid between the pericardial membranes is called *serous fluid*. Normally only a small amount of fluid is present because the rates of fluid production and absorption are about the same. Many abnormal conditions can result in the buildup of fluid within the pericardium. Specific tests are usually ordered in addition to a common battery of tests used to distinguish a transudate from an exudate. *Transudates* are effusions that form as a result of a systemic disorder that disrupts the regulation of fluid balance, such as a suspected perforation. *Exudates* are caused by conditions involving the tissue of the membrane itself, such as an infection or malignancy. Fluid is withdrawn from the pericardium by needle aspiration and tested as listed in the previous and following tables. ■

Characteristic	Transudate	Exudate
Appearance	Clear	Cloudy or turbid
Specific gravity	Less than 1.015	Greater than 1.015
Total protein	Less than 2.5 g/dL	Greater than 3.0 g/dL
Fluid-to-serum protein ratio	Less than 0.5	Greater than 0.5
LDH	Parallels serum value	Less than 200 U/L
Fluid-to-serum LDH ratio	Less than 0.6	Greater than 0.6
Fluid cholesterol	Less than 55 mg/dL	Greater than 55 mg/dL
White blood cell count	Less than 100/mm^3	Greater than 1000/mm^3

LDH = lactate dehydrogenase.

INDICATIONS:

• Evaluate effusion of unknown etiology

• Investigate suspected hemorrhage, immune disease, malignancy, or infection

RESULT

Increased in (condition/test showing increased result):

• Bacterial pericarditis (red blood cell [RBC] count, white blood cell [WBC] count with a predominance of neutrophils)

• Hemorrhagic pericarditis (RBC count, WBC count)

• Malignancy (RBC count, abnormal cytology)

• Postmyocardial infarction syndrome, also called Dressler's syndrome (RBC count, WBC count with a predominance of neutrophils)

• Rheumatoid disease or systemic lupus erythematosus (RBC count, WBC count)

• Tuberculous or fungal pericarditis (RBC count, WBC count with a predominance of lymphocytes)

• Viral pericarditis (RBC count, WBC count with a predominance of neutrophils)

Decreased in (condition/test showing decreased result):

• Bacterial pericarditis (glucose)

• Malignancy (glucose)

• Rheumatoid disease or systemic lupus erythematosus (glucose)

CRITICAL VALUES: N/A

INTERFERING FACTORS:

• Bloody fluid may be the result of a traumatic tap.

• Unknown hyperglycemia or hypoglycemia may be misleading in the comparison of fluid and serum glucose levels. Therefore, it is advisable to collect comparative serum samples a few hours before performing pericardiocentesis.

Nursing Implications and Procedure • • • • • • • • • • •

Pretest:

➤ Obtain a history of the patient's complaints, including a list of known allergens.

➤ Obtain a history of the patient's cardiovascular and immune systems, as well as results of previously performed tests and procedures. For related tests refer to the cardiovascular and immune system tables.

➤ Obtain a list of the medications the patient is taking, including herbs, nutritional supplements, and nutraceuticals. The requesting health care practitioner and laboratory should be advised if the patient regularly uses these products so that their effects can be taken into consideration when reviewing results.

➤ Restrict food and fluids for 6 to 8 hours before the procedure, as directed.

➤ The requesting health care practitioner may request that anticoagulants and aspirin be withheld.

➤ Review the procedure with the patient. Inform the patient where the test will be performed (some procedures are performed in a cardiac laboratory).

➤ Explain the importance of remaining still during the procedure.

➤ Inform the patient that an intravenous infusion will be started before and during the procedure.

➤ Inform the patient that a local anesthetic will be administered at the needle insertion site immediately before the procedure to reduce discomfort during needle aspiration. Explain that the anesthetic injection may cause a stinging sensation. Explain that after the skin has been anesthetized, a large needle will be inserted through the chest to obtain the fluid.

➤ Assess whether the patient has an allergy to local anesthetic, and inform the health care practitioner accordingly.

➤ *Obtain written and informed consent before administering any medications prior to the procedure.*

➤ Have the patient void before the procedure.

➤ Inform the patient that specimen collection takes approximately 30 minutes.

Intratest:

➤ Ensure that the patient has complied with dietary preparations and other pretesting restrictions.

➤ Assist the patient into a supine position with the head elevated 45° to 60°.

➤ Direct the patient to breathe normally and to avoid unnecessary movement.

➤ Take and record baseline vital signs.

➤ Observe standard precautions and follow the general guidelines in Appendix A.

➤ Cleanse the skin with an antiseptic solution, and protect the area with a sterile drape. The skin at the injection site is anesthetized.

➤ The precordial (V) cardiac lead wire is attached to the cardiac needle with an alligator clip. The cardiac needle is inserted just below and to the left of the breastbone, and fluid is removed.

➤ Monitor vital signs every 15 minutes for signs of hypovolemia or shock. Monitor electrocardiogram for needle-tip positioning to indicate accidental puncture of the right atrium.

➤ The needle is withdrawn and slight pressure applied to the site. If there is no evidence of bleeding or drainage, a sterile dressing is applied to the site.

➤ If there is no sign of arrhythmia, the cardiac monitor can be removed.

➤ Fill the appropriate collection containers with fluid for analysis.

➤ Label the specimens, and promptly transport them to the laboratory.

Post-test:

➤ Instruct the patient to resume usual diet and medication, if withheld and as directed by the requesting health care practitioner.

➤ Observe the patient for signs of respiratory and cardiac distress, such as shortness of breath, cyanosis, or rapid pulse.

➤ Inform the patient that 1 hour or more of bed rest is required after the procedure.

➤ Take vital signs every 15 minutes for the first hour, every 30 minutes for the next 2 hours, every hour for the next 4 hours, and every 4 hours for the next 24 hours. Take the patient's temperature every 4 hours for 24 hours. Monitor intake and output for 24 hours.

➤ Continue intravenous fluids until vital signs are stable and the patient can resume fluid intake independently.

➤ Assess the puncture site for bleeding or drainage and signs of inflammation each time vital signs are taken and daily thereafter for several days.

➤ Administer antibiotics, as ordered, and instruct the patient in the importance of completing the entire course of antibiotic therapy even if no symptoms are present.

➤ Evaluate test results in relation to the patient's symptoms and other tests performed. Related tests include α_1-fetoprotein, bacterial culture, CA 15-3, CA 19-9, CA 125, carcinoembryonic antigen, fungal culture, mycobacterial culture, and viral culture.

PERITONEAL FLUID ANALYSIS

· ·

SYNONYM/ACRONYM: Ascites fluid analysis.

SPECIMEN: Peritoneal fluid (5 mL) collected in a red- or green-top (heparin) tube for amylase, glucose, and alkaline phosphatase; lavender-top (ethylenediaminetetra-acetic acid [EDTA]) tube for cell count; sterile containers for microbiology specimens; 200 to 500 mL of fluid in a clear container with anticoagulant for cytology.

REFERENCE VALUE: (Method: Spectrophotometry for glucose, amylase, and alkaline phosphatase; automated or manual cell count, macroscopic examination of cultured organisms, and microscopic examination of specimen for microbiology and cytology; microscopic examination of cultured microorganisms)

Peritoneal Fluid	Reference Value
Appearance	Clear
Color	Pale yellow
Amylase	Parallel serum values
Alkaline phosphatase	Parallel serum values
Glucose	Parallel serum values
Red blood cell count	Less than 100,000/mm^3

(Continued on the following page)

Peritoneal Fluid	Reference Value
White blood cell count	Less than 300/mm^3
Culture	No growth
Acid-fast stain	No organisms seen
Gram stain	No organisms seen
Cytology	No abnormal cells seen

DESCRIPTION: The peritoneal cavity and organs within it are lined with a protective membrane. The fluid between the membranes is called *serous fluid.* Normally only a small amount of fluid is present because the rates of fluid production and absorption are about the same. Many abnormal conditions can result in the buildup of fluid within the peritoneal cavity. Specific tests are usually ordered in addition to a common battery of tests used to distinguish a transudate from an exudate. *Transudates* are effusions that form as a result of a systemic disorder that disrupts the regulation of fluid balance, such as a suspected perforation. *Exudates* are caused by conditions involving the tissue of the membrane itself, such as an infection or malignancy. Fluid is withdrawn from the peritoneal cavity by needle aspiration and tested as listed in the previous and following tables. ∎

Characteristic	Transudate	Exudate
Appearance	Clear	Cloudy or turbid
Specific gravity	Less than 1.015	Greater than 1.015
Total protein	Less than 2.5 g/dL	Greater than 3.0 g/dL
Fluid-to-serum protein ratio	Less than 0.5	Greater than 0.5
LDH	Parallels serum value	Less than 200 U/L
Fluid-to-serum LDH ratio	Less than 0.6	Greater than 0.6
Fluid cholesterol	Less than 55 mg/dL	Greater than 55 mg/dL
White blood cell count	Less than 100/mm^3	Greater than 1000/mm^3

LDH = lactate dehydrogenase.

INDICATIONS:

- Evaluate ascites of unknown cause

- Investigate suspected peritoneal rupture, perforation, malignancy, or infection

RESULT

Increased in (condition/test showing increased result):

- Abdominal malignancy (red blood cell [RBC] count, carcinoembryonic antigen, abnormal cytology)

- Abdominal trauma (RBC count greater than 100,000/mm^3)

- Ascites caused by cirrhosis (white blood cell [WBC] count, neutrophils greater than 25 percent but less than 50 percent, absolute granulocyte count greater than 250/mm^3)

- Bacterial peritonitis (WBC count,

neutrophils greater than 50 percent, absolute granulocyte count greater than $250/mm^3$)

- Peritoneal effusion due to gastric strangulation, perforation, or necrosis (amylase, ammonia, alkaline phosphatase)

- Peritoneal effusion due to pancreatitis, pancreatic trauma, or pancreatic pseudocyst (amylase)

- Rupture or perforation of urinary bladder (ammonia, creatinine, urea)

- Tuberculous effusion (elevated lymphocyte count, positive acid-fast bacillus smear and culture [25 to 50 percent of cases])

Decreased in (condition/test showing decreased result):
- Abdominal malignancy (glucose)
- Tuberculous effusion (glucose)

CRITICAL VALUES: N/A

INTERFERING FACTORS:
- Bloody fluids may result from a traumatic tap.
- Unknown hyperglycemia or hypoglycemia may be misleading in the comparison of fluid and serum glucose levels. Therefore, it is advisable to collect comparative serum samples a few hours before performing paracentesis.

Nursing Implications and Procedure · · · · · · · · · · ·

Pretest:

➤ Obtain a history of the patient's complaints, including a list of known allergens.

➤ Obtain a history of the patient's gastrointestinal and immune systems, as well as results of previously performed tests and procedures. For related tests, refer to the gastrointestinal and immune system tables.

➤ Obtain a list of the medications the patient is taking, including herbs, nutritional supplements, and nutraceuticals. The requesting health care practitioner and laboratory should be advised if the patient regularly uses these products so that their effects can be taken into consideration when reviewing results.

➤ There are no food or fluid restrictions unless by medical direction.

➤ The requesting health care practitioner may request that anticoagulants and aspirin be withheld.

➤ If patient has ascites, obtain weight and measure abdominal girth.

➤ Review the procedure with the patient. Explain the importance of remaining still during the procedure.

➤ Inform the patient that a local anesthetic will be administered at the abdominal needle insertion site immediately before the procedure to reduce discomfort during aspiration. Explain that the anesthetic injection may cause a stinging sensation. Explain that after the skin has been anesthetized, a large needle will be inserted through the abdominal wall and a "popping" sensation may be experienced as the needle penetrates the peritoneum.

➤ Assess whether the patient has an allergy to local anesthetics, and inform the health care practitioner accordingly.

➤ *Obtain written and informed consent before administering any medications prior to the procedure.*

➤ Have the patient void or catheterize the patient to avoid accidental puncture of the bladder if he or she is unable to void.

➤ Inform the patient that specimen collection takes approximately 30 minutes.

Intratest:

➤ Assist the patient to a seated position with feet and back supported or in high Fowler's position.

➤ Direct the patient to breathe

normally and to avoid unnecessary movement.

➤ Take and record baseline vital signs.

➤ Observe standard precautions and follow the general guidelines in Appendix A.

➤ Cleanse the skin with an antiseptic solution, and protect the area with a sterile drape. The skin at the injection site is anesthetized.

➤ The paracentesis needle is inserted 1 to 2 inches below the umbilicus, and fluid is removed. If lavage fluid is required (helpful if malignancy is suspected), saline or Ringer's lactate can be infused via the needle over a 15- to 20-minute period before the lavage fluid is removed. Monitor vital signs every 15 minutes for signs of hypovolemia or shock.

➤ No more than 1500 to 2000 mL should be removed at a time, even in the case of a therapeutic paracentesis, because of the risk of hypovolemia and shock.

➤ The needle is withdrawn and slight pressure applied to the site. If there is no evidence of bleeding or drainage, a sterile dressing is applied to the site.

➤ Fill the appropriate collection containers with fluid for analysis.

➤ Label the specimens, and promptly transport them to the laboratory.

Post-test:

➤ Instruct the patient to resume usual medication as directed by the requesting health care practitioner.

➤ Inform the patient that 1 hour or more of bed rest is required after the procedure.

➤ Take vital signs every 15 minutes for the first hour, every 30 minutes for the next 2 hours, every hour for the next 4 hours and every 4 hours for the next 24 hours. Take the patient's temperature every 4 hours for 24 hours. Monitor intake and output for 24 hours.

➤ Assess the puncture site for bleeding or drainage and signs of inflammation each time vital signs are taken and daily thereafter for several days.

➤ If a large amount of fluid was removed, obtain weight and measure abdominal girth.

➤ Instruct the patient to immediately report severe abdominal pain (*note*: rigidity of abdominal muscles indicates developing peritonitis).

➤ Administer antibiotics, as ordered, and instruct the patient in the importance of completing the entire course of antibiotic therapy even if no symptoms are present.

➤ Evaluate test results in relation to the patient's symptoms and other tests performed. Related laboratory tests include bacterial culture, CA 15-3, CA 19-9, CA 125, carcinoembryonic antigen, fungal culture, mycobacterial culture, and viral culture.

PHOSPHORUS, SERUM

SYNONYMS/ACRONYM: Inorganic phosphorus, phosphate, PO_4.

SPECIMEN: Serum (1 mL) collected in a red- or tiger-top tube. Plasma (1 mL) collected in green-top (heparin) tube is also acceptable.

REFERENCE VALUE: (Method: Spectrophotometry)

Age	Conventional Units	SI Units (Conversion Factor ×0.323)
0–5 d	4.6–8.0 mg/dL	1.5–2.6 mmol/L
1–3 y	3.9–6.5 mg/dL	1.3–2.1 mmol/L
4–6 y	4.0–5.4 mg/dL	1.3–1.7 mmol/L
7–11 y	3.7–5.6 mg/dL	1.2–1.8 mmol/L
12–13 y	3.3–5.4 mg/dL	1.1–1.7 mmol/L
14–15 y	2.9–5.4 mg/dL	0.9–1.7 mmol/L
16–19 y	2.8–4.6 mg/dL	0.9–1.5 mmol/L
Adult	2.5–4.5 mg/dL	0.8–1.4 mmol/L

DESCRIPTION: Phosphorus, in the form of phosphate, is distributed throughout the body. Approximately 85 percent of the body's phosphorus is stored in bones; the remainder is found in cells and body fluids. It is the major intracellular anion and plays a crucial role in cellular metabolism, maintenance of cellular membranes, and formation of bones and teeth. Phosphorus also indirectly affects the release of oxygen from hemoglobin by affecting the formation of 2,3-bisphosphoglycerate. Levels of phosphorus are dependent on dietary intake.

Phosphorus excretion is regulated by the kidneys. Calcium and phosphorus are interrelated with respect to absorption and metabolic function. They have an inverse relationship with respect to concentration: serum phosphorus is increased when serum calcium is decreased. Hyperphosphatemia can result in an infant fed only cow's milk during the first few weeks of life because of the combination of a high phosphorus content in cow's milk and the inability of infants' kidneys to clear the excess phosphorus. ∎

INDICATIONS:

• Assist in establishing a diagnosis of hyperparathyroidism

• Assist in the evaluation of renal failure

RESULT

Increased in:

• Acromegaly

• Bone metastases

• Diabetic ketoacidosis

• Excessive levels of vitamin D

• Hyperthermia

• Hypocalcemia

• Hypoparathyroidism

• Lactic acidosis

• Milk alkali syndrome

• Pulmonary embolism

• Pseudohypoparathyroidism

• Renal failure

• Respiratory acidosis

Decreased in:

• Acute gout

• Alcohol withdrawal

• Gram-negative bacterial septicemia

- Growth hormone deficiency
- Hyperalimentation therapy
- Hypercalcemia
- Hyperinsulinism
- Hyperparathyroidism
- Hypokalemia
- Impaired renal absorption
- Malabsorption syndromes
- Malnutrition
- Osteomalacia
- Parathyroid hormone–producing tumors
- Primary hyperparathyroidism
- Renal tubular acidosis
- Renal tubular defects
- Respiratory alkalosis
- Respiratory infections
- Rickets
- Salicylate poisoning
- Severe burns
- Severe vomiting and diarrhea
- Vitamin D deficiency

CRITICAL VALUES: ⚠ Values less than 1.0 mg/dL may have significant effects on the neuromuscular, gastrointestinal, cardiopulmonary, and skeletal systems. Interventions including intravenous (IV) replacement therapy with sodium or potassium phosphate may be necessary. Close monitoring of both phosphorus and calcium is important during replacement therapy.

INTERFERING FACTORS:
- Drugs that may increase phosphorus levels include anabolic steroids, β-adrenergic blockers, ergocalciferol, furosemide, hydrochlorothiazide, methicillin (occurs with nephrotoxicity), oral contraceptives, parathy-roid extract, phosphates, sodium etidronate, tetracycline (occurs with nephrotoxicity), and vitamin D.
- Drugs that may decrease phosphorus levels include acetazolamide, albuterol, aluminum salts, amino acids (via IV hyperalimentation), anesthetic agents, anticonvulsants, calcitonin, epinephrine, fibrin hydrolysate, fructose, glucocorticoids, glucose, insulin, mannitol, oral contraceptives, pamidronate, phenothiazine, phytate, and plicamycin.
- Serum phosphorus levels are subject to diurnal variation: They are highest in late morning and lowest in the evening; therefore serial samples should be collected at the same time of day for consistency in interpretation.
- Hemolysis will falsely increase phosphorus values.
- Specimens should never be collected above an IV because of the potential for dilution when the specimen and the IV solution combine in the collection container, thereby falsely decreasing the result. There is also the potential of contaminating the sample with the substance of interest, contained in the IV solution, thereby falsely increasing the result.

Nursing Implications and Procedure • • • • • • • • • • •

Pretest:

➤ Obtain a history of the patient's complaints, including a list of known allergens.

➤ Obtain a history of the patient's endocrine, gastrointestinal, genitourinary, and musculoskeletal systems, as well as results of previously performed tests and procedures. For related tests, refer to the endocrine, gastrointestinal, genitourinary, and musculoskeletal system tables.

➤ Obtain a list of the medications the patient is taking, including herbs, nutritional supplements, and nutraceuticals. The requesting health care practitioner and laboratory should be advised if the patient regularly uses these products so that their effects can be taken into consideration when reviewing results.

➤ There are no food, fluid, or medication restrictions unless by medical direction.

➤ Review the procedure with the patient.

➤ Inform the patient that specimen collection takes approximately 5 to 10 minutes.

Intratest:

➤ Direct the patient to breathe normally and to avoid unnecessary movement.

➤ Observe standard precautions and follow the general guidelines in Appendix A. Perform a venipuncture, and collect the specimen in a 5-mL red- or tiger-top tube.

➤ Label the specimen, and promptly transport it to the laboratory.

Post-test:

➤ Observe venipuncture site for bleeding or hematoma formation. Apply pressure bandage.

➤ Severe hypophosphatemia is common in elderly patients or patients who have been hospitalized for long periods of time. Good dietary sources of phosphorus include meat, dairy products, nuts, and legumes.

➤ To decrease phosphorus levels to normal in the patient with hyperphosphatemia, dietary restriction may be recommended. Other interventions may include the administration of phosphate binders or administration of calcitriol (the activated form of vitamin D).

➤ Evaluate test results in relation to the patient's symptoms and other tests performed. Related laboratory tests include calcitonin, calcium, collagen crosslinked N-telopeptides, growth hormone, kidney stone analysis, osteocalcin, parathyroid hormones, and vitamin D.

PHOSPHORUS, URINE

SYNONYM/ACRONYM: Urine phosphate.

SPECIMEN: Urine (5 mL) from an unpreserved random or timed specimen collected in a clean, plastic collection container.

REFERENCE VALUE: (Method: Spectrophotometry) Reference values are dependent on phosphorus and calcium intake. Phosphate excretion exhibits diurnal variation and is significantly higher at night.

Conventional Units	SI Units (Conversion Factor ×32.3)
0.4–1.3 g/24 h	12.9–42.0 g/24 h

DESCRIPTION: Phosphorus, in the form of phosphate, is distributed throughout the body. Approximately 85 percent of the body's phosphorus is stored in bones; the remainder is found in cells and body fluids. It is the major intracellular anion and plays a crucial role in cellular metabolism, maintenance of cellular membranes, and formation of bones and teeth. Phosphorus also indirectly affects the release of oxygen from hemoglobin by affecting the formation of 2,3-bisphosphoglycerate. Levels of phosphorus are dependent on dietary intake.

Analyzing urinary phosphorus levels can provide important clues to the functioning of the kidneys and other major organs. Tests for phosphorus in urine usually involve timed urine collections over a 12- or 24-hour period. Measurement of random specimens may also be requested. Children with thalassemia may have normal phosphorus absorption but increased excretion, which may result in a phosphorus deficiency. ∎

INDICATIONS:
- Assist in the diagnosis of hyperparathyroidism
- Assist in the evaluation of calcium and phosphorus balance
- Assist in the evaluation of nephrolithiasis
- Assist in the evaluation of renal tubular disease

RESULT

Increased in:
- Abuse of diuretics
- Primary hyperparathyroidism
- Renal tubular acidosis

- Vitamin D deficiency

Decreased in:
- Hypoparathyroidism
- Pseudohypoparathyroidism
- Vitamin D intoxication

CRITICAL VALUES: N/A

INTERFERING FACTORS:
- Drugs and vitamins that can cause an increase in urine phosphorus levels include acetazolamide, acetylsalicylic acid, alanine, bismuth salts, calcitonin, corticosteroids, dihydrotachysterol, glycine, hydrochlorothiazide, metolazone, parathyroid extract, parathyroid hormone, phosphates, tryptophan, valine, and vitamin D.

- Drugs that can cause a decrease in urine phosphorus levels include aluminum-containing antacids.

- Urine phosphorus levels are subject to diurnal variation: Output is highest in the afternoon, which is why 24-hour urine collections are recommended.

- All urine voided for the timed collection period must be included in the collection or else falsely decreased values may be obtained. Compare output records with volume collected to verify that all voids were included in the collection.

Nursing Implications and Procedure

Pretest:
➤ Obtain a history of the patient's complaints, including a list of known allergens.

➤ Obtain a history of the patient's endocrine and genitourinary systems, as well as results of previously performed tests and procedures. For related tests, refer to the endocrine and genitourinary system tables.

➤ Obtain a list of the medications the patient is taking, including herbs, nutritional supplements, and nutraceuticals. The requesting health care practitioner and laboratory should be advised if the patient regularly uses these products so that their effects can be taken into consideration when reviewing results.

➤ There are no food, fluid, or medication restrictions unless by medical direction.

➤ Instruct the patient to avoid excessive exercise and stress during the 24-hour collection of urine.

➤ Review the procedure with the patient. Provide a nonmetallic urinal, bedpan, or toilet-mounted collection device.

➤ Usually a 24-hour time frame for urine collection is ordered. Inform the patient that all urine must be saved during that 24-hour period. Instruct the patient not to void directly into the laboratory collection container. Instruct the patient to avoid defecating in the collection device and to keep toilet tissue out of the collection device to prevent contamination of the specimen. Place a sign in the bathroom to remind the patient to save all urine.

➤ Instruct the patient to void all urine into the collection device and then to pour the urine into the laboratory collection container. Alternatively the specimen can be left in the collection device for a health care staff member to add to the laboratory collection container.

Intratest:

➤ Observe standard precautions and follow the general guidelines in Appendix A.

Random specimen (collect in early morning):

Clean-catch specimen:

➤ Instruct the male patient to (1) thor-oughly wash his hands, (2) cleanse the meatus, (3) void a small amount into the toilet, and (4) void directly into the specimen container.

➤ Instruct the female patient to (1) thoroughly wash her hands; (2) cleanse the labia from front to back; (3) while keeping the labia separated, void a small amount into the toilet; and (4) without interrupting the urine stream, void directly into the specimen container.

Timed specimen:

➤ Obtain a clean 3-L urine specimen container, toilet-mounted collection device, and plastic bag (for transport of the specimen container). The specimen must be refrigerated or kept on ice throughout the entire collection period. If an indwelling urinary catheter is in place, the drainage bag must be kept on ice.

➤ Begin the test between 6 and 8 a.m., if possible. Collect first voiding and discard. Record the time the specimen was discarded as the beginning of the timed collection period. The next morning, ask the patient to void at the same time the collection was started and add this last voiding to the container.

➤ If an indwelling catheter is in place, replace the tubing and container system at the start of the collection time. Keep the container system on ice during the collection period, or empty the urine into a larger container periodically during the collection period; monitor to ensure continued drainage, and conclude the test the next morning at the same hour the collection was begun.

➤ At the conclusion of the test, compare the quantity of urine with the urinary output record for the collection; if the specimen contains less than what was recorded as output, some urine may have been discarded, invalidating the test.

➤ Label the specimen, and promptly

transport it to the laboratory. Include on the label the amount of urine, test start and stop times, and ingestion of any foods or medications that can affect test results.

Post-test:

➤ Increased urine phosphorus levels may be associated with the formation of kidney stones. Educate the patient, if appropriate, on the importance of drinking a sufficient amount of water when kidney stones are suspected.

➤ Evaluate test results in relation to the patient's symptoms and other tests performed. Related laboratory tests include calcitonin, kidney stone analysis, parathyroid hormone, phosphorus, serum and urine calcium, and urinalysis.

PLASMINOGEN

SYNONYM/ACRONYM: Profibrinolysin, PMG.

SPECIMEN: Plasma (1 mL) collected in blue-top (sodium citrate) tube.

REFERENCE VALUE: (Method: Chromogenic substrate) 80 to 120 percent of normal for plasma.

DESCRIPTION: Plasminogen is a plasma glycoprotein. It is the circulating, inactive precursor to plasmin. Damaged tissues release a substance called *plasminogen activator* that initiates the conversion of plasminogen to plasmin. Plasmin participates in fibrinolysis and is capable of degrading fibrin, factor I (fibrinogen), factor V, and factor VIII. (For more information on fibrin degradation, see monograph titled "Fibrinogen.") ∎

INDICATIONS: Evaluate the level of circulating plasminogen in patients with thrombosis or disseminated intravascular coagulation (DIC)

RESULT

Increased in:
• Pregnancy (late)

Decreased in:
• DIC

• Fibrinolytic therapy with tissue plasminogen activators such as streptokinase or urokinase

• Postsurgical period

• Hereditary deficiency

• Liver disease

• Neonatal hyaline membrane disease

CRITICAL VALUES: N/A

INTERFERING FACTORS: Drugs that may decrease plasminogen levels include streptokinase and urokinase.

Nursing Implications and Procedure • • • • • • • • • • •

Pretest: ■

➤ Obtain a history of the patient's complaints, including a list of known allergens.

➤ Obtain a history of the patient's hematopoietic system and results of previously performed tests and procedures. For related tests, refer to the hematopoietic system table.

➤ Obtain a list of the medications the patient is taking, including herbs, nutritional supplements, and nutraceuticals. The requesting health care practitioner and laboratory should be advised if the patient regularly uses these products so that their effects can be taken into consideration when reviewing results.

➤ There are no food, fluid, or medication restrictions unless by medical direction.

➤ Review the procedure with the patient.

➤ Inform the patient that specimen collection takes approximately 5 to 10 minutes.

Intratest: ■

➤ Direct the patient to breathe normally and to avoid unnecessary movement.

➤ Observe standard precautions and follow the general guidelines in Appendix A. Perform a venipuncture, and collect the specimen in a 5-mL

blue-top tube. *Important note*: Two different concentrations of sodium citrate preservative are currently added to blue-top tubes for coagulation studies: 3.2% and 3.8%. The National Committee for Clinical Laboratory Standards (NCCLS) guideline for sodium citrate is 3.2%. Laboratories establish reference ranges for coagulation testing based on numerous factors, including sodium citrate concentration, test equipment, and test reagents. It is important to inquire from the laboratory which concentration it recommends, because each concentration will have its own specific reference range.

➤ When multiple specimens are drawn, the blue-top tube should be collected after sterile (i.e., blood culture) and red-top tubes. When coagulation testing is the only work to be done, an extra red-top tube should be collected before the blue-top tube to avoid contaminating the specimen with tissue thromboplastin, which can falsely decrease values.

➤ Label the specimen, and promptly transport it to the laboratory. The NCCLS recommendation for processed and unprocessed specimens stored in unopened tubes is that testing should be completed within 1 to 4 hours of collection.

Post-test: ■

➤ Observe venipuncture site for bleeding or hematoma formation. Apply pressure bandage.

➤ Evaluate test results in relation to the patient's symptoms and other tests performed. Related laboratory tests include factor assays, fibrinogen, and fibrin degradation products.

PLATELET ANTIBODIES

SYNONYMS/ACRONYMS: Antiplatelet antibody, platelet-bound IgG/IgM direct and indirect.

SPECIMEN: Serum (1 mL) collected in a red-top tube for indirect IgG antibody. Whole blood (7 mL) collected in lavender-top (ethylenediaminetetraacetic acid [EDTA]) tube for direct antibody.

REFERENCE VALUE: (Method: Solid-phase hemagglutination and flow cytometry) Negative.

DESCRIPTION: Platelet antibodies can be formed by autoimmune response, or they can be acquired in reaction to transfusion products. Platelet autoantibodies are immunoglobulins of autoimmune origin (i.e., immunoglobulin G), and they are present in various autoimmune disorders, including thrombocytopenias. Platelet alloantibodies develop in patients who become sensitized to platelet antigens of transfused blood. As a result, destruction of both donor and native platelets occurs along with a shortened survival time of platelets in the transfusion recipient. The platelet antibody detection test is also used for platelet typing, which allows compatible platelets to be transfused to patients with disorders such as aplastic anemia and cancer. Platelet typing decreases the alloimmunization risk resulting from repeated transfusions from random donors. Platelet typing may also provide additional support for a diagnosis of post-transfusional purpura. ∎

INDICATIONS:
- Assist in the detection of platelet alloimmune disorders
- Determine platelet type for refractory patients

RESULT

Increased in:
- Acquired immunodeficiency syndrome (AIDS)
- Acute myeloid leukemia
- Idiopathic thrombocytopenia purpura
- Immune complex diseases
- Multiple blood transfusions
- Multiple myeloma
- Neonatal immune thrombocytopenia
- Paroxysmal hemoglobinuria
- Rheumatoid arthritis
- Systemic lupus erythematosus
- Thrombocytopenias provoked by drugs (see monograph titled "Platelet Count")

Decreased in: N/A

CRITICAL VALUES: N/A

INTERFERING FACTORS: Hemolyzed or clotted specimens will affect results.

Nursing Implications and Procedure • • • • • • • • • •

Pretest:

➤ Obtain a history of the patient's complaints, including a list of known allergens.

➤ Obtain a history of the patient's hematopoietic and immune systems, a history of any bleeding disorders, and results of previously performed tests and procedures, especially bleeding time, complete blood count, clotting time, partial thromboplastin time, prothrombin time, and platelets. For related tests, refer to the hematopoietic and immune system tables.

➤ Obtain a list of the medications the patient is taking to include anticoagulant therapy, acetylsalicylic acid, herbals, and nutraceuticals known to affect coagulation. It is recommended that use be discontinued 14 days before dental or surgical procedures. The requesting health care practitioner and laboratory should be advised if the patient regularly uses these products so that their effects can be taken into consideration when reviewing results.

➤ There are no food, fluid, or medication restrictions unless by medical direction.

➤ Review the procedure with the patient.

➤ Inform the patient that specimen collection takes approximately 5 to 10 minutes.

Intratest:

➤ Direct the patient to breathe normally and to avoid unnecessary movement.

➤ Observe standard precautions and follow the general guidelines in Appendix A. Perform a venipuncture, and collect the specimen in a 5-mL red-top and a 7-mL lavender-top tube.

➤ Label the specimen, and promptly transport it to the laboratory.

Post-test:

➤ Observe venipuncture site for bleeding or hematoma formation. Apply pressure bandage.

➤ Note the patient's response to platelet transfusions.

➤ Instruct the patient to report severe bruising or bleeding from any areas of the skin or mucous membranes.

➤ Inform the patient who has developed platelet antibodies of the importance of taking precautions against bruising and bleeding, including the use of a soft bristle toothbrush, use of an electric razor, avoidance of constipation, avoidance of acetylsalicylic acid and similar products, and avoidance of intramuscular injections.

➤ Evaluate test results in relation to the patient's symptoms and other tests performed. Related laboratory tests include clot retraction and platelet count.

PLATELET COUNT

• •

SYNONYM/ACRONYM: Thrombocytes.

SPECIMEN: Whole blood from one full lavender-top (ethylenediaminetetra-acetic acid [EDTA]) tube.

REFERENCE VALUE: (Method: Automated, computerized multichannel analyzers that sort and size cells on the basis of either changes in electrical impedance or light pulses as the cells pass in front of a laser)

Age	Platelet Count*	SI Units (Conversion Factor $\times 10^6$)	MPV (fl)
1–5 y	217–497 $\times$ 10³/µL/mm³	217–497 $\times$ 10⁹/L	7.2–10.0
Adult	150–450 $\times$ 10³/µL/mm³	181–521 $\times$ 10⁹/L	7.0–10.2

Note: Platelet counts decrease with age.
* Conventional units.
MPV = mean platelet volume.

DESCRIPTION: *Platelets* are non-nucleated, cytoplasmic, round or oval disks formed by budding off of large, multinucleated cells (megakaryocytes). Platelets have an essential function in coagulation, hemostasis, and blood thrombus formation. *Thrombocytosis* is an increase in platelet count. In reactive thrombocytosis, the increase is transient and short lived, and it usually does not pose a health risk. One exception may be reactive thrombocytosis occurring after coronary bypass surgery. This circumstance has been identified as an important risk factor for postoperative infarction and thrombosis. The term *thrombocythemia* is used to describe platelet increases associated with chronic myeloproliferative disorders. *Thrombocytopenia* is used to describe platelet counts of less than 140 $\times$ 10⁶/µL. Decreased platelet counts occur whenever the body's need for platelets exceeds the rate of platelet production; this circumstance will arise if production rate decreases or platelet loss increases. The severity of bleeding is related to platelet count as well as platelet function. Platelet counts can be within normal limits, but the patient may exhibit signs of internal bleeding; this circumstance usually indicates an anomaly in platelet function. Abnormal scatterplot findings by automated cell counters may indicate the need to review a smear of peripheral blood for platelet estimate. Abnormally large or giant platelets may result in underestimated automated counts by 30 to 50 percent. A large discrepancy between the automated count and the estimate requires that a manual count be performed. The significance of platelet sizing is becoming more widely known, as modern cell counters are capable of reporting platelet indexes that are analogous to red blood cell (RBC) indices. Platelet size, reflected by mean platelet volume (MPV) and cellular age, are inversely related; that is, younger platelets tend to be larger. An increase in MPV indicates an increase in platelet turnover. Therefore, in a normal patient the platelet count and MPV have an inverse relationship. Abnormal platelet size may also indicate the presence of a disorder. MPV and platelet distribution width (PDW) are both increased in idiopathic thrombocytopenic purpura. MPV is also increased in May-Hegglin anomaly, Bernard-Soulier syndrome, myeloproliferative disorders, hyperthyroidism, and preeclampsia. MPV is decreased in Wiskott-Aldrich syndrome, septic thrombocytopenia, and hypersplenism. ∎

INDICATIONS:
- Confirm a low platelet count (thrombocytopenia), which can be associated with bleeding
- Confirm an elevated platelet count (thrombocytosis), which can cause increased clotting
- Identify the possible cause of abnormal bleeding, such as epistaxis, hematoma, gingival bleeding, hematuria, and menorrhagia
- Provide screening as part of a complete blood count in a general physical examination, especially upon admission to a health care facility or before surgery

RESULT

Increased in:
- Acute infections
- After exercise (transient)
- Anemias (posthemorrhagic, hemolytic, iron-deficiency)
- Chronic heart disease
- Cirrhosis
- Essential thrombocythemia
- Leukemias (chronic)
- Malignancies (carcinoma, Hodgkin's, lymphomas)
- Pancreatitis (chronic)
- Polycythemia vera
- Rebound recovery from thrombocytopenia

- Rheumatic fever (acute)
- Rheumatoid arthritis
- Splenectomy (2 months postprocedure)
- Surgery (2 weeks postprocedure)
- Trauma
- Tuberculosis
- Ulcerative colitis

Decreased in (as a result of megakaryocytic hypoproliferation):
- Alcohol toxicity
- Aplastic anemia
- Congenital states (Fanconi's, May-Hegglin, Bernard-Soulier, Wiskott-Aldrich, Gaucher's, Chédiak-Higashi syndromes)
- Drug toxicity
- Prolonged hypoxia

Decreased in (as a result of ineffective thrombopoiesis):
- Ethanol abuse without malnutrition
- Iron-deficiency anemia
- Megaloblastic anemia (B_{12}/folate deficiency)
- Paroxysmal nocturnal hemoglobinuria
- Thrombopoietin deficiency
- Viral infection

Decreased in (as a result of bone marrow replacement):
- Lymphoma
- Granulomatous infections
- Metastatic carcinoma
- Myelofibrosis

Increased destruction in (as a result of increased loss/consumption):
- Contact with foreign surfaces (dialysis

membranes, artificial organs, grafts, prosthetic devices)

- Disseminated intravascular coagulation

- Extensive transfusion

- Severe hemorrhage

- Thrombotic thrombocytopenic purpura

- Uremia

Increased destruction in (as a result of immune reaction):
- Antibody/human leukocyte antigen reactions

- Hemolytic disease of the newborn (target is platelets instead of RBCs)

- Idiopathic thrombocytopenic purpura

- Refractory reaction to platelet transfusion

Increased destruction in (as a result of immune reaction secondary to infection):
- Bacterial infections

- Burns

- Congenital infections (cytomegalovirus, herpes, syphilis, toxoplasmosis)

- Histoplasmosis

- Malaria

- Rocky Mountain spotted fever

Increased destruction in (as a result of other causes):
- Radiation

- Splenomegaly caused by liver disease

CRITICAL VALUES:

Less than 50,000 K/µL or mm³
Greater than 1,000,000 K/µL or mm³
Possible interventions for decreased platelet count may include transfusion of platelets.

INTERFERING FACTORS:

- Drugs that may decrease platelet counts include acetohexamide, acetophenazine, amphotericin B, antazoline, anticonvulsants, antimony compounds, apronalide, arsenicals, azathioprine, barbiturates, benzene, busulfan, butaperazine, chlordane, chlorophenothane, chlortetracycline, dactinomycin, dextromethorphan, diethylstilbestrol, ethinamate, ethoxzolamide, floxuridine, hexachlorobenzene, hydantoin derivatives, hydroflumethiazide, hydroxychloroquine, iproniazid, mechlorethamine, mefenamic acid, mepazine, miconazole, mitomycin, nitrofurantoin, novobiocin, nystatin, phenolphthalein, phenothiazine, pipamazine, plicamycin, procarbazine, pyrazolones, streptomycin, sulfonamides, tetracycline, thiabendazole, thiouracil, tolazamide, tolazoline, tolbutamide, trifluoperazine, and urethane.

- Drugs that may increase platelet counts include glucocorticoids.

- X-ray therapy may also decrease platelet counts.

- The results of blood counts may vary depending on the patient's position. Platelet counts can decrease when the patient is recumbent, as a result of hemodilution, and can increase when the patient rises, as a result of hemoconcentration.

- Platelet counts normally increase under a variety of stressors, such as high altitudes or strenuous exercise.

- Platelet counts are normally decreased before menstruation and during pregnancy.

- Leaving the tourniquet in place for longer than 60 seconds can affect the results.

- Traumatic venipunctures may lead to erroneous results as a result of activation of the coagulation sequence.

- Failure to fill the tube sufficiently (i.e., tube less than three-quarters full) may yield inadequate sample volume for automated analyzers and may be reason for specimen rejection.

- Hemolysis or clotted specimens are reasons for rejection.

- Complete blood count should be carefully evaluated after transfusion or acute blood loss because the value may appear to be normal.

- A white blood cell count greater than 100,000 per mm^3, severe RBC fragmentation, and extraneous particles in the fluid used to dilute the sample can alter test results.

Nursing Implications and Procedure

Pretest:

➤ Obtain a history of the patient's complaints, including a list of known allergens.

➤ Obtain a history of the patient's hematopoietic and immune systems, a history of any bleeding disorders, and results of previously performed tests and procedures, especially bleeding time, complete blood count, clotting time, partial thromboplastin time, prothrombin time, and platelets. For related tests, refer to the hematopoietic and immune system tables.

➤ Obtain a list of the medications the patient is taking to include anticoagulant therapy, acetylsalicylic acid, herbals, and nutraceuticals known to affect coagulation. It is recommended that use be discontinued 14 days before dental or surgical procedures. The requesting health care practitioner and laboratory should be advised if the patient regularly uses these products so that their effects can be taken into consideration when reviewing results.

➤ Note any recent procedures that can interfere with test results.

➤ There are no food, fluid, or medication restrictions unless by medical direction.

➤ Review the procedure with the patient.

➤ Inform the patient that specimen collection takes approximately 5 to 10 minutes.

Intratest:

➤ Direct the patient to breathe normally and to avoid unnecessary movement.

➤ Observe standard precautions and follow the general guidelines in Appendix A. Perform a venipuncture, and collect the specimen in a 5-mL lavender-top tube. The specimen should be mixed gently by inverting the tube 10 times. The specimen should be analyzed within 6 hours when stored at room temperature or within 24 hours if stored at refrigerated temperature. In addition, if it is anticipated that the specimen will not be analyzed within 4 to 6 hours, two blood smears should be made immediately after the venipuncture and should be submitted with the blood sample.

➤ Label the specimen, and promptly transport it to the laboratory.

Post-test:

➤ Observe venipuncture site for bleeding or hematoma formation. Apply pressure bandage.

➤ Instruct the patient to report bleeding from any areas of the skin or mucous membranes.

➤ Inform the patient with a decreased platelet count of the importance of taking precautions against bruising and bleeding, including the use of a soft bristle toothbrush, use of an electric razor, avoidance of constipation, avoidance of acetylsalicylic acid and similar products, and avoidance of intramuscular injections.

➤ Inform the patient of the importance of periodic laboratory testing if he or she is taking an anticoagulant.

> Evaluate test results in relation to the patient's symptoms and other tests performed. Related laboratory tests include bleeding time, clot

retraction, complete blood count, RBC morphology and inclusions, platelet antibodies, and white blood cell count and differential.

PLETHYSMOGRAPHY

. . . .

SYNONYM/ACRONYM: Impedance plethysmography, PVR.

AREA OF APPLICATION: Veins, arteries, and lungs.

CONTRAST: Done without contrast.

DESCRIPTION: Plethysmography is a noninvasive diagnostic manometric study used to measure changes in the size of blood vessels by determining volume changes in the blood vessels of the eye, extremities, and neck; or gas volume changes in the lungs.

Arterial plethysmography assesses arterial circulation in an upper or lower limb; it is used to diagnose extremity arteriosclerotic disease and to rule out occlusive disease. The test requires a normal extremity for comparison of results. The test is performed by applying a series of three blood pressure cuffs to the extremity. The amplitude of each pulse wave is then recorded.

Venous plethysmography, done with a series of cuffs, measures changes in venous capacity and outflow (volume and rate of outflow); it is used to diagnose a thrombotic condition that causes obstruction of the major veins of the extremity.

When the cuffs are applied to an extremity in patients with venous obstruction, no initial increase in leg volume is recorded because the venous volume of the leg cannot dissipate quickly.

Body plethysmography measures the total amount (volume) of air within the thorax, whether or not the air is in ventilatory communication with the lung; the elasticity (compliance) of the lungs; and the resistance to airflow in the respiratory tree. It is used in conjunction with pulmonary stress testing and pulmonary function testing.

Impedance plethysmography is widely used to detect acute deep vein thrombosis (DVT) of the leg, but it can also be used in the arm, abdomen, neck, or thorax. Doppler flow studies now are used to identify DVT, but ultrasound studies are less accurate in examinations below the knee. ■

INDICATIONS

Arterial Plethysmography:

- Evaluate suspected arterial occlusive disease

- Determine changes in toe or finger pressures when ankle pressures are elevated as a result of arterial calcifications

- Determine the effect of trauma on the arteries in an extremity

- Determine peripheral small-artery changes (ischemia) caused by diabetes, and differentiate these changes from neuropathy

- Detect vascular changes associated with Raynaud's phenomenon and disease

- Locate and determine the degree of arterial atherosclerotic obstruction and vessel patency in peripheral atherosclerotic disease, as well as inflammatory changes causing obliteration in the vessels in thromboangiitis obliterans

- Confirm suspected acute arterial embolization

Venous Plethysmography:

- Detect partial or total venous thrombotic obstruction

- Determine valve competency in conjunction with Doppler ultrasonography in the diagnosis of varicose veins

Body Plethysmography:

- Detect or determine the status of chronic obstructive pulmonary disease (COPD), such as emphysema, asthma, or chronic bronchitis

- Detect or determine the status of restrictive pulmonary disease, such as fibrosis

- Differentiate between obstructive and restrictive pulmonary pathology

- Detect acute pulmonary disorders, such as atelectasis

- Detect infectious pulmonary diseases, such as pneumonia

- Determine baseline pulmonary status before pulmonary rehabilitation to determine potential therapeutic benefit

Impedance Plethysmography:

- Detect and evaluate DVT

- Act as a diagnostic screen for patients at risk for DVT

- Evaluate patients with suspected pulmonary embolism (most pulmonary emboli are complications of DVT in the leg)

- Evaluate degree of resolution of DVT after treatment

RESULT

Normal Findings:

- Arterial plethysmography:

  Normal arterial pulse waves: steep up-slope, more gradual down-slope with narrow pointed peaks

  Normal pressure: less than 20 mm Hg systolic difference between the lower and upper extremities; toe pressure greater than or equal to 80 percent of ankle pressure, and finger pressure greater than or equal to 80 percent of wrist pressure

- Venous plethysmography:

  Normal venous blood flow in the extremities

  Venous filling times greater than 20 seconds

- Body plethysmography:

  Thoracic gas volume: 2400 mL

  Compliance: 0.2 L/cm H_2O

  Airway resistance: 0.6 to 2.5 cm H_2O/L per second

- Impedance plethysmography:

  Sharp rise in volume with temporary occlusion

  Rapid venous outflow with release of the occlusion

Abnormal Findings:

- DVT (arterial, venous, or impedance plethysmography)

- Incompetent valves, thrombosis, or thrombotic obstruction in a major vein in an extremity

- COPD, restrictive lung disease, lung infection, or atelectasis (body plethysmography)

- Small-vessel diabetic changes

- Vascular disease (Raynaud's phenomenon)

- Vascular trauma

CRITICAL VALUES: N/A

INTERFERING FACTORS

Arterial Plethysmography:

Factors that may impair results of the examination:

- Cigarette smoking 2 hours before the study, which causes inaccurate results because the nicotine constricts the arteries

- Alcohol consumption

- Low cardiac output

- Shock

- Compression of pelvic veins (tumors or external compression by dressings)

- Environmental temperatures (hot or cold)

- Arterial occlusion proximal to the extremity to be examined, which can prevent blood flow to the limb

Venous Plethysmography:

Factors that may impair results of the examination:

- Environmental temperature or cold extremity, which constricts the vessels

- High anxiety level or muscle tenseness

- Venous thrombotic occlusion proximal

to the extremity to be examined, which can affect blood flow to the limb

Body Plethysmography:

Factors that may impair results of the examination:

- Inability of the patient to follow breathing instructions during the procedure

Impedance Plethysmography:

Factors that may impair results of the examination:

- Movement of the extremity during electrical impedance recording, poor electrode contact, or nonlinear electrical output, which can cause false-positive impedance plethysmography results

- Constricting clothing or bandages

Nursing Implications and Procedure

Pretest:

➤ Explain to the patient the purpose of the procedure and how it is performed; assess for compliance with directions given for rest, positioning, and activity before and during the procedure. For body plethysmography, explain that the procedure measures the amount of air contained in the chest, the elasticity of the lungs, and the occurrence of restrictive breathing in the bronchioles.

➤ Explain that the procedure is generally performed in a specialized area by a technologist or at bedside and usually takes 30 to 60 minutes.

➤ Obtain a history of signs and symptoms of vascular disorders, known or suspected peripheral vascular disease (for arterial and vascular plethysmography), known or suspected diseases of the pulmonary system (for body plethysmography), signs or symptoms of DVT or circulatory changes (for impedance plethysmography), results of previous diagnostic tests and procedures, and medical regimens. For related tests, refer to the cardiovascular system table.

➤ Obtain a list of the medications the patient is taking.

➤ Obtain pertinent history of other diagnostic procedure results, laboratory test results, present cardiac conditions or vascular abnormalities, surgeries, and therapy received.

➤ Determine date of last menstrual period and possibility of pregnancy in perimenopausal women.

➤ Ensure that the patient has refrained from smoking for 2 hours before the procedure.

➤ For body plethysmography, record the patient's weight, height, and gender. Determine whether the patient is claustrophobic.

➤ Explain that the procedure is painless and carries no risks.

➤ Ask the patient to notify medical personnel if he or she has ill effects or unexpected symptoms during the test.

➤ Do not restrict food, fluid, or medications.

➤ Obtain and record baseline vital signs.

Intratest:

➤ Ask the patient to void before the procedure. Have the patient put on a hospital gown.

Arterial plethysmography:

➤ Explain to the patient that cuffs are applied to the extremity to measure and compare blood flow.

➤ Place the patient in a semi-Fowler position on the examining table or bed.

➤ Apply three blood pressure cuffs to the extremity and attach a pulse volume recorder (plethysmograph), which records the amplitude of each pulse wave.

➤ Inflate the cuffs to 65 mm Hg to measure the pulse waves of each cuff. When compared with a normal limb, these measurements determine the presence of arterial occlusive disease.

➤ Explain to the patient that it is essential to remain still during the procedure.

Venous plethysmography:

➤ Explain to the patient that cuffs are applied to the extremity to measure and compare blood flow.

➤ Place the patient in a semi-Fowler position on an examining table or in bed.

➤ Apply two cuffs to the extremity one on the proximal part of the extremity (occlusion cuff) and the other on the distal part of the extremity (recorder cuff). Attach a third cuff to the pulse volume recorder.

➤ Inflate the recorder cuff to 10 mm Hg, and evaluate the effects of respiration on venous volume: Absence of changes during respirations indicates venous thrombotic occlusion.

➤ Inflate the occlusion cuff to 50 mm Hg, and record venous volume on the pulse monitor. Deflate the occlusion cuff after the highest volume is recorded in the recorder cuff. A delay in the return to preocclusion volume indicates venous thrombotic occlusion.

➤ Explain to the patient that it is essential to remain still during the procedure.

Body plethysmography:

➤ Place the patient in a sitting position on a chair in the body box.

➤ Position a nose clip to prevent breathing through the nose, and connect a mouthpiece to a measuring instrument.

➤ Ask the patient to breathe through the mouthpiece.

➤ Close the door to the box, and record the start time of the procedure. At the beginning of the study, ask the patient to pant rapidly and shallowly, without allowing the glottis to close.

➤ For compliance testing, a double-lumen nasoesophageal catheter is inserted, and the bag is inflated with air. Intraesophageal pressure is recorded during normal breathing.

Impedance plethysmography:

➤ Place the patient on his or her back with the leg being tested above the heart level.

➤ Flex the patient's knee slightly, and rotate the hips by shifting weight to the same side as the leg being tested.

➤ Apply conductive gel and electrodes.

➤ Inflate the pressure cuff attached to the thigh temporarily to occlude venous return without interfering with arterial blood flow. Expect the blood volume in the other calf to increase.

➤ A tracing of changes in electrical impedance occurring during inflation and for 15 seconds after cuff deflation is recorded.

➤ With DVT, blood volume increases less than expected because the veins are already at capacity.

Post-test:

➤ Remove conductive gel and electrodes, as applied.

➤ Instruct the patient to continue normal activity and diet, unless otherwise indicated.

➤ Note severe ischemia, ulcers, and pain of the extremity after arterial, venous, or impedance plethysmography, and handle the extremity gently.

➤ Note respiratory pattern after body plethysmography, and allow the patient time to resume a normal breathing pattern.

➤ A physician specializing in this branch of medicine sends a written report to the ordering provider, who discusses the results with the patient.

➤ Inform the patient that further examinations may be necessary to evaluate progression of the disease process or to determine the need for a change in therapy.

➤ Note test results in relation to the patient's symptoms and any related tests performed.

PLEURAL FLUID ANALYSIS

SYNONYM/ACRONYM: Thoracentesis fluid analysis.

SPECIMEN: Pleural fluid (5 mL) collected in a green-top (heparin) tube for amylase, cholesterol, glucose, lactate dehydrogenase (LDH), pH, protein, and triglycerides; lavender-top (ethylenediaminetetra-acetic acid [EDTA]) tube for cell count; sterile containers for microbiology specimens; equal amounts of fixative and fluid in plastic containers for cytology.

REFERENCE VALUE: (Method: Spectrophotometry for amylase, cholesterol, glucose, LDH, protein, and triglycerides; ion-selective electrode for pH; automated or manual cell count; macroscopic and microscopic examination of cultured microorganisms; microscopic examination of specimen for microbiology and cytology.)

Pleural Fluid	Reference Value
Appearance	Clear
Color	Pale yellow
Amylase	Parallel serum values
Cholesterol	Parallel serum values
Glucose	Parallel serum values
LDH	Less than 200 U/L
Fluid LDH–to–serum LDH ratio	0.6 or less
Protein	3.0 g/dL
Fluid protein–to–serum protein ratio	0.5 or less
Triglycerides	Parallel serum values
pH	7.37–7.43
RBC count	Less than 1000/mm^3
WBC count	Less than 1000/mm^3
Culture	No growth
Gram stain	No organisms seen
Cytology	No abnormal cells seen

LDH = lactate dehydrogenase; RBC = red blood cell; WBC = white blood cell.

DESCRIPTION: The pleural cavity and organs within it are lined with a protective membrane. The fluid between the membranes is called *serous fluid.* Normally only a small amount of fluid is present because the rates of fluid production and absorption are about the same. Many abnormal conditions can result in the buildup of fluid within the pleural cavity. Specific tests are usually ordered in addition to a common battery of tests used to distinguish a transudate from an exudate. *Transudates* are effusions that form as a result of a systemic disorder that disrupts the regulation of fluid balance, such as a suspected perforation. *Exudates* are caused by conditions involving the tissue of the membrane itself, such as an infection or malignancy. Fluid is withdrawn from the pleural cavity by needle aspiration and tested as listed in the previous and following tables. ■

Characteristic	Transudate	Exudate
Appearance	Clear	Cloudy or turbid
Specific gravity	Less than 1.015	Greater than 1.015
Total protein	Less than 2.5 g/dL	Greater than 3.0 g/dL
Fluid protein–to–serum protein ratio	Less than 0.5	Greater than 0.5
LDH	Parallels serum value	Less than 200 U/L
Fluid LDH–to–serum LDH ratio	Less than 0.6	Greater than 0.6
Fluid cholesterol	Less than 55 mg/dL	Greater than 55 mg/dL
WBC count	Less than 100/mm^3	Greater than 1000/mm^3

LDH = lactate dehydrogenase; WBC = white blood cell.

INDICATIONS:

- Differentiate transudates from exudates

- Evaluate effusion of unknown cause

- Investigate suspected rupture, immune disease, malignancy, or infection

RESULT:

- *Bacterial or tuberculous empyema:* Red blood cell (RBC) count 5000/mm³, white blood cell (WBC) count 25,000 to 100,000/mm³ with a predominance of neutrophils, increased protein-to-serum ratio, increased LDH-to-serum ratio, decreased glucose, pH less than 7.3

- *Chylous pleural effusion:* Marked increase in both triglycerides (two to three times serum level) and chylomicrons

- *Effusion caused by pneumonia:* RBC count 5000/mm³, WBC count 5000 to 25,000/mm³ with a predominance of neutrophils and some eosinophils, increased protein-to-serum ratio, increased LDH-to-serum ratio, pH less than 7.4 (and decreased glucose if bacterial pneumonia)

- *Esophageal rupture:* Significantly decreased pH (6.0) and elevated amylase

- *Hemothorax:* Bloody appearance, increased RBC count, elevated hematocrit

- *Malignancy:* RBC count 1000 to 100,000/mm³, WBC count 5000 to 10,000/mm³ with a predominance of lymphocytes, abnormal cytology, increased protein-to-serum ratio, increased LDH-to-serum ratio, deceased glucose, pH less than 7.3

- *Pancreatitis:* RBC count 1000 to 10,000/mm³, WBC count 5000 to 20,000/mm³ with a predominance of neutrophils, pH greater than 7.3, increased protein-to-serum ratio, increased LDH-to-serum ratio, increased amylase

- *Pulmonary infarction:* RBC count 10,000 to 100,000/mm³, WBC count 5000 to 15,000/mm³ with a predominance of neutrophils, pH greater than 7.3, normal glucose, increased fluid protein-to-serum protein ratio, and increased fluid LDH-to-serum LDH ratio.

- *Pulmonary tuberculosis:* RBC count 10,000/mm³, WBC count 5000 to 10,000/mm³ with a predominance of lymphocytes, positive acid-fast bacillus stain and culture, increased protein, decreased glucose, pH less than 7.3

- *Rheumatoid disease:* Normal RBC count, WBC count 1000 to 20,000/mm³ with a predominance of either lymphocytes or neutrophils, pH less than 7.3, decreased glucose, increased protein-to-serum ratio, increased LDH-to-serum ratio, increased immunoglobulins

- *Systemic lupus erythematosus:* Similar findings as with rheumatoid disease, except that glucose is usually not decreased

CRITICAL VALUES: N/A

INTERFERING FACTORS:

- Bloody fluids may be the result of a traumatic tap.

- Unknown hyperglycemia or hypoglycemia may be misleading in the comparison of fluid and serum glucose levels. It is advisable to collect comparative serum samples a few hours before thoracentesis.

Nursing Implications and Procedure

Pretest:

▶ Obtain a history of the patient's

complaints, including a list of known allergens.

➤ Obtain a history of the patient's immune and respiratory systems, as well as results of previously performed tests and procedures. For related tests, refer to the immune and respiratory system tables.

➤ Obtain a list of medications the patient is taking, including herbs, nutritional supplements, and nutraceuticals. The requesting health care practitioner and laboratory should be advised if the patient regularly uses these products so that their effects can be taken into consideration when reviewing results.

➤ There are no food or fluid restrictions unless by medical direction.

➤ The requesting health care practitioner may request that a cough suppressant be given before the procedure.

➤ Anticoagulants and aspirin may be withheld by medical direction.

➤ Review the procedure with the patient. Explain the importance of remaining still during the procedure.

➤ Inform the patient that a local anesthetic will be administered at the chest needle-insertion site immediately before the procedure. Explain that the anesthetic injection may cause a stinging sensation.

➤ Assess if the patient has an allergy to local anesthetics, and inform the health care practitioner accordingly.

➤ *Obtain written and informed consent before medication is administered prior to the procedure.*

➤ Have the patient void before the procedure.

➤ Inform the patient that specimen collection takes approximately 20 minutes and is performed by a health care practitioner.

Intratest: ■

➤ Assist the patient into a sitting or side-lying position.

➤ Direct the patient to breathe normally and to avoid unnecessary movement.

➤ Record baseline vital signs.

➤ Observe standard precautions and follow the general guidelines in Appendix A.

➤ Cleanse the skin with an antiseptic solution, and protect area with sterile drape. The skin at the injection site is anesthetized.

➤ The thoracentesis needle is inserted, and fluid is removed.

➤ The needle is withdrawn, and slight pressure is applied to the site. If there is no evidence of bleeding or drainage, a sterile dressing is applied to the site.

➤ Label the specimen, and promptly transport it to the laboratory.

Post-test: ■

➤ Instruct the patient to resume usual medications, as directed by the requesting health care practitioner.

➤ Inform the patient that 1 hour or more of bed rest (lying on the unaffected side) is required after the procedure. Elevate the patient's head for comfort.

➤ Observe the patient for signs of respiratory distress or skin color changes.

➤ Assess vital signs every 15 minutes for the first hour, every 30 minutes for the next 2 hours, every hour for the next 4 hours, and every 4 hours for the next 24 hours. Take temperature every 4 hours for 24 hours. Monitor intake and output for 24 hours.

➤ Prepare the patient for a chest x-ray, if ordered, to ensure that a pneumothorax has not occurred as a result of the procedure.

➤ Assess the puncture site for bleeding or drainage and signs of inflammation each time vital signs are assessed and daily for several days thereafter.

➤ Administer antibiotics, as ordered, and instruct the patient in the importance of completing the entire course of antibiotic therapy even if no symptoms are present.

➤ Evaluate test results in relation to the patient's symptoms and other tests performed. Related laboratory tests include bacterial culture, CA 15-3, CA 19-9, CA 125, carcinoembryonic antigen, fungal culture, mycobacterial culture, and viral culture.

PORPHYRINS, URINE

· ·

SYNONYMS/ACRONYM: Coproporphyrin, porphobilinogen, urobilinogen, and other porphyrins.

SPECIMEN: Urine (10 mL) from a random or timed specimen collected in a clean, amber-colored, plastic collection container with sodium carbonate as a preservative.

REFERENCE VALUE: (Method: Chromatography for uroporphyrins; spectrophotometry for δ-aminolevulinic acid, urobilinogen, and porphobilinogen)

Test	Conventional Units	SI Units
Total porphyrins	Less than 320 μg/24 h	
		(Conversion Factor × 1.53)
Coproporphyrin *Tetracarboxylcoproporphyrin*		
Male	Less than 96 μg/24 h	Less than 147 nmol/24 h
Female	Less than 60 μg/24 h	Less than 92 nmol/24 h
		(Conversion Factor × 1.43)
Uroporphyrins *Pentacarboxylporphyrin*		
Male	Less than 4 μg/24 h	Less than 6 nmol/24 h
Female	Less than 3 μg/24 h	Less than 4 nmol/24 h
		(Conversion Factor × 1.34)
Hexacarboxylporphyrin		
Male	Less than 5 μg/24 h	Less than 7 nmol/24 h
Female	Less than 3 μg/24 h	Less than 4 nmol/24 h

(Continued on the following page)

Test	Conventional Units	SI Units
		(Conversion Factor ✕ 1.27)
Heptacarboxyl-porphyrin		
Male	Less than 13 μg/24 h	Less than 17 nmol/24 h
Female	Less than 9 μg/24 h	Less than 11 nmol/24 h
		(Conversion Factor ✕ 4.42)
Porphobilinogen	Less than 2.0 mg/24 h	Less than 8.8 μmol/24 h
		(Conversion Factor ✕ 1)
Urobilinogen	0.5–4.0 EU/24 h	0.5–4.0 EU/24 h
		(Conversion Factor ✕ 7.626)
δ-Aminolevulinic acid	1.5–7.5 mg/24 h	11.4–57.2 μmol/24 h

DESCRIPTION: Porphyrins are produced during the synthesis of heme. If heme synthesis is disturbed, these precursors accumulate and are excreted in the urine in excessive amounts. Conditions producing increased levels of heme precursors are called *porphyrias*. The two main categories of genetically determined porphyrias are erythropoietic porphyrias, in which major abnormalities occur in red blood cell chemistry, and hepatic porphyrias, in which heme precursors are found in urine and feces. Erythropoietic and hepatic porphyrias are rare. Acquired porphyrias are characterized by greater accumulation of precursors in urine and feces than in red blood cells. Lead poisoning is the most common cause of acquired porphyrias. Porphyrins are reddish fluorescent compounds. Depending on the type of porphyrin present, the urine may be reddish, resembling port wine. Porphobilinogen is excreted as a colorless compound. A color change may occur in an acidic sample containing porphobilinogen if the sample is exposed to air for several hours. ■

INDICATIONS:
- Assist in the diagnosis of congenital or acquired porphyrias, characterized by abdominal pain, tachycardia, emesis, fever, leukocytosis, and neurologic abnormalities
- Detect suspected lead poisoning, as indicated by elevated porphyrins

RESULT

Increased in:
- Acute hepatic porphyrias
- Congenital or acquired porphyrias
- Heavy metal, benzene, or carbon tetrachloride toxicity
- Variegated porphyrias

Decreased in: N/A

CRITICAL VALUES: N/A

INTERFERING FACTORS:
- Drugs that may increase urine porphyrin levels include acriflavine, aminopyrine, ethoxazene, griseofulvin, hexachlorobenzene, oxytetracycline, and sulfonmethane.
- Numerous drugs are suspected as potential initiators of acute attacks, but

drugs classified as unsafe for high-risk individuals include antipyrine, aminopyrine, aminoglutethimide, barbiturates, carbamazepine, carbromal, chlorpropamide, danazol, dapsone, diclofenac, diphenylhydantoin, ergot preparations, ethchlorvynol, ethinamate, glutethimide, griseofulvin, N-isopropyl meprobamate, mephenytoin, meprobamate, methyprylon, N-butylscopolammoniumine bromide, novobiocin, phenylbutazone, primidone, pyrazolone preparations, succinimides, sulfonamide antibiotics, sulfonethylmethane, sulfonmethane, synthetic estrogens and progestins, tolazamide, tolbutamide, trimethadione, and valproic acid.

- Exposure of the specimen to light can falsely decrease values.

- Screening methods are not well standardized and can produce false-negative results.

- Failure to collect all urine and store specimen properly during the 24-hour test period will interfere with results.

Nursing Implications and Procedure

Pretest:

➤ Obtain a history of the patient's complaints, including a list of known allergens.

➤ Obtain a history of the patient's hematopoietic system and results of previously performed tests and procedures. For related tests, refer to the hematopoietic system table.

➤ Obtain a list of medications the patient is taking, including herbs, nutritional supplements, and nutraceuticals. The requesting health care practitioner and laboratory should be advised if the patient regularly uses these products so that their effects can be taken into consideration when reviewing results.

➤ There are no food, fluid, or medication restrictions unless by medical direction.

➤ Review the procedure with the patient. Provide a nonmetallic urinal, bedpan, or toilet-mounted collection device.

➤ Usually a 24-hour time frame for urine collection is ordered. Inform the patient that all urine must be saved during that 24-hour period. Instruct the patient not to void directly into the laboratory collection container. Instruct the patient to avoid defecating in the collection device and to keep toilet tissue out of the collection device to prevent contamination of the specimen. Place a sign in the bathroom to remind the patient to save all urine.

➤ Instruct the patient to void all urine into the collection device and then to pour the urine into the laboratory collection container. Alternatively the specimen can be left in the collection device for a health care staff member to add to the laboratory collection container.

Intratest:

➤ Observe standard precautions and follow the general guidelines in Appendix A.

Random specimen (collect in early morning):

Clean-catch specimen:

➤ Instruct the male patient to (1) thoroughly wash his hands, (2) cleanse the meatus, (3) void a small amount into the toilet, and (4) void directly into the specimen container.

➤ Instruct the female patient to (1) thoroughly wash her hands; (2) cleanse the labia from front to back; (3) while keeping the labia separated, void a small amount into the toilet; and (4) without interrupting the urine stream, void directly into the specimen container.

Indwelling catheter:

➤ Put on gloves. Empty drainage tube

of urine. It may be necessary to clamp off the catheter for 15 to 30 minutes before specimen collection. Cleanse specimen port with antiseptic swab, and then aspirate 5 mL of urine with a 21- to 25-gauge needle and syringe. Transfer urine to a sterile container.

Timed specimen:

➤ Obtain a clean 3-L urine specimen container, toilet-mounted collection device, and plastic bag (for transport of the specimen container). The specimen must be refrigerated or kept on ice throughout the entire collection period. If an indwelling urinary catheter is in place, the drainage bag must be kept on ice.

➤ Begin the test between 6 and 8 a.m., if possible. Collect first voiding and discard. Record the time the specimen was discarded as the beginning of the timed collection period. The next morning, ask the patient to void at the same time the collection was started and add this last voiding to the container.

➤ If an indwelling catheter is in place, replace the tubing and container system at the start of the collection

time. Keep the container system on ice during the collection period, or empty the urine into a larger container periodically during the collection period; monitor to ensure continued drainage, and conclude the test the next morning at the same hour the collection was begun.

➤ At the conclusion of the test, compare the quantity of urine with the urinary output record for the collection; if the specimen contains less than what was recorded as output, some urine may have been discarded, invalidating the test.

➤ Label the specimen, and promptly transport it to the laboratory. Include on the label the amount of urine, test start and stop times, and ingestion of any foods or medications that can affect test results.

Post-test:

➤ Evaluate test results in relation to the patient's symptoms and other tests performed. Related laboratory tests include δ-aminolevulinic acid, erythrocyte protoporphyrin, and lead.

POSITRON EMISSION TOMOGRAPHY, BRAIN

SYNONYM/ACRONYM: PET scan of the brain.

AREA OF APPLICATION: Brain.

CONTRAST: Intravenous radioactive material.

DESCRIPTION: Positron emission tomography (PET) combines the biochemical properties of nuclear medicine with the accuracy of computed tomography (CT). PET uses positron emissions from specific radionuclides (oxygen, nitrogen, carbon, and fluorine) to produce detailed functional images within the body. After the radionuclide becomes concentrated in the brain, PET images of blood flow or metabolic processes at the cellular level can be obtained. Fluorine-18, in the form of fluorodeoxyglucose (FDG), is one of the more commonly used radionuclides. FDG is a glucose analogue, and because every cell uses glucose, the metabolic activity occurring in neurologic conditions can be measured. There is little localization of FDG in normal tissue, allowing rapid detection of abnormal disease states. The brain uses oxygen and glucose almost exclusively to meet its energy needs, and therefore the brain's metabolism has been studied widely with PET.

The positron radiopharmaceuticals generally have short half-lives, ranging from a few seconds to a few hours, and therefore they must be produced in a cyclotron located near where the test is being done. The PET scanner translates the emissions from the radioactivity as the positron combines with the negative electrons from the tissues and forms gamma rays that can be detected by the scanner. This information is transmitted to the computer, which determines the location and its distribution and translates the emissions as color-coded images for viewing, quantitative measurements, activity changes in relation to time, and three-dimensional computer-aided analysis. Each radionuclide tracer is designed to measure a specific body process, such as glucose metabolism, blood flow, or brain tissue perfusion. The radionuclide can be administered intravenously or inhaled as a gas. PET has had the greatest clinical impact in patients with epilepsy, dementia, neurodegenerative diseases, inflammation, cerebrovascular disease (indirectly), and brain tumors.

The expense of the study and the limited availability of radiopharmaceuticals limit the use of PET, even though it is more sensitive than traditional nuclear scanning and single photon emission computed tomography (SPECT). Changes in reimbursement and the advent of mobile technology have increased the availability of this procedure in the community setting. ■

INDICATIONS:

- Identify focal seizures, as evidenced by decreased metabolism between seizures

- Evaluate Alzheimer's disease and differentiate it from other causes of dementia, as evidenced by decreased cerebral flow and metabolism

- Identify cerebrovascular accident or aneurysm, as evidenced by decreased blood flow and oxygen use

- Detect Parkinson's disease and Huntington's disease, as evidenced by decreased metabolism

- Evaluate cranial tumors preoperatively and postoperatively and determine stage and appropriate treatment or procedure

- Determine physiologic changes in psychosis and schizophrenia

- Determine the effectiveness of therapy, as evidenced by biochemical activity of normal and abnormal tissues

- Differentiate between tumor recurrence and radiation necrosis

RESULT

Normal Findings:

- Normal patterns of tissue metabolism, blood flow, and radionuclide distribution

Abnormal Findings:
- Alzheimer's disease
- Cerebrovascular accident
- Cerebral metastases
- Creutzfeldt-Jakob disease
- Dementia
- Head trauma
- Huntington's disease
- Migraine
- Parkinson's disease
- Schizophrenia
- Seizure disorders
- Tumors

CRITICAL VALUES: N/A

INTERFERING FACTORS

This procedure is contraindicated for:
- Patients who are pregnant or suspected of being pregnant, unless the potential benefits of the procedure far outweigh the risks to the fetus and mother

Factors that may impair clear imaging:
- Inability of the patient to cooperate or remain still during the procedure because of age, significant pain, or mental status
- Patients who are very obese, who may exceed the weight limit for the equipment
- Incorrect positioning of the patient, which may produce poor visualization of the area to be examined
- Drugs that alter glucose metabolism, such as tranquilizers or insulin, because hypoglycemia can alter PET results
- The use of alcohol, tobacco, or caffeine-containing drinks at least 24 hours before the study, because the effects of these substances would make it difficult to evaluate the patient's true physiologic state (e.g., alcohol is a vasoconstrictor and would decrease blood flow to the target organ)
- Metallic objects within the examination field (e.g., jewelry or body rings), which may inhibit organ visualization and can produce unclear images

Other considerations:
- Improper injection of the radionuclide that allows the tracer to seep deep into the muscle tissue produces erroneous hot spots.
- False-positive findings may occur as a result of normal gastrointestinal tract uptake and uptake in areas of infection or inflammation.
- Consultation with a physician should occur before the procedure for radiation safety concerns regarding infants of patients who are lactating.
- Risks associated with radiographic overexposure can result from frequent x-ray procedures. Personnel in the room with the patient should stand behind a shield or leave the area while the examination is being done. Personnel working in the area where the examination is being done should wear badges that reveal their level of exposure to radiation.

Nursing Implications and Procedure

Pretest:

➤ Inform the patient that the procedure assesses blood flow to the brain and brain tissue metabolism.

➤ Inform the patient that the procedure is performed in a special department by a technologist and takes approximately 30 to 120 minutes.

➤ Restrict alcohol, tobacco, or caffeine-containing drinks for 24 hours before the study or as per physician order.

➤ Instruct the insulin-dependent patient to take insulin as usual on the day of the procedure, to have a meal 4 hours before the procedure, and then to refrain from food or liquids.

➤ Obtain a list of medications the patient is taking.

➤ Obtain a history of neurologic tests, other diagnostic procedure results, laboratory test results, present neurologic conditions or abnormalities, and therapy received. For related tests, refer to the musculoskeletal system table.

➤ Determine date of last menstrual period and possibility of pregnancy in perimenopausal women.

➤ Reassure the patient that the radionuclide poses minimal radioactive hazard because of its short half-life and rarely produces side effects.

➤ *Obtain a written, informed consent for the procedure from the patient.*

➤ Sometimes fluorodeoxyglucose (FDG) examinations are done after blood has been drawn to determine circulating blood glucose levels. If blood glucose levels are high, insulin may be given.

➤ Obtain and record baseline electrocardiogram and vital signs.

Intratest:

➤ Ensure that emergency equipment is readily available during the procedure.

➤ Ask the patient to void before the procedure.

➤ Make sure jewelry and any other metallic objects have been removed from the brain area.

➤ Ask the patient to lie still during the procedure because movement produces unclear images.

➤ Place the patient supine on the imaging table with the head resting in a supportive device to minimize motion artifacts.

➤ An intravenous or arterial line may be started.

➤ The radionuclide is injected, and imaging is started 30 minutes later.

➤ If comparative studies are indicated, additional injections may be needed.

➤ The patient may be asked to perform different cognitive activities (e.g., reading) to measure changes in brain activity during reasoning or remembering.

➤ The patient may be blindfolded or asked to use earplugs to decrease auditory and visual stimuli.

➤ Wear gloves during the radionuclide injection and while handling the patient's urine.

Post-test:

➤ Monitor electrocardiogram tracings and blood pressures and compare with baseline readings until the patient is stable.

➤ Observe the injection site for redness, swelling, or hematoma.

➤ Observe the patient for 30 minutes after the procedure for possible reaction to the radionuclide or other procedure complications.

➤ Instruct the patient to resume normal activity and diet, unless otherwise indicated.

➤ If the patient must return for further imaging, advise the patient to rest in the interim and restrict diet to liquids before further studies.

➤ Advise patient to drink increased amounts of fluids for 24 hours to eliminate the radionuclide from the body, unless contraindicated. Tell the patient that radionuclide is eliminated from the body within 6 to 24 hours.

➤ Instruct the patient to flush the toilet immediately after each voiding following the procedure and to wash hands meticulously with soap and water after each voiding for 24 hours after the procedure.

➤ Tell all caregivers to wear gloves when discarding urine for 24 hours after the procedure. Wash gloved hands with soap and water before removing gloves. Then wash hands after the gloves are removed.

➤ A physician specializing in this branch of medicine sends a written report to the ordering provider, who discusses the results with the patient.

➤ Inform the patient that abnormalities

of the brain scan may indicate the need for additional studies.

➤ Evaluate test results in relation to the patient's symptoms and other tests performed.

➤ Related diagnostic tests include electroencephalogram, CT and magnetic resonance imaging of the brain, and Doppler ultrasound.

POSITRON EMISSION TOMOGRAPHY, HEART

· ·

SYNONYMS/ACRONYM: PET scan of the heart.

AREA OF APPLICATION: Heart, chest/thorax, vascular system.

CONTRAST: Intravenous radioactive material.

DESCRIPTION: Positron emission tomography (PET) combines the biochemical properties of nuclear medicine with the accuracy of computed tomography (CT). PET uses positron emissions from specific radionuclides (oxygen, nitrogen, carbon, and fluorine) to produce detailed functional images within the body. After the radionuclide becomes concentrated in the heart, PET images of blood flow or metabolic processes at the cellular level can be obtained. Fluorine-18, in the form of fluorodeoxyglucose (FDG), is one of the more commonly used radionuclides. FDG is a glucose analogue, and because every cell uses glucose, the metabolic activity occurring in heart conditions such as myocardial viability can be measured. There is

little localization of FDG in normal tissue, allowing rapid detection of abnormal disease states.

The positron radiopharmaceuticals generally have short half-lives, ranging from a few seconds to a few hours, and therefore they must be produced in a cyclotron located near where the test is being done. The PET scanner translates the emissions from the radioactivity as the positron combines with the negative electrons from the tissues and forms gamma rays that can be detected by the scanner. This information is transmitted to the computer, which determines the location and its distribution and translates the emissions as color-coded images for viewing, quantitative measurements, activity changes in relation to time, and three-dimensional computer-aided analysis. Each radionuclide tracer is designed to measure a specific body process, such as glucose metabolism, blood flow, or tissue perfusion. The radionuclide can be administered intravenously or inhaled as a gas.

The expense of the study and the limited availability of radiopharmaceuticals limit the use of PET, even though it is more sensitive than traditional nuclear scanning and single photon emission computed tomography (SPECT). Changes in reimbursement and the advent of mobile technology have increased the availability of this procedure in the community setting. ■

INDICATIONS:

• Assess tissue permeability

• Determine the size of heart infarcts

• Determine localization of areas of heart metabolism

• Determine the effects of therapeutic drugs on malfunctioning or diseased tissue

• Identify cerebrovascular accident or aneurysm, as evidenced by decreasing blood flow and oxygen use

• Determine the presence of coronary artery disease, as evidenced by metabolic state during ischemia and after angina

RESULT

Normal Findings:

• Normal patterns of tissue metabolism, blood flow, and radionuclide distribution

Abnormal Findings:

• Chronic obstructive pulmonary disease (COPD)

• Decreased blood flow and decreased glucose concentration, indicating necrotic, scarred tissue

• Enlarged left ventricle

• Heart chamber disorder

• Myocardial infarction, indicating increased radionuclide uptake in the myocardium

• Pulmonary edema

• Reduced blood flow but increased glucose concentration, indicating ischemia

CRITICAL VALUES: N/A

INTERFERING FACTORS:

This procedure is contraindicated for:

• Patients who are pregnant or suspected of being pregnant, unless the potential benefits of the procedure far outweigh the risks to the fetus and mother

Factors that may impair clear imaging:

• Inability of the patient to cooperate or remain still during the procedure because of age, significant pain, or mental status

• Patients who are very obese, who may exceed the weight limit for the equipment

• Incorrect positioning of the patient, which may produce poor visualization of the area to be examined

• Drugs that alter glucose metabolism, such as tranquilizers or insulin, because hypoglycemia can alter PET results

• The use of alcohol, tobacco, or caffeine-containing drinks at least 24 hours before the study, because the effects of these substances would make it difficult to evaluate the patient's true physiologic state (e.g., alcohol is a vasoconstrictor and would decrease blood flow to the target organ)

• Metallic objects within the examination field (e.g., jewelry or body rings), which may inhibit organ visualization and can produce unclear images

Other considerations:
• Improper injection of the radionuclide that allows the tracer to seep deep into the muscle tissue produces erroneous hot spots.

• False-positive findings may occur as a result of normal gastrointestinal tract uptake and uptake in areas of infection or inflammation.

• Consultation with a physician should occur before the procedure for radiation safety concerns regarding infants of patients who are lactating.

• Risks associated with radiographic overexposure can result from frequent x-ray procedures. Personnel in the room with the patient should stand behind a shield or leave the area while the examination is being done. Personnel working in the area where the examination is being done should wear badges that reveal their level of exposure to radiation.

Nursing Implications and Procedure

Pretest:

➤ Inform the patient that the procedure assesses blood flow to the heart.

➤ Inform the patient that the procedure is performed in a special department by a technologist and takes approximately 30 to 180 minutes.

➤ Restrict alcohol, tobacco, or caffeine-containing drinks for 24 hours before the study or as per physician order.

➤ Instruct the insulin-dependent patient to take insulin as usual on the day of the procedure, to have a meal 4 hours before the procedure, and then to refrain from food or liquids.

➤ Obtain a list of medications the patient is taking.

➤ Obtain a history of cardiac tests, other diagnostic procedure results, laboratory test results, present cardiac conditions or abnormalities, and therapy received for cardiac conditions. For related tests, refer to the cardiovascular system table.

➤ Determine date of last menstrual period and possibility of pregnancy in perimenopausal women.

➤ Reassure the patient that the radionuclide poses minimal radioactive hazard because of its short half-life and rarely produces side effects.

➤ *Obtain a written, informed consent for the procedure from the patient.*

➤ Sometimes fluorodeoxyglucose (FDG) examinations are done after blood has been drawn to determine circulating blood glucose levels. If blood glucose levels are high, insulin may be given.

Intratest:

➤ Ensure that emergency equipment is readily available during the procedure.

➤ Ask the patient to void before the procedure. Have the patient put on a hospital gown.

➤ Make sure jewelry, chains, and any other metallic objects have been removed from the chest area.

➤ Ask the patient to lie still during the procedure because movement produces unclear images.

➤ Expose the chest, and attach the electrocardiogram leads for simultaneous tracings. Apply a blood pressure cuff.

➤ An intravenous or arterial line may be started.

➤ The radionuclide is injected; imaging is done at periodic intervals, and continuous scanning is done for 1 hour.

➤ If comparative studies are indicated, additional injections may be needed.

➤ Wear gloves during the radionuclide

injection and while handling the patient's urine.

Post-test: ■

➤ Monitor electrocardiogram tracings and compare blood pressures with baseline readings until the patient is stable.

➤ Observe the injection site for redness, swelling, or hematoma.

➤ Observe the patient for 60 minutes after the procedure for possible reaction to the radionuclide or other procedure complications.

➤ Instruct the patient to resume normal activity and diet, unless otherwise indicated.

➤ If the patient must return for further imaging, advise the patient to rest in the interim and restrict diet to liquids before further studies.

➤ Advise patient to drink increased amounts of fluids for 24 hours to eliminate the radionuclide from the body, unless contraindicated. Tell the patient that radionuclide is eliminated from the body within 6 to 24 hours.

➤ Instruct the patient to flush the toilet immediately after each voiding following the procedure and to wash hands meticulously with soap and water after each voiding for 24 hours after the procedure.

➤ Tell all caregivers to wear gloves when discarding urine for 24 hours after the procedure. Wash gloved hands with soap and water before removing gloves. Then wash hands after the gloves are removed.

➤ Inform the patient that abnormalities of the heart scan may indicate the need for additional studies, including cardiac catheterization for cardiac abnormalities.

➤ A physician specializing in this branch of medicine sends a written report to the ordering provider, who discusses the results with the patient.

➤ Evaluate test results in relation to the patient's symptoms and other tests performed.

➤ Related diagnostic tests include echocardiogram, electrocardiogram, myocardial perfusion scan, and CT and magnetic resonance imaging of the chest.

POSITRON EMISSION TOMOGRAPHY, PELVIS

• •

SYNONYM/ACRONYM: PET scan of the pelvis.

AREA OF APPLICATION: Pelvis.

CONTRAST: Intravenous radioactive material.

DESCRIPTION: Positron emission tomography (PET) combines the biochemical properties of nuclear medicine with the accuracy of computed tomography (CT). PET uses positron emissions from specific radionuclides (oxygen, nitrogen, carbon, and fluorine) to produce detailed functional images within the body. After the radionuclide becomes concentrated in the pelvis, PET images of blood flow or metabolic processes at the cellular level can be obtained. Colorectal tumor detection, tumor staging, evaluation of the effects of therapy, detection of recurrent disease, and detection of metastases are the main reasons to do a pelvic PET scan. Fluorine-18, in the form of fluorodeoxyglucose (FDG), is one of the more commonly used radionuclides. FDG is a glucose analogue, and because every cell uses glucose, the metabolic activity occurring in pelvic conditions such as colorectal cancer can be measured. There is little localization of FDG in normal tissue, allowing rapid detection of abnormal disease states.

The positron radiopharmaceuticals generally have short half-lives, ranging from a few seconds to a few hours, and therefore they must be produced in a cyclotron located near where the test is being done. The PET scanner translates the emissions from the radioactivity as the positron combines with the negative electrons from the tissues and forms gamma rays that can be detected by the scanner. This information is transmitted to the computer, which determines the location and its distribution and translates the emissions as color-coded images for viewing, quantitative measurements, activity changes in relation to time, and three-dimensional computer-aided analysis. Each radionuclide tracer is designed to measure a specific body process, such as glucose metabolism, blood flow, or tissue perfusion.

The expense of the study and the limited availability of radiopharmaceuticals limit the use of PET, even though it is more sensitive than traditional nuclear scanning and single photon emission computed tomography (SPECT). Changes in reimbursement and the advent of mobile technology have increased the availability of this procedure in the community setting. ■

INDICATIONS:
- Determine the presence of colorectal cancer
- Determine the recurrence of tumor or cancer
- Determine the presence of metastases of a cancerous tumor
- Determine the effects of therapy
- Identify the site for biopsy

RESULT

Normal Findings:
- Normal patterns of tissue metabolism, blood flow, and radionuclide distribution
- No focal uptake of radionuclide

Abnormal Findings:
- Focal uptake of the radionuclide in pelvis
- Focal uptake in abnormal lymph nodes
- Focal uptake in tumor
- Focal uptake in metastases

CRITICAL VALUES: N/A

INTERFERING FACTORS:

This procedure is contraindicated for:
- Patients who are pregnant or suspected of being pregnant, unless the potential

benefits of the procedure far outweigh the risks to the fetus and mother

Factors that may impair clear imaging:

- Inability of the patient to cooperate or remain still during the procedure because of age, significant pain, or mental status

- Patients who are very obese, who may exceed the weight limit for the equipment

- Incorrect positioning of the patient, which may produce poor visualization of the area to be examined

- Metallic objects within the examination field (e.g., jewelry or body rings), which may inhibit organ visualization and can produce unclear images

- Drugs that alter glucose metabolism, such as tranquilizers or insulin, because hypoglycemia can alter PET results

Other considerations:

- Improper injection of the radionuclide that allows the tracer to seep deep into the muscle tissue produces erroneous hot spots.

- False-positive findings may occur as a result of normal gastrointestinal tract uptake and uptake in areas of infection or inflammation.

- Consultation with a physician should occur before the procedure for radiation safety concerns regarding infants of patients who are lactating.

- Risks associated with radiographic overexposure can result from frequent x-ray procedures. Personnel in the room with the patient should wear a protective lead apron, stand behind a shield, or leave the area while the examination is being done. Personnel working in the area where the examination is being done should wear badges that reveal their level of exposure to radiation.

Nursing Implications and Procedure • • • • • • • • • • •

Pretest: ■

➤ Inform the patient that the procedure assesses the pelvis and its contents for abnormal organ function.

➤ Inform the patient that the procedure is performed in a special department by a technologist and takes approximately 30 to 50 minutes.

➤ Restrict alcohol, tobacco, or caffeine-containing drinks for 24 hours before the study or as per physician order.

➤ Instruct the insulin-dependent patient to take insulin as usual on the day of the procedure, to have a meal 4 hours before the procedure, and then to refrain from food or liquids.

➤ Obtain a list of medications the patient is taking.

➤ Obtain a history of pelvic tests, other diagnostic procedure results, laboratory test results, present conditions or abnormalities, surgeries, and therapy received. For related tests, refer to the reproductive and gastrointestinal system tables.

➤ Determine date of last menstrual period and possibility of pregnancy in perimenopausal women.

➤ Reassure the patient that radioactive material poses minimal radioactive hazard because of its short half-life and rarely produces side effects.

➤ *Obtain a written, informed consent for the procedure from the patient.*

➤ Sometimes fluorodeoxyglucose (FDG) examinations are done after blood has been drawn to determine circulating blood glucose levels. If blood glucose levels are high, insulin may be given.

Intratest: ■

➤ Ensure that emergency equipment is readily available during the procedure.

➤ Ask the patient to void before the procedure. Have the patient put on a hospital gown.

➤ Make sure jewelry, watches, chains, belts, and any other metallic objects have been removed from the pelvic area.

➤ Ask the patient to lie still during the procedure because movement produces unclear images.

➤ An intravenous line may be started.

➤ The radionuclide is injected, and imaging is started after a 45-minute delay. Continuous scanning may be done for 1 hour after the patient is placed in the supine position on a scanning table. If comparative studies are indicated, additional injections of radionuclide may be needed.

➤ If required, the bladder may need to be lavaged via a urinary catheter with 2 L of 0.9% saline solution to remove concentrated radionuclide.

➤ Wear gloves during the radionuclide injection and while handling the patient's urine.

Post-test:

➤ Observe the injection site for redness, swelling, or hematoma.

➤ Observe the patient for 60 minutes after the procedure for possible reaction to the radionuclide or other procedure complications.

➤ Instruct the patient to resume normal activity and diet, unless otherwise indicated.

➤ If the patient must return for further imaging, advise the patient to rest in the interim and restrict diet to liquids before further studies.

➤ Advise patient to drink increased amounts of fluids for 24 hours to eliminate the radionuclide from the body, unless contraindicated. Tell the patient that radionuclide is eliminated from the body within 6 to 24 hours.

➤ Instruct the patient to flush the toilet immediately after each voiding following the procedure and to wash hands meticulously with soap and water after each voiding for 24 hours after the procedure.

➤ Tell all caregivers to wear gloves when discarding urine for 24 hours after the procedure. Wash gloved hands with soap and water before removing gloves. Then wash hands after the gloves are removed.

➤ Inform the patient that abnormalities of the pelvic scan may indicate the need for additional studies.

➤ A physician specializing in this branch of medicine sends a written report to the ordering provider, who discusses the results with the patient.

➤ Evaluate test results in relation to the patient's symptoms and other tests performed. Related diagnostic tests include computed tomography; magnetic resonance imaging; and kidney, ureter, and bladder (KUB) film.

POTASSIUM, SERUM

SYNONYM/ACRONYM: Serum K$^+$.

SPECIMEN: Serum (1 mL) collected in a red- or tiger-top tube. Plasma (1 mL) collected in green-top (heparin) tube is also acceptable.

REFERENCE VALUE: (Method: Ion-selective electrode)

Serum	SI Units (Conversion Factor ×1)
Newborn	3.7–5.9 mmol/L or mEq/L
Infant	4.1–5.3 mmol/L or mEq/L
Child	3.4–4.7 mmol/L or mEq/L
Adult	3.5–5.0 mmol/L or mEq/L

Note : Serum values are 0.1 mmol/L higher than plasma values, and reference ranges should be adjusted accordingly. It is important that serial measurements be collected using the same type of collection container to reduce variability of results from collection to collection.

DESCRIPTION: Electrolytes dissociate into electrically charged ions when dissolved. Cations, including potassium, carry a positive charge. Body fluids contain approximately equal numbers of anions and cations, although the nature of the ions and their mobility differs between the intracellular and extracellular compartments. Both types of ions affect the electrical and osmolar functions of the body. Electrolyte quantities and the balance among them are controlled by oxygen and carbon dioxide exchange in the lungs; absorption, secretion, and excretion of many substances by the kidneys; and secretion of regulatory hormones by the endocrine glands. Potassium is the most abundant intracellular cation. It is essential for the transmission of electrical impulses in cardiac and skeletal muscle. It also functions in enzyme reactions that transform glucose into energy and amino acids into proteins. Potassium helps maintain acid-base equilibrium, and it has a significant and inverse relationship to pH: A decrease in pH of 0.1 increases the potassium level by 0.6 mEq/L.

Abnormal potassium can be caused by a number of contributing factors, which can be categorized as follows:

Altered renal excretion: Normally, 80 to 90 percent of the body's potassium is filtered out through the kidneys each day (the remainder is excreted in sweat and stool); renal disease can result in abnormally high potassium levels.

Altered dietary intake: A severe potassium deficiency can be caused by an inadequate intake of dietary potassium.

Altered cellular metabolism: Damaged red blood cells (RBCs) release potassium into the circulating fluid, resulting in increased potassium levels. ■

INDICATIONS:

• Assess a known or suspected disorder associated with renal disease, glucose metabolism, trauma, or burns

• Assist in the evaluation of electrolyte imbalances; this test is especially indicated in elderly patients, patients receiving hyperalimentation supplements, patients on hemodialysis, and patients with hypertension

• Evaluate cardiac arrhythmia to determine whether altered potassium levels are contributing to the problem, especially during digitalis therapy, which leads to ventricular irritability

- Evaluate the effects of drug therapy, especially diuretics

- Evaluate the response to treatment for abnormal potassium levels

- Monitor known or suspected acidosis, because potassium moves from RBCs into the extracellular fluid in acidotic states

- Routine screen of electrolytes in acute and chronic illness

RESULT

Increased in:
- Acidosis
- Acute renal failure
- Addison's disease
- Asthma
- Burns
- Chronic interstitial nephritis
- Dehydration
- Dialysis
- Diet (excessive intake of salt substitutes or potassium salts of medications)
- Excessive theophylline administration
- Exercise
- Hemolysis (massive)
- Hyperventilation
- Hypoaldosteronism
- Insulin deficiency
- Ketoacidosis
- Leukocytosis
- Muscle necrosis
- Near-drowning
- Pregnancy

- Prolonged periods of standing
- Tissue trauma
- Transfusion of old banked blood
- Tubular unresponsiveness to aldosterone
- Uremia

Decreased in:
- Alcoholism
- Alkalosis
- Anorexia nervosa
- Bradycardia
- Chronic, excessive licorice ingestion (from licorice root)
- Congestive heart failure
- Crohn's disease
- Cushing's syndrome
- Diet deficient in meat and vegetables
- Excess insulin
- Familial periodic paralysis
- Gastrointestinal loss due to vomiting, diarrhea, nasogastric suction, or intestinal fistula
- Hyperaldosteronism
- Hypertension
- Hypomagnesemia
- Intravenous (IV) therapy with inadequate potassium supplementation
- Laxative abuse
- Malabsorption
- Pica (clay eating)
- Renal tubular acidosis
- Stress
- Sweating
- Thyrotoxicosis
- Toxic shock syndrome

CRITICAL VALUES:

Newborns:

Less than 2.5 mmol/L
Greater than 7.0 mmol/L

Adults:

Less than 2.5 mmol/L
Greater than 6.5 mmol/L

Note and report increased or decreased values and symptoms of fluid imbalance to the requesting health care practitioner. Symptoms of hyperkalemia include irritability, diarrhea, cramps, oliguria, difficulty speaking, and cardiac arrhythmias (peaked T waves and ventricular fibrillation). Continuous cardiac monitoring is indicated. Administration of sodium bicarbonate or calcium chloride may be requested. If the patient is receiving an IV supplement, verify that the patient is voiding.

Symptoms of hypokalemia include malaise, thirst, polyuria, anorexia, weak pulse, low blood pressure, vomiting, decreased reflexes, and electrocardiographic changes (depressed T waves and ventricular ectopy). Replacement therapy is indicated.

INTERFERING FACTORS:

- Drugs that can cause an increase in potassium levels include dexamethasone, enalapril, mannitol, methicillin, metoprolol, nonsteroidal anti-inflammatory drugs, some drugs with potassium salts, propranolol, spironolactone, and succinylcholine.
- Drugs that can cause a decrease in potassium levels include acetazolamide, alanine, albuterol, aldosterone, ammonium chloride, amphotericin B, acetylsalicylic acid, bicarbonate, bisacodyl, captopril, carbenicillin, cathartics, cisplatin, clorexolone, desoxycorticosterone, dexamethasone, digoxin, diuretics, enalapril, furosemide, hydrocortisone, hydroflumethiazide, laxatives, moxalactam (common when coadministered with amikacin), large doses of any IV penicillin, phenolphthalein (with chronic laxative abuse), phosphates, IV theophylline, thiazides, and triamterene. A number of these medications initially increase the serum potassium level, but they also have a diuretic effect, which promotes potassium loss in the urine except in cases of renal insufficiency.

- Leukocytosis, as seen in leukemia, causes elevated potassium levels.

- False elevations can occur with vigorous pumping of the hand during venipuncture. Hemolysis of the sample and high platelet counts also increase potassium levels, as follows: (1) Because potassium is an intracellular ion and concentrations are approximately 150 times extracellular concentrations, even a slight amount of hemolysis can cause a significant increase in levels. (2) Platelets release potassium during the clotting process, and therefore serum samples collected from patients with elevated platelet counts may produce spuriously high potassium levels. Plasma would be the specimen of choice in patients known to have elevated platelet counts.

- False increases are seen in unprocessed samples left at room temperature because a significant amount of potassium leaks out of the cells within a few hours. Plasma or serum should be separated from cells within 4 hours of collection.

- Storage of unprocessed blood causes potassium levels to increase because a significant amount of potassium leaks out of the cells within a few hours. Plasma or serum should be separated from cells within 4 hours of collection.

- Specimens should never be collected above an IV line because of the potential for dilution when the specimen and the IV solution combine in the collection container, falsely decreasing the result. There is also the potential of contaminating the sample with the substance of interest, contained in the IV solution, falsely increasing the result.

Nursing Implications and Procedure • • • • • • • • • • • •

Pretest:

➤ Obtain a history of the patient's complaints, and especially note weakness and confusion. Obtain a list of known allergens.

➤ Obtain a history of the patient's cardiovascular, endocrine, gastrointestinal, genitourinary, immune, and respiratory systems, as well as results of previously performed tests and procedures. For related tests, refer to the cardiovascular, endocrine, gastrointestinal, genitourinary, immune, and respiratory system tables.

➤ Obtain a list of medications the patient is taking.

➤ There are no food, fluid, or medication restrictions unless by medical direction.

➤ Review the procedure with the patient.

➤ Inform the patient that specimen collection takes approximately 5 to 10 minutes.

Intratest:

➤ Direct the patient to breathe normally and to avoid unnecessary movement. Instruct patient not to clench and unclench the fist immediately before or during specimen collection.

➤ Observe standard precautions and follow the general guidelines in Appendix A. Perform a venipuncture, and collect the specimen in a 5-mL red-, tiger-, or green-top (heparin) tube.

➤ Label the specimen, and promptly transport it to the laboratory.

Post-test:

➤ Observe venipuncture site for bleeding or hematoma formation. Apply pressure bandage.

➤ There are no recommended dietary allowances established for potassium, but the estimated minimum intake for adults is 200 mEq/d. Potassium is present in all plant and animal cells, making dietary replacement simple to achieve in the potassium-deficient patient.

➤ Observe the patient for signs and symptoms of fluid-volume excess related to excess potassium intake, fluid-volume deficit related to active loss, or risk of injury related to an alteration in body chemistry. Symptoms include dehydration, diarrhea, vomiting, or prolonged anorexia. Instruct the patient in electrolyte replacement therapy and changes in dietary intake that affect electrolyte levels.

➤ Increased potassium levels may be associated with dehydration. Evaluate the patient for signs and symptoms of dehydration. Dehydration is a significant and common finding in geriatric patients and other patients in whom renal function has deteriorated.

➤ Patients receiving digoxin or diuretics should have potassium levels monitored carefully because cardiac arrhythmias can occur.

➤ Evaluate test results in relation to the patient's symptoms and other tests performed. Related laboratory tests include aldosterone, arterial/alveolar oxygen ratio, anion gap, blood gases, calcium, digoxin, electrolytes, and osmolality.

POTASSIUM, URINE

SYNONYM/ACRONYM: Urine K^+.

SPECIMEN: Urine (5 mL) from an unpreserved random or timed specimen collected in a clean, plastic collection container.

REFERENCE VALUE: (Method: Ion-selective electrode)

Age	Conventional Units	SI Units (Conversion Factor ×1)
6–10 y		
Male	17–54 mEq/24 h	17–54 mmol/24 h
Female	8–37 mEq/24 h	8–37 mmol/24 h
10–14 y		
Male	22–57 mEq/24 h	22–57 mmol/24 h
Female	18–58 mEq/24 h	18–58 mmol/24 h
Adult	26–123 mEq/24 h	26–123 mmol/24 h

Note: Reference values depend on potassium intake and diurnal variation. Excretion is significantly higher at night.

DESCRIPTION: Electrolytes dissociate into electrically charged ions when dissolved. Cations, including potassium, carry a positive charge. Body fluids contain approximately equal numbers of anions and cations, although the nature of the ions and their mobility differs between the intracellular and extracellular compartments. Both types of ions affect the electrical and osmolar functions of the body. Electrolyte quantities and the balance among them are controlled by oxygen and carbon dioxide exchange in the lungs; absorption, secretion, and excretion of many substances by the kidneys; and secretion of regulatory hormones by the endocrine glands. Potassium is the most abundant intracellular cation. It is essential for the transmission of electrical impulses in cardiac and skeletal muscle. It also functions in enzyme reactions that transform glucose into energy and amino acids into proteins. Potassium helps maintain acid-base equilibrium, and it has a significant and inverse relationship to pH: A decrease in pH of 0.1 increases the potassium level by 0.6 mEq/L.

Abnormal potassium can be caused by a number of contributing factors, which can be categorized as follows:
Altered renal excretion: Normally, 80 to 90 percent of the body's potassium is filtered out through the kidneys each day (the remainder is excreted in sweat and stool); renal disease can result in abnormally high potassium levels.

Altered dietary intake: A severe potassium deficiency can be caused by an inadequate intake of dietary potassium.

Altered cellular metabolism: Damaged red blood cells (RBCs) release potassium into the circulating fluid, resulting in increased potassium levels.

Regulating electrolyte balance is one of the major functions of the kidneys. In normally functioning kidneys, urine potassium levels increase when serum levels are high and decrease when serum levels are low to maintain homeostasis. The kidneys respond to alkalosis by excreting potassium to retain hydrogen ions and increase acidity. In acidosis, the body excretes hydrogen ions and retains potassium. Analyzing these urinary levels can provide important clues to the functioning of the kidneys and other major organs. Urine potassium tests usually involve timed urine collections over a 12- or 24-hour period. Measurement of random specimens also may be requested. ∎

INDICATIONS:

- Determine the potential cause of renal calculi

- Evaluate known or suspected endocrine disorder

- Evaluate known or suspected renal disease

- Evaluate malabsorption disorders

RESULT

Increased in:
- Albright-type renal disease

- Hyperaldosteronism

- Cushing's syndrome

- Diabetic ketoacidosis

- Diuretic therapy

- Starvation (onset)

- Vomiting

Decreased in:
- Addison's disease

- Potassium deficiency (chronic)

- Renal failure with decreased urine flow

CRITICAL VALUES: N/A

INTERFERING FACTORS:

- Drugs and substances that can cause an increase in urine potassium levels include acetazolamide, acetylsalicylic acid, ammonium chloride, bendroflumethiazide, carbenoxolone, chlorthalidone, citrates, clopamide, corticosteroids, cortisone, desoxycorticosterone, dexamethasone, diuretics, dopamine, ethacrynic acid, glycyrrhiza, intra-amniotic saline, mefruside, niacinamide, some oral contraceptives, thiazides, triflocin, and viomycin.

- Drugs that can cause a decrease in urine potassium levels include alanine, amiloride, anesthetic agents, cyclosporine, felodipine, levarterenol, and ramipril.

- A dietary deficiency or excess of potassium can lead to spurious results.

- Diuretic therapy with excessive loss of electrolytes into the urine may falsely elevate results.

- All urine voided for the timed collection period must be included in the collection or else falsely decreased values may be obtained. Compare output records with volume collected to verify that all voids were included in the collection.

- Potassium levels are subject to diurnal variation (output being highest at night), which is why 24-hour collections are recommended.

Nursing Implications and Procedure • • • • • • • • • • • •

➤ Obtain a history of the patient's complaints, including a list of known allergens.

➤ Obtain a history of the patient's endocrine, gastrointestinal, and genitourinary systems, as well as results of previously performed tests and procedures. For related tests, refer to the endocrine, gastrointestinal, and genitourinary system tables.

➤ Obtain a list of the medications the patient is taking, including herbs, nutritional supplements, and nutraceuticals. The requesting health care practitioner and laboratory should be advised if the patient regularly uses these products so that their effects can be taken into consideration when reviewing results.

➤ There are no food, fluid, or medication restrictions unless by medical direction.

➤ Review the procedure with the patient. Provide a nonmetallic urinal, bedpan, or toilet-mounted collection device.

➤ Usually a 24-hour time frame for urine collection is ordered. Inform the patient that all urine must be saved during that 24-hour period. Instruct the patient not to void directly into the laboratory collection container. Instruct the patient to avoid defecating in the collection device and to keep toilet tissue out of the collection device to prevent contamination of the specimen. Place a sign in the bathroom to remind the patient to save all urine.

➤ Instruct the patient to void all urine into the collection device and then to pour the urine into the laboratory collection container. Alternatively the specimen can be left in the collection device for a health care staff member to add to the laboratory collection container.

➤ Observe standard precautions and follow the general guidelines in Appendix A.

Random specimen (collect in early morning):

Clean-catch specimen:

➤ Instruct the male patient to (1) thoroughly wash his hands, (2) cleanse the meatus, (3) void a small amount into the toilet, and (4) void directly into the specimen container.

➤ Instruct the female patient to (1) thoroughly wash her hands; (2) cleanse the labia from front to back; (3) while keeping the labia separated, void a small amount into the toilet; and (4) without interrupting the urine stream, void directly into the specimen container.

Indwelling catheter:

➤ Put on gloves. Empty drainage tube of urine. It may be necessary to clamp off the catheter for 15 to 30 minutes before specimen collection. Cleanse specimen port with antiseptic swab, and then aspirate 5 mL of urine with a 21- to 25-gauge needle and syringe. Transfer urine to a sterile container.

Timed specimen:

➤ Obtain a clean 3-L urine specimen container, toilet-mounted collection device, and plastic bag (for transport of the specimen container). The specimen must be refrigerated or kept on ice throughout the entire collection period. If an indwelling urinary catheter is in place, the drainage bag must be kept on ice.

➤ Begin the test between 6 and 8 a.m., if possible. Collect first voiding and discard. Record the time the specimen was discarded as the beginning of the timed collection period. The next morning, ask the patient to void at the same time the collection was started and add this last voiding to the container.

➤ If an indwelling catheter is in place, replace the tubing and container system at the start of the collection time. Keep the container system on ice during the collection period, or empty the urine into a larger container periodically during the collection period; monitor to ensure continued drainage, and conclude the test the next morning at the same hour the collection was begun.

➤ At the conclusion of the test, compare the quantity of urine with the urinary output record for the collection; if the specimen contains less than what was recorded as output, some urine may have been discarded, invalidating the test.

➤ Label the specimen, and promptly transport it to the laboratory. Include on the label the amount of urine, test start and stop times, and ingestion of any foods or medications that can affect test results.

Post-test:

➤ There are no recommended dietary allowances established for potassium, but the estimated minimum intake for adults is 200 mEq/d. Potassium is present in all plant and animal cells, making dietary replacement simple to achieve in the potassium-deficient patient.

➤ Observe the patient for signs and symptoms of fluid-volume excess related to excess potassium intake, fluid-volume deficit related to active loss, or risk of injury related to an alteration in body chemistry.

➤ Increased potassium levels may be associated with dehydration. Evaluate the patient for signs and symptoms of dehydration. Dehydration is a significant and common finding in geriatric patients and other patients in whom renal function has deteriorated.

➤ Patients receiving digoxin or diuretics should have potassium levels monitored carefully because cardiac arrhythmias can occur.

➤ Observe the patient for signs and symptoms of fluid-volume excess related to excess potassium intake, fluid-volume deficit related to active loss, or risk of injury related to an alteration in body chemistry. Symptoms include dehydration, diarrhea, vomiting, or prolonged anorexia. Instruct the patient in electrolyte replacement therapy and changes in dietary intake that affect electrolyte levels.

➤ Increased urine potassium levels may be associated with the formation of kidney stones. Educate the patient, if appropriate, on the importance of drinking a sufficient amount of water when kidney stones are suspected.

➤ Evaluate test results in relation to the patient's symptoms and other tests performed. Related laboratory tests include aldosterone, kidney stone analysis, osmolality, serum potassium, renin, and serum and urine sodium.

PREALBUMIN

SYNONYM/ACRONYM: Transthyretin.

SPECIMEN: Serum (1 mL) collected in a red- or tiger-top tube.

REFERENCE VALUE: (Method: Nephelometry)

Age	Conventional Units	SI Units (Conversion Factor ×10)
Newborn–1 mo	7.0–39.0 mg/dL	70–390 mg/L
1–6 mo	8.3–34.0 mg/dL	83–340 mg/L
6 mo–4 y	2.0–36.0 mg/dL	20–360 mg/L
5–6 y	12.0–30.0 mg/dL	120–300 mg/L
6 y–adult	12.0–42.0 mg/dL	120–420 mg/L

DESCRIPTION: Prealbumin is a protein primarily produced by the liver. It is the major transport protein for triiodothyronine and thyroxine. It is also important in the metabolism of retinol-binding protein, which is needed for transporting vitamin A (retinol). Prealbumin has a short biological half-life of 2 days. This makes it a good indicator of protein status and an excellent marker for malnutrition. Prealbumin is often measured simultaneously with transferrin and albumin. ∎

INDICATIONS: Evaluate nutritional status

RESULT

Increased in:
• Alcoholism

• Chronic renal failure

• Patients receiving steroids

Decreased in:
• Acute-phase inflammatory response

• Diseases of the liver

• Hepatic damage

• Malnutrition

• Tissue necrosis

CRITICAL VALUES: N/A

INTERFERING FACTORS:
• Drugs that may increase prealbumin

levels include anabolic steroids, anticonvulsants, danazol, oral contraceptives, prednisolone, prednisone, and propranolol.

• Drugs that may decrease prealbumin levels include amiodarone and diethylstilbestrol.

• Fasting 4 hours before specimen collection is highly recommended. Reference ranges are often based on fasting populations to provide some level of standardization for comparison. The presence of lipids in the blood may also interfere with the test method; fasting eliminates this potential source of error, especially if the patient has elevated lipid levels.

Nursing Implications and Procedure • • • • • • • • • • •

Pretest: ∎

➤ Obtain a history of the patient's complaints, including a list of known allergens.

➤ Obtain a history of the patient's endocrine, gastrointestinal, and hepatobiliary systems, as well as results of previously performed tests and procedures. For related tests, refer to the endocrine, gastrointestinal, and hepatobiliary system tables.

➤ Obtain a list of medications the patient is taking, including herbs, nutritional supplements, and nutraceuticals. The requesting health care practitioner and laboratory should be advised if the patient regularly uses these products so that their effects can be taken into consideration when reviewing results.

➤ Instruct the patient to fast for 4 hours before specimen collection.

➤ There are no fluid or medication restrictions unless by medical direction.

➤ Review the procedure with the patient.

➤ Inform the patient that specimen collection takes approximately 5 to 10 minutes.

Intratest:

➤ Direct the patient to breathe normally and to avoid unnecessary movement.

➤ Ensure that the patient has complied with dietary preparations and other pretesting restrictions.

➤ Observe standard precautions and follow the general guidelines in Appendix A. Perform a venipuncture,

and collect the specimen in a 5-mL red- or tiger-top tube.

➤ Label the specimen, and promptly transport it to the laboratory.

Post-test:

➤ Observe venipuncture site for bleeding or hematoma formation. Apply pressure bandage.

➤ Nutritional therapy may be indicated for patients with decreased prealbumin levels. Educate the patient, as appropriate, that good dietary sources of complete protein (containing all eight essential amino acids) include meat, fish, eggs, and dairy products; and that good sources of incomplete protein (lacking one or more of the eight essential amino acids) include grains, nuts, legumes, vegetables, and seeds.

➤ Evaluate test results in relation to the patient's symptoms and other tests performed. Related laboratory tests include albumin, chloride, ferritin, iron/total iron-binding capacity, potassium, protein, and sodium.

PROCTOSIGMOIDOSCOPY

· ·

SYNONYMS/ACRONYM: Anoscopy (anal canal), proctoscopy (rectum), sigmoidoscopy (sigmoid colon), flexible fiberoptic sigmoidoscopy, flexible proctosigmoidoscopy.

AREA OF APPLICATION: Anus, rectum, colon.

CONTRAST: Air.

DESCRIPTION: Proctosigmoidoscopy allows direct visualization of the mucosa of the anal canal (anoscopy), rectum (proctoscopy), and distal sigmoid colon (sigmoidoscopy). The procedure can be performed using a rigid or flexible fiberoptic endoscope, but the flexible instrument is generally preferred. The endoscope is a multichannel device allowing visualization of the mucosal lining of the colon, instillation of air, removal of fluid and foreign objects, obtaining of tissue biopsy specimens, and use of a laser for the destruction of tissue and control of bleeding. The endoscope is advanced approximately 60 cm into the colon. This procedure is commonly used in patients with lower abdominal and perineal pain; changes in bowel habits; rectal prolapse during defecation; or passage of blood, mucus, or pus in the stool. Proctosigmoidoscopy can also be a therapeutic procedure, allowing removal of polyps or hemorrhoids or reduction of a volvulus. Biopsy specimens of suspicious sites may be obtained during the procedure. This procedure is recommended for patients who are more than 50 years old as part of a routine screening for colorectal cancer. ∎

INDICATIONS:

- Screen and excise polyps

- Examine the distal colon before barium enema x-ray to obtain improved visualization of the area, and after a barium enema when x-ray findings are inconclusive

- Evaluate the cause of blood, pus, or mucus in the stool

- Determine the cause of pain and rectal prolapse during defecation

- Determine the cause of rectal itching, pain, or burning

- Confirm the diagnosis of diverticular disease

- Confirm the diagnosis of Hirschsprung's disease and colitis in children

- Evaluate postoperative anastomosis of the colon

- Reduce volvulus of the sigmoid colon

- Remove hemorrhoids by laser therapy

- Screen for colon cancer

RESULT

Normal Findings:

- Normal mucosa of the anal canal, rectum, and sigmoid colon

Abnormal Findings:

- Anal fissure or fistula

- Anorectal abscess

- Bleeding sites

- Benign lesions

- Bowel infection or inflammation

- Crohn's disease

- Diverticula

- Hypertrophic anal papillae

- Internal and external hemorrhoids

- Polyps

- Tumors

- Ulcerative colitis

- Vascular abnormalities

- Rectal prolapse

CRITICAL VALUES: N/A

INTERFERING FACTORS:

This procedure is contraindicated for:

- Patients with bleeding disorders, especially disorders associated with uremia and cytotoxic chemotherapy

- Patients with cardiac conditions or arrhythmias

- Patients with bowel perforation, acute peritonitis, ischemic bowel necrosis, toxic megacolon, diverticulitis, recent bowel surgery, advanced pregnancy, severe cardiac or pulmonary disease, recent myocardial infarction, known or suspected pulmonary embolus, large abdominal aortic or iliac aneurysm, and coagulation abnormality

Factors that may impair clear imaging:

• Inability of the patient to cooperate or remain still during the procedure because of age, significant pain, or mental status

• Patients who are very obese, who may exceed the weight limit for the equipment

• Incorrect positioning of the patient, which may produce poor visualization of the area to be examined

• Strictures or other abnormalities preventing passage of the scope

• Barium swallow or upper gastrointestinal (GI) series within the preceding 48 hours

• Severe lower GI bleeding or the presence of feces, barium, blood, or blood clots

Other considerations:

• Failure to follow dietary restrictions before the procedure may cause the procedure to be canceled or repeated.

• Use of bowel preparations that include laxatives or enemas should be avoided in pregnant patients or patients with inflammatory bowel disease, unless specifically directed by a physician.

Nursing Implications and Procedure • • • • • • • • • •

Pretest:

➤ Explain to the patient the purpose of the procedure and how it is performed.

➤ Explain that the procedure is generally performed in an endoscopy suite by a physician and support staff and usually takes 15 to 30 minutes.

➤ Obtain a list of medications the patient is taking, including herbs, nutritional supplements, and nutraceuticals.

➤ Obtain a history of GI disorders, noting any information relating to lower bowel, anal, rectal, or coagulation disorders and use of drugs that affect bleeding, such as aspirin and other salicylates. For related tests, refer to the gastrointestinal system table.

➤ Obtain the results of laboratory tests (particularly hematologic or coagulation tests), treatments, surgeries, and procedures done to diagnose or treat disorders of the intestinal system.

➤ *Obtain a written, informed consent for the procedure from the patient.*

➤ Determine date of last menstrual period and possibility of pregnancy in perimenopausal women.

➤ Inform the patient that the urge to defecate may be experienced when the scope is passed. Encourage slow, deep breathing through the mouth to help alleviate the feeling.

➤ Inform the patient that flatus may be expelled during and after the procedure owing to air that is injected into the scope to improve visualization.

➤ Note intake of oral iron preparations 1 week before the procedure because these cause black, sticky feces that are difficult to remove with bowel preparation.

➤ Note recent administration of barium because it can obscure the area to be examined.

➤ Inform the patient that it is important the bowel be cleaned thoroughly so that the physician can visualize the colon and that the patient will have to take laxatives and receive enemas before the test. Ensure that ordered laxative has been administered late in the afternoon of the day before the procedure.

➤ Restrict the diet to clear liquids for 48 hours before beginning oral bowel preparation.

➤ Ask the patient to void before the procedure. Have the patient put on a hospital gown.

➤ Two small-volume enemas are administered 1 hour before the procedure.

➤ The patient is placed on an examination table in the left lateral decubitus position or the knee-chest position and draped with the buttocks exposed. The buttocks are placed at or extending slightly beyond the edge of the examination table or bed, preferably on a special examining table that tilts the patient into the desired position.

➤ The physician visually inspects the perianal area and then performs a digital rectal examination with a well-lubricated, gloved finger. A fecal specimen may be obtained from the glove when the finger is removed from the rectum.

➤ A lubricated anoscope (7 cm in length) is inserted, and the anal canal is inspected (anoscopy). The anoscope is removed, and a lubricated proctoscope (27 cm in length) or flexible sigmoidoscope (35 to 60 cm in length) is inserted.

➤ The scope is manipulated gently to facilitate passage, and air may be insufflated through the scope to improve visualization. Suction and cotton swabs also are used to remove materials that hinder visualization. Examination is done as the scope is gradually withdrawn.

➤ The patient is instructed to take deep breaths to aid in movement of the scope downward through the ascending colon to the cecum and into the terminal portion of the ileum.

➤ Air is insufflated to distend the GI tract, as needed. Biopsy specimens, cultures, or any exudate may be obtained.

➤ Polyps or tissue is removed and placed in appropriate specimen containers, labeled properly, and sent to the laboratory.

➤ Photographs are obtained for future reference.

➤ At the end of the procedure, the scope is completely withdrawn, and residual lubricant is cleansed from the anal area.

➤ Wear gloves and gowns throughout the procedure.

➤ Instruct the patient to resume normal activity, medication, and diet after the procedure, unless otherwise indicated.

➤ Monitor for any rectal bleeding. Instruct the patient to expect slight rectal bleeding for 2 days after removal of polyps or biopsy specimens, but that heavy rectal bleeding must be immediately reported to the physician.

➤ Emphasize that any abdominal pain, tenderness, or distention; pain on defecation; or fever must be reported to the physician immediately.

➤ Inform the patient that any bloating or flatulence is the result of air insufflation.

➤ Encourage the patient to drink several glasses of water to help replace fluid lost during test preparation.

➤ A physician specializing in this branch of medicine sends a written report to the ordering provider, who discusses the results with the patient.

➤ Inform the patient that further examinations may be necessary to evaluate progression of the disease process or to determine the need for a change in therapy.

➤ Evaluate test results in relation to the patient's symptoms and other tests performed. Related diagnostic tests include kidney, ureter, and bladder (KUB) film; and ultrasound, positron emission tomography, computed tomography, and magnetic resonance imaging of the pelvis.

PROGESTERONE

· ·

SYNONYM/ACRONYM: N/A.

SPECIMEN: Serum (1 mL) collected in a red- or tiger-top tube.

REFERENCE VALUE: (Method: Radioimmunoassay)

Hormonal State	Conventional Units	SI Units (Conversion Factor ×0.0318)
Prepubertal males and females	Less than 20 ng/dL	Less than 0.6 nmol/L
Men	10–50 ng/dL	0.3–1.6 nmol/L
Women		
Follicular phase	Less than 50 ng/dL	Less than 1.6 nmol/L
Luteal phase	300–2500 ng/dL	9.5–79.5 nmol/L
Pregnancy, first trimester	725–4400 ng/dL	23.0–139.9 nmol/L
Pregnancy, second trimester	1950–8250 ng/dL	62.0–262.3 nmol/L
Pregnancy, third trimester	6500–22,900 ng/dL	206.7–728.2 nmol/L
Postmenopausal period	Less than 40 ng/dL	Less than 1.3 nmol/L

DESCRIPTION: Progesterone is a female sex hormone. Its function is to prepare the uterus for pregnancy and the breasts for lactation. Progesterone testing can be used to confirm that ovulation has occurred and to assess the functioning of the corpus luteum. Serial measurements can be performed to help determine the day of ovulation. ■

INDICATIONS:

• Assist in the diagnosis of luteal phase defects (performed in conjunction with endometrial biopsy)

• Evaluate patients at risk for early or spontaneous abortion

• Identify patients at risk for ectopic pregnancy and assessment of corpus luteum function

• Monitor patients ovulating during human chorionic gonadotropin (HCG), human menopausal gonadotropin, follicle-stimulating hormone/luteinizing hormone–releasing hormone, or clomiphene induction (serial measurements can assist in pinpointing the day of ovulation)

• Monitor patients receiving progesterone-replacement therapy

RESULT

Increased in:

- Chorioepithelioma of the ovary
- Congenital adrenal hyperplasia
- Hydatidiform mole
- Lipoid ovarian tumor
- Theca lutein cyst

Decreased in:

- Galactorrhea-amenorrhea syndrome
- Primary or secondary hypogonadism
- Short luteal phase syndrome
- Threatened abortion

CRITICAL VALUES: N/A

INTERFERING FACTORS:

- Drugs that may increase progesterone levels include clomiphene, corticotropin, hydroxyprogesterone, ketoconazole, mifepristone, progesterone, tamoxifen, and valproic acid.
- Drugs that may decrease progesterone levels include ampicillin, epostane, goserelin, leuprolide, and prostaglandin F_2.
- Recent radioactive scans or radiation within 1 week before the test can interfere with test results when radioimmunoassay is the test method.

Nursing Implications and Procedure

Pretest:

- ➤ Obtain a history of the patient's complaints, including a list of known allergens.
- ➤ Obtain a history of the patient's endocrine and reproductive systems, as well as results of previously performed tests and procedures. For related tests, refer to the endocrine and reproductive system tables.
- ➤ Obtain a list of the medications the patient is taking, including herbs, nutritional supplements, and nutraceuticals. The requesting health care practitioner and laboratory should be advised if the patient regularly uses these products so that their effects can be taken into consideration when reviewing results.
- ➤ Note any recent procedures that may interfere with test results.
- ➤ There are no food, fluid, or medication restrictions unless by medical direction.
- ➤ Review the procedure with the patient. Inform the patient that multiple specimens may be required.
- ➤ Inform the patient that specimen collection takes approximately 5 to 10 minutes.

Intratest:

- ➤ Direct the patient to breathe normally and to avoid unnecessary movement.
- ➤ Observe standard precautions and follow the general guidelines in Appendix A. Perform a venipuncture, and collect the specimen in a 5-mL red- or tiger-top tube.
- ➤ Label the specimen, and promptly transport it to the laboratory.

Post-test:

- ➤ Observe venipuncture site for bleeding or hematoma formation. Apply pressure bandage.
- ➤ Recognize anxiety related to test results and provide support. Provide teaching and information regarding the clinical implications of the test results, as appropriate. Inform the patient, as appropriate, of the potential outcome based on test results and offer grief counseling. Encourage the patient to discuss additional alternatives for becoming a parent with her health care provider.
- ➤ Evaluate test results in relation to the patient's symptoms and other tests performed. Related laboratory tests include HCG, estradiol, and prolactin.

PROLACTIN

· ·

SYNONYMS/ACRONYMS: Luteotropic hormone, lactogenic hormone, lactogen, HPRL, PRL.

SPECIMEN: Serum (1 mL) collected in a red- or tiger-top tube. Specimen should be transported tightly capped and in an ice slurry.

REFERENCE VALUE: (Method: Immunoassay)

Age	Conventional Units	SI Units (Conversion Factor ×1)
Prepubertal males and females	3.2–20.0 ng/mL	3.2–20.0 µg/L
Men	2.4–13.8 ng/mL	2.4–13.8 µg/L
Women	3.3–26.7 ng/mL	3.3–26.7 µg/L
Pregnant	5.3–215.3 ng/mL	5.3–215.3 µg/L
Postmenopausal	2.4–24.0 ng/mL	2.4–24.0 µg/L

DESCRIPTION: Prolactin is secreted by the pituitary gland. It is unique among hormones in that it responds to inhibition by the hypothalamus rather than to stimulation. The only known function of prolactin is to induce milk production in female breasts that are already stimulated by high estrogen levels. When milk production is established, lactation can continue without elevated prolactin levels. Prolactin levels rise late in pregnancy, peak with the initiation of lactation, and surge each time a woman breastfeeds. The function of prolactin in males is unknown. ■

INDICATIONS:
• Assist in the diagnosis of primary hypothyroidism, as indicated by elevated levels

• Assist in the diagnosis of suspected tumor involving the lungs or kidneys (elevated levels indicating ectopic prolactin production)

• Evaluate failure of lactation in the postpartum period

• Evaluate suspected postpartum hypophyseal infarction (Sheehan's syndrome), as indicated by decreased levels

• Evaluate sexual dysfunction of unknown cause in men and women

RESULT

Increased in:
• Adrenal insufficiency

• Amenorrhea

• Anorexia nervosa

• Breastfeeding

- Chiari-Frommel and Argonz–Del Castillo syndromes

- Chest wall injury

- Chronic renal failure

- Ectopic prolactin-secreting tumors (e.g., lung, kidney)

- Galactorrhea

- Hypothalamic and pituitary disorders

- Hypothyroidism (primary)

- Insulin-induced hypoglycemia

- Liver failure

- Pituitary tumor

- Polycystic ovary (Stein-Leventhal) syndrome

- Pregnancy

- Surgery (pituitary stalk section)

Decreased in:
- Sheehan's syndrome

CRITICAL VALUES: N/A

INTERFERING FACTORS:
- Drugs and hormones that may increase prolactin levels include amitryptyline, amoxapine, arginine, azosemide, benserazide, butaperazine, butorphanol, carbidopa, chlorophenylpiperazine, chlorpromazine, cimetidine, clomipramine, desipramine, diethylstilbestrol, β-endorphin, enflurane, fenfluramine, fenoldopam, flunarizine, fluphenazine, growth hormone–releasing hormone, imipramine, insulin, interferon-β, labetalol, loxapine, megestrol, mestranol, methyldopa, metoclopramide, molindone, morphine, nitrous oxide, oral contraceptives, oxcarbazepine, parathyroid hormone, pentagastrin, perphenazine, phenothiazines, phenytoin, pimozide, prochlorperazine, promazine, ranitidine, remoxipride, reserpine, sulpiride, sultopride, thiethylperazine, thioridazine, thiothixene, thyrotropin-releasing hormone, trifluoperazine, trimipramine, tumor necrosis factor, veralipride, verapamil, and zometapine.

- Drugs and hormones that may decrease prolactin levels include anticonvulsants, apomorphine, bromocriptine, cabergoline, calcitonin, cyclosporine, dexamethasone, dopamine, D-Trp-6-LHRH, levodopa, metoclopramide, morphine, nifedipine, octreotide, pergolide, ranitidine, rifampin, ritanserin, ropinirole, secretin, thyroid hormones, and terguride.

- Episodic elevations can occur in response to sleep, stress, exercise, hypoglycemia, and breastfeeding.

- Venipuncture can cause falsely elevated levels.

- Prolactin secretion is subject to diurnal variation, with highest levels occurring in the morning.

Nursing Implications and Procedure

Pretest:

➤ Obtain a history of the patient's complaints, including a list of known allergens.

➤ Obtain a history of the patient's endocrine and reproductive systems, as well as results of previously performed tests and procedures. For related tests, refer to the endocrine and reproductive system tables.

➤ Obtain a list of medications the patient is taking, including herbs, nutritional supplements, and nutraceuticals. The requesting health care practitioner and laboratory should be advised if the patient regularly uses these products so that their effects can be taken into consideration when reviewing results.

➤ There are no fluid or medication restrictions unless by medical direction.

➤ The patient should fast for 12 hours before specimen collection.

➤ Review the procedure with the patient.

➤ Inform the patient that specimen collection takes approximately 5 to 10 minutes.

➤ Prepare an ice slurry in a cup or plastic bag to have on hand for immediate transport of the specimen to the laboratory.

Appendix A. Perform a venipuncture, and collect the specimen in a prechilled 5-mL red- or tiger-top tube.

➤ Label the specimen, and promptly transport it to the laboratory. The specimen should be placed in an ice slurry immediately after collection. Information on the specimen label can be protected from water in the ice slurry if the specimen is first placed in a protective plastic bag.

Intratest:

➤ Specimen collection should occur between 8 and 10 a.m.

➤ Ensure that the patient has complied with dietary preparations and other pretesting restrictions.

➤ Direct the patient to breathe normally and to avoid unnecessary movement.

➤ Observe standard precautions and follow the general guidelines in

Post-test:

➤ Observe venipuncture site for bleeding or hematoma formation. Apply pressure bandage.

➤ Evaluate test results in relation to the patient's symptoms and other tests performed. Related laboratory tests include dehydroepiandrosterone, estradiol, follicle-stimulating hormone, human chorionic gonadotropin, and luteinizing hormone.

PROSTATE-SPECIFIC ANTIGEN

· ·

SYNONYM/ACRONYM: PSA.

SPECIMEN: Serum (1 mL) collected in a red- or tiger-top tube.

REFERENCE VALUE: (Method: Immunoassay)

Sex	Conventional Units	SI Units (Conversion Factor ×1)
Male	Less than 4 ng/mL	Less than 4 µg/L
Female	Less than 0.5 ng/mL	Less than 0.5 µg/L

DESCRIPTION: Prostate-specific antigen (PSA) is produced exclusively by the epithelial cells of the prostate, periurethral, and perirectal glands. Used in conjunction with the digital rectal examination, PSA is a useful test for monitoring adenocarcinoma of the prostate. PSA circulates in a free and bound (complexed) form. A low ratio of free to complexed PSA (i.e., less than 10 percent) is suggestive of prostate cancer; a ratio of greater than 30 percent is rarely associated with prostate cancer. Serial measurements are often performed before and after surgery. *Important note:* When following patients using serial testing, use the same method of measurement consistently. ■

INDICATIONS:

- Evaluate the effectiveness of treatment for prostate cancer (prostatectomy): Levels decrease if treatment is effective; rising levels are associated with recurrence and a poor prognosis.

- Investigate or evaluate an enlarged prostate gland, especially if prostate cancer is suspected.

- Stage prostate cancer.

RESULT

Increased in:

- Benign prostatic hypertrophy

- Prostate cancer

- Prostatic infarct

- Urinary retention

Decreased in: N/A

CRITICAL VALUES: N/A

INTERFERING FACTORS:

- Drugs that decrease PSA levels include buserelin, finasteride, and flutamide.

- Specimens should not be collected for at least 4 weeks after digital rectal examination, biopsy, or other manipulation of the prostate or else results may be falsely increased.

Nursing Implications and Procedure • • • • • • • • • •

Pretest:

- Obtain a history of the patient's complaints, including a list of known allergens.

- Obtain a history of the patient's genitourinary, immune, and reproductive systems, as well as results of previously performed tests and procedures. For related tests, refer to the genitourinary, immune, and reproductive system tables.

- Obtain a list of medications the patient is taking, including herbs, nutritional supplements, and nutraceuticals. The requesting health care practitioner and laboratory should be advised if the patient regularly uses these products so that their effects can be taken into consideration when reviewing results.

- There are no food, fluid, or medication restrictions unless by medical direction.

- Review the procedure with the patient.

- Inform the patient that specimen collection takes approximately 5 to 10 minutes.

Intratest:

- Direct the patient to breathe normally and to avoid unnecessary movement.

- Observe standard precautions and follow the general guidelines in Appendix A. Perform a venipuncture, and collect the specimen in a 5-mL red- or tiger-top tube.

- Label the specimen, and promptly transport it to the laboratory.

Post-test:

- Observe venipuncture site for bleeding or hematoma formation. Apply pressure bandage.

➤ Recognize anxiety related to test results and offer support. Provide teaching and information regarding the clinical implications of the test results. Educate the patient regarding access to counseling services, as appropriate. Counsel the patient, as appropriate, that sexual dysfunction related to altered body function, drugs, or radiation may occur.

➤ Evaluate test results in relation to the patient's symptoms and other tests performed. Related laboratory tests include prostate biopsy and prostatic acid phosphatase.

PROTEIN C

SYNONYMS/ACRONYM: Protein C antigen, protein C functional.

SPECIMEN: Plasma (1 mL) collected in blue-top (sodium citrate) tube.

REFERENCE VALUE: (Method: Chromogenic) 70 to 140 percent activity (0.7–1.4 U/mL). Values are significantly reduced in children (0.4 to 1.1 U/mL) because of liver immaturity.

DESCRIPTION: Protein C is a vitamin K–dependent protein that originates in the liver and circulates in plasma. Protein C activation occurs on thrombomodulin receptors on the endothelial cell surface. Thrombin bound to thrombomodulin receptors preferentially activates protein C. Freely circulating thrombin mainly converts fibrinogen to fibrin. Other steps in the activation process require calcium and protein S cofactor binding (see monographs titled "Protein S" and "Fibrinogen"). Activated protein C exhibits potent anticoagulant effects by degrading activated factors V and VIII. There are two types of protein C deficiency:

Type I: Decreased antigen and function, detected by functional and antigenic assays

Type II: Normal antigen but decreased function, detected only by a functional assay

Functional assays are recommended for initial evaluation because of their greater sensitivity. ■

INDICATIONS:
• Differentiate inherited deficiency from acquired deficiency

• Investigate the mechanism of idiopathic venous thrombosis

RESULT

Increased in: N/A

Decreased in:
• Congenital deficiency

• Liver disease

• Oral anticoagulant therapy

CRITICAL VALUES: N/A

INTERFERING FACTORS:

• Drugs that may increase protein C levels include desmopressin and oral contraceptives.

• Drugs that may decrease protein C levels include warfarin (Coumadin) and coumarin.

• Placement of tourniquet for longer than 1 minute can result in venous stasis and changes in the concentration of plasma proteins to be measured. Platelet activation may also occur under these conditions, causing erroneous results.

• Vascular injury during phlebotomy can activate platelets and coagulation factors, causing erroneous results.

• Hemolyzed specimens must be rejected because hemolysis is an indication of platelet and coagulation factor activation.

• Incompletely filled tubes contaminated with heparin or clotted specimens must be rejected.

• Icteric or lipemic specimens interfere with optical testing methods, producing erroneous results.

Nursing Implications and Procedure

Pretest:

➤ Obtain a history of the patient's complaints, including a list of known allergens.

➤ Obtain a history of the patient's hematopoietic and hepatobiliary systems, as well as results of previously performed tests and procedures. For related tests, refer to the hematopoietic and hepatobiliary system tables.

➤ Obtain a list of medications the patient is taking, including herbs, nutritional supplements, and

nutraceuticals. The requesting health care practitioner and laboratory should be advised if the patient regularly uses these products so that their effects can be taken into consideration when reviewing results.

➤ There are no food, fluid, or medication restrictions unless by medical direction.

➤ Review the procedure with the patient.

➤ Inform the patient that specimen collection takes approximately 5 to 10 minutes.

Intratest:

➤ Direct the patient to breathe normally and to avoid unnecessary movement.

➤ Observe standard precautions and follow the general guidelines in Appendix A. Perform a venipuncture, and collect the specimen in a 5-mL blue-top tube. *Important note*: Two different concentrations of sodium citrate preservative are currently added to blue-top tubes for coagulation studies: 3.2% and 3.8%. The National Committee for Clinical Laboratory Standards (NCCLS) guideline for sodium citrate is 3.2%. Laboratories establish reference ranges for coagulation testing based on numerous factors, including sodium citrate concentration, test equipment, and test reagents. It is important to inquire from the laboratory which concentration it recommends, because each concentration will have its own specific reference range.

➤ When multiple specimens are drawn, the blue-top tube should be collected after sterile (i.e., blood culture) and red-top tubes. When coagulation testing is the only work to be done, an extra red-top tube should be collected before the blue-top tube to avoid contaminating the specimen with tissue thromboplastin, which can falsely decrease values.

➤ Label the specimen, and promptly

transport it to the laboratory. The NCCLS recommendation for processed and unprocessed specimens stored in unopened tubes is that testing should be completed within 1 to 4 hours of collection.

Post-test:

> Observe venipuncture site for bleed-ing or hematoma formation. Apply pressure bandage.

➤ Evaluate test results in relation to the patient's symptoms and other tests performed. Related laboratory tests include anticardiolipin antibody, antithrombin III, complete blood count, factor V, fibrin degradation products, fibrinogen, lupus anticoagulant, and protein S.

PROTEIN S

· ·

SYNONYMS/ACRONYM: Protein S antigen, protein S functional.

SPECIMEN: Plasma (1 mL) collected in blue-top (sodium citrate) tube.

REFERENCE VALUE: (Method: Clot detection)

	Conventional Units	SI Units (Conversion Factor ×.01)
Total protein S	70–140% activity	0.7–1.4 U/mL
Free protein S	60–120% activity	0.6–1.2 U/mL

The low end of "normal" is lower in children younger than age 16 years because of the immaturity of the liver.

DESCRIPTION: Protein S is a vitamin K–dependent protein that originates in the liver and circulates in plasma. It is a cofactor required for the activation of protein C (see monographs titled "Protein C" and "Fibrinogen"). Protein S exists in two forms, free (biologically active) and bound. Approximately 40 percent of protein S circulates in the free form; the remainder is bound and is functionally inactive. There are two types of protein S deficiency:

Type I: Decreased antigen and function, detected by functional and antigenic assays

Type II: Normal antigen but decreased function, detected only by a functional assay

Functional assays are recommended for initial evaluation because of their greater sensitivity. ∎

INDICATIONS: Investigate the cause of hypercoagulable states

RESULT

Increased in: N/A

Decreased in:

- Chronic renal failure due to hypertension
- Congenital deficiency
- Coumarin-induced skin necrosis
- Diabetic neuropathy
- Disseminated intravascular coagulation
- Liver disease
- Oral anticoagulant therapy

CRITICAL VALUES: N/A

INTERFERING FACTORS:

- Drugs that may decrease protein S levels include oral contraceptives, warfarin (Coumadin), and coumarin.
- Placement of tourniquet for longer than 1 minute can result in venous stasis and changes in the concentration of plasma proteins to be measured. Platelet activation may also occur under these conditions, causing erroneous results.
- Vascular injury during phlebotomy can activate platelets and coagulation factors, causing erroneous results.
- Hemolyzed specimens must be rejected because hemolysis is an indication of platelet and coagulation factor activation.
- Incompletely filled tubes contaminated with heparin or clotted specimens must be rejected.
- Icteric or lipemic specimens interfere with optical testing methods, producing erroneous results.

Nursing Implications and Procedure . . . .

Pretest:

➤ Obtain a history of the patient's complaints, including a list of known allergens.

➤ Obtain a history of the patient's hematopoietic and hepatobiliary systems, as well as results of previously performed tests and procedures. For related tests, refer to the hematopoietic and hepatobiliary system tables.

➤ Obtain a list of medications the patient is taking, including herbs, nutritional supplements, and nutraceuticals. The requesting health care practitioner and laboratory should be advised if the patient regularly uses these products so that their effects can be taken into consideration when reviewing results.

➤ There are no food, fluid, or medication restrictions unless by medical direction.

➤ Review the procedure with the patient.

➤ Inform the patient that specimen collection takes approximately 5 to 10 minutes.

Intratest:

➤ Direct the patient to breathe normally and to avoid unnecessary movement.

➤ Observe standard precautions and follow the general guidelines in Appendix A. Perform a venipuncture, and collect the specimen in a 5-mL blue-top tube. *Important note:* Two different concentrations of sodium citrate preservative are currently added to blue-top tubes for coagulation studies: 3.2% and 3.8%. The National Committee for Clinical Laboratory Standards (NCCLS) guideline for sodium citrate is 3.2%. Laboratories establish reference ranges for coagulation testing based on numerous factors, including sodium citrate concentration, test equipment, and test reagents. It is important to inquire from the laboratory which concentration it recommends, because each concentration will have its own specific reference range.

➤ When multiple specimens are drawn, the blue-top tube should be collected after sterile (i.e., blood culture) and red-top tubes. When coagulation testing is the only work to be done, an extra red-top tube should be collected before the blue-top tube to avoid contaminating the specimen with tissue thromboplastin, which can falsely decrease values.

➤ Label the specimen, and promptly transport it to the laboratory. The NCCLS recommendation for processed and unprocessed specimens stored in unopened tubes is that testing should be completed within 1 to 4 hours of collection.

Post-test:

➤ Observe venipuncture site for bleeding or hematoma formation. Apply pressure bandage.

➤ Evaluate test results in relation to the patient's symptoms and other tests performed. Related laboratory tests include anticardiolipin antibody, antithrombin III, complete blood count, fibrin degradation products, fibrinogen, lupus anticoagulant, and protein C.

PROTEIN, URINE: TOTAL QUANTITATIVE AND FRACTIONS

SYNONYM/ACRONYM: N/A.

SPECIMEN: Urine (5 mL) from an unpreserved random or timed specimen collected in a clean, plastic collection container.

REFERENCE VALUE: (Method: Spectrophotometry for total protein, electrophoresis for protein fractions)

	Conventional Units	SI Units (Conversion Factor ×0.001)
Total protein	10–140 mg/24 h	0.01–0.14 g/24 h

Electrophoresis for fractionation is qualitative: No monoclonal gammopathy detected. (Urine protein electrophoresis should be ordered along with serum protein electrophoresis.)

DESCRIPTION: Most proteins, with the exception of the immunoglobulins, are synthesized and catabolized in the liver, where they are broken down into amino acids. The amino acids are converted to ammonia and ketoacids. Ammonia is converted to urea via the urea cycle. Urea is excreted in the urine. ∎

INDICATIONS:
• Assist in the diagnosis of myeloma,

Waldenström's macroglobulinemia, lymphoma, and amyloidosis

- Assist in the detection of Bence Jones proteins (light chains)

- Evaluate kidney function

RESULT

Increased in:

- Postexercise period

- Diabetic nephropathy

- Fanconi's syndrome

- Heavy metal poisoning

- Malignancies of the urinary tract

- Monoclonal gammopathies

- Multiple myeloma

- Nephrotic syndrome

- Other myeloproliferative and lymphoproliferative disorders

- Sarcoidosis

- Sickle cell disease

- Urinary tract infections

Decreased in: N/A

CRITICAL VALUES: N/A

INTERFERING FACTORS:
- Drugs and substances that may increase urine protein levels include acetaminophen, aminosalicylic acid, amphotericin B, ampicillin, antimony compounds, antipyrine, arsenicals, ascorbic acid, bacitracin, bismuth subsalicylate, bromate, capreomycin, captopril, carbamazepine, carbarsone, carbenoxolone, carbutamide, cephaloglycin, cephaloridine, chlorpromazine, chlorpropamide, chlorthalidone, chrysarobin, colistimethate, colistin, corticosteroids, cyclosporine, demeclocycline, 1,2-diaminopropane, diatrizoic acid, dihydrotachysterol, doxycycline, enalapril, gentamicin,

gold, hydrogen sulfide, iodoalphionic acid, iodopyracet, iopanoic acid, iophenoxic acid, ipodate, kanamycin, corn oil (Lipomul), lithium, mefenamic acid, melarsonyl, melarsoprol, mercury compounds, methicillin, methylbromide, meziocillin, mitomycin, nafcillin, naphthalene, neomycin, nonsteroidal anti-inflammatory drugs, oxacillin, paraldehyde, penicillamine, penicillin, phenols, phenolphthalein, phensuximide, phosphorus, picric acid, piperacillin, plicamycin, polymyxin, probenecid, promazine, pyrazolones, quaternary ammonium compounds, radiographic agents, rifampin, sodium bicarbonate, streptokinase, sulfisoxazole, suramin, tetracyclines, thallium, thiosemicarbazones, tolbutamide, tolmetin, triethylenemelamine, and vitamin D.

- Drugs that may decrease urine protein levels include captopril, cyclosporine, diltiazem, enalapril, fosinopril, interferon, lisinopril, prednisolone, and quinapril.

- All urine voided for the timed collection period must be included in the collection or else falsely decreased values may be obtained. Compare output records with volume collected to verify that all voids were included in the collection.

Nursing Implications and Procedure • • • • • • • • • • •

Pretest: ■

➤ Obtain a history of the patient's complaints, including a list of known allergens.

➤ Obtain a history of the patient's genitourinary and immune systems, as well as results of previously performed tests and procedures. For related tests, refer to the genitourinary and immune system tables.

➤ Obtain a list of medications the

patient is taking, including herbs, nutritional supplements, and nutraceuticals. The requesting health care practitioner and laboratory should be advised if the patient regularly uses these products so that their effects can be taken into consideration when reviewing results.

➤ There are no food, fluid, or medication restrictions unless by medical direction.

➤ Review the procedure with the patient. Provide a nonmetallic urinal, bedpan, or toilet-mounted collection device.

➤ Usually a 24-hour time frame for urine collection is ordered. Inform the patient that all urine must be saved during that 24-hour period. Instruct the patient not to void directly into the laboratory collection container. Instruct the patient to avoid defecating in the collection device and to keep toilet tissue out of the collection device to prevent contamination of the specimen. Place a sign in the bathroom to remind the patient to save all urine.

➤ Instruct the patient to void all urine into the collection device and then to pour the urine into the laboratory collection container. Alternatively the specimen can be left in the collection device for a health care staff member to add to the laboratory collection container.

Intratest:

➤ Observe standard precautions and follow the general guidelines in Appendix A.

Random specimen (collect in early morning):

Clean-catch specimen:

➤ Instruct the male patient to (1) thoroughly wash his hands, (2) cleanse the meatus, (3) void a small amount into the toilet, and (4) void directly into the specimen container.

➤ Instruct the female patient to (1) thoroughly wash her hands; (2) cleanse the labia from front to back; (3) while keeping the labia separated, void a small amount into the toilet; and (4) without interrupting the urine stream, void directly into the specimen container.

Indwelling catheter:

➤ Put on gloves. Empty drainage tube of urine. It may be necessary to clamp off the catheter for 15 to 30 minutes before specimen collection. Cleanse specimen port with antiseptic swab, and then aspirate 5 mL of urine with a 21- to 25-gauge needle and syringe. Transfer urine to a sterile container.

Timed specimen:

➤ Obtain a clean 3-L urine specimen container, toilet-mounted collection device, and plastic bag (for transport of the specimen container). The specimen must be refrigerated or kept on ice throughout the entire collection period. If an indwelling urinary catheter is in place, the drainage bag must be kept on ice.

➤ Begin the test between 6 and 8 a.m., if possible. Collect first voiding and discard. Record the time the specimen was discarded as the beginning of the timed collection period. The next morning, ask the patient to void at the same time the collection was started and add this last voiding to the container.

➤ If an indwelling catheter is in place, replace the tubing and container system at the start of the collection time. Keep the container system on ice during the collection period, or empty the urine into a larger container periodically during the collection period; monitor to ensure continued drainage, and conclude the test the next morning at the same hour the collection was begun.

➤ At the conclusion of the test, compare the quantity of urine with the urinary output record for the collection; if the specimen contains less than what was recorded as output, some urine may have been discarded, invalidating the test.

➤ Label the specimen, and promptly transport it to the laboratory. Include on the label the amount of urine, test start and stop times, and ingestion of any foods or medications that can affect test results.

Post-test:

➤ Evaluate test results in relation to the patient's symptoms and other tests performed. Related laboratory tests include glucose, glycated hemoglobin, serum and urine immunofixation electrophoresis, microalbumin, serum and urine osmolality, serum protein and fractions, and urinalysis.

PROTHROMBIN TIME AND INTERNATIONAL NORMALIZED RATIO

SYNONYM/ACRONYM: Pro-time, PT.

SPECIMEN: Plasma (1 mL) collected in a completely filled blue-top (sodium citrate) tube.

REFERENCE VALUE: (Method: Clot detection) 10 to 13 seconds.
International normalized ratio (INR) = 2.0 to 3.0 for patients receiving treatment for venous thrombosis, pulmonary embolism, and valvular heart disease.
INR = 2.5 to 3.5 for patients with mechanical heart valves and/or receiving treatment for recurrent systemic embolism.

DESCRIPTION: Prothrombin time (PT) is a coagulation test performed to measure the time it takes for a firm fibrin clot to form after tissue thromboplastin (factor III) and calcium are added to the sample. It is used to evaluate the extrinsic pathway of the coagulation sequence in patients receiving oral warfarin or coumarin-type anticoagulants. Prothrombin is a vitamin K–dependent protein produced by the liver; measurement is reported as time in seconds or percentage of normal activity. PT evaluation can now be based on an

INR using a standardized thromboplastin reagent to assist in making decisions regarding oral anticoagulation therapy. Some inferences of factor deficiency can be made by comparison of results obtained from the activated partial thromboplastin time (APTT) and PT tests. A normal APTT with a prolonged PT can occur only with factor VII deficiency. A prolonged APTT with a normal PT could indicate a deficiency in factors XII, XI, IX, and VIII as well as VIII:C (von Willebrand factor). Factor deficiencies can also be identified by correction or substitution studies using normal serum. These studies are easy to perform and are accomplished by adding plasma from a normal patient to a sample from a suspected factor-deficient patient. When the PT is repeated and corrected, or within reference range, it can be assumed that the prolonged PT is due to a factor deficiency (see monograph titled "Coagulation Factors"). ■

INDICATIONS:

• Differentiate between deficiencies of clotting factors II, V, VII, and X, which prolong the PT; and congenital coagulation disorders, such as hemophilia A (factor VIII) and hemophilia B (factor IX), which do not alter the PT

• Evaluate the response to anticoagulant therapy with coumarin derivatives and determine dosage required to achieve therapeutic results

• Identify the possible cause of abnormal bleeding, such as epistaxis, hematoma, gingival bleeding, hematuria, and menorrhagia

• Identify individuals who may be prone to bleeding during surgical, obstetric, dental, or invasive diagnostic procedures

• Monitor the effects of conditions such as liver disease, protein deficiency, and fat malabsorption on hemostasis

• Screen for prothrombin deficiency

• Screen for vitamin K deficiency

RESULT

Increased in:

• Afibrinogenemia, dysfibrinogenemia, or hypofibrinogenemia

• Biliary obstruction

• Disseminated intravascular coagulation

• Hereditary deficiencies of factors II, V, VII, and X

• Intravascular coagulation

• Liver disease

• Poor fat absorption (tropical sprue, celiac disease, chronic diarrhea)

• Presence of circulating anticoagulant

• Systemic lupus erythematosus

• Vitamin K deficiency

Decreased in:

• Ovarian hyperfunction

• Regional enteritis or ileitis

CRITICAL VALUES:

Greater than 20 seconds (uncoagulated)

Three times normal control (anticoagulated)

Important signs to note are prolonged bleeding, hematoma at the puncture site, hemorrhage, blood in stool, bleeding gums, and shock. Monitoring vital signs and neurologic changes until PT is within normal range is indicated. Administration of vitamin K, a potent anticoagulant, may be requested.

INTERFERING FACTORS:

• Drugs that may increase PT in patients receiving anticoagulation therapy include acetaminophen, amiodarone, anabolic steroids, anisindione, anistreplase, antibiotics, antipyrine, acetylsalicylic acid (high doses), carbenicillin, cathartics, chlorthalidone, cholestyramine, clofibrate, corticotropin, demeclocycline, dextrothyroxine, diazoxide, diflunisal, diuretics, doxycycline, erythromycin, glucagon, hydroxyzine, indomethacin, laxatives, mercaptopurine, miconazole, nalidixic acid, neomycin, niacin, oxyphenbutazone, phenytoin, quinine, sulfachlorpyridazine, and thyroxine.

• Drugs that may decrease PT in patients receiving anticoagulation therapy include amobarbital, anabolic steroids, antacids, antihistamines, barbiturates, carbamazepine, chloral hydrate, chlordane, colchicine, corticosteroids, diuretics, oral contraceptives, penicillin, primidone, rifampin, simethicone, spironolactone, tolbutamide, and vitamin K.

- Traumatic venipunctures can activate the coagulation sequence by contaminating the sample with tissue thromboplastin, and producing falsely shortened PT.

- Failure to fill the tube sufficiently to yield proper blood-to-anticoagulant ratio may cause a falsely lengthened PT; an incompletely filled tube is reason for specimen rejection.

- Excessive agitation causing sample hemolysis can falsely shorten the PT because the hemolyzed cells activate plasma-clotting factors.

Nursing Implications and Procedure • • • • • • • • • •

Pretest: ■

➤ Obtain a history of the patient's complaints, including a list of known allergens.

➤ Obtain a history of the patient's cardiovascular, hematopoietic, and hepatobiliary systems, any bleeding disorders, and results of previously performed tests and procedures, especially bleeding time, complete blood count, clotting time, partial thromboplastin time, prothrombin time, and platelets. For related tests, refer to the cardiovascular, hematopoietic, and hepatobiliary system tables.

➤ Obtain a list of medications the patient is taking, including anticoagulant therapy, acetylsalicylic acid, herbals, and nutraceuticals known to affect coagulation. It is recommended that use be discontinued 14 days before dental or surgical proce-

dures. The requesting health care practitioner and laboratory should be advised if the patient regularly uses these products so that their effects can be taken into consideration when reviewing results.

➤ There are no food, fluid, or medication restrictions unless by medical direction.

➤ Review the procedure with the patient.

➤ Inform the patient that specimen collection takes approximately 5 to 10 minutes.

Intratest: ■

➤ Direct the patient to breathe normally and to avoid unnecessary movement.

➤ Observe standard precautions and follow the general guidelines in Appendix A. Perform a venipuncture, and collect the specimen in a 5-mL blue-top tube. Fill tube completely. *Important note*: Two different concentrations of sodium citrate preservative are currently added to blue-top tubes for coagulation studies: 3.2% and 3.8%. The National Committee for Clinical Laboratory Standards (NCCLS) guideline for sodium citrate is 3.2%. Laboratories establish reference ranges for coagulation testing based on numerous factors, including sodium citrate concentration, test equipment, and test reagents. It is important to inquire from the laboratory which concentration it recommends, because each concentration will have its own specific reference range.

➤ When multiple specimens are drawn, the blue-top tube should be collected after sterile (i.e., blood culture) and red-top tubes. When coagulation testing is the only work to be done, an extra red-top tube should be collected before the blue-top tube to avoid contaminating the specimen with tissue thromboplastin, which can falsely shorten PT.

➤ Label the specimen, and promptly transport it to the laboratory. The

NCCLS recommendation for processed and unprocessed samples stored in unopened tubes is that testing should be completed within 1 to 4 hours of collection.

Post-test:

➤ Observe venipuncture site for bleeding or hematoma formation. Apply pressure bandage.

➤ Instruct the patient to report bleeding from any areas of the skin or mucous membranes.

➤ Inform the patient with prolonged PT of the importance of taking precautions against bruising and bleeding, including the use of a soft bristle toothbrush, use of an electric razor, avoidance of constipation, avoidance of aspirin products, and avoidance of intramuscular injections.

➤ Inform the patient of the importance of periodic laboratory testing while taking an anticoagulant.

➤ Evaluate test results in relation to the patient's symptoms and other tests performed. Related laboratory tests include alanine aminotransferase, aspartate aminotransferase, bilirubin, factor assays, γ-glutamyl transpeptidase, platelet count, and vitamin K.

PSEUDOCHOLINESTERASE AND DIBUCAINE NUMBER

• •

SYNONYMS/ACRONYMS: CHS, PCHE, AcCHS.

SPECIMEN: Plasma (1 mL) collected in a lavender-top (ethylenediaminetetra-acetic acid [EDTA]) tube. Serum (1 mL) collected in a red-top tube is also acceptable.

REFERENCE VALUE: (Method: Spectrophotometry, kinetic)

Test	Conventional Units	SI Units (Conversion Factor ×1)
Pseudocholinesterase	2–11 U/mL	2–11 kU/L

Dibucaine Number	Fraction (%) of Activity Inhibited	SI Units (Conversion Factor ×0.01)
Normal homozygote	79–84%	0.79–0.84 kU/L
Heterozygote	55–70%	0.55–0.70 kU/L
Abnormal homozygote	16–28%	0.16–0.28 kU/L

DESCRIPTION: There are two types of cholinesterase: *acetylcholinesterase*, which is found in red blood cells, lung, and brain (nerve) tissue (see monograph titled "Red Blood Cell Cholinesterase"); and *cholinesterase*, which is found mainly in the plasma, liver, and heart. Pseudocholinesterase is a nonspecific enzyme that hydrolyzes acetylcholine and noncholine esters; carbamate and organophosphate insecticides (e.g., parathion, malathion) inhibit its activity.

Patients with inherited pseudocholinesterase deficiency are at risk during anesthesia if succinylcholine is administered as an anesthetic. Succinylcholine, a short-acting muscle relaxant, is a reversible inhi-bitor of acetylcholinesterase and is hydrolyzed by cholinesterase. Succinylcholine-sensitive patients may be unable to metabolize the anesthetic quickly, resulting in prolonged or unrecoverable apnea. Abnormal genotypes of pseudocholinesterase are detected using the dibucaine and fluoride inhibition tests because, in normal individuals, these chemicals inhibit pseudocholinesterase activity. The prevalence of succinylcholate sensitivity is 1 in 1500 patients. Widespread preoperative screening is not routinely performed. ∎

INDICATIONS:

• Assist in the evaluation of liver function

• Screen for abnormal genotypes of pseudocholinesterase in patients with a family history of succinylcholate sensitivity who are about to undergo anesthesia using succinylcholate.

RESULT

Increased in:

• Diabetes

• Hyperthyroidism

• Nephrotic syndrome

• Obesity

Decreased in:

• Acute infection

• Anemia (severe)

• Carcinomatosis

• Cirrhosis

• Congenital deficiency

• Hepatic carcinoma

• Hepatocellular disease

• Infectious hepatitis

• Insecticide exposure (organic phosphate)

• Malnutrition

• Muscular dystrophy

• Myocardial infarction

• Plasmapheresis

• Succinylcholine hypersensitivity

• Tuberculosis

• Uremia

CRITICAL VALUES: ⚠
Notify the anesthesiologist if the test result is positive and surgery is scheduled. A positive result indicates that the patient is at risk for prolonged or unrecoverable apnea related to the inability to metabolize succinylcholine.

INTERFERING FACTORS:

• Drugs and substances that may decrease pseudocholinesterase levels include ambenonium, barbiturates, cyclophosphamide, echothiophate, edrophonium, fluorides, ibuprofen, iodipamide, iopanoic acid, isoflurophate, neostigmine, parathion, procainamide, physostigmine, pyridostigmine, estrogens, and oral contraceptives.

- Drugs that may increase pseudocholinesterase levels include carbamazepine, phenytoin, and valproic acid.

- Pregnancy decreases pseudocholinesterase levels by about 30 percent.

- Improper anticoagulant; fluoride interferes with the measurement and causes a falsely decreased value.

Nursing Implications and Procedure • • • • • • • • • • •

Pretest:

➤ Obtain a history of the patient's complaints, including a list of known allergens. Particularly important to report is exposure to pesticides causing symptoms including blurred vision, muscle weakness, nausea, vomiting, headaches, pulmonary edema, salivation, sweating, or convulsions.

➤ Obtain a history of the patient's hepatobiliary and musculoskeletal systems, as well as results of previously performed tests and procedures. For related tests, refer to the hepatobiliary and musculoskeletal system tables.

➤ Obtain a list of medications the patient is taking, including herbs, nutritional supplements, and nutraceuticals. The requesting health care practitioner and laboratory should be advised if the patient regularly uses these products so that their effects can be taken into consideration when reviewing results.

➤ There are no food, fluid, or medication restrictions unless by medical direction.

➤ Review the procedure with the patient.

➤ Inform the patient that specimen collection takes approximately 5 to 10 minutes.

Intratest:

➤ Direct the patient to breathe normally and to avoid unnecessary movement.

➤ Observe standard precautions and follow the general guidelines in Appendix A. Perform a venipuncture, and collect the specimen in a 5-mL lavender- or red-top tube.

➤ Label the specimen, and promptly transport it to the laboratory.

Post-test:

➤ Observe venipuncture site for bleeding or hematoma formation. Apply pressure bandage.

➤ The patient with decreased values should be observed for signs of fluid volume excess related to compromised regulatory mechanisms, decreased cardiac output related to decreased myocardial contractility or arrhythmias, and pain related to inflammation or ischemia.

➤ Evaluate test results in relation to the patient's symptoms and other tests performed. Related laboratory tests include alanine aminotransferase and aspartate aminotransferase.

PULMONARY FUNCTION STUDIES

• •

SYNONYM/ACRONYM: Pulmonary function tests (PFTs).

AREA OF APPLICATION: Lungs, respiratory system.

CONTRAST: None.

DESCRIPTION: Pulmonary function studies provide information about the volume, pattern, and rates of airflow involved in respiratory function. These studies may also include tests involving the diffusing capabilities of the lungs (i.e., volume of gases diffusing across a membrane). A complete pulmonary study profile includes the determination of all lung volumes, spirometry, diffusing capacity, maximum voluntary ventilation, flow-volume loop (Fig. 1–1), and maximum expiratory and inspiratory pressures. Other studies include small airway volumes.

Pulmonary function studies are classified according to lung volumes and capacities, rates of flow, and gas exchange. The exception is the diffusion test, which records the movement of a gas during inspiration and expiration. Lung volumes and capacities constitute the amount of air inhaled or exhaled from the lungs; this value is compared to normal reference values specific for the patient's age, height, and sex. The following are volumes and capacities measured by spirometry that do not require timed testing. ■

TIDAL VOLUME: Total amount of air inhaled and exhaled with one breath.

RESIDUAL VOLUME: Amount of air remaining in the lungs after a maximum expiration effort (not measured by spirometry, but can be calculated from the functional residual capacity [FRC] minus the expiratory reserve volume [ERV]). This indirect type of measurement can be done by body plethysmography (see monograph titled "Plethysmography").

INSPIRATORY RESERVE VOLUME: Maximum amount of air inhaled after normal inspirations.

EXPIRATORY RESERVE VOLUME: Maximum amount of air exhaled after a resting expiration (can be calculated by the vital capacity [VC] minus the inspiratory capacity [IC]).

VITAL CAPACITY: Maximum amount of air exhaled after a maximum inspiration (can be calculated by adding the IC and the expiratory reserve volume [ERV]).

TOTAL LUNG CAPACITY: Total amount of air that the lungs can hold after maximal inspiration (can be calculated by adding the VC and the residual volume [RV]).

INSPIRATORY CAPACITY: Maximum amount of air inspired after normal expiration (can be calculated by adding the inspiratory RV and tidal volume).

FUNCTIONAL RESIDUAL CAPACITY: Volume of air that remains in the lungs after normal expiration (can be calculated by adding the RV and ERV).

The volumes, capacities, and rates of flow measured by spirometry that do require timed testing include the following:

FORCED VITAL CAPACITY IN 1 SECOND: Maximum amount of air that can be forcefully exhaled after a full inspiration.

FORCED EXPIRATORY VOLUME: Amount of air exhaled in the first second (can also be determined at 2 or 3 seconds) of forced vital capacity (FVC, which is the amount of air exhaled in seconds, expressed as a percent).

MAXIMAL MIDEXPIRATORY FLOW: Also

known as forced expiratory flow rate (FEF$_{25-75}$), maximal rate of air flow during a forced expiration.

FORCED INSPIRATORY FLOW RATE: Volume inspired from the RV at a point of measurement (can be expressed as a percent to identify the corresponding volume pressure and inspired volume).

PEAK INSPIRATORY FLOW RATE: Maximum airflow during a forced maximal inspiration.

PEAK EXPIRATORY FLOW RATE: Maximum airflow expired during FVC.

FLOW-VOLUME LOOPS: Flows and volumes recorded during forced expiratory volume (FEV) and forced inspiratory vital capacity (FIVC) procedures (Fig. 1–2).

MAXIMAL INSPIRATORY-EXPIRATORY PRESSURES: Measures the strength of the respiratory muscles in neuromuscular disorders.

MAXIMAL VOLUNTARY VENTILATION: Maximal volume of air inspired and expired in 1 minute (may be done for shorter periods and multiplied to equal 1 minute).

Other studies for gas-exchange capacity, small airway abnormalities, and allergic responses in hyperactive airway disorders can be performed during the conventional pulmonary function study. These include the following:

DIFFUSING CAPACITY OF THE LUNGS: Rate of transfer of carbon monoxide through the alveolar and capillary membrane in 1 minute.

CLOSING VOLUME: Measures the closure of small airways in the lower alveoli by monitoring volume and percent of alveolar nitrogen after inhalation of 100 percent oxygen.

ISOFLOW VOLUME: Flow-volume loop test followed by inhalation of a mix of helium and oxygen to determine small airway disease.

BODY PLETHYSMOGRAPHY: Measures thoracic gas volume and airway resistance.

BRONCHIAL PROVOCATION: Quantifies airway response after inhalation of methacholine.

ARTERIAL BLOOD GASES: Measures oxygen, pH, and carbon dioxide in arterial blood.

Values are expressed in units of mL, %, L, L/sec, and L/min, depending on the test performed.

INDICATIONS:

• Detect chronic obstructive pulmonary disease (COPD) and/or restrictive pulmonary diseases that affect the chest wall (e.g., neuromuscular disorders, kyphosis, scoliosis) and lungs, as evidenced by abnormal air flows and volumes

• Determine the presence of lung disease when other studies, such as x-rays, do not provide a definitive diagnosis or determine the progression and severity of known COPD and restrictive pulmonary disease

• Evaluate the cause of dyspnea occurring with or without exercise

• Determine the effectiveness of therapy regimens, such as bronchodilators, for pulmonary disorders

• Evaluate the respiratory system to determine the patient's ability to tolerate procedures such as surgery or diagnostic studies

• Screen high-risk populations for early detection of pulmonary conditions (e.g., patients with exposure to occupational or environmental hazards, smokers, patients with a hereditary predisposition)

- Evaluate pulmonary function after surgical pneumonectomy, lobectomy, or segmental lobectomy

- Evaluate pulmonary disability for legal or insurance claims

- Determine airway response to inhalants in patients with an airway-reactive disorder

- Evaluate lung compliance to determine changes in elasticity evidenced by changes in lung volumes (decreased in restrictive pulmonary disease, increased in COPD and in elderly patients)

- Determine the diffusing capacity of the lungs (DCOL)

RESULT

Normal Findings:

- Normal respiratory volume and capacities, gas diffusion, and distribution

- No evidence of COPD or restrictive pulmonary disease

TV	500 mL at rest
RV	1200 mL (approximate)
IRV	3000 mL (approximate)
ERV	1100 mL (approximate)
VC	4600 mL (approximate)
TLC	5800 mL (approximate)
IC	3500 mL (approximate)
FRC	2300 mL (approximate)
FVC	3000–5000 mL (approximate)
FEV_1/FVC	81–83%
MMEF	25–75%
FIF	25–75%
MVV	25–35% or 170 L/min
PIFR	300 L/min
PEFR	450 L/min
F-V loop	Normal curve
DCOL	25 mL/min per mm Hg (approximate)
CV	10–20% of VC
V_{iso}	Based on age formula
Bronchial provocation	No change, or less than 20% reduction in FEV_1

Note: Normal values listed are estimated values for adults. Actual pediatric and adult values are based on age, height, and gender. These normal values are included on the patient's pulmonary function laboratory report.
TV = tidal volume; RV = residual volume; IRV = inspiratory reserve volume; ERV = expiratory reserve volume; VC = vital capacity; TLC = total lung capacity; IC = inspiratory capacity; FRC = functional residual capacity; FVC = forced vital capacity in 1 second; FEV_1 = forced expiratory volume in 1 second; MMEF = maximal midexpiratory flow (also known as $FEF_{25-75\%}$); FIF = forced inspiratory flow rate; MVV = maximal voluntary ventilation; PIFR = peak inspiratory flow rate; PEFR = peak expiratory flow rate; F-V loop = flow-volume loop; DCOL = diffusing capacity of the lungs; CV = closing volume; V_{iso} = isoflow volume.

Normal adult lung volumes, capacities, and flow rates are as follows:

Abnormal Findings:

- Allergy
- Asbestosis
- Asthma
- Bronchiectasis
- Chest trauma
- Chronic bronchitis
- Curvature of the spine
- Emphysema
- Myasthenia gravis
- Obesity
- Pulmonary fibrosis
- Pulmonary tumors
- Respiratory infections
- Sarcoidosis

INTERFERING FACTORS:

- The aging process can cause decreased values (FVC, DCOL) depending on the study done.

- Inability of the patient to put forth the necessary breathing effort affects the results.

- Medications such as brochodilators can affect results.

- Improper placement of the nose clamp or mouthpiece that allows for leakage can affect volume results.

- Confusion or inability to understand instructions or cooperate during the study can cause inaccurate results.

- Testing is contraindicated in patients with cardiac insufficiency, recent myocardial infarction, and presence of chest pain that affects inspiration or expiration ability.

- Exercise caution with patients who have upper respiratory infections, such as a cold or acute bronchitis.

Nursing Implications and Procedure

Pretest:

➤ Explain the purpose of the study, and inform the patient that it will not cause any pain.

➤ Explain that the procedure is generally performed in a specially equipped room or in a physician's office by a technologist and usually lasts 1 hour.

➤ Measure the patient's height and weight.

➤ Assess medication history for recent administration of analgesics that may depress respiratory function. Ensure that medications such as bronchodilators (oral or inhalant) are withheld at least 4 hours before the study.

➤ Obtain a history of suspected or known pulmonary conditions, respiratory status and patterns, medications (oral, inhalant, other), smoking history, and previously performed tests and procedures. For related tests, refer to the respiratory system table.

➤ Ensure that the patient has refrained from smoking tobacco or eating a heavy meal for 4 to 6 hours.

Intratest:

➤ Obtain an inhalant bronchodilator to treat any bronchospasms that can occur with testing.

➤ Ask patient to void and loosen any restrictive clothing.

➤ Place the patient in a sitting position on a chair near the spirometry equipment.

➤ Place a soft clip on the patient's nose to restrict nose breathing, and instruct the patient to breathe through the mouth.

> Place a mouthpiece in the mouth and tell the patient to close his or her lips around it to form a seal.

> Tubing from the mouthpiece is connected to a cylinder that is connected to a computer that measures, records, and calculates the values for the tests done.

> Instruct the patient to inhale deeply and then to quickly exhale as much air as possible into the mouthpiece.

> Additional breathing maneuvers are performed on inspiration and expiration (normal, forced, and breathholding).

Post-test:

> Assess the patient for dizziness or weakness after the testing.

> Allow the patient to rest as long as needed to recover.

> Compare new pulmonary function test values with previous values to determine response to medical problem or treatment.

> Tell patient to resume medications withheld before the test was ordered or to contact the provider ordering the test if he or she has any questions.

> Determine if the patient or family members have any further questions or concerns.

> A physician specializing in this branch of medicine sends a written report to the ordering provider, who discusses the results with the patient.

> Evaluate test results in relation to the patient's symptoms and other tests performed. Related diagnostic tests include x-ray, computed tomography, magnetic resonance imaging, and positron emission tomography of the chest; and electrocardiography.

FIGURE 1–1

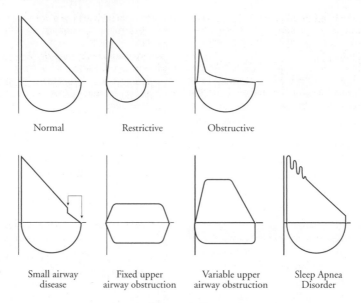

Normal Restrictive Obstructive

Small airway Fixed upper Variable upper Sleep Apnea
disease airway obstruction airway obstruction Disorder

FIGURE 1–2

PULSE OXIMETRY

SYNONYMS/ACRONYM: Oximetry, Pulse Ox.

AREA OF APPLICATION: Earlobe, fingertip; for infants, use the large toe, top or bottom of the foot, or sides of the ankle.

CONTRAST: None.

DESCRIPTION: Pulse oximetry is a noninvasive study that provides continuous readings of arterial blood oxygen saturation (SPO_2) using a sensor site (earlobe or fingertip). The SPO_2 equals the ratio of the amount of O_2 contained in the hemoglobin to the maximum amount of O_2 contained with hemoglobin expressed as a percent. The results obtained may compare favorably with O_2 saturation levels obtained by arterial blood gas (ABG) analysis without the need to perform successive arterial punctures. The device used is a clip or probe that produces a light beam with two different wavelengths. A sensor on the opposite side measures the absorption of each of the wavelengths of light to determine the O_2 saturation reading. The displayed result is a ratio, expressed as a percent, between the actual O_2 content of the hemoglobin and the potential maximum O_2-carrying capacity of the hemoglobin. ∎

INDICATIONS:

- Monitor oxygenation perioperatively and during acute illnesses

- Monitor oxygenation status in patients on a ventilator, during surgery, and during bronchoscopy

- Evaluate suspected nocturnal hypoxemia in chronic obstructive pulmonary disease (COPD)

- Monitor O_2 saturation during activities such as pulmonary exercise stress testing or pulmonary rehabilitation exercises to determine optimal tolerance

- Determine the effectiveness of pulmonary gas exchange function

- Monitor response to pulmonary drug regimens, especially flow and O_2 content

- Monitor oxygenation during testing for sleep apnea

RESULT

Normal Findings:
- Greater than or equal to 95 percent

Abnormal Findings:
- Abnormal gas exchange

- Hypoxemia with levels less than 95 percent

- Impaired cardiopulmonary function

INTERFERING FACTORS:

This procedure is contraindicated for:
- Patients who smoke or have suffered

carbon monoxide inhalation, because O_2 levels may be falsely elevated

Factors that may result in incorrect values:
- Patients with anemic conditions reflecting a reduction in hemoglobin, the O_2-carrying component in the blood

- Excessive light surrounding the patient, such as from surgical lights

- Impaired cardiopulmonary function

- Lipid emulsion therapy and presence of certain dyes

- Movement of the finger or ear or improper placement of probe or clip

- Nail polish, false fingernails, and skin pigmentation when a finger probe is used

- Vasoconstriction from cool skin temperature, drugs, hypotension, or vessel obstruction causing a decrease in blood flow

Other considerations:
- Accuracy for most units is plus or minus 4 percent with a standard deviation of 1 percent.

Nursing Implications and Procedure • • • • • • • • • •

Pretest: ■

➤ Inform the patient that the procedure is generally performed at the bedside, in the operating room during a surgical procedure, or in a physician's office.

➤ Explain that the procedure lasts as long as the monitoring is needed and could be continuous.

➤ Explain that no pain is associated with the procedure.

➤ Obtain a history of pulmonary disorders, respiratory and cardiac status, reason for monitoring procedure, and ABG results. For related tests, refer to the respiratory system table.

➤ Ensure that the patient does not have false fingernails and that nail polish has been removed.

➤ Instruct the patient not to smoke for 24 hours before the test.

➤ If a finger probe is used, instruct the patient not to grip treadmill rail or bedrail tightly; doing so restricts blood flow.

➤ When used in the presence of flammable gases, the equipment must be approved for that specific use.

➤ There are no food, fluid, or medication restrictions.

Intratest:

➤ Massage or apply a warm towel to the upper earlobe or finger to increase the blood flow.

➤ The index finger is normally used, but if the patient's finger is too large for the probe, a smaller finger can be used.

➤ If the earlobe is used, make sure good contact is achieved.

➤ With infants, the big toe, top or bottom of the foot, or sides of the heel may be used.

➤ Place the photodetector probe over the finger in such a way that the light beams and sensors are opposite each other. Turn the power switch to the oximeter monitor, which will display information about heart rate and SaO₂.

➤ Remove the clip for monitoring when the test is complete.

Post-test:

➤ Compare new value with previous value to determine response to medical problem or treatment.

➤ Consider test results as they relate to ABGs.

➤ Closely observe SPO₂, and report if it decreases to 90 percent.

➤ Determine if the patient or family members have any further questions or concerns.

➤ Evaluate test results in relation to the patient's symptoms and other tests performed. Related diagnostic tests include electrocardiogram, x-ray, computed tomography, and magnetic resonance imaging of the chest; and pulmonary function tests.

PYRUVATE KINASE

SYNONYM/ACRONYM: PK assay.

SPECIMEN: Whole blood collected in yellow-top (acid-citrate-dextrose [ACD]) tube. Specimens collected in a lavender-top (ethylenediaminetetraacetic acid [EDTA]) or green-top (heparin) tube also may be acceptable in some laboratories.

REFERENCE VALUE: (Method: Spectrophotometry) 9–22 U/g hemoglobin.

DESCRIPTION: Pyruvate kinase is an enzyme that forms pyruvate and adenosine diphosphate (ADP) during glycolysis. Deficiency of this enzyme can be acquired by ingestion of a drug or as an effect of liver disease.

There is also a hereditary form of pyruvate kinase deficiency that can be transmitted as an autosomal-recessive trait. Red blood cells lacking this enzyme have a membrane defect resulting from low levels of adenosine triphosphate (ATP) and are more susceptible to hemolysis. ■

INDICATIONS: Evaluate chronic hemolytic anemia

RESULT

Increased in:
• Carriers of Duchenne's muscular dystrophy

• Muscle disease

• Myocardial infarction

Decreased in:
• Hereditary pyruvate kinase deficiency: Congenital nonspherocytic hemolytic anemia

• Acquired pyruvate kinase deficiency: Acute leukemia
   Other anemias
   Aplasias

CRITICAL VALUES: N/A

INTERFERING FACTORS:
• Testing after blood transfusion may produce a falsely normal result.

• The enzyme is unstable. The specimen should be refrigerated immediately after collection.

Nursing Implications and Procedure • • • • • • • • •

Pretest:

➤ Obtain a history of the patient's complaints, including a list of known allergens.

➤ Obtain a history of the patient's hematopoietic system as well as results of previously performed tests and procedures. For related tests, refer to the hematopoietic system table.

➤ Obtain a list of medications the patient is taking, including herbs, nutritional supplements, and nutraceuticals. The requesting health care practitioner and laboratory should be advised if the patient is regularly using these products so that their effects can be taken into consideration when reviewing results.

➤ Note any recent procedures that can interfere with test results.

➤ There are no food, fluid, or medication restrictions unless by medical direction.

➤ Review the procedure with the patient.

➤ Inform the patient that specimen collection takes approximately 5- to 10 minutes.

Intratest:

➤ Direct the patient to breathe normally and to avoid unnecessary movement.

➤ Observe standard precautions and follow the general guidelines in Appendix A. Perform a venipuncture, and collect the specimen in a 5-mL yellow-top tube.

➤ Label the specimen, and promptly transport it to the laboratory.

Post-test:

➤ Observe venipuncture site for bleeding or hematoma formation. Apply pressure bandage.

➤ Evaluate test results in relation to the patient's symptoms and other tests performed. Related laboratory tests include complete blood count, osmotic fragility test, glucose-6-phosphate dehydrogenase, and paroxysmal nocturnal hemoglobinuria test.

RADIOACTIVE IODINE UPTAKE

SYNONYM/ACRONYM: Thyroid uptake, RAIU.

AREA OF APPLICATION: Thyroid.

CONTRAST: Oral radioactive iodine.

DESCRIPTION: Radioactive iodine uptake (RAIU) is a nuclear medicine study used for evaluating thyroid function. It directly measures the ability of the thyroid gland to concentrate and retain circulating iodide for the synthesis of thyroid hormone. RAIU assists in the diagnosis of both hyperthyroidism and hypothyroidism, but it is more useful in the diagnosis of hyperthyroidism.

A very small dose of radioactive iodine-123 (I-123) or I-131 is administered orally and at specified intervals after the initial dose is administered. The radionuclide emits gamma radiation, which allows external measurement. The uptake of radionuclide in the thyroid gland is measured as the percentage of radionuclide absorbed in a specific amount of time. The iodide not used is excreted in the urine. The thyroid gland does not distinguish between radioactive and nonradioactive iodine. Uptake values are used in conjunction with measurements of circulating thyroid hormone levels to differentiate primary and secondary thyroid disease, and serial measurements are helpful in long-term management of thyroid disease and its treatment. ■

INDICATIONS:

• Evaluate hyperthyroidism and/or hypothyroidism

• Evaluate thyroiditis, goiter, or pituitary failure

• Monitor response to therapy for thyroid disease

• Evaluate neck pain

• Evaluate the patient as part of a complete thyroid evaluation for symptomatic patients (e.g., swollen neck, neck pain, extreme sensitivity to heat or cold, jitters, sluggishness)

RESULT

Normal Findings:

• Variations in normal ranges of iodine uptake can occur with differences in dietary intake, geographic location, and protocols among laboratories:

Iodine Uptake	Percentage of Radionuclide
2-hour absorption	1–13%
6-hour absorption	2–25%
24-hour absorption	15–45%

Abnormal Findings:

• Decreased iodine intake or increased iodine excretion

• Graves' disease

- Hypoalbuminemia

- Iodine-deficient goiter

- Hashimoto's thyroiditis (early)

- Hyperthyroidism, increased uptake of:

Iodine Uptake	Percentage of Radionuclide
1-h absorption	20%
6-h absorption	25%
24-h absorption	45%

Rebound thyroid hormone withdrawal

Drugs and hormones such as barbiturates, diuretics, estrogens, lithium carbonate, phenothiazines, and thyroid-stimulating hormone

- Decreased uptake:

Hypothyroidism, with a response of decreased uptake of 0 to 10 percent over a 24-hour period

- Thyrotoxicosis as a result of ectopic thyroid metastasis

- Subacute thyroiditis

- Renal failure

- Malabsorption

INTERFERING FACTORS:

This procedure is contraindicated for:

- Patients who are pregnant or suspected of being pregnant, unless the potential benefits of the procedure far outweigh the risks to the fetus and mother

Factors that may impair clear imaging:

- Inability of the patient to cooperate or remain still during the procedure because of age, significant pain, or mental status

- Patients who are very obese, who may exceed the weight limit for the equipment

- Incorrect positioning of the patient, which may produce poor visualization of the area to be examined

- Recent use of iodinated contrast medium for radiographic studies (within the last 4 weeks) or nuclear medicine procedures done within the previous 24 to 48 hours

- Iodine deficiency (e.g., patients with inadequate dietary intake, patients on phenothiazine therapy), which can increase radionuclide uptake

- Certain drugs and other external sources of excess iodine, which can decrease radionuclide uptake, as follows:

Foods containing iodine (e.g., iodized salt)

Drugs such as aminosalicylic acid, antihistamines, antithyroid medications (e.g., propylthiouracil, iodothiouracil), corticosteroids, cough syrup, isoniazid, levothyroxine sodium/T4, Lugol's solution, nitrates, penicillins, potassium iodide, propylthiouracil, saturated solution of potassium iodide (SSKI), sulfonamides, thiocyanate, thyroid extract, L-triiodothyronine, tolbutamide, and warfarin

Multivitamins containing minerals

- Vomiting, severe diarrhea, and gastroenteritis, which can affect absorption of the oral radionuclide dose

- Metallic objects within the examination field (e.g., jewelry or body rings), which may inhibit organ visualization and can produce unclear images

Other considerations:

- Failure to follow dietary restrictions before the procedure may cause the procedure to be canceled or repeated.

- Consultation with a physician should occur before the procedure for radiation safety concerns regarding infants of patients who are lactating.

Nursing Implications and Procedure • • • • • • • • • • • •

➤ Inform the patient that the procedure assesses thyroid function.

➤ Inform the patient that the procedure is performed in a special nuclear medicine department by a technologist and usually takes approximately 30 minutes, and that delayed images are needed 24 hours later. The patient may leave the department and return later to undergo delayed imaging.

➤ Obtain a history of the patient's complaints, including a list of known allergens.

➤ Obtain a history of the patient's thyroid system and results of previously performed laboratory tests, surgical procedures, and thyroid therapy. For related tests, refer to the endocrine system table.

➤ Obtain a list of the medications the patient is taking, including herbs, nutritional supplements, and nutraceuticals.

➤ All thyroid blood tests should be taken before the procedure.

➤ Determine date of last menstrual period and possibility of pregnancy in perimenopausal women.

➤ Ensure that the patient has fasted for 8 to 12 hours before the uptake, but the patient may eat 4 hours after the test begins, unless otherwise indicated.

➤ All radiographic procedures using iodinated contrast medium should be done after this procedure is complete.

➤ Make sure jewelry and any other

metallic objects have been removed from the neck area.

➤ Administer the I-123 orally (pill form).

➤ At 2, 6, and 24 hours, place the patient in a sitting or supine position in front of a radionuclide detector that will determine the thyroid gland's ability to bind iodine.

➤ Ask the patient to hold very still during the procedure because movement will produce unclear images.

➤ Wear gloves during the radionuclide administration and while handling the patient's urine.

➤ Instruct the patient to resume normal activity, medications, and diet, unless otherwise indicated.

➤ Advise patient to drink increased amounts of fluids for 24 hours to eliminate the radionuclide from the body, unless contraindicated. Tell the patient that radionuclide is eliminated from the body within 24 to 48 hours.

➤ Instruct the patient to flush the toilet immediately after each voiding following the procedure and to wash hands meticulously with soap and water after each voiding for 24 hours after the procedure.

➤ Tell all caregivers to wear gloves when discarding urine for 24 hours after the procedure. Wash gloved hands with soap and water before removing gloves. Then wash hands after the gloves are removed.

➤ A physician specializing in this branch of medicine sends a written report to the ordering provider, who discusses the results with the patient.

➤ Evaluate test results in relation to the patient's symptoms and other tests performed. Related diagnostic tests include ultrasound of the thyroid, upper gastrointestinal series, and computed tomography of the spine.

RADIOGRAPHY, BONE

SYNONYM/ACRONYM: Bone x-rays, hand x-rays, foot x-rays, wrist x-rays, arm x-rays.

AREA OF APPLICATION: Skeleton.

CONTRAST: None.

DESCRIPTION: Skeletal x-rays are used to evaluate extremity pain or discomfort due to trauma, bone abnormalities, or fluid within a joint. Serial skeletal x-rays are used to evaluate growth pattern. Radiation emitted from the x-ray machine passes through the patient onto a photographic plate or x-ray film. X-rays pass through air freely and are mostly absorbed by the photographic media. Bones and tissues absorb the x-rays in varying degrees, thereby causing white and shades of gray on the x-ray–recording media: Bones are very dense and therefore absorb most of the x-ray and appear white; organs are denser than air but not as dense as bone, so they appear in shades of gray. All metals absorb x-rays. Because the x-ray is absorbed or blocked, metal appears totally white on the film and thus facilitates the search for foreign bodies in the patient. ■

INDICATIONS:
• Detect bone fracture, dislocation, deformity, and degeneration

• Monitor fracture-healing process

• Evaluate growth pattern

• Identify abnormalities of bones, joints, and surrounding tissues

• Evaluate for child abuse

RESULT

Normal Findings:
• *Infants and children:* Thin plate of cartilage, known as growth plate or epiphyseal plate, between the shaft and both ends

• *Adolescents and adults:* By age 17, calcification of cartilage plate; no evidence of fracture, congenital abnormalities, tumors, or infection

Abnormal Findings:

• Arthritis

• Bone degeneration

• Bone spurs

• Foreign bodies

• Fracture

• Genetic disturbance (achondroplasia, dysplasia, dyostosis)

• Hormonal disturbance

• Infection, including osteomyelitis

• Injury

• Joint dislocation or effusion

• Nutritional or metabolic disturbances

- Osteoporosis or osteopenia

- Soft tissue abnormalities

- Tumor or neoplastic disease (osteogenic sarcoma, Paget's disease, myeloma)

INTERFERING FACTORS:

This procedure is contraindicated for:

- Patients who are pregnant or suspected of being pregnant, unless the potential benefits of the procedure far outweigh the risks to the fetus and mother

Factors that may impair clear imaging:

- Inability of the patient to cooperate or remain still during the procedure because of age, significant pain, or mental status

- Improper adjustment of the radiographic equipment to accommodate obese or thin patients, which can cause overexposure or underexposure and poor-quality study

- Patients who are very obese, who may exceed the weight limit for the equipment

- Incorrect positioning of the patient, which may produce poor visualization of the area to be examined

- Prior barium studies, which can diminish the full radiographic visualization of some of the bones surrounding the abdominal cavity

- Metallic objects within the examination field (e.g., jewelry or body rings), which may inhibit organ visualization and can produce unclear images

Other considerations:

- Consultation with a physician should occur before the procedure for radiation safety concerns regarding infants of patients who are lactating.

- Risks associated with radiographic

overexposure can result from frequent x-ray procedures. Personnel in the room with the patient should stand behind a shield or leave the area while the examination is being done. Personnel working in the area where the examination is being done should wear badges that reveal their level of exposure to radiation.

Nursing Implications and Procedure • • • • • • • • • •

Pretest: ■

➤ Inform the patient that the procedure assesses bone discomfort, injury, or healing and lasts 10 to 20 minutes.

➤ Obtain a history of injury, as well as any known congenital bone, metabolic, or genetic problems that could affect the bones. For related tests, refer to the musculoskeletal system table.

➤ Obtain a list of the medications the patient is taking, including herbs, nutritional supplements, and nutraceuticals.

➤ Obtain previous x-rays of the injured site, if available.

➤ Determine date of last menstrual period and possibility of pregnancy in perimenopausal women.

➤ Inform the patient that no pain is associated with the study.

➤ There are no food or fluid restrictions.

Intratest: ■

➤ Make sure clothing, jewelry, watches, chains, belts, and any other metallic objects have been removed from the area to be examined.

➤ Have the patient put on a hospital gown, as appropriate.

➤ Place patient in a standing, sitting, or recumbent position in front of the x-ray film holder or electronic receiver.

➤ Instruct the patient to inhale deeply and hold his or her breath while the x-ray is taken and then to exhale after the film is taken. Warn the patient that the extremity's position during the procedure may be uncomfortable, but ask the patient to hold very still during the procedure because movement will produce unclear images.

➤ Numerous x-rays may be taken depending on the bones or joint affected.

Post-test:

➤ Tell the patient to contact the physician if the injured area does not improve.

➤ Determine whether the patient or family members have any further questions or concerns.

➤ A physician specializing in this branch of medicine sends a written report to the ordering provider, who discusses the results with the patient.

➤ Inform the patient that further examinations may be necessary to evaluate progression of the disease process or to determine the need for a change in therapy.

➤ Evaluate test results in relation to the patient's symptoms and other tests performed. Related diagnostic tests include bone scan, magnetic resonance imaging, and computed tomography of the suspected area.

RED BLOOD CELL CHOLINESTERASE

SYNONYMS/ACRONYMS: acetylcholinesterase (ACE), RBC.

SPECIMEN: Whole blood (1 mL) collected in a lavender-top (ethylenedi-aminetetra-acetic acid [EDTA]) tube.

REFERENCE VALUE: (Method: Spectrophotometry, kinetic)

Test	Conventional Units	SI Units (Conversion Factor ×1)
RBC cholinesterase	5–10 U/mL	5–10 kU/L

DESCRIPTION: There are two types of cholinesterase: *acetylcholinesterase*, which is found in red blood cells (RBCs), lung, and brain (nerve) tissue; and *cholinesterase*, which is mainly found in the plasma, liver, and heart. RBC cholinesterase is used to assist in the diagnosis of chronic carbamate or organophosphate insecticide (e.g., parathion, malathion) toxicity. Organophosphate pesticides bind irreversibly with cholinesterase, inhibiting normal enzyme activity. Carbamate insecticides bind reversibly. Serum or plasma pseudocholinesterase is used more frequently to measure acute pesticide toxicity.

Patients with inherited cholinesterase deficiency are at risk during anesthesia if succinylcholine is administered as an anesthetic. Succinyl-choline, a short-acting muscle relaxant, is a reversible inhibitor of acetyl-cholinesterase and is hydrolyzed by cholinesterase. Succinylcholine-sensitive patients may be unable to metabolize the anesthetic quickly, resulting in prolonged or unrecoverable apnea. This test, along with the pseudocholinesterase test, is also used to identify individuals with atypical forms of the enzyme cholinesterase (see monograph titled "Pseudo-cholinesterase"). The prevalence of succinylcholate sensitivity is 1 in 1500 patients. Widespread preoperative screening is not routinely performed. ■

INDICATIONS:
• Verify suspected exposure to organic phosphate insecticides

• Monitor cumulative exposure to organic phosphate insecticides

RESULT

Increased in:
• Sickle cell anemia

Decreased in:
• Insecticide exposure (organic phosphate)

• Late pregnancy

• Paroxysmal nocturnal hemoglobinuria

• Relapse of megaloblastic anemia

CRITICAL VALUES: N/A

INTERFERING FACTORS:
• Drugs and substances that may increase RBC cholinesterase levels include echothiophate, parathion, and antiepileptic drugs such as carbamazepine, phenobarbital, phenytoin, and valproic acid.

• Improper anticoagulant; fluoride interferes with the measurement and causes a falsely decreased value.

Nursing Implications and Procedure • • • • • • • • • • •

Pretest: ■

➤ Obtain a history of the patient's complaints, including a list of known allergens. Particularly important to report is exposure to pesticides causing symptoms including blurred vision, muscle weakness, nausea, vomiting, headaches, pulmonary edema, salivation, sweating, or convulsions.

➤ Obtain a history of exposure to occupational hazards and medication regimen.

➤ Obtain a history of the patient's hematopoietic system and results of previously performed tests and procedures. For related tests refer to the hematopoietic system table.

➤ Obtain a list of the medications the patient is taking, including herbs, nutritional supplements, and nutraceuticals. The requesting health care practitioner and laboratory should be advised if the patient regularly uses these products so that their effects can be taken into consideration when reviewing results.

➤ There are no food, fluid, or medication restrictions unless by medical direction.

➤ Review the procedure with the patient.

➤ Inform the patient that specimen collection takes approximately 5 to 10 minutes.

Intratest: ■

➤ Direct the patient to breathe normally and to avoid unnecessary movement.

➤ Observe standard precautions and follow the general guidelines in Appendix A. Perform a venipuncture, and collect the specimen in a 5-mL lavender-top tube.

➤ Label the specimen, and promptly transport it to the laboratory.

Post-test: ■

▷ Observe venipuncture site for bleed-

ing or hematoma formation. Apply pressure bandage.

➤ Evaluate test results in relation to the patient's symptoms and other tests. Related laboratory tests include complete blood count and pseudocholinesterase.

RED BLOOD CELL COUNT

· ·

SYNONYM/ACRONYM: RBC.

SPECIMEN: Whole blood (1 mL) collected in a lavender-top (ethylenedi-aminetetra-acetic acid [EDTA]) tube.

REFERENCE VALUE: (Method: Automated, computerized, multichannel analyzers that sort and size cells on the basis of changes in either electrical impedance or light pulses as the cells pass in front of a laser)

Age	Conventional Units	SI Units (Conversion Factor ×1)
Cord Blood	$4.14–4.69 \times 10^6$ cells/mm^3	$4.14–4.69 \times 10^{12}$ cells/L
1 d	$5.33–5.47 \times 10^6$ cells/mm^3	$5.33–5.47 \times 10^{12}$ cells/L
2 wk	$4.32–4.98 \times 10^6$ cells/mm^3	$4.32–4.98 \times 10^{12}$ cells/L
1 mo	$3.75–4.95 \times 10^6$ cells/mm^3	$3.75–4.95 \times 10^{12}$ cells/L
6 mo	$3.71–4.25 \times 10^6$ cells/mm^3	$3.71–4.25 \times 10^{12}$ cells/L
1 y	$4.40–4.48 \times 10^6$ cells/mm^3	$4.40–4.48 \times 10^{12}$ cells/L
10 y	$4.75–4.85 \times 10^6$ cells/mm^3	$4.75–4.85 \times 10^{12}$ cells/L
Adult male	$4.71–5.14 \times 10^6$ cells/mm^3	$4.71–5.14 \times 10^{12}$ cells/L
Adult female	$4.20–4.87 \times 10^6$ cells/mm^3	$4.20–4.87 \times 10^{12}$ cells/L

DESCRIPTION: A component of the complete blood count (CBC), the red blood cell (RBC) count determines the number of RBCs per cubic millimeters (expressed as the number of RBCs per liter of blood according to the international system of units [SI]). Because RBCs contain hemoglobin (Hgb), which is responsible for the transport and exchange of oxygen, the number of circulating RBCs is important. Although the life span of the normal RBC is 120 days, other factors besides cell age and decreased production can cause decreased values; examples are abnormal destruction due to intravascular trauma caused by atherosclerosis or to an enlarged spleen caused by leukemia. The main sites of RBC production in healthy adults include the bone marrow of the vertebrae, pelvis, ribs, sternum, skull, and proximal ends of the femur and humerus. The main sites of RBC destruction are the spleen and liver. Erythropoietin, a hormone produced by the kidneys, regulates RBC production. Normal RBC development and function are also dependent on adequate levels of vitamin B_{12}, folic acid, and iron. A deficiency in vitamin E (α-tocopherol), which is needed to protect the RBC membrane from oxidizers, can result in increased cellular destruction.

Polycythemia is a term used in conjunction with conditions resulting from an abnormal increase in Hgb, hematocrit (Hct), and RBC count. *Anemia* is a term associated with conditions resulting from an abnormal decrease in Hgb, Hct, and RBC count. Results of the Hgb, Hct, and RBC count should be evaluated simultaneously because the same underlying conditions affect this triad of tests similarly. The RBC count multiplied by three should approximate the Hgb concentration. The Hct should be within three times the Hgb if the RBC population is normal in size and shape. The Hct plus six should approximate the first two figures of the RBC count within three (e.g., Hct is 40 percent; therefore 40 + 6 = 46, and the RBC count should be 4.3–4.9). (See monographs titled "Hematocrit," "Hemoglobin," and "Red Blood Cell Indices.") ∎

INDICATIONS:

- Detect a hematologic disorder involving RBC destruction (e.g., hemolytic anemia)

- Determine the presence of hereditary hematologic abnormality

- Monitor the effects of acute or chronic blood loss

- Monitor patients with disorders associated with elevated erythrocyte counts (e.g., polycythemia vera, chronic obstructive pulmonary disease [COPD])

- Monitor the effects of physical or emotional stress

- Monitor the progression of nonhematologic disorders associated with elevated erythrocyte counts, such as COPD, liver disease, hypothyroidism, adrenal dysfunction, bone marrow failure, malabsorption syndromes, cancer, and renal disease

- Monitor the response to drugs or chemotherapy and evaluate undesired reactions to drugs that may cause blood dyscrasias

- Provide screening as part of a CBC in a general physical examination, especially upon admission to a health care facility or before surgery

RESULT

Increased in:
- Bone marrow failure
- Anxiety or stress
- Dehydration with hemoconcentration
- High altitude
- Erythremic erythrocytosis
- Polycythemia vera
- COPD with hypoxia and secondary polycythemia

Decreased in:
- Chemotherapy
- Dietary deficiencies
- Hemoglobinopathy
- Hemolytic anemia

- Hemorrhage

- Hodgkin's disease

- Chronic inflammatory diseases

- Leukemia

- Multiple myeloma

- Organ failure

- Overhydration

- Pregnancy (normal dilutional effect)

- Subacute endocarditis

CRITICAL VALUES: ⚠ The presence of abnormal cells, other morphologic characteristics, or cellular inclusions may signify a potentially life-threatening or serious health condition and should be investigated. Examples are the presence of sickle cells, moderate numbers of spherocytes, marked schistocytosis, oval macrocytes, basophilic stippling, nucleated RBCs (if the patient is not an infant), or malarial organisms.

INTERFERING FACTORS:

- Drugs and substances that may decrease RBC count include those causing hemolysis resulting from drug sensitivity or enzyme deficiency, such as acetaminophen, aminopyrine, aminosalicylic acid, amphetamine, antipyrine, arsenicals, benzene, busulfan, anticonvulsants, carbenicillin, cephalothin, chemotherapy, chlorate, chloroquine, chlorothiazide, chlorpromazine, colchicine, diphenhydramine, dipyrone, glucosulfone, gold, hydroflumethiazide, indomethacin, mephenytoin, nalidixic acid, neomycin, nitrofurantoin, penicillin, phenacemide, phenazopyridine, and phenothiazine.

- Drugs that may decrease RBC count include those that result in anemia, such as miconazole, penicillamine, phenylhydrazine, primaquine, probenecid, pyrazolones, pyrimethamine, quinines, streptomycin, sulfamethi-

zole, sulfamethoxypyridine, sulfisoxazole, suramin, thioridazine, tolbutamide trimethadione, and tripelennamine.

- Drugs that may decrease RBC count include those causing bone marrow suppression such as amphotericin B, floxuridine, and phenylbutazone.

- Drugs and vitamins that may increase the RBC count include glucocorticosteroids, pilocarpine, and vitamin B_{12}.

- Use of the neutraceutical liver extract is strongly contraindicated in patients with iron-storage disorders such as hemochromatosis because it is rich in heme (the iron-containing pigment in Hgb).

- Hemodilution (e.g., excessive administration of intravenous fluids, normal pregnancy) in the presence of a normal number of RBCs may lead to false decreases in RBC count.

- Cold agglutinins may falsely increase the mean corpuscular volume (MCV) and decrease the RBC count. This can be corrected by warming the blood or diluting the sample with warmed saline and repeating the analysis.

- Excessive exercise, anxiety, pain, and dehydration may cause false elevations in RBC count.

- A grossly elevated white blood cell count (greater than 500,000 × $10^3/mm^3$) will cause a falsely elevated RBC count. This can be corrected by diluting the sample with saline to obtain an accurate white blood cell count and then correcting the RBC mathematically.

- Care in evaluating the CBC after transfusion should be taken into consideration.

- RBC counts can vary depending on the patient's position, decreasing when the patient is recumbent as a result of hemodilution and increasing when the patient rises as a result of hemoconcentration.

• Venous stasis can falsely elevate RBC counts; therefore the tourniquet should not be left on the arm for longer than 60 seconds.

• Failure to fill the tube sufficiently (i.e., tube less than three-quarters full) may yield inadequate sample volume for automated analyzers and may be reason for specimen rejection.

• Hemolyzed or clotted specimens should be rejected for analysis.

Nursing Implications and Procedure

Pretest:

➤ Obtain a history of the patient's complaints, including a list of known allergens.

➤ Obtain a history of the patient's gastrointestinal, hematopoietic, hepatobiliary, immune, and respiratory systems, as well as results of previously performed tests and procedures. For related tests refer to the gastrointestinal, hematopoietic, hepatobiliary, immune, and respiratory system tables.

➤ Obtain a list of the medications the patient is taking, including herbs, nutritional supplements, and nutraceuticals. The requesting health care practitioner and laboratory should be advised if the patient regularly uses these products so that their effects can be taken into consideration when reviewing results.

➤ Note any recent procedures that can interfere with test results.

➤ There are no food, fluid, or medication restrictions unless by medical direction.

➤ Review the procedure with the patient.

➤ Inform the patient that specimen collection takes approximately 5 to 10 minutes.

Intratest:

➤ Direct the patient to breathe normally and to avoid unnecessary movement.

➤ Perform a venipuncture, and collect the specimen in a 5-mL lavender-top (EDTA) tube. Observe standard precautions and follow the general guidelines in Appendix A. Handle the specimen gently to avoid hemolysis. The specimen should be mixed gently by inverting the tube 10 times. It is stable when stored for up to 6 hours at room temperature or 24 hours if stored refrigerated. In addition, if it is anticipated that the specimen will not be analyzed within 4 to 6 hours, two blood smears should be made immediately after the venipuncture and submitted with the blood sample.

➤ Label the specimen, and promptly transport it to the laboratory.

Post-test:

➤ Observe venipuncture site for bleeding or hematoma formation. Apply pressure bandage. Iron deficiency is the most common nutrient deficiency in the United States. Patients at risk (e.g., children, pregnant women and women of childbearing age, low-income populations) should be instructed to include foods that are high in iron in their diet, such as meats (especially liver), eggs, grains, vegetables, and multivitamins with iron. Iron absorption is affected by numerous factors (see monograph titled "Iron").

➤ Patients at risk for vitamin B_{12} or folate deficiency include those with the following conditions: malnourishment (inadequate intake), pregnancy (increased need), infancy, malabsorption syndromes (inadequate absorption/increased metabolic rate), infections, cancer, hyperthyroidism, serious burns, excessive blood loss, and gastrointestinal damage. These patients should be instructed, as appropriate, to ingest food sources rich in vitamin B_{12} such as meats, milk, cheese, eggs, and fortified soy milk products. Sources of folate are meats (especially liver), kidney beans, beets, vegetables in the cabbage family, oranges, cantaloupe, and green leafy vegetables such as spinach, asparagus, and broccoli.

➤ A diet deficient in vitamin E puts the patient at risk for increased RBC destruction, which could lead to anemia. Nutritional therapy may be indicated for these patients. Vitamin E is found in many of the previously mentioned foods, as well as in vegetable oils and wheat germ. Supplemental vitamin E may also be

taken, but the danger of toxicity should be explained to the patient. Very large supplemental doses, in excess of 600 mg of vitamin E over a period of 1 year, may result in excess bleeding. Vitamin E is heat stable but is very negatively affected by light.

➤ Evaluate test results in relation to the patient's symptoms and other tests performed. Related laboratory tests include the other tests included in a CBC, erythropoietin, ferritin, folate, iron/total iron-binding capacity, RBC morphology and inclusions, reticulocyte count, and vitamin B_{12}.

RED BLOOD CELL INDICES

SYNONYMS/ACRONYMS: mean corpuscular hemoglobin (MCH), mean corpuscular volume (MCV), mean corpuscular hemoglobin concentration (MCHC), red blood cell distribution width (RDW).

SPECIMEN: Whole blood (1 mL) collected in a lavender-top (ethylenedi-aminetetra-acetic acid [EDTA]) tube.

REFERENCE VALUE: (Method: Automated, computerized, multichannel analyzers that sort and size cells on the basis of changes in either electrical impedance or light pulses as the cells pass in front of a laser)

Age	MCV (fl)	MCH (pg/cell)	MCHC (g/dL)	RDW
Cord blood	107–119	35–39	32–34	14.9–18.7
1 d	104–116	35–39	32–34	14.9–18.7
2 wk	95–117	29–35	28–32	14.9–18.7
1 mo	93–115	29–35	28–34	14.9–18.7
6 mo	82–100	24–30	28–32	14.9–18.7
1 y	81–95	25–29	29–31	11.6–14.8
10 y	75–87	25–31	33–35	11.6–14.8
Adult male	85–95	28–32	33–35	11.6–14.8
Adult female	85–95	28–32	33–35	11.6–14.8

MCV = mean corpuscular volume; MCH = mean corpuscular hemoglobin; MCHC = mean corpuscular hemoglobin concentration; RDW = red blood cell distribution width.

DESCRIPTION: Red blood cell (RBC) indices provide information about the mean corpuscular volume (MCV), mean corpuscular hemoglobin (MCH), mean corpuscular hemoglobin concentration (MCHC), and RBC distribution width (RDW). The hematocrit, RBC count, and total hemoglobin tests are used to determine the RBC indices. MCV is determined by dividing the hematocrit by the total RBC count and is helpful in classifying anemias. MCH is determined by dividing the total hemoglobin concentration by the RBC count. MCHC is determined by dividing total hemoglobin by hematocrit. Hemoglobin content is indicated as normochromic, hypochromic, and hyperchromic. The RDW is a measurement of cell size distribution over the entire RBC population measured. It is an indication of anisocytosis or excessive variations in cell size. Cell size is indicated as normocytic, microcytic, and macrocytic. (See monographs titled "Hemoglobin," "Hematocrit," "Red Blood Cell Count," and "Red Blood Cell Morphology and Inclusions.") ■

INDICATIONS:

• Assist in the diagnosis of anemia

• Detect a hematologic disorder, neoplasm or immunologic abnormality

• Determine the presence of a hereditary hematologic abnormality

• Monitor the effects of physical or emotional stress

• Monitor the progression of nonhematologic disorders such as chronic obstructive pulmonary disease (COPD), malabsorption syndromes, cancer, and renal disease

• Monitor the response to drugs or chemotherapy, and evaluate undesired reactions to drugs that may cause blood dyscrasias

• Provide screening as part of a complete blood count (CBC) in a general physical examination, especially upon admission to a health care facility or before surgery

RESULT

MCV increased in:

• Alcoholism

• Antimetabolite therapy

• Liver disease

• Pernicious anemia

• Vitamin B_{12}/folate anemia

MCV decreased in:

• Iron-deficiency anemia

• Thalassemias

MCH increased in:

• Macrocytic anemias

MCH decreased in:

• Hypochromic anemias

• Microcytic anemias

MCHC increased in:

• Thalassemia

• Spherocytosis

MCHC decreased in:

• Iron-deficiency anemia

RDW increased in:

• Anemias with heterogeneous cell size

RDW decreased in:

• N/A

CRITICAL VALUES: N/A

INTERFERING FACTORS:

- Drugs and substances that may decrease MCHC include styrene (occupational exposure).

- Drugs that may decrease MCV include nitrofurantoin.

- Drugs that may increase MCV include colchicine, pentamidine, pyrimethamine, and triamterene.

- Drugs that may increase the MCH and MCHC include oral contraceptives (long-term use).

- Diseases that cause agglutination of RBCs will alter test results.

- Cold agglutinins may falsely increase the MCV and decrease the RBC count. This can be corrected by warming the blood or diluting the sample with warmed saline and then correcting the RBC count mathematically.

- RBC counts can vary depending on the patient's position, decreasing when the patient is recumbent as a result of hemodilution and increasing when the patient rises as a result of hemoconcentration.

- Care in evaluating the CBC after transfusion should be taken into consideration.

- Venous stasis can falsely elevate RBC counts; therefore the tourniquet should not be left on the arm for longer than 60 seconds.

- Failure to fill the tube sufficiently (i.e., tube less than three-quarters full) may yield inadequate sample volume for automated analyzers and may be reason for specimen rejection.

- Hemolyzed or clotted specimens should be rejected.

- Lipemia and elevated white blood cell count (greater than 50,000/mm^3) will falsely increase the hemoglobin measurement, also affecting the MCV and MCH.

Nursing Implications and Procedure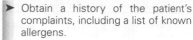

Pretest: ■

➤ Obtain a history of the patient's complaints, including a list of known allergens.

➤ Obtain a history of the patient's gastrointestinal, hematopoietic, immune, and respiratory systems, as well as results of previously performed tests and procedures. For related tests, refer to the gastrointestinal, hematopoietic, immune, and respiratory system tables.

➤ Obtain a list of the medications the patient is taking, including herbs, nutritional supplements, and nutraceuticals. The requesting health care practitioner and laboratory should be advised if the patient regularly uses these products so that their effects can be taken into consideration when reviewing results.

➤ Note any recent procedures that can interfere with test results.

➤ There are no food, fluid, or medication restrictions unless by medical direction.

➤ Review the procedure with the patient.

➤ Inform the patient that specimen collection takes approximately 5 to 10 minutes.

Intratest: ■

➤ Direct the patient to breathe normally and to avoid unnecessary movement.

➤ Observe standard precautions and follow the general guidelines in Appendix A. Perform a venipuncture, and collect the specimen in a 5-mL lavender-top (EDTA) tube. The specimen should be mixed gently by inverting the tube 10 times. It is stable when stored for up to 6 hours at room temperature or 24 hours if stored refrigerated. In addition, if it is anticipated that the specimen will not be analyzed within 4 to 6 hours, two blood smears should be made immediately after the venipuncture and submitted with the blood sample.

➤ Label the specimen, and promptly transport it to the laboratory.

Post-test:

➤ Observe venipuncture site for bleed-

ing or hematoma formation. Apply pressure bandage.

➤ Evaluate test results in relation to the patient's symptoms and other tests performed. Related laboratory tests include the other tests included in a CBC, erythropoietin, ferritin, iron/total iron-binding capacity, RBC morphology and inclusions, and reticulocyte count.

RED BLOOD CELL MORPHOLOGY AND INCLUSIONS

SYNONYM/ACRONYM: N/A.

SPECIMEN: Whole blood from one full lavender-top (ethylenediaminetetraacetic acid [EDTA]) tube or Wright's-stained, thin-film peripheral blood smear. The laboratory should be consulted as to the necessity of thick-film smears for the evaluation of malarial inclusions.

REFERENCE VALUE: (Method: Microscopic, manual review of stained blood smear)

Red Blood Cell Morphology	Within Normal Limits	1+	2+	3+	4+
Size					
Anisocytosis	0–5+	5–10	10–20	20–50	Greater than 50
Macrocytes	0–5+	5–10	10–20	20–50	Greater than 50
Microcytes	0–5+	5–10	10–20	20–50	Greater than 50
Shape					
Poikilocytes	0–2+	3–10	10–20	20–50	Greater than 50
Burr cells	0–2+	3–10	10–20	20–50	Greater than 50
Acanthocytes	Less than 1+	2–5	5–10	10–20	Greater than 20
Schistocytes	Less than 1+	2–5	5–10	10–20	Greater than 20
Dacryocytes (teardrop cells)	0–2+	2–5	5–10	10–20	Greater than 20
Codocytes (target cells)	0–2+	2–10	10–20	20–50	Greater than 50
Spherocytes	0–2+	2–10	10–20	20–50	Greater than 50
Ovalocytes	0–2+	2–10	10–20	20–50	Greater than 50
Stomatocytes	0–2+	2–10	10–20	20–50	Greater than 50

(Continued on the following page)

Red Blood Cell Morphology	Within Normal Limits	1+	2+	3+	4+
Drepanocytes (sickle cells)	Absent	Reported as present or absent			
Helmet cells	Absent	Reported as present or absent			
Agglutination	Absent	Reported as present or absent			
Rouleaux	Absent	Reported as present or absent			
Hemoglobin (Hgb) content					
Hypochromia	0–2+	3–10	10–50	50–75	Greater than 75
Polychromasia					
Adult	Less than 1+	2–5	5–10	10–20	Greater than 20
Newborn	1–6+	7–15	15–20	20–50	Greater than 50
Inclusions					
Cabot rings	Absent	Reported as present or absent			
Basophilic stippling	0–1+	1–5	5–10	10–20	Greater than 20
Howell-Jolly bodies	Absent	1–2	3–5	5–10	Greater than 10
Heinz bodies	Absent	Reported as present or absent			
Hgb C crystals	Absent	Reported as present or absent			
Pappenheimer bodies	Absent	Reported as present or absent			
Intracellular parasites (e.g., Plasmodium, Babesia, Trypanosoma)	Absent	Reported as present or absent			

DESCRIPTION: The decision to manually review a peripheral blood smear for abnormalities in red blood cell (RBC) shape or size is made based on criteria established by the reporting laboratory. Cues in the results of the complete blood count (CBC) will point to specific abnormalities that can be confirmed visually, by microscopic review of the sample on a stained blood smear. ▪

INDICATIONS:

- Assist in the diagnosis of anemia

- Detect a hematologic disorder, neoplasm, or immunologic abnormality

- Determine the presence of a hereditary hematologic abnormality

- Monitor the effects of physical or emotional stress

- Monitor the progression of nonhematologic disorders, such as chronic obstructive pulmonary disease (COPD), malabsorption syndromes, cancer, and renal disease

- Monitor the response to drugs or chemotherapy, and evaluate undesired reactions to drugs that may cause blood dyscrasias

- Provide screening as part of a CBC in a general physical examination, especially upon admission to a health care facility or before surgery

RESULT

Red Blood Cell Size

Cell size increased in:
- Alcoholism

- Aplastic anemia

- Chemotherapy

- Chronic hemolytic anemia

- Grossly elevated glucose (hyperosmotic)

- Hemolytic disease of the newborn

- Hypothyroidism

- Leukemia

- Lymphoma

- Metastatic carcinoma

- Myelofibrosis

- Myeloma

- Refractory anemia

- Sideroblastic anemia

- Vitamin B_{12}/folate deficiency

Cell size decreased in:
- Hemoglobin C disease

- Hemolytic anemias

- Hereditary spherocytosis

- Inflammation

- Iron-deficiency anemia

- Thalassemias

Red Blood Cell Shape

Variations in cell shape are the result of hereditary conditions such as elliptocytosis, sickle cell anemia, spherocytosis, thalassemias, or hemoglobinopathies (e.g., hemoglobin C disease). Irregularities in cell shape can also result from acquired conditions, such as physical/mechanical cellular trauma, exposure to chemicals, or reactions to medications.

- Acquired spherocytosis can result from Heinz body hemolytic anemia, microangiopathic hemolytic anemia, secondary isoimmunohemolytic anemia, and transfusion of old banked blood.

- Acanthocytes are associated with acquired conditions such as alcoholic cirrhosis with hemolytic anemia, disorders of lipid metabolism, hepatitis of newborns, malabsorptive diseases, metastatic liver disease, postsplenectomy, and pyruvate kinase deficiency.

• Burr cells are commonly seen in acquired renal insufficiency, burns, cardiac valve disease, disseminated intravascular coagulation (DIC), intravenous fibrin deposition, hypertension, metastatic malignancy, normal neonatal period, and uremia.

• Codocytes are seen in hemoglobinopathies, iron-deficiency anemia, obstructive liver disease, and postsplenectomy.

• Dacryocytes are most commonly associated with metastases to the bone marrow, myelofibrosis, myeloid metaplasia, pernicious anemia, and tuberculosis.

• Schistocytes are seen in burns, cardiac valve disease, DIC, glomerulonephritis, hemolytic anemia, microangiopathic hemolytic anemia, renal graft rejection, thrombotic thrombocytopenic purpura, uremia, and vasculitis.

Red Blood Cell Hemoglobin Content

RBCs with a normal hemoglobin (Hgb) level have a clear central pallor and are referred to as *normochromic.*

• Cells with low Hgb and lacking in central pallor are referred to as *hypochromic.* Hypochromia is associated with iron-deficiency anemia, thalassemias, and sideroblastic anemia.

• Cells with excessive Hgb levels are referred to as *hyperchromic,* even though they technically lack a central pallor. Hyperchromia is usually associated with an elevated mean corpuscular Hgb concentration as well as hemolytic anemias.

• Cells referred to as *polychromic* are young erythrocytes that still contain ribonucleic acid (RNA). The RNA is picked up by the Wright's stain.

Polychromasia is indicative of premature release of RBCs from bone marrow secondary to increased erythropoietin stimulation.

Red Blood Cell Inclusions

RBC inclusions can result from certain types of anemia, abnormal Hgb precipitation, or parasitic infection.

• Cabot rings may be seen in megaloblastic and other anemias, lead poisoning, and conditions in which RBCs are destroyed before they are released from bone marrow.

• Basophilic stippling is seen whenever there is altered Hgb synthesis, as in thalassemias, megaloblastic anemias, alcoholism, and lead or arsenic intoxication.

• Howell-Jolly bodies are seen in sickle cell anemia, other hemolytic anemias, megaloblastic anemia, congenital absence of the spleen, and the postsplenectomy period.

• Pappenheimer bodies may be seen in cases of sideroblastic anemia, thalassemias, refractory anemia, dyserythropoietic anemias, hemosiderosis, and hemochromatosis.

• Heinz bodies are most often seen in the blood of patients who have ingested drugs known to induce the formation of these inclusion bodies. They are also seen in patients with hereditary glucose-6-phosphate dehydrogenase (G-6-PD) deficiency.

• Hgb C crystals can often be identified in stained peripheral smears of patients with hereditary hemoglobin C disease.

• Parasites such as *Plasmodium* (transmitted by mosquitoes and causing malaria) and *Babesia* (transmitted by ticks), known to invade human RBCs, can be visualized with Wright's stain and other special stains of the peripheral blood.

CRITICAL VALUES: ⚠ The presence of sickle cells or parasitic inclusions should be brought to the immediate attention of the requesting health care practitioner.

INTERFERING FACTORS:

• Drugs and substances that may increase Heinz body formation as an initial precursor to significant hemolysis include acetanilid, acetylsalicylic acid, aminopyrine, antimalarials, antipyretics, furadaltone, furazolidone, methylene blue, naphthalene, and nitrofurans.

• Care in evaluating the CBC after transfusion should be taken into consideration.

• Leaving the tourniquet in place for longer than 60 seconds can affect the results.

• Morphology can be evaluated to some extent via indices; therefore failure to fill the tube sufficiently (i.e., tube less than three-quarters full) may yield inadequate sample volume for automated analyzers and may be reason for specimen rejection.

• Hemolyzed or clotted specimens should be rejected.

Nursing Implications and Procedure • • • • • • • • • • •

Pretest: ■

➤ Obtain a history of the patient's complaints, including a list of known allergens.

➤ Obtain a history of the patient's hematopoietic, hepatobiliary, and immune systems, as well as results of previously performed tests and procedures. For related tests, refer to the hematopoietic, hepatobiliary, and immune system tables.

➤ Obtain a list of the medications the patient is taking, including herbs, nutritional supplements, and nutraceuticals. The requesting health care

practitioner and laboratory should be advised if the patient regularly uses these products so that their effects can be taken into consideration when reviewing results.

➤ Note any recent procedures that can interfere with test results.

➤ There are no food, fluid, or medication restrictions unless by medical direction.

➤ Review the procedure with the patient.

➤ Inform the patient that specimen collection takes approximately 5 to 10 minutes.

Intratest: ■

➤ Direct the patient to breathe normally and to avoid unnecessary movement.

➤ Observe standard precautions and follow the general guidelines in Appendix A. Perform a venipuncture, and collect the specimen in a 5-mL lavender-top (EDTA) tube. The specimen should be mixed gently by inverting the tube 10 times. It is stable when stored for up to 6 hours at room temperature or 24 hours if stored refrigerated. In addition, if it is anticipated that the specimen will not be analyzed within 4 to 6 hours, two blood smears should be made immediately after the venipuncture and submitted with the blood sample.

➤ Label the specimen, and promptly transport it to the laboratory.

Post-test: ■

➤ Observe venipuncture site for bleeding or hematoma formation. Apply pressure bandage.

➤ Evaluate test results in relation to the patient's symptoms and other tests performed. Related laboratory tests include the other tests included in a CBC, δ-aminolevulinic acid, erythropoietin, ferritin, G-6-PD, Hgb electrophoresis, iron/total iron-binding capacity, lead, reticulocyte count, and white blood cell count and differential.

RENIN

· ·

SYNONYM/ACRONYM: Plasma renin activity (PRA).

SPECIMEN: Plasma (3 mL) collected in a lavender-top (ethylenediaminete-tra-acetic acid [EDTA]) tube.

REFERENCE VALUE: (Method: Radioimmunoassay)

Age and Position	Conventional Units	SI Units (Conversion Factor ×1)
Newborn	2.0–35.0 ng/mL per hour	2.0–35.0 µg/L per hour
Supine, normal sodium diet		
1–12 mo	2.4–37.0 ng/mL per hour	2.4–37.0 µg/L per hour
1–3 y	1.7–112 ng/mL per hour	1.7–112 µg/L per hour
3–5 y	1.0–6.5 ng/mL per hour	1.0–6.5 µg/L per hour
5–10 y	0.5–5.9 ng/mL per hour	0.5–5.9 µg/L per hour
10–15 y	0.5–3.3 ng/mL per hour	0.5–3.3 µg/L per hour
Adult	0.2–1.6 ng/mL per hour	0.2–1.6 µg/L per hour
Upright, normal sodium diet		
Adult	0.7–3.3 ng/mL per hour	0.7–3.3 µg/L per hour

Values vary according to the laboratory performing the test, as well as the patient's age, gender, dietary pattern, state of hydration, posture, and physical activity.

DESCRIPTION: Renin is an enzyme that activates the renin-angiotensin system. It is released into the renal veins by the juxtaglomerular apparatus in response to sodium depletion and hypovolemia. Renin converts angiotensinogen to angiotensin I. Angiotensin I is converted to angiotensin II, the biologically active form. Angiotensin II is a powerful vasoconstrictor that stimulates aldosterone production in the adrenal cortex. Angiotensin II and aldosterone increase blood pressure. Excessive amounts of angiotensin II cause renal hypertension. The renin assay screens for essential, renal, or renovascular hypertension. Plasma renin is expressed as the rate of angiotensin I formation per unit of time. The random collection of specimens without prior dietary preparations does not provide clinically significant information. Values should also be evaluated along with simultaneously collected aldosterone levels. (See monographs titled "Aldosterone" and "Angiotensin-Converting Enzyme.") ∎

INDICATIONS:

* Assist in the identification of primary hyperaldosteronism resulting from aldosterone-secreting adrenal adenoma

* Assist in monitoring patients on mineralocorticoid therapy

* Assist in the screening of the origin of essential, renal, or renovascular hypertension

RESULT

Increased in:

* Addison's disease

* Bartter's syndrome

* Cirrhosis

* Congestive heart failure

* Gastrointestinal disorders with electrolyte loss

* Hepatitis

* Hypokalemia

* Malignant hypertension

* Nephritis

* Nephropathies with sodium or potassium wasting

* Pheochromocytoma

* Pregnancy

* Renin-producing renal tumors

* Renovascular hypertension

Decreased in:

* Cushing's syndrome

* Essential hypertension

* Primary hyperaldosteronism

CRITICAL VALUES: N/A

INTERFERING FACTORS:

* Drugs that may increase renin levels include albuterol, amiloride, azosemide, benazepril, bendroflumethiazide, captopril, chlorthalidone, cilazapril, cromakalim, desmopressin, diazoxide, dihydralazine, doxazosin, enalapril, endralazine, felodipine, fenoldopam, fosinopril, furosemide, hydralazine, hydrochlorothiazide, laxatives, lisinopril, lithium, methyclothiazide, metolazone, muzolimine, nicardipine, nifedipine, opiates, oral contraceptives, perindopril, ramipril, spironolactone, triamterene, and xipamide.

* Drugs and substances that may decrease renin levels include angiotensin, angiotensin II, acetylsalicylic acid, atenolol, bopindolol, bucindolol, carbenoxolone, carvedilol, clonidine, cyclosporine A, dexfenfluramine, glycyrrhiza, ibuprofen, indomethacin, levodopa, metoprolol, naproxen, nicardipine, nonsteroidal antiinflammatory drugs (NSAIDs), oral contraceptives, oxprenolol, propranolol, sulindac, and vasopressin.

* Upright body posture, stress, and strenuous exercise can increase renin levels.

* Recent radioactive scans or radiation can interfere with test results when radioimmunoassay is the test method.

* Diet can significantly affect results (e.g., low-sodium diets stimulate the release of renin).

* Hyperkalemia, acute increase in blood pressure, and increased blood volume may suppress renin secretion.

Nursing Implications and Procedure · · · · · · · · · · ·

Pretest:

➤ Obtain a history of the patient's complaints, including a list of known allergens.

➤ Obtain a history of the patient's endocrine and genitourinary systems, as well as results of previously performed tests and procedures. For related tests, refer to the endocrine and genitourinary system tables.

➤ Obtain a list of the medications the patient is taking, including herbs, nutritional supplements, and nutraceuticals. The requesting health care practitioner and laboratory should be advised if the patient regularly uses these products so that their effects can be taken into consideration when reviewing results.

➤ Note any recent procedures that can interfere with test results.

➤ The patient should be on a normal sodium diet (1 to 2 g sodium per day) for 2 to 4 weeks before the test.

➤ By medical direction, the patient should avoid diuretics, antihypertensive drugs, herbals, cyclic progestogens, and estrogens for 2 to 4 weeks before the test.

➤ Review the procedure with the patient. Inform the patient that multiple specimens may be required.

➤ Inform the patient or family member that the position required (supine or upright) must be maintained for 2 hours before specimen collection.

➤ Inform the patient that each specimen collection takes approximately 5 to 10 minutes.

Intratest:

➤ Ensure that the patient has complied with dietary preparations and other pretesting restrictions.

➤ Direct the patient to breathe normally and to avoid unnecessary movement.

➤ Observe standard precautions and follow the general guidelines in Appendix A. Perform a venipuncture after the patient has been in the upright (sitting or standing) position for 2 hours. If a supine specimen is requested on an inpatient, the specimen should be collected early in the morning before the patient rises. Collect the specimen in a 5-mL lavender-top (EDTA) tube.

➤ Label the specimen, and promptly transport it to the laboratory on ice. Specify patient position (upright or supine) and exact source of specimen (peripheral vs. arterial).

Post-test:

➤ Observe venipuncture site for bleeding or hematoma formation. Apply pressure bandage.

➤ Instruct the patient to resume usual medication, if withheld and as directed by the requesting health care practitioner.

➤ Instruct the patient to notify the requesting health care practitioner of any signs and symptoms of dehydration or fluid overload related to abnormal renin levels or compromised sodium regulatory mechanisms. Fluid loss or dehydration is signaled by the thirst response. Decreased skin turgor, dry mouth and multiple longitudinal furrows in the tongue are symptoms of dehydration. Fluid overload may be signaled by a loss of appetite and nausea. Excessive fluid also causes pitting edema: When firm pressure is placed on the skin over a bone (e.g., the ankle) the indentation will remain after 5 seconds.

➤ Educate patients of the importance of proper water balance. There is no recommended daily allowance (RDA) for water. Adults need 1 mL/kcal per day; infants need more because their basal metabolic heat production is much higher. In buildings with hard water, untreated tap water contains minerals such as calcium, magnesium, and iron. Water-softening systems replace these minerals with sodium, and therefore patients on a low-sodium diet should avoid drinking treated tap water and drink bottled water instead.

➤ Renin levels affect the regulation of fluid balance and electrolytes. If appropriate, educate patients with low sodium levels that the major source of dietary sodium is found in table salt. Many foods, such as milk and other dairy products, are also good sources of dietary sodium. Most other dietary sodium is available through the consumption of processed foods. Patients on low-sodium diets should be advised to avoid beverages such as colas, ginger ale, sports drinks, lemon-lime sodas, and root beer. Many over-the-counter medications including antacids, laxatives, analgesics, sedatives, and antitussives contain significant amounts of sodium. The best advice is to emphasize the importance of reading all food, beverage, and medicine labels. In 1989, the Subcommittee on the 10th Edition of the RDA established 500 mg as the recommended maximum daily intake for dietary intake of sodium. The requesting health care practitioner or nutritionist should be consulted before the patient on a low-sodium diet begins using salt substitutes. There are no RDAs established for potassium, but the estimated minimum intake for adults is 200 mEq/day. Potassium is present in all plant and animal cells, making dietary replacement fairly simple to achieve.

➤ Evaluate test results in relation to the patient's symptoms and other tests performed. Related laboratory tests include aldosterone, creatinine, kidney biopsy, serum and urine potassium, urine protein, serum and urine sodium, blood urea nitrogen, and urinalysis.

RENOGRAM

SYNONYMS/ACRONYM: Renocystography, renocystogram, radioactive renogram, renal scintigraphy.

AREA OF APPLICATION: Kidneys.

CONTRAST: Intravenous radioactive material.

DESCRIPTION: A renogram is a nuclear medicine study performed to assist in diagnosing renal disorders, such as abnormal blood flow, collecting-system defects, and excretion dysfunction. Because renography uses no iodinated contrast medium, it is safe to use in patients who have iodine allergies or compromised renal function.

After intravenous administration of the radioisotope, information about the structures of the kidneys is obtained. The radioactive material is detected by a gamma camera, which can detect the gamma rays emitted by the radionuclide in the kidney. Renography simultaneously tracks the rate at which the radionuclide flows into (*vascular phase*), through (*tubular phase*), and out of (*excretory phase*) the kidneys. The times are plotted on a graph and compared to normal parameters of organ function. Differential estimates of left and right kidney contributions to glomerular filtration rate and effective renal plasma flow can be calculated. With the use of diuretic stimulation during the excretory phase, it is possible to differentiate between anatomic obstruction and nonobstructive residual dilation from previous hydronephrosis. All information obtained is stored in a computer to be used for further interpretation and computations. Renal function can be monitored by serially repeating this test and comparing results. ∎

INDICATIONS:
- Aid in the diagnosis of renal artery stenosis resulting from renal dysplasia or atherosclerosis and causing arterial hypertension and reduced glomerular filtration rate
- Aid in the diagnosis of renal vein thrombosis resulting from dehydration in infants or obstruction of blood flow in the presence of renal tumors in adults
- Aid in the diagnosis of renal artery embolism or renal infarction causing obstruction
- Evaluate obstruction caused by stones or tumor
- Determine the presence and effects of renal trauma, such as arterial injury, renal contusion, hematoma, rupture, arteriovenous fistula, or urinary extravasation
- Detect renal infectious or inflammatory diseases, such as acute or chronic pyelonephritis, renal abscess, or nephritis
- Evaluate chronic urinary tract infections, especially in children
- Determine the presence, location, and cause of obstructive uropathy, such as calculi, neoplasm, congenital disorders, scarring, or inflammation
- Evaluate acute and chronic renal failure

- Evaluate kidney transplant for acute or chronic rejection

RESULT

Normal Findings:
- Normal shape, size, position, symmetry, vasculature, perfusion, and function of the kidneys
- Radionuclide material circulates bilaterally, symmetrically, and without interruption through the renal parenchyma, ureters, and urinary bladder, with 50 percent of the radionuclide excreted within the first 10 minutes

Abnormal Findings:
- Acute tubular necrosis
- Congenital anomalies (e.g., absence of a kidney)
- Decreased renal function
- Diminished blood supply
- Infection or inflammation (pyelonephritis, glomerulonephritis)
- Masses
- Obstructive uropathy
- Renal failure, infarction, cyst, or abscess
- Renal vascular disease including renal artery stenosis or renal vein thrombosis
- Trauma

CRITICAL VALUES: N/A

INTERFERING FACTORS:

This procedure is contraindicated for:
- Patients who are pregnant or suspected of being pregnant, unless the potential benefits of the procedure far outweigh the risks to the fetus and mother

Factors that may impair clear imaging:
- Inability of the patient to cooperate or

remain still during the procedure because of age, significant pain, or mental status

- Patients who are very obese, who may exceed the weight limit for the equipment

- Incorrect positioning of the patient, which may produce poor visualization of the area to be examined

- Serum creatinine levels greater than or equal to 3 mg/dL (depending on the radionuclide used), which can decrease renal perfusion

- Other nuclear scans done within the previous 24 to 48 hours

- Medications such as antihypertensives, angiotensin-converting enzyme (ACE) inhibitors, and beta blockers taken within 24 hours of the test, which can affect the results (depending on the reason for the study)

- Dehydration, which can accentuate abnormalities; or overhydration, which can mask abnormalities

- Metallic objects within the examination field (e.g., jewelry or body rings), which may inhibit organ visualization and can produce unclear images

Other considerations:

- Failure to follow dietary restrictions before the procedure may cause the procedure to be canceled or repeated.

- Consultation with a physician should occur before the procedure for radiation safety concerns regarding infants of patients who are lactating.

- Risks associated with radiographic overexposure can result from frequent x-ray procedures. Personnel in the room with the patient should stand behind a shield or leave the area while the examination is being done. Personnel working in the area where the examination is being done should wear badges that reveal their level of exposure to radiation.

- Inaccurate timing of imaging after the radionuclide injection can affect the results.

Nursing Implications and Procedure • • • • • • • • • • •

Pretest:

➤ Inform the patient that the procedure assesses the renal system.

➤ Inform the patient that the procedure is performed in a special nuclear medicine department by a technologist and usually takes approximately 60 to 90 minutes, and that delayed images are needed 2 to 24 hours later. The patient may leave the department and return later to undergo delayed imaging.

➤ Obtain a history of the patient's complaints, including a list of known allergens. Assess for allergy to the radionuclide.

➤ Obtain a history of the patient's renal and urinary systems, as well as results of previously performed tests and surgical procedures. For related tests, refer to the genitourinary/renal system table.

➤ Obtain a list of the medications the patient is taking.

➤ Determine date of last menstrual period and possibility of pregnancy in perimenopausal women.

➤ There are no food or fluid restrictions, unless otherwise indicated. Inform the patient that he or she will be asked to drink several glasses of fluid before the study for hydration, unless the patient has a restricted fluid intake for other reasons.

Intratest:

➤ Ask the patient to void before the procedure. Have the patient put on a hospital gown.

➤ Administer sedative to a child or to an uncooperative adult, as ordered.

➤ Ask the patient to lie still during the procedure because movement produces unclear images. Make sure jewelry, watches, chains, belts, and any other metallic objects have been removed from the renal area.

➤ Place the patient in a supine position on a flat table with foam wedges to help maintain position and immobilization.

➤ The radionuclide is administered intravenously, and the kidney area is scanned immediately with images taken every minute for 30 minutes.

➤ During the flow and static imaging, the diuretic furosemide (Lasix) or ACE inhibitor (captopril) can be administered intravenously and images obtained.

➤ Renogram curves can be plotted concurrently with flow studies in which blood flow is imaged and recorded as it occurs.

➤ Urine and blood laboratory studies are done after the renogram to correlate findings before diagnosis.

➤ If a study for vesicoureteral reflux is done, the patient is asked to void and a catheter is placed into the bladder. The radionuclide is instilled into the bladder, and multiple images are obtained during bladder filling. The patient is then requested to void, with the catheter in place or after catheter removal, depending on department policy. Imaging is continued during and after voiding. Reflux is determined by calculating the urine volume and counts obtained by imaging.

➤ Wear gloves during the radionuclide administration and while handling the patient's urine.

Post-test: ■

➤ Instruct the patient to resume normal activity, medications, and diet, unless otherwise indicated.

➤ Advise patient to drink increased amounts of fluids for 24 hours to eliminate the radionuclide from the body, unless contraindicated. Tell the patient that radionuclide is eliminated from the body within 6 to 24 hours.

➤ Instruct the patient to flush the toilet immediately after each voiding following the procedure and to wash hands meticulously with soap and water after each voiding for 24 hours after the procedure.

➤ Tell all caregivers to wear gloves when discarding urine for 24 hours after the procedure. Wash gloved hands with soap and water before removing gloves. Then wash hands after the gloves are removed.

➤ A physician specializing in this branch of medicine sends a written report to the ordering provider, who discusses the results with the patient.

➤ Evaluate test results in relation to the patient's symptoms and other tests performed. Related diagnostic tests include intravenous pyelogram, as well as computed tomography, ultrasonography, and magnetic resonance imaging of the abdomen.

RETICULOCYTE COUNT

SYNONYM/ACRONYM: Retic count.

SPECIMEN: Whole blood (1 mL) collected in lavender-top (ethylenediaminetetra-acetic acid [EDTA]) tube.

REFERENCE VALUE: (Method: Microscopic examination of specially stained peripheral blood smear or automated analyzer)

Age	Total Erythrocyte Count*
Newborn	3–7%
1–12 mo	0.2–2.8%
Adult	1.5–2.5%

* Values are expressed as percentage of the red blood cell count.

DESCRIPTION: Normally, as it matures, the red blood cell (RBC) loses its nucleus. The remaining ribonucleic acid (RNA) will produce a characteristic color when special stains are used, making these cells easy to identify and enumerate. The presence of reticulocytes is an indication of the level of erythropoietic activity in the bone marrow. In abnormal conditions, reticulocytes are prematurely released into circulation. (See monographs titled "Red Blood Cell Count" and "Red Blood Cell Morphology and Inclusions.") ■

INDICATIONS:

• Evaluate erythropoietic activity

• Monitor response to therapy for anemias

RESULT: The reticulocyte production index (RPI) is a good estimate of RBC production. The calculation corrects the count for anemia and for the premature release of reticulocytes into the peripheral blood during periods of hemolysis or significant bleeding. The RPI also takes the maturation time of large polychromatophilic cells or nucleated RBCs seen on the peripheral smear into consideration.

RPI = % reticulocytes × [patient hematocrit (Hct)/normal Hct] × (1/maturation time)

As the formula shows, the RPI is inversely proportional to Hct, as follows:

Hematocrit (%)	Maturation Time (days)
45	1.0
35	1.5
25	2.0
15	2.5

Increased in:

• Blood loss

• Hemolytic anemias

• Iron-deficiency anemia

• Megaloblastic anemia

Decreased in:

• Alcoholism

• Anemia of chronic disease

• Aplastic anemia

• Bone marrow replacement

• Endocrine disease

• RBC aplasia

• Renal disease

• Sideroblastic anemia

CRITICAL VALUES: N/A

INTERFERING FACTORS:

• Drugs that may increase reticulocyte counts include acetanilid, acetylsalicylic acid, amyl nitrate, antimalarials, antipyretics, antipyrine, arsenicals, corticotropin, dimercaprol, furaltadone, furazolidone, levodopa, methyldopa, nitrofurans, penicillin, procainamide, and sulfones.

• Drugs that may decrease reticulocyte counts include azathioprine, dactinomycin, hydroxyurea, methotrexate, and zidovudine.

• Reticulocyte count may be falsely increased by the presence of RBC inclusions (Howell-Jolly bodies, Heinz bodies, and Pappenheimer bodies) that stain with methylene blue.

• Reticulocyte count may be falsely decreased after a recent blood transfusion, as a result of the dilutional effect.

Nursing Implications and Procedure · · · · · · · · · · ·

Pretest: ▪

➤ Obtain a history of the patient's complaints, including a list of known allergens.

➤ Obtain a history of the patient's hematopoietic system and results of previously performed tests and procedures. For related tests, refer to the hematopoietic system table.

➤ Obtain a list of the medications the patient is taking, including herbs, nutritional supplements, and nutraceuticals. The requesting health care practitioner and laboratory should be advised if the patient regularly uses these products so that their effects can be taken into consideration when reviewing results.

➤ Note any recent procedures that can interfere with test results.

➤ There are no food, fluid, or medication restrictions unless by medical direction.

➤ Review the procedure with the patient.

➤ Inform the patient that specimen collection takes approximately 5 to 10 minutes.

Intratest: ▪

➤ Direct the patient to breathe normally and to avoid unnecessary movement.

➤ Observe standard precautions and follow the general guidelines in Appendix A. Perform a venipuncture, and collect the specimen in a 5-mL lavender-top tube.

➤ Label the specimen, and promptly transport it to the laboratory.

Post-test: ▪

➤ Observe venipuncture site for bleeding or hematoma formation. Apply pressure bandage.

➤ Evaluate test results in relation to the patient's symptoms and other tests performed. Related laboratory tests include complete blood count and RBC morphology and inclusions.

RETROGRADE URETEROPYELOGRAPHY

· ·

SYNONYM/ACRONYM: Retrograde.

AREA OF APPLICATION: Renal calyces, ureter.

CONTRAST: Radiopaque iodine-based contrast medium.

DESCRIPTION: Retrograde ureteropyelography uses a contrast medium introduced through a ureteral catheter during cystography and radiographic visualization to view the renal collecting system (calyces, renal pelvis, and urethra). During a cystoscopic examination, a catheter is advanced through the ureters and into the kidney; contrast medium is injected through the catheter into the kidney. This procedure is primarily used in patients who are known to be hypersensitive to intravenously injected iodine-based contrast medium and when excretory ureterography does not adequately reveal the renal collecting system. The incidence of allergic reaction to the contrast medium is reduced because there is less systemic absorption of the contrast medium when injected into the kidney than when injected intravenously. Retrograde ureteropyelography sometimes provides more information about the anatomy of the different parts of the collecting system than can be obtained by excretory ureteropyelography. The procedure is not hampered by impaired renal function, but it carries the risk of urinary tract infection and sepsis. ■

INDICATIONS:
• Evaluate known or suspected ureteral obstruction

• Evaluate the presence of calculi in the kidneys, ureters, or bladder

• Evaluate the structure and integrity of the renal collecting system

• Evaluate the renal collecting system when excretory urography is unsuccessful

• Evaluate space-occupying lesions or congenital anomalies of the urinary system

• Evaluate the effects of urinary system trauma

• Evaluate placement of a ureteral stent or catheter

RESULT

Normal Findings:
• Normal outline and opacification of renal pelvis and calyces

• Symmetrical and bilateral outline of structures

• Normal size and uniform filling of the ureters

Abnormal Findings:
• Congenital renal or urinary tract abnormalities

• Hydronephrosis

• Neoplasms

• Obstruction as a result of tumor, blood clot, stricture, or calculi

• Obstruction of ureteropelvic junction

• Perinephric abscess

• Perinephric inflammation or suppuration

• Polycystic kidney disease

• Prostatic enlargement

• Tumor of the kidneys or the collecting system

CRITICAL VALUES: N/A

INTERFERING FACTORS:

This procedure is contraindicated for:
• Patients with allergies to shellfish or iodinated dye. The contrast medium used may cause a life-threatening allergic reaction. Patients with a known hypersensitivity to the contrast medium may benefit from premedication with corticosteroids or the use of nonionic contrast medium.

- Patients who are pregnant or suspected of being pregnant, unless the potential benefits of the procedure far outweigh the risks to the fetus and mother

- Elderly and other patients who are ⚠ chronically dehydrated before the test, because of their risk of contrast-induced renal failure.

- ⚠ Patients who are in renal failure.

- Patients with renal insufficiency, indicated by a blood urea nitrogen ⚠ (BUN) value greater than 40 mg/dL, because contrast medium can complicate kidney function.

Factors that may impair clear imaging:

- Inability of the patient to cooperate or remain still during the procedure because of age, significant pain, or mental status

- Improper adjustment of the radiographic equipment to accommodate obese or thin patients, which can cause overexposure or underexposure and poor-quality study

- Patients who are very obese, who may exceed the weight limit for the equipment

- Incorrect positioning of the patient, which may produce poor visualization of the area to be examined

- Gas or feces in the gastrointestinal (GI) tract resulting from inadequate cleansing or failure to restrict food intake before the study

- Retained barium from a previous radiologic procedure

- Metallic objects within the examination field (e.g., jewelry or body rings), which may inhibit organ visualization and can produce unclear images

Other considerations:

- Failure to follow dietary restrictions before the procedure may cause the procedure to be canceled or repeated.

- Consultation with a physician should occur before the procedure for radiation safety concerns regarding infants of patients who are lactating.

- Risks associated with radiographic overexposure can result from frequent x-ray procedures. Personnel in the room with the patient should stand behind a shield or leave the area while the examination is being done. Personnel working in the area where the examination is being done should wear badges that reveal their level of exposure to radiation.

Nursing Implications and Procedure • • • • • • • • • • •

Pretest: ■

➤ Inform the patient that the procedure assesses the renal collecting system. Inform the patient that the procedure is done by a urologist and support staff during a cystoscopic examination in the surgical department and takes approximately 60 minutes.

➤ Obtain a history of the patient's complaints, including a history of allergies or sensitivities to contrast medium or shellfish.

➤ Patients receiving metformin (Glucophage) for non–insulin-dependent (type 2) diabetes should discontinue the drug on the day of the test and continue to withhold it for 48 hours after the test. Failure to do so may result in lactic acidosis.

➤ Obtain a history of the patient's genitourinary and abdominal systems, as well as results of previously performed tests and procedures, especially BUN and creatinine. For related tests, refer to the genitourinary system table.

➤ Determine date of last menstrual period and possibility of pregnancy in perimenopausal women.

➤ *Obtain a written, informed consent before administering any medications prior to the procedure.*

➤ Inform the patient that if a local anesthetic is used, the patient may feel (1) some pressure in the kidney area as the catheter is introduced and contrast medium injected, or (2) the urgency to void.

➤ Inform the patient that he or she may receive a laxative the night before the test, an enema, or a cathartic the morning of the test, as ordered.

➤ Instruct the patient to increase fluid intake the day before the test, but to withhold food and fluids for 8 hours before the test.

➤ Schedule GI or any barium studies after this study.

➤ Obtain and record baseline vital signs.

Intratest:

➤ Have the patient put on a hospital gown.

➤ Make sure jewelry, watches, chains, belts, and any other metallic objects have been removed from the abdominal area.

➤ Remove any wires connected to electrodes, if allowed.

➤ Place patient on the table in a supine position in the lithotomy position.

➤ A kidney, ureter, and bladder (KUB) or plain film is taken to ensure that no barium or stool will obscure visualization of the urinary system. Ask the patient to lie still during the procedure because movement produces unclear images. The patient may be asked to hold his or her breath to facilitate visualization.

➤ While the patient is anesthetized, a cystoscopic examination is performed and the bladder is inspected.

➤ A catheter is inserted, and the renal pelvis is emptied by gravity. Contrast medium is introduced into the catheter. Inform the patient that the contrast medium may cause a temporary flushing of the face, a feeling of warmth, or nausea.

➤ X-ray exposures are made and the results processed. Inform the

patient that additional views may be necessary to visualize the area in question.

➤ Additional contrast medium is injected through the catheter to outline the ureters as the catheter is withdrawn.

➤ Additional x-ray exposures are taken 10 to 15 minutes after the catheter is removed to evaluate retention of the contrast medium, indicating urinary stasis.

➤ The catheter may be kept in place and attached to a gravity drainage unit until urinary flow has returned or is corrected.

Post-test:

➤ Monitor vital and neurologic signs until they return to preprocedure levels.

➤ Instruct the patient to resume usual diet and medications, unless otherwise indicated. Renal function should be assessed before metformin is restarted.

➤ Monitor fluid intake and urinary output following the procedure. Decreased urine output may indicate impending renal failure or edema caused by instrumentation.

➤ Monitor for signs of sepsis and severe pain in the kidney area.

➤ Maintain the patient on adequate hydration after the procedure. Encourage the patient to drink lots of fluids to prevent stasis and to prevent the buildup of bacteria.

➤ Determine whether the patient or family members have any further questions or concerns.

➤ A physician specializing in this branch of medicine sends a written report to the ordering health care provider, who discusses the results with the patient.

➤ Inform the patient that further examinations may be necessary to evaluate progression of the disease process or to determine the need for a change in therapy.

➤ Evaluate test results in relation to the patient's symptoms and other tests performed. Related diagnostic tests include renogram, intravenous pyelogram, renal ultrasound, and

computed tomography and magnetic resonance imaging of the abdomen.

RHEUMATOID FACTOR

SYNONYMS/ACRONYMS: RF, RA.

SPECIMEN: Serum (1 mL) collected in a red-top tube

REFERENCE VALUE: (Method: Nephelometry) 0 to 20 IU/mL.

DESCRIPTION: Individuals with rheumatoid arthritis harbor a macroglobulin-type antibody called *rheumatoid factor* (RF) in their blood. Patients with other diseases (e.g., systemic lupus erythematosus [SLE] and occasionally tuberculosis, chronic hepatitis, infectious mononucleosis, and subacute bacterial endocarditis) may also test positive for RF. RF antibodies are usually immunoglobulin M (IgM) but may also be IgG or IgA. ∎

INDICATIONS: Assist in the diagnosis of rheumatoid arthritis, especially when clinical diagnosis is difficult

RESULT

Increased in:
- Chronic hepatitis
- Chronic viral infections
- Cirrhosis
- Dermatomyositis
- Infectious mononucleosis
- Leishmaniasis

- Leprosy
- Malaria
- Rheumatoid arthritis
- Sarcoidosis
- Scleroderma
- Sjögren's syndrome
- SLE
- Syphilis
- Tuberculosis
- Waldenström's macroglobulinemia

Decreased in: N/A

CRITICAL VALUES: N/A

INTERFERING FACTORS:
- Older patients may have higher values.
- Recent blood transfusion, multiple vaccinations or transfusions, or an inadequately activated complement may affect results.
- Serum with cryoglobulin or high lipid levels may cause a false-positive test and may require that the test be repeated after a fat-restriction diet.

Nursing Implications and Procedure • • • • • • • • • •

Pretest: ■

➤ Obtain a history of the patient's complaints, including a list of known allergens.

➤ Obtain a history of the patient's immune and musculoskeletal systems, as well as results of previously performed tests and procedures. For related tests, refer to the immune and musculoskeletal system tables.

➤ Obtain a list of the medications the patient is taking, including herbs, nutritional supplements, and nutraceuticals. The requesting health care practitioner and laboratory should be advised if the patient regularly uses these products so that their effects can be taken into consideration when reviewing results.

➤ There are no food, fluid, or medication restrictions unless by medical direction.

➤ Review the procedure with the patient.

➤ Inform the patient that specimen collection takes approximately 5 to 10 minutes.

Intratest: ■

➤ Direct the patient to breathe normally and to avoid unnecessary movement.

➤ Observe standard precautions and follow the general guidelines in Appendix A. Perform a venipuncture, and collect the specimen in a 5-mL red-top tube.

➤ Label the specimen, and promptly transport it to the laboratory.

Post-test: ■

➤ Observe venipuncture site for bleeding or hematoma formation. Apply pressure bandage.

➤ Advise the patient, as appropriate, that additional studies may be undertaken to determine treatment regimen or to determine the possible causes of symptoms if the test is negative for rheumatoid arthritis.

➤ Recognize anxiety related to test results and offer support and information regarding the clinical implications of the test results. Provide support for anxiety related to anticipated chronic pain resulting from joint inflammation, impairment in mobility, musculoskeletal deformity, and loss of independence. Educate the patient regarding access to counseling services, as appropriate.

➤ Evaluate test results in relation to the patient's symptoms and other tests performed. Related laboratory tests include antinuclear antibodies, C-reactive protein, erythrocyte sedimentation rate, synovial fluid analysis, and uric acid.

RUBELLA ANTIBODIES

• •

SYNONYM/ACRONYM: German measles serology.

SPECIMEN: Serum (1 mL) collected in a red-top tube.

REFERENCE VALUE: (Method: Indirect immunofluorescence) Immune or less than a fourfold increase in titer.

DESCRIPTION: Rubella, commonly known as German measles, is a communicable viral disease transmitted by contact with respiratory secretions and aerosolized droplets of the secretions. The incubation period is 14 to 21 days. This disease produces a pink, macular rash that disappears in 2 to 3 days. Rubella infection induces immunoglobulin G (IgG) and IgM antibody production. This test can determine current infection or immunity from past infection. Rubella serology is part of the TORCH (*tox*oplasmosis, *ru*bella, *cy*tomegalovirus, *he*rpes simplex type 2) panel routinely performed on pregnant women. Fetal infection during the first trimester can cause spontaneous abortion or congenital defects. Ideally the immune status of women of childbearing age should be ascertained before pregnancy, when vaccination can be administered to provide lifelong immunity. The presence of IgM antibodies indicates acute infection. The presence of IgG antibodies indicates current or past infection. Susceptibility to rubella is indicated by a negative reaction. Many laboratories use a qualitative assay that detects the presence of both IgM and IgG rubella antibodies. IgM- and IgG-specific enzyme immunoassays are also available to help distinguish acute infection from immune status. A rise in titer greater than fourfold in paired specimens is an indication of current infection. ∎

INDICATIONS:

• Assist in the diagnosis of rubella infection

• Determine presence of rubella antibodies

• Determine susceptibility to rubella, particularly in pregnant women

• Perform as part of routine prenatal serologic testing

RESULT

Positive findings in: Rubella infection (past or present)

CRITICAL VALUES: N/A

INTERFERING FACTORS: N/A

Nursing Implications and Procedure ● ● ● ● ● ● ● ● ● ●

Pretest: ∎

➤ Obtain a history of the patient's complaints, including a list of known allergens. Obtain a history of exposure to rubella.

➤ Obtain a history of the patient's immune and reproductive systems, as well as results of previously performed tests and procedures. For related tests, refer to the immune and reproductive system tables.

➤ Obtain a list of the medications the patient is taking, including herbs, nutritional supplements, and nutraceuticals. The requesting health care practitioner and laboratory should be advised if the patient regularly uses these products so that their effects can be taken into consideration when reviewing results.

➤ There are no food, fluid, or medication restrictions unless by medical direction.

➤ Review the procedure with the patient. Inform the patient that several tests may be necessary to confirm diagnosis. Any individual positive result should be repeated in 7 to 14 days to monitor a change in titer.

➤ Inform the patient that each specimen collection takes approximately 5 to 10 minutes.

Intratest:

➤ Direct the patient to breathe normally and to avoid unnecessary movement.

➤ Observe standard precautions and follow the general guidelines in Appendix A. Perform a venipuncture, and collect the specimen in a 5-mL red-top tube.

➤ Label the specimen, and promptly transport it to the laboratory.

Post-test:

➤ Observe venipuncture site for bleeding or hematoma formation. Apply pressure bandage.

➤ Recognize anxiety related to test results and provide emotional support if results are positive and the patient is pregnant. Encourage the family to seek counseling if concerned with pregnancy termination. Provide teaching and information regarding the clinical implications of the test results, as appropriate. Decisions regarding elective abortion should take place in the presence of both parents. Provide a nonjudgmental, nonthreatening atmosphere for discussing the risks and difficulties of delivering and raising an abnormal infant, as well as exploring other options (e.g., termination of pregnancy or adoption). Educate the patient regarding access to counseling services, as appropriate.

➤ Instruct the patient in isolation precautions during time of communicability or contagion.

➤ Emphasize the need to return to have a convalescent blood sample taken in 7 to 14 days.

➤ Evaluate test results in relation to the patient's symptoms and other tests performed. Related laboratory tests include cytomegalovirus, herpes simplex, and *Toxoplasma*.

RUBEOLA ANTIBODIES

• •

SYNONYM/ACRONYM: Measles serology.

SPECIMEN: Serum (1 mL) collected in a red-top tube.

REFERENCE VALUE: (Method: Indirect immunofluorescence) Negative or less than a fourfold increase in titer.

DESCRIPTION: Measles is caused by a single-stranded ribonucleic acid (RNA) paramyxovirus that invades the respiratory tract and lymphoreticular tissues. It is transmitted by respiratory secretions and aerosolized droplets of the secretions. The incubation period is 10 to 11 days. Symptoms initially include conjunctivitis, cough, and fever. Koplik's spots develop 4 to 5 days later, followed by papular eruptions, body rash, and lymphadenopathy. The presence of immunoglobulin M (IgM) antibodies indicates acute infection. The presence of IgG antibodies indicates current or past infection. Susceptibility to measles is indicated by a negative reaction. Many laboratories use a qualitative assay that detects the presence of both IgM and IgG rubeola antibodies. IgM- and IgG-specific enzyme immunoassays are also available to help distinguish acute infection from immune status. A rise in titer greater than fourfold in paired specimens is an indication of current infection. ∎

INDICATIONS:

• Determine resistance to or protection against measles virus

• Differential diagnosis of viral infection, especially in pregnant women with a history of exposure to measles

RESULT

Positive findings in: Measles infection

CRITICAL VALUES: N/A

INTERFERING FACTORS: N/A

Nursing Implications and Procedure • • • • • • • • • • •

Pretest:

➤ Obtain a history of the patient's complaints, including a list of known allergens. Obtain a history of exposure to measles.

➤ Obtain a history of the patient's immune and reproductive systems, as well as results of previously performed tests and procedures. For related tests, refer to the immune and reproductive system tables.

➤ Obtain a list of the medications the patient is taking, including herbs, nutritional supplements, and nutraceuticals. The requesting health care practitioner and laboratory should be advised if the patient regularly uses these products so that their effects can be taken into consideration when reviewing results.

➤ There are no food, fluid, or medication restrictions unless by medical direction.

➤ Review the procedure with the patient. Inform the patient that several tests may be necessary to confirm the diagnosis. Any individual positive result should be repeated in 7 to 14 days to monitor a change in titer.

➤ Inform the patient that each specimen collection takes approximately 5 to 10 minutes.

Intratest:

➤ Direct the patient to breathe normally and to avoid unnecessary movement.

➤ Observe standard precautions and follow the general guidelines in Appendix A. Perform a venipuncture, and collect the specimen in a 5-mL red-top tube.

➤ Label the specimen, and promptly transport it to the laboratory.

Post-test:

➤ Observe venipuncture site for bleeding or hematoma formation. Apply pressure bandage.

➤ Instruct the patient in isolation precautions during time of communicability or contagion.

➤ Emphasize the need to return to have a convalescent blood sample taken in 7 to 14 days.

➤ Evaluate test results in relation to the patient's symptoms and other tests performed. A related laboratory test is rubella.

SEMEN ANALYSIS

· ·

SYNONYM/ACRONYM: N/A.

SPECIMEN: Semen from ejaculate specimen collected in a clean, dry, glass container known to be free of detergent. The specimen container should be kept at body temperature (37°C) during transportation.

REFERENCE VALUE: (Method: Macroscopic and microscopic examination)

Volume	2–5 mL
Color	White or opaque
Appearance	Viscous (pours in droplets not clumps or strings)
Clotting and liquefaction	Complete in 20–30 minutes
pH	7.5–8.5
Sperm count	20–200 million/mL
Motility	At least 60%
Morphology	At least 70% normal oval-headed forms

DESCRIPTION: Semen analysis is a valid measure of overall male fertility. Semen contains a combination of elements produced by various parts of the male reproductive system. Spermatozoa are produced in the testes and account for only a small volume of seminal fluid. Fructose and other nutrients are provided by fluid produced in the seminal vesicles. The prostate gland provides acid phosphatase and other enzymes required for coagulation and liquefaction of semen. Sperm motility depends on the presence of a sufficient level of ionized calcium. If the specimen has an abnormal appearance (e.g., bloody, oddly colored, turbid), the patient may have an infection. Specimens can be tested with a leukocyte esterase strip to detect the presence of white blood cells. ■

INDICATIONS:

• Assist in the diagnosis of azoospermia and oligospermia

• Evaluate infertility

• Evaluate vasectomy effectiveness

• Support or disprove sterility in paternity suit

RESULT: There is marked intraindividual variation in sperm count. Indications of suboptimal fertility should be investigated by serial analysis of two to three samples collected over several months. If abnormal results are obtained, additional testing may be requested.

Abnormality	Test Ordered	Normal Result
Decreased count	Fructose	Present (greater than 150 mg/dL)
Decreased motility with clumping	Male antisperm antibodies	Absent
Normal semen analysis with infertility	Female antisperm antibodies	Absent

Increased in: N/A

Decreased in:

- Hyperpyrexia

- Obstruction of ejaculatory system

- Orchitis

- Postvasectomy period

- Primary and secondary testicular failure

- Testicular atrophy (e.g., recovery from mumps)

- Varicocele

CRITICAL VALUES: N/A

INTERFERING FACTORS:

- Drugs and substances that may decrease sperm count include arsenic, azathioprine, cannabis, cimetidine, cocaine, cyclophosphamide, estrogens, fluoxymesterone, ketoconazole, lead, methotrexate, methyltestosterone, nitrofurantoin, nitrogen mustard, procarbazine, sulfasalazine, and vincristine.

- Testicular radiation may decrease sperm counts.

- Cigarette smoking is associated with decreased production of semen.

- Caffeine consumption is associated with increased sperm density and number of abnormal forms.

- Delays in transporting the specimen and failure to keep the specimen warm during transportation are the most common reasons for specimen rejection.

Nursing Implications and Procedure

Pretest:

➤ Obtain a history of the patient's complaints, including a list of known allergens.

➤ Obtain a history of the patient's reproductive system as well as results of previously performed tests and procedures. For related tests, refer to the reproductive system table.

➤ Obtain a list of medications the patient is taking, including herbs, nutritional supplements, and nutraceuticals. The requesting health care practitioner and laboratory should be advised if the patient regularly uses these products so that their effects can be taken into consideration when reviewing results.

➤ Note any recent procedures that can interfere with test results.

➤ There are no food, fluid, or medication restrictions unless by medical direction.

➤ The requesting health care practitioner usually provides the patient with instructions for specimen collection.

➤ Review the procedure with the patient. Sensitivity to cultural and social issues, as well as concern for modesty, is important in providing psychological support.

➤ Instruct the patient to refrain from

any sexual activity for 3 days before specimen collection. Instruct the patient to bring the specimen to the laboratory within 30 to 60 minutes of collection and to keep the specimen warm (close to body temperature) during transportation.

Intratest:

➤ Observe standard precautions and follow the general guidelines in Appendix A.

Ejaculated specimen:

➤ Ideally, the specimen is obtained by masturbation in a private location close to the laboratory. In cases in which the patient expresses psychological or religious concerns about masturbation, the specimen can be obtained during coitus interruptus, through the use of a condom, or through postcoital collection of samples from the cervical canal and vagina of the patient's sexual partner. The patient should be warned about the possible loss of the sperm-rich portion of the sample if coitus interruptus is the collection approach. If a condom is used, the patient must be carefully instructed to wash and dry the condom completely before use to prevent contamination of the specimen with spermicides.

Cervical vaginal specimen:

➤ Assist the patient to the lithotomy position on the examination table. A speculum is inserted, and the specimen is obtained by direct smear or aspiration of saline lavage.

Specimens collected from skin or clothing:

➤ Dried semen may be collected by sponging the skin with a gauze soaked in saline or soaking the material in a saline solution.

Post-test:

➤ Provide a supportive, nonjudgmental environment when assisting a patient through the process of fertility testing. Provide teaching and information regarding the clinical implications of the test results, as appropriate.

➤ Provide a supportive, nonjudgmental environment when assisting a patient through the process of fertility testing. Recognize anxiety related to test results, and encourage the patient or family to seek counseling and other support services if concerned with infertility.

➤ Evaluate test results in relation to the patient's symptoms and other tests performed. Related laboratory tests include antisperm antibodies, estradiol, and testosterone.

SICKLE CELL SCREEN

SYNONYM/ACRONYM: Sickle cell test.

SPECIMEN: Whole blood (1 mL) collected in a lavender-top (ethylenediaminetetra-acetic acid [EDTA]) tube.

REFERENCE VALUE: (Method: Hemoglobin high-salt solubility) Negative.

DESCRIPTION: The sickle cell screen is one of several screening tests for a group of hereditary hemoglobinopathies. The test is positive in the presence of rare sickling hemoglobin (Hgb) variants such as Hgb S and Hgb C Harlem. Hgb S results from an amino acid substitution during Hgb synthesis whereby valine replaces glutamic acid. Hemoglobin C Harlem results from the substitution of lysine for glutamic acid. Individuals with sickle cell disease have chronic anemia because the abnormal Hgb is unable to carry oxygen. The red blood cells of affected individuals are also abnormal in shape, resembling a crescent or sickle rather than the normal disk shape. This abnormality, combined with cell-wall rigidity, prevents the cells from passing through smaller blood vessels. Blockages in blood vessels result in hypoxia, damage, and pain. Individuals with the sickle cell trait do not have the clinical manifestations of the disease but may pass the disease on to children if the other parent has the trait (or the disease) as well. ■

INDICATIONS:
• Detect sickled red blood cells
• Evaluate hemolytic anemias

RESULT

Positive findings in:
• Combination of Hgb S with other hemoglobinopathies
• Hgb C Harlem anemia
• Sickle cell anemia
• Sickle cell trait
• Thalassemias

Negative findings in: N/A

CRITICAL VALUES: N/A

INTERFERING FACTORS:
• Drugs that may increase sickle cells *in vitro* include prostaglandins.

• A positive test does not distinguish between the sickle trait and sickle cell anemia; to make this determination, follow-up testing by Hgb electrophoresis should be performed.

• False-negative results may occur in children younger than 3 months of age.

• False-negative results may occur in patients who have received a recent blood transfusion before specimen collection, as a result of the dilutional effect.

• False-positive results may occur in patients without the trait or disease who have received a blood transfusion from a sickle cell–positive donor; this effect can last for 4 months after the transfusion.

• Test results are unreliable if the patient has pernicious anemia or polycythemia.

Nursing Implications and Procedure ● ● ● ● ● ● ● ● ● ● ●

Pretest: ■

➤ Obtain a history of the patient's complaints, including a list of known allergens.

➤ Obtain a history of the patient's hematopoietic system as well as results of previously performed tests and procedures. For related tests, refer to the hematopoietic system table.

➤ Obtain a list of medications the patient is taking, including herbs, nutritional supplements, and nutraceuticals. The requesting health care

practitioner and laboratory should be advised if the patient regularly uses these products so that their effects can be taken into consideration when reviewing results.

➤ There are no food, fluid, or medication restrictions unless by medical direction.

➤ Review the procedure with the patient. Sensitivity to cultural and social issues is important in providing psychological support.

➤ Inform the patient that specimen collection takes approximately 5 to 10 minutes.

Intratest:

➤ Direct the patient to breathe normally and to avoid unnecessary movement.

➤ Observe standard precautions and follow the general guidelines in Appendix A. Perform a venipuncture, and collect the specimen in a 5-mL lavender-top tube.

➤ Label the specimen, and promptly transport it to the laboratory.

Post-test:

➤ Observe venipuncture site for bleeding or hematoma formation. Apply pressure bandage.

➤ Inform the patient that further testing may be indicated if results are positive.

➤ Recognize anxiety related to test results and offer support, as appropriate. Provide teaching and information regarding the clinical implications of the test results, as appropriate. Educate the patient regarding access to counseling services.

➤ Advise the patient with sickle cell disease to avoid situations in which hypoxia may occur, such as strenuous exercise, staying at high altitudes, or traveling in an unpressurized aircraft. Maternity and surgical patients with sickle cell anemia are at risk for hypoxia and therefore require close observation: Maternity patients are at risk for hypoxia during the stress of labor and delivery, and surgical patients may become hypoxic while under general anesthesia.

➤ Evaluate test results in relation to the patient's symptoms and other tests performed. Related laboratory tests include complete blood count and Hgb electrophoresis.

SODIUM, SERUM

SYNONYM/ACRONYM: Serum Na^+.

SPECIMEN: Serum (1 mL) collected in a red- or tiger-top tube. Plasma (1 mL) collected in green-top (heparin) tube is also acceptable.

REFERENCE VALUE: (Method: Ion-selective electrode)

Age	Conventional Units	SI Units (Conversion Factor ×1)
Newborn	133–146 mEq/L	133–146 mmol/L
Infant	133–144 mEq/L	133–144 mmol/L
Child	135–145 mEq/L	135–145 mmol/L
Adult	135–145 mEq/L	135–145 mmol/L

DESCRIPTION: Sodium is the most abundant cation in the extracellular fluid and, together with the accompanying chloride and bicarbonate anions, accounts for 92 percent of serum osmolality. Sodium plays a major role in maintaining homeostasis in a variety of ways, including maintaining the osmotic pressure of extracellular fluid, regulating renal retention and excretion of water, maintaining acid-base balance, regulating potassium and chloride levels, stimulating neuromuscular reactions, and maintaining systemic blood pressure. *Hypernatremia* (elevated sodium level) occurs when there is excessive water loss or abnormal retention of sodium. *Hyponatremia* (low sodium level) occurs when there is inadequate sodium retention or inadequate intake. ■

INDICATIONS:
- Determine whole-body stores of sodium, because the ion is predominantly extracellular
- Monitor the effectiveness of drug therapy, especially diuretics, on serum sodium levels

RESULT

Increased in:
- Azotemia
- Burns
- Cushing's disease
- Dehydration

- Diabetes
- Diarrhea (water loss in excess of salt loss)
- Excessive intake
- Excessive saline therapy
- Excessive sweating
- Fever
- Hyperaldosteronism
- Lactic acidosis
- Nasogastric feeding with inadequate fluid
- Vomiting

Decreased in:
- Central nervous system disease
- Congestive heart failure
- Cystic fibrosis
- Excessive antidiuretic hormone production
- Excessive use of diuretics
- Hepatic failure
- Hypoproteinemia
- Insufficient intake
- Intravenous (IV) glucose infusion
- Metabolic acidosis
- Mineralocorticoid deficiency (Addison's disease)
- Nephrotic syndrome

CRITICAL VALUES:

Hyponatremia: Less than 120 mmol/L

Hypernatremia: Greater than 160 mmol/L

Note and report increased or decreased values and symptoms of fluid imbalance to the requesting health care practitioner. Signs and symptoms of hyponatremia include confusion, irritability, convulsions, tachycardia, nausea, vomiting, and loss of consciousness. Possible interventions include maintenance of airway, monitoring for convulsions, fluid restriction, and performance of hourly neurologic checks. Administration of saline for replacement requires close attention to serum and urine osmolality. Signs and symptoms of hypernatremia include restlessness, intense thirst, weakness, swollen tongue, seizures, and coma. Possible interventions include treatment of the underlying cause of water loss or sodium excess, which includes sodium restriction and administration of diuretics combined with IV solutions of 5% dextrose in water (D$_5$W).

INTERFERING FACTORS:

- Drugs that may increase serum sodium levels include anabolic steroids, angiotensin, bicarbonate, carbenoxolone, cisplatin, corticotropin, cortisone, gamma globulin, and mannitol.

- Drugs that may decrease serum sodium levels include amphotericin B, bicarbonate, cathartics (excessive use), chlorpropamide, chlorthalidone, diuretics, ethacrynic acid, fluoxetine, furosemide, laxatives (excessive use), methyclothiazide, metolazone, nicardipine, quinethazone, theophylline (IV infusion), thiazides, and triamterene.

- Specimens should never be collected above an IV line because of the potential for dilution when the specimen and the IV solution combine in the collection container, falsely decreasing the result. There is also the potential of contaminating the sample with the substance of interest, contained in the IV solution, falsely increasing the result.

Nursing Implications and Procedure · · · · · · · · · · ·

Pretest:

➤ Obtain a history of the patient's complaints, including a list of known allergens.

➤ Obtain a history of the patient's endocrine and genitourinary systems, as well as results of previously performed tests and procedures. For related tests, refer to the endocrine and genitourinary system tables.

➤ Obtain a list of medications the patient is taking, including herbs, nutritional supplements, and nutraceuticals. The requesting health care practitioner and laboratory should be advised if the patient regularly uses these products so that their effects can be taken into consideration when reviewing results.

➤ There are no food, fluid, or medication restrictions unless by medical direction.

➤ Review the procedure with the patient.

➤ Inform the patient that specimen collection takes approximately 5 to 10 minutes.

Intratest:

➤ Direct the patient to breathe normally and to avoid unnecessary movement.

➤ Observe standard precautions and follow the general guidelines in Appendix A. Perform a venipuncture, and collect the specimen in a 5-mL red- or tiger-top tube.

➤ Label the specimen, and promptly transport it to the laboratory.

Post-test:

➤ Observe venipuncture site for bleeding or hematoma formation. Apply pressure bandage.

➤ Evaluate the patient for signs and

symptoms of dehydration. Decreased skin turgor, dry mouth, and multiple longitudinal furrows in the tongue are symptoms of dehydration. Dehydration is a significant and common finding in geriatric and other patients in whom renal function has deteriorated.

➤ If appropriate, educate patients with low sodium levels that the major source of dietary sodium is found in table salt. Many foods, such as milk and other dairy products, are also good sources of dietary sodium. Most other dietary sodium is available through the consumption of processed foods. Patients on low-sodium diets should be advised to avoid beverages such as colas, ginger ale, sports drinks, lemon-lime

sodas, and root beer. Many over-the-counter medications including antacids, laxatives, analgesics, sedatives, and antitussives contain significant amounts of sodium. The best advice is to emphasize the importance of reading all food, beverage, and medicine labels. In 1989, the Subcommittee on the 10th Edition of the RDA established 500 mg as the recommended maximum daily intake for dietary intake of sodium.

➤ Evaluate test results in relation to the patient's symptoms and other tests performed. Related laboratory tests include aldosterone, anion gap, chloride, kidney stone analysis, serum and urine osmolality, serum and urine potassium, renin, and urine sodium.

SODIUM, URINE

SYNONYMS/ACRONYM: Urine Na$^+$.

SPECIMEN: Urine (5 mL) from an unpreserved random or timed specimen collected in a clean, plastic collection container.

REFERENCE VALUE: (Method: Ion-selective electrode)

Age	Conventional Units	SI Units (Conversion Factor ×1)
6–10 y		
Male	41–115 mEq/24 h	41–115 mmol/24 h
Female	20–69 mEq/24 h	20–69 mmol/24 h
10–14 y		
Male	63–177 mEq/24 h	63–177 mmol/24 h
Female	48–168 mEq/24 h	48–168 mmol/24 h
Adult	27–287 mEq/24 h	27–287 mmol/24 h

Values vary markedly depending on dietary intake and hydration state.

DESCRIPTION: Regulating electrolyte balance is a major function of the kidneys. In normally functioning

kidneys, urine sodium levels increase when serum levels are high and decrease when serum levels are low to maintain homeostasis. Analyzing these urinary levels can provide important clues to the functioning of the kidneys and other major organs. There is diurnal variation in excretion of sodium, with values lower at night. Urine sodium tests usually involve timed urine collections over a 12- or 24-hour period. Measurement of random specimens may also be requested. ∎

INDICATIONS:
- Determine potential cause of renal calculi
- Evaluate known or suspected endocrine disorder
- Evaluate known or suspected renal disease
- Evaluate malabsorption disorders

RESULT

Increased in:
- Adrenal failure
- Alkalosis
- Diabetes
- Diuretic therapy
- Excessive intake
- Renal tubular acidosis
- Salt-losing nephritis

Decreased in:
- Adrenal hyperfunction
- Congestive heart failure
- Diarrhea
- Excessive sweating
- Extrarenal sodium loss with adequate hydration
- Insufficient intake
- Postoperative period (first 24 to 48 hours)

- Prerenal azotemia
- Sodium retention (premenstrual)

CRITICAL VALUES: N/A

INTERFERING FACTORS:
- Drugs that may increase urine sodium levels include acetazolamide, amiloride, ammonium chloride, acetyl-salicylic acid, azosemide, benzthiazide, bumetanide, calcitonin, chlorothiazide, clopamide, cyclothiazide, diapamide, dopamine, ethacrynic acid, furosemide, hydrocortisone, hydroflumethiazide, isosorbide, levodopa, mercurial diuretics, methylclothiazide, metolazone, polythiazide, quinethazone, spironolactone, sulfates, tetracycline, thiazides, torasemide, triamterene, trichlormethiazide, triflocin, verapamil, and vincristine.
- Drugs that may decrease urine sodium levels include aldosterone, anesthetics, angiotensin, corticosteroids, cortisone, etodolac, indomethacin, levarterenol, lithium, and propranolol.
- Sodium levels are subject to diurnal variation (output being lowest at night), which is why 24-hour collections are recommended.

Nursing Implications and Procedure • • • • • • • • • • •

Pretest:

➤ Obtain a history of the patient's complaints, including a list of known allergens.

➤ Obtain a history of the patient's endocrine and genitourinary systems, as well as results of previously performed tests and procedures. For related tests, refer to the endocrine and genitourinary system tables.

➤ Obtain a list of medications the patient is taking, including herbs, nutritional supplements, and nutraceuticals. The requesting health care practitioner and laboratory should be advised if the patient regularly uses these products so that their effects can be taken into consideration when reviewing results.

➤ There are no food, fluid, or medication restrictions unless by medical direction.

➤ Review the procedure with the patient. Provide a nonmetallic urinal, bedpan, or toilet-mounted collection device.

➤ Usually a 24-hour time frame for urine collection is ordered. Inform the patient that all urine must be saved during that 24-hour period. Instruct the patient not to void directly into the laboratory collection container. Instruct the patient to avoid defecating in the collection device and to keep toilet tissue out of the collection device to prevent contamination of the specimen. Place a sign in the bathroom to remind the patient to save all urine.

➤ Instruct the patient to void all urine into the collection device and then to pour the urine into the laboratory collection container. Alternatively the specimen can be left in the collection device for a health care staff member to add to the laboratory collection container.

Intratest:

➤ Observe standard precautions and follow the general guidelines in Appendix A.

Random specimen (collect in early morning):

Clean-catch specimen:

➤ Instruct the male patient to (1) thoroughly wash his hands, (2) cleanse the meatus, (3) void a small amount into the toilet, and (4) void directly into the specimen container.

➤ Instruct the female patient to (1) thoroughly wash her hands; (2) cleanse the labia from front to back; (3) while keeping the labia sepa-

rated, void a small amount into the toilet; and (4) without interrupting the urine stream, void directly into the specimen container.

Timed specimen:

➤ Obtain a clean 3-L urine specimen container, toilet-mounted collection device, and plastic bag (for transport of the specimen container). The specimen must be refrigerated or kept on ice throughout the entire collection period. If an indwelling urinary catheter is in place, the drainage bag must be kept on ice.

➤ Begin the test between 6 and 8 a.m., if possible. Collect first voiding and discard. Record the time the specimen was discarded as the beginning of the timed collection period. The next morning, ask the patient to void at the same time the collection was started and add this last voiding to the container.

➤ If an indwelling catheter is in place, replace the tubing and container system at the start of the collection time. Keep the container system on ice during the collection period, or empty the urine into a larger container periodically during the collection period; monitor to ensure continued drainage, and conclude the test the next morning at the same hour the collection was begun.

➤ At the conclusion of the test, compare the quantity of urine with the urinary output record for the collection; if the specimen contains less than what was recorded as output, some urine may have been discarded, invalidating the test.

➤ Label the specimen, and promptly transport it to the laboratory. Include on the label the amount of urine, test start and stop times, and ingestion of any foods or medications that can affect test results.

Post-test:

➤ If appropriate, educate patients with low sodium levels that the major source of dietary sodium is found in table salt. Many foods, such as milk and other dairy products, are also good sources of dietary sodium. Most other dietary sodium is available through the consumption of processed foods. Patients on low-sodium diets should be advised to avoid beverages such as colas, ginger ale, sports drinks, lemon-lime sodas, and root beer. Many over-the-counter medications including antacids, laxatives, analgesics, sedatives, and antitussives contain significant amounts of sodium. The best advice is to emphasize the importance of reading all food, beverage, and medicine labels. In 1989, the Subcommittee on the 10th Edition of the RDA established 500 mg as the recommended maximum daily intake for dietary intake of sodium.

➤ Evaluate test results in relation to the patient's symptoms and other tests performed. Related laboratory tests include aldosterone, kidney stone analysis, serum and urine osmolality, potassium, urine potassium, renin, and sodium.

SYNOVIAL FLUID ANALYSIS

SYNONYMS/ACRONYM: Arthrocentesis, joint fluid analysis, knee fluid analysis.

SPECIMEN: Synovial fluid collected in a red-top tube for antinuclear antibodies (ANAs), complement, crystal examination, protein, rheumatoid factor (RF), and uric acid; sterile (red-top) tube for microbiologic testing; lavender-top (ethylenediaminetetra-acetic acid [EDTA]) tube for complete blood count (CBC) and differential; gray-top (sodium fluoride [NaFl]) tube for glucose; green-top (heparin) tube for lactic acid and pH.

REFERENCE VALUE: (Method: Macroscopic evaluation of appearance; spectrophotometry for glucose, lactic acid, protein, and uric acid; Gram stain, acid-fast stain, and culture for microbiology; microscopic examination of fluid for cell count and evaluation of crystals; ion-selective electrode for pH; nephelometry for RF and C3; indirect fluorescence for ANAs)

Color	Colorless to pale yellow
Clarity	Clear
Viscosity	High
ANA	Parallels serum level
C3	Parallels serum level
Glucose	Less than 10 mg/dL of blood level
Lactic acid	5–20 mg/dL
pH	7.2–7.4
Protein	Less than 3 g/dL

(Continued on the following page)

RF	Parallels serum level
Uric acid	Parallels serum level
Crystals	None present
RBC count	None
WBC count	Less than 200/mm³
Neutrophils	Less than 25%
WBC morphology	No abnormal cells or inclusions
Gram stain and culture	No organisms present
AFB smear and culture	No AFB present

ANA = antinuclear antibodies; C3 = complement; RF = rheumatoid factor; RBC = red blood cell; WBC = white blood cell; AFB = acid-fast bacilli.

DESCRIPTION: Synovial fluid analysis is performed via arthrocentesis, an invasive procedure involving insertion of a needle into the joint space. Synovial effusions are associated with disorders or injuries involving the joints. The most commonly aspirated joint is the knee, although samples also can be obtained from the shoulder, hip, elbow, wrist, and ankle, if clinically indicated. Joint disorders can be classified into five categories: noninflammatory, inflammatory, septic, crystal-induced, and hemorrhagic. ■

INDICATIONS:
• Assist in the evaluation of joint effusions
• Differentiate gout from pseudogout

RESULT

Fluid values increased in:
• *Acute bacterial arthritis:* White blood cell (WBC) count 10,000 to 200,000/mm³, marked predominance of neutrophils (90 percent of cases), positive Gram stain (50 percent of cases), positive cultures (30 to 80 percent of cases), possible presence of Rice bodies, increased lactic acid, and complement levels paralleling those found in serum (may be elevated or decreased)
• *Gout:* WBC count 500 to 200,000/mm³ with a predominance

of neutrophils (approximately 70 percent), presence of monosodium urate crystals, increased uric acid, and complement levels paralleling those of serum (may be elevated or decreased)

• *Osteoarthritis, degenerative joint disease:* WBC count less than 5000/mm³ with a normal differential and the presence of cartilage cells

• *Pseudogout:* Presence of calcium pyrophosphate crystals

• *Rheumatoid arthritis:* WBC count 2000 to 100,000/mm³ with a predominance of neutrophils (30 to 50 percent), presence of ragocyte cells and possibly Rice bodies, presence of cholesterol crystals if effusion is chronic, increased protein, increased lactic acid, and presence of rheumatoid factor (60 percent of cases)

• *Systemic lupus erythematosus (SLE):* WBC count 2000 to 100,000/mm³ with a predominance of neutrophils (30 to 40 percent), presence of SLE cells, and presence of antinuclear antibodies (20 percent of cases)

• *Trauma, joint tumors, or hemophilic arthritis:* Elevated RBC count, increased protein level, and presence of fat droplets (if trauma involved)

• *Tuberculous arthritis:* WBC count 2000 to 100,000/mm³ with a predominance of neutrophils (30 to 60 percent), possible presence of Rice bodies, presence of cholesterol crystals if effusion is chronic, in some cases a positive culture and smear for acid-fast bacilli (results frequently negative), and lactic acid

Fluid values decreased in (analytes in parentheses are decreased):

* Acute bacterial arthritis (glucose and pH)

* Gout (glucose)

* Rheumatoid arthritis (glucose, pH, and complement)

* SLE (glucose, pH, and complement)

* Tuberculous arthritis (glucose and pH)

CRITICAL VALUES: N/A

INTERFERING FACTORS:

* Blood in the sample from traumatic arthrocentesis may falsely elevate the RBC count.

* Undetected hypoglycemia or hyperglycemia may produce misleading glucose values.

* Refrigeration of the sample may result in an increase in monosodium urate crystals secondary to decreased solubility of uric acid; exposure of the sample to room air with a resultant loss of carbon dioxide and rise in pH encourages the formation of calcium pyrophosphate crystals.

Nursing Implications and Procedure • • • • • • • • • •

Pretest: ■

➤ Obtain a history of the patient's complaints, including a list of known allergens.

➤ Obtain a history of the patient's immune and musculoskeletal systems as well as results of previously performed tests and procedures. For related tests, refer to the immune and musculoskeletal system tables.

➤ Obtain a list of medications the patient is taking, including herbs,

nutritional supplements, and nutraceuticals. The requesting health care practitioner and laboratory should be advised if the patient regularly uses these products so that their effects can be taken into consideration when reviewing results.

➤ There are no fluid restrictions unless by medical direction. Fasting for at least 12 hours before the procedure is recommended if fluid glucose measurements are included in the analysis.

➤ Ensure that anticoagulant medications and aspirin have been withheld, as ordered.

➤ Review the procedure with the patient. Inform the patient that it may be necessary to shave the site before specimen collection.

➤ Inform the patient that a local anesthetic will be administered before the procedure.

➤ Assess if the patient has an allergy to local anesthetics, and inform the health care practitioner accordingly.

➤ *Obtain written and informed consent before administering any medications prior to the procedure.*

➤ Inform the patient that the procedure will be performed by a physician specializing in this branch of medicine (possibly an orthopedic surgeon) and can take approximately 20 minutes to complete.

Intratest: ■

➤ Direct the patient to breathe normally and to avoid unnecessary movement.

➤ Record baseline vital signs.

➤ Observe standard precautions and follow the general guidelines in Appendix A.

➤ Assemble the necessary equipment, including an arthrocentesis tray with solution for skin preparation, local anesthetic, a 20-mL syringe, needles of various sizes, sterile drapes, sterile gloves, and specimen collection tubes and containers for the tests to be performed.

➤ Assist the patient to the sitting or supine position, as appropriate; cleanse the skin with antiseptic solution using sterile technique; and protect the site with sterile drapes. Inform the patient that injection of the anesthetic can cause a stinging sensation. Also inform the patient that some pain may be experienced as the aspirating needle is inserted into the joint space and the fluid withdrawn. After the local anesthetic is administered, the needle is inserted at the collection site, and fluid is removed by syringe. Manual pressure may be applied to facilitate fluid removal.

➤ If medication is injected into the joint, the syringe containing the sample is detached from the needle and replaced with the one containing the drug. The medication is injected with gentle pressure. The needle is withdrawn, and digital pressure is applied to the site for a few minutes. If there is no evidence of bleeding, a sterile dressing is applied to the site. An elastic bandage can be applied to the joint.

➤ Label the specimens, place them in the appropriate containers, and promptly transport them to the laboratory. If bacterial culture and sensitivity tests are to be performed, record on the specimen containers any antibiotic therapy the patient is receiving.

Post-test:

➤ Instruct the patient to resume usual diet and medication, if withheld and as directed by the requesting health care practitioner.

➤ Compare vital signs with baseline values.

➤ Assess puncture site for bleeding, bruising, inflammation, and excessive drainage of synovial fluid approximately every 4 hours for 24 hours and daily thereafter for several days.

➤ Instruct the patient or caregiver to handle linen and dispose of dressings cautiously, especially if septic arthritis is suspected.

➤ Instruct the patient to apply an ice pack to the site for 24 to 48 hours, and administer ordered analgesics as needed.

➤ Instruct the patient to avoid excessive use of the joint for several days to prevent pain and swelling.

➤ Instruct the patient to report excessive pain, bleeding, or swelling to the requesting health care practitioner immediately and to return for a follow-up visit as scheduled.

➤ Evaluate test results in relation to the patient's symptoms and other tests performed. Related laboratory tests include rheumatoid factor and uric acid.

SYPHILIS SEROLOGY

SYNONYMS/ACRONYMS: Automated reagin testing (ART), fluorescent treponemal antibody testing (FTA-ABS), microhemagglutination–*Treponema pallidum* (MHA-TP), rapid plasma reagin (RPR), treponemal studies, Venereal Disease Research Laboratory (VDRL) testing.

SPECIMEN: Serum (1 mL) collected in a red- or tiger-top tube.

REFERENCE VALUE: (Method: Darkfield microscopy, rapid plasma reagin, enzyme-linked immunosorbent assay [ELISA], microhemagglutination, fluorescence) Nonreactive or absence of treponemal organisms.

DESCRIPTION: There are numerous methods for detecting *Treponema pallidum,* the organism known to cause syphilis. Syphilis serology is routinely ordered as part of a prenatal workup and is required for evaluating donated blood units before release for transfusion. Selection of the proper testing method is important. Automated reagin testing (ART), rapid plasma reagin (RPR), and Venereal Disease Research Laboratory (VDRL) testing should be used for screening purposes. Fluorescent treponemal antibody testing (FTA-ABS) and microhemagglutination–*Treponema pallidum* (MHA-TP) are confirmatory methods for samples that screen positive or reactive. Cerebrospinal fluid should be tested only by the FTA-ABS method. Cord blood should not be submitted for testing by any of the aforementioned methods; instead, the mother's serum should be tested to establish whether the infant should be treated. ■

INDICATIONS:

- Screen for and confirm the presence of syphilis
- Monitor effectiveness of treatment for syphilis

RESULT

Positive or reactive findings in:

- Syphilis

False-positive or false-reactive findings in screening (RPR, VDRL) tests:

- Infectious:
  Bacterial endocarditis
  Chancroid
  Chickenpox
  Human immunodeficiency virus
  Infectious mononucleosis
  Leprosy
  Leptospirosis
  Lymphogranuloma venereum
  Malaria
  Measles
  Mumps
  Mycoplasma pneumoniae
  Pneumococcal pneumonia
  Psittacosis
  Rickettsial disease
  Relapsing fever
  Scarlet fever
  Trypanosomiasis
  Tuberculosis
  Vaccinia (live or attenuated)
  Viral hepatitis

- Noninfectious:
  Advanced cancer
  Advancing age
  Chronic liver disease
  Connective tissue diseases
  Intravenous drug use
  Multiple myeloma and other immunologic disorders
  Multiple blood transfusions
  Narcotic addiction
  Pregnancy

False-positive or false-reactive findings in confirmatory (FTA-ABS, MHA-TP) tests:

- Infectious:
  Infectious mononucleosis
  Leprosy
  Leptospirosis
  Lyme disease
  Malaria
  Relapsing fever

- Noninfectious:
  Systemic lupus erythematosus

Negative or nonreactive findings in: N/A

CRITICAL VALUES: N/A

INTERFERING FACTORS: N/A

Nursing Implications and Procedure • • • • • • • • • • •

Pretest: ■

➤ Obtain a history of the patient's complaints, including a list of known allergens. Obtain a history of exposure.

➤ Obtain a history of the patient's immune and reproductive systems, as well as results of previously performed tests and procedures. For related tests, refer to the immune and reproductive system tables.

➤ Obtain a list of medications the patient is taking, including herbs, nutritional supplements, and nutraceuticals. The requesting health care practitioner and laboratory should be advised if the patient regularly uses these products so that their effects can be taken into consideration when reviewing results.

➤ There are no food, fluid, or medication restrictions unless by medical direction.

➤ Review the procedure with the patient.

➤ Inform the patient that specimen collection takes approximately 5 to 10 minutes.

Intratest: ■

➤ Direct the patient to breathe normally and to avoid unnecessary movement.

➤ Observe standard precautions and follow the general guidelines in Appendix A. Perform a venipuncture, and collect the specimen in a 5-mL red- or tiger-top tube.

➤ Label the specimen, and promptly transport it to the laboratory.

Post-test: ■

➤ Observe venipuncture site for bleeding or hematoma formation. Apply pressure bandage.

➤ Recognize anxiety related to test results and offer support. Provide teaching and information regarding the clinical implications of the test results, as appropriate. Educate the patient regarding access to counseling services.

➤ Counsel the patient, as appropriate, regarding the risk of transmission and proper prophylaxis, and reinforce the importance of strict adherence to the treatment regimen.

➤ Inform the patient that positive findings must be reported to local health department officials, who will question him or her regarding sexual partners.

➤ Offer support, as appropriate, to patients who may be the victim of rape or sexual assault. Educate the patient regarding access to counseling services. Provide a nonjudgmental, nonthreatening atmosphere for a discussion during which risks of sexually transmitted diseases are explained. It is also important to discuss problems the patient may experience (e.g., guilt, depression, anger).

➤ Inform the patient that repeat testing may be needed at 3-month intervals for 1 year to monitor the effectiveness of treatment.

➤ Evaluate test results in relation to the patient's symptoms and other tests performed. Related laboratory tests include related cultures and serologies for sexually transmitted diseases.

TESTOSTERONE, TOTAL

SYNONYM/ACRONYM: N/A.

SPECIMEN: Serum (1 mL) collected in a red- or tiger-top tube. Plasma (1 mL) collected in green-top (heparin) tube is also acceptable.

REFERENCE VALUE: (Method: Radioimmunoassay)

Age	Conventional Units	SI Units (Conversion Factor × 0.0347)
Cord blood		
Male	13–55 ng/dL	0.45–1.91 nmol/L
Female	5–45 ng/dL	0.17–1.56 nmol/L
Newborn		
Male	75–400 ng/dL	2.6–13.9 nmol/L
Female	20–64 ng/dL	0.69–2.22 nmol/L
1–5 mo		
Male	1–177 ng/dL	0.03–6.14 nmol/L
Female	1–5 ng/dL	0.03–0.17 nmol/L
6–11 mo		
Male	2–7 ng/dL	0.07–0.24 nmol/L
Female	2–5 ng/dL	0.07–0.17 nmol/L
1–5 y		
Male	2–25 ng/dL	0.07–0.87 nmol/L
Female	2–10 ng/dL	0.07–0.35 nmol/L
6–9 y		
Male	3–30 ng/dL	0.10–1.04 nmol/L
Female	2–20 ng/dL	0.07–0.35 nmol/L
10–11 y		
Male	5–50 ng/dL	0.17–1.73 nmol/L
Female	5–25 ng/dL	0.17–0.87 nmol/L
12–14 y		
Male	10–572 ng/dL	0.35–19.83 nmol/L
Female	10–40 ng/dL	0.35–1.39 nmol/L
15–17 y		
Male	220–800 ng/dL	7.63–27.74 nmol/L
Female	5–40 ng/dL	0.17–1.39 nmol/L
Adult		
Male	280–1100 ng/dL	9.71–38.14 nmol/L
Female	15–70 ng/dL	0.52–2.43 nmol/L

DESCRIPTION: Testosterone is the major androgen responsible for sexual differentiation. In males, testosterone is made by the Leydig cells in the testicles and is responsible for spermatogenesis and the development of secondary sex characteristics. In females, the ovary and adrenal gland secrete small amounts of this hormone; however, most of the testosterone in females comes from the metabolism of androstenedione. In males, a testicular, adrenal, or pituitary tumor can cause an overabundance of testosterone, triggering precocious puberty. In females, adrenal tumors, hyperplasia, and medications can cause an overabundance of this hormone, resulting in masculinization or hirsutism. ■

INDICATIONS:
- Assist in the diagnosis of hypergonadism
- Assist in the diagnosis of male sexual precocity before age 10
- Distinguish between primary and secondary hypogonadism
- Evaluate hirsutism
- Evaluate male infertility

RESULT

Increased in:
- Adrenal hyperplasia
- Adrenocortical tumors
- Hirsutism
- Hyperthyroidism
- Idiopathic sexual precocity
- Polycystic ovaries
- Syndrome of androgen resistance
- Testicular or extragonadal tumors
- Trophoblastic tumors during pregnancy
- Virilizing ovarian tumors

Decreased in:
- Anovulation
- Cryptorchidism
- Delayed puberty
- Down's syndrome
- Excessive alcohol intake
- Hepatic insufficiency
- Impotence
- Klinefelter's syndrome
- Malnutrition
- Myotonic dystrophy
- Orchiectomy
- Primary and secondary hypogonadism
- Primary and secondary hypopituitarism
- Uremia

CRITICAL VALUES: N/A

INTERFERING FACTORS:
- Drugs that may increase testosterone levels include barbiturates, bromocriptine, cimetidine, flutamide, gonadotropin, levonorgestrel, mifepristone, moclobemide, nafarelin (males), nilutamide, oral contraceptives, rifampin, and tamoxifen.
- Drugs that may decrease testosterone levels include cyclophosphamide, cyproterone, danazol, dexamethasone, diethylstilbestrol, digoxin, D-Trp-6-LHRH, fenoldopam, goserelin, ketoconazole, leuprolide, magnesium sulfate, medroxyprogesterone, methylprednisone, nandrolone, oral contraceptives, pravastatin, prednisone, pyridoglutethimide, spironolactone, stanozolol, tetracycline, and thioridazine.

• Recent radioactive scans or radiation within 1 week before the test can interfere with test results when radioimmunoassay is the test method.

Nursing Implications and Procedure • • • • • • • • • • •

Pretest: ■

➤ Obtain a history of the patient's complaints, including a list of known allergens.

➤ Obtain a history of the patient's endocrine and reproductive systems, as well as results of previously performed tests and procedures. For related tests, refer to the endocrine and reproductive system tables.

➤ Obtain a list of medications the patient is taking, including herbs, nutritional supplements, and nutraceuticals. The requesting health care practitioner and laboratory should be advised if the patient regularly uses these products so that their effects can be taken into consideration when reviewing results.

➤ Note any recent procedures that can interfere with test results.

➤ There are no food, fluid, or medication restrictions unless by medical direction.

➤ Review the procedure with the patient.

➤ Inform the patient that specimen collection takes approximately 5 to 10 minutes.

Intratest: ■

➤ Direct the patient to breathe normally and to avoid unnecessary movement.

➤ Observe standard precautions and follow the general guidelines in Appendix A. Perform a venipuncture, and collect the specimen in a 5-mL red- or tiger-top tube.

➤ Label the specimen, and promptly transport it to the laboratory.

Post-test: ■

➤ Observe venipuncture site for bleeding or hematoma formation. Apply pressure bandage.

➤ Recognize anxiety related to test results and offer support, as appropriate. Educate the patient regarding access to counseling services.

➤ Evaluate test results in relation to the patient's symptoms and other tests performed. Related laboratory tests include adrenocorticotropic hormone, cortisol, dehydroepiandrosterone sulfate, follicle-stimulating hormone, and luteinizing hormone.

THYROGLOBULIN

• •

SYNONYM/ACRONYM: Tg.

SPECIMEN: Serum (1 mL) collected in a red- or tiger-top tube.

REFERENCE VALUE: (Method: Radioimmunoassay)

Age	Conventional Units	SI Units (Conversion Factor ×1)
Cord blood	20.7–28.1 ng/mL	20.7–28.1 µg/L
1 h	25.5–33.9 ng/mL	25.5–33.9 µg/L
48 h	36.1–47.7 ng/mL	36.1–47.7 µg/L
Adult	3.0–42.0 ng/mL	3.0–42.0 µg/L
Athyrotic patient	Less than 5 ng/mL	Less than 5 µg/L

DESCRIPTION: Thyroglobulin is an iodinated glycoprotein secreted by follicular epithelial cells of the thyroid gland. It is the storage form of the thyroid hormones thyroxine (T_4) and triiodothyronine (T_3). When thyroid hormones are released into the bloodstream, they split from thyroglobulin in response to thyroid-stimulating hormone. Values greater than 50 ng/mL are indicative of tumor recurrence in athyrotic patients. ∎

INDICATIONS:
- Assist in the diagnosis of subacute thyroiditis
- Assist in the diagnosis of suspected disorders of excess thyroid hormone
- Management of differentiated or metastatic cancer of the thyroid
- Monitor response to treatment of goiter
- Monitor T_4 therapy in patients with solitary nodules

RESULT

Increased in:
- Differentiated thyroid cancer
- Graves' disease (untreated)
- Neonates
- Pregnancy
- Surgery or irradiation of the thyroid (elevated levels indicate residual or disseminated carcinoma)
- T_4-binding globulin deficiency
- Thyroiditis
- Thyrotoxicosis

Decreased in:
- Administration of thyroid hormone
- Congenital athyrosis (neonates)
- Thyrotoxicosis factitia

CRITICAL VALUES: N/A

INTERFERING FACTORS:
- Drugs that may decrease thyroglobulin levels include neomycin and T_4.
- Autoantibodies to thyroglobulin can cause decreased values.
- Recent radioactive scans or radiation can interfere with test results when radioimmunoassay is the test method.
- Recent thyroid surgery or needle biopsy can interfere with test results.

Nursing Implications and Procedure • • • • • • • • • • •

Pretest:
➤ Obtain a history of the patient's complaints, including a list of known allergens.
➤ Obtain a history of the patient's endocrine system as well as results of previously performed tests and procedures. For related tests, refer to the endocrine system table.
➤ Obtain a list of medications the patient is taking, including herbs, nutritional supplements, and nutraceuticals. The requesting health care practitioner and laboratory should be advised if the patient is regularly using these products so

that their effects can be taken into consideration when reviewing results.

➤ Note any recent procedures that can interfere with test results.

➤ There are no food, fluid, or medication restrictions unless by medical direction.

➤ Review the procedure with the patient.

➤ Inform the patient that specimen collection takes approximately 5 to 10 minutes.

Intratest: ■

➤ Direct the patient to breathe normally and to avoid unnecessary movement.

➤ Observe standard precautions and follow the general guidelines in Appendix A. Perform a venipuncture, and collect the specimen in a 5-mL red- or tiger-top tube.

➤ Label the specimen and promptly transport to the laboratory.

Post-test: ■

➤ Observe venipuncture site for bleeding or hematoma formation. Apply pressure bandage.

➤ Evaluate test results in relation to the patient's symptoms and other tests performed. Related laboratory tests include thyroid-stimulating hormone, T_4, free T_4, T_3, and free T_3.

THYROID-BINDING INHIBITORY IMMUNOGLOBULIN

· ·

SYNONYMS/ACRONYM: Thyrotropin-receptor antibodies, thyrotropin-binding inhibitory immunoglobulin, TBII.

SPECIMEN: Serum (1 mL) collected in a red-top tube.

REFERENCE VALUE: (Method: Radioreceptor) Less than 10 percent inhibition. (*Note*: In patients with Graves' disease, inhibition is expected to be 10 to 100 percent.)

DESCRIPTION: There are two functional types of thyroid-receptor immunoglobulins: *thyroid-stimulating immunoglobulin* (TSI) and *thyroid-binding inhibitory immunoglobulin* (TBII). TSI reacts with the receptors, activates intracellular enzymes, and promotes epithelial cell activity that operates outside the feedback regulation for thyroid-stimulating hormone (TSH; see monograph titled "Thyroid-Stimulating Immunoglobulin"); TBII blocks the action of TSH and is believed to cause certain types of hyperthyroidism. These antibodies were formerly known as *long-acting thyroid stimulators*. High levels in pregnancy may have some predictive value for neonatal thyrotoxicosis:

A positive result indicates that the antibodies are stimulating (TSI); a negative result indicates that the antibodies are blocking (TBII). TBII testing measures thyroid-receptor immunoglobulin levels in the evaluation of thyroid disease. ∎

INDICATIONS:

• Evaluate suspected acute toxic goiter

• Investigate suspected neonatal thyroid disease secondary to maternal thyroid disease

• Monitor hyperthyroid patients at risk for relapse or remission

RESULT

Increased in:
• Graves' disease

• Hyperthyroidism (various forms)

• Toxic goiter

• Maternal thyroid disease

• Neonatal thyroid disease

Decreased in: N/A

CRITICAL VALUES: N/A

INTERFERING FACTORS:
• Lithium may cause false-positive results.

• Recent radioactive scans or radiation within 1 week before the test can interfere with test results when radioimmunoassay is the test method.

Nursing Implications and Procedure • • • • • • • • •

Pretest: ■

➤ Obtain a history of the patient's complaints, including a list of known allergens.

➤ Obtain a history of the patient's endocrine system as well as results of previously performed tests and procedures. For related tests, refer to the endocrine system table.

➤ Obtain a list of medications the patient is taking, including herbs, nutritional supplements, and nutraceuticals. The requesting health care practitioner and laboratory should be advised if the patient regularly uses these products so that their effects can be taken into consideration when reviewing results.

➤ Note any recent procedures that can interfere with test results.

➤ There are no food, fluid, or medication restrictions unless by medical direction.

➤ Review the procedure with the patient.

➤ Inform the patient that specimen collection takes approximately 5 to 10 minutes.

Intratest: ■

➤ Direct the patient to breathe normally and to avoid unnecessary movement.

➤ Observe standard precautions and follow the general guidelines in Appendix A. Perform a venipuncture, and collect the specimen in a 5-mL red-top tube.

➤ Label the specimen, and promptly transport it to the laboratory.

Post-test: ■

➤ Observe venipuncture site for bleeding or hematoma formation. Apply pressure bandage.

➤ Evaluate test results in relation to the patient's symptoms and other tests performed. Related laboratory tests include TSH and thyroid-stimulating immunoglobulins.

THYROID SCAN

. . . .

SYNONYMS/ACRONYM: Thyroid scintiscan, iodine thyroid scan, technetium thyroid scan.

AREA OF APPLICATION: Thyroid.

CONTRAST: Oral radioactive iodine or intravenous technetium-99m pertechnetate.

DESCRIPTION: The thyroid scan is a nuclear medicine study performed to assess thyroid size, shape, position, and function; it is useful for evaluating thyroid nodules, multinodular goiter, and thyroiditis; assisting in the differential diagnosis of masses in the neck, base of the tongue, and mediastinum; and ruling out possible ectopic thyroid tissue in these areas. Thyroid scanning is performed after oral administration of radioactive iodine-123 (I-123) or I-131, or intravenous (IV) injection of technetium-99m (Tc-99m). Increased or decreased uptake by the thyroid gland and surrounding area and tissue is noted: Areas of increased radionuclide uptake ("hot spots") are caused by hyperfunctioning thyroid nodules, which are usually nonmalignant; areas of decreased uptake ("cold spots") are caused by hypofunctioning nodules, which are more likely to be malignant. Ultrasound imaging may be used to determine if the cold spot is a solid, semicystic lesion or a pure cyst (cysts are rarely cancerous). To determine whether the cold spot depicts a malignant neoplasm, however, a biopsy must be performed. ▪

INDICATIONS:
- Assess the presence of a thyroid nodule or enlarged thyroid gland
- Detect thyroid dysfunction
- Detect benign or malignant thyroid tumors
- Assess palpable nodules and differentiate between a benign tumor or cyst and a malignant tumor
- Detect causes of neck or substernal masses
- Differentiate between Graves' disease and Plummer's disease, both of which cause hyperthyroidism
- Evaluate thyroid function in hyperthyroidism and hypothyroidism (analysis combined with interpretation of laboratory tests, thyroid function panel including thyroxine and triiodothyronine, and thyroid uptake tests)
- Detect forms of thyroiditis (e.g., acute, chronic, Hashimoto's)

RESULT

Normal Findings:
- Normal size, contour, position, and function of the thyroid gland with homogeneous uptake of the radionuclide

Abnormal Findings:

- Adenoma

- Cysts

- Fibrosis

- Goiter

- Graves' disease (diffusely enlarged, hyperfunctioning gland)

- Hematoma

- Metastasis

- Plummer's disease (nodular hyperfunctioning gland)

- Tumors, benign or malignant

- Thyroiditis (Hashimoto's)

- Thyrotoxicosis

CRITICAL VALUES: N/A

INTERFERING FACTORS:

This procedure is contraindicated for:

- Patients who are pregnant or suspected of being pregnant, unless the potential benefits of the procedure far outweigh the risks to the fetus or mother

Factors that may impair clear imaging:

- Inability of the patient to cooperate or remain still during the procedure because of age, significant pain, or mental status

- Improper adjustment of the radiographic equipment to accommodate obese or thin patients, which can cause overexposure or underexposure and a poor-quality study

- Patients who are very obese, who may exceed the weight limit for the equipment

- Incorrect positioning of the patient, which may produce poor visualization of the area to be examined

- Other nuclear scans done within the previous 24 to 48 hours

- Ingestion of foods containing iodine (iodized salt), medications containing iodine (cough syrup, potassium iodide, vitamins, Lugol's solution, thyroid replacement medications), which can decrease the uptake of the radionuclide

- Antithyroid medications (propylthiouracil), corticosteroids, antihistamines, warfarin, sulfonamides, nitrates, corticosteroids, thyroid hormones, and isoniazid, which can decrease the uptake of the radionuclide

- Increased uptake of iodine in persons with an iodine-deficient diet or who are on phenothiazine therapy

- Vomiting and severe diarrhea, which could affect absorption of orally administered radionuclide

- Gastroenteritis, which can interfere with absorption of orally administered radionuclide

- Metallic objects within the examination field (e.g., jewelry or body rings), which may inhibit organ visualization and can produce unclear images

Other considerations:

- Improper injection of the radionuclide that allows the tracer to seep deep into the muscle tissue can produce erroneous hot spots.

- Recent use of iodinated contrast medium for radiographic studies or recently performed nuclear medicine procedures can affect the uptake of the radionuclide.

- Consultation with a physician should occur before the procedure for radiation safety concerns regarding infants of patients who are lactating.

- Risks associated with radiographic overexposure can result from frequent x-ray procedures. Personnel in the room with the patient should wear a protective lead apron, stand behind a shield, or leave the area while the examination is being done. Personnel working in the area where the examination is being done should wear badges that reveal their level of exposure to radiation.

Nursing Implications and Procedure • • • • • • • • • • • •

Pretest: ■

➤ Inform the patient that the procedure assesses thyroid function and structure.

➤ Inform the patient that the procedure is performed in a special nuclear medicine department by a technologist and usually takes approximately 30 minutes.

➤ Obtain a history of the patient's complaints, including a list of known allergens.

➤ Obtain a history of the patient's thyroid system as well as results of previously performed laboratory tests, surgical procedures, thyroid therapy, and other radiologic procedures. For related tests, refer to the endocrine system table.

➤ Obtain a list of medications the patient is taking, including herbs, nutritional supplements, and nutraceuticals.

➤ All thyroid blood tests should be done before doing this test.

➤ Determine date of last menstrual period and possibility of pregnancy in perimenopausal women.

➤ All radiographic procedures done with iodinated contrast medium should be scheduled after this procedure and after radioactive iodine uptake is completed.

➤ Ensure that the patient fasted for 8 to 12 hours before the procedure, unless otherwise indicated.

Intratest: ■

➤ Ask the patient to void before the procedure. Have the patient put on a hospital gown.

➤ Administer sedative to a child or to an uncooperative adult, as ordered.

➤ Ask the patient to lie still during the procedure because movement produces unclear images. Make sure jewelry and any other metallic objects have been removed from the neck area.

➤ Administer oral I-123 24 hours before scanning or IV technetium-99m 20 minutes before scanning. Place the patient in a supine position on a flat table. Scanning is performed over the anterior neck area, and the images are recorded on film or stored electronically for recall and postprocedural interpretation by a physician.

➤ Wear gloves during the radionuclide administration and while handling the patient's urine.

Post-test: ■

➤ Instruct the patient to resume normal activity, medications, and diet, unless otherwise indicated.

➤ Advise patient to drink increased amounts of fluids for 24 to 48 hours to eliminate the radionuclide from the body, unless contraindicated. Tell the patient that radionuclide is eliminated from the body within 6 to 24 hours.

➤ Instruct the patient to flush the toilet immediately after each voiding following the procedure and to wash hands meticulously with soap and water after each voiding for 24 hours after the procedure.

➤ Tell all caregivers to wear gloves when discarding urine for 24 hours after the procedure. Wash gloved hands with soap and water before removing gloves. Then wash hands after the gloves are removed.

➤ A physician specializing in this branch of medicine sends a written report to the ordering provider, who discusses the results with the patient.

➤ Evaluate test results in relation to the patient's symptoms and other tests performed. Related diagnostic tests include thyroid uptake and thyroid ultrasound.

THYROID-STIMULATING HORMONE

· ·

SYNONYM/ACRONYM: Thyrotropin, TSH.

SPECIMEN: Serum (1 mL) collected in a red- or tiger-top tube; for a neonate, use filter paper.

REFERENCE VALUE: (Method: Immunoassay)

Age	Conventional Units	SI Units (Conversion Factor ×1)
Neonates–3 d	Less than 20 µIU/mL	Less than 20 mIU/L
Adults	0.4–4.2 µIU/mL	0.4–4.2 mIU/L

DESCRIPTION: Thyroid-stimulating hormone (TSH) is produced by the pituitary gland in response to stimulation by thyrotropin-releasing hormone (TRH), a hypothalamic-releasing factor. TRH regulates the release and circulating levels of thyroid hormones in response to variables such as cold, stress, and increased metabolic need. Thyroid and pituitary function can be evaluated by TSH measurement. TSH exhibits diurnal variation, peaking between midnight and 4 a.m. and troughing between 5 and 6 p.m. TSH values are high at birth but reach adult levels in the first week of life. Elevated TSH levels combined with decreased thyroxine (T_4) levels indicate hypothyroidism and thyroid gland dysfunction. In general, decreased TSH and T_4 levels indicate secondary congenital hypothyroidism and pituitary hypothalamic dysfunction. A normal TSH level and a depressed T_4 level may indicate (1) hypothyroidism owing to a congeni-

tal defect in T_4-binding globulin, or (2) transient congenital hypothyroidism owing to hypoxia or prematurity. Early diagnosis and treatment in the neonate are crucial for the prevention of cretinism and mental retardation. ■

INDICATIONS:

• Assist in the diagnosis of congenital hypothyroidism

• Assist in the diagnosis of hypothyroidism or hyperthyroidism or suspected pituitary or hypothalamic dysfunction

• Differentiate functional euthyroidism from true hypothyroidism in debilitated individuals

RESULT

Increased in:

• Congenital hypothyroidism in the neonate (filter paper test)

• Ectopic TSH-producing tumors (lung, breast)

• Primary hypothyroidism

- Secondary hyperthyroidism owing to pituitary hyperactivity

- Thyroid hormone resistance

- Thyroiditis (Hashimoto's autoimmune disease)

Decreased in:

- Excessive thyroid hormone replacement

- Graves' disease

- Primary hyperthyroidism

- Secondary hypothyroidism (pituitary involvement)

- Tertiary hypothyroidism (hypothalamic involvement)

CRITICAL VALUES: N/A

INTERFERING FACTORS:

- Drugs and hormones that may increase TSH levels include amiodarone, benserazide, erythrosine, flunarizine (males), iobenzamic acid, iodides, lithium, methimazole, metoclopramide, morphine, propranolol, radiographic agents, TRH, and valproic acid.

- Drugs and hormones that may decrease TSH levels include amiodarone, anabolic steroids, acetylsalicylic acid, carbamazepine, corticosteroids, dopamine, glucocorticoids, hydrocortisone, insulin-like growth factor-I, interferon-alfa-2b, iodamide, josamycin, levodopa, levothyroxine, methergoline, nifedipine, pyridoxine, T_4, and triiodothyronine (T_3).

- Failure to let the filter paper sample dry may affect test results.

Nursing Implications and Procedure . . . .

➤ Obtain a history of the patient's

complaints, including a list of known allergens.

➤ Obtain a history of the patient's endocrine system and results of previously performed tests and procedures. For related tests, refer to the endocrine system table.

➤ Obtain a list of medications the patient is taking, including herbs, nutritional supplements, and nutraceuticals. The requesting health care practitioner and laboratory should be advised if the patient regularly uses these products so that their effects can be taken into consideration when reviewing results.

➤ There are no food, fluid, or medication restrictions unless by medical direction.

➤ Review the procedure with the patient.

➤ Inform the patient that specimen collection takes approximately 5 to 10 minutes.

Intratest:

➤ Direct the patient to breathe normally and to avoid unnecessary movement.

➤ Observe standard precautions and follow the general guidelines in Appendix A. Perform a venipuncture, and collect the specimen in a 5-mL red- or tiger-top tube. Label the specimen, and promptly transport it to the laboratory.

Filter paper test (neonate):

➤ Obtain kit and cleanse heel with antiseptic. Observe standard precautions and follow the general guidelines in Appendix A. Use gauze to dry the stick area completely. Perform heel stick, gently squeeze infant's heel, and touch filter paper to the puncture site. Completely fill the circles on the filter paper, saturating the filter paper with blood. Apply pressure to the heel stick with a gauze pad to stop the bleeding. Allow the filter paper to dry thoroughly, label the specimen, and promptly transport it to the laboratory. Alternatively, if a specimen collection kit is used, follow instructions for labeling and mailing to the testing laboratory.

Post-test:

➤ Observe venipuncture site for bleed-

ing or hematoma formation. Apply pressure bandage.

➤ Evaluate test results in relation to the patient's symptoms and other tests performed. Related laboratory tests include adrenocorticotropic hormone, TRH stimulation test, T_4, free T_4, and T_3.

THYROID-STIMULATING IMMUNOGLOBULIN

SYNONYM/ACRONYM: Thyrotropin-receptor antibodies, TSI.

SPECIMEN: Serum (1 mL) collected in a red-top tube.

REFERENCE VALUE: (Method: Radioimmunoassay) Less than 130 percent of basal activity.

DESCRIPTION: There are two functional types of thyroid-receptor immunoglobulins: *thyroid-stimulating immunoglobulin* (TSI) and *thyroid-binding inhibitory immunoglobulin* (TBII). TSI reacts with the receptors, activates intracellular enzymes, and promotes epithelial cell activity that operates outside the feedback regulation for thyroid-stimulating hormone (TSH; see monograph titled "Thyroid-Stimulating Immunoglobulin"); TBII blocks the action of TSH and is believed to cause certain types of hyperthyroidism. These antibodies were formerly known as *long-acting thyroid stimulators.* High levels in pregnancy may have some predictive value for neonatal thyrotoxicosis: A positive result indicates that the

antibodies are stimulating (TSI); a negative result indicates that the antibodies are blocking (TBII). TSI testing measures thyroid-receptor immunoglobulin levels in the evaluation of thyroid disease. ■

INDICATIONS:

• Follow-up to positive TBII assay in differentiating antibody stimulation from neutral or suppressing activity

• Monitor hyperthyroid patients at risk for relapse or remission

RESULT

Increased in: Graves' disease

Decreased in: N/A

CRITICAL VALUES: N/A

INTERFERING FACTORS:

- Lithium may cause false-positive TBII results.

- Recent radioactive scans or radiation can interfere with test results when radioimmunoassay is the test method.

Nursing Implications and Procedure • • • • • • • • • • •

Pretest: ◼

➤ Obtain a history of the patient's complaints, including a list of known allergens.

➤ Obtain a history of the patient's endocrine system as well as results of previously performed tests and procedures. For related tests, refer to the endocrine system table.

➤ Obtain a list of medications the patient is taking, including herbs, nutritional supplements, and nutraceuticals. The requesting health care practitioner and laboratory should be advised if the patient regularly uses these products so that their effects can be taken into consideration when reviewing results.

➤ Note any recent procedures that can interfere with test results.

➤ There are no food, fluid, or medication restrictions unless by medical direction.

➤ Review the procedure with the patient.

➤ Inform the patient that specimen collection takes approximately 5 to 10 minutes.

Intratest: ◼

➤ Direct the patient to breathe normally and to avoid unnecessary movement.

➤ Observe standard precautions and follow the general guidelines in Appendix A. Perform a venipuncture, and collect the specimen in a 5-mL red-top tube.

➤ Label the specimen, and promptly transport it to the laboratory.

Post-test: ◼

➤ Observe venipuncture site for bleeding or hematoma formation. Apply pressure bandage.

➤ Evaluate test results in relation to the patient's symptoms and other tests performed. Related laboratory tests include thyroglobulin, TBII, and TSH.

THYROTROPIN-RELEASING HORMONE STIMULATION TEST

• •

SYNONYM/ACRONYM: TRH stimulation.

SPECIMEN: Serum (1 mL) collected in a red- or tiger-top tube.

REFERENCE VALUE: (Method: Immunoassay) Minimal rise of 1 to 2 mIU/L above baseline; typical response is a 5- to 10-fold increase above baseline.

DESCRIPTION: In the thyrotropin-releasing hormone (TRH) stimulation test, TRH is administered intravenously after collection of a baseline measurement of thyroid-stimulating hormone (TSH). Subsequent specimens are collected for TSH measurement at 30- and 60-minute intervals. An exaggerated response is an indication of abnormal thyroid gland function or disorders of the hypothalamic pituitary axis. Third-generation or "sensitive" TSH assays are now preferred over TRH stimulation. ■

INDICATIONS:
• Assist in the diagnosis and treatment of hypothalamic and pituitary disorders

• Differentiation of mania from schizophrenia

RESULT

Increased in:
• Pregnancy

• Primary hypothyroidism

Decreased in:
• Major depressive illnesses

• Primary hyperthyroidism

• Secondary hypothyroidism

CRITICAL VALUES: N/A

INTERFERING FACTORS: N/A

Nursing Implications and Procedure · · · · · · · · · · ·

Pretest: ■

➤ Obtain a history of the patient's complaints, including a list of known allergens.

➤ Obtain a history of the patient's endocrine system and results of previously performed tests and procedures. For related tests, refer to the endocrine system table.

➤ Obtain a list of medications the patient is taking, including herbs, nutritional supplements, and nutraceuticals. The requesting health care practitioner and laboratory should be advised if the patient regularly uses these products so that their effects can be taken into consideration when reviewing results.

➤ There are no food, fluid, or medication restrictions unless by medical direction.

➤ The test should be performed in the morning because of the diurnal variation in TSH secretion.

➤ Review the procedure with the patient. Inform the patient that multiple specimens will be collected.

➤ Inform the patient that each specimen collection takes approximately 5 to 10 minutes.

Intratest: ■

➤ Direct the patient to breathe normally and to avoid unnecessary movement.

➤ Inform the patient that he or she may experience temporary nausea (mild), flushing, dizziness, peculiar taste, rise in blood pressure, and an urge to urinate as the infusion begins.

➤ Observe standard precautions and follow the general guidelines in Appendix A. Perform a venipuncture, and collect the specimen in a 5-mL red- or tiger-top tube.

➤ Begin intravenous infusion of 500 µg of protirelin (Thypinone), and collect specimens at 30- and 60-minute intervals.

➤ Monitor the patient's blood pressure if dizziness or other unusual symptoms are reported.

➤ Label the specimen, and promptly transport it to the laboratory.

the patient's symptoms and other tests performed. Related laboratory tests include adrenocorticotropin hormone, follicle-stimulating hormone, growth hormone, luteinizing hormone, thyroxine, and free thyroxine.

THYROXINE-BINDING GLOBULIN

SYNONYM/ACRONYM: TBG.

SPECIMEN: Serum (1 mL) collected in a red- or tiger-top tube.

REFERENCE VALUE: (Method: Radioimmunoassay)

Age	Conventional Units	SI Unit (Conversion Factor ×10)
0–1 wk	3–8 mg/dL	30–80 mg/L
1–12 mo	1.6–3.6 mg/dL	16–36 mg/L
14 y–adult	1.2–2.5 mg/dL	12–25 mg/L
Adult		
Pregnancy, third trimester	4.7–5.9 mg/dL	47–59 mg/L
Oral contraceptives	1.5–5.5 mg/dL	15–55 mg/L

DESCRIPTION: Thyroxine-binding globulin (TBG) is the predominant protein carrier for circulating thyroxine (T_4) and triiodothyronine (T_3). T_4-binding prealbumin and T_4-binding albumin are the other transport proteins. Conditions that affect TBG levels and binding capacity also affect free T_3 and free T_4 levels. ∎

INDICATIONS:

• Differentiate elevated T_4 due to hyperthyroidism from increased TBG binding in euthyroid patients

• Evaluate hypothyroid patients

• Identify deficiency or excess TBG due to hereditary abnormality

RESULT

Increased in:

• Acute intermittent porphyria

• Genetically high TBG

• Hypothyroidism

• Infectious hepatitis and other liver diseases

• Neonates

• Pregnancy

Decreased in:

• Acromegaly

• Chronic hepatic disease

• Genetically low TBG

• Marked hypoproteinemia, malnutrition

• Major illness

• Nephrotic syndrome

• Ovarian hypofunction

• Surgical stress

• Testosterone-producing tumors

CRITICAL VALUES: N/A

INTERFERING FACTORS:

• Drugs and hormones that may increase TBG levels include estrogens, oral contraceptives, tamoxifen, and perphenazine.

• Drugs that may decrease TBG levels include anabolic steroids, androgens, asparaginase, corticosteroids, corticotropin, danazol, phenytoin, and propranolol.

• Recent radioactive scans or radiation within 1 week before the test can interfere with test results when radioimmunoassay is the test method.

Nursing Implications and Procedure • • • • • • • • • •

Pretest: ▪

➤ Obtain a history of the patient's complaints, including a list of known allergens.

➤ Obtain a history of the patient's

endocrine system as well as results of previously performed tests and procedures. For related tests, refer to the endocrine system table.

➤ Obtain a list of medications the patient is taking, including herbs, nutritional supplements, and nutraceuticals. The requesting health care practitioner and laboratory should be advised if the patient regularly uses these products so that their effects can be taken into consideration when reviewing results.

➤ Note any recent procedures that can interfere with test results.

➤ There are no food, fluid, or medication restrictions unless by medical direction.

➤ Review the procedure with the patient.

➤ Inform the patient that specimen collection takes approximately 5 to 10 minutes.

Intratest: ▪

➤ Direct the patient to breathe normally and to avoid unnecessary movement.

➤ Observe standard precautions and follow the general guidelines in Appendix A. Perform a venipuncture, and collect the specimen in a 5-mL red- or tiger-top tube.

➤ Label the specimen, and promptly transport it to the laboratory.

Post-test: ▪

➤ Observe venipuncture site for bleeding or hematoma formation. Apply pressure bandage.

➤ Evaluate test results in relation to the patient's symptoms and other tests performed. Related tests include T_4, free T_4, T_3, and free T_3.

THYROXINE, FREE

• •

SYNONYMS/ACRONYM: Free T_4, FT_4.

SPECIMEN: Serum (1 mL) collected in a red- or tiger-top tube. Plasma (1 mL) collected in green-top (heparin) tube is also acceptable.

REFERENCE VALUE: (Method: Immunoassay)

Age	Conventional Units	SI Units (Conversion Factor ×12.9)
Newborn	0.8–2.8 ng/dL	10–36 pmol/L
1–12 mo	0.8–2.0 ng/dL	10–26 pmol/L
1–18 y	0.8–1.7 ng/dL	10–22 pmol/L
Adult	0.8–1.5 ng/dL	10–19 pmol/L

DESCRIPTION: Thyroxine (T_4) is a hormone produced and secreted by the thyroid gland. Newborns are commonly tested for decreased T_4 levels by a filter paper method (see monograph titled "Thyroxine, Total"). Most T_4 in the serum (99.97 percent) is bound to thyroxine-binding globulin (TBG), prealbumin, and albumin. The remainder (0.03 percent) circulates as unbound or free T_4, which is the physiologically active form. Levels of free T_4 are proportional to levels of total T_4. The advantage of measuring free T_4 instead of total T_4 is that, unlike total T_4 measurements, free T_4 levels are not affected by fluctuations in TBG levels; as a result, free T_4 levels are considered the most accurate indicator of T_4 and its thyrometabolic activity. Free T_4 measurements are useful in evaluating thyroid disease when thyroid-stimulating hormone (TSH) levels alone provide insuffi-

cient information. Free T_4 and TSH levels are inversely proportional. Measurement of free T_4 is also recommended during treatment for hyperthyroidism, until symptoms have abated and levels have decreased into the normal range. ■

INDICATIONS:
• Evaluate signs of hypothyroidism or hyperthyroidism

• Monitor response to therapy for hypothyroidism or hyperthyroidism

RESULT

Increased in:
• Hyperthyroidism

• Hypothyroidism treated with T_4

Decreased in:
• Hypothyroidism

• Hypothyroidism treated with triiodothyronine (T_3)

• Pregnancy (late)

CRITICAL VALUES: N/A

INTERFERING FACTORS:
- Drugs that may increase free T_4 levels include amiodarone, acetylsalicylic acid, halofenate, heparin, iopanoic acid, levothyroxine, methimazole, and radiographic agents.

- Drugs that may decrease free T_4 levels include amiodarone, anabolic steroids, asparaginase, methadone, methimazole, oral contraceptives, and phenylbutazone.

Nursing Implications and Procedure

Pretest:

➤ Obtain a history of the patient's complaints, including a list of known allergens.

➤ Obtain a history of the patient's endocrine system as well as results of previously performed tests and procedures. For related tests, refer to the endocrine system table.

➤ Obtain a list of medications the patient is taking, including herbs, nutritional supplements, and nutraceuticals. The requesting health care practitioner and laboratory should be advised if the patient regularly uses these products so that their effects can be taken into consideration when reviewing results.

➤ There are no food, fluid, or medication restrictions unless by medical direction.

➤ Review the procedure with the patient.

➤ Inform the patient that specimen collection takes approximately 5 to 10 minutes.

Intratest:

➤ Direct the patient to breathe normally and to avoid unnecessary movement.

➤ Observe standard precautions and follow the general guidelines in Appendix A. Perform a venipuncture, and collect the specimen in a 5-mL red- or tiger-top tube.

➤ Label the specimen, and promptly transport it to the laboratory.

Post-test:

➤ Observe venipuncture site for bleeding or hematoma formation. Apply pressure bandage.

➤ Evaluate test results in relation to the patient's symptoms and other tests performed. Related laboratory tests include antithyroglobulin and antiperoxidase antibodies, thyroid-stimulating immunoglobulins, thyroid-binding inhibitory immunoglobulins, TSH, T_4, T_3, and free T_3.

THYROXINE, TOTAL

SYNONYMS/ACRONYM: T_4.

SPECIMEN: Serum (1 mL) collected in a red- or tiger-top tube. Plasma (1 mL) collected in green-top (heparin) tube is also acceptable.

REFERENCE VALUE: (Method: Immunoassay)

Age	Conventional Units	SI Units (Conversion Factor ×12.9)
1–3 d	11.8–22.6 μg/dL	152–292 nmol/L
1–2 wk	9.8–16.6 μg/dL	126–214 nmol/L
1–4 mo	7.2–14.4 μg/dL	93–186 nmol/L
5–12 mo	7.8–16.5 μg/dL	101–213 nmol/L
1–5 y	7.3–15.0 μg/dL	94–194 nmol/L
5–10 y	6.4–13.3 μg/dL	83–172 nmol/L
10–15 y	5.6–11.7 μg/dL	72–151 nmol/L
Adult		
Man	4.6–10.5 μg/dL	59–135 nmol/L
Woman	5.5–11.0 μg/dL	71–142 nmol/L
Pregnant woman	5.5–16.0 μg/dL	71–155 nmol/L
Over 60 y	5.0–10.7 μg/dL	65–138 nmol/L

DESCRIPTION: Thyroxine (T_4) is a hormone produced and secreted by the thyroid gland. Newborns are commonly tested for decreased T_4 levels by a filter paper method. Most T_4 in the serum (99.97 percent) is bound to thyroxine-binding globulin (TBG), prealbumin, and albumin. The remainder (0.03 percent) circulates as unbound or free T_4, which is the physiologically active form. Levels of free T_4 are proportional to levels of total T_4. The advantage of measuring free T_4 instead of total T_4 is that, unlike total T_4 measurements, free T_4 levels are not affected by fluctuations in TBG levels; as a result, free T_4 levels are considered the most accurate indicator of T_4 and its thyrometabolic activity. (See monograph titled "Thyroxine, Free.") ■

INDICATIONS:
- Evaluate signs of hypothyroidism or hyperthyroidism and neonatal screening for congenital hypothyroidism (required in many states)
- Evaluate thyroid response to protein deficiency associated with severe illnesses
- Monitor response to therapy for hypothyroidism or hyperthyroidism

RESULT

Increased in:
- Acute psychiatric illnesses
- Excessive intake of iodine
- Hepatitis
- Hyperemesis gravidarum
- Hyperthyroidism
- Obesity
- Thyrotoxicosis factitia
- Thyrotoxicosis due to Graves' disease

Decreased in:
- Decreased TBG (nephrotic syndrome, liver disease, gastrointestinal protein loss, malnutrition)
- Hypothyroidism
- Panhypopituitarism
- Strenuous exercise

CRITICAL VALUES: ⚠️

Hypothyroidism: Less than 2.0 μg/dL

Hyperthyroidism: Greater than 20.0 μg/dL

At levels less than 2.0 µg/dL, the patient is at risk for myxedema coma. Signs and symptoms of severe hypothyroidism include hypothermia, hypotension, bradycardia, hypoventilation, lethargy, and coma. Possible interventions include airway support, hourly monitoring for neurologic function and blood pressure, and administration of intravenous thyroid hormone.

At levels greater than 20.0 µg/dL, the patient is at risk for thyroid storm. Signs and symptoms of severe hyperthyroidism include hyperthermia, diaphoresis, vomiting, dehydration, and shock. Possible interventions include supportive treatment for shock, fluid and electrolyte replacement for dehydration, and administration of antithyroid drugs (propylthiouracil and Lugol's solution).

INTERFERING FACTORS:

• Drugs that may increase T_4 levels include amiodarone, amphetamines, corticosteroids, ether, fluorouracil, glucocorticoids, halofenate, insulin, iobenzamic acid, iopanoic acid, ipodate, levarterenol, levodopa, levothyroxine, opiates, oral contraceptives, phenothiazine, and prostaglandins.

• Drugs, substances, and treatments that may decrease T_4 levels include aminoglutethimide, aminosalicylic acid, amiodarone, anabolic steroids, anticonvulsants, asparaginase, acetylsalicylic acid, barbiturates, carbimazole, chlorpromazine, chlorpropamide, cholestyramine, clofibrate, cobalt, colestipol, corticotropin, cortisone, cotrimoxazole, cytostatic therapy, danazol, dehydroepiandrosterone, dexamethasone, diazepam, diazo dyes, dinitrophenol, ethionamide, Evans blue, fenclofenac, halofenate, hydroxyphenylpyruvic acid, interferon alfa-2b, iothiouracil, iron, isotretinoin, liothyronine, lithium, lovastatin, methimazole, methylthiouracil, mitotane, norethindrone, penicillamine, penicillin, phenylacetic acid derivatives, phenylbutazone, potassium iodide, propylthiouracil, reserpine, salicylate, sodium nitroprusside, stanozolol, sulfonylureas, tetrachlorothyronine, tolbutamide, and triiodothyronine (T_3).

Nursing Implications and Procedure

Pretest:

➤ Obtain a history of the patient's complaints.

➤ Obtain a history of the patient's endocrine system and results of previously performed tests and procedures. For related tests, refer to the endocrine system table.

➤ Obtain a list of medications the patient is taking, including herbs, nutritional supplements, and nutraceuticals. The requesting health care practitioner and laboratory should be advised if the patient regularly uses these products so that their effects can be taken into consideration when reviewing results.

➤ There are no food, fluid, or medication restrictions unless by medical direction.

➤ Review the procedure with the patient.

➤ Inform the patient that specimen collection takes approximately 5 to 10 minutes.

Intratest:

➤ Direct the patient to breathe normally and to avoid unnecessary movement.

➤ Observe standard precautions and follow the general guidelines in Appendix A. Perform a venipuncture, and collect the specimen in a 5-mL red- or tiger-top tube.

➤ Label the specimen, and promptly transport it to the laboratory.

tests include adrenocorticotropic hormone, antithyroglobulin and antithyroid peroxidase antibodies, thyroid-binding inhibitory immunoglobulin, thyroxine-binding globulin, thyroid-stimulating hormone, thyroid-stimulating immunoglobulin, free T_4, T_3, and free T_3.

TOTAL PROTEIN AND FRACTIONS

SYNONYMS/ACRONYMS: TP, SPEP (fractions include albumin, α_1-globulin, α_2-globulin, β-globulin, and γ-globulin).

SPECIMEN: Serum (1 mL) collected in a red- or tiger-top tube.

REFERENCE VALUE: (Method: Spectrophotometry for total protein, electrophoresis for protein fractions)

Total Protein

Age	Conventional Units	SI Units (Conversion Factor ×10)
Newborn–5 d	3.8–6.2 g/dL	38–62 g/L
1–3 y	5.9–7.0 g/dL	59–70 g/L
4–6 y	5.9–7.8 g/dL	59–78 g/L
7–9 y	6.2–8.1 g/dL	62–81 g/L
10–19 y	6.3–8.6 g/dL	63–86 g/L
Adult	6.0–8.0 g/dL	60–80 g/L

Protein Fractions

	Conventional Units	SI Units (Conversion Factor ×10)
Albumin	3.4–4.8 g/dL	34–48 g/L
α_1-Globulin	0.2–0.4 g/dL	2–4 g/L
α_2-Globulin	0.4–0.8 g/dL	4–8 g/L
β-Globulin	0.5–1.0 g/dL	5–10 g/L
γ-Globulin	0.6–1.2 g/dL	6–12 g/L

DESCRIPTION: Protein is essential to all physiologic functions. Proteins consist of amino acids, the building blocks of blood and body tissues. Protein is also required for the regulation of metabolic processes, immunity, and proper water balance. Total protein includes albumin and globulins. α_1-Globulin includes α_1-antitrypsin, α_1-fetoprotein, α_1-acid glycoprotein, α_1-antichymotrypsin, inter-α_1-trypsin inhibitor, high-density lipoproteins, and group-specific component (vitamin D–binding protein). α_2-Globulin includes haptoglobin, ceruloplasmin, and α_2-macroglobulin. β-Globulin includes transferrin, hemopexin, very-low-density lipoproteins, low-density lipoproteins, β_2-microglobulin, fibrinogen, complement, and C-reactive protein. γ-Globulin includes immunoglobulin G (IgG), IgA, IgM, IgD, and IgE. After an acute infection or trauma, many of the liver-derived proteins increase, whereas albumin decreases; these conditions may not reflect an abnormal total protein determination. ∎

INDICATIONS:
- Evaluation of edema, as seen in patients with low total protein and low albumin levels
- Evaluation of nutritional status

RESULT

Increased:
- α_1-Globulin proteins in acute and chronic inflammatory diseases
- α_2-Globulin proteins occasionally in diabetes, pancreatitis, and hemolysis
- β-Globulin proteins in hyperlipoproteinemias and monoclonal gammopathies
- γ-Globulin proteins in chronic liver diseases, chronic infections, autoimmune disorders, hepatitis, cirrhosis, and lymphoproliferative disorders
- Total protein:
  Dehydration
  Monoclonal and polyclonal gammopathies
  Myeloma
  Sarcoidosis
  Some types of chronic liver disease
  Tropical diseases (e.g., leprosy)
  Waldenström's macroglobulinemia

Decreased:
- α_1-Globulin proteins in hereditary deficiency
- α_2-Globulin proteins in nephrotic syndrome, malignancies, numerous subacute and chronic inflammatory disorders, recovery stage of severe burns
- β-Globulin proteins in hypo-β-lipoproteinemias and IgA deficiency
- γ-Globulin proteins in immune deficiency or suppression
- Total protein
  Administration of intravenous fluids
  Burns
  Chronic alcoholism
  Chronic ulcerative colitis
  Cirrhosis
  Crohn's disease
  Glomerulonephritis
  Heart failure
  Hyperthyroidism
  Malabsorption
  Malnutrition
  Neoplasms
  Nephrotic syndrome
  Pregnancy
  Prolonged immobilization
  Protein-losing enteropathies
  Severe skin disease
  Starvation

CRITICAL VALUES: N/A

INTERFERING FACTORS:

• Drugs that may increase protein levels include amino acids (if given intravenously), anabolic steroids, angiotensin, anticonvulsants, carbenicillin, corticosteroids, corticotropin, digitalis, furosemide, insulin, isotretinoin, levonorgestrel, oral contraceptives, progesterone, radiographic agents, and thyroid agents.

• Drugs and substances that may decrease protein levels include arginine, acetylsalicylic acid, benzene, carvedilol, citrates, floxuridine, laxatives, mercury compounds, oral contraceptives, pentastarch, phosgene, pyrazinamide, rifampin, trimethadione, and valproic acid.

• Values are significantly lower (5 to 10 percent) in recumbent patients.

• Hemolysis can falsely elevate results.

• Venous stasis can falsely elevate results; the tourniquet should not be left on the arm for longer than 60 seconds.

Nursing Implications and Procedure • • • • • • • • • • •

Pretest:

➤ Obtain a history of the patient's complaints, including a list of known allergens.

➤ Obtain a history of the patient's gastrointestinal, hepatobiliary, and immune systems, as well as results of previously performed tests and procedures. For related tests, refer to the gastrointestinal, hepatobiliary, and immune system tables.

➤ Obtain a list of medications the patient is taking, including herbs, nutritional supplements, and nutraceuticals. The requesting health care practitioner and laboratory should be advised if the patient regularly uses these products so that their effects can be taken into consideration when reviewing results.

➤ There are no food, fluid, or medication restrictions unless by medical direction.

➤ Review the procedure with the patient.

➤ Inform the patient that specimen collection takes approximately 5 to 10 minutes.

Intratest:

➤ Direct the patient to breathe normally and to avoid unnecessary movement.

➤ Observe standard precautions and follow the general guidelines in Appendix A. Perform a venipuncture, and collect the specimen in a 5-mL red- or tiger-top tube.

➤ Label the specimen, and promptly transport it to the laboratory.

Post-test:

➤ Observe venipuncture site for bleeding or hematoma formation. Apply pressure bandage.

➤ Educate the patient, as appropriate, that good dietary sources of complete protein (containing all eight essential amino acids) include meat, fish, eggs, and dairy products; and that good sources of incomplete protein (lacking one or more of the eight essential amino acids) include grains, nuts, legumes, vegetables, and seeds.

➤ Evaluate test results in relation to the patient's symptoms and other tests performed. Related laboratory tests include albumin, complete blood count, urine protein electrophoresis, serum and urine immunofixation electrophoresis, IgA, IgG, IgM, and urine protein.

TOXOPLASMA ANTIBODY

SYNONYMS/ACRONYM: Toxoplasmosis serology, toxoplasmosis titer.

SPECIMEN: Serum (1 mL) collected in a red-top tube.

REFERENCE VALUE: (Method: Indirect fluorescent antibody) Negative or less than a fourfold increase in titer.

DESCRIPTION: Toxoplasmosis is a severe, generalized granulomatous central nervous system disease caused by the protozoan *Toxoplasma gondii.* Transmission to humans occurs by ingesting undercooked meat or handling contaminated matter such as cat litter. Immunoglobulin M (IgM) antibodies develop approximately 5 days after infection and can remain elevated for 3 weeks to several months. IgG antibodies develop 1 to 2 weeks after infection and can remain elevated for months or years. *Toxoplasma* serology is part of the TORCH (*to*xoplasmosis, *ru*bella, *c*ytomegalovirus, *h*erpes simplex type 2) panel routinely performed on pregnant women. Fetal infection during the first trimester can cause spontaneous abortion or congenital defects. Immunocompromised individuals are also at high risk for serious complications if infected. The presence of IgM antibodies indicates acute or congenital infection; the presence of IgG antibodies indicates current or past infection. ∎

INDICATIONS:
• Assist in establishing a diagnosis of toxoplasmosis

• Document past exposure or immunity
• Serologic screening during pregnancy

RESULT

Positive findings in: Toxoplasma infection

CRITICAL VALUES: N/A

INTERFERING FACTORS: N/A

Nursing Implications and Procedure

Pretest:

➤ Obtain a history of the patient's complaints, including a list of known allergens. Obtain a history of exposure.

➤ Obtain a history of the patient's immune and reproductive systems, dietary history, and history of other potential sources of exposure; as well as results of previously performed tests and procedures. For related tests, refer to the immune and reproductive system tables.

➤ Obtain a list of medications the patient is taking, including herbs, nutritional supplements, and nutraceuticals. The requesting health care practitioner and laboratory should be advised if the patient regularly uses these products so that their effects can be taken into consideration when reviewing results.

➤ There are no food, fluid, or medication restrictions unless by medical direction.

➤ Review the procedure with the patient.

➤ Inform the patient that several tests may be necessary to confirm the diagnosis. Any individual positive result should be repeated in 3 weeks to monitor a change in titer.

➤ Inform the patient that each specimen collection takes approximately 5 to 10 minutes.

Intratest:

➤ Direct the patient to breathe normally and to avoid unnecessary movement.

➤ Observe standard precautions and follow the general guidelines in Appendix A. Perform a venipuncture, and collect the specimen in a 5-mL red-top tube.

➤ Label the specimen, and promptly transport it to the laboratory.

Post-test:

➤ Observe venipuncture site for bleeding or hematoma formation. Apply pressure bandage.

➤ Instruct the patient in isolation precautions during time of communicability or contagion.

➤ Emphasize the need to return to have a convalescent blood sample taken in 3 weeks.

➤ Recognize anxiety related to test results and provide emotional support if results are positive and the patient is pregnant and/or immunocompromised. Provide teaching and information regarding the clinical implications of the test results, as appropriate. Educate the patient regarding access to counseling services.

➤ Evaluate test results in relation to the patient's symptoms and other tests performed. Related laboratory tests include cytomegalovirus, herpes simplex, and rubella.

TRANSFERRIN

SYNONYM/ACRONYM: Siderophilin, TRF.

SPECIMEN: Serum (1 mL) collected in a red- or tiger-top tube.

REFERENCE VALUE: (Method: Nephelometry)

Age	Conventional Units	SI Units (Conversion Factor ×0.01)
Newborn	130–275 mg/dL	1.3–2.75 g/L
Adult		
Male	215–365 mg/dL	2.2–3.6 g/L
Female	250–380 mg/dL	2.5–3.8 g/L

DESCRIPTION: Transferrin is a glycoprotein formed in the liver. It transports circulating iron obtained from dietary intake and red blood cell breakdown. Transferrin carries 50 to 70 percent of the body's iron; normally it is approximately one-third saturated. Inadequate transferrin levels can lead to impaired hemoglobin synthesis and anemia. Transferrin is subject to diurnal variation, and it is responsible for the variation in levels of serum iron throughout the day. (See monograph titled "Iron-Binding Capacity [Total], Transferrin, and Iron Saturation.") ∎

INDICATIONS:

• Determine the iron-binding capacity of the blood

• Evaluate iron metabolism in iron-deficiency anemia

• Evaluate nutritional status

• Screen for hemochromatosis

RESULT

Increased in:
• Iron-deficiency anemia

Decreased in:
• Acute or chronic infection

• Cancer (especially of the gastrointestinal tract)

• Excessive protein loss from renal disease

• Hepatic damage

• Malnutrition

• Hereditary atransferrinemia

CRITICAL VALUES: N/A

INTERFERING FACTORS:
• Drugs that may increase transferrin

levels include carbamazepine, danazol, mestranol, and oral contraceptives.

• Drugs that may decrease transferrin levels include cortisone and dextran.

• Transferrin levels are subject to diurnal variation and should be collected in the morning, when levels are highest.

Nursing Implications and Procedure • • • • • • • • • • •

Pretest: ■

➤ Obtain a history of the patient's complaints, including a list of known allergens.

➤ Obtain a history of the patient's hematopoietic system and results of previously performed tests and procedures. For related tests, refer to the hematopoietic system table.

➤ Obtain a list of medications the patient is taking, including herbs, nutritional supplements, and nutraceuticals. The requesting health care practitioner and laboratory should be advised if the patient regularly uses these products so that their effects can be taken into consideration when reviewing results.

➤ There are no fluid or medication restrictions unless by medical direction.

➤ Review the procedure with the patient. Instruct the patient to fast for at least 12 hours before specimen collection.

➤ Inform the patient that specimen collection takes approximately 5 to 10 minutes.

Intratest: ■

➤ Ensure that the patient has complied with dietary preparations and other pretesting restrictions.

➤ Direct the patient to breathe normally and to avoid unnecessary movement.

➤ Observe standard precautions and follow the general guidelines in Appendix A. Perform a venipuncture, and collect the specimen in a 5-mL red- or tiger-top tube.

➤ Label the specimen, and promptly transport it to the laboratory.

Post-test: ■

➤ Observe venipuncture site for bleed-ing or hematoma formation. Apply pressure bandage.

➤ Instruct the patient to resume usual diet as directed by the requesting health care practitioner.

➤ Evaluate test results in relation to the patient's symptoms and other tests performed. Related laboratory tests include ferritin and iron/total iron-binding capacity.

TRIGLYCERIDES

• •

SYNONYM/ACRONYM: Trigs, TG.

SPECIMEN: Serum (1 mL) collected in a red- or tiger-top tube. Plasma (1 mL) collected in green-top (heparin) tube is also acceptable.

REFERENCE VALUE: (Method: Spectrophotometry)

Age	Conventional Units	SI Units (Conversion Factor ×0.0113)	Risk
0–9 y			
Male	30–100 mg/dL	0.34–1.13 mmol/L	
Female	35–110 mg/dL	0.40–1.24 mmol/L	
10–20 y			
Male	32–148 mg/dL	0.36–1.67 mmol/L	
Female	37–124 mg/dL	0.42–1.40 mmol/L	
Adult	Less than 150 mg/dL	Less than 1.70 mmol/L	Normal
	150–199 mg/dL	1.70–2.25 mmol/L	Borderline high
	200–499 mg/dL	2.26–5.64 mmol/L	High
	Greater than 500 mg/dL	Greater than 5.65 mmol/L	Very high

DESCRIPTION: Triglycerides are a combination of three fatty acids and one glycerol molecule. They are necessary to provide energy for various metabolic processes. Excess triglycerides are stored in adipose tissue, and the fatty acids provide the raw materials needed for conversion to glucose (gluconeogenesis) or for direct use as an energy source. Although fatty acids originate in the diet, many are also derived from unused glucose and amino acids that the liver converts into stored energy. Triglyceride levels vary by age, sex, weight, and race:

Levels increase with age.

Levels are higher in men than in women (among women, those who take oral contraceptives have levels that are 20 to 40 mg/dL higher compared to those who do not).

Levels are higher in overweight and obese populations compared to those with normal weight.

Levels in African-Americans are approximately 10 to 20 mg/dL lower compared to Caucasians. ■

INDICATIONS:

- Evaluate known or suspected disorders associated with altered triglyceride levels

- Identify hyperlipoproteinemia (hyperlipidemia) in patients with a family history of the disorder

- Monitor the response to drugs known to alter triglyceride levels

- Screen adults who are either over 40 years of age or obese to estimate the risk for atherosclerotic cardiovascular disease

RESULT

Increased in:
- Acute myocardial infarction
- Alcoholism
- Anorexia nervosa
- Chronic ischemic heart disease
- Cirrhosis

- Glycogen storage disease
- Gout
- Hyperlipoproteinemia
- Hypertension
- Hypothyroidism
- Impaired glucose tolerance
- Nephrotic syndrome
- Obesity
- Pancreatitis (acute and chronic)
- Pregnancy
- Renal failure
- Respiratory distress syndrome
- Stress
- Viral hepatitis
- Werner's syndrome

Decreased in:
- Brain infarction
- Chronic obstructive lung disease (COPD)
- End-stage liver disease
- Hyperparathyroidism
- Hyperthyroidism
- Hypolipoproteinemia and a-β-lipoproteinemia
- Intestinal lymphangiectasia
- Malabsorption disorders
- Malnutrition

CRITICAL VALUES: N/A

INTERFERING FACTORS:

- Drugs that may increase triglyceride levels include acetylsalicylic acid, aldatense, atenolol, bendroflumethiazide, cyclosporine, danazol, glucocorticoids, oral contraceptives, oxprenolol, pindolol, prazosin, propranolol, tamoxifen, and timolol.

• Drugs and substances that may decrease triglyceride levels include ascorbic acid, bezafibrate, captopril, carvedilol, celiprolol, chenodeoxycholic acid, cholestyramine, cilazapril, ciprofibrate, clofibrate, colestipol, dextrothyroxine, doxazosin, enalapril, eptastatin, fenofibrate, flaxseed oil, gemfibrozil, glucagon, halofenate, insulin, levonorgestrel, lovastatin, medroxyprogesterone, metformin, nafenopin, niacin, niceritrol, pinacidil, pindolol, pravastatin, prazosin, probucol, simvastatin, and verapamil.

Nursing Implications and Procedure • • • • • • • • • • •

Pretest:

➤ Obtain a history of the patient's complaints, including a list of known allergens.

➤ Obtain a history of the patient's cardiovascular and gastrointestinal systems, as well as results of previously performed tests and procedures. For related tests, refer to the cardiovascular and gastrointestinal system tables.

➤ Obtain a list of medications the patient is taking, including herbs, nutritional supplements, and nutraceuticals. The health care practitioner and laboratory should be advised if the patient regularly uses these products so that their effects can be taken into consideration when reviewing results.

➤ The patient should fast for 12 hours before specimen collection. Ideally the patient should be on a stable diet for 3 weeks and avoid alcohol consumption for 3 days before specimen collection.

➤ There are no fluid or medication restrictions unless by medical direction.

➤ Review the procedure with the patient.

➤ Inform the patient that specimen collection takes approximately 5 to 10 minutes.

Intratest:

➤ Ensure that the patient has complied with dietary preparations and other pretesting restrictions.

➤ Direct the patient to breathe normally and to avoid unnecessary movement.

➤ Observe standard precautions and follow the general guidelines in Appendix A. Perform a venipuncture, and collect the specimen in a 5-mL red- or tiger-top tube.

➤ Label the specimen, and promptly transport it to the laboratory.

Post-test:

➤ Observe venipuncture site for bleeding or hematoma formation. Apply pressure bandage.

➤ Instruct the patient to resume usual diet as directed by the requesting health care practitioner.

➤ Increased triglyceride levels may be associated with atherosclerosis and coronary artery disease.

➤ Nutritional therapy is recommended for individuals identified to be at high risk for developing coronary artery disease. If overweight, these patients should be encouraged to achieve a normal weight. The American Heart Association has Step 1 and Step 2 diets that may be helpful in achieving a goal of lowering total cholesterol and triglyceride levels. The Step 1 diet emphasizes a reduction in foods high in saturated fats and cholesterol. Red meats, eggs, and dairy products are the major sources of saturated fats and cholesterol. If triglycerides are also elevated, patients should be advised to eliminate or reduce alcohol and simple carbohydrates from their diet. The Step 2 diet recommends stricter reductions.

➤ Numerous studies point to the increased prevalence of excess body weight in American children and adolescents. Experts estimate that

25 percent of American children aged 6 to 11 years are obese. The medical, social, and emotional consequences of excess body weight are significant.

➤ Special attention should be given to instructing the pediatric patient and caregiver regarding health risks and weight control.

➤ Evaluate test results in relation to the patient's symptoms and other tests performed. Related laboratory tests include apolipoprotein A and B, cholesterol, high-density lipoprotein cholesterol, low-density lipoprotein cholesterol, homocysteine, and lipoprotein electrophoresis.

TRIIODOTHYRONINE, FREE

SYNONYMS/ACRONYMS: Free T_3, FT_3.

SPECIMEN: Serum (1 mL) collected in a red- or tiger-top tube.

REFERENCE VALUE: (Method: Immunoassay)

Age	Conventional Units	SI Units (Conversion Factor ×0.0154)
Children and adults	260–480 pg/dL	4.0–7.4 pmol/L
Pregnant women (4–9 mo gestation)	196–338 pg/dL	3.0–5.2 pmol/L

DESCRIPTION: Unlike the thyroid hormone thyroxine (T_4), most T_3 is converted enzymatically from T_4 in the tissues rather than being produced directly by the thyroid gland. (See monograph titled "Thyroxine, Total.") Approximately one-third of T_4 is converted to T_3. Most T_3 in the serum (99.97 percent) is bound to thyroxine-binding globulin (TBG), prealbumin, and albumin. The remainder (0.03 percent) circulates as unbound or free T_3, which is the physiologically active form. Levels of free T_3 are proportional to levels of total T_3. The advantage of measuring free T_3 instead of total T_3 is that, unlike total T_3 measurements, free T_3 levels are not affected by fluctuations in TBG levels. T_3 is four to five times more biologically potent than T_4. This hormone, along with T_4, is responsible for maintaining a euthyroid state. Free T_3 measurements are rarely required, but they are indicated in the diagnosis of T_3 toxicosis and when certain drugs are being administered that interfere with the conversion of T_4 to T_3. ■

INDICATIONS:

* Adjunctive aid to thyroid-stimulating hormone (TSH) and free T_4 assessment

* Assist in the diagnosis of T_3 toxicosis

RESULT

Increased in:

* High altitude

* Hyperthyroidism

* T_3 toxicosis

Decreased in:

* Hypothyroidism

* Malnutrition

* Nonthyroidal chronic diseases

* Pregnancy (late)

CRITICAL VALUES: N/A

INTERFERING FACTORS:

* Drugs that may increase free T_3 include amiodarone, acetylsalicylic acid, and levothyroxine.

* Drugs that may decrease free T_3 include amiodarone, methimazole, phenytoin, propranolol, and radiographic agents.

Nursing Implications and Procedure · · · · · · · · · · · ·

Pretest:

➤ Obtain a history of the patient's complaints, including a list of known allergens.

➤ Obtain a history of the patient's endocrine system and results of previously performed tests and procedures. For related tests, refer to the endocrine system table.

➤ Obtain a list of medications the patient is taking, including herbs, nutritional supplements, and nutraceuticals. The requesting health care practitioner and laboratory should be advised if the patient regularly uses these products so that their effects can be taken into consideration when reviewing results.

➤ There are no food, fluid, or medication restrictions unless by medical direction.

➤ Review the procedure with the patient.

➤ Inform the patient that specimen collection takes approximately 5 to 10 minutes.

Intratest:

➤ Direct the patient to breathe normally and to avoid unnecessary movement.

➤ Observe standard precautions and follow the general guidelines in Appendix A. Perform a venipuncture, and collect the specimen in a 5-mL red- or tiger-top tube.

➤ Label the specimen, and promptly transport it to the laboratory.

Post-test:

➤ Observe venipuncture site for bleeding or hematoma formation. Apply pressure bandage.

➤ Evaluate test results in relation to the patient's symptoms and other tests performed. Some related laboratory tests include TSH, T_4, free T_4, and total T_3.

TRIIODOTHYRONINE, TOTAL

SYNONYM/ACRONYM: T_3.

SPECIMEN: Serum (1 mL) collected in a red- or tiger-top tube. Plasma (1 mL) collected in green-top (heparin) tube is also acceptable.

REFERENCE VALUE: (Method: Immunoassay)

Age	Conventional Units	SI Units (Conversion Factor ×0.0154)
1–3 d	100–740 ng/dL	1.54–11.40 nmol/L
1–12 mo	105–245 ng/dL	1.62–3.77 nmol/L
1–5 y	105–269 ng/dL	1.62–4.14 nmol/L
6–10 y	94–241 ng/dL	1.45–3.71 nmol/L
16–20 y	80–210 ng/dL	1.20–3.20 nmol/L
Adult	70–204 ng/dL	1.08–3.14 nmol/L
Pregnant woman (last 4 mo gestation)	116–247 ng/dL	1.79–3.80 nmol/L

DESCRIPTION: Unlike the thyroid hormone thyroxine (T_4), most T_3 is converted enzymatically from T_4 in the tissues rather than being produced directly by the thyroid gland. (See monograph titled "Thyroxine, Total.") Approximately one-third of T_4 is converted to T_3. Most T_3 in the serum (99.97 percent) is bound to thyroxine-binding globulin (TBG), prealbumin, and albumin. The remainder (0.03 percent) circulates as unbound or free T_3, which is the physiologically active form. Levels of free T_3 are proportional to levels of total T_3. The advantage of measuring free T_3 instead of total T_3 is that, unlike total T_3 measurements, free T_3 levels are not affected by fluctuations in TBG levels. T_3 is four to five times more biologically potent than T_4. This hormone, along with T_4, is responsible for maintaining a euthyroid state. ∎

INDICATIONS: Adjunctive aid to thyroid-stimulating hormone (TSH) and free T_4 assessment

RESULT

Increased in:
- Conditions with increased TBG
- Early thyroid failure
- Hyperthyroidism
- Iodine-deficiency goiter
- Pregnancy
- T_3 toxicosis
- Thyrotoxicosis factitia

• Treated hyperthyroidism

Decreased in:

• Acute and subacute nonthyroidal disease

• Conditions with decreased TBG

• Hypothyroidism

CRITICAL VALUES: N/A

INTERFERING FACTORS:

• Drugs that may increase total T_3 levels include amiodarone, amphetamine, benziodarone, clofibrate, fenoprofen, fluorouracil, halofenate, insulin, levothyroxine, methadone, opiates, oral contraceptives, phenytoin, prostaglandins, T_3, and valproic acid.

• Drugs that may decrease total T_3 levels include amiodarone, anabolic steroids, asparaginase, acetylsalicylic acid, carbamazepine, cholestyramine, clomiphene, colestipol, cotrimoxazole, dexamethasone, fenclofenac, furosemide, glucocorticoids, hydrocortisone, interferon alfa-2b, iobenzamic acid, iodides, ipodate, isotretinoin, lithium, methimazole, neomycin, netilmicin, oral contraceptives, penicillamine, phenobarbital, phenylacetic acid derivatives, phenylbutazone, phenytoin, potassium iodide, prednisone, propranolol, propylthiouracil, radiographic agents, salicylate, sodium ipodate, sulfonylureas, and tyropanoic acid.

Nursing Implications and Procedure

Pretest:

➤ Obtain a history of the patient's complaints, including a list of known allergens.

➤ Obtain a history of the patient's endocrine system and results of previously performed tests and procedures. For related tests, refer to the endocrine system table.

➤ Obtain a list of medications the patient is taking, including herbs, nutritional supplements, and nutraceuticals. The requesting health care practitioner and laboratory should be advised if the patient regularly uses these products so that their effects can be taken into consideration when reviewing results.

➤ There are no food, fluid, or medication restrictions unless by medical direction.

➤ Review the procedure with the patient.

➤ Inform the patient that specimen collection takes approximately 5 to 10 minutes.

Intratest:

➤ Direct the patient to breathe normally and to avoid unnecessary movement.

➤ Observe standard precautions and follow the general guidelines in Appendix A. Perform a venipuncture, and collect the specimen in a 5-mL red- or tiger-top tube.

➤ Label the specimen, and promptly transport it to the laboratory.

Post-test:

➤ Observe venipuncture site for bleeding or hematoma formation. Apply pressure bandage.

➤ Evaluate test results in relation to the patient's symptoms and other tests performed. Some related laboratory tests include TSH hormone, T_4, free T_4, and free T_3.

TROPONINS I AND T

• •

SYNONYMS/ACRONYMS: Cardiac troponin, cardiac troponin I (cTnI), cardiac troponin T (cTnT).

SPECIMEN: Serum (1 mL) collected in a red- or tiger-top tube. Plasma (1 mL) collected in green-top (heparin) tube is also acceptable. Serial sampling is highly recommended. Care must be taken to use the same type of collection container if serial measurements are to be taken.

REFERENCE VALUE: (Method: Enzyme immunoassay)

Troponin I	Less than 0.35 ng/mL
Troponin T	Less than 0.20 μg/L

DESCRIPTION: Troponin is a complex of three contractile proteins that regulate the interaction of actin and myosin. Troponin C is the calcium-binding subunit; it does not have a cardiac muscle–specific subunit. Troponin I and troponin T, however, do have cardiac muscle–specific subunits. They are detectable a few hours to 7 days after the onset of symptoms. Troponin I is thought to be a more specific marker of cardiac damage than troponin T. Cardiac troponin I begins to rise 2 to 6 hours after myocardial infarction (MI). It has a biphasic peak: It initially peaks at 15 to 24 hours after MI and then exhibits a lower peak after 60 to 80 hours. Cardiac troponin T levels rise 2 to 6 hours after MI and remain elevated. Both proteins return to the reference range 7 days after MI. ∎

INDICATIONS:
• Assist in establishing a diagnosis of MI
• Evaluate myocardial cell damage

RESULT

Increased in:
• Acute MI
• Minor myocardial damage
• Myocardial damage after coronary artery bypass graft surgery or percutaneous transluminal coronary angioplasty
• Unstable angina pectoris

Decreased in: N/A

CRITICAL VALUES: N/A

INTERFERING FACTORS: N/A

Nursing Implications and Procedure • • • • • • • • • • •

Pretest:

➤ Obtain a history of the patient's complaints, including a list of known allergens.

> Obtain a history of the patient's cardiovascular system and results of previously performed tests and procedures. For related tests, refer to the cardiovascular system table.

> Obtain a list of medications the patient is taking, including herbs, nutritional supplements, and nutraceuticals. The requesting health care practitioner and laboratory should be advised if the patient regularly uses these products so that their effects can be taken into consideration when reviewing results.

> There are no food, fluid, or medication restrictions unless by medical direction.

> Review the procedure with the patient. Inform the patient that a number of samples will be collected. Collection at time of admission, 2 to 4 hours, 6 to 8 hours, and 12 hours after admission are the minimal recommendations. Additional samples may be requested.

> Inform the patient that specimen collection takes approximately 5 to 10 minutes.

Intratest: ■

> Direct the patient to breathe normally and to avoid unnecessary movement.

> Observe standard precautions and follow the general guidelines in Appendix A. Perform a venipuncture, and collect the specimen in a 5-mL red- or tiger-top tube.

> Label the specimen, and promptly transport it to the laboratory.

Post-test: ■

> Observe venipuncture site for bleeding or hematoma formation. Apply pressure bandage.

> Increased troponin levels are associated with coronary artery disease. Nutritional therapy is recommended for individuals identified to be at high risk for developing coronary artery disease. If overweight, these patients should be encouraged to achieve a normal weight. The American Heart Association has Step 1 and Step 2 diets that may be helpful in achieving a goal of lowering total cholesterol and triglyceride levels. The Step 1 diet emphasizes a reduction in foods high in saturated fats and cholesterol. Red meats, eggs, and dairy products are the major sources of saturated fats and cholesterol. If triglycerides are also elevated, patients should be advised to eliminate or reduce alcohol and simple carbohydrates from their diet. The Step 2 diet recommends stricter reductions.

> Evaluate test results in relation to the patient's symptoms and other tests performed. Related laboratory tests include calcium, creatine kinase and isoenzymes, digoxin, lactate dehydrogenase and isoenzymes, homocysteine, magnesium, myoglobin, and potassium.

TUBERCULIN SKIN TESTS

. . . .

SYNONYMS/ACRONYMS: TB tine test, PPD, Mantoux skin test.

SPECIMEN: N/A.

REFERENCE VALUE: (Method: Intradermal skin test) Negative.

DESCRIPTION: Tuberculin skin tests are done to determine past or present exposure to tuberculosis. The multipuncture or tine test, a screening technique, uses either purified protein derivative (PPD) of tuberculin or old tuberculin. A positive response at the puncture site indicates cell-mediated immunity to the organism or a delayed hypersensitivity caused by interaction of the sensitized T lymphocytes. Verification of the patient's positive response to the multipuncture is done with the more definitive Mantoux test using Aplisol or Tubersol administered by intradermal injection. The Mantoux test is the test of choice in symptomatic patients. It is also used in some settings as a screening test. A negative result is judged if there is no sign of redness or induration at the site of the injection or if the zone of redness and induration is less than 5 mm in diameter. A positive result is evidenced by an area of erythema and induration at the injection site that is greater than 10 mm. A positive result does not distinguish between active and dormant infection. A positive response to the Mantoux test is followed up with chest radiography and bacteriologic sputum testing to confirm diagnosis. ▪

INDICATIONS:
• Evaluate cough, weight loss, fatigue, hemoptysis, and abnormal x-rays to determine if the cause of symptoms is tuberculosis

• Evaluate known or suspected exposure to tuberculosis, with or without symptoms, to determine if tuberculosis is present

• Evaluate patients with medical conditions placing them at risk for tuberculosis (e.g., acquired immunodeficiency syndrome [AIDS], lymphoma, diabetes)

• Screen infants with the tine test at the time of first immunizations to determine tuberculosis exposure

• Screen populations at risk for developing tuberculosis (e.g., health care practitioners, nursing home residents, correctional facility personnel, prison inmates, and residents of the inner city living in poor hygienic conditions)

RESULT

Positive findings in: Pulmonary tuberculosis

CRITICAL VALUES: N/A

INTERFERING FACTORS:
• Drugs such as immunosuppressive agents or steroids can alter results.

• Diseases such as hematologic cancers or sarcoidosis can alter results.

• Recent or present bacterial, fungal, or viral infections may affect results. False-positive results may be caused by the presence of nontuberculous mycobacteria or by serial testing.

• False-negative results can occur if sensitized T cells are temporarily decreased. False-negative results also can occur in the presence of bacterial infections, immunologic deficiencies, immunosuppressive agents, live-virus vaccinations (e.g., measles, mumps, polio, rubella), malnutrition, old age, overwhelming tuberculosis, renal failure, and active viral infections (e.g., chickenpox, measles, mumps).

• Improper storage of the tuberculin solution (e.g., with respect to temperature, exposure to light, and stability on opening) may affect the results.

- Improper technique when performing the intradermal injection (e.g., injecting into subcutaneous tissue) may cause false-negative results.

- Incorrect amount or dilution of antigen injected or delayed injection after drawing the antigen up into the syringe may affect the results.

- Incorrect reading of the measurement of response or timing of the reading may interfere with results.

- It is not known whether the test has ⚠ teratogenic effects or reproductive implications; the test should be administered to pregnant women only when clearly indicated.

- The test should not be administered ⚠ to a patient with a previously positive tuberculin skin test because of the danger of severe reaction, including vesiculation, ulceration, and necrosis.

- The test does not distinguish between current and past infection.

Nursing Implications and Procedure • • • • • • • • • • •

Pretest: ■

➤ Obtain a history of the patient's complaints, including a list of known allergens.

➤ Obtain a history of tuberculosis or tuberculosis exposure, signs and symptoms indicating possible tuberculosis, other diagnostic procedures and results, and other skin test or vaccinations and sensitivities.

➤ Obtain a history of the patient's immune and respiratory systems as well as results of previously performed tests and procedures. For related tests, refer to the immune and respiratory system tables.

➤ Obtain a list of medications the

patient is taking, including herbs, nutritional supplements, and nutraceuticals. The requesting health care practitioner and laboratory should be advised if the patient regularly uses these products so that their effects can be taken into consideration when reviewing results.

➤ There are no food, fluid, or medication restrictions unless by medical direction.

➤ Ensure that the patient does not have tuberculosis and has not had a positive skin test previously before beginning the test.

➤ Do not administer the test if the patient has a skin rash or other eruptions at the test site.

➤ Review the procedure with the patient. Inform the patient that a moderate amount of pain may be experienced when the intradermal injection is performed.

➤ Inform the patient that the procedure takes approximately 5 minutes.

➤ Emphasize to the patient that the area should not be scratched or disturbed after the injection and before the reading.

Intratest: ■

➤ Have epinephrine hydrochloride solution (1:1000) available in the event of anaphylaxis.

➤ Observe standard precautions and follow the general guidelines in Appendix A.

➤ Cleanse the skin site on the lower anterior forearm with alcohol swabs and allow to air-dry.

Multipuncture test:

➤ Remove the cap covering the tines and stretch the forearm skin taut. Firmly press the device into the prepared site, hold it in place for 1 second, and then remove it. Four punctures should be visible. Record the site, and remind the patient to return in 48 to 72 hours to have the test read. At the time of the reading, use a plastic ruler to measure the diameter of the largest indurated area, making sure the room is sufficiently lighted to perform the reading. A palpable induration greater than or equal to 2 mm at one or more of the punctures indicates a positive test result.

Mantoux (intradermal) test:

➤ Prepare PPD or old tuberculin in a tuberculin syringe with a short, 26-gauge needle attached. Prepare the appropriate dilution and amount for the most commonly used intermediate strength (5 tuberculin units in 0.1 mL) or a first strength usually used for children (1 tuberculin unit in 0.1 mL). Inject the preparation intradermally at the prepared site as soon as it is drawn up into the syringe. When properly injected, a bleb or wheal 6 to 10 mm in diameter is formed within the layers of the skin. Record the site, and remind the patient to return in 48 to 72 hours to have the test read. At the time of the reading, use a plastic ruler to measure the diameter of the largest indurated area, making sure the room is sufficiently lighted to perform the reading. Palpate for thickening of the tissue; a positive result is indicated by a reaction of 5 mm or more with erythema and edema.

Post-test: ■

➤ Emphasize to the patient the need to return and have the test results read within the specified time frame of 48 to 72 hours after injection.

➤ Inform the patient that the effects from a positive response at the site can remain for 1 week.

➤ Educate the patient that a positive result may put him or her at risk for infection related to impaired primary defenses, impaired gas exchange related to decrease in effective lung surface, and intolerance to activity related to an imbalance between oxygen supply and demand.

➤ Recognize anxiety related to test results and offer support. Provide teaching and information regarding the clinical implications of the test results, as appropriate. Reinforce information about additional testing needed, answer questions, or direct questions to the appropriate professionals.

➤ Educate the patient regarding access to counseling services.

➤ Evaluate test results in relation to the patient's symptoms and other tests performed. Related laboratory tests include relevant acid-fast cultures and smears.

ULTRASOUND, ARTERIAL DOPPLER, CAROTID STUDIES

• • • • • • • • • • • • • • • ➤ • • • • • • • • • • • • • • •

SYNONYMS/ACRONYM: Carotid Doppler, carotid ultrasound, arterial ultrasound.

AREA OF APPLICATION: Arteries.

CONTRAST: Done without contrast.

DESCRIPTION: Ultrasound procedures are diagnostic, noninvasive, and relatively inexpensive. They take a short time to complete, do not use radiation, and cause no harm to the patient. Using the duplex scanning method, carotid ultrasound records sound waves to obtain information about the carotid arteries. The amplitude and waveform of the carotid pulse are measured, resulting in a two-dimensional image of the artery. Carotid arterial sites used for the studies include the common carotid, external carotid, and internal carotid. Blood flow direction, velocity, and the presence of flow disturbances can be readily assessed. The sound waves hit the moving red blood cells and are reflected back to the transducer, a flashlight-shaped device. The sound that is emitted by the equipment corresponds to the velocity of the blood flow through the vessel. The result is the visualization of the artery to assist in the diagnosis (i.e., presence, amount, location) of plaques causing vessel stenosis or atherosclerotic occlusion affecting the flow of blood to the brain. Depending on the degree of stenosis causing a reduction in vessel diameter, additional testing can be performed to determine the effect of stenosis on the hemodynamic status of the artery. ∎

INDICATIONS:

- Detect plaque or stenosis of the carotid artery, evidenced by turbulent blood flow or changes in Doppler signals indicating occlusion

- Detect irregularities in the structure of the carotid arteries

- Aid in the diagnosis of carotid artery occlusive disease, evidenced by visualization of blood flow disruption

RESULT

Normal Findings:
- Normal blood flow through the carotid arteries with no evidence of occlusion or narrowing

Abnormal Findings:
- Carotid artery occlusive disease (atherosclerosis)

- Plaque or stenosis of carotid artery

- Reduction in vessel diameter of more than 16 percent, indicating stenosis

CRITICAL VALUES: N/A

INTERFERING FACTORS

Factors that may impair clear imaging:
- Inability of the patient to cooperate or remain still during the procedure because of age, significant pain, or mental status

- Incorrect placement of the transducer over the desired test site

- An abnormally large neck, which may make direct examination difficult

Nursing Implications and Procedure ⋅ ⋅ ⋅ ⋅ ⋅ ⋅ ⋅ ⋅ ⋅ ⋅ ⋅

Pretest:

➤ Inform the patient that the procedure assesses the arteries.

➤ Inform the patient that the procedure is performed in a special nuclear medicine department by a technologist and usually takes approximately 30 to 60 minutes.

➤ Obtain a history of previous arterial studies, presence of disorders predisposing the patient to arterial thrombosis, or therapy received for arterial abnormalities.

➤ Assess the presence of disorders

predisposing the patient to cerebral arterial vascular problems.

➤ Obtain the results of other tests, treatments, therapies, surgeries, medication usage, and other procedures done to diagnose disorders of the cardiovascular system. For related tests, refer to the cardiovascular system table.

➤ Inform the patient that the procedure is painless and carries no risks.

➤ Obtain and record baseline vital signs to use for comparison after the procedure, if needed.

Intratest:

➤ Place the patient in a supine position on a table or examining cart.

➤ Expose the area to be examined and support the head to prevent movement.

➤ Apply conductive gel to the skin, and slowly move the transducer over the site in the area of the common carotid artery to the bifurcation and then to areas of the internal and external carotids. Ask the patient to lie still during the proce-

dure because movement produces unclear images.

Post-test:

➤ When the study is completed, remove the gel from the area examined.

➤ Instruct the patient to resume normal activity and diet, unless otherwise indicated.

➤ Instruct the patient to report dizziness, syncope, or blurred vision caused by impaired circulation to the brain (transient ischemic attacks).

➤ A physician specializing in this branch of medicine sends a written report to the ordering provider, who discusses the results with the patient.

➤ Inform the patient that an abnormal examination may indicate the need for further studies.

➤ Evaluate test results in relation to the patient's symptoms and other tests performed. Related diagnostic tests include computed tomography and magnetic resonance angiography.

ULTRASOUND, ARTERIAL DOPPLER, LOWER EXTREMITY STUDIES

· ·

SYNONYMS/ACRONYM: Arterial leg ultrasound, leg sonogram.

AREA OF APPLICATION: Arteries of the lower extremities.

CONTRAST: Done without contrast.

DESCRIPTION: Ultrasound procedures are diagnostic, noninvasive, and relatively inexpensive. They take a short time to complete, do not use radiation, and cause no harm to the

patient. Using the duplex scanning method, arterial leg ultrasound records sound waves to obtain information about the arteries of the lower extremities from the common femoral artery and their branches as they extend into the calf area. The amplitude and waveform of the pulses are measured, resulting in a two-dimensional image of the artery. Blood flow direction, velocity, and the presence of flow disturbances can be readily assessed, and for diagnostic studies, the technique is done bilaterally. The sound waves hit the moving red blood cells and are reflected back to the transducer, a flashlight-shaped device. The sound that is emitted by the equipment corresponds to the velocity of the blood flow through the vessel. The result is the visualization of the artery to assist in the diagnosis and presence, amount, and location of plaques causing vessel stenosis or occlusion and to help determine the cause of claudication. Arterial reconstruction and graft condition and patency can also be evaluated. ∎

INDICATIONS:

- Detect plaque or stenosis of the lower extremity artery, evidenced by turbulent blood flow or changes in Doppler signals indicating occlusion

- Detect irregularities in the structure of the arteries

- Aid in the diagnosis of ischemia, arterial calcification, or plaques, evidenced by visualization of blood flow disruption

- Aid in the diagnosis of aneurysm, pseudoaneurysm, hematoma, arteriovenous malformation, or hemangioma

RESULT

Normal Findings:

- Normal blood flow through the lower extremity arteries with no evidence of vessel occlusion or narrowing

Abnormal Findings:

- Aneurysm

- Arterial calcification or plaques

- Graft diameter reduction

- Hemangioma

- Hematoma

- Ischemia

- Pseudoaneurysm

- Reduction in vessel diameter of more than 16 percent, indicating stenosis

- Vessel occlusion or stenosis

CRITICAL VALUES: N/A

INTERFERING FACTORS:

Factors that may impair clear imaging:

- Inability of the patient to cooperate or remain still during the procedure because of age, significant pain, or mental status

- Incorrect placement of the transducer over the desired test site

- Cold extremities, resulting in vasoconstriction that can cause inaccurate measurements

- Occlusion proximal to the site being studied, which would affect blood flow to the area

- Open wound or incision overlying the area to be examined

- Cigarette smoking, because nicotine can cause constriction of the peripheral vessels

- An abnormally large leg, making direct examination difficult.

Nursing Implications and Procedure ∙ ∙ ∙ ∙ ∙ ∙ ∙ ∙ ∙ ∙ ∙

Pretest:

➤ Inform the patient that the procedure assesses the arteries of the leg.

➤ Inform the patient that the procedure is performed in a special nuclear medicine department by a technologist and usually takes approximately 30 to 60 minutes.

➤ Obtain a history of previous arterial studies, presence of disorders predisposing the patient to arterial thrombosis, or therapy received for arterial abnormalities. For related tests, refer to the cardiovascular system table.

➤ Assess the presence of disorders predisposing the patient to peripheral vascular problems.

➤ Inform the patient that the procedure is painless and carries no risks.

➤ Obtain and record baseline vital signs to use for comparison after the procedure, if needed.

Intratest:

➤ Ask the patient to void before the procedure. Have the patient put on a hospital gown.

➤ Place the patient in a supine position on a table or examining cart, and allow the patient to rest for a minimum of 10 minutes before the examination is started.

➤ Expose the area to be examined and support the leg to prevent movement.

➤ Apply conductive gel to the skin, and slowly move the transducer over the site in the area of the iliac artery. Ask the patient to lie still during the procedure because movement produces unclear images.

➤ For segmental blood pressure assessment, place numerous blood pressure cuffs on the extremity from the thigh to the ankle. Inflate the cuffs and record pressure readings.

Post-test:

➤ When the study is completed, remove the gel from the area examined.

➤ Instruct the patient to resume normal activity and diet, unless otherwise indicated.

➤ A physician specializing in this branch of medicine sends a written report to the ordering provider, who discusses the results with the patient.

➤ Inform the patient that an abnormal examination may indicate the need for additional studies.

➤ Evaluate test results in relation to the patient's symptoms and other tests performed. Related diagnostic tests found in this publication include venous Doppler ultrasound, computed tomography angiography, and magnetic resonance angiography.

ULTRASOUND, BLADDER

SYNONYM/ACRONYM: Bladder sonography.

AREA OF APPLICATION: Bladder.

CONTRAST: Done without contrast.

DESCRIPTION: Ultrasound procedures are diagnostic, noninvasive, and relatively inexpensive. They take a short time to complete, do not use radiation, and cause no harm to the patient. Bladder ultrasound evaluates disorders of the bladder, such as masses or lesions. Bladder position, structure, and size are examined with the use of high-frequency waves of various intensities delivered by a transducer, a flashlight-shaped device. Methods for imaging include the transrectal, transurethral, and transvaginal approach. The waves are bounced back, converted to electrical energy, amplified by the transducer, and displayed on a monitor to evaluate the structure and position of the contents of the bladder. The examination is helpful for monitoring patient response to therapy for bladder disease. Bladder images can be included in ultrasonography of the kidneys, ureters, bladder, urethra, and gonads in diagnosing renal/neurologic disorders. Bladder ultrasound may be the diagnostic examination of choice because there is no radiation used and in most cases the accuracy is sufficient to make the diagnosis without any further imaging procedures. ■

INDICATIONS:
- Detect tumor of the bladder wall or pelvis, evidenced by distorted position or changes in bladder contour
- Assess residual urine after voiding to diagnose urinary tract obstruction causing overdistention
- Determine end-stage malignancy of the bladder caused by extension of a primary tumor of the ovary or other pelvic organ
- Measure urinary bladder volume by transurethral or transvaginal approach

- Evaluate the cause of urinary tract infection, urine retention, and flank pain
- Evaluate hematuria, urinary frequency, dysuria, and suprapubic pain

RESULT

Normal Findings:
- Normal size, position, and contour of the bladder

Abnormal Findings:
- Bladder diverticulum
- Cyst
- Cystitis
- Malignancy of the bladder
- Tumor
- Urinary tract obstruction
- Ureterocele

INTERFERING FACTORS:

This procedure is contraindicated for:
- Patients with latex allergies, if an internal examination is required

Factors that may impair clear imaging:
- Inability of the patient to cooperate or remain still during the procedure because of age, significant pain, or mental status
- Incorrect placement of the transducer over the desired test site
- Incorrect positioning of the patient, which may produce poor visualization of the area to be examined
- Patients who are very obese, who may exceed the weight limit for the equipment
- Retained gas or barium from a previous radiologic procedure

Nursing Implications and Procedure ∙ ∙ ∙ ∙ ∙ ∙ ∙ ∙ ∙ ∙ ∙

Pretest: ■

➤ Inform the patient that the procedure assesses the bladder.

➤ Inform the patient that the procedure is performed in a specialized area by a technologist and usually takes approximately 30 minutes.

➤ Determine whether the patient is allergic to latex.

➤ Obtain a history of suspected or existing disorders of the bladder.

➤ Obtain the results of other tests and procedures done to diagnose bladder disorders, as well as a history of previous treatments, therapies, or surgery performed for these disorders. For related tests, refer to the genitourinary system table.

➤ Assure the patient that his or her privacy will be maintained.

➤ Instruct the patient to administer an enema 1 hour before this examination.

➤ Inform the patient that the procedure is painless and carries no risks.

➤ Do not restrict food or fluids before the procedure. Offer three to four glasses of water within 2 hours before the test and instruct the patient to refrain from voiding.

Intratest: ■

➤ Ask the patient to disrobe below the waist and put on a hospital gown.

➤ Place the patient in a supine position on the examining table.

➤ Expose the lower abdomen and drape the patient.

➤ Place the transducer over the bladder and pelvic sites; the sound wave images are projected on the screen and stored electronically for future viewing or reproduced on a film. Ask the patient to lie still during the procedure because movement produces unclear images.

➤ If the patient is to be examined for residual urine volume, ask the patient to empty the bladder; repeat the procedure and calculate the volume.

Post-test: ■

➤ When the study is completed, remove the gel from the bladder area.

➤ Instruct the patient to resume normal activity, medication, and diet, unless otherwise indicated.

➤ A physician specializing in this branch of medicine sends a written report to the ordering provider, who discusses the results with the patient.

➤ Inform the patient that an abnormal examination may indicate the need for additional studies.

➤ Evaluate test results in relation to the patient's symptoms and other tests performed. Related diagnostic tests include kidney, ureter, and bladder (KUB) film; intravenous pyelography; cystoscopy; and computed tomography and magnetic resonance imaging of the pelvis.

ULTRASOUND, BREAST

∙ ∙

SYNONYM/ACRONYM: Mammographic ultrasound.

AREA OF APPLICATION: Breast.

CONTRAST: Done without contrast.

DESCRIPTION: Ultrasound procedures are diagnostic, noninvasive, and relatively inexpensive. They take a short time to complete, do not use radiation, and cause no harm to the patient. When used in conjunction with mammography and clinical examination, breast ultrasound is indispensable in the diagnosis and management of benign and malignant process. Both breasts are usually examined during this procedure. The examination uses high-frequency waves of various intensities delivered by a transducer, a flashlight-shaped device, pressed against the skin. The waves are bounced back, converted to electrical energy, amplified by the transducer, and displayed on a monitor to determine the presence of palpable and nonpalpable masses, their size, and structure. This procedure is useful in patients with an abnormal mass on a mammogram because it can determine whether the abnormality is cystic or solid; that is, it can differentiate between a palpable, fluid-filled cyst and a palpable, solid breast lesion (benign or malignant). It is especially useful in patients with dense breast tissue and in those with silicone prostheses, because the ultrasound beam easily penetrates in these situations, allowing routine examination that cannot be performed with x-ray mammography. The procedure can be done as an adjunct to mammography, or it can be done in place of mammography in patients who refuse having x-ray exposure or those in whom it is contraindicated (e.g., pregnant women, women less than 25 years old). The procedure is indicated as a guide for biopsy or other interventional procedure and as a means of monitoring disease progression or the effects of treatment. ■

INDICATIONS:

- Determine the presence of nonpalpable abnormalities viewed on mammography of dense breast tissue, and monitor changes in these abnormalities

- Differentiate among types of breast masses (e.g., cyst, solid tumor, other lesions) in dense breast tissue

- Detect very small tumors in combination with mammography for diagnostic validation

- Evaluate palpable masses in young (less than age 25), pregnant, and lactating patients

- Identify an abscess in a patient with mastitis

- Guide interventional procedures such as cyst aspiration, large-needle core biopsy, fine-needle aspiration biopsy, abscess drainage, presurgical localization, and galactography

RESULT

Normal Findings:

- Normal subcutaneous, mammary, and retromammary layers of tissue in both breasts; no evidence of pathologic lesions (cyst or tumor) in either breast

Abnormal Findings:

- Abscess

- Breast solid tumor, lesions

- Cancer (ductal carcinoma, infiltrating lobular carcinoma, medullary carcinoma, tubular carcinoma, and papillary carcinoma)

- Cystic breast disease
- Fibroadenoma
- Focal fibrosis
- Galactocele
- Hamartoma (fibroadenolipoma)
- Hematoma
- Papilloma
- Phyllodes tumor
- Radial scar

INTERFERING FACTORS

Factors that may impair clear imaging:
- Inability of the patient to cooperate or remain still during the procedure because of age, significant pain, or mental status
- Incorrect placement of the transducer over the desired test site
- Incorrect positioning of the patient, which may produce poor visualization of the area to be examined
- Patients who are very obese, who may exceed the weight limit for the equipment
- Excessively large breasts

Nursing Implications and Procedure • • • • • • • • • •

Pretest: ■

➤ Inform the patient that the procedure assesses the breasts.

➤ Inform the patient that the procedure is performed in a specialized area by a technologist and usually takes approximately 30 to 60 minutes.

➤ Obtain a history of suspected or existing disease of the breast.

➤ Obtain the results of other tests and procedures done to diagnose and/or monitor disorders of or treatments to the breast region. For related tests, refer to the reproductive system table.

➤ Ensure that the patient has not applied lotions, bath powder, or other substances to the chest and breast area before the examination.

➤ Inform the patient that the procedure is painless and carries no risks.

➤ Do not restrict food before the procedure.

Intratest: ■

➤ Ask the patient to put on a hospital gown.

➤ Place the patient in a supine position on the examining table; other positions may be used during the examination.

➤ Expose the breast and drape the patient.

➤ Apply conductive gel to the area, and move a handheld transducer over the skin; the sound wave images are projected on the screen and stored electronically for future viewing or reproduced on a film. Ask the patient to lie still during the procedure because movement produces unclear images. *Note:* Women with back problems or limited flexibility may have difficulty maintaining the appropriate positions for this procedure.

Post-test: ■

➤ When the study is completed, remove the gel from the skin.

➤ Instruct the patient in the monthly breast self-examination procedure, and ask the patient to demonstrate the technique of breast self-examination.

➤ A physician specializing in this branch of medicine sends a written report to the ordering provider, who discusses the results with the patient.

➤ Inform the patient that an abnormal examination may indicate the need for additional studies.

➤ Evaluate test results in relation to the patient's symptoms and any related tests performed.

ULTRASOUND, KIDNEY

SYNONYM/ACRONYM: Renal ultrasound, renal sonography.

AREA OF APPLICATION: Kidney.

CONTRAST: Done without contrast.

DESCRIPTION: Ultrasound procedures are diagnostic, noninvasive, and relatively inexpensive. They take a short time to complete, do not use radiation, and cause no harm to the patient. Renal ultrasound is used to evaluate renal system disorders. It is valuable for determining the internal components of renal masses (solid versus cystic) and for evaluating other renal diseases, renal parenchyma, perirenal tissues, and obstruction. Ultrasound uses high-frequency waves of various intensities delivered by a transducer, a flashlight-shaped device, pressed against the skin. The waves are bounced back, converted to electrical energy, amplified by the transducer, and displayed on a monitor to evaluate the structure, size, and position of the kidney. Renal ultrasound can be performed on the same day as a radionuclide scan or other radiologic procedure, and is especially valuable in patients who are in renal failure, have hypersensitivity to contrast medium, have a kidney that did not visualize on intravenous pyelography (IVP), or are pregnant. It does not rely on renal function or the injection of contrast medium to obtain a diagnosis. The procedure is indicated for evaluation after a kidney transplant and is used as a guide for biopsy or other interventional procedures, abscess drainage, and nephrostomy tube placement. Renal ultrasound may be the diagnostic examination of choice because there is no radiation used and in most cases the accuracy is sufficient to make the diagnosis without any further imaging procedures. ■

INDICATIONS:

• Detect masses and differentiate between cysts or solid tumors, evidenced by specific waveform patterns or absence of sound waves

• Provide the location and size of renal masses in patients who are unable to undergo IVP because of poor renal function or an allergy to iodinated contrast medium

• Determine the presence and location of renal or ureteral calculi and obstruction

• Determine an accumulation of fluid in the kidney caused by backflow of urine, hemorrhage, or perirenal fluid

• Monitor kidney development in children, when renal disease has been diagnosed

• Determine the size, shape, and position of a nonfunctioning kidney to identify the cause

• Aid in the diagnosis of the effect of chronic glomerulonephritis and end-stage chronic renal failure on the kidneys (e.g., decreasing size)

• Locate the site and guide percutaneous renal biopsy, aspiration needle insertion, or nephrostomy tube insertion

• Evaluate renal transplantation for changes in kidney size

• Evaluate or plan therapy for renal tumors

RESULT

Normal Findings:

• Normal size, position, and shape of the kidneys and associated structures

• Absence of calculi, cysts, hydronephrosis, obstruction, or tumor

Abnormal Findings:

• Acute glomerulonephritis

• Acute pyelonephritis

• Congenital anomalies, such as absent, horseshoe, ectopic, or duplicated kidney

• Hydronephrosis

• Obstruction of ureters

• Perirenal abscess or hematoma

• Polycystic kidney

• Rejection of renal transplant

• Renal calculi

• Renal cysts, hypertrophy, or tumors

• Ureteral obstruction

INTERFERING FACTORS

Factors that may impair clear imaging:

• Inability of the patient to cooperate or remain still during the procedure because of age, significant pain, or mental status

• Incorrect placement of the transducer over the desired test site

• Incorrect positioning of the patient, which may produce poor visualization of the area to be examined

• Patients who are very obese, who may exceed the weight limit for the equipment

• Retained gas or barium from a previous radiologic procedure

Nursing Implications and Procedure

Pretest:

➤ Inform the patient that the procedure assesses the kidneys.

➤ Inform the patient that the procedure is performed in a specialized area by a technologist and usually takes approximately 30 minutes.

➤ Obtain a history of suspected or existing renal disease.

➤ Obtain the results of other tests and procedures done to diagnose disorders of or treatments to the renal system. For related tests, refer to the genitourinary system table.

➤ Inform the patient that the procedure is painless and carries no risks.

➤ Note recent administration of barium because residual barium can obscure the organ to examined. There should be 24 hours between administration of barium and this test.

➤ Do not restrict food or fluids before the procedure.

Intratest:

➤ Ask the patient to put on a hospital gown and void.

➤ Place the patient in a supine position on the examining table; other positions may be used during the examination.

➤ Expose the abdomen/kidney area and drape the patient.

➤ Apply a conductive gel to the skin, and move the transducer over the area to obtain several images of the area of interest; the sound wave images are projected on the screen and stored electronically for future viewing or reproduced on a film. Ask the patient to lie still during the procedure because movement produces unclear images.

➤ If necessary for better visualization of the upper portions of the kidneys, ask the patient to inhale deeply and hold his or her breath.

Post-test:

➤ When the study is completed, remove the gel from the skin.

➤ Instruct the patient to resume normal activity, medication, and diet, unless otherwise indicated.

➤ A physician specializing in this branch of medicine sends a written report to the ordering provider, who discusses the results with the patient.

➤ Inform the patient that an abnormal examination may indicate the need for additional studies.

➤ Evaluate test results in relation to the patient's symptoms and other tests performed. Related diagnostic tests include IVP; renal angiogram; renogram; kidney, ureter, and bladder (KUB) film; and computed tomography and magnetic resonance imaging of the abdomen.

ULTRASOUND, LIVER AND BILIARY SYSTEM

SYNONYMS/ACRONYM: Gallbladder ultrasound, liver ultrasound, hepato-biliary sonography.

AREA OF APPLICATION: Liver, gallbladder, bile ducts.

CONTRAST: Done without contrast.

DESCRIPTION: Ultrasound procedures are diagnostic, noninvasive, and relatively inexpensive. They take a short time to complete, do not use radiation, and cause no harm to the patient. Hepatobiliary ultrasound uses high-frequency waves of various intensities delivered by a transducer, a flashlight-shaped device, pressed against the skin. The waves are bounced back, converted to electrical energy, amplified by the transducer, and displayed on a monitor to evalu-ate the structure, size, and position of the liver and gallbladder in the right upper quadrant (RUQ) of the abdomen. The gallbladder and biliary system collects, stores, concentrates, and transports bile to the intestines to aid in digestion. This procedure allows visualization of the gallbladder and bile ducts when the patient may have impaired liver function, and it is especially helpful when done on patients whose gallbladder is unable to visualize gallstones with oral or intravenous radiologic studies. Liver ultrasound can be done in combination with a nuclear scan to obtain information about liver function and density differences in the liver. The procedure is indicated as a guide for biopsy or other interventional procedures. Hepatobiliary ultrasound may be the diagnostic examination of choice because there is no radiation used and in most cases the accuracy is sufficient to make the diagnosis without any further imaging procedures. ∎

INDICATIONS:

• Detect hepatic lesions, evidenced by density differences and echo-pattern changes

• Determine patency and diameter of the hepatic duct for dilation or obstruction

• Differentiate between obstructive and nonobstructive jaundice by determining the cause

• Determine the cause of unexplained hepatomegaly and abnormal liver function tests

• Detect gallstones or inflammation when oral cholecystography is inconclusive

• Detect cysts, polyps, hematoma, abscesses, hemangioma, adenoma, metastatic disease, hepatitis, or solid tumor of the liver or gallbladder evidenced by echoes specific to tissue density and sharply or poorly defined masses

• Determine cause of unexplained RUQ pain

• Evaluate response to therapy for tumor, evidenced by a decrease in size of the organ

• Guide catheter placement into the gallbladder for stone dissolution and gallbladder fragmentation

• Guide biopsy or tube placement

RESULT

Normal Findings:

• Normal size, position, and shape of the liver and gallbladder, as well as patency of the cystic and common bile ducts

Abnormal Findings:

• Biliary or hepatic duct obstruction/dilation

• Cirrhosis

• Gallbladder inflammation, stones, carcinoma, polyps

• Hematoma or trauma

• Hepatic tumors, metastasis, cysts, hemangioma, hepatitis

• Hepatocellular disease, adenoma

• Hepatomegaly

• Intrahepatic abscess

• Subphrenic abscesses

CRITICAL VALUES: N/A

INTERFERING FACTORS

Factors that may impair clear imaging:

• Attenuation of the sound waves by the ribs, which can impair clear imaging of the right lobe of the liver

• Inability of the patient to cooperate or remain still during the procedure because of age, significant pain, or mental status

• Incorrect placement of the transducer over the desired test site

• Incorrect positioning of the patient, which may produce poor visualization of the area to be examined

• Patients who are very obese, who may exceed the weight limit for the equipment

• Retained gas or barium from a previous radiologic procedure

Other considerations:

• Failure to follow dietary restrictions before the procedure may cause the procedure to be canceled or repeated.

Nursing Implications and Procedure • • • • • • • • • • •

Pretest:

➤ Inform the patient that the procedure assesses the hepatobiliary system.

➤ Inform the patient that the procedure is performed in a specialized area by a technologist and usually takes approximately 30 minutes.

➤ Obtain a history of suspected or existing disease of the liver or gallbladder and duct system.

➤ Obtain the results of other tests and procedures done to diagnose disorders of or treatments to the liver, gallbladder, and duct system. For related tests, refer to the hepatobiliary system table.

➤ Note recent administration of barium because residual barium can obscure the organ to examined. There should be 24 hours between administration of barium and this test.

➤ Endoscopy, endoscopic retrograde cholangiopancreatography (ERCP), colonoscopy, and computed tomography (CT) of the abdomen, if ordered, should be scheduled after this procedure.

➤ Restrict food, fluid, smoking, and gum chewing for 6 to 8 hours before the procedure.

Intratest:

➤ Ask the patient to put on a hospital gown and void.

➤ Administer an enema before the study, if ordered, to remove any remaining barium.

➤ Place the patient in a supine position on the examining table; other positions may be used during the examination. The right- or left-side-up position allows gravity to reposition the liver, gas, and fluid to facilitate better organ visualization.

➤ Expose the abdomen and drape the patient.

➤ Apply a conductive gel to the skin of the RUQ, and move the transducer over the area to obtain several images of the area of interest, including the liver, gallbladder, and bile ducts (cystic and common); the sound wave images are projected on the screen and stored electronically for future viewing or reproduced on a film. Ask the patient to lie still during the procedure because movement produces unclear images.

➤ If necessary for better organ visualization, ask the patient to inhale deeply and hold his or her breath.

➤ Gallbladder contractibility is viewed by scanning after administration of a pharmaceutical that induces gallbladder contraction or after administration of a fatty meal.

Post-test:

➤ When the study is completed, remove the gel from the skin.

➤ Instruct the patient to resume normal activity, medication, and diet, unless otherwise indicated.

➤ A physician specializing in this branch of medicine sends a written report to the ordering provider, who discusses the results with the patient.

➤ Inform the patient that an abnormal examination may indicate the need for additional studies.

➤ Evaluate test results in relation to the patient's symptoms and other tests performed. Related diagnostic tests include ERCP, endoscopy, colonoscopy, hepatobiliary scan, and CT scan of the abdomen.

ULTRASOUND, LYMPH NODES AND RETROPERITONEUM

SYNONYM/ACRONYM: Lymph node sonography.

AREA OF APPLICATION: Abdomen, pelvis, and retroperitoneum.

CONTRAST: Done without contrast.

DESCRIPTION: Ultrasound procedures are diagnostic, noninvasive, and relatively inexpensive. They take a short time to complete, do not use radiation, and cause no harm to the patient. Lymph node ultrasound uses high-frequency waves of various intensities delivered by a transducer, a flashlight-shaped device, pressed against the skin. The waves are bounced back, converted to electrical energy, amplified by the transducer, and displayed on a monitor to evaluate the structure, size, and position of the lymph nodes to examine the retroperitoneum and surrounding tissues. This procedure is used for the evaluation of retroperitoneal pathology, usually lymph node enlargement. Ultrasound is the preferred diagnostic method because this area is inaccessible to conventional radiography in diagnosing lymphadenopathy, although it can be used in combination with lymphangiography, magnetic resonance imaging, and computed tomography (CT) to confirm the diagnosis. The procedure may be used for monitoring the effect of radiation or chemotherapy on the lymph nodes. Lymph node ultrasound may be the diagnostic examination of choice because there is no radiation used and in most cases the accuracy is sufficient to make the diagnosis without any further imaging procedures. ■

INDICATIONS:
• Determine the size or enlargement of aortic and iliac lymph nodes

• Detect lymphoma

• Determine the location of enlarged nodes to plan radiation and other therapy

• Evaluate the effects of medical, radiation, or surgical therapy on the size of nodes or tumors, evidenced by shrinkage or continued presence of the mass or nodes

RESULT

Normal Findings:
• Normal retroperitoneal and intrapelvic node size of 1.5 cm in diameter

Abnormal Findings:
• Infection or abscess

• Lymphoma

• Retroperitoneal tumor

INTERFERING FACTORS:

Factors that may impair clear imaging:

- Inability of the patient to cooperate or remain still during the procedure because of age, significant pain, or mental status

- Incorrect placement of the transducer over the desired test site

- Incorrect positioning of the patient, which may produce poor visualization of the area to be examined

- Patients who are dehydrated, resulting in failure to demonstrate the boundaries between organs and tissue structures

- Patients who are very obese, who may exceed the weight limit for the equipment

- Retained gas or barium from a previous radiologic procedure

Other considerations:

- Ensure that the patient maintains a full bladder if scanning is to be performed below the umbilicus.

- Ensure that the procedure is performed before endoscopy, endoscopic retrograde cholangiopancreatography (ERCP), barium studies, and colonoscopy.

Nursing Implications and Procedure • • • • • • • • • • • •

Pretest:

➤ Inform the patient that the procedure assesses the lymph nodes and retroperitoneum.

➤ Inform the patient that the procedure is performed in a specialized area by a technologist and usually takes approximately 45 minutes.

➤ Obtain a history of suspected or existing tumor or lymphoma.

➤ Obtain the results of other tests and procedures done to diagnose disorders of or treatments to the lymphatic system or retroperitoneum. For related tests, refer to the hematopoietic system.

➤ Inform the patient that the procedure is painless and carries no risks.

➤ Ensure that the patient has abstained from smoking several hours before the procedure to prevent swallowing of air.

➤ Note recent administration of barium because residual barium can obscure the organ to be examined. There should be 24 hours between administration of barium and this test.

➤ Restrict food and fluids 12 hours before the procedure, but inform the patient that clear liquids will be given the morning of the procedure to fill the bladder and aid the study.

Intratest:

➤ Ask the patient to put on a front-opening hospital gown.

➤ Place the patient in a supine position on the examining table; other positions may be used during the examination.

➤ Expose the abdomen/pelvic area and drape the patient.

➤ Apply a conductive gel to the skin, and move the transducer over the flank, pelvis, and abdominal areas to obtain several images of the area of interest; the sound wave images are projected on the screen and stored electronically for future viewing or reproduced on a film. Ask the patient to lie still during the procedure because movement produces unclear images.

Post-test:

➤ When the study is completed, remove the gel from the skin.

➤ Instruct the patient to resume normal activity, medication, and diet, unless otherwise indicated.

➤ A physician specializing in this branch of medicine sends a written report to the ordering provider, who discusses the results with the patient.

➤ Inform the patient that an abnormal examination may indicate the need for additional studies.

➤ Evaluate test results in relation to the patient's symptoms and other tests performed. Related diagnostic tests include CT and magnetic resonance imaging of the abdomen and pelvis.

ULTRASOUND, OBSTETRIC

· ·

SYNONYMS/ACRONYM: OB sonography, fetal age sonogram, gestational age sonogram, pregnancy ultrasound, pregnancy echo, pregnant uterus ultrasonography.

AREA OF APPLICATION: Pelvis and abdominal region.

CONTRAST: Done without contrast.

DESCRIPTION: Ultrasound procedures are diagnostic, noninvasive, and relatively inexpensive. They take a short time to complete, do not use radiation, and cause no harm to the patient. Obstetric ultrasound uses high-frequency waves of various intensities delivered by a transducer, a flashlight-shaped device, pressed against the skin or inserted into the vagina. The waves are bounced back, converted to electrical energy, amplified by the transducer, and displayed on a monitor to visualize the fetus and placenta. This procedure is done by a transabdominal or transvaginal approach, depending on when the procedure is performed (e.g., first trimester [transvaginal], second trimester [transabdominal]). It is the safest method of examination to evaluate the uterus and determine fetal size, growth, position, fetal structural abnormalities, ectopic pregnancy, placenta position, amount of amniotic fluid, and multiple gestation. Obstetric ultrasound is used to secure different types of information regarding the fetus, varying with the trimester during which the procedure is done. This procedure can also be used in combination with Doppler monitoring of the fetal heart or respiratory movements to detect high-risk pregnancy. The procedure is indicated as a guide for amniocentesis, cordocentesis, fetoscopy, aspiration of multiple oocytes for *in vitro* fertilization, and other intrauterine interventional procedures. Because the pregnant uterus is filled with amniotic fluid, ultrasonography is an ideal method of evaluating the fetus and placenta; it is also the diagnostic examination of choice because there is no radiation used and in most cases the accuracy is sufficient to make the diagnosis without any further imaging procedures. ■

INDICATIONS:

- Determine and confirm pregnancy or multiple gestation by determining the number of gestational sacs in the first trimester

- Determine fetal heart and body movements and detect high-risk pregnancy by monitoring fetal heart and respiratory movements in combination with Doppler ultrasound or real-time gray scale scanning

- Measure fetal gestational age and evaluate umbilical artery, uterine artery, and fetal aorta by Doppler examination to determine fetal intrauterine growth retardation (IUGR)

- Determine fetal gestational age by uterine size and measurements of crown-rump length, biparietal diameter, fetal extremities, head, and other parts of the anatomy at key phases of fetal development

- Determine fetal structural anomalies, usually at 20th week or later

- Detect fetal death, evidenced by absence of movement and fetal heart tones

- Blighted ovum (missed abortion), evidenced by empty gestational sac

- Determine cause of bleeding such as placenta previa or abruptio placentae

- Determine the placental size, location, and site of implantation

- Monitor placental growth and amniotic fluid volume

- Detect fetal position before birth, such as breech or transverse presentations

- Guide the needle during amniocentesis and fetal transfusion

- Determine fetal effects of Rh incompatibility

- Detect tubal and other forms of ectopic pregnancy

- Differentiate a tumor (hydatidiform mole) from a normal pregnancy

RESULT

Normal Findings:

- Normal age, size, viability, position, and functional capacities of the fetus

- Normal placenta size, position, and structure; adequate volume of amniotic fluid

Abnormal Findings:

- Abruptio placentae

- Cardiac abnormalities

- Ectopic pregnancy

- Fetal malpresentation (breech, transverse)

- Fetal hydrops

- Fetal death

- Hydrocephalus

- Intestinal atresia

- Myelomeningocele

- Multiple pregnancy

- Placenta previa

- Renal or skeletal defects

CRITICAL VALUES: N/A

INTERFERING FACTORS:

This procedure is contraindicated for:

- Patients with latex allergy; the vaginal probe requires the probe to be covered with a condom-like sac, usually made from latex.

Factors that may impair clear imaging:

- Inability of the patient to cooperate or remain still during the procedure because of age, significant pain, or mental status

- Incorrect placement of the transducer over the desired test site

- Incorrect positioning of the patient,

which may produce poor visualization of the area to be examined

• Patients who are dehydrated, resulting in failure to demonstrate the boundaries between organs and tissue structures

• Patients who are very obese, exceeding the weight limit for the equipment and preventing the sound beam from penetrating to the site

• Retained gas or barium from a previous radiologic procedure

• Insufficiently full bladder, which fails to push the bowel from the pelvis and the uterus from the symphysis pubis, thereby prohibiting clear imaging of the pregnant uterus in transabdominal imaging

Nursing Implications and Procedure • • • • • • • • • • • •

Pretest: ■

➤ Inform the patient that the procedure assesses the pelvis and abdominal region.

➤ Inform the patient that the procedure is performed in a specialized area by a technologist and usually takes approximately 30 to 60 minutes.

➤ Assess whether the patient is allergic to latex. If the patient is allergic to latex, consult with the ordering physician before the patient has the examination.

➤ Obtain a history of menstrual dates, previous pregnancy, and treatment received for high-risk pregnancy. Obtain the results of other tests, treatments, and procedures done to diagnose and treat conditions of the pregnancy. For related tests, refer to the reproductive system tables.

➤ Inform the patient that the procedure is painless and carries no risks to the patient or fetus.

➤ For the transvaginal approach, inform the patient that a latex or sterile sheath-covered probe will be inserted into the vagina.

➤ Note recent administration of barium because residual barium can obscure the organ to examined. There should be 24 hours between administration of barium and this test.

➤ Do not restrict food or fluids before the procedure. Inform the patient receiving transabdominal ultrasound that the procedure requires a full bladder; instruct the patient to drink five to six glasses of fluid and not to void before the procedure. Patients receiving transvaginal ultrasound do not need to have a full bladder.

Intratest: ■

➤ Ask the patient to put on a hospital gown.

➤ Place the patient in a supine position on the examining table; other positions may be used during the examination.

➤ Expose the abdomen and drape the patient.

➤ *Transabdominal approach*: Apply conductive gel to the area, and move the transducer over the skin while the bladder is distended; the sound wave images are projected on the screen and stored electronically for future viewing or reproduced on a film. Ask the patient to lie still during the procedure because movement produces unclear images.

➤ *Transvaginal approach*: A covered and lubricated probe is inserted into the vagina and moved to different levels. Images are obtained and recorded. A full bladder is not required for transvaginal ultrasound.

Post-test: ■

➤ Allow the patient to void, as needed.

➤ When the study is completed, remove the gel from the skin or the probe from the abdomen or vagina.

➤ Instruct the patient to resume normal activity, medication, and diet, unless otherwise indicated.

➤ A physician specializing in this branch of medicine sends a written report to the ordering provider, who discusses the results with the patient.

➤ Inform the patient that there may be a need for additional studies.

➤ Evaluate test results in relation to the patient's symptoms and any related tests performed.

ULTRASOUND, PANCREAS

SYNONYM/ACRONYM: Pancreatic ultrasonography.

AREA OF APPLICATION: Pancreas and upper abdomen.

CONTRAST: Done without contrast.

DESCRIPTION: Ultrasound procedures are diagnostic, noninvasive, and relatively inexpensive. They take a short time to complete, do not use radiation, and cause no harm to the patient. Pancreatic ultrasound uses high-frequency waves of various intensities delivered by a transducer, a flashlight-shaped device, pressed against the skin. The waves are bounced back, converted to electrical energy, amplified by the transducer, and displayed on a monitor to determine the size, shape, and position of the pancreas; determine the presence of masses or other abnormalities of the pancreas; and examine the surrounding viscera. The procedure is indicated as a guide for biopsy, aspiration, or other interventional procedures. Pancreatic ultrasound may be the diagnostic examination of choice because there is no radiation used and in most cases the accuracy is sufficient to make the diagnosis without any further imaging procedures;

however, it is usually done in combination with computed tomography (CT) or magnetic resonance imaging of the pancreas. ■

INDICATIONS:

• Detect pancreatitis, evidenced by pancreatic enlargement with increased echoes

• Detect pancreatic cancer, evidenced by a poorly defined mass or a mass in the head of the pancreas that obstructs the pancreatic duct

• Detect pseudocysts, evidenced by a well-defined mass with absence of echoes from the interior

• Monitor therapeutic response to tumor treatment

• Provide guidance for percutaneous aspiration and fine-needle biopsy of the pancreas

• Detect anatomic abnormalities as a consequence of pancreatitis

RESULT

Normal Findings:
• Normal size, position, contour, and texture of the pancreas

Abnormal Findings:
• Acute pancreatitis

• Calculi

• Pancreatic duct obstruction

• Pancreatic tumor

• Pseudocysts

CRITICAL VALUES: N/A

INTERFERING FACTORS:

Factors that may impair clear imaging:
• Inability of the patient to cooperate or remain still during the procedure because of age, significant pain, or mental status

• Incorrect placement of the transducer over the desired test site

• Incorrect positioning of the patient, which may produce poor visualization of the area to be examined

• Patients who are very obese, who may exceed the weight limit for the equipment

• Retained gas, feces, or barium from a previous radiologic procedure, inadequate cleansing, or failure to restrict food intake before the study

Other considerations:
• Failure to follow dietary restrictions before the procedure may cause the procedure to be canceled or repeated.

Nursing Implications and Procedure • • • • • • • • • • •

Pretest:

➤ Inform the patient that the procedure assesses the pancreas.

➤ Inform the patient that the procedure is performed in a specialized area by a technologist and usually takes approximately 30 to 60 minutes. The room may be darkened for better visualization of the pancreas.

➤ Obtain a history of suspected or existing disease of the pancreas.

➤ Obtain the results of tests and procedures done to diagnose disorders of or treatments to the pancreas. For related tests, refer to the endocrine system table.

➤ Inform the patient that the procedure is painless and carries no risks.

➤ Note recent administration of barium because residual barium can obscure the organ to be examined. There should be a 24-hour waiting period between administration of barium and this test.

➤ Inform the patient to withhold food for 8 hours, but to drink increased amounts of fluids to distend the stomach before and during the procedure.

Intratest:

➤ Ask the patient to put on a hospital gown.

➤ Place the patient in a supine position on the examining table; other positions may be used during the examination.

➤ Expose the abdomen and drape the patient.

➤ Apply conductive gel to the epigastric area, and move the transducer over the skin; the sound wave images are projected on the screen and stored electronically for future viewing or reproduced on a film. Ask the patient to lie still during the procedure because movement produces unclear images.

➤ If necessary for better visualization of the pancreas and abdominal organs, ask the patient to inhale deeply, regulate breathing, hold his or her breath, or drink water.

ULTRASOUND, PELVIS (GYNECOLOGIC, NONOBSTETRIC)

SYNONYMS/ACRONYM: Pelvic sonography, lower abdomen ultrasound, pelvic gynecologic (GYN) sonogram.

AREA OF APPLICATION: Pelvis and appendix region.

CONTRAST: Done without contrast.

DESCRIPTION: Ultrasound procedures are diagnostic, noninvasive, and relatively inexpensive. They take a short time to complete, do not use radiation, and cause no harm to the patient. Gynecologic ultrasound uses high-frequency waves of various intensities delivered by a transducer, a flashlight-shaped device, pressed against the skin or inserted into the vagina. The waves are bounced back, converted to electrical energy, amplified by the transducer, and displayed on a monitor in order to:

Determine the presence, size, and structure of masses and cysts; and determine the position of

an intrauterine contraceptive device (IUD)

Evaluate postmenopausal bleeding

Examine other abnormalities of the uterus, ovaries, fallopian tubes, and vagina

This procedure is done by a transabdominal or transvaginal approach. The transabdominal approach provides a view of the pelvic organs posterior to the bladder. It requires a full bladder, thereby allowing a window for transmission of the ultrasound waves, pushing the uterus away from the pubic symphysis, pushing the bowel out of the pelvis, and acting as a reference for comparison in the evaluation of the internal structures of a mass or cyst being examined. The transvaginal approach focuses on the female reproductive organs and is often used to monitor ovulation over a period of days in patients undergoing fertility assessment. This approach is also used in obese patients or in patients with retroversion of the uterus because the sound waves are better able to reach the organ from the vaginal site. Transvaginal images are significantly more accurate compared to anterior transabdominal images in identifying paracervical, endometrial, and ovarian pathology, and the transvaginal approach does not require a full bladder. The procedure is indicated as a guide for biopsy or other interventional procedures. Pelvic ultrasound may be the diagnostic examination of choice because there is no radiation used and in most cases the accuracy is sufficient to make the diagnosis without any further imaging procedures. ■

INDICATIONS:
- Monitor placement and location of an IUD
- Detect masses in the pelvis and differentiate them from cysts or solid tumors, evidenced by differences in sound-wave patterns
- Detect the presence of ovarian cysts and malignancy and determine the type, if possible, evidenced by size, outline, and change in position of other pelvic organs
- Detect and monitor the treatment of pelvic inflammatory disease (PID) when done in combination with other laboratory tests
- Evaluate the effectiveness of tumor therapy, evidenced by a reduction in mass size

- Detect pelvic abscess or peritonitis caused by a ruptured appendix or diverticulitis
- Detect bleeding into the pelvis resulting from trauma to the area or ascites associated with tumor metastasis
- Evaluate the thickness of the uterine wall
- Monitor follicular size associated with fertility studies or to remove follicles for *in vitro* transplantation
- Detect pregnancy, including ectopic pregnancy
- Evaluate suspected fibroid tumor or bladder tumor

RESULT

Normal Findings:
- Normal size, position, location, and structure of pelvic organs (e.g., uterus, ovaries, fallopian tubes, vagina); IUD properly positioned within the uterine cavity

Abnormal Findings:
- Endometrioma
- Fibroids (leiomyoma)
- Nonovarian cyst
- Ovarian cysts
- Pelvic abscess
- Peritonitis
- PID
- Uterine tumor or adnexal tumor

CRITICAL VALUES: N/A

INTERFERING FACTORS:

This procedure is contraindicated for:
- Patients with latex allergy; the vaginal probe requires the probe to be covered with a condom-like sac, usually made from latex.

Factors that may impair clear imaging:

- Inability of the patient to cooperate or remain still during the procedure because of age, significant pain, or mental status

- Incorrect placement of the transducer over the desired test site

- Incorrect positioning of the patient, which may produce poor visualization of the area to be examined

- Patients who are dehydrated, resulting in failure to demonstrate the boundaries between organs and tissue structures

- Patients who are very obese, exceeding the weight limit for the equipment and preventing the sound beam from penetrating to the site

- Retained gas, feces, or barium from a previous radiologic procedure, inadequate cleansing, or failure to restrict food intake before the study

- Insufficiently full bladder, which fails to push the bowel from the pelvis and the uterus from the symphysis pubis, thereby prohibiting clear imaging of the pelvic organs in transabdominal imaging

Nursing Implications and Procedure •••••••••••

Pretest:

➤ Inform the patient that the procedure assesses the pelvis and abdominal region.

➤ Inform the patient that the procedure is performed in a specialized area by a technologist and usually takes approximately 30 to 60 minutes.

➤ Assess whether the patient is allergic to latex. If the patient is allergic to latex, consult the ordering physician before ordering the examination.

➤ Obtain a history of suspected or existing disease of the pelvic organs.

➤ Obtain the results of tests and procedures done to diagnose disorders of or treatments to the pelvic region and organs. For related tests, refer to the genitourinary and reproductive systems tables.

➤ Inform the patient that the procedure is painless and carries no risks to the patient or fetus.

➤ For the transvaginal approach, inform the patient that a latex or sterile sheath-covered probe will be inserted into the vagina.

➤ Note recent administration of barium because residual barium can obscure the organ to examined. There should be a 24-hour waiting period between administration of barium and this test.

➤ Do not restrict food or fluids before the procedure. Inform the patient receiving transabdominal ultrasound that the procedure requires a full bladder; instruct the patient to drink five to six glasses of fluid and not to void before the procedure. Patients receiving transvaginal ultrasound do not need to have a full bladder.

Intratest:

➤ Ask the patient to put on a hospital gown.

➤ Place the patient in a supine position on the examining table; other positions may be used during the examination.

➤ Expose the abdomen and drape the patient.

➤ *Transabdominal approach*: Apply conductive gel to the area, and move the transducer over the skin while the bladder is distended; the sound wave images are projected on the screen and stored electronically for future viewing or reproduced on a film. Ask the patient to lie still during the procedure because movement produces unclear images.

➤ *Transvaginal approach*: A covered

and lubricated probe is inserted into the vagina and moved to different levels. Images are obtained and recorded. A full bladder is not required for transvaginal ultrasound.

Post-test:

➤ Allow the patient to void, as needed.

➤ When the study is completed, remove the gel from the skin or the probe from the vagina.

➤ Instruct the patient to resume

normal activity, medication, and diet, unless otherwise indicated.

➤ A physician specializing in this branch of medicine sends a written report to the ordering provider, who discusses the results with the patient.

➤ Inform the patient that an abnormal examination may indicate the need for additional studies.

➤ Evaluate test results in relation to the patient's symptoms and any related tests performed.

ULTRASOUND, PERIPHERAL DOPPLER

· ·

SYNONYMS/ACRONYM: Doppler, venous ultrasound, arterial ultrasound, duplex scan.

AREA OF APPLICATION: Veins and arteries.

CONTRAST: Done without contrast.

DESCRIPTION: Ultrasound procedures are diagnostic, noninvasive, and relatively inexpensive. They take a short time to complete, do not use radiation, and cause no harm to the patient. Peripheral Doppler ultrasound studies can be used to identify narrowing or occlusions of the veins or arteries. In venous Doppler studies, the Doppler identifies moving red blood cells (RBCs) within the vein. The ultrasound beam is directed at the vein and through the Doppler transducer while the RBCs reflect the beam back to the transducer. The reflected sound waves or echoes can be transformed by a computer into scans, graphs, or audible sounds.

Blood flow direction, velocity, and the presence of flow disturbances can be readily assessed. The velocity of the blood flow is transformed as a "swishing" noise, audible through the audio speaker. If the vein is occluded, no swishing sound is heard.

In arterial Doppler studies, arteriosclerotic disease of the peripheral vessels can be detected by slowly deflating blood pressure cuffs that are placed on an extremity such as the calf, ankle, or upper extremity. The systolic pressure of the various arteries of the extremities can be measured. The Doppler transducer can detect the first sign of blood flow through the cuffed artery, even the most minimal blood flow, as evidenced by a swishing noise. There is normally a reduction in systolic blood pressure from the arteries of the arms to the arteries of the legs; a reduction exceeding 20 mm Hg is indicative of occlusive disease (deep vein thrombosis [DVT]) proximal to the area being tested. This procedure may also be used to monitor the patency of a graft, status of previous corrective surgery, vascular status of the blood flow to a transplanted organ, blood flow to a mass, or the extent of vascular trauma. ■

INDICATIONS:

- Aid in the diagnosis of venous occlusion secondary to thrombosis or thrombophlebitis
- Aid in the diagnosis of small- or large-vessel arterial occlusive disease
- Aid in the diagnosis of spastic arterial disease, such as Raynaud's phenomenon
- Aid in the diagnosis of embolic arterial occlusion
- Evaluate the origin of pain related to vascular inflammation
- Determine the patency of a vascular graft, stent, or previous surgery
- Evaluate possible arterial trauma

RESULT

Normal venous findings:
- Normal Doppler venous signal that occurs spontaneously with the client's respiration
- Normal venous system, with no evidence of occlusion

Normal arterial findings:
- No evidence of arterial occlusion
- Normal arterial systolic and diastolic Doppler signals

- Normal reduction in systolic blood pressure (i.e., less than 20 mm Hg) when compared to a normal extremity
- Normal ankle-to-brachial arterial blood pressure (ankle pressure [A] divided by brachial [B] pressure; normal AB pressure index is greater than 0.85)

Abnormal venous findings:
- Venous narrowing or occlusion secondary to thrombosis or thrombophlebitis

Abnormal arterial findings:
- Large- or small-vessel arterial occlusive disease
- Embolic arterial occlusion
- Spastic arterial occlusive disease, such as Raynaud's phenomenon
- AB pressure index less than 0.85, indicating significant arterial occlusive disease within the extremity

CRITICAL VALUES: N/A

INTERFERING FACTORS:

This procedure is contraindicated for:
- Patients with an open or draining lesion

Factors that may alter test results:
- Cigarette smoking
- Inability of the patient to cooperate or remain still during the procedure because of age, significant pain, or mental status
- Incorrect placement of the transducer over the desired test site
- Incorrect positioning of the patient, which may produce poor visualization of the area to be examined
- Patients who are very obese, who may

exceed the weight limit for the equipment

• Venous or arterial occlusive disease proximal to the site being tested

Nursing Implications and Procedure • • • • • • • • • • •

Pretest:

➤ Inform the patient that the procedure assesses the veins and arteries.

➤ Inform the patient that the procedure is performed in a specialized area by a technologist and usually takes approximately 30 to 60 minutes.

➤ Obtain a history of previous arterial studies, presence of disorders predisposing the patient to DVT, or therapy received for arterial abnormalities. For related tests, refer to the cardiovascular system table.

➤ Inform the patient that the procedure is painless and carries no risks.

➤ Obtain and record baseline vital signs to use for comparison after the procedure, if needed.

Intratest:

➤ Ask the patient to put on a hospital gown and void.

Venous studies:

➤ Place the patient in a supine position on a table or examining cart.

➤ Expose the area to be examined.

➤ Inform the patient that movement during the procedure will affect the results and make interpretation difficult.

➤ Apply conductive gel to the skin, and slowly move the transducer over the site. A swishing sound is heard in a vein that is patent; absence of sound indicates venous occlusion or incorrect placement of the transducer.

Arterial Doppler studies:

➤ Place blood pressure cuffs on the thigh, calf, and ankle.

➤ Apply a conductive get to the skin over the area distal to the cuff.

➤ Inflate the proximal cuff to a level above the patient's systolic pressure found in the normal extremity.

➤ Place the Doppler transducer to the inflated cuff, and slowly release the pressure in the cuff.

➤ When the swishing sound is heard, record it at the highest level audible. The test is repeated at each successive level.

Post-test:

➤ When the study is completed, remove the gel from the leg.

➤ Instruct the patient to resume normal activity, medication, and diet, unless otherwise indicated.

➤ A physician specializing in this branch of medicine sends a written report to the ordering provider, who discusses the results with the patient.

➤ Inform the patient that an abnormal examination may indicate the need for additional studies.

➤ Note test results in relation to other test performed and the patient's symptoms. Related diagnostic tests include venous Doppler ultrasound, computed tomographic angiography, and magnetic resonance angiography.

ULTRASOUND, PROSTATE (TRANSRECTAL)

SYNONYM/ACRONYM: Prostate sonography.

AREA OF APPLICATION: Prostate, seminal vesicles.

CONTRAST: Done without contrast.

DESCRIPTION: Ultrasound procedures are diagnostic, noninvasive, and relatively inexpensive. They take a short time to complete, do not use radiation, and cause no harm to the patient. Prostate ultrasound is used for the evaluation of disorders of the prostate, especially in response to an elevated concentration of prostate-specific antigen (PSA) on a blood test and as a complement to a digital rectal examination. It uses high-frequency waves of various intensities delivered by a transducer, a candle-shaped device, which is lubricated, sheathed with a condom, and inserted a few inches into the rectum. The waves are bounced back, converted to electrical energy, amplified by the transducer, and displayed on a monitor to evaluate the structure, size, and position of the contents of the prostate (e.g., masses), as well as other prostate pathology. It aids in the diagnosis of prostatic cancer by evaluating palpable nodules and is useful as a guide to biopsy. This procedure can evaluate prostate tissue, the seminal vesicles, and surrounding perirectal tissue. It can also be used to stage carcinoma and to assist in radiation seed placement.

The examination is helpful in monitoring patient response to therapy for prostatic disease. Micturition disorders can also be evaluated by this procedure. Prostate ultrasound may be the diagnostic examination of choice because there is no radiation used and in most cases the accuracy is sufficient to make the diagnosis without any further imaging procedures. ■

INDICATIONS:
• Aid in prostate cancer diagnosis

• Assess prostatic calcifications

• Determine prostatic cancer staging

• Detect prostatitis

• Aid in the diagnosis of micturition disorders

• Assist in guided needle biopsy of a suspected tumor

• Assist in radiation seed placement

RESULT

Normal Findings:
• Normal size, consistency, and contour of the prostate gland

Abnormal Findings:
• Benign prostatic hypertrophy or hyperplasia

- Micturition disorders
- Perirectal abscess
- Perirectal tumor
- Prostate abscess
- Prostate cancer
- Prostatitis
- Rectal tumor
- Seminal vesicle tumor

CRITICAL VALUES: N/A

INTERFERING FACTORS:

This procedure is contraindicated for:
- Patients with latex allergy; the rectal probe requires the probe to be covered with a condom, usually made from latex.

Factors that may impair clear imaging:
- Inability of the patient to cooperate or remain still during the procedure because of age, significant pain, or mental status
- Incorrect placement of the transducer over the desired test site
- Incorrect positioning of the patient, which may produce poor visualization of the area to be examined
- Patients who are very obese, who may exceed the weight limit for the equipment
- Retained gas or barium from a previous radiologic procedure, inadequate cleansing, or failure to restrict food intake before the study

---

Nursing Implications and Procedure • • • • • • • • • •

Pretest: ◼

➤ Inform the patient that the procedure assesses the prostate.

➤ Inform the patient that the procedure is performed in a specialized area by a technologist and usually takes approximately 30 minutes.

➤ Determine whether the patient is allergic to latex. If the patient is allergic to latex, consult with the ordering physician before the patient has the examination.

➤ Obtain a history of suspected or existing disorder of the prostate gland.

➤ Obtain the results of other tests and procedures done to diagnose disorders of or treatments to the prostate gland. For related tests, refer to the genitourinary system table.

➤ Inform the patient that the procedure is painless and carries no risks.

➤ Assure the patient that his privacy will be maintained.

➤ Instruct the patient to administer an enema 1 hour before this examination.

➤ Do not restrict food or fluids before the procedure.

Intratest: ◼

➤ Ask the patient to put on a hospital gown and void.

➤ Place the patient on the examining table on his left side with his knees bent toward the chest.

➤ To ensure that no feces remain in the rectum, perform a digital rectal examination.

➤ Cover the rectal probe with a lubricated condom and insert it into the rectum. Inform the patient that he may feel slight pressure as the transducer is inserted. Water may be introduced through the sheath surrounding the transducer. The scan is performed at several levels. Ask the patient to lie still during the procedure because movement produces unclear images.

Post-test: ◼

➤ When the study is completed, remove the gel from the rectal and genital areas.

➤ Instruct the patient to resume

normal activity, medication, and diet, unless otherwise indicated.

➤ A physician specializing in this branch of medicine sends a written report to the ordering provider, who discusses the results with the patient.

➤ Inform the patient that an abnormal examination may indicate the need for additional studies.

➤ Evaluate test results in relation to the patient's symptoms and any related tests performed.

ULTRASOUND, SCROTAL

· ·

SYNONYM/ACRONYM: Scrotal sonography, ultrasound of the testes, testicular ultrasound.

AREA OF APPLICATION: Scrotum.

CONTRAST: Done without contrast.

DESCRIPTION: Ultrasound procedures are diagnostic, noninvasive, and relatively inexpensive. They take a short time to complete, do not use radiation, and cause no harm to the patient. Scrotal ultrasound is used for the evaluation of disorders of the scrotum. It is valuable in determining the internal components of masses (solid versus cystic) and for the evaluation of the testicle, extratesticular and intrascrotal tissues, benign and malignant tumors, and other scrotal pathology. It uses high-frequency waves of various intensities delivered by a transducer, a flashlight-shaped device, which is pressed against the skin. The waves are bounced back, converted to electrical energy, amplified by the transducer, and displayed on a monitor to evaluate the structure, size, and position of the contents of the scrotum. Scrotal ultrasound can be performed before or after a radionuclide scan for further clarification of a testicular mass. Extratesticular lesions such as hydrocele, hematocele (blood in the scrotum), pyocele (pus in the scrotum) can be identified, as well as cryptorchidism (undescended testicles). Scrotal ultrasound may be the diagnostic examination of choice because there is no radiation used and in most cases the accuracy is sufficient to make the diagnosis without any further imaging procedures. ■

INDICATIONS:
• Aid in the diagnosis of a mass and differentiate between a cyst and a solid tumor, evidenced by specific waveform patterns or the absence of sound waves, respectively

• Determine the cause of chronic scrotal swelling or pain

• Aid in the diagnosis of scrotal or testicular size, abnormality, or pathology

• Aid in the diagnosis of a chronic

inflammatory condition such as epididymitis

- Determine the presence of a hydrocele, pyocele, spermatocele, or hernia before surgery

- Aid in the diagnosis of testicular torsion and associated testicular infarction

- Evaluate the effectiveness of treatment for testicular infections

- Locate an undescended testicle

- Assist ultrasound-guided needle biopsy of a suspected testicle tumor

RESULT

Normal Findings:
- Normal size, position, and shape of the scrotum and structure of the testes

Abnormal Findings:
- Abscess

- Epididymal cyst

- Epididymitis

- Hematoma

- Hydrocele

- Infarction

- Microlithiasis

- Orchitis

- Pyocele

- Scrotal hernia

- Spermatocele

- Torsion

- Tumor, benign or malignant

- Tunica albuginea cyst

- Undescended testicle (cryptorchidism).

- Varicocele

CRITICAL VALUES: N/A

INTERFERING FACTORS:

Factors that may impair clear imaging:
- Inability of the patient to cooperate or remain still during the procedure because of age, significant pain, or mental status

- Incorrect placement of the transducer over the desired test site

- Incorrect positioning of the patient, which may produce poor visualization of the area to be examined

- Patients who are very obese, who may exceed the weight limit for the equipment

Nursing Implications and Procedure • • • • • • • • • •

Pretest:
➤ Inform the patient that the procedure assesses the scrotum.

➤ Inform the patient that the procedure is performed in a specialized area by a technologist and usually takes approximately 30 minutes.

➤ Obtain a history of suspected or existing disorder of the scrotum or testes.

➤ Obtain the results of tests and procedures done to diagnose disorders of or treatments to the scrotum or testes. For related tests, refer to the genitourinary system table.

➤ Inform the patient that the procedure is painless and carries no risks.

➤ Assure the patient that his privacy will be maintained.

➤ Do not restrict food or fluids before the procedure.

Intratest:
➤ Ask the patient to put on a hospital gown and void.

➤ Place the patient in a supine position with the patient's legs apart on the examining table.

> Expose the scrotal area and drape the patient.

> Lift the penis upward and gently tape it to the lower part of the abdomen. Elevate the scrotum with a rolled towel or sponge for immobilization. Display particular sensitivity toward the patient regarding any embarrassment he may feel during this part of the procedure.

> Apply a conductive gel to the skin, and move the transducer over the area to obtain several images of the area of interest; the sound wave images are projected on the screen and stored electronically for future viewing or reproduced on a film. Ask the patient to lie still during the procedure because movement produces unclear images.

Post-test:

> When the study is completed, remove the gel from the scrotal area.

> Instruct the patient to resume normal activity, medication, and diet, unless otherwise indicated.

> A physician specializing in this branch of medicine sends a written report to the ordering provider, who discusses the results with the patient.

> Inform the patient that an abnormal examination may indicate the need for additional studies. Evaluate test results in relation to the patient's symptoms and any related tests performed.

ULTRASOUND, SPLEEN

· ·

SYNONYM/ACRONYM: Spleen ultrasonography.

AREA OF APPLICATION: Spleen/left upper quadrant.

CONTRAST: Done without contrast.

DESCRIPTION: Ultrasound procedures are diagnostic, noninvasive, and relatively inexpensive. They take a short time to complete, do not use radiation, and cause no harm to the patient. Spleen ultrasound uses high-frequency waves of various intensities delivered by a transducer, a flashlight-shaped device, pressed against the skin. The waves are bounced back, converted to electrical energy, amplified by the transducer, and displayed on a monitor to evaluate the structure, size, and position of the spleen. This test is valuable for determining the internal components of splenic masses (solid versus cystic) and evaluating other splenic pathology, splenic trauma, and left upper quadrant perisplenic tissues. It can be performed to supplement a radionuclide scan or computed tomography (CT). It is especially valuable in patients who are in renal failure, are hypersensitive to contrast medium, or are pregnant because it does not rely on adequate renal function or the injection of contrast medium to obtain a diagnosis. The procedure may also be used as a guide for biopsy, other interventional procedures, or abscess drainage. Spleen ultrasound may be the diagnostic examination of choice because there is no radiation used and in most cases the accuracy is sufficient to make the diagnosis without any further imaging procedures. ■

INDICATIONS:

• Detect splenic masses; differentiate between cysts or solid tumors (in combination with CT), evidenced by specific waveform patterns or absence of sound waves, respectively; and determine whether they are intrasplenic or extrasplenic

• Determine the presence of splenomegaly, and assess the size and volume of the spleen in these cases, evidenced by increased echoes and visibility of the spleen

• Detect the presence of a subphrenic abscess after splenectomy

• Evaluate the extent of abdominal trauma and spleen involvement, including enlargement or rupture, after a recent trauma

• Differentiate spleen trauma from blood or fluid accumulation between the splenic capsule and parenchyma

• Evaluate the spleen before splenectomy performed for thrombocytopenic purpura

• Determine late-stage sickle cell disease, evidenced by decreased spleen size and presence of echoes

• Evaluate the effect of medical or surgical therapy on the progression or resolution of splenic disease

RESULT

Normal Findings:

• Normal size, position, and contour of the spleen and associated structures

Abnormal Findings:

• Abscesses

• Accessory or ectopic spleen

• Infection

• Lymphatic disease, lymph node enlargement

• Splenic calcifications

• Splenic masses, tumors, cysts, or infarction

• Splenic trauma

• Splenomegaly

CRITICAL VALUES: N/A

INTERFERING FACTORS

Factors that may impair clear imaging:

• Attenuation of the sound waves by the ribs and an aerated left lung, which can impair clear imaging of the spleen

• Inability of the patient to cooperate or remain still during the procedure because of age, significant pain, or mental status

• Incorrect placement of the transducer over the desired test site

• Incorrect positioning of the patient, which may produce poor visualization of the area to be examined

• Masses near the testing site, which can displace the spleen and cause inaccurate results if confused with splenomegaly

• Patients who are dehydrated, resulting in failure to demonstrate the boundaries between organs and tissue structures

- Patients who are very obese, exceeding the weight limit for the equipment and preventing the sound beam from penetrating to the site

- Retained gas, feces, or barium from a previous radiologic procedure, inadequate cleansing, or failure to restrict food intake before the study

Other considerations:
- Ensure that the examination is performed before endoscopy, endoscopic retrograde cholangiopancreatography (ERCP), barium studies, and colonoscopy.

Nursing Implications and Procedure • • • • • • • • • • • •

Pretest:

➤ Inform the patient that the procedure assesses the spleen.

➤ Inform the patient that the procedure is performed in a specialized area by a technologist and usually takes approximately 45 minutes.

➤ Obtain a history of suspected or existing disease of or trauma to the spleen.

➤ Obtain the results of tests and procedures done to diagnose disorders of or treatments to the splenic system. For related tests, refer to the hematopoietic and gastrointestinal system tables.

➤ Ensure that the patient has abstained from smoking several hours before the procedure to prevent the swallowing of air.

➤ Inform the patient that the procedure is painless and carries no risks to the patient or fetus.

➤ Note recent administration of barium because residual barium can obscure the organ to be examined. There should be a 24-hour waiting period between administration of barium and this test.

➤ Restrict food and fluids 12 hours before the procedure.

Intratest:

➤ Ask the patient to put on a front-opening hospital gown and void.

➤ Place the patient in a supine position on the examining table; other positions may be used during the examination.

➤ Expose the abdomen/splenic area and drape the patient.

➤ Apply a conductive gel to the skin, and move the transducer over the skin; the sound wave images are projected on the screen and stored electronically for future viewing or reproduced on a film. Ask the patient to lie still during the procedure because movement produces unclear images. The patient may be requested to inhale deeply and hold his or her breath to obtain better views of the spleen.

Post-test:

➤ When the study is completed, remove the gel from the skin.

➤ Instruct the patient to resume normal activity, medication, and diet, unless otherwise indicated.

➤ A physician specializing in this branch of medicine sends a written report to the ordering provider, who discusses the results with the patient.

➤ Inform the patient that an abnormal examination may indicate the need for additional studies.

➤ Evaluate test results in relation to the patient's symptoms and other tests performed. Related diagnostic tests include abdominal angiogram, CT and magnetic resonance angiography, and CT and magnetic resonance imaging of the abdomen.

ULTRASOUND, THYROID AND PARATHYROID

· ·

SYNONYMS/ACRONYM: Thyroid sonography, parathyroid sonography, thyroid echo.

AREA OF APPLICATION: Thyroid, parathyroid, and anterior neck region.

CONTRAST: Done without contrast.

DESCRIPTION: Ultrasound procedures are diagnostic, noninvasive, and relatively inexpensive. They take a short time to complete, do not use radiation, and cause no harm to the patient. Thyroid and parathyroid ultrasound uses high-frequency waves of various intensities delivered by a transducer, a flashlight-shaped device, pressed against the skin. The waves are bounced back, converted to electrical energy, amplified by the transducer, and displayed on a monitor to determine the position, size, shape, weight, presence of masses of the thyroid gland, enlargement of the parathyroid glands, and other abnormalities of the thyroid and parathyroid glands and surrounding tissues. The primary purpose of this procedure is to determine whether a nodule is a fluid-filled cyst (usually benign) or a solid tumor (possibly malignant). This procedure is useful in evaluating the glands' response to medical treatment or assessing the remaining tissue after surgical resection. The procedure may be indicated as a guide for biopsy, aspiration, or other interventional procedures.

Thyroid and parathyroid ultrasound may be the diagnostic examination of choice because there is no radiation used and in most cases the accuracy is sufficient to make the diagnosis without any further imaging procedures; it is clearly the procedure of choice when examining the glands of pregnant patients. This procedure is usually done in combination with nuclear medicine imaging procedures and computed tomography (CT) of the neck. Despite the advantages of the procedure, in some cases it may not detect small nodules and lesions (less than 1 cm), leading to false-negative findings. ■

INDICATIONS:
• Aid in determining the presence of a tumor, evidenced by an irregular border and shadowing at the distal edge, peripheral echoes, or high- and low-amplitude echoes, depending on the density of the tumor mass; and diagnosing tumor type (e.g., benign, adenoma, carcinoma)

• Aid in diagnosing the presence of a cyst, evidenced by a smoothly outlined, echo-free amplitude except at the far borders of the mass

- Differentiate among a nodule, solid tumor, or fluid-filled cyst

- Aid in diagnosis in the presence of a parathyroid enlargement indicating a tumor or hyperplasia, evidenced by an echo pattern of lower amplitude than that for a thyroid tumor

- Evaluate the effect of a therapeutic regimen for a thyroid mass or Graves' disease by determining the size and weight of the gland

- Determine the need for surgical biopsy of a tumor or fine-needle biopsy of a cyst

- Evaluate thyroid abnormalities during pregnancy

RESULT

Normal Findings:
- Normal size, position, contour, and structure of the thyroid and parathyroid glands with uniform echo patterns throughout the glands; no evidence of tumor cysts or nodules in the glands

Abnormal Findings:
- Glandular enlargement

- Goiter

- Graves' disease

- Parathyroid tumor or hyperplasia

- Thyroid cysts

- Thyroid tumors (benign or malignant)

INTERFERING FACTORS

Factors that may impair clear imaging:
- Inability of the patient to cooperate or remain still during the procedure because of age, significant pain, or mental status

- Incorrect placement of the transducer over the desired test site

- Incorrect positioning of the patient, which may produce poor visualization of the area to be examined

- Patients who are very obese, who may exceed the weight limit for the equipment

Other considerations:
- Nodules less than 1 cm in diameter may not be detected.

- Nonthyroid cysts may appear the same as thyroid cysts.

Nursing Implications and Procedure • • • • • • • • • •

Pretest:

➤ Inform the patient that the procedure assesses the thyroid and parathyroid glands.

➤ Inform the patient that the procedure is performed in a specialized area by a technologist and usually takes approximately 30 to 60 minutes. The room may be darkened for better visualization of the glands.

➤ Obtain a history of suspected or existing disease of the thyroid and parathyroid glands.

➤ Obtain the results of tests and procedures done to diagnose disorders of or treatments to the thyroid and parathyroid glands. For related tests, refer to the endocrine system table.

➤ Inform the patient that the procedure is painless and carries no risks.

➤ Do not restrict food or fluids before the procedure.

Intratest:

➤ Ask the patient to remove clothing from the waist up, to put on a hospital gown with the opening in the front, and to void.

➤ Make sure jewelry, chains, and any other metallic objects have been removed from the neck area.

➤ Place the patient in a supine position

on the examining table; other positions may be used during the examination.

➤ Hyperextend the neck and place a pillow under the patient's shoulders to maintain a comfortable position.

➤ Apply the conductive gel to the neck, and move the transducer over the entire thyroid site; the sound wave images are projected on the screen and stored electronically for future viewing or reproduced on a film. Ask the patient to lie still during the procedure because movement produces unclear images. (An alternative method of imaging includes the use of a bag filled with water or gel placed over the neck area; the bag serves as a transmitter of the waves from the transducer to the thyroid.)

Post-test:

➤ When the study is completed, remove the gel from the skin.

➤ Instruct the patient to resume normal activity, medication, and diet, unless otherwise indicated.

➤ A physician specializing in this branch of medicine sends a written report to the ordering provider, who discusses the results with the patient.

➤ Inform the patient that an abnormal examination may indicate the need for additional studies.

➤ Evaluate test results in relation to the patient's symptoms and other tests performed. Related diagnostic tests include biopsy, thyroid scan, thyroid uptake, magnetic resonance imaging of the neck, and CT of the spine.

ULTRASOUND, VENOUS DOPPLER, EXTREMITY STUDIES

SYNONYMS/ACRONYM: Venous ultrasound, venous sonogram, venous ultrasonography, venous duplex.

AREA OF APPLICATION: Veins of the upper and lower extremities.

CONTRAST: Done without contrast.

DESCRIPTION: Ultrasound procedures are diagnostic, noninvasive, and relatively inexpensive. They take a short time to complete, do not use radiation, and cause no harm to the patient. Venous Doppler ultrasound records sound waves to obtain information about the patency of the venous vasculature in the upper and lower extremities. Ultrasound waves are sent into the body by a small transducer pressed against the body. The transducer sends the sound waves into the body and also receives the returning sound waves, which are deflected back as they bounce off various structures. The transducer converts and amplifies the returning sound waves into electric signals that are transformed by a computer into audible sounds, graphic readings, and gray-scale images. Blood flow direction and velocity can be readily assessed; and the presence of blood flow disturbances, which are proportional to blood flow velocity, can be determined.

For diagnostic studies, the procedure is done bilaterally. The sound waves hit the moving red blood cells and are reflected back to the transducer. The sound emitted by the equipment corresponds to the velocity of the blood flow through the vessel occurring with spontaneous respirations. Changes in these sounds during respirations indicate the possibility of abnormal venous flow secondary to occlusive disease; the absence of sound indicates complete obstruction. Compression with a transducer augments a vessel for evaluation of thrombosis. Noncompressibility of the vessel indicates a thrombosis. Plethysmography may be performed to determine the filling time of calf veins to diagnose thrombotic disorder of a major vein and to identify incompetent valves in the venous system. An additional method used to evaluate incompetent valves is the Valsalva technique combined with venous duplex imaging. ■

INDICATIONS:

- Detect chronic venous insufficiency, evidenced by reverse blood flow indicating incompetent valves
- Aid in the diagnosis of superficial thrombosis or deep vein thrombosis (DVT) leading to venous occlusion or obstruction, evidenced by absence of venous flow, especially upon augmentation of the extremity; variations in

flow during respirations; or failure of the veins to compress completely when the extremity is compressed

- Determine the source of emboli when pulmonary embolism is suspected or diagnosed
- Determine venous damage after trauma to the site
- Evaluate the patency of the venous system in patients with a swollen painful leg
- Differentiate between primary and secondary varicose veins
- Determine if further diagnostic procedures are needed to make or confirm a diagnosis
- Monitor the effectiveness of therapeutic interventions

RESULT

Normal Findings:
- Normal blood flow through the veins of the extremities with no evidence of vessel occlusion

Abnormal Findings:
- Chronic venous insufficiency
- Primary varicose veins
- Secondary varicose veins
- Superficial thrombosis or DVT
- Venous trauma
- Venous occlusion
- Recannulization in the area of an old thrombus

CRITICAL VALUES: N/A

INTERFERING FACTORS:
- Inability of the patient to maintain a stable position during the procedure
- Inability of the patient to cooperate or remain still during the procedure because of age, significant pain, or mental status

- Incorrect placement of the transducer over the desired test site

- Cold extremities, resulting in vasoconstriction that can cause inaccurate measurements

- Occlusion proximal to the site being studied, which would affect blood flow to the area

- Open wound or incision overlying the area to be examined

- Cigarette smoking, because nicotine can cause constriction of the peripheral vessels

- An abnormally large or swollen leg, making sonic penetration difficult.

Nursing Implications and Procedure

Pretest:

➤ Inform the patient that the procedure assesses the veins of the leg.

➤ Inform the patient that the procedure is performed in a special ultrasound or vascular department by a technologist and usually takes approximately 30 to 60 minutes.

➤ Report the presence of a lesion that is open or draining; maintain clean, dry dressing for the ulcer; protect the limb from trauma.

➤ Obtain a history of previous venous studies, presence of disorders predisposing to venous thrombosis or other peripheral vascular problems, or therapy received for venous abnormalities. For related tests, refer to the cardiovascular system table.

➤ Ensure that the patient has refrained from smoking for at least 30 minutes before the test.

➤ Inform the patient that the procedure is painless and carries no risks.

➤ Obtain and record baseline vital signs to use for comparison after the procedure, if needed.

➤ Do not restrict food or fluids before the procedure.

Intratest:

➤ Ask the patient to put on a hospital gown and void.

➤ Place the patient in a supine position on a table or examining cart, and allow the patient to rest for a minimum of 10 minutes before starting the examination.

➤ Expose the area to be examined and support the extremity to prevent movement. Ask the patient to lie still during the procedure because movement produces unclear images.

➤ Apply conductive gel to the skin, and slowly move the transducer over the site and in the area of the vein. Waveforms are visualized and recorded with variations in respirations. Images with and without compression are performed proximally or distally to an obstruction to obtain information about a venous occlusion or obstruction. The procedure can be performed for both arms and legs to obtain bilateral blood flow determination.

➤ Do not place the transducer on an ulcer site when there is evidence of venous stasis or ulcer.

Post-test:

➤ When the study is completed, remove the gel from the skin.

➤ Instruct the patient to resume normal activity, medications, and diet, unless otherwise indicated.

➤ Instruct the patient to report skin lesions (open or draining) and skin discoloration.

➤ A physician specializing in this branch of medicine sends a written report to the ordering provider, who discusses the results with the patient.

➤ Inform the patient that an abnormal examination may indicate the need for additional studies.

➤ Evaluate test results in relation to the patient's symptoms and other tests performed. Related diagnostic tests include computed tomographic angiography and magnetic resonance angiography.

UPPER GASTROINTESTINAL AND SMALL BOWEL SERIES

· ·

SYNONYMS/ACRONYMS: Stomach series, gastric radiography, small bowel study, upper GI series, UGI.

AREA OF APPLICATION: Esophagus, stomach, and small intestine.

CONTRAST: Barium sulfate.

DESCRIPTION: The upper gastrointestinal (GI) series is a radiologic examination of the esophagus, stomach, and small intestine after ingestion of barium sulfate, which is a milkshakelike, radiopaque substance. A combination of x-ray and fluoroscopy techniques is used to record the study. Air may be instilled to provide double contrast and better visualization of the lumen of the esophagus, stomach, and duodenum. If perforation or obstruction is suspected, a water-soluble iodinated contrast medium is used. This test is especially useful in the evaluation of patients experiencing dysphagia, regurgitation, gastroesophageal reflux (GER), epigastric pain, hematemesis, melena, and unexplained weight loss. This test is also used to evaluate the results of gastric surgery, especially when an anastomotic leak is suspected. When a small bowel series is included, the test detects disorders of the jejunum and ileum. The patient's position is changed during the examination to allow visualization of the various structures and their function. The images are visualized on a fluoroscopic screen, recorded, and stored electronically or on x-ray film for review by a physician. Drugs such as glucagon may be given during an upper GI series to relax the GI tract; drugs such as metoclopramide (Reglan) may be given to accelerate the passage of the barium through the stomach and small intestine.

When the small bowel series is performed separately, the patient may be asked to drink several glasses of barium or enteroclysis may be used to instill the barium. With enteroclysis, a catheter is passed through the nose or mouth and advanced past the pylorus and into the duodenum. Barium, followed by methylcellulose solution, is instilled via the catheter directly into the small bowel. ■

INDICATIONS:

• Determine the cause of regurgitation or epigastric pain

• Evaluate unexplained weight loss or anemia

• Determine the presence of neoplasms, ulcers, diverticula, obstruction, foreign body, and hiatal hernia

• Identify and locate the origin of hematemesis

- Evaluate suspected GER, inflammatory process, congenital anomaly, motility disorder, or structural change

RESULT

Normal Findings:
- Normal size, shape, position, and functioning of the esophagus, stomach, and small bowel

Abnormal Findings:
- Achalasia
- Cancer of the esophagus
- Chalasis
- Congenital abnormalities
- Duodenal cancer, diverticula, and ulcers
- Esophageal diverticula, motility disorders, ulcers, varices, and inflammation
- Gastric cancer, tumors, and ulcers
- Gastritis
- Hiatal hernia
- Perforation of the esophagus, stomach, or small bowel
- Polyps
- Small bowel tumors
- Strictures

CRITICAL VALUES: N/A

INTERFERING FACTORS

This procedure is contraindicated for:
- Patients who are pregnant or suspected of being pregnant, unless the potential benefits of the procedure far outweigh the risks to the fetus and mother
- Patients with an intestinal obstruction
- Patients suspected of upper GI perforation, in whom barium should not be used

Factors that may impair clear imaging:
- Inability of the patient to cooperate or remain still during the procedure because of age, significant pain, or mental status
- Patients who are very obese, who may exceed the weight limit for the equipment
- Incorrect positioning of the patient, which may produce poor visualization of the area to be examined
- Improper adjustment of the radiographic equipment to accommodate obese or thin patients, which can cause overexposure or underexposure and poor-quality study
- Metallic objects within the examination field (e.g., jewelry or body rings), which may inhibit organ visualization and can produce unclear images

Other considerations:
- Failure to follow dietary restrictions before the procedure may cause the procedure to be canceled or repeated.
- Patients with swallowing problems may aspirate the barium, which could interfere with the procedure and cause patient complications.
- Possible constipation or partial bowel obstruction caused by retained barium in the small bowel or colon may affect test results.
- This procedure should be done after a kidney x-ray (intravenous pyelography) or computed tomography (CT) of the abdomen or pelvis.
- Risks associated with radiographic overexposure can result from frequent x-ray procedures. Personnel in the room with the patient should stand behind a shield or leave the area while the examination is being done. Personnel working in the area where the examination is being done should wear badges that reveal their level of exposure to radiation.

Nursing Implications and Procedure • • • • • • • • • • •

Pretest:

➤ Inform the patient that the procedure assesses the upper GI system and/or small bowel.

➤ Explain to the patient that he or she will be asked to drink a milkshakelike solution that has a chalky taste.

➤ Inform the patient that the procedure is done by a physician and/or technologist and takes 30 to 60 minutes for the stomach images and as long as 5 hours for the small bowel images.

➤ Determine whether the patient has any allergies or sensitivities to contrast medium, shellfish, or barium.

➤ Obtain a history of the patient's complaints and medications the patient is taking.

➤ Obtain a history of the patient's upper GI system and the results of previously performed tests, surgeries, therapies, and procedures. For related tests, refer to the gastrointestinal system table.

➤ Determine date of last menstrual period and possibility of pregnancy in perimenopausal women.

➤ Withhold food and fluids for 8 hours before the test.

Intratest:

➤ Ask the patient to put on a hospital gown.

➤ Make sure jewelry, chains, and any other metallic objects have been removed from the chest area.

➤ Remove any wires connected to electrodes, if allowed.

Upper gastrointestinal series:

➤ Place the patient on the x-ray table in a supine position, or ask the patient to stand in front of an x-ray fluoroscopy screen.

➤ Instruct the patient to take several swallows of the barium mixture through a straw while images are taken of the pharyngeal motion. Drinking through a straw allows some air to be introduced into the abdomen. This permits detailed examination of the stomach's lining. This same effect can be achieved by administering an effervescent agent.

➤ While the patient continues to drink the barium solution, images of the esophageal area are recorded from a variety of angles.

➤ Instruct the patient to finish the barium mixture while images are taken at different angles and positions to aid in the evaluation of stomach filling and emptying into the duodenum.

Small bowel series:

➤ If the small bowel is to be examined after the upper GI series, instruct the patient to drink an additional glass of barium while the small intestine is observed for passage of barium. Images are taken at 30- to 60-minute intervals until the barium reaches the ileocecal valve. This process can last up to 5 hours, with a follow-up film taken at 24 hours.

Post-test:

➤ Instruct the patient to resume food, fluids, and medications withheld before the procedure.

➤ Inform the patient that further examinations may be necessary to evaluate progression of the disease process or to determine the need for a change in therapy.

➤ Monitor for reaction to iodinated contrast medium including tachycardia, hyperpnea, hypertension, or palpitations, if iodine is used.

➤ Instruct the patient to take a mild laxative and increase fluid intake (four glasses) to aid in the elimination of barium, unless contraindicated.

➤ Inform the patient that his or her stool will be white or light in color for 2 to 3 days. If the patient is unable to eliminate the barium, or if the stool does not return to normal color, the patient should notify the physician.

➤ Determine whether the patient or family members have any further questions or concerns.

➤ A physician specializing in this branch of medicine sends a written report to the ordering provider, who discusses the results with the patient.

➤ Evaluate test results in relation to the patient's symptoms and other tests performed. Related diagnostic tests include endoscopic retrograde cholangiopancreatography (ERCP); kidney, ureter, and bladder (KUB) film; and CT and magnetic resonance imaging of the abdomen.

UREA NITROGEN, BLOOD

• •

SYNONYM/ACRONYM: BUN.

SPECIMEN: Serum (1 mL) collected in a red- or tiger-top tube. Plasma (1 mL) collected in green-top (heparin) tube is also acceptable.

REFERENCE VALUE: (Method: Spectrophotometry)

Age	Conventional Units	SI Units (Conversion Factor ×0.357)
Newborn–3 y	5–17 mg/dL	1.8–6.0 mmol/L
4–13 y	7–17 mg/dL	2.5–6.0 mmol/L
14 y–adult	8–21 mg/dL	2.9–7.5 mmol/L
Adult older than 90 y	10–31 mg/dL	3.6–11.1 mmol/L

DESCRIPTION: Urea is a nonprotein nitrogen compound formed in the liver from ammonia as an end product of protein metabolism. Urea diffuses freely into extracellular and intracellular fluid and is ultimately excreted by the kidneys. Blood urea nitrogen (BUN) levels reflect the balance between the production and excretion of urea. BUN and creatinine values are commonly evaluated together. The normal BUN/creatinine ratio is 15:1 to 24:1. (e.g., if a patient has a BUN of 15 mg/dL, the creatinine should be approximately 0.6 to 1.0 mg/dL). BUN is used in the following calculation to estimate serum osmolality:

$$[(2[Na^+]) + (glucose/18) + (BUN/2.8)]$$ ∎

INDICATIONS:
• Evaluate renal function
• Evaluate liver function
• Evaluate hydration
• Monitor the effects of drugs known to be nephrotoxic or hepatotoxic

- Evaluate hemodialysis therapy

- Assess nutritional support

- Evaluate patients with lymphoma after chemotherapy (tumor lysis)

RESULT

Increased in:

- Acute renal failure

- Chronic glomerulonephritis

- Congestive heart failure

- Decreased renal perfusion

- Diabetes

- Excessive protein ingestion

- Gastrointestinal (GI) bleeding (excessive blood protein in the GI tract)

- Hyperalimentation

- Hypovolemia

- Ketoacidosis

- Muscle wasting from starvation

- Neoplasms

- Nephrotoxic agents

- Pyelonephritis

- Shock

- Urinary tract obstruction

Decreased in:

- Inadequate dietary protein

- Low-protein/high-carbohydrate diet

- Malabsorption syndromes

- Pregnancy

- Severe liver disease

CRITICAL VALUES: ⚠ Potential critical value is greater than 100 mg/dL (except in the case of renal dialysis patients). A patient with a grossly elevated BUN may have signs and symptoms including acidemia, agitation, confusion, fatigue, nausea, vomiting, and coma. Possible interventions include treatment of the cause, administration of intravenous bicarbonate, a low-protein diet, hemodialysis, and caution with respect to prescribing and continuing nephrotoxic medications.

INTERFERING FACTORS:

- Drugs, substances, and vitamins that may increase BUN levels include acetaminophen, alanine, aldatense, alkaline antacids, amphotericin B, antimony compounds, arsenicals, bacitracin, bismuth subsalicylate, capreomycin, carbenoxolone, carbutamide, cephalosporins, chloral hydrate, chloramphenicol, chlorthalidone, colistimethate, colistin, cotrimoxazole, dexamethasone, dextran, diclofenac, doxycycline, ethylene glycol, gentamicin, guanethidine, guanoxan, ibuprofen, ifosfamide, ipodate, kanamycin, mephenesin, metolazone, mitomycin, neomycin, phosphorus, plicamycin, tertatolol, tetracycline, triamterene, triethylenemelamine, viomycin, and vitamin D.

- Drugs that may decrease BUN levels include acetohydroxamic acid, chloramphenicol, fluorides, paramethasone, phenothiazine, and streptomycin.

Nursing Implications and Procedure • • • • • • • • • • •

Pretest: ■

➤ Obtain a history of the patient's complaints, including a list of known allergens.

➤ Obtain a history of the patient's genitourinary and hepatobiliary systems, as well as results of previously performed tests and procedures. For related tests, refer to the genitourinary and hepatobiliary system tables.

➤ Obtain a list of medications the patient is taking, including herbs, nutritional supplements, and nutraceuticals. The requesting health care practitioner and laboratory should be advised if the patient is regularly using these products so that their effects can be taken into consideration when reviewing results.

➤ There are no food, fluid, or medication restrictions unless by medical direction.

➤ Review the procedure with the patient.

➤ Inform the patient that specimen collection takes approximately 5 to 10 minutes.

Intratest:

➤ Direct the patient to breathe normally and to avoid unnecessary movement.

➤ Observe standard precautions and follow the general guidelines in Appendix A. Perform a venipuncture, and collect the specimen in a 5-mL red- or tiger-top tube.

➤ Label the specimen, and promptly transport it to the laboratory.

Post-test:

➤ Observe venipuncture site for bleeding or hematoma formation. Apply pressure bandage.

➤ Monitor intake and output for fluid imbalance in renal dysfunction and dehydration.

➤ Nitrogen balance is commonly used as a nutritional assessment tool to indicate protein change. In healthy individuals, protein anabolism and catabolism are in equilibrium. During various disease states, nutritional intake decreases, resulting in a negative balance. During recovery from illness and with proper nutritional support, the nitrogen balance becomes positive. BUN is an important analyte to measure during administration of total parenteral nutrition (TPN). Educate the patient, as appropriate, in dietary adjustments required to maintain proper nitrogen balance. Inform the patient that the requesting health care practitioner may prescribe TPN as part of the treatment plan.

➤ Evaluate test results in relation to the patient's symptoms and other tests performed. Related laboratory tests include anion gap, blood and urine creatinine, creatinine clearance, blood and urine electrolytes, gentamicin, kidney stone analysis, microalbumin, blood and urine osmolality, tobramycin, urine urea nitrogen, BUN/creatinine ratio, blood and urine uric acid, and vancomycin.

UREA NITROGEN, URINE

SYNONYM/ACRONYM: N/A.

SPECIMEN: Urine (5 mL) from an unpreserved random or timed specimen collected in a clean plastic collection container.

REFERENCE VALUE: (Method: Spectrophotometry)

Conventional Units	SI Units (Conversion Factor ×35.7)
12–20 g/24 h	428–714 mmol/24 h

DESCRIPTION: Urea is a nonprotein nitrogen compound formed in the liver from ammonia as an end product of protein metabolism. Urea diffuses freely into extracellular and intracellular fluid and is ultimately excreted by the kidneys. Urine urea nitrogen levels reflect the balance between the production and excretion of urea. ∎

INDICATIONS:

• Evaluate renal disease

• Predict the impact that other conditions, such as diabetes and liver disease, will have on the kidneys

RESULT

Increased in:

• Diabetes

• Hyperthyroidism

• Increased dietary protein

• Postoperative period

Decreased in:

• Liver disease

• Low-protein/high-carbohydrate diet

• Normal-growing pediatric patients

• Pregnancy

• Renal disease

• Toxemia

CRITICAL VALUES: N/A

INTERFERING FACTORS:

• Drugs that may increase urine urea nitrogen levels include alanine and glycine.

• Drugs that may decrease urine urea nitrogen levels include furosemide, growth hormone, insulin, and testosterone.

• All urine voided for the timed collection period must be included in the collection or else falsely decreased values may be obtained. Compare output records with volume collected to verify that all voids were included in the collection.

Nursing Implications and Procedure • • • • • • • • • • •

Pretest: ∎

➤ Obtain a history of the patient's complaints, including a list of known allergens.

➤ Obtain a history of the patient's genitourinary and hepatobiliary systems, as well as results of previously performed tests and procedures. For related tests, refer to the genitourinary and hepatobiliary system tables.

➤ Obtain a list of medications the patient is taking, including herbs, nutritional supplements, and nutraceuticals. The requesting health care practitioner and laboratory should be advised if the patient regularly uses these products so that their effects can be taken into consideration when reviewing results.

➤ There are no food, fluid, or medication restrictions unless by medical direction.

➤ Review the procedure with the patient. Provide a nonmetallic urinal, bedpan, or toilet-mounted collection device.

➤ Usually a 24-hour time frame for

urine collection is ordered. Inform the patient that all urine must be saved during that 24-hour period. Instruct the patient not to void directly into the laboratory collection container. Instruct the patient to avoid defecating in the collection device and to keep toilet tissue out of the collection device to prevent contamination of the specimen.

➤ Place a sign in the bathroom to remind the patient to save all urine.

➤ Instruct the patient to void all urine into the collection device and then to pour the urine into the laboratory collection container. Alternatively the specimen can be left in the collection device for a health care staff member to add to the laboratory collection container.

Intratest: ■

➤ Observe standard precautions and follow the general guidelines in Appendix A.

Random specimen (collect in early morning):

Clean-catch specimen:

➤ Instruct the male patient to (1) thoroughly wash his hands, (2) cleanse the meatus, (3) void a small amount into the toilet, and (4) void directly into the specimen container.

➤ Instruct the female patient to (1) thoroughly wash her hands; (2) cleanse the labia from front to back; (3) while keeping the labia separated, void a small amount into the toilet; and (4) without interrupting the urine stream, void directly into the specimen container.

Timed specimen:

➤ Obtain a clean 3-L urine specimen container, toilet-mounted collection device, and plastic bag (for transport of the specimen container). The specimen must be refrigerated or kept on ice throughout the entire collection period. If an indwelling urinary catheter is in place, the drainage bag must be kept on ice.

➤ Begin the test between 6 and 8 a.m., if possible. Collect first voiding and discard. Record the time the specimen was discarded as the beginning of the timed collection period. The next morning, ask the patient to void at the same time the collection was started and add this last voiding to the container.

➤ If an indwelling catheter is in place, replace the tubing and container system at the start of the collection time. Keep the container system on ice during the collection period, or empty the urine into a larger container periodically during the collection period; monitor to ensure continued drainage, and conclude the test the next morning at the same hour the collection was begun.

➤ At the conclusion of the test, compare the quantity of urine with the urinary output record for the collection; if the specimen contains less than what was recorded as output, some urine may have been discarded, invalidating the test.

➤ Label the specimen, and promptly transport it to the laboratory. Include on the label the amount of urine, test start and stop times, and ingestion of any medications that can affect test results.

Post-test: ■

➤ Evaluate test results in relation to the patient's symptoms and other tests performed.

➤ Related laboratory tests include anion gap, blood and urine creatinine, creatinine clearance, blood and urine electrolytes, gentamicin, kidney stone analysis, microalbumin, blood urea nitrogen (BUN), BUN/creatinine ratio, blood and urine osmolality, tobramycin, blood and urine uric acid, urinalysis, and vancomycin.

URETHROGRAPHY, RETROGRADE

· ·

SYNONYM/ACRONYM: None.

AREA OF APPLICATION: Urethra.

CONTRAST: Radiopaque contrast medium.

DESCRIPTION: Retrograde urethrography is performed almost exclusively in male patients. It uses contrast medium, either injected or instilled via a catheter into the urethra, to visualize the membranous, bulbar, and penile portions, particularly after surgical repair of the urethra to assess the success of the surgery. The posterior portion of the urethra is visualized better when the procedure is performed with voiding cystourethrography. In women, it may be performed after surgical repair of the urethra to assess the success of the surgery and to assess structural abnormalities in conjunction with an evaluation for voiding dysfunction. ∎

INDICATIONS: Aid in the diagnosis of urethral strictures, lacerations, diverticula, and congenital anomalies

RESULT

Normal Findings:
• Normal size, shape, and course of the membranous, bulbar, and penile portions of the urethra in male patients
• If the prostatic portion can be visualized, it also should appear normal

Abnormal Findings:
• Congenital anomalies, such as urethral valves and perineal hypospadias
• False passages in the urethra
• Prostatic enlargement
• Tumors of the urethra
• Urethral calculi
• Urethral diverticula
• Urethral fistulas
• Urethral strictures and lacerations

CRITICAL VALUES: N/A

INTERFERING FACTORS:

This procedure is contraindicated for:
• Patients with allergies to shellfish or iodinated dye. The contrast medium used may cause a life-threatening allergic reaction. Patients with a known hypersensitivity to the contrast medium may benefit from premedication with corticosteroids or the use of nonionic contrast medium.

• Patients who are pregnant or suspected of being pregnant, unless the potential benefits of the procedure far outweigh the risks to the fetus and mother.

- Elderly and other patients who are ⚠ chronically dehydrated before the test, because of their risk of contrast-induced renal failure.

- ⚠ Patients who are in renal failure.

Factors that may impair clear imaging:

- Inability of the patient to cooperate or remain still during the procedure because of age, significant pain, or mental status

- Patients who are very obese, who may exceed the weight limit for the equipment

- Incorrect positioning of the patient, which may produce poor visualization of the area to be examined

- Improper adjustment of the radiographic equipment to accommodate obese or thin patients, which can cause overexposure or underexposure and a poor-quality study

- Metallic objects within the examination field (e.g., jewelry or body rings), which may inhibit organ visualization and can produce unclear images

Other considerations:

- Consultation with a physician should occur before the procedure for radiation safety concerns regarding infants of patients who are lactating.

- Risks associated with radiographic overexposure can result from frequent x-ray procedures. Personnel in the room with the patient should stand behind a shield or leave the area while the examination is being done. Personnel working in the area where the examination is being done should wear badges that reveal their level of exposure to radiation.

Nursing Implications and Procedure • • • • • • • • • • •

Pretest: ▮

➤ Inform the patient that the procedure assesses the urethra

➤ Inform the patient that the procedure is performed in a cystoscopy room by a urologist and takes approximately 30 minutes.

➤ Obtain a history of known or suspected hypersensitivity to radiographic contrast medium or shellfish.

➤ Obtain a history of the patient's complaints.

➤ Obtain a history of the patient's genitourinary system and the results of previously performed tests and procedures, specifically blood urea nitrogen and creatinine. For related tests, refer to the genitourinary system table.

➤ Patients receiving metformin (Glucophage) for non–insulin-dependent (type 2) diabetes should discontinue the drug on the day of the test and continue to withhold it for 48 hours after the test. Failure to do so may result in lactic acidosis.

➤ *Obtain a written, informed consent for the procedure from the patient, if needed.*

➤ If the contrast medium is instilled through a catheter, inform the patient that some pressure may be experienced when the catheter is inserted and contrast medium is instilled.

➤ Determine date of last menstrual period and possibility of pregnancy in perimenopausal women.

➤ Do not withhold food and fluids before the test.

Intratest: ▮

➤ Ask the patient to put on a hospital gown.

➤ Make sure jewelry, watches, chains,

belts, and any other metallic objects have been removed from the abdominal area.

➤ Place the patient on the table in a supine position in the recumbent position. Ask the patient to lie still during the procedure because movement produces unclear images.

➤ A single plain film is taken of the bladder and urethra.

➤ A catheter is filled with contrast medium to eliminate air pockets and is inserted until the balloon reaches the meatus. Inform the patient that the contrast medium may cause a temporary flushing of the face, a feeling of warmth, urticaria, headache, vomiting, or nausea.

➤ The patient is placed in the right posterior oblique position with the thigh drawn up to a 90° angle; in male patients, the penis is placed parallel to the leg.

➤ After three-fourths of the contrast medium is injected, another exposure is taken while the remainder of the contrast medium is injected.

➤ Left lateral and oblique exposures may be taken.

➤ The procedure may be done on female patients using a double balloon to occlude the bladder neck from above and below the external meatus.

➤ Wear gloves during the radionuclide administration and while handling the patient's urine.

Post-test: ■

➤ Monitor vital and neurologic signs until they return to preprocedure levels.

➤ Instruct the patient to resume usual diet and medications, as directed by the physician. Renal function should be assessed before metformin is restarted.

➤ Monitor fluid intake and urinary output for 24 hours after the procedure. Decreased urine output may indicate impending renal failure.

➤ Monitor for signs and symptoms of sepsis, including fever, chills, and severe pain in the kidney area.

➤ Maintain the patient on adequate hydration after the procedure. Encourage the patient to drink lots of fluids to prevent stasis and to prevent the buildup of bacteria.

➤ Advise patient to drink increased amounts of fluids for 24 to 48 hours to eliminate the radionuclide from the body, unless contraindicated. Tell the patient that radionuclide is eliminated from the body within 6 to 24 hours.

➤ Instruct the patient to immediately flush the toilet after each voiding after the procedure and to meticulously wash hands with soap and water after each voiding for 24 hours after the procedure.

➤ Tell all caregivers to wear gloves when discarding urine for 24 hours after the procedure. Wash gloved hands with soap and water before removing gloves. Then wash ungloved hands after the gloves are removed.

➤ Determine whether the patient or family members have any further questions or concerns.

➤ A physician specializing in this branch of medicine sends a written report to the ordering provider, who discusses the results with the patient.

➤ Inform the patient that further examinations may be necessary to evaluate progression of the disease process or to determine the need for a change in therapy.

➤ Evaluate test results in relation to the patient's symptoms and other tests performed. Related diagnostic tests include cystoscopy and intravenous pyelography.

URIC ACID, BLOOD

. . . .

SYNONYM/ACRONYM: Urate.

SPECIMEN: Serum (1 mL) collected in a red- or tiger-top tube. Plasma (1 mL) collected in green-top (heparin) tube is also acceptable.

REFERENCE VALUE: (Method: Spectrophotometry)

Age	Conventional Units	SI Units (Conversion Factor ×0.059)
Child less than 12 y	2.0–5.5 mg/dL	0.12–0.32 mmol/L
Adult younger than 60 y		
Male	4.4–7.6 mg/dL	0.26–0.45 mmol/L
Female	2.3–6.6 mg/dL	0.14–0.39 mmol/L
Adult older than 60 y		
Male	4.2–8.0 mg/dL	0.25–0.48 mmol/L
Female	3.5–7.3 mg/dL	0.21–0.43 mmol/L

DESCRIPTION: Uric acid is the end product of purine metabolism. Purines are important constituents of nucleic acids; purine turnover occurs continuously in the body, producing substantial amounts of uric acid even in the absence of purine intake from dietary sources such as organ meats (e.g., liver, thymus gland and/or pancreas [sweetbread], kidney), legumes, and yeasts. Uric acid is filtered, absorbed, and secreted by the kidneys and is a common constituent of urine. Serum urate levels are affected by the amount of uric acid produced and by the efficiency of renal excretion. ■

INDICATIONS:
• Assist in the diagnosis of gout when there is a family history (autosomal-dominant genetic disorder) or signs and symptoms of gout, indicated by elevated uric acid levels

• Determine the cause of known or suspected renal calculi

• Evaluate the extent of tissue destruction in infection, starvation, excessive exercise, malignancies, chemotherapy, or radiation therapy

• Evaluate possible liver damage in eclampsia, indicated by elevated uric acid levels

• Monitor the effects of drugs known to alter uric acid levels, either as a side effect or as a therapeutic effect

RESULT

Increased in:
• Acute tissue destruction as a result of starvation or excessive exercise

- Alcoholism
- Chemotherapy and radiation therapy
- Chronic lead toxicity
- Congestive heart failure
- Diabetes
- Down's syndrome
- Eclampsia
- Excessive dietary purines
- Glucose-6-phosphate dehydrogenase deficiency
- Gout
- Hyperparathyroidism
- Hypertension
- Hypoparathyroidism
- Lactic acidosis
- Lead poisoning
- Lesch-Nyhan syndrome
- Multiple myeloma
- Pernicious anemia
- Polycystic kidney disease
- Polycythemia
- Psoriasis
- Sickle cell anemia
- Type III hyperlipidemia

Decreased in:
- Fanconi's syndrome
- Low-purine diet
- Severe liver disease
- Wilson's disease

CRITICAL VALUES: N/A

INTERFERING FACTORS:
- Drugs and substances that may increase uric acid levels include acetylsalicylic acid (low doses), aldatense, aminothiadiazole, anabolic steroids, antineoplastic agents, ascorbic acid, chlorambucil, chlorthalidone, cisplatin, corn oil, cyclosporine, cyclothiazide, cytarabine, diapamide, diazoxide, diuretics, ergothioneine, ethacrynic acid, ethambutol, ethoxzolamide, etoposide, flumethiazide, hydroflumethiazide, hydroxyurea, ibufenac, ibuprofen, levarterenol, levodopa, mefruside, mercaptopurine, methicillin, methotrexate, methoxyflurane, methyclothiazide, mitomycin, morinamide, polythiazide, prednisone, pyrazinamide, salicylate, spironolactone, theophylline, thiazide diuretics, thioguanine, thiotepa, thiouric acid, triamterene, trichlormethiazide, vincristine, warfarin, and xylitol.

- Drugs that may decrease uric acid levels include allopurinol, aspirin (high doses), azathioprine, acetohexamide, benzbromaron, benziodarone, canola oil, chlorothiazide (given intravenously), chlorpromazine, chlorprothixene, cinchophen, corticotropin, corticosteroids, clofibrate, coumarin, diatrizoic acid, dicumarol, dipyrone, enalapril, fenofibrate, flufenamic acid, guaifenesin, hydralazine, iodipamide, iodopyracet, iopanoic acid, ipodate, lisinopril, mefenamic acid, mersalyl, methotrexate, oxyphenbutazone, phenindione, phenolsulfonphthalein, probenecid, seclazone, sulfinpyrazone, and verapamil.

Nursing Implications and Procedure . . . .

Pretest: ◼

➤ Obtain a history of the patient's complaints, including a list of known allergens. Especially note pain and edema in joints and great toe (caused by precipitation of sodium urates), headache, fatigue, decreased urinary output, and hypertension.

➤ Obtain a history of the patient's genitourinary, hepatobiliary, and musculoskeletal systems, as well as results of previously performed tests and procedures. For related tests, refer to the genitourinary, hepatobiliary, and musculoskeletal system tables.

➤ Obtain a list of medications the patient is taking, including herbs, nutritional supplements, and nutraceuticals. The requesting health care practitioner and laboratory should be advised if the patient is regularly using these products so that their effects can be taken into consideration when reviewing results.

➤ There are no food, fluid, or medication restrictions unless by medical direction.

➤ Review the procedure with the patient.

➤ Inform the patient that specimen collection takes approximately 5 to 10 minutes.

Intratest: ■

➤ Direct the patient to breathe normally and to avoid unnecessary movement.

➤ Observe standard precautions and follow the general guidelines in Appendix A. Perform a venipuncture, and collect the specimen in a 5-mL red- or tiger-top tube.

➤ Label the specimen, and promptly transport it to the laboratory.

Post-test: ■

➤ Observe venipuncture site for bleeding or hematoma formation. Apply pressure bandage.

➤ Increased uric acid levels may be associated with the formation of kidney stones. Educate the patient, if appropriate, on the importance of drinking a sufficient amount of water when kidney stones are suspected.

➤ Increased uric acid levels may be associated with gout. Nutritional therapy may be appropriate for some patients identified as having gout. Educate the patient that foods high in oxalic acid include caffeinated beverages, raw blackberries, gooseberries and plums, whole-wheat bread, beets, carrots, beans, rhubarb, spinach, dry cocoa, and Ovaltine. Foods high in purines include organ meats. In other cases, the requesting health care practitioner may not prescribe a low-purine or purine-restricted diet for treatment of gout because medications can control the condition easily and effectively.

➤ Evaluate test results in relation to the patient's symptoms and other tests performed. Related laboratory tests include complete blood count, creatinine, creatinine clearance, kidney stone analysis, synovial fluid analysis, and urine uric acid.

URIC ACID, URINE

. . . .

SYNONYM/ACRONYM: Urine urate.

SPECIMEN: Urine (5 mL) from a random or timed specimen collected in a clean plastic, unrefrigerated collection container. Sodium hydroxide preservative may be recommended to prevent precipitation of urates.

REFERENCE VALUE: (Method: Spectrophotometry)

Gender	Conventional Units*	SI Units (Conversion Factor ×0.0059)*
Male	250–800 mg/24 h	1.48–4.72 mmol/24 h
Female	250–750 mg/24 h	1.48–4.43 mmol/24 h

* Values reflect average purine diet.

DESCRIPTION: Uric acid is the end product of purine metabolism. Purines are important constituents of nucleic acids; purine turnover occurs continuously in the body, producing substantial amounts of uric acid even in the absence of purine intake from dietary sources such as organ meats (e.g., liver, thymus gland and/or pancreas [sweetbread], kidney), legumes, and yeasts. Uric acid is filtered, absorbed, and secreted by the kidneys and is a common constituent of urine. ■

INDICATIONS:
- Compare urine and serum uric acid levels to provide an index of renal function
- Detect enzyme deficiencies and metabolic disturbances that affect the body's production of uric acid
- Monitor the response to therapy with uricosuric drugs
- Monitor urinary effects of disorders that cause hyperuricemia

RESULT

Increased in:
- Disorders associated with impaired renal tubular absorption, such as Fanconi's syndrome and Wilson's disease
- Disorders of purine metabolism
- Excessive dietary intake of purines
- Gout
- Neoplastic disorders, such as leukemia, lymphosarcoma, and multiple myeloma

- Pernicious anemia
- Polycythemia vera
- Sickle cell anemia

Decreased in:
- Folic acid deficiency
- Lead toxicity
- Severe renal damage (possibly resulting from chronic glomerulonephritis, collagen disorders, diabetic glomerulosclerosis, lactic acidosis, ketoacidosis, and alcohol abuse)

CRITICAL VALUES: N/A

INTERFERING FACTORS:
- Drugs that may increase urine uric acid levels include acetaminophen, acetohexamide, ampicillin, ascorbic acid, azapropazone, benzbromarone, chlorpromazine, chlorprothixene, corticotropin, coumarin, cytotoxics, diatrizoic acid, dicumarol, ethyl biscoumacetate, glycine, iodipamide, iodopyracet, iopanoic acid, ipodate, levodopa, mannose, merbarone, mercaptopurine, mersalyl, methotrexate, niacinamide, phenindione, phenolsulfonphthalein, phenylbutazone, phloridzin, probenecid, salicylates (long-term, large doses), seclazone, sulfinpyrazone, theophylline, verapamil, and xylitol.

- Drugs that may decrease urine uric acid levels include acetylsalicylic acid (small doses), ascorbic acid, azathioprine, benzbromaron, bumetanide, chlorothiazide, chlorthalidone, citrates, ethacrynic acid, ethambutol, ethoxzolamide, hydrochlorothiazide, levarterenol, niacin, pyrazinoic acid, and thiazide diuretics.

- All urine voided for the timed collection period must be included in the collection or else falsely decreased values may be obtained. Compare output records with volume collected to verify that all voids were included in the collection.

Nursing Implications and Procedure • • • • • • • • • • • • •

Pretest:

➤ Obtain a history of the patient's complaints, including a list of known allergens.

➤ Obtain a history of the patient's genitourinary system and results of previously performed tests and procedures. For related tests, refer to the genitourinary system table.

➤ Obtain a list of medications the patient is taking, including herbs, nutritional supplements, and nutraceuticals. The requesting health care practitioner and laboratory should be advised if the patient regularly uses these products so that their effects can be taken into consideration when reviewing results.

➤ There are no food, fluid, or medication restrictions unless by medical direction.

➤ Review the procedure with the patient. Provide a nonmetallic urinal, bedpan, or toilet-mounted collection device.

➤ Usually a 24-hour time frame for urine collection is ordered. Inform the patient that all urine must be saved during that 24-hour period. Instruct the patient not to void directly into the laboratory collection container. Instruct the patient to avoid defecating in the collection device and to keep toilet tissue out of the collection device to prevent contamination of the specimen. Place a sign in the bathroom to remind the patient to save all urine.

➤ Instruct the patient to void all urine into the collection device and then to pour the urine into the laboratory collection container. Alternatively the specimen can be left in the collection device for a health care staff member to add to the laboratory collection container.

Intratest:

➤ Observe standard precautions and follow the general guidelines in Appendix A.

Random specimen (collect in early morning):

Clean-catch specimen:

➤ Instruct the male patient to (1) thoroughly wash his hands, (2) cleanse the meatus, (3) void a small amount into the toilet, and (4) void directly into the specimen container.

➤ Instruct the female patient to (1) thoroughly wash her hands; (2) cleanse the labia from front to back; (3) while keeping the labia separated, void a small amount into the toilet; and (4) without interrupting the urine stream, void directly into the specimen container.

Timed specimen:

➤ Obtain a clean 3-L urine specimen container, toilet-mounted collection device, and plastic bag (for transport of the specimen container). The specimen must be refrigerated or kept on ice throughout the entire collection period. If an indwelling urinary catheter is in place, the drainage bag must be kept on ice.

➤ Begin the test between 6 and 8 a.m., if possible. Collect first voiding and discard. Record the time the specimen was discarded as the beginning of the timed collection period. The next morning, ask the patient to void at the same time the collection was started and add this last voiding to the container.

➤ If an indwelling catheter is in place, replace the tubing and container system at the start of the collection time. Keep the container system on ice during the collection period, or empty the urine into a larger container periodically during the collection period; monitor to ensure continued drainage, and conclude the test the next morning at the same hour the collection was begun.

➤ At the conclusion of the test, compare the quantity of urine with the urinary output record for the collection; if the specimen contains less than what was recorded as output, some urine may have been discarded, invalidating the test.

➤ Label the specimen, and promptly transport it to the laboratory. Include on the label the amount of urine, test start and stop times, and ingestion of any medications that can affect test results.

Post-test:

➤ Instruct the patient to resume usual diet as directed by the requesting health care practitioner.

➤ Increased uric acid levels may be associated with the formation of kidney stones. Educate the patient, if appropriate, on the importance of drinking a sufficient amount of water when kidney stones are suspected.

➤ Increased uric acid levels may be associated with gout. Nutritional therapy may be appropriate for some patients identified as having gout. Educate the patient that foods high in oxalic acid include caffeinated beverages, raw blackberries, gooseberries and plums, whole-wheat bread, beets, carrots, beans, rhubarb, spinach, dry cocoa, and Ovaltine. Foods high in purines include organ meats. In other cases, the requesting health care practitioner may not prescribe a low-purine or purine-restricted diet for treatment of gout because medications can control the condition easily and effectively.

➤ Evaluate test results in relation to the patient's symptoms and other tests performed. Related laboratory tests include urine calcium, complete blood count, urine creatinine, kidney stone analysis, urine oxalate, blood uric acid, and urinalysis.

URINALYSIS

. . . .

SYNONYM/ACRONYM: UA.

SPECIMEN: Urine (15 mL) from an unpreserved, random specimen collected in a clean, plastic collection container.

REFERENCE VALUE: (Method: Macroscopic evaluation by dipstick and microscopic examination) Urinalysis comprises a battery of tests including a description of the color and appearance of urine; measurement of specific gravity and pH; and semiquantitative measurement of protein, glucose, ketones, urobilinogen, bilirubin, hemoglobin, nitrites, and leukocyte esterase. Urine sediment may also be examined for the presence of crystals, casts, renal epithelial cells, transitional epithelial cells, squamous epithelial cells, white blood cells (WBCs), red blood cells (RBCs), bacteria, yeast, sperm, and any other substances excreted in the urine that may have clinical significance. Examination of urine sediment is performed microscopically under high power, and results are reported as the number seen per high-power field (hpf). The color of normal urine ranges from light yellow to deep amber. The color depends on the patient's state of hydration (more concentrated samples are darker in color), diet, medication regimen, and exposure to other substances that may contribute to unusual color or odor. The appearance of normal urine is clear. Cloudiness is sometimes attributable to the presence of amorphous phosphates or urates as well as blood, WBCs, fat, or bacteria. Normal specific gravity is 1.001 to 1.035.

Dipstick

pH	5.0–9.0
Protein	Less than 20 mg/dL
Glucose	Negative
Ketones	Negative
Hemoglobin	Negative
Bilirubin	Negative
Urobilinogen	Up to 1 mg/dL
Nitrite	Negative
Leukocyte esterase	Negative

Microscopic Examination

Red blood cells	Less than 5/hpf
White blood cells	Less than 5/hpf
Renal cells	None seen
Transitional cells	None seen
Squamous cells	Rare; usually no clinical significance
Casts	Rare hyaline; otherwise, none seen
Crystals in acid urine	Uric acid, calcium oxalate, amorphous urates
Crystals in alkaline urine	Triple phosphate, calcium phosphate, ammonium biurate, calcium carbonate, amorphous phosphates
Bacteria, yeast, parasites	None seen

DESCRIPTION: Routine urinalysis, one of the most widely ordered laboratory procedures, is used for basic screening purposes. It is a group of tests that evaluate the kidneys' ability to selectively excrete and reabsorb substances while maintaining proper water balance. The results can provide valuable information regarding the overall health of the patient and the patient's response to disease and treatment. The urine dipstick has a number of pads on it to indicate various biochemical markers. Urine pH is an indication of the kidneys' ability to help maintain balanced hydrogen ion concentration in the blood. Specific gravity is a reflection of the concentration ability of the kidneys. Urine protein is the most common indicator of renal disease, although there are conditions that can cause benign proteinuria. Glucose is used as an indicator of diabetes. The presence of ketones indicates impaired carbohydrate metabolism. Hemoglobin indicates the presence of blood, which is associated with renal disease. Bilirubin is used to assist in the detection of liver disorders. Urobilinogen indicates hepatic or hematopoietic conditions. Nitrites and leukocytes are used to test for bacteriuria and other sources of urinary tract infections (UTIs). Most laboratories have established criteria for the microscopic examination of urine based on patient population (e.g., pediatric, oncology, urology), unusual appearance, and biochemical reactions. ∎

INDICATIONS:

• Determine the presence of a genitourinary infection or abnormality

• Monitor the effects of physical or emotional stress

• Monitor fluid imbalances or treatment for fluid imbalances

• Monitor the response to drug therapy and evaluate undesired reactions to drugs that may impair renal function

• Provide screening as part of a general physical examination, especially on admission to a health care facility or before surgery

RESULT

Unusual Color

Color	Presence of
Deep yellow	Riboflavin
Orange	Bilirubin, chrysophanic acid, pyridium, santonin
Pink	Beet pigment, hemoglobin, myoglobin, porphyrin, rhubarb
Red	Beet pigment, hemoglobin, myoglobin, porphyrin, uroerythrin
Green	Oxidized bilirubin, Clorets (breath mint)
Blue	Diagnex, indican, methylene blue
Brown	Bilirubin, hematin, methemoglobin, metronidazole, nitrofurantoin, metabolites of rhubarb, senna
Black	Homogentisic acid, melanin
Smokey	Red blood cells

Test	Increased in	Decreased in
pH	Ingestion of citrus fruits Metabolic and respiratory alkalosis Vegetarian diets	High-protein diets Ingestion of fruits (e.g., cranberries) Metabolic or respiratory acidosis

(Continued on the following page)

Test	Increased in	Decreased in
Protein	Benign proteinuria owing to stress, physical exercise, exposure to cold, or standing Diabetic nephropathy Glomerulonephritis Nephrosis Toxemia of pregnancy	N/A
Glucose	Diabetes	N/A
Ketones	Diabetes Fever Fasting Postanesthesia period High-protein diets Isopropanol intoxication Starvation Vomiting	N/A
Hemoglobin	Diseases of the bladder Exercise (March hemoglobinuria) Glomerulonephritis Hemolytic anemia or other causes of hemolysis (e.g., drugs, parasites, transfusion reaction) Malignancy Menstruation Paroxysmal cold hemoglobinuria Paroxysmal nocturnal hemoglobinuria Pyelonephritis Snake or spider bites Trauma Tuberculosis Urinary tract infections Urolithiasis	N/A
Urobilinogen	Cirrhosis Heart failure Hemolytic anemia Hepatitis Infectious mononucleosis Malaria Pernicious anemia	Antibiotic therapy (suppresses normal intestinal flora) Obstruction of the bile duct
Bilirubin	Cirrhosis Hepatic tumor Hepatitis	N/A

(Continued on the following page)

Test	Increased in	Decreased in
Nitrites	Presence of nitrite-forming bacteria (e.g., *Citrobacter, Enterobacter, Escherichia coli, Klebsiella, Proteus, Pseudomonas, Salmonella,* and some species of *Staphylococcus*)	N/A
Leukocyte esterase	Bacterial infection Calculus formation Fungal or parasitic infection Glomerulonephritis Interstitial nephritis Tumor	N/A

Formed Elements in Urine Sediment

Cellular Elements:

- Clue cells (cell wall of the bacteria causes adhesion to epithelial cells) are present in nonspecific vaginitis caused by *Gardnerella vaginitis, Mobiluncus cortisii,* and *Mobiluncus mulieris.*

- RBCs are present in glomerulonephritis, lupus nephritis, focal glomerulonephritis, calculus, malignancy, infection, tuberculosis, infarction, renal vein thrombosis, trauma, hydronephrosis, polycystic kidney, urinary tract disease, prostatitis, pyelonephritis, appendicitis, salpingitis, diverticulitis, gout, scurvy, subacute bacterial endocarditis, infectious mononucleosis, hemoglobinopathies, coagulation disorders, heart failure, and malaria.

- Renal cells that have absorbed cholesterol and triglycerides are also known as *oval fat bodies.*

- Renal cells come from the lining of the collecting ducts, and increased numbers indicate acute tubular damage as seen in acute tubular necrosis, pyelonephritis, malignant nephrosclerosis, acute glomerulonephritis, acute drug or substance (salicylate, lead, or ethylene glycol) intoxication, or chemotherapy, resulting in desquamation, urolithiasis, and kidney transplant rejection.

- Squamous cells line the vagina and distal portion of the urethra. The presence of normal squamous epithelial cells in female urine is generally of no clinical significance. Abnormal cells with enlarged nuclei indicate the need for cytologic studies to rule out malignancy.

- Transitional cells line the renal pelvis, ureter, bladder, and proximal portion of the urethra. Increased numbers are seen with infection, trauma, and malignancy.

- WBCs are present in acute UTI, tubulointerstitial nephritis, lupus nephritis, pyelonephritis, kidney transplant rejection, fever, and strenuous exercise.

Casts:

- Granular casts are formed from protein or by the decomposition of cellular elements. They may be seen in renal disease, viral infections, or lead intoxication.

- Large numbers of hyaline casts may be seen in renal diseases, hypertension, congestive heart failure, nephrotic syndrome, and in more benign conditions such as fever, exposure to cold temperatures, exercise, or diuretic use.

- RBC casts may be found in acute glomerulonephritis, lupus nephritis, and subacute bacterial endocarditis.

- Waxy casts are seen in chronic renal failure or conditions such as kidney transplant rejection, in which there is renal stasis.

- WBC casts may be seen in lupus nephritis, acute glomerulonephritis, interstitial nephritis, and acute pyelonephritis.

Crystals:
- Crystals found in freshly voided urine have more clinical significance than crystals seen in a urine sample that has been standing for more than 2 to 4 hours.

- Calcium oxalate crystals are found in ethylene glycol poisoning, urolithiasis, high dietary intake of oxalates, and Crohn's disease.

- Cystine crystals are seen in patients with cystinosis or cystinuria.

- Leucine or tyrosine crystals may be seen in patients with severe liver disease.

- Large numbers of uric acid crystals are seen in patients with urolithiasis, gout, high dietary intake of foods rich in purines, or receiving chemotherapy (see monograph titled "Uric Acid, Urine").

CRITICAL VALUES: ⚠ Possible critical values are the presence of uric acid, cystine, leucine, or tyrosine crystals. The combination of grossly elevated urine glucose and ketones is also considered significant.

INTERFERING FACTORS:
- Certain foods, such as onion, garlic, and asparagus, contain substances that

may give urine an unusual odor. An ammonia-like odor may be produced by the presence of bacteria. Urine with a maple syrup–like odor may indicate a congenital metabolic defect (maple syrup urine disease).

- The various biochemical strips are subject to interference that may produce false-positive or false-negative results. Consult the laboratory for specific information regarding limitations of the method in use and a listing of interfering drugs.

- The dipstick method for protein detection is mostly sensitive to the presence of albumin; light-chain or Bence Jones proteins may not be detected by this method. Alkaline pH may produce false-positive protein results.

- Large amounts of ketones or ascorbic acid may produce false-negative or decreased color development on the glucose pad. Contamination of the collection container or specimen with chlorine, sodium hypochlorite, or peroxide may cause false-positive glucose results.

- False-positive ketone results may be produced in the presence of ascorbic acid, levodopa metabolites, valproic acid, phenazopyridine, phenylketones, or phthaleins.

- The hemoglobin pad may detect myoglobin, intact RBCs, and free hemoglobin. Contamination of the collection container or specimen with sodium hypochlorite or iodine may cause false-positive hemoglobin results. Negative or decreased hemoglobin results may occur in the presence of formalin, elevated protein, nitrite, ascorbic acid, or high specific gravity.

- False-negative nitrite results are common. Negative or decreased results may be seen in the presence of ascorbic acid and high specific gravity. Other causes of false-negative values relate to the amount of time the urine was in the bladder before voiding or the presence of pathogenic organisms that do not reduce nitrates to nitrites.

- False-positive leukocyte esterase reactions result from specimens contaminated by vaginal secretions. The presence of high glucose, protein, or ascorbic acid concentrations may cause false-negative results. Specimens with high specific gravity may also produce false-negative results. Patients with neutropenia (e.g., oncology patients) may also have false-negative results because they do not produce enough WBCs to exceed the sensitivity of the biochemical reaction.

- Specimens that cannot be delivered to the laboratory or tested within 1 hour should be refrigerated or should have a preservative added that is recommended by the laboratory. Specimens collected more than 2 hours before submission may be rejected for analysis.

- Because changes in the urine specimen occur over time, prompt and proper specimen processing, storage, and analysis are important to achieve accurate results. Changes that may occur over time include:

- Production of a stronger odor and an increase in pH (bacteria in the urine break urea down to ammonia)

- A decrease in clarity (as bacterial growth proceeds or precipitates form)

- A decrease in bilirubin and urobilinogen (oxidation to biliverdin and urobilin)

- A decrease in ketones (lost through volatilization)

- Decreased glucose (consumed by bacteria)

- An increase in bacteria (growth over time)

- Disintegration of casts, WBCs, and RBCs

- An increase in nitrite (overgrowth of bacteria)

Nursing Implications and Procedure • • • • • • • • • • • •

Pretest:

➤ Obtain a history of the patient's complaints, including a list of known allergens.

➤ Obtain a history of the patient's endocrine, genitourinary, immune, hematopoietic, hepatobiliary, and reproductive systems, as well as results of previously performed tests and procedures. For related tests, refer to the endocrine, genitourinary, immune, hematopoietic, hepatobiliary, and reproductive system tables.

➤ Obtain a list of medications the patient is taking, including herbs, nutritional supplements, and nutraceuticals. The requesting health care practitioner and laboratory should be advised if the patient is regularly using these products so that their effects can be taken into consideration when reviewing results.

➤ There are no food, fluid, or medication restrictions unless by medical direction.

➤ Review the procedure with the patient. If a catheterized specimen is to be collected, explain this procedure to the patient, and obtain a catheterization tray.

➤ Inform the patient that specimen collection takes approximately 5 to 10 minutes.

Intratest:

➤ Observe standard precautions and follow the general guidelines in Appendix A.

Random specimen (collect in early morning):

Clean-catch specimen:

➤ Instruct the male patient to (1) thoroughly wash his hands, (2) cleanse the meatus, (3) void a small amount into the toilet, and (4) void directly into the specimen container.

➤ Instruct the female patient to (1) thoroughly wash her hands; (2) cleanse the labia from front to back; (3) while keeping the labia separated, void a small amount into the toilet; and (4) without interrupting the urine stream, void directly into the specimen container.

Pediatric urine collector:

➤ Put on gloves. Appropriately cleanse the genital area and allow the area to dry. Remove the covering over the adhesive strips on the collector bag and apply over the genital area. Diaper the child. When specimen is obtained, place the entire collection bag in a sterile urine container.

Indwelling catheter:

➤ Put on gloves. Empty drainage tube of urine. It may be necessary to clamp off the catheter for 15 to 30 minutes before specimen collection. Cleanse specimen port with antiseptic swab, and then aspirate 5 mL of urine with a 21- to 25-gauge needle and syringe. Transfer urine to a sterile container.

Urinary catheterization:

➤ Place female patient in lithotomy position or male patient in supine position. Using sterile technique, open the straight urinary catheterization kit and perform urinary catheterization. Place the retained urine in a sterile specimen container.

Suprapubic aspiration:

➤ Place the patient in a supine position. Cleanse the area with antiseptic and drape with sterile drapes. Using sterile technique, insert needle and remove sterile sample. Place the returned sample in a sterile specimen container. Place a dry sterile dressing over the site.

➤ Do not collect urine from the pouch from the patient with a urinary diversion (e.g., ilieal conduit). Instead perform catheterization through the stoma.

General:

➤ Label the specimen, indicate whether the specimen is clean catch or catheter, and promptly transport it to the laboratory. Indicate on the label the date and time of collection and any medications that may interfere with test results.

Post-test:

➤ Instruct the patient to report symptoms, such as pain related to tissue inflammation, pain or irritation during void, bladder spasms, or alterations in urinary elimination.

➤ Observe for signs of inflammation if the specimen is obtained by suprapubic aspiration.

➤ Instruct the patient to begin antibiotic therapy, as prescribed, and instruct the patient in the importance of completing the entire course of antibiotic therapy even if symptoms are no longer present.

➤ Instruct the patient with a UTI, as appropriate, on the proper technique for wiping the perineal area (front to back) after a bowel movement.

➤ UTIs are more common in women who use diaphragm/spermicide contraception. These patients can be educated, as appropriate, in the proper insertion and removal of the contraceptive device to avoid recurrent UTIs.

➤ Evaluate test results in relation to the patient's symptoms and other tests performed. Related laboratory tests include blood and urine amino acids, anti–glomerular basement membrane antibody, bladder biopsy, kidney biopsy, bladder cancer marker, urine calcium, complete blood count, blood and urine creatinine, relevant cultures, blood and urine electrolytes, glucose, glycated hemoglobin, blood and urine ketones, kidney stone analysis, microalbumin, urine osmolality, urine oxalate, urine protein, blood and urine protein immunofixation electrophoresis, urine phosphorus, blood and urine urea nitrogen, and blood and urine uric acid.

VANILLYLMANDELIC ACID, URINE

SYNONYM/ACRONYM: VMA.

SPECIMEN: Urine (25 mL) from a timed specimen collected in a clean plastic collection container with 6N hydrochloric acid as a preservative.

REFERENCE VALUE: (Method: High-pressure liquid chromatography)

Age	Conventional Units	SI Units (Conversion Factor ×5.05)
3–6 y	1.0–2.6 mg/24 h	5–13 μmol/24 h
6–10 y	2.0–3.2 mg/24 h	10–16 μmol/24 h
10–16 y	2.3–5.2 mg/24 h	12–26 μmol/24 h
16–83 y	1.4–6.5 mg/24 h	7–33 μmol/24 h

DESCRIPTION: Vanillylmandelic acid (VMA) is a major metabolite of epinephrine and norepinephrine. It is elevated in conditions that also are marked by overproduction of catecholamines. Creatinine is usually measured simultaneously to ensure adequate collection and to calculate an excretion ratio of metabolite to creatinine. ■

INDICATIONS:
• Assist in the diagnosis of neuroblastoma, ganglioneuroma, or pheochromocytoma

• Evaluate hypertension of unknown cause

RESULT

Increased in:
• Ganglioneuroma

• Hypertension

• Neuroblastoma

• Pheochromocytoma

Decreased in: N/A

CRITICAL VALUES: N/A

INTERFERING FACTORS:
• Drugs that may increase VMA levels include ajmaline, chlorpromazine, glucagon, guaifenesin, guanethidine, isoproterenol, methyldopa, nitroglycerin, oxytetracycline, phenazopyridine, phenolsulfonphthalein, prochlorperazine, rauwolfia, reserpine, sulfobromophthalein, and syrosingopine.

• Drugs that may decrease VMA levels include brofaromine, guanethidine, guanfacine, imipramine, isocarboxazid, monoamine oxidase inhibitors, methyldopa, morphine, nialamide (in schizophrenics), and reserpine.

• Stress, hypoglycemia, hyperthyroidism, strenuous exercise, smoking, and drugs can produce elevated catecholamines.

• Failure to collect all urine and store 24-hour specimen properly will result in a falsely low result.

Nursing Implications and Procedure • • • • • • • • • • • •

➤ Obtain a history of the patient's complaints, including a list of known allergens.

➤ Obtain a history of the patient's endocrine system and results of previously performed tests and procedures. For related tests, refer to the endocrine system table.

➤ Obtain a list of medications the patient is taking, including herbs, nutritional supplements, and nutraceuticals. The requesting health care practitioner and laboratory should be advised if the patient regularly uses these products so that their effects can be taken into consideration when reviewing results.

➤ There are no fluid restrictions unless by medical direction.

➤ Instruct the patient to abstain from smoking tobacco for 24 hours before testing.

➤ Inform the patient of the following dietary, medication, and activity restrictions in preparation for the test:

The patient should not consume foods high in amines for 48 hours before testing (bananas, avocados, beer, aged cheese, chocolate, cocoa, coffee, fava beans, grains, tea, vanilla, walnuts, and Chianti wine).

The patient should avoid self-prescribed medications (especially aspirin) and prescribed medications (especially pyridoxine, levodopa, amoxicillin, carbidopa, reserpine, and disulfiram) for 2 weeks before testing and as directed.

The patient should continue to avoid excessive exercise and stress during the 24-hour collection of urine.

➤ Review the procedure with the patient. Provide a nonmetallic urinal, bedpan, or toilet-mounted collection device.

➤ Usually a 24-hour time frame for urine collection is ordered. Inform the patient that all urine must be saved during that 24-hour period. Instruct the patient not to void directly into the laboratory collection container. Instruct the patient to avoid defecating in the collection device and to keep toilet tissue out of the collection device to prevent contamination of the specimen. Place a sign in the bathroom to remind the patient to save all urine.

➤ Instruct the patient to void all urine into the collection device and then to pour the urine into the laboratory collection container. Alternatively the specimen can be left in the collection device for a health care staff member to add to the laboratory collection container.

➤ Ensure that the patient has complied with dietary preparations and other pretesting restrictions.

➤ Observe standard precautions and follow the general guidelines in Appendix A.

Timed specimen:

➤ Obtain a clean 3-L urine specimen container, toilet-mounted collection device, and plastic bag (for transport of the specimen container). The specimen must be refrigerated or kept on ice throughout the entire collection period. If an indwelling urinary catheter is in place, the drainage bag must be kept on ice.

➤ Begin the test between 6 and 8 a.m., if possible. Collect first voiding and discard. Record the time the specimen was discarded as the beginning of the timed collection period. The next morning, ask the patient to void at the same time the collection was started and add this last voiding to the container.

➤ If an indwelling catheter is in place, replace the tubing and container system at the start of the collection time. Keep the container system on ice during the collection period, or empty the urine into a larger container periodically during the collection period; monitor to ensure continued drainage, and conclude the test the next morning at the same hour the collection was begun.

➤ At the conclusion of the test, compare the quantity of urine with the urinary output record for the collection; if the specimen contains less than what was recorded as output, some urine may have been discarded, invalidating the test.

➤ Label the specimen, and promptly transport it to the laboratory. Include on the label the amount of urine, test start and stop times, and ingestion of any foods or medications that can affect test results.

Post-test:

➤ Instruct the patient to resume usual diet, medications, and activity, as appropriate and as directed by the requesting health care practitioner.

➤ Evaluate test results in relation to the patient's symptoms and other tests performed. Related laboratory tests include catecholamines, homovanillic acid, and metanephrines.

VARICELLA ANTIBODIES

SYNONYMS/ACRONYM: Varicella zoster antibodies, chickenpox, VZ.

SPECIMEN: Serum (1 mL) collected in a red-top tube.

REFERENCE VALUE: (Method: Indirect fluorescent antibody) Negative or less than a fourfold increase in titer.

DESCRIPTION: Varicella zoster is a double-stranded DNA herpesvirus that is responsible for two clinical syndromes, chickenpox and shingles. The incubation period is 2 to 3 weeks, and it is highly contagious for about 2 weeks beginning 2 days before a rash develops. It is transmitted in respiratory secretions. The primary exposure to the highly contagious virus usually occurs in susceptible school-age children. Adults without prior exposure and who become infected may have severe complications, including pneumonia. Neonatal infection from the mother is possible if exposure occurs during the last 3 weeks of gestation. Shingles results when the presumably latent virus is reactivated. The presence of immunoglobulin M (IgM) antibodies indicates acute infection. The presence of IgG antibodies indicates current or past infection. A reactive varicella antibody result indicates immunity but does not protect an individual from shingles. ■

INDICATIONS: Determine susceptibility or immunity to chickenpox

RESULT

Positive findings in: Varicella infection

Negative findings in: N/A

CRITICAL VALUES: N/A

INTERFERING FACTORS: N/A

Nursing Implications and Procedure · · · · · · · · · · ·

Pretest: ▪

➤ Obtain a history of the patient's complaints, including a list of known allergens. Obtain a history of exposure to varicella.

➤ Obtain a history of the patient's immune and reproductive systems, as well as results of previously performed tests and procedures. For related tests, refer to the immune and reproductive system tables.

➤ Obtain a list of medications the patient is taking, including herbs, nutritional supplements, and nutraceuticals. The requesting health care practitioner and laboratory should be advised if the patient is regularly using these products so that their effects can be taken into consideration when reviewing results.

➤ There are no food, fluid, or medication restrictions unless by medical direction.

➤ Review the procedure with the patient.

➤ Inform the patient that several tests may be necessary to confirm diagnosis. Any individual positive result should be repeated in 7 to 14 days to monitor a change in titer.

➤ Inform the patient that each specimen collection takes approximately 5 to 10 minutes.

Intratest: ▪

➤ Direct the patient to breathe normally and to avoid unnecessary movement.

➤ Observe standard precautions and follow the general guidelines in Appendix A. Perform a venipuncture, and collect the specimen in a 5-mL red-top tube.

➤ Label the specimen, and promptly transport it to the laboratory.

Post-test: ▪

➤ Observe venipuncture site for bleeding or hematoma formation. Apply pressure bandage.

➤ Instruct the patient in isolation precautions during the time of communicability or contagion.

➤ Emphasize the need to return to have a convalescent blood sample taken in 7 to 14 days.

➤ Recognize anxiety related to test results and provide emotional support if results are positive and the patient is pregnant. Provide teaching and information regarding the clinical implications of the test results, as appropriate. Educate the patient regarding access to counseling services. Inform the patient with shingles regarding access to pain management.

➤ Evaluate test results in relation to the patient's symptoms and other tests performed.

VENOGRAPHY, LOWER EXTREMITY STUDIES

SYNONYMS/ACRONYM: Phlebography, lower limb venography, venogram.

AREA OF APPLICATION: Veins of the lower extremities.

CONTRAST: Iodine based.

DESCRIPTION: Venography allows x-ray visualization of the venous vasculature system of the extremities after injection of an iodinated contrast medium. Lower extremity studies identify and locate thrombi within the venous system of the lower limbs. After injection of the contrast medium, x-ray films are taken at timed intervals. Usually both extremities are studied, and the unaffected side is used for comparison for the side suspected of having deep vein thrombosis (DVT) or other venous abnormalities, such as congenital malformations or incompetent valves. Thrombus formation usually occurs in the deep calf veins and at the venous junction and its valves. If DVT is not treated, it can lead to femoral and iliac venous occlusion, or the thrombus can become an embolus, causing a pulmonary embolism. Venography is accurate for thrombi in veins below the knee. ■

INDICATIONS:
- Confirm a diagnosis of DVT
- Distinguish clot formation from venous obstruction
- Evaluate congenital venous malformations

- Assess deep vein valvular competence
- Locate a vein for arterial bypass graft surgery
- Determine the cause of extremity swelling or pain
- Determine the source of pulmonary emboli

RESULT

Normal Findings: No obstruction to flow or filling defects after injection of radiopaque dye; steady opacification of superficial and deep vasculature with no filling defects

Abnormal Findings: Abnormal results may indicate DVT, deep vein valvular incompetence, or venous obstruction

CRITICAL VALUES: N/A

INTERFERING FACTORS:

This procedure is contraindicated for:
- Patients with allergies to shellfish or iodinated dye. The contrast medium used may cause a life-threatening allergic reaction. Patients with a known hypersensitivity to the contrast medium may benefit from premedication with corticosteroids or the use of nonionic contrast medium.

- Patients who are pregnant or suspected of being pregnant, unless the potential benefits of the procedure far outweigh the risks to the fetus and mother.

- Elderly and other patients who are chronically dehydrated before the test, because of their risk of contrast-induced renal failure.

- Patients who are in renal failure.

- Patients with bleeding disorders.

Factors that may impair clear imaging:

- Inability of the patient to cooperate or remain still during the procedure because of age, significant pain, or mental status

- Patients who are very obese, who may exceed the weight limit for the equipment

- Incorrect positioning of the patient, which may produce poor visualization of the area to be examined

- Improper adjustment of the radiographic equipment to accommodate obese or thin patients, which can cause overexposure or underexposure and a poor-quality study

- Metallic objects within the examination field (e.g., jewelry or body rings), which may inhibit organ visualization and can produce unclear images

- Movement of the leg being tested, excessive tourniquet constriction, insufficient injection of contrast medium, and delay between injection and the x-ray

- Severe edema of the legs, making venous access impossible

- Weight bearing on the leg being tested, which prevents the contrast medium from filling the veins

Other considerations:

- Improper injection of the radionuclide

that allows the tracer to seep deep into the muscle tissue can produce erroneous hot spots.

- Consultation with a physician should occur before the procedure for radiation safety concerns regarding infants of patients who are lactating.

- Risks associated with radiographic overexposure can result from frequent x-ray procedures. Personnel in the room with the patient should wear a protective lead apron, stand behind a shield, or leave the area while the examination is being done. Personnel working in the area where the examination is being done should wear badges that reveal their level of exposure to radiation.

Nursing Implications and Procedure

Pretest:

➤ Inform the patient that the procedure assesses the venous system of the lower extremities.

➤ Inform the patient that the procedure is performed by a physician and takes approximately 60 minutes.

➤ Obtain a history of known or suspected hypersensitivity to radiographic contrast medium or shellfish.

➤ Obtain a history pertinent to the venogram to be performed. For related tests, refer to the cardiovascular system table.

➤ Determine previous abnormalities in laboratory tests and diagnostic procedures. Ascertain recent coagulation times, blood urea nitrogen (BUN), creatinine, and renal function values, as ordered.

➤ Withhold anticoagulant medication or reduce dosage before the procedure, as ordered.

➤ Patients receiving metformin (Glucophage) for non–insulin-dependent (type 2) diabetes should discontinue the drug on the day of the test and continue to withhold it for 48 hours after the test. Failure to do so may result in lactic acidosis.

➤ *Obtain a written, informed consent for the procedure from the patient, if needed.*

➤ Determine date of last menstrual period and possibility of pregnancy in perimenopausal women.

➤ Restrict food and fluids for at least 4 hours before the procedure.

➤ Obtain and record baseline vital signs to use for comparison after the procedure.

Intratest:

➤ Administer a mild sedative as ordered.

➤ Ask the patient to put on a hospital gown and void.

➤ Make sure jewelry and any other metallic objects have been removed from the lower extremities.

➤ Make sure emergency equipment is readily accessible.

➤ If the patient has a history of severe allergic reactions to various substances or drugs, administer ordered prophylactic steroids or antihistamines before the procedure. Use nonionic contrast medium for the procedure.

➤ Using a pen, mark the site of the patient's peripheral pulses before angiography; this permits quicker and more consistent assessment of pulses after the procedure.

➤ Place electrocardiographic electrodes on the patient for cardiac monitoring. Establish a baseline rhythm; determine whether the patient has ventricular arrhythmias.

➤ Place the patient in the supine position on an x-ray table. Cleanse the selected vein, and cover with a sterile drape.

➤ Establish intravenous (IV) fluid line for the injection of contrast medium.

➤ After the contrast medium is injected into a vein, x-rays are taken following the course of the contrast

medium into the veins of the leg. A tourniquet may be used on the leg to prevent the dye from traveling to the superficial saphenous vein, thus allowing all of the contrast medium to go to the deep venous system. Inform the patient that the contrast medium may cause a temporary flushing of the face, a feeling of warmth, urticaria, headache, vomiting, or nausea.

➤ Monitor the patient for complications related to the contrast medium (e.g., allergic reaction, anaphylaxis, bronchospasm, dyspnea).

➤ Observe the injection site for signs of contrast medium infiltration, such as redness, edema, warmth, or tenderness.

➤ Report signs of vein perforation, embolism, and extravasation of contrast medium, including chills; fever; rapid pulse and respiratory rates; hypotension; dyspnea; and chest, abdominal, or flank pain.

➤ Report to the physician any complaints of paresthesia or pain in the catheterized limb, such as symptoms of nerve irritation or vascular compromise.

➤ Remove the IV line, and apply a pressure dressing over the puncture site.

Post-test:

➤ Observe injection site for bleeding or hematoma formation. Apply a warm compress to ease discomfort if a hematoma develops.

➤ Instruct the patient to resume usual diet, medications, and activity, as directed by the physician. Renal function should be assessed before metformin is restarted.

➤ Instruct the patient to increase fluid intake to counteract the diuretic effects of contrast medium.

➤ Observe for a delayed allergic reaction to contrast, including flushing, hives, urticaria, laryngeal stridor, rash, tightening of throat, or difficulty breathing, and advise the patient to immediately report any of these symptoms.

➤ Monitor for complications after venography, including bacteremia, cellulitis, embolism, and thrombophlebitis.

➤ Check pulse rate on the dorsalis pedis, popliteal, and femoral arteries after the procedure.

➤ Assess peripheral color, motion, temperature, and sensation of the lower extremities on a regular basis in accordance with hospital protocol.

➤ A physician specializing in this branch of medicine sends a written report to the ordering provider, who discusses the results with the patient.

➤ Evaluate test results in relation to the patient's symptoms and other tests performed. Related diagnostic tests include angiography of the leg, magnetic resonance angiography, and computed tomography angiography.

VITAMIN B₁₂

. . . .

SYNONYM/ACRONYM: Cyanocobalamin.

SPECIMEN: Serum (1 mL) collected in a red- or tiger-top tube.

REFERENCE VALUE: (Method: Radioimmunoassay)

Age	Conventional Units	SI Units (Conversion Factor ×0.738)
Newborn	160–1300 pg/mL	118–959 pmol/L
Adult	200–900 pg/mL	148–664 pmol/L

DESCRIPTION: Vitamin B_{12} has a ringed crystalline structure that surrounds an atom of cobalt. It is essential in DNA synthesis, hematopoiesis, and central nervous system integrity. It is derived solely from dietary intake. Animal products are the richest source of vitamin B_{12}. Its absorption depends on the presence of intrinsic factor. Circumstances that may result in a deficiency of this vitamin include the presence of stomach or intestinal disease as well as insufficient dietary intake of foods containing vitamin B_{12}. A significant increase in red blood cell (RBC) mean corpuscular volume may be an important indicator of vitamin B_{12} deficiency. ▪

INDICATIONS:
• Assist in the diagnosis of central nervous system disorders

• Assist in the diagnosis of megaloblastic anemia

• Evaluate alcoholism

• Evaluate malabsorption syndromes

RESULT

Increased in:
• Chronic granulocytic leukemia

- Chronic renal failure

- Chronic obstructive pulmonary disease (COPD)

- Diabetes

- Leukocytosis

- Liver cell damage (hepatitis, cirrhosis)

- Obesity

- Polycythemia vera

- Protein malnutrition

- Severe congestive heart failure

- Some carcinomas

Decreased in:

- Abnormalities of cobalamin transport or metabolism

- Bacterial overgrowth

- Crohn's disease

- Dietary deficiency (e.g., in vegetarians)

- *Diphyllobothrium* (fish tapeworm) infestation

- Gastric or small intestine surgery

- Hypochlorhydria

- Inflammatory bowel disease

- Intestinal malabsorption

- Intrinsic factor deficiency

- Late pregnancy

- Pernicious anemia

CRITICAL VALUES: N/A

INTERFERING FACTORS:

- Drugs that may increase vitamin B$_{12}$ levels include chloral hydrate.

- Drugs that may decrease vitamin B$_{12}$ levels include alcohol, aminosalicylic acid, anticonvulsants, ascorbic acid, cholestyramine, cimetidine, colchicine, metformin, neomycin, oral contraceptives, ranitidine, and triamterene.

- Hemolysis or exposure of the specimen to light invalidates results.

- Recent radioactive scans or radiation within 1 week before the test can interfere with test results when radioimmunoassay is the test method.

- Specimen collection soon after blood transfusion can falsely increase vitamin B$_{12}$ levels.

Nursing Implications and Procedure · · · · · · · · · · ·

Pretest:

➤ Obtain a history of the patient's complaints, including a list of known allergens.

➤ Obtain a history of the patient's gastrointestinal and hematopoietic systems as well as results of previously performed tests and procedures. For related tests, refer to the gastrointestinal and hematopoietic system tables.

➤ Obtain a list of medications the patient is taking, including herbs, nutritional supplements, and nutraceuticals. The requesting health care practitioner and laboratory should be advised if the patient is regularly using these products so that their effects can be taken into consideration when reviewing results.

➤ Note any recent procedures that can interfere with test results.

➤ Instruct the patient to fast at least 12 hours before specimen collection.

➤ There are no fluid or medication restrictions unless by medical direction.

➤ Review the procedure with the patient.

➤ Inform the patient that specimen collection takes approximately 5 to 10 minutes.

Intratest:

➤ Ensure that the patient has complied with dietary preparations and other pretesting restrictions.

➤ Direct the patient to breathe

normally and to avoid unnecessary movement.

➤ Observe standard precautions and follow the general guidelines in Appendix A. Perform a venipuncture, and collect the specimen in a 5-mL red- or tiger-top tube.

➤ Label the specimen, protect it from light, and promptly transport it to the laboratory.

Post-test:

➤ Observe venipuncture site for bleeding or hematoma formation. Apply pressure bandage.

➤ Instruct the patient to resume usual diet and medication, if withheld and as directed by the requesting health care practitioner.

➤ Instruct the patient with a deficiency of vitamin B_{12}, as appropriate, in the use of vitamin supplements. Inform the patient, as appropriate, that the best dietary sources of vitamin B_{12} are meats, fish, poultry, eggs, and milk.

➤ Evaluate test results in relation to the patient's symptoms and other tests performed. Related laboratory tests include complete blood count, folate, homocysteine, intrinsic factor antibodies, peripheral blood smear for RBC morphology and presence of hypersegmented neutrophils, and RBC indices for mean corpuscular volume.

VITAMIN D

• •

SYNONYMS/ACRONYM: Cholecalciferol, vitamin D,25-dihydroxy.

SPECIMEN: Serum (1 mL) collected in a red-top tube. Plasma (1 mL) collected in green-top (heparin) tube is also acceptable.

REFERENCE VALUE: (Method: Radiobinding assay for vitamin D 25-dihydroxy, radioreceptor assay for vitamin D 1,25-dihydroxy)

Form	Conventional Units	SI Units (Conversion Factor ×2.496)
Vitamin D 25-dihydroxy	9–52 ng/mL	22.5–129.8 nmol/L
Vitamin D 1,25-dihydroxy	15–60 pg/mL	37.4–149.8 pmol/L

DESCRIPTION: There are two metabolically active forms of vitamin D. Ergocalciferol (vitamin D_2) is formed when ergosterol in plants is exposed to sunlight. Ergocalciferol is absorbed by the stomach and intestine when orally ingested. Cholecalciferol (vitamin D_3) if formed when the skin is exposed to sunlight or ultraviolet light. Vitamins D_2 and D_3 enter the bloodstream after absorption. Vitamin D_3 is converted to vitamin

D 25-hydroxy by the liver and is the major circulating form of the vitamin. Vitamin D₂ is converted to vitamin D 1,25-dihydroxy by the kidneys and is the more biologically active form. Vitamin D acts with parathyroid hormone and calcitonin to regulate calcium metabolism and osteoblast function. ∎

INDICATIONS:

- Differential diagnosis of disorders of calcium and phosphorus metabolism
- Evaluate deficiency or suspected toxicity
- Investigate bone diseases
- Investigate malabsorption

RESULT

Increased in:
- Vitamin D intoxication

Decreased in:
- Bowel resection
- Celiac disease
- Inflammatory bowel disease
- Malabsorption
- Osteitis fibrosa cystica
- Osteomalacia
- Pancreatic insufficiency
- Rickets
- Thyrotoxicosis

CRITICAL VALUES: ⚠ Vitamin toxicity can be as significant as problems brought about by vitamin deficiencies. The potential for toxicity is especially important to consider with respect to fat-soluble vitamins, which are not eliminated from the body as quickly as water-soluble vitamins and can accumulate in the body. Most cases of toxicity are brought about by oversupplementing and

can be avoided by consulting a qualified nutritionist for recommended daily dietary and supplemental allowances. Signs and symptoms of vitamin D toxicity include nausea, loss of appetite, vomiting, polyuria, muscle weakness, and constipation.

INTERFERING FACTORS:

- Drugs that may increase vitamin D levels include etidronate disodium and pravastatin.

- Drugs and substances that may decrease vitamin D levels include aluminum hydroxide, anticonvulsants, cholestyramine, colestipol, glucocorticoids, isoniazid, mineral oil, and rifampin.

- Recent radioactive scans or radiation within 1 week before the test can interfere with test results when radioimmunoassay is the test method.

Nursing Implications and Procedure · · · · · · · · · · ·

Pretest: ∎

➤ Obtain a history of the patient's complaints, including a list of known allergens.

➤ Obtain a history of the patient's gastrointestinal and musculoskeletal systems, as well as results of previously performed tests and procedures. For related tests, refer to the gastrointestinal and musculoskeletal system tables.

➤ Obtain a list of medications the patient is taking, including herbs, nutritional supplements, and nutraceuticals. The requesting health care practitioner and laboratory should be advised if the patient regularly uses these products so that their effects can be taken into consideration when reviewing results.

➤ There are no food, fluid, or medication restrictions unless by medical direction.

➤ Review the procedure with the patient.

➤ Inform the patient that specimen collection takes approximately 5 to 10 minutes.

Intratest:

➤ Direct the patient to breathe normally and to avoid unnecessary movement.

➤ Observe standard precautions and follow the general guidelines in Appendix A. Perform a venipuncture, and collect the specimen in a 5-mL red-top tube.

➤ Label the specimen, and promptly transport it to the laboratory.

Post-test:

➤ Observe venipuncture site for bleeding or hematoma formation. Apply pressure bandage.

➤ Educate the patient with vitamin D deficiency, as appropriate, that the main dietary sources of vitamin D are fortified dairy foods and cod liver oil. Explain to the patient that vitamin D is also synthesized by the body, in the skin, and is activated by sunlight.

➤ Evaluate test results in relation to the patient's symptoms and other tests performed. Related laboratory tests include calcium, urine calcium, kidney stone analysis, osteocalcin, and phosphorus.

VITAMIN E

· ·

SYNONYM/ACRONYM: α-Tocopherol.

SPECIMEN: Serum (1 mL) collected in a red- or tiger-top tube.

REFERENCE VALUE: (Method: High-performance liquid chromatography)

Age	Conventional Units	SI Units (Conversion Factor ×23.22)
1–12 y	0.3–0.9 mg/dL	7–21 μmol/L
13–19 y	0.6–1.0 mg/dL	14–23 μmol/L
Adult	0.5–1.8 mg/dL	12–42 μmol/L

DESCRIPTION: Vitamin E is a powerful fat-soluble antioxidant that prevents the oxidation of unsaturated fatty acids, which can combine with polysaccharides to form deposits in tissue. For this reason, vitamin E is believed to reduce the risk of coronary artery disease. Vitamin E reserves in lung tissue provide a barrier against air pollution and protect red blood cell membrane integrity from oxidation. Oxidation of fatty acids in red blood cell membranes can result in irreversible membrane damage and hemolysis. Studies are in progress to confirm the suspicion that oxidation also contributes to the formation of cataracts and macular degeneration of the retina. Because vitamin E is found in a wide variety of foods, a deficiency secondary to inadequate dietary intake is rare. ■

INDICATIONS:

- Evaluate neuromuscular disorders in premature infants and adults

- Evaluate patients with malabsorption disorders

- Evaluate suspected hemolytic anemia in premature infants and adults

- Monitor patients on long-term parenteral nutrition

RESULT

Increased in:

- Obstructive liver disease

- Vitamin E intoxication

Decreased in:

- A-β-lipoproteinemia

- Hemolytic anemia

- Malabsorption disorders, such as biliary atresia, cirrhosis, cystic fibrosis, chronic pancreatitis, pancreatic carcinoma, and chronic cholestasis

CRITICAL VALUES: ⚠ Vitamin toxicity can be as significant as problems brought about by vitamin deficiencies. The potential for toxicity is especially important to consider with respect to fat-soluble vitamins, which are not eliminated from the body as quickly as water-soluble vitamins and can accumulate in the body. Most cases of toxicity are brought about by oversupplementing and can be avoided by consulting a qualified nutritionist for recommended daily dietary and supplemental allowances. *Note:* Excessive supplementation (greater than 60 times the Recommended Dietary Allowance over a period of 1 year or longer) can result in excessive bleeding, delayed healing of wounds, and depression.

INTERFERING FACTORS:

- Drugs that may increase vitamin E levels include anticonvulsants (in women).

- Drugs that may decrease vitamin E levels include anticonvulsants (in men).

- Exposure of the specimen to light decreases vitamin E levels, resulting in a falsely low result.

Nursing Implications and Procedure • • • • • • • • • • •

Pretest: ■

➤ Obtain a history of the patient's complaints, including a list of known allergens.

➤ Obtain a history of the patient's cardiovascular, gastrointestinal, hematopoietic, and hepatobiliary systems, as well as results of previously performed tests and procedures. For related tests, refer to the cardiovascular, gastrointestinal, hematopoietic, and hepatobiliary system tables.

➤ Obtain a list of medications the patient is taking, including herbs, nutritional supplements, and nutraceuticals. The requesting health care practitioner and laboratory should be advised if the patient regularly uses these products so that their effects can be taken into consideration when reviewing results.

➤ There are no food, fluid, or medication restrictions unless by medical direction.

➤ Review the procedure with the patient.

➤ Inform the patient that specimen collection takes approximately 5 to 10 minutes.

Intratest: ■

➤ Direct the patient to breathe normally and to avoid unnecessary movement.

➤ Observe standard precautions and

follow the general guidelines in Appendix A. Perform a venipuncture, and collect the specimen in a 5-mL red- or tiger-top tube.

➤ Label the specimen, and promptly transport it to the laboratory.

Post-test:

➤ Observe venipuncture site for bleeding or hematoma formation. Apply pressure bandage.

➤ Educate the patient with a vitamin E deficiency, if appropriate, that the main dietary sources of vitamin E are vegetable oils, whole grains, wheat germ, milk, eggs, meats, fish, and green leafy vegetables. Vitamin E is fairly stable at most cooking temperatures (except frying) and when exposed to acidic foods.

➤ Evaluate test results in relation to the patient's symptoms and other tests performed.

VITAMIN K

SYNONYMS/ACRONYM: Phylloquinone, phytonadione.

SPECIMEN: Serum (1 mL) collected in a red-top tube.

REFERENCE VALUE: (Method: High-performance liquid chromatography)

Conventional Units	SI Units (Conversion Factor ×2.22)
0.13–1.19 ng/mL	0.29–2.64 nmol/L

DESCRIPTION: Vitamin K is one of the fat-soluble vitamins. It is essential for the formation of prothrombin; factors VII, IX, and X; and proteins C and S. Vitamin K also works with vitamin D in synthesizing bone protein and regulating calcium levels (see monograph titled "Vitamin D.") Vitamin K levels are not often requested, but vitamin K is often prescribed as a medication. Approximately one-half of the body's vitamin K is produced by intestinal bacteria; the other half is obtained from dietary sources. There are three forms of vitamin K: vitamin K_1, or phylloquinone, which is found in foods; vitamin K_2, or menaquinone, which is synthesized by intestinal bacteria; and vitamin K_3, or menadione, which is the synthetic, water-soluble, pharmaceutical form of the vitamin. Vitamin K_3 is two to three times more potent than the naturally occurring forms. ∎

INDICATIONS: Evaluation of bleeding of unknown cause (e.g., frequent nosebleeds, bruising)

RESULT

Increased in:

• Excessive administration of vitamin K

Decreased in:

- Antibiotic therapy (by decreasing intestinal flora)

- Chronic fat malabsorption

- Cystic fibrosis

- Diarrhea (in infants)

- Gastrointestinal disease

- Hemorrhagic disease of the newborn

- Hypoprothrombinemia

- Liver disease

- Obstructive jaundice

- Pancreatic disease

CRITICAL VALUES: Vitamin toxicity can be as significant as problems brought about by vitamin deficiencies. The potential for toxicity is especially important to consider with respect to fat-soluble vitamins, which are not eliminated from the body as quickly as water-soluble vitamins and can accumulate in the body. The naturally occurring forms, vitamin K_1 and K_2, do not cause toxicity. Signs and symptoms of vitamin K_3 toxicity include bleeding and jaundice. Possible interventions include withholding the source.

INTERFERING FACTORS: Drugs and substances that may decrease vitamin K levels include antibiotics, cholestyramine, coumarin, mineral oil, and warfarin.

Nursing Implications and Procedure

Pretest:

➤ Obtain a history of the patient's complaints, including a list of known allergens.

➤ Obtain a history of the patient's hematopoietic and hepatobiliary systems, as well as results of previously performed tests and procedures. For related tests, refer to the hematopoietic and hepatobiliary system tables.

➤ Obtain a list of medications the patient is taking, including herbs, nutritional supplements, and nutraceuticals. The requesting health care practitioner and laboratory should be advised if the patient regularly uses these products so that their effects can be taken into consideration when reviewing results.

➤ There are no food, fluid, or medication restrictions unless by medical direction.

➤ Review the procedure with the patient.

➤ Inform the patient that specimen collection takes approximately 5 to 10 minutes.

Intratest

➤ Direct the patient to breathe normally and to avoid unnecessary movement.

➤ Observe standard precautions and follow the general guidelines in Appendix A. Perform a venipuncture, and collect the specimen in a 5-mL red-top tube.

➤ Label the specimen, and promptly transport it to the laboratory.

Post-test:

➤ Observe venipuncture site for bleeding or hematoma formation. Apply pressure bandage.

➤ Inform the patient with a vitamin K deficiency, as appropriate, that the main dietary sources of vitamin K are cabbage, cauliflower, spinach and other green leafy vegetables, pork, liver, soybeans, and vegetable oils.

➤ Instruct the patient to report bleeding from any areas of the skin or mucous membranes.

➤ Inform the patient of the importance of taking precautions against bleeding or bruising, including the use of a soft bristle toothbrush, use of an electric razor, avoidance of constipation, avoidance of aspirin products, and avoidance of intramuscular injections.

➤ Evaluate test results in relation to

the patient's symptoms and other tests performed. Related laboratory tests include antithrombin III and prothrombin time.

VITAMINS A, B₁, B₆, AND C

SYNONYMS/ACRONYMS: Vitamin A: retinol, carotene; vitamin B_1: thiamine; vitamin B_6: niacin, pyroxidine, P-5'-P, pyridoxyl-5-phosphate; vitamin C: ascorbic acid.

SPECIMEN: Serum (1 mL) collected in a red-top tube each for vitamins A and C; plasma (1 mL) collected in a lavender-top (ethylenediaminetetra-acetic acid [EDTA]) tube each for vitamins B_1 and B_6.

REFERENCE VALUE: (Method: Chromatography for vitamins A, B_1, and B_6; capillary electrophoresis for vitamin C)

Vitamin	Age	Conventional Units	SI Units
			(Conversion Factor ×0.0349)
Vitamin A	1–6 y	20–43 µg/dL	0.70–1.50 µmol/L
	7–12 y	26–49 µg/dL	0.91–1.71 µmol/L
	13–19 y	26–72 µg/dL	0.91–2.51 µmol/L
	Adult	30–80 µg/dL	1.05–2.80 µmol/L
			(Conversion Factor ×29.6)
Vitamin B₁		0.21–0.43 µg/dL	6.2–12.8 µmol/L
			(Conversion Factor ×4.046)
Vitamin B₆		5–30 ng/mL	20–121 nmol/L
			(Conversion Factor ×56.78)
Vitamin C		0.2–1.9 mg/dL	11.4–107.9 µmol/L

DESCRIPTION: Vitamin assays are used in the measurement of nutritional status. Low levels indicate inadequate oral intake, poor nutritional status, or malabsorption problems. High levels indicate excessive intake, vitamin intoxication, or absorption problems. Vitamin A is a fat-soluble nutrient that promotes normal vision and prevents night blindness; contributes to growth of bone, teeth, and soft tissues; supports thyroxine formation; maintains epithelial cell membranes, skin, and mucous membranes; and acts as an anti-infection agent. Vitamins B_1, B_6, and C are water soluble. Vitamin B_1 acts as an enzyme and plays an important role in the Krebs cycle. Vitamin B_6 is important in heme synthesis and functions as a coenzyme in amino acid metabolism and glycogenolysis. It includes pyridoxine, pyridoxal, and pyridoxamine. Vitamin C promotes collagen synthesis, maintains capillary strength, facilitates release of iron from ferritin to form hemoglobin, and functions in the stress response. ∎

INDICATIONS

Vitamin A:

* Assist in the diagnosis of night blindness

* Evaluate skin disorders

* Investigate suspected vitamin A deficiency

Vitamin B₁:

* Investigate suspected beriberi

* Monitor the effects of chronic alcoholism

Vitamin B₆:

* Investigate suspected vitamin B₆ deficiency

* Investigate suspected malabsorption or malnutrition

Vitamin C:

* Investigate suspected metabolic or malabsorptive disorders

* Investigate suspected scurvy

RESULT

Increases in:

* Vitamin A:
  Chronic kidney disease
  Idiopathic hypercalcemia in infants
  Vitamin A toxicity

Decreases in:

* Vitamin A:
  A-β-lipoproteinemia

Carcinoid syndrome
Chronic infections
Cystic fibrosis
Disseminated tuberculosis
Hypothyroidism
Infantile blindness
Liver, gastrointestinal, or pancreatic disease
Night blindness
Protein malnutrition
Sterility and teratogenesis
Zinc deficiency

* Vitamin B₁:
  Alcoholism
  Carcinoid syndrome
  Hartnup's disease
  Pellagra

* Vitamin B₆:
  Alcoholism
  Asthma
  Carpal tunnel syndrome
  Gestational diabetes
  Lactation
  Malabsorption
  Malnutrition
  Neonatal seizures
  Normal pregnancies
  Occupational exposure to hydrazine compounds
  Pellagra
  Preeclamptic edema
  Renal dialysis
  Uremia

* Vitamin C:
  Alcoholism
  Anemia
  Cancer
  Hemodialysis
  Hyperthyroidism
  Malabsorption
  Pregnancy
  Rheumatoid disease
  Scurvy

CRITICAL VALUES: ⚠ Vitamin toxicity can be as significant as problems brought about by vitamin deficiencies. The potential for toxicity is especially important to consider with respect to fat-soluble vitamins, which are not eliminated from the body as quickly as water-soluble vitamins and can accumulate in the body. Most cases of toxicity are brought about by oversupplementing and can be avoided by consulting a qualified nutritionist for recommended daily dietary and supplemental allowances. Signs and symptoms of vitamin A toxicity may include headache, blurred vision, bone pain, joint pain, dry skin, and loss of appetite.

INTERFERING FACTORS:

• Drugs and substances that may increase vitamin A levels include probucol, alcohol (moderate intake), and oral contraceptives.

• Drugs and substances that may decrease vitamin A levels include alcohol (chronic intake, alcoholism), allopurinol, cholestyramine, colestipol, mineral oil, and neomycin.

• Drugs that may decrease vitamin B_1 levels include glibenclamide, isoniazid, and valproic acid.

• Drugs that may decrease vitamin B_6 levels include amiodarone, anticonvulsants, cycloserine, disulfiram, ethanol, hydralazine, isoniazid, levodopa, oral contraceptives, penicillamine, pyrazinoic acid, and theophylline.

• Drugs and substances that may decrease vitamin C levels include aminopyrine, acetylsalicylic acid, barbiturates, estrogens, heavy metals, oral contraceptives, nitrosamines, and paraldehyde.

• Various diseases may affect vitamin levels (see Results section).

• Diets high in freshwater fish and tea,

which are thiamine antagonists, may cause decreased vitamin B_1 levels.

• Long-term hyperalimentation may result in decreased vitamin levels.

• Exposure of the specimen to light decreases vitamin levels, resulting in a falsely low results.

• Chronic tobacco smoking decreases vitamin C levels.

Nursing Implications and Procedure • • • • • • • • • •

Pretest: ■

➤ Obtain a history of the patient's complaints, including a list of known allergens.

➤ Obtain a history of the patient's gastrointestinal, genitourinary, hepatobiliary, immune, and musculoskeletal systems, as well as results of previously performed tests and procedures. For related tests, refer to the gastrointestinal, genitourinary, hepatobiliary, immune, and musculoskeletal system tables.

➤ Obtain a list of medications the patient is taking, including herbs, nutritional supplements, and nutraceuticals. The requesting health care practitioner and laboratory should be advised if the patient regularly uses these products so that their effects can be taken into consideration when reviewing results.

➤ Instruct the patient to fast at least 12 hours before specimen collection for vitamin A.

➤ There are no fluid or medication restrictions unless by medical direction.

➤ Review the procedure with the patient.

➤ Inform the patient that specimen collection takes approximately 5 to 10 minutes.

Intratest: ■

➤ Ensure that the patient has complied with dietary preparations and other pretesting restrictions before specimen collection for vitamin A level.

➤ Direct the patient to breathe normally and to avoid unnecessary movement.

➤ Observe standard precautions and follow the general guidelines in Appendix A. Perform a venipuncture, and collect the specimen in a 5-mL red- or lavender-top tube.

➤ Label the specimen, and promptly transport it to the laboratory.

Post-test: ■

➤ Observe venipuncture site for bleeding or hematoma formation. Apply pressure bandage.

➤ Instruct the patient to resume usual diet, as directed by the requesting health care practitioner.

➤ Educate the patient with a specific vitamin deficiency, as appropriate, regarding dietary sources of these vitamins. Advise the patient to ask a nutritionist to develop a diet plan recommended for his or her specific needs.

Vitamin A:

➤ The main source of vitamin A comes from carotene, a yellow pigment noticeable in most fruits and vegetables, especially carrots, sweet potatoes, squash, apricots, and cantaloupe. It is also present in spinach, collards, broccoli, and cabbage. This vitamin is fairly stable at most cooking temperatures, but it is destroyed easily by light and oxidation.

Vitamin B₁:

➤ Vitamin B₁ is the most stable to environmental elements. It is found in meats, coffee, peanuts, and legumes. The body is also capable of making some vitamin B₁ by converting the amino acid tryptophan to niacin.

Vitamin B₆:

➤ Good sources of vitamin B₆ include meats (especially beef and pork), whole grains, wheat germ, legumes, potatoes, oatmeal, and bananas. As with other water-soluble vitamins, it is best preserved by rapid cooking, although it is relatively stable at most cooking temperatures (except frying) and when exposed to acidic foods. This vitamin is destroyed rapidly by light and alkalis.

Vitamin C:

➤ Citrus fruits are excellent dietary sources of vitamin C. Other good sources are green and red peppers, tomatoes, white potatoes, cabbage, broccoli, chard, kale, turnip greens, asparagus, berries, melons, pineapple, and guava. Vitamin C is destroyed by exposure to air, light, heat, or alkalis. Boiling water before cooking eliminates dissolved oxygen that destroys vitamin C in the process of boiling. Vegetables should be crisp and cooked as quickly as possible.

➤ Evaluate test results in relation to the patient's symptoms and other tests performed.

WHITE BLOOD CELL COUNT AND CELL DIFFERENTIAL

SYNONYMS/ACRONYM: WBC with diff, leukocyte count, white cell count.

SPECIMEN: Whole blood from one full lavender-top (ethylenediaminetetra-acetic acid [EDTA]) tube.

REFERENCE VALUE: (Method: Automated, computerized, multichannel analyzers that sort and size cells on the basis of changes in either electrical impedance or light pulses as the cells pass in front of a laser. Many of these analyzers are capable of determining a five-part WBC differential.) The WBC count and differential enumerates and identifies granulocytes, lymphocytes, monocytes, eosinophils, basophils, and platelets.

Age	SI Units (Conversion Factor ×10 cells/L)*	Neutrophils		
		Total (Absolute) and %	Bands (Absolute) and %	Segments (Absolute) and %
Birth	9.0–30.0	(6.0–26.0) 61%	(1.65) 9.1%	(9.4) 52%
1 d	9.4–34.0	(5.0–21.0) 61%	(1.75) 9.2%	(9.8) 52%
2 wk	5.0–20.0	(1.0–9.5) 40%	(0.63) 5.5%	(3.9) 34%
1 mo	5.0–19.5	(1.0–9.0) 35%	(0.49) 4.5%	(3.3) 30%
6 mo	6.0–17.5	(1.0–8.5) 32%	(0.45) 3.8%	(3.3) 28%
1 y	6.0–17.5	(1.5–8.5) 31%	(0.35) 3.1%	(3.2) 28%
10 y	4.5–13.5	(1.8–8.0) 54%	(0–1.0) 3.0%	(1.8–7.0) 51%
Adult	4.5–11.0	(1.8–7.7) 59%	(0–0.7) 3.0%	(1.8–7.0) 56%

* WBC × 10^3/mm^3 or cells/µL.

DESCRIPTION: White blood cells (WBCs) constitute the body's primary defense system against foreign organisms, tissues, and other substances. The life span of a normal WBC is 13 to 20 days. Old WBCs are destroyed by the lymphatic system and excreted in the feces. The main WBC types are neutrophils, eosinophils, basophils, monocytes, and lymphocytes. They are produced in the bone marrow, although lymphocytes can be produced in other sites as well. The WBC count can be performed alone with the differential cell count or as part of the complete blood count (CBC). An increased WBC count is termed *leukocytosis,* and a decreased WBC count is termed *leukopenia.* A total WBC count indicates the degree of response to a pathologic process, but a more complete evaluation for specific diagnoses for any one disorder is provided by the differential count. The WBCs in the count and differential are reported as an absolute value and as a percentage. The relative percentages of cell types are arrived at by basing the enumeration of each cell type on a 100-cell count. The absolute value is obtained by multiplying the relative percentage value of each cell type by the total WBC count.

Acute leukocytosis is initially accompanied by changes in the WBC count population, followed by changes within the individual WBCs. Leukocytosis usually occurs by way of increase in a single WBC family rather than a proportional increase in all cell types. Toxic granulation and vacuolation are commonly seen in leukocytosis accompanied by a *shift to the left,* or increase in the percentage of immature band neutrophils to mature segmented neutrophils. These changes are most commonly associated with an infectious process, usually bacterial, but they can occur in healthy individuals who are under stress, such as women in childbirth and very young infants. The WBC

Lymphocytes (Absolute) and %	Monocytes (Absolute) and %	Eosinophils (Absolute) and %	Basophils (Absolute) and %
(2.0–11) 31%	(0.4–3.1) 5.8%	(0.02–0.85) 2.2%	(0–0.64) 0.6%
(2.0–11.5) 31%	(0.2–3.1) 5.8%	(0.02–0.95) 2.0%	(0–0.30) 0.5%
(2.0–17.0) 48%	(0.2–2.4) 8.8%	(0.07–1.0) 3.1%	(0–0.23) 0.4%
(2.5–16.5) 56%	(0.15–2.0) 6.5%	(0.07–0.90) 2.8%	(0–0.20) 0.5%
(4.0–13.5) 61%	(0.1–1.3) 4.8%	(0.07–0.75) 2.5%	(0–0.20) 0.4%
(4.0–10.5) 61%	(0.05–1.1) 4.8%	(0.05–0.70) 2.6%	(0–0.20) 0.4%
(1.5–6.5) 38%	(0–0.8) 4.3%	(0–0.60) 2.4%	(0–0.20) 0.5%
(1.0–4.8) 34%	(0–0.8) 4.0%	(0–0.45) 2.7%	(0–0.20) 0.5%

count and differential of an actively crying infant may show an overall increase in WBCs with a shift to the left. Any stressful situation causing production of epinephrine results in a rapid increase in WBC count. Before initiating any kind of intervention, it is important to determine whether an increased WBC count is the result of a normal condition involving physiologic stress versus a pathologic processes. The use of multiple specimen types may confuse the interpretation of results in infants. Multiple samples from the same collection site (i.e., capillary versus venous) may be necessary to obtain an accurate assessment of the WBC picture in these young patients.

Neutrophils are normally found as the predominant WBC type in the circulating blood. Also called *polymorphonuclear cells,* they are the body's first line of defense through the process of phagocytosis. They also contain enzymes and pyogens, which combat foreign invaders. Lymphocytes are agranular, mononuclear blood cells that are smaller than granulocytes. They are found in the next highest percentage in normal circulation.

Lymphocytes are classified as B cells and T cells. Both types are formed in the bone marrow, but B cells mature in the bone marrow and T cells mature in the thymus. Lymphocytes play a major role in the body's natural defense system. B cells differentiate into immunoglobulin-synthesizing plasma cells. T cells function as cellular mediators of immunity and comprise helper/inducer (CD4) lymphocytes, delayed hypersensitivity lymphocytes, cytotoxic (CD8 or CD4) lympho-cytes, and suppressor (CD8) lympho-cytes.

Monocytes are mononuclear cells similar to lymphocytes, but they are related more closely to granulocytes in terms of their function. They are formed in the bone marrow from the same cells as those that produce neutrophils. The major function of monocytes is phagocytosis. Monocytes stay in the peripheral blood for about 70 hours, after which they migrate into the tissues and become macrophages.

The function of eosinophils is phagocytosis of antigen-antibody complexes. They become active in the later stages of inflammation. Eosinophils respond to allergic and parasitic diseases: They have granules that contain histamine used to kill foreign cells in the body and proteolytic enzymes that damage parasitic worms (see monograph titled "Eosinophil Count").

Basophils are found in small numbers in the circulating blood. They have a phagocytic function and, similar to eosinophils, contain numerous specific granules. Basophilic granules contain heparin, histamines, and serotonin. Basophils may also be found in tissue and as such are classified as mast cells. Basophilia is noted in conditions such as leukemia, Hodgkin's disease, polycythemia vera, ulcerative colitis, nephrosis, and chronic hypersensitivity states. ∎

INDICATIONS:

• Assist in confirming suspected bone marrow depression

• Assist in determining the cause of an elevated WBC count (e.g., infection, inflammatory process)

- Detect hematologic disorder, neoplasm, or immunologic abnormality

- Determine the presence of a hereditary hematologic abnormality

- Monitor the effects of physical or emotional stress

- Monitor the progression of nonhematologic disorders, such as chronic obstructive pulmonary disease

(COPD), malabsorption syndromes, cancer, and renal disease

- Monitor the response to drugs or chemotherapy, and evaluate undesired reactions to drugs that may cause blood dyscrasias

- Provide screening as part of a CBC in a general physical examination, especially on admission to a health care facility or before surgery

RESULT

WBC Abnormalities	Associated Condition
Alder-Reilly cytoplasmic granulations	Hereditary condition, ucopolysaccharidosis
Auer bodies or Auer rods	Acute myelocytic leukemia, yelomonocytic leukemia
Chédiak-Higashi lysosomal granulations	Hereditary condition, albinism, leukopenia, thrombocytopenia
Döhle bodies	Infections, inflammatory conditions, burns, myelocytic leukemia
Hypersegmented neutrophils	Megaloblastic anemia
Systemic lupus erythematosus (SLE) cells	SLE and other collagen diseases, drug reactions, chronic hepatitis
Left shift	Infections, intoxication, tissue necrosis, leukemia, pernicious anemia
Leukemic cells (immature blast forms)	Leukemia, leukemoid reaction, severe infection, myeloproliferative disorders, intoxication, malignancy, recovery from bone marrow suppression
May-Hegglin anomaly	Hereditary condition with thrombocytopenia and giant platelets
Smudge cells	Leukemias
Pelger-Huët cells	Hereditary condition, myelocytic leukemia, myeloproliferative disorders
Tart cell	Drug reactions
Toxic granulation	Infections, inflammatory conditions

Increased in (leukocytosis):
- Normal physiologic and environmental conditions:
  Early infancy
  Emotional stress
  Exposure to cold

Increased epinephrine secretion

Menstruation

Pregnancy and labor

Strenuous exercise

Ultraviolet light

- Pathologic conditions:
  Acute hemolysis, transfusion
    reactions
  All types of infections
  Anemias
  Appendicitis
  Collagen disorders
  Cushing's disease
  Inflammatory disorders
  Leukemias and other malignancies
  Parasitic infestations
  Polycythemia vera

Decreased in (leukopenia):
- Normal physiologic conditions:
  Diurnal rhythms

- Pathologic conditions:
  Alcoholism
  Anemias
  Bone marrow depression
  SLE and other autoimmune
    disorders
  Malaria
  Malnutrition
  Radiation
  Rheumatoid arthritis
  Toxic and antineoplastic drugs
  Viral infections

*Neutrophils increased
(neutrophilia):*
- Acute hemolysis

- Acute hemorrhage

- Extremes in temperature

- Infectious diseases

- Inflammatory conditions (rheumatic
  fever, gout, rheumatoid arthritis,
  vasculitis, myositis)

- Malignancies

- Metabolic disorders (uremia, eclampsia, diabetic ketoacidosis, thyroid
  storm, Cushing's syndrome)

- Myelocytic leukemia

- Physiologic stress (e.g., allergies,
  asthma, exercise, childbirth, surgery)

- Tissue necrosis (burns, crushing
  injuries, abscesses, myocardial infarction)

- Tissue poisoning with toxins and
  venoms

*Neutrophils decreased
(neutropenia):*
- Acromegaly

- Addison's disease

- Anaphylaxis

- Anorexia nervosa, starvation, malnutrition

- Vitamin B_{12} or folate deficiency

- Bone marrow depression (viruses, toxic
  chemicals, overwhelming infection,
  radiation, Gaucher's disease)

- Disseminated SLE

- Thyrotoxicosis

- Viral infection (mononucleosis, hepatitis, influenza)

*Lymphocytes increased
(lymphocytosis):*
- Addison's disease

- Felty's syndrome

- Infections

- Lymphocytic leukemia

- Lymphomas

- Lymphosarcoma

- Malnutrition

- Myeloma

- Rickets

- Thyrotoxicosis

- Ulcerative colitis

- Waldenström's macroglobulinemia

Lymphocytes decreased (lymphopenia):
- Antineoplastic drugs
- Aplastic anemia
- Bone marrow failure
- Burns
- Gaucher's disease
- Hemolytic disease of the newborn
- High doses of adrenocorticosteroids
- Hodgkin's disease
- Hypersplenism
- Immunodeficiency diseases
- Pernicious anemia
- Pneumonia
- Radiation
- Rheumatic fever
- Septicemia
- Thrombocytopenic purpura
- Toxic chemical exposure
- Transfusion reaction

Monocytes increased (monocytosis):
- Carcinomas
- Cirrhosis
- Collagen diseases
- Gaucher's disease
- Hemolytic anemias
- Hodgkin's disease
- Infections
- Lymphomas
- Monocytic leukemia
- Polycythemia vera
- Radiation

- Sarcoidosis
- SLE
- Thrombocytopenic purpura
- Ulcerative colitis

CRITICAL VALUES:

Less than 2500 WBC/mm^3 (on admission)

Greater than 30,000 WBC/mm^3 (on admission)

The presence of abnormal cells, other morphologic characteristics, or cellular inclusions may signify a potentially life-threatening or serious health condition and should be investigated. Examples are hypersegmented neutrophils, agranular neutrophils, blasts or other immature cells, Auer rods, Döhle bodies, marked toxic granulation, or plasma cells.

INTERFERING FACTORS:
- Drugs that may decrease the overall WBC count include acetyldigitoxin, acetylsalicylic acid, aminoglutethimide, aminopyrine, aminosalicylic acid, ampicillin, amsacrine, antazoline, anticonvulsants, antineoplastic agents (therapeutic intent), antipyrine, barbiturates, busulfan, carbutamide, carmustine, chlorambucil, chloramphenicol, chlordane, chlorophenothane, chlortetracycline, chlorthalidone, cisplatin, colchicine, colistimethate, cycloheximide, cyclophosphamide, cytarabine, dacarbazine, dactinomycin, diaprim, diazepam, diethylpropion, digitalis, dipyridamole, dipyrone, fumagillin, glaucarubin, glucosulfone, hexachlorobenzene, hydroflumathiazide, hydroxychloroquine, iothiouracil, iproniazid, lincomycin, local anesthetics, mefenamic acid, mepazine, meprobamate, mercaptopurine, methotrexate, methylpromazine, mitomycin, paramethadione, parathion, penicillin, phenacemide, phenindione, phenothiazine, pipamazine, pred-

nisone (by Coulter S method), primaquine, procainamide, procarbazine, prochlorperazine, promazine, promethazine, pyrazolones, quinacrine, quinines, radioactive compounds, razoxane, ristocetin, sulfa drugs, tamoxifen, tetracycline, thenalidine, thioridazine, tolazamide, tolazoline, tolbutamide, trimethadione, and urethan.

• A significant decrease in basophil count occurs rapidly after intravenous injection of propanidid and thiopental.

• A significant decrease in lymphocyte count occurs rapidly after administration of corticotropin, mechlorethamine, methylsergide, and x-ray therapy; and after megadoses of niacin, pyradoxine, and thiamine.

• Drugs that may increase the overall WBC count include amphetamine, amphotericin B, chloramphenicol, chloroform (normal response to anesthesia), colchicine (leukocytosis follows leukopenia), corticotropin, erythromycin, ether (normal response to anesthesia), fluroxene (normal response to anesthesia), isoflurane (normal response to anesthesia), niacinamide, phenylbutazone, prednisone, and quinine.

• Drug allergies may have a significant effect on eosinophil count and may affect the overall WBC count. Refer to the specific monograph for a detailed listing of interfering drugs.

• The WBC count may vary depending on the patient's position, decreasing when the patient is recumbent owing to hemodilution and increasing when the patient rises owing to hemoconcentration.

• Venous stasis can falsely elevate results; the tourniquet should not be left on the arm for longer than 60 seconds.

• Failure to fill the tube sufficiently (i.e., tube less than three-quarters full) may yield inadequate sample volume for automated analyzers and may be reason for specimen rejection.

• Hemolyzed or clotted specimens should be rejected for analysis.

• The presence of nucleated red blood cells or giant or clumped platelets affects the automated WBC, requiring a manual correction of the WBC count.

• Care should be taken in evaluating the CBC during the first few hours after transfusion.

• Patients with cold agglutinins or monoclonal gammopathies may have a falsely decreased WBC count as a result of cell clumping.

Nursing Implications and Procedure · · · · · · · · · · ·

Pretest: ▮

➤ Obtain a history of the patient's complaints, including a list of known allergens.

➤ Obtain a history of the patient's hematopoietic, immune, and respiratory systems, as well as results of previously performed tests and procedures. For related tests, refer to the hematopoietic, immune, and respiratory system tables.

➤ Obtain a list of medications the patient is taking, including herbs, nutritional supplements, and nutraceuticals. The requesting health care practitioner and laboratory should be advised if the patient regularly uses these products so that their effects can be taken into consideration when reviewing results.

➤ Note any recent procedures that can interfere with test results.

➤ There are no food, fluid, or medication restrictions unless by medical direction.

➤ Review the procedure with the patient.

➤ Inform the patient that specimen collection takes approximately 5 to 10 minutes.

Intratest:

➤ Direct the patient to breathe normally and to avoid unnecessary movement.

➤ Observe standard precautions and follow the general guidelines in Appendix A. Perform a venipuncture, and collect the specimen in a 5-mL lavender-top tube. The specimen should be mixed gently by inverting the tube 10 times. It is stable when stored for up to 6 hours at room temperature or 24 hours if stored refrigerated. In addition, if it is anticipated that the specimen will not be analyzed within 4 to 6 hours, two blood smears should be made immediately after the venipuncture and submitted with the blood sample.

➤ Label the specimen, and promptly transport it to the laboratory.

Post-test:

➤ Observe venipuncture site for bleeding or hematoma formation. Apply pressure bandage.

➤ Infection, fever, sepsis, and trauma can result in an impaired nutritional status. Malnutrition can occur for many reasons, including fatigue, lack of appetite, and gastrointestinal distress.

➤ Adequate intake of vitamins A and C are also important for regenerating body stores depleted by the effort exerted in fighting infections. Educate the patient or caregiver regarding the importance of following the prescribed diet.

➤ Evaluate test results in relation to the patient's symptoms and other tests performed. Related laboratory tests include anti–cytoplasmic neutrophilic antibody, lymph node biopsy, bone marrow biopsy, infectious mononucleosis, other tests included in a CBC, eosinophil count, peripheral blood smear, leukocyte alkaline phosphatase, and zinc.

WHITE BLOOD CELL SCAN

SYNONYMS/ACRONYM: WBC imaging, inflammatory scan, labeled leukocyte scan, infection scintigraphy, labeled autologous leukocytes.

AREA OF APPLICATION: Whole body.

CONTRAST: Intravenous radionuclide combined with white blood cells.

DESCRIPTION: Because white blood cells (WBCs) naturally accumulate in areas of inflammation, the WBC scan uses radiolabeled WBCs to help determine the site of an acute infection or confirm the presence or absence of infection or inflammation at a suspected site. A gamma camera detects the radiation emitted from the injected radionuclide, and a representative image of the radionuclide distribution is obtained and recorded on film or stored electronically. Because of its better image resolution and greater specificity for acute infections, the WBC scan has replaced scanning with gallium-67 citrate (Ga-67). Some chronic infections associated with pulmonary disease, however, may be better imaged with Ga-67. The WBC scan is especially helpful in detecting postoperative infection sites and in documenting lack of residual infection after a course of therapy. ∎

INDICATIONS:
- Aid in the diagnosis of infectious or inflammatory diseases

- Evaluate patients with fever of unknown origin

- Evaluate suspected osteomyelitis

- Differentiate infectious from noninfectious process

- Evaluate the effects of treatment

- Evaluate postsurgical sites and wound infections

- Evaluate inflammatory bowel disease

- Evaluate suspected infection of an orthopedic prostheses

RESULT

Normal Findings:
- No focal localization of the radionuclide, along with some slight localization of the radionuclide within the reticuloendothelial system (liver, spleen, and bone marrow)

Abnormal Findings:
- Abscess

- Arthritis

- Infection

- Inflammation

- Inflammatory bowel disease

- Osteomyelitis

CRITICAL VALUES: N/A

INTERFERING FACTORS:

This procedure is contraindicated for:
- Patients who are pregnant or suspected of being pregnant, unless the potential benefits of the procedure far outweigh the risks to the fetus and mother

Factors that may impair clear imaging:
- Inability of the patient to cooperate or remain still during the procedure because of age, significant pain, or mental status

- Patients who are very obese, who may exceed the weight limit for the equipment

- Incorrect positioning of the patient, which may produce poor visualization of the area to be examined

- Retained barium from a previous radiologic procedure, which may inhibit visualization of an abdominal lesion

- Other nuclear scans done within 48 hours and Ga-67 scans within 4 weeks before the procedure

- Lesions smaller than 1 to 2 cm, which may not be detectable

- A distended bladder, which may obscure pelvic detail

Other considerations:
- Improper injection of the radionuclide that allows the tracer to seep deep into the muscle tissue produces erroneous hot spots.

- Patients with a low WBC count may need donor WBCs to complete the radionuclide labeling process; otherwise, Ga-67 scanning should be performed instead.

- False-negative images may be a result of hemodialysis, hyperglycemia, hyperalimentation, steroid therapy, and antibiotic therapy.

- The presence of multiple myeloma or thyroid cancer can result in a false-negative scan for bone abnormalities.

- Consultation with a physician should occur before the procedure for radiation safety concerns regarding infants of patients who are lactating.

- Risks associated with radiographic overexposure can result from frequent x-ray procedures. Personnel in the room with the patient should stand behind a shield or leave the area while the examination is being done. Personnel working in the area where the examination is being done should wear badges that reveal their level of exposure to radiation.

Nursing Implications and Procedure

Pretest: ■

➤ Inform the patient that the procedure assesses the presence of inflammation or infection.

➤ Inform the patient that the procedure is performed in a special nuclear medicine department by a technologist and usually takes approximately 60 minutes, and that delayed images are needed 24 hours later. The patient may leave the department and return later to undergo delayed imaging.

➤ Obtain a list of known allergens.

➤ Obtain a medical history of the patient's complaints as well as results of previously performed tests, treatments, and surgical procedures. For related tests, refer to the immunologic system table.

➤ Obtain a list of medications the patient is taking.

➤ Assure the patient and family members that radiation exposure is minimal and similar to that involved in other nuclear medicine procedures.

➤ Determine date of last menstrual period and possibility of pregnancy in perimenopausal women.

➤ Do not restrict food or fluids unless otherwise indicated.

Intratest: ■

➤ Ask the patient to void before the procedure. Have the patient put on a hospital gown.

➤ Administer sedative to a child or to an uncooperative adult, as ordered.

➤ Ask the patient to lie still during the procedure because movement produces unclear images. Make sure jewelry, watches, chains, belts, and any other metallic objects have been removed from the area to be scanned.

➤ On the day of the test, draw a 40- to 60-mL sample of blood for an *in vitro* process of labeling and separating the WBCs from the blood. An injection of radionuclide-labeled autologous WBCs is administered. Delayed views may be taken 4 to 24 hours after the injection.

➤ If abdominal abscess or infection is suspected, laxatives or enemas may be ordered before delayed imaging.

➤ Wear gloves during the radionuclide administration and while handling the patient's urine.

Post-test: ■

➤ Instruct the patient to resume normal activity, medications, and diet after imaging is complete, unless otherwise indicated.

➤ Advise patient to drink increased amounts of fluids for 24 hours to eliminate the radionuclide from the body, unless contraindicated. Tell the patient that radionuclide is eliminated from the body within 48 to 72 hours.

➤ Instruct the patient to flush the toilet immediately after each voiding following the procedure and to wash hands meticulously with soap and water after each voiding for 24 hours after the procedure.

➤ Tell all caregivers to wear gloves when discarding urine for 24 hours after the procedure. Wash gloved hands with soap and water before removing gloves. Then wash hands after the gloves are removed.

➤ A physician specializing in this branch of medicine sends a written report to the ordering provider, who discusses the results with the patient.

➤ Evaluate test results in relation to the patient's symptoms and other tests performed. Related diagnostic tests include kidney, ureter, and bladder (KUB) film; Ga-67 scan; ultrasound of the pelvis; and computed tomography and magnetic resonance imaging of the abdomen.

ZINC

SYNONYM/ACRONYM: Zn.

SPECIMEN: Serum (1 mL) collected in a trace element–free, royal blue–top tube.

REFERENCE VALUE: (Method: Atomic absorption spectrophotometry)

Age	Conventional Units	SI Units (Conversion Factor ×0.153)
Newborn–6 mo	26–141 µg/dL	4.0–21.6 µmol/L
6–11 mo	29–131 µg/dL	4.5–20.1 µmol/L
1–4 y	31–115 µg/dL	4.8–17.6 µmol/L
4–5 y	48–119 µg/dL	7.4–18.2 µmol/L
6–9 y	48–129 µg/dL	7.3–19.7 µmol/L
10–13 y	25–148 µg/dL	3.9–22.7 µmol/L
14–17 y	46–130 µg/dL	7.1–19.9 µmol/L
Adult	70–120 µg/dL	10.7–18.4 µmol/L

DESCRIPTION: Zinc is found in all body tissues, but the highest concentrations are found in the eye, bone, and male reproductive organs. Zinc is involved in RNA and DNA synthesis and is essential in the process of tissue repair. It is also required for the formation of collagen and the production of active vitamin A (for the visual pigment rhodopsin). Zinc also functions as a chelating agent to protect the body from lead and cadmium poisoning. Zinc is absorbed from the small intestine. Its absorption and excretion seem to be through the same sites as those for iron and copper. The body does not store zinc as it does copper and iron. Untreated zinc deficiency in infants may result in a condition called acrodermatitis enteropathica. Symptoms include growth retardation, diarrhea, impaired wound healing, and frequent infections. Adolescents and adults with zinc deficiency exhibit similar adverse effects on growth, sexual development, and immune function, as well as altered taste and smell, emotional instability, impaired adaptation to darkness, impaired night vision, tremors, and a bullous, pustular rash over the extremities. ■

INDICATIONS:

- Assist in confirming acrodermatitis enteropathica

- Evaluate nutritional deficiency

- Evaluate possible toxicity

- Monitor replacement therapy in individuals with identified deficiencies

- Monitor therapy of individuals with Wilson's disease

RESULT

Increased in:
- Anemia

- Arteriosclerosis

- Coronary heart disease

- Primary osteosarcoma of the bone

Decreased in:
- Acrodermatitis enteropathica

- Acute infections

- Acute stress

- Acquired immunodeficiency syndrome (AIDS)

- Burns

- Cirrhosis

- Conditions that decrease albumin

- Diabetes

- Long-term total parenteral nutrition

- Malabsorption

- Myocardial infarction

- Nephrotic syndrome

- Nutritional deficiency

- Pulmonary tuberculosis

- Pregnancy

CRITICAL VALUES: N/A

INTERFERING FACTORS:

- Drugs that may increase zinc levels include auranofin, chlorthalidone, corticotropin, oral contraceptives, and penicillamine.

- Drugs that may decrease zinc levels include anticonvulsants, cisplatin, citrates, corticosteroids, estrogens, interferon, and oral contraceptives.

Nursing Implications and Procedure

Pretest:

➤ Obtain a history of the patient's complaints, including a list of known allergens.

➤ Obtain a history of the patient's gastrointestinal, hepatobiliary, immune, and musculoskeletal systems, as well as results of previously performed tests and procedures. For related tests, refer to the gastrointestinal, immune, hepatobiliary, and musculoskeletal system tables.

➤ Obtain a list of medications the patient is taking, including herbs, nutritional supplements, and nutraceuticals. The requesting health care practitioner and laboratory should be advised if the patient regularly uses these products so that their effects can be taken into consideration when reviewing results.

➤ There are no food, fluid, or medication restrictions unless by medical direction.

➤ Review the procedure with the patient.

➤ Inform the patient that specimen collection takes approximately 5 to 10 minutes.

Intratest:

➤ Direct the patient to breathe normally and to avoid unnecessary movement.

➤ Observe standard precautions and follow the general guidelines in Appendix A. Perform a venipuncture, and collect the specimen in a 5-mL royal blue–top tube.

➤ Label the specimen, and promptly transport it to the laboratory.

Post-test:

➤ Observe venipuncture site for bleeding or hematoma formation. Apply pressure bandage.

➤ Instruct the patient to resume usual diet and medication, if withheld and as directed by the requesting health care practitioner.

➤ Topical or oral supplementation may be ordered for patients with zinc deficiency. Dietary sources high in zinc include shellfish, red meat, wheat germ, and processed foods such as canned pork and beans and canned chili. Patients should be informed that diets high in phytates from whole grains, coffee, cocoa, or tea bind zinc and prevent it from being absorbed. Decreases in zinc also can be induced by increased intake of iron, copper, or manganese. Vitamin and mineral supplements with a greater than 3:1 iron/zinc ratio inhibit zinc absorption.

➤ Evaluate test results in relation to the patient's symptoms and other tests performed. Related laboratory tests include albumin, iron, and copper.

B-TYPE NATRIURETIC PEPTIDE AND PRO-B-TYPE NATRIURETIC PEPTIDE

SYNONYMS/ACRONYMS: BNP and Pro-BNP

SPECIMEN: Plasma (1 mL) collected in a plastic, lavender-top (ethylenediaminetetraacetic acid [EDTA]) tube.

REFERENCE VALUE: (Method: (Immunochemiluminometric for BNP; immuno(electro)chemiluminescence for Pro-BNP).)

	BNP	Pro-BNP (N-Terminal)
Male	Less than 100 pg/mL.	Less than or equal to 60 pg/mL
Female	Less than 100 pg/mL.	12–150 pg/mL

DESCRIPTION: The peptides (B-type natriuretic peptide [BNP] and atrial natriuretic peptide [ANP]) assist in the regulation of fluid balance and blood pressure. BNP, Pro-BNP, and ANP are useful markers in the diagnosis of congestive heart failure. BNP, first isolated in the brain of pigs, is a neurohormone synthesized primarily in the ventricles of the human heart in response to increases in ventricular pressure and volume. Circulating levels of BNP and Pro-BNP increase in proportion to the severity of heart failure. ■

INDICATIONS:

- Assist in the diagnosis of heart failure
- Assist in differentiating heart failure from pulmonary disease
- To screen for left ventricular dysfunction and therefore need for echocardiography for further assessment
- Assist in determining the prognosis and therapy of patients with heart failure

RESULT

Increased in:

- Cardiac inflammation (myocarditis, cardiac allograft rejection)
- Cirrhosis
- Cushing's syndrome
- Heart failure
- Kawasaki's disease
- Left ventricular hypertrophy
- Myocardial infarction
- Primary hyperaldosteronism
- Primary pulmonary hypertension

- Renal failure
- Ventricular dysfunction

Decreased in: N/A

CRITICAL VALUES: N/A

INTERFERING FACTORS: N/A

Nursing Implications and Procedure · · · · · · · · · · ·

Pretest:

➤ Obtain a history of the patient's complaints, including a list of known allergens.

➤ Obtain a history of the patient's cardiovascular system, as well as results of previously performed tests and procedures. For related tests, refer to the cardiovascular system table.

➤ Obtain a list of the medications the patient is taking, including herbs, nutritional supplements, and nutraceuticals. The requesting health care practitioner should be advised if the patient regularly uses these products so that their effects can be taken into consideration when reviewing results.

➤ There are no food, fluid, or medication restrictions unless by medical direction.

➤ Review the procedure with the patient.

➤ Inform the patient that specimen collection takes approximately 5 to 10 minutes.

Intratest:

➤ Direct the patient to breathe normally and to avoid unnecessary movement.

➤ Observe standard precautions and follow the general guidelines in Appendix A.

➤ Perform a venipuncture, and collect the specimen in a 5-mL plastic, lavender-top tube.

➤ Label the specimen and promptly transport it to the laboratory.

Post-test:

➤ Observe venipuncture site for bleeding or hematoma formation. Apply pressure bandage.

➤ Evaluate test results in relation to the patient's symptoms and other tests performed. Related laboratory tests include atrial natriuretic factor, aspartate aminotranspeptidase, calcium, C-reactive protein, creatine kinase and isoenzymes, ionized calcium, homocysteine, lactate dehydrogenase and isoenzymes, magnesium, myoglobin, and tropinin.

A Rapid BNP immunoassay point-of-care assay may be performed, in which a venous blood sample is collected, placed on a strip, and inserted into a device that measures BNP. Results are completed in 10 to 15 minutes.

SYSTEM TABLES

CARDIOVASCULAR SYSTEM

Laboratory Tests Associated with the Cardiovascular System

Anion gap 81
Apolipoprotein A 133
Apolipoprotein B 136
Aspartate aminotranspeptidase 143
Atrial natriuretic factor 146
Blood gases 216
C-reactive protein 247
Calcium, serum 259
Calcium, ionized 256
Chloride 293
Cholesterol, HDL, LDL 310
Cholesterol, total 314
Creatine kinase and isoenzymes 401
D-Dimer 439
Digoxin 84
Disopyramide 84
Fibrin degradation products 509
Flecainide 84
Hematocrit 562

Hemoglobin 566
Homocysteine and methylmalonic acid 592
International normalized ratio (INR) 837
Lactate dehydrogenase and isoenzymes 645
Lactic acid 648
Lidocaine 84
Lipoprotein electrophoresis 668
Magnesium, serum 689
Myoglobin 743
Pericardial fluid analysis 769
Potassium, serum 810
Procainamide 84
Prothrombin time and INR 837
Quinidine 84
Triglycerides 931
Troponins I and T 938
Vitamin E 1016

Diagnostic Tests Associated with the Cardiovascular System

Angiography, coronary 64
Angiography, magnetic
  resonance 68
Blood pool imaging 231
Chest x-ray 289
Computed tomography,
  angiography 351
Echocardiography 450
Echocardiography,
  transesophageal 453
Electrocardiogram 456
Exercise stress test 493
Holter monitoring 590
Magnetic resonance imaging,
  chest 701

Myocardial scan 736
Plethysmography 789
Positron emission tomography,
  heart 804
Stress echocardiography 493
Ultrasound, arterial Doppler,
  carotid 942
Ultrasound, arterial Doppler,
  lower extremity studies 944
Ultrasound, peripheral Doppler
  966
Ultrasound, venous Doppler,
  extremity studies 978
Venography, lower extremity
  studies 1009

ENDOCRINE SYSTEM

Laboratory Tests Associated with the Endocrine System

Adrenocorticotropic hormone
  (and challenge tests) 7
Albumin 14
Aldosterone 19
Amylase 51
Angiotensin-converting enzyme
  78
Anion gap 81
Antibodies, antithyroglobulin
  and antithyroid peroxidase 103
Antidiuretic hormone 122
Biopsy, thyroid 210
C-peptide 244
Calcitonin 253
Calcium, ionized 256
Calcium, urine 263
Catecholamines, urine 277
Chloride, serum 293

Chloride, sweat 297
Cortisol and challenge tests 7
Dehydroepiandrosterone sulfate
  444
Dexamethasone suppression test
  398
Estradiol 485
Estrogen and progesterone
  receptor assays 487
Follicle-stimulating hormone 515
Fructosamine 517
Gastrin and gastrin stimulation
  test 527
Glucagon 534
Glucose (random, 2-hour
  postprandial) 537
Glucose tolerance tests 542
Glycated hemoglobin A_1C 549

(*Continued on the following page*)

Laboratory Tests Associated with the Endocrine System

Growth hormone, stimulation
and suppression tests 554
Homovanillic acid 594
Human chorionic gonadotropin
597
5-Hydroxyindoleacetic acid 605
Insulin and insulin response to
glucose 624
Insulin antibodies 627
Ketones, blood and urine 638
Lactic acid 648
Luteinizing hormone 681
Magnesium, serum 689
Magnesium, urine 691
Metanephrines 724
Metyrapone stimulation 398
Microalbumin 729
Osmolality, serum and urine 744
Parathyroid hormone: Intact,
C-terminal, and N-terminal 759
Phosphorus, serum 775
Phosphorus, urine 778
Potassium, serum 810

Potassium, urine 815
Prealbumin 818
Progesterone 824
Prolactin 826
Renin 872
Sodium, serum 893
Sodium, urine 896
Testosterone, total 905
Thyroglobulin 907
Thyroid-binding inhibitory
antibodies 909
Thyroid-stimulating hormone
914
Thyroid-stimulating
immunoglobulins 916
Thyrotropin-releasing hormone
917
Thyroxine-binding globulin 919
Thyroxine, free 921
Thyroxine, total 922
Triiodothyronine, free 934
Triiodothyronine, total 936
Vanillylmandelic acid 1005

Diagnostic Tests Associated with the Endocrine System

Adrenal gland scan 4
Angiography, adrenal 60
Computed tomography, pancreas
367
Computed tomography, pituitary
374
Magnetic resonance imaging,
pancreas 714

Magnetic resonance imaging,
pituitary 707
Parathyroid scan 761
Radioactive iodine uptake 852
Thyroid scan 911
Ultrasound, pancreas 961
Ultrasound, thyroid and
parathyroid 976

GASTROINTESTINAL SYSTEM

Laboratory Tests Associated with the Gastrointestinal System

Albumin and albumin/globulin
   ratio 14
Ammonia 45
Amylase 51
Anion gap 81
Antibodies, anticytoplasmic
   neutrophilic 94
Antibodies, gliadin
   (immunoglobulin G and
   immunoglobulin A) 106
Bacterial culture, stool 160
Biopsy, intestinal 191
CA 19-9 252
Calcium, serum 259
Carcinoembryonic antigen 272
Chloride, serum 293
Cholesterol, total 314
Complete blood count 340
Culture, viral 419
D-Xylose tolerance test 441
Fecal analysis 496
Fecal fat 498
Folate 513
Fructosamine 517
Gastric acid stimulation test 522
Gastrin and gastrin stimulation
   test 527
Gram stain 551
Helicobacter pylori 561

Hematocrit 562
Hemoglobin 566
5-Hydroxyindoleacetic acid 605
Immunoglobulins A, E, G,
   and M 616
Intrinsic factor antibodies 632
Lactose tolerance test 650
Lipase 666
Magnesium, serum 689
Magnesium, urine 691
Ova and parasites 751
Oxalate 753
Peritoneal fluid analysis 772
Phosphorus, serum 775
Potassium, serum 810
Potassium, urine 815
Prealbumin 818
Red blood cell count 859
Red blood cell indices 863
Total protein and fractions 834
Triglycerides 931
Vitamin A 1020
Vitamin B_1 1020
Vitamin B_6 1020
Vitamin B_{12} 1012
Vitamin C 1020
Vitamin D 1014
Vitamin E 1016
Zinc 1034

Diagnostic Tests Associated with the Gastrointestinal System

Barium enema 167
Barium swallow 170
Cholangiography, percutaneous
   transhepatic 301

Cholangiography, postoperative
   304
Cholangiopancreatography,
   endoscopic retrograde 307

(*Continued on the following page*)

Diagnostic Tests Associated with the Gastrointestinal System

Colonoscopy 330
Computed tomography, abdomen 347
Computed tomography, pancreas 367
Esophageal manometry 479
Esophagogastroduodenoscopy 482
Gastric emptying scan 524
Gastroesophageal reflux scan 529
Gastrointestinal blood loss scan 531

Hepatobiliary imaging 582
Kidney, ureter, and bladder study 641
Laparoscopy 652
Liver scan 671
Magnetic resonance imaging, abdomen 694
Proctosigmoidoscopy 820
Ultrasound, liver and biliary system 953
Upper gastrointestinal and small bowel series 981

GENITOURINARY SYSTEM

Laboratory Tests Associated with the Genitourinary System

Acetaminophen 54
Acid phosphatase, prostatic 2
Albumin and albumin/globulin ratio 14
Aldosterone 19
Amikacin 90
Ammonia 45
Anion gap 81
Antibodies, anticytoplasmic neutrophilic 94
Antibodies, anti–glomerular basement membrane 95
Antidiuretic hormone 122
Bacterial culture, urine 164
Biopsy, bladder 176
Biopsy, kidney 193
Bladder cancer markers, urine 212
Calcitonin and calcitonin stimulation tests 253
Calcium, ionized 256
Calcium, serum 259
Calcium, urine 263
Calculus, kidney stone panel 266

Carbon dioxide 267
Chloride, serum 293
Creatinine, serum 404
Creatinine, urine, and creatinine clearance, urine 407
Culture, viral 419
Cyclosporine 619
Cytology, urine 435
Erythropoietin 477
Gentamicin 90
Gram stain 551
Lithium 126
Magnesium, serum 689
Magnesium, urine 691
Methotrexate 619
Microalbumin 729
β_2-Microglobulin 732
Osmolality, serum and urine 744
Oxalate, urine 753
Phosphorus, serum 775
Phosphorus, urine 778
Potassium, serum 810
Potassium, urine 815
Prostate-specific antigen 828

(Continued on the following page)

Laboratory Tests Associated with the Genitourinary System

Protein, urine 834	Urea nitrogen, blood 984
Renin 872	Urea nitrogen, urine 986
Salicylate 54	Uric acid, blood 992
Sodium, serum 893	Uric acid, urine 994
Sodium, urine 896	Urinalysis 997
Tobramycin 90	Vancomycin 90

Diagnostic Tests Associated with the Genitourinary System

Angiography, renal 74	Renogram 875
Computed tomography, renal 377	Ultrasound, bladder 946
Cystometry 422	Ultrasound, kidney 951
Cystoscopy 425	Ultrasound, pelvis 963
Cystourethrography, voiding 428	Ultrasound, prostate 969
Intravenous pyelography 628	Ultrasound, scrotum 971
Kidney, ureter, and bladder study 641	Urethrography, retrograde 989

HEMATOPOIETIC SYSTEM

Laboratory Tests Associated with the Hematopoietic System

δ-Aminolevulinic acid 43	Coombs' antiglobulin, direct 391
Anion gap 81	Coombs' antiglobulin, indirect 393
Antithrombin III 128	Copper 395
Antibody, cardiolipin, immunoglobulin G and immunoglobulin M 105	D-Dimer 439
	Eosinophil count 470
Biopsy, bone marrow 181	Erythrocyte protoporphyrin, free 472
Bleeding time 214	
Blood groups and antibodies 227	Erythrocyte sedimentation rate 474
Calcium, serum 259	
Cholesterol, total 314	Erythropoietin 477
Clot retraction 320	Ferritin 501
Coagulation factor assays 322	Fibrin degradation products 509
Complete blood count 340	Fibrinogen 511

(*Continued on the following page*)

Laboratory Tests Associated with the Hematopoietic System

Folate 513
Glucose-6-phosphate
  dehydrogenase 540
Ham's test for paroxysmal
  nocturnal hemoglobinuria 557
Haptoglobin 559
Hematocrit 562
Hemoglobin 566
Hemoglobin electrophoresis 570
Hemosiderin 573
Homocysteine and
  methylmalonic acid 592
Immunoglobulins A, E, G, and
  M 616
Immunofixation electrophoresis,
  serum and urine 612
International normalized ratio
  (INR) 837
Intrinsic factor antibodies 632
Iron 633
Iron-binding capacity (total),
  transferrin, and iron saturation
  636
Kleihauer-Betke test 644
Lactate dehydrogenase and
  isoenzymes 645
Lead 660
Leukocyte alkaline phosphatase
  664

Lupus anticoagulant antibodies
  679
Methemoglobin 727
Osmotic fragility 748
Partial thromboplastin time
  764
Plasminogen 781
Platelet antibodies 783
Platelet count 784
Porphyrins, urine 797
Protein C 830
Protein S 832
Prothrombin time and INR 837
Pyruvate kinase 850
Red blood cell cholinesterase
  857
Red blood cell count 859
Red blood cell indices 863
Red blood cell morphology and
  inclusions 866
Reticulocyte count 878
Sickle cell screen 891
Transferrin 929
Vitamin B_{12} 1012
Vitamin E 1016
Vitamin K 1018
White blood cell count and cell
  differential 1024

Diagnostic Tests Associated with the Hematopoietic System

Angiography, abdomen 56
Computed tomography, spleen
  384
Gastrointestinal blood loss scan
  531
Lymphangiography 685

Meckel's diverticulum scan 719
Liver and spleen scan 671

Ultrasound, lymph nodes and
  retroperitoneum 956
Ultrasound, spleen 973

HEPATOBILIARY SYSTEM

Laboratory Tests Associated with the Hepatobiliary System

Acetaminophen 54
Acetylsalicylic acid 54
Alanine aminotransferase 12
Albumin 14
Aldolase 17
Alkaline phosphatase and
  isoenzymes 22
α_1-Antitrypsin and α_1-antitrypsin
  phenotyping 130
Amitryptyline 118
Ammonia 45
Amylase 51
Antibodies, anticytoplasmic
  neutrophilic 94
Antibody, antimitochondrial 108
Antibody, anti–smooth muscle
  109
Aspartate aminotranspeptidase
  143
Bilirubin and bilirubin fractions
  173
Biopsy, liver 196
Calcium, serum 259
Carbamazepine 112
Ceruloplasmin 287
Cholesterol, total 314
Coagulation factor assays 322
Copper 395
Desipramine 118
Diazepam 118
Doxepin 118
Ethosuximide 112
Fibrinogen 511
δ-Glutamyltransferase 547
Haloperidol 126
Haptoglobin 559
Hematocrit 562
Hemoglobin 566

Hepatitis A, antibody 574
Hepatitis B, core antibody 577
Hepatitis B, surface antibody 577
Hepatitis B, surface antigen 576
Hepatitis Be, antibody and
  antigen 576
Hepatitis C, antibody 579
Hepatitis D, antibody 581
Infectious mononucleosis screen
  622
Imipramine 118
International normalized ratio
  (INR) 837
Lactate dehydrogenase and
  isoenzymes 645
Lactic acid 648
Lipase 666
Nortriptyline 118
Partial thromboplastin time 764
Phenobarbital 112
Phenytoin 112
Prealbumin 818
Primidone 112
Protein C 830
Protein S 832
Protein, total and fractions 834
Prothrombin time and INR 837
Pseudocholinesterase 840
Red blood cell count 859
Red blood cell morphology and
  inclusions 866
Urea nitrogen, blood 984
Uric acid, blood 992
Valproic acid 112
Vitamin E 1016
Vitamin K 1018
Zinc 1034

Diagnostic Tests Associated with the Hepatobiliary System

Angiography, abdomen 56
Angiography, magnetic
resonance 68
Cholangiography, percutaneous
transhepatic 301
Cholangiography, postoperative
304
Cholangiopancreatography,
endoscopic retrograde 307

Computed tomography, liver 354
Computed tomography,
angiography 351
Hepatobiliary scan 582

Magnetic resonance imaging,
abdomen 694
Ultrasound, liver and biliary
system 953

IMMUNE SYSTEM

Laboratory Tests Associated with the Immune System

Acid phosphatase, prostatic 2
Allergen-specific immunoglobulin
E 27
Amikacin 90
Angiotensin-converting enzyme
78
Anion gap 81
Antibodies, anticytoplasmic
neutrophilic 94
Antibodies, anti–glomerular
basement membrane 95
Antibodies, antinuclear, anti-
DNA, and anticentromere 97
Antibodies, antiscleroderma 99
Antibodies, antisperm 100
Antibodies, antistreptolysin O
102
Antibodies, antithyroglobin and
antithyroid peroxidase 103
Antibodies, cardiolipin,
immunoglobulin G and
immunoglobulin M 105
Antibodies, gliadin 106
Antibody, antimitochondrial 108

Antibody, anti–smooth muscle
109
Antibody, Jo-1 111
Antideoxyribonuclease-B,
streptococcal 116
Antigens/antibodies,
anti–extractable nuclear 124
Bacterial culture, anal/genital,
ear, eye, skin, and wound 148
Bacterial culture, blood 153
Bacterial culture, sputum 156
Bacterial culture, stool 160
Bacterial culture, throat or nasal
pharyngeal 162
Bacterial culture, urine 164
Biopsy, bladder 176
Biopsy, bone 179
Biopsy, bone marrow 181
Biopsy, breast 185
Biopsy, cervical 187
Biopsy, intestinal 191
Biopsy, kidney 193
Biopsy, liver 196
Biopsy, lung 198

(Continued on the following page)

Laboratory Tests Associated with the Immune System

(Continued on the following page)

Laboratory Tests Associated with the Immune System

Parvovirus B19 immunoglobulin G and immunoglobulin M antibody 767
Pericardial fluid analysis 769
Peritoneal fluid analysis 772
Platelet antibodies 783
Platelet count 784
Pleural fluid analysis 793
Potassium 810
Prostate-specific antigen 828
Protein, total and fractions 834
Protein, urine, total quantitative and fractions 834
Red blood cell count 859
Red blood cell morphology and inclusions 866

Red blood cell indices 863
Rheumatoid factor 884
Rubella 885
Rubeola 887
Streptococcal screen, rapid 553
Synovial fluid analysis 899
Syphilis serology 902
Tobramycin 90
Toxoplasma antibody 928
Tuberculin skin tests 939
Vancomycin 90
Varicella 1007
White blood cell count and cell differential 1024
Zinc 1034

Diagnostic Tests Associated with the Immune System

Gallium scan 519

White blood cell scan 1031

MUSCULOSKELETAL SYSTEM

Laboratory Tests Associated with the Musculoskeletal System

Acetylcholine receptor antibody 1
Aldolase 17
Alkaline phosphatase and isoenzymes 22
Angiotensin-converting enzyme 78
Antibodies, anticytoplasmic neutrophilic 94
Antibodies, antinuclear, anti-DNA, and anticentromere 97
Antibodies, antiscleroderma 99
Antibody, Jo-1 111

Antigens/antibodies, anti–extractable nuclear 124
Biopsy, bone 179
Biopsy, lymph node 201
Biopsy, muscle 204
Biopsy, skin 208
Calcitonin and calcitonin stimulation tests 253
Calcium, serum 259
Calcium, urine 263
Cerebrospinal fluid analysis 282
Collagen crosslinked N-telopeptides 327

(Continued on the following page)

Laboratory Tests Associated with the Musculoskeletal System

Creatine kinase and isoenzymes 401
Creatinine, serum 404
Hematocrit 562
Hemoglobin 566
Human leukocyte antigen B27 601
Immunoglobulins A, D, G, and M 616
Lactate dehydrogenase and isoenzymes 645
Lactic acid 648
Lupus anticoagulant antibodies 679

Lyme antibody 684
Myoglobin 743
Osteocalcin 749
Phosphorus 775
Pseudocholinesterase and dibucaine number 840
Rheumatoid factor 884
Synovial fluid analysis 899
Uric acid, blood 992
Vitamin D 1014
Zinc 1034

Diagnostic Tests Associated with the Musculoskeletal System

Arthrogram 138
Bone mineral density 234
Bone scan 238
Computed tomography, brain 357
Computed tomography, spine 381
Electroencephalography 460
Electromyography 463

Electromyography, pelvic floor sphincter 466
Electroneurography 468
Evoked brain potentials 489
Magnetic resonance imaging, musculoskeletal 704
Radiography, bone 855
Positron emission tomography, brain 800

REPRODUCTIVE SYSTEM

Laboratory Tests Associated with the Reproductive System

Acid phosphatase, prostatic 2
Amino acid screen, blood 34
Amino acid screen, urine 38
Amniotic fluid analysis 47
Antibodies, antisperm 100

Antibodies, cardiolipin, immunoglobulin G and immunoglobulin M 105
Bacterial culture, anal/genital 148
Biopsy, breast 185

(Continued on the following page)

Laboratory Tests Associated with the Reproductive System

Biopsy, cervical 187
Biopsy, chorionic villus 189
Biopsy, prostate 206
CA 125 249
CA 15-3 250
Carcinoembryonic antigen 272
Chlamydia group antibody 291
Chromosome analysis, blood 317
Collagen crosslinked
  N-telopeptides 327
Culture, viral 419
Cytomegalovirus,
  immunoglobulin G and
  immunoglobulin M 437
Estradiol 485
Estrogen and progesterone
  receptor assays 487
Fetal fibronectin 503
α_1-Fetoprotein 505
Follicle-stimulating hormone 515
Gram stain 551
Her-2/neu oncoprotein 585
Hexosaminidase A and B 587

Human chorionic gonadotropin
  597
Human immunodeficiency virus
  type 1 and type 2 antibodies
  599
Kleihauer-Betke test 644
Lecithin/sphingomyelin ratio 661
Lupus anticoagulant antibodies
  679
Luteinizing hormone 681
Magnesium 689
Papanicolaou smear 756
Progesterone 824
Prolactin 826
Prostate-specific antigen 828
Rubeola 885
Rubella 887
Semen analysis 889
Syphilis serology 902
Testosterone, total 905
Toxoplasma antibody 928
Urinalysis 997
Varicella 1007

Diagnostic Tests Associated with the Reproductive System

Colposcopy 333
Computed tomography, pelvis
  370
Hysterosalpingography 609
Laparoscopy, abdominal 652
Laparoscopy, gynecologic 655
Magnetic resonance imaging,
  pelvis 710

Mammography 717
Positron emission tomography,
  pelvis 807
Ultrasound, obstetric 958
Ultrasound, pelvic 963
Ultrasound, scrotal 971

RESPIRATORY SYSTEM

Laboratory Tests Associated with the Respiratory System

Allergen-specific immunoglobulin E 27
Alveolar/arterial gradient and arterial/alveolar oxygen ratio 29
Angiotensin-converting enzyme 78
Anion gap 81
Antibodies, anti–glomerular basement membrane 95
α_1-Antitrypsin and α_1-antitrypsin phenotyping 130
Bacterial culture, sputum 156
Bacterial culture, throat 162
Biopsy, lung 198
Blood gases 216
Carbon dioxide 267
Carboxyhemoglobin 270
Chloride 293
Chloride, sweat 297
Cold agglutinin titer 325
Complete blood count 340
Culture and smear, mycobacteria 412

Culture, viral 419
Cytology, sputum 431
D-Dimer 439
Eosinophil count 470
Erythrocyte sedimentation rate 474
Fecal fat 498
Gram stain 551
Hematocrit 562
Hemoglobin 566
Hypersensitivity pneumonitis 607
Immunoglobulin E 614
Lactic acid 648
Lecithin/sphingomyelin ratio 661
Pleural fluid analysis 793
Potassium 810
Rapid streptococcal screen 553
Red blood cell count 859
Red blood cell indices 863
Tuberculin skin tests 939
White blood cell count and cell differential 1024

Diagnostic Tests Associated with the Respiratory System

Angiography, pulmonary 71
Bronchoscopy 241

Chest x-ray 289
Computed tomography, chest 388
Lung perfusion scan 674

Lung ventilation scan 677
Magnetic resonance imaging, chest 701
Mediastinoscopy 722
Pulmonary function studies 842
Pulse oximetry 848

THERAPEUTIC DRUG MONITORING AND TOXICOLOGY

Laboratory Tests Associated with Therapeutic Drug Monitoring and Toxicology

Acetaminophen 54
Acetylsalicylic acid 54
Albumin 14
Alcohol, ethyl 447
Amikacin 90
Amitryptyline 118
Amphetamines 447
Barbiturates 447
Benzodiazepines 447
Cannabinoids 447
Carbamazepine 112
Cocaine 447
Cyclosporine 619
Desipramine 118
Diazepam 118
Digoxin 84
Disopyramide 84
Doxepin 118
Ethanol 447
Ethosuximide 112

Flecainide 84
Gentamicin 90
Haloperidol 126
Imipramine 118
Lead 660
Lidocaine 84
Lithium 126
Methotrexate 619
Nortriptyline 118
Opiates 447
Phencyclidine 447
Phenobarbital 112
Phenytoin 112
Primidone 112
Procainamide 84
Quinidine 84
Tobramycin 90
Tricyclic antidepressants 118
Valproic acid 112
Vancomycin 90

Patient Preparation Before Diagnostic and Laboratory Procedures

The first step in any laboratory or diagnostic procedure is patient preparation or patient teaching before the performance of the procedure. This pretesting explanation to the patient or caregiver follows essentially the same pattern for all sites and types of studies and includes the following:

- *Statement of the purpose of the study.* The level of detail provided to patients about the test purpose depends on numerous factors and should be individualized appropriately in each particular setting.
- *Description of the procedure, including site and method.* It is a good idea to explain to the patient that you will be wearing gloves throughout the procedure. The explanation should help the patient understand that the use of gloves is standard practice established for his or her protection as well as yours. Many institutions require hand washing at the beginning and end of each specimen collection encounter and between each patient.
- *Description of the sensations, including discomfort and pain, the patient may experience during the specimen collection procedure.* Address concerns about pain related to the procedure and suggest breathing or visualization techniques to promote relaxation. For pediatric patients, a doll may be used to "show" the procedure. Where appropriate, the use of anesthetizing agents may assist in allaying anxiety the patient may experience that is related to anticipation of pain associated with the procedure. Sensitivity to cultural and social issues, as well as concern for modesty is important in providing psychological support.
- *Instruction regarding pretesting preparations related to diet, liquids, medications, and activity as well as any restrictions regarding diet, liquids, medications, activity, known allergies, therapies, or other procedures that might affect test results.* To increase patient compliance, the instructions should include an explanation of why strict adherence to the instructions is required.
- *Recognition of anxiety related to test results.* Provide a compassionate, reassuring environment. Be prepared to educate the patient regarding access to the appropriate counseling services. Encourage the patient to ask questions and verbalize his or her concerns.

Specific collection techniques and patient preparation vary by site, study required, and level of invasiveness. These techniques are described in the individual monographs.

Blood Specimens

Most laboratory tests that require a blood specimen use venous blood. Venous blood can be collected directly from the vein or by way of capillary puncture. Capillary blood can be obtained from the fingertips or earlobes of adults and small children. Capillary blood can also be obtained from the heel of infants. The circumstances in which the capillary method would be selected over direct venipuncture include cases in which:

- The patient has poor veins.
- The patient has small veins.
- The patient has a limited number of available veins.
- The patient has significant anxiety about the venipuncture procedure.

Venous blood also can be obtained from vascular access devices, such as heparin locks and central venous catheters. Examples of central venous catheters include the triple-lumen subclavian, Hickman, and Groshong catheters.

Fetal blood samples can be obtained, when warranted, by a qualified health care practitioner from the scalp or from the umbilical cord.

Arterial blood can be collected from the radial, brachial, or femoral artery if blood gas analysis is requested.

There are some general guidelines one should follow in the procurement and handling of blood specimens:

- It is essential that the patient be positively and properly identified. Specimens should always be labeled with the patient's name, medical record number (or some other unique identifier), date collected, time collected, and initials of the person collecting the sample.
- Requisitions should be completed accurately and submitted per laboratory policy.
- The practice of an overnight fast before specimen collection is a general recommendation. Reference ranges are often based on fasting populations to provide some level of standardization for comparison. Some test results are dramatically affected by foods, however, and fasting is a pretest requirement. The presence of lipids in the blood also may interfere with the test method; fasting eliminates this potential source of error, especially if the patient already has elevated lipid levels. The laboratory should always be consulted if there is a question as to whether fasting is a requirement or a recommendation.
- Gloves and any other additional personal protective equipment indicated by the patient's condition should always be worn during the specimen collection process. Appendix F can be consulted for a more detailed description of standard precautions.
- Stress can cause variations in some test results. A sleeping patient should be gently wakened and allowed the opportunity to become oriented before collection site selection. The comatose or unconscious patient should be greeted in

the same gentle manner because although they are unable to respond, they may be capable of hearing and understanding. Anticipate instances where patient cooperation may be an issue. Enlist the assistance of a second person to assist with specimen collection to ensure a safe, quality collection experience for all involved.

- Localized activity such as the application of a tourniquet or clenching the hand to assist in visualizing the vein can cause variations in some test results. It is important to be aware of affected studies before specimen collection.
- Hemoconcentration may cause variations in some test results. The tourniquet should never be left in place for longer than 1 minute.
- Previous puncture sites should be avoided when accessing a blood vessel by any means, to reduce the potential for infection.
- Specimens should never be collected above an intravenous (IV) line because of the potential for dilution when the specimen and the IV solution combine in the collection container, falsely decreasing the result. It is also possible that substances in the IV solution could contaminate the specimen and result in falsely elevated test results.
- Changes in posture from supine to erect or long-term maintenance of a supine posture causes variations in some test results. It is important to be aware of this effect when results are interpreted and compared with previous values.
- Collection times for therapeutic drug (peak and trough) or other specific monitoring (e.g., chemotherapy, glucose, insulin, or potassium) should be documented carefully in relation to the time of medication administration. It is essential that this information be communicated clearly and accurately to avoid misunderstanding of the dose time in relation to the collect time. Miscommunication between the individual administering the medication and the individual collecting the specimen is the most frequent cause of subtherapeutic levels, toxic levels, and misleading information used in the calculation of future therapies.
- The laboratory should be consulted regarding minimum specimen collection requirements when multiple tube types or samples are required. The amount of serum or plasma collected can be estimated using assumptions of packed cell volume or hematocrit. The packed cell volume of a healthy woman is usually 38 to 44 percent of the total blood volume. If a full 5-mL red-top tube is collected, and the hematocrit is 38 to 44 percent, approximately 2.8 to 3.1 mL of the total blood volume should be serum $[5 - (5 \times 0.44)]$ to $[5 - (5 \times 0.38)]$. Factors that invalidate estimation include conditions such as anemia, polcythemia, dehydration, or overhydration.
- The laboratory should be consulted regarding the preferred specimen container before specimen collection. Specific analytes may vary in concentration depending on whether the sample is serum or plasma. It is recommended that when serial measurements are to be carried out, the same type of collection container be used so that fluctuations in values caused by variations in specimen type are not misinterpreted as changes in clinical status. Consultation regarding collection containers is also important because some laboratory methods are optimized for a specific specimen type (serum versus plasma).

Also, preservatives present in collection containers, such as sodium fluoride, may exhibit a chemical interference with test reagents that can cause underestimation or overestimation of measured values. Other preservatives, such as ethylenediaminetetra-acetic acid (EDTA), can block the analyte of interest in the sample from participating in the test reaction, invalidating test results. Finally, it is possible that some high-throughput, robotic equipment systems require specific and standardized collection containers.

• Prompt and proper specimen processing, storage, and analysis are important to achieve accurate results. Specimens collected in containers with solid or liquid preservatives or with gel separators should be mixed by inverting the tube 10 times immediately after the tube has been filled. Handle the specimen gently to avoid hemolysis. Specimens should always be transported to the laboratory as quickly as possible after collection.

Results that are evaluated outside the entire context of the preparatory, collection, and handling process may be interpreted erroneously if consideration is not given to the above-listed general guidelines.

Site Selection

Capillary Puncture: Assess the selected area. It should be free of lesions and calluses, there should be no edema, and the site should feel warm. If the site feels cool or if the site appears pale or cyanotic, warm compresses can be applied over 3 to 5 minutes to dilate the capillaries. For finger sticks, the central, fleshy, distal portions of the third or fourth fingers are the preferred collection sites (Fig. A–1). For neonatal heel sticks, the medial and lateral surfaces of the plantar area are preferred to avoid direct puncture of the heel bone, which could result in osteomyelitis (Fig. A–2).

Venipuncture: Assess the arm for visibly accessible veins. The selected area should not be burned or scarred, have a tattoo, or have hematoma present. Even after the tourniquet is applied, not all patients have a prominent median cubital, cephalic, or basilic vein. Both arms should be observed because some patients have accessible veins in one arm and not the other. The median cubital vein in the antecubital fossa is the preferred venipuncture site. The patient may be able to provide the best information regarding venous access if he or she has had previous venipuncture experience (Fig. A–3). Alternative techniques to increase visibility of veins may include warming the arm, allowing the arm to dangle downward for a minute or two, tapping the antecubital area with the index finger, or massaging the arm upward from wrist to elbow. The condition of the vein also should be assessed before venipuncture. Sclerotic (hard, scarred) veins or veins in which phlebitis previously occurred should be avoided. Arms with a functioning hemodialysis access site should not be used. The arm on the affected side of a mastectomy should be avoided. In the case of a double mastectomy, the requesting health care practitioner should be consulted before specimen collection.

Venipuncture of Hand and Wrist: If no veins in the arms are available, hands and wrists should be examined as described previously. Consideration should be given to the venipuncture equipment selected because the veins in these areas are much smaller. Pediatric-sized collection containers and needles with a larger gauge may be more appropriate.

Figure Appendix A–1

Figure Appendix A–2

Venipuncture of Legs and Feet: The veins in the legs and feet can be accessed as with sites located on the arm, hand, or wrist. These extremities should be used only on the approval of the requesting health care practitioner because veins in these locations are more prone to infection and formation of blood clots, especially in patients with diabetes, cardiac disease, and bleeding disorders.

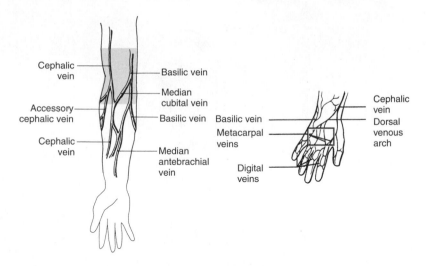

FIGURE Appendix A–3

Radial Arterial Puncture: The radial artery is the artery of choice for obtaining arterial blood gas specimens because it is close to the surface of the wrist and does not require a deep puncture. Its easy access also allows for more effective compression after the needle has been removed. The nearby ulnar artery can provide sufficient collateral circulation to the hand during specimen collection and postcollection compression (Fig. A–4).

Percutaneous Umbilical Cord Sampling: The blood is aspirated from the umbilical cord under the guidance of ultrasonography and using a 20- or 22-gauge spinal needle inserted through the mother's abdomen.

Postnatal Umbilical Cord Sampling: The blood is aspirated from the umbilical cord using a 20- or 22-gauge needle and transferred to the appropriate collection container.

Fetal Scalp Sampling: The requesting health care practitioner makes a puncture in the fetal scalp using a microblade, and the specimen is collected in a long capillary tube. The tube is usually capped on both ends immediately after specimen collection.

Locks and Catheters: These devices are inserted sometimes to provide a means for the administration of fluids or medications and to obtain blood specimens without the need for frequent venipuncture. The device first should be assessed for patency. The need for heparinization, irrigation, or clot removal depends on the type of device in use and the institution-specific or health care practitioner–specific protocols in use. Care should be taken to use sterile technique because these devices provide direct access to the patient's bloodstream. When IV fluids are being administered via a device at the time of specimen collection, blood should be obtained from the opposite side of the body. If this is not possible, the flow should be stopped for 5 minutes before specimen collection. The first 5 mL of blood collected should be discarded.

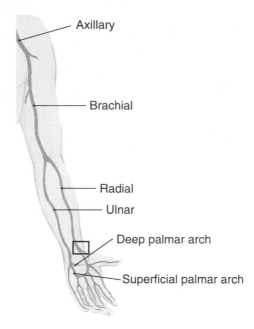

Axillary

Brachial

Radial

Ulnar

Deep palmar arch

Superficial palmar arch

FIGURE Appendix A–4

Selection of Blood Collection Equipment

In many cases when a blood sample is required, serum is the specimen type of choice. Plasma also may be frequently substituted, however. Specimen processing is more rapid for plasma samples than serum samples because the anticoagulated sample does not need to clot before centrifugation. Plasma samples also require less centrifugation time to achieve adequate separation. Consult with the testing laboratory regarding recommended specimen types. The basic blood collection tubes are shown on the inside cover of this book. Consider latex allergy when selecting the collection equipment appropriate for each patient. Equipment used in specimen collection includes:

- Gloves and other personal protective equipment depending on the situation
- Tourniquet
- Materials to cleanse or disinfect the collection site (alcohol preparations [70% alcohol], povidone-iodine solution [Betadine], or green soap are the most commonly used materials)
- Gauze (to wipe collection site dry after cleansing)
- Sterile lancet (capillary puncture)
- Syringe and needle (arterial puncture or venipuncture)
- Vial of heparin and syringe or heparin unit dose
- Sterile normal saline in 50-mL syringe (for indwelling devices such as Groshong catheter)
- Sterile cap or hub (for indwelling devices when the cap or hub will be replaced after specimen procurement)
- Needle and holder for vacuumized collection tube system (arterial puncture or venipuncture)

- Butterfly or winged infusion set (venipuncture)
- Collection container (vacuumized collection tube, capillary tube, or Microtainer)
- Bandage (to cover puncture site after specimen collection)

Collection Procedure

The procedures outlined here are basic in description. A phlebotomy or other text should be consulted for specific details regarding specimen collection and complications encountered during various types of blood collection.

Capillary: Place the patient in a comfortable position either sitting or lying down. Assess whether the patient has allergies to the disinfectant or to latex if latex gloves or tourniquet will be used in the collection procedure. Use gloved hands to select the collection site as described in the site selection section. Cleanse the skin with the appropriate disinfectant and dry the area. Pull the skin tightly by moving the thumb and index finger in opposite directions. Puncture the skin with a sterile lancet to a depth of approximately 2 mm, using a quick, firm motion. Wipe the first drop of blood away using the gauze. If flow is poor, the site should not be squeezed or the specimen may become contaminated with tissue fluid. Do not allow the collection container to touch the puncture site. Collect the sample in the capillary tube or Microtainer. The capillary tube should be held in a horizontal position to avoid the introduction of air bubbles into the sample. Microtainer tubes should be held in a downward slanted direction to facilitate the flow of blood into the capillary scoop of the collection device. If a smear is required, allow a drop of blood to fall onto a clean microscope slide. Gently spread the drop across the slide using the edge of another slide. Apply slight pressure to the puncture site with a clean piece of gauze until bleeding stops, and then apply a bandage. Safely dispose of the sharps. Properly label the specimens and transport immediately to the laboratory.

Venipuncture Using a Syringe or Vacuumized Needle and Holder System: Place the patient in a comfortable position either sitting or lying down. Assess whether the patient has allergies to the disinfectant or to latex if latex gloves or tourniquet will be used in the collection procedure. Use gloved hands to select the collection site as described in the site selection section. Locate the vein visually, then by palpation using the index finger. The thumb should not be used because it has a pulse beat and may cause confusion in site selection or differentiating a vein from an artery. Select the appropriate collection materials (needle size, butterfly, syringe, collection container size) based on the vein size, vein depth, appearance of the collection site, patient's age, and anticipated level of cooperation. Cleanse the skin with the appropriate disinfectant and dry the area. Select the appropriate collection tubes. If blood cultures are to be collected, disinfect the top of the collection containers as directed by the testing laboratory. Be sure to have extra tubes within easy reach in case the vacuum in a collection tube is lost and a substitute is required. Apply the tourniquet 3 to 4 inches above the selected collection site. Remove the sterile needle cap, and inspect the tip of the needle for defects. Pull the skin tightly by placing the thumb of the nondominant hand 1 or 2 inches below the puncture site and moving the thumb in the opposite direction. The thumb is placed below the puncture site to help avoid an accidental needle stick if the patient should suddenly move. Ensure that the needle is bevel up and held at an angle of approximately 15° to 30° (depending on the depth of the vein) (Fig. A–5).

Figure Appendix A–5

Puncture the skin with smooth, firm motion using a sterile needle held by the dominant hand. A reduction in pressure is achieved when the needle has penetrated the vein
successfully. Be sure to release the tourniquet within 1 minute of application. Fill the
vacuumized collection containers in the prescribed order of draw for the studies
ordered. Tubes with anticoagulants can be gently mixed with the free nondominant
hand as they are filled. When the required containers have been filled, withdraw the
needle and apply pressure to the collection site until the bleeding stops. In most cases,
a piece of gauze can be placed on the collection site and the arm bent upward to hold
it in place while attention is given to disposing of the sharps safely and labeling the
collection tubes properly. In cases in which a syringe is used, the barrel of the syringe
should be gently pulled back during specimen collection and gently pushed in during
the transfer to collection tubes. The vacuum in the collection container should not be
allowed to suck the sample into the container, but rather the speed of entry should be
controlled by the pressure applied to the barrel. The blood should gently roll down the
side of the tube to prevent hemolysis.

Radial Artery Puncture: Place the patient in a comfortable position either sitting or
lying down. Assess whether the patient has allergies to the disinfectant or to latex if
latex gloves or tourniquet will be used in the collection procedure. Assess if the patient
has an allergy to local anesthetics, and inform the health care practitioner accordingly.
Glove the hands, and select the collection site as described in the site selection section.
Ensure that the patient has adequate collateral circulation to the hand if thrombosis of
the radial artery occurs after arterial puncture by performing an Allen test before puncture. The Allen test is performed by occlusion of the ulnar and radial arteries on the
palmar surface of the wrist with two fingers. The thumb should not be used to locate
these arteries because it has a pulse. Compress both arteries, and ask the patient to
open and close the fist several times until the palm turns pale. Release pressure only on
the ulnar artery. Color should return to the palm within 5 seconds if the ulnar artery
is functioning. If coloring returns above the wrist, the Allen test is positive. The Allen
test also should be performed on the opposite hand. The wrist to which color is
restored fastest has better circulation and should be selected as the site for blood gas
collection. Be sure to explain to the patient that an arterial puncture is painful. The
site may be anesthetized with 1% to 2% lidocaine (Xylocaine) before puncture. The
index finger of the nondominant hand is placed over the site where the needle will
enter the artery, not the site where the needle will penetrate the skin. The specimen is
collected in an air-free heparinized syringe, which is held like a dart in the dominant
hand and inserted slowly, bevel up, about 5 to 10 mm below the palpating finger at a
45° to 60° angle. When blood enters the needle hub, arterial pressure should cause
blood to pump into the syringe. When enough specimen has been collected, the needle
is withdrawn from the arm, and pressure is applied to the collection site for a mini-

mum of 5 to 10 minutes. Immediately after the needle has been withdrawn safely from the arm, the exposed end of the syringe should be stoppered.

Samples should be gently and well mixed to ensure proper mixing of the heparin with the sample. The heparin prevents formation of small clots that result in rejection of the sample. The tightly capped sample should be placed in an ice slurry immediately after collection. Information on the specimen label can be protected from water in the ice slurry if the specimen is first placed in a protective plastic bag.

Indwelling Devices: Indwelling devices are either heparinized or irrigated after specimen collection. Before specimen collection, prepare the heparin in a syringe, if required. Allow the heparin (unit dose or prepared solution in the syringe) to equilibrate at room temperature during specimen collection. Cleanse the catheter cap or hub with povidone-iodine and 70% alcohol over 2 minutes. Using sterile gloves, remove the cap and attach a 5- or 10-mL syringe to the connector. Withdraw 5 mL of blood to be discarded. Clamp the catheter. The Groshong catheter does not require clamping because it has a special valve that eliminates the need for clamping. Attach another 5- or 10-mL syringe and begin collecting blood for transfer to the collection tubes. After the required specimen has been withdrawn, the device is heparinized. The device is heparinized by slowly injecting the heparin into the cap or hub of the device. Clamp the device 2 inches from the cap, remove the needle, and unclamp the device. Attach a new sterile cap or hub if the old one has been discarded. Groshong catheters are irrigated rather than heparinized. Irrigation of a Groshong catheter is accomplished by gently injecting 20 to 30 mL of sterile normal saline through the cap with moderate force. Remove the needle using some positive pressure (pressing down on the plunger) to prevent the solution from backing up into the syringe.

Order of Draw

- Blood culture and other tests requiring sterile specimen
- Red or red/gray (gel)
- Light blue (citrated) (If this is the only tube to be collected, draw a 5-mL red-top tube specimen first and discard the red-top tube. This is done to eliminate contamination of the specimen with tissue thromboplastin.)
- Green (heparin)
- Lavender (EDTA)
- Gray (oxalate/fluoride)

Urine Specimens

The patient should be informed that improper collection, storage, and transport are the primary reasons for specimen rejection and subsequent requests for recollection. If the specimen is to be collected at home, it should be collected in a clean plastic container (preferably a container from the testing laboratory). Many studies require refrigeration after collection. If the collection container includes a preservative, the patient should be made aware of the contents and advised as to what the precaution labels mean (caution labels such as caustic, corrosive, acid, and base should be affixed to the container as appropriate). When a preservative or fixative is included in the container, the patient should be advised not to remove it. The patient also should be told not to void directly into the container. The patient should be given a collection device, if indicated, and instructed to void into the collection device. The specimen should be carefully transferred into the collection container. Some laboratories provide preprinted collection instructions tailored to their methods. The specimen should be transported promptly to the laboratory after collection.

Wear gloves and any other additional personal protective equipment indicated by the patient's condition. See Appendix F for a more detailed description of standard precautions.

Random: These samples are mainly used for routine screening and can be collected at any time of the day. The patient should be instructed to void either directly into the collection container (if there is no preservative) or into a collection device for transfer into the specimen container.

First Morning: Urine on rising in the morning is very concentrated. These specimens are indicated when screening for substances that may not be detectable in a more dilute random sample. These specimens are also necessary for testing conditions such as orthostatic proteinuria, in which levels vary with changes in posture.

Second Voided: In some cases, it is desirable to test freshly produced urine to evaluate the patient's current status, as with glucose and ketones. Explain to the patient that he or she should first void and then drink a glass of water. The patient should be instructed to wait 30 minutes and then void either directly into the collection container or into a collection device for transfer into the collection container.

Clean Catch: These midstream specimens are generally used for microbiologic or cytologic studies. They also may be requested for routine urinalysis to provide a specimen that is least contaminated with urethral cells, microorganisms, mucus, or other substances that may affect the interpretation of results. Instruct the male patient first to wash hands thoroughly, then cleanse the meatus, void a small amount into the toilet, and void either directly into the specimen container or into a collection device for transfer into the specimen container. Instruct the female patient first to wash hands thoroughly, and then to cleanse the labia from front to back. While keeping the labia separated, the patient should void a small amount into the toilet, and then without interrupting the urine stream, void either directly into the specimen container or into a collection device for transfer into the specimen container.

Catheterized Random or Clean Catch: "Straight catheterization" is indicated when the patient is unable to void, when the patient is unable to prepare properly for clean-catch specimen collection, or when the patient has an indwelling catheter in place and from which a urine sample may be obtained. Before collecting a specimen from the catheter, observe the drainage tube to ensure that it is empty, and then clamp the tube distal to the collection port 15 minutes before specimen collection. Cleanse the port with an antiseptic swab such as 70% alcohol and allow the port to dry. Use a needle and syringe (sterile if indicated) to withdraw the required amount of specimen. Unclamp the tube.

Timed: To quantify substances in urine, 24-hour urine collections are used. They are also used to measure substances whose level of excretion varies over time. The use of preservatives and the handling of specimens during the timed collection may be subject to variability among laboratories. The testing laboratory should be consulted regarding specific instructions before starting the test. Many times the specimen must be refrigerated or kept on ice throughout the entire collection period. Explain to the patient that it is crucial for *all* urine to be included in the collection. The test should begin between 6 and 8 a.m., if possible. Instruct the patient to collect the first void of the day and discard it. The start time of the collection period begins at the time the first voided specimen was discarded and should be recorded along with the date on the collection container. The patient should be instructed to void at the same time the following morning and to add this last voiding to the container. This is the end time of the collection and should be recorded along with the date on the container. For patients who are in the hospital, the urinary output should be compared with the volume measured in the completed collection container. Discrepancies between the two volumes indicate that a collection might have been discarded. Many times a creatinine level is requested along with the study of interest to evaluate the completeness of the collection.

Catheterized Timed: Instructions for this type of collection are basically the same as those for timed specimen collection. The test should begin by changing the tubing and drainage bag. If a preservative is required, it can be placed directly in the drainage bag, or the specimen can be removed at frequent intervals (every 2 hours) and transferred to the collection container to which the preservative has been added. The drainage bag must be kept on ice or emptied periodically into the collection container during the entire collection period if indicated by the testing laboratory. The tubing should be monitored throughout the collection period to ensure continued drainage.

Suprapubic Aspiration: This procedure is performed by inserting a needle directly into the bladder. Because the bladder is normally sterile, the urine collected should also be free from any contamination caused by the presence of microorganisms. First the skin in the suprapubic region is cleansed with an antiseptic solution and draped with sterile drapes. A local anesthetic may be administered before insertion of the needle. After the sample has been collected, a sterile dressing is applied to the site. The site must be observed for signs of inflammation or infection.

Pediatric: Specimen collection can be achieved by any of the above-described methods using collection devices specifically designed for pediatric patients. Appropriately cleanse the genital area and allow the area to dry. For a random collection, remove the covering of the adhesive strips on the collector bag and apply over the genital area. Diaper the child. When the specimen is obtained, place the entire collection bag in the specimen container (use a sterile container as appropriate for the requested study). Some laboratories may have specific preferences for the submission of urine specimens for culture. Consult the laboratory before collection to avoid specimen rejection.

Body Fluid, Stool, and Tissue

Wear gloves and any other additional personal protective equipment indicated by the patient's condition. See Appendix F for a more detailed description of standard precautions. Assess whether the patient has allergies to the disinfectant, anesthetic, or to latex if latex gloves will be used in the procedure.

Specific collection techniques vary by site, study required, and level of invasiveness. These techniques are described in the individual monographs.

Diagnostic Testing

Wear gloves and any other additional personal protective equipment indicated by the patient's condition. See Appendix F for a more detailed description of standard precautions. Assess whether the patient has allergies to the disinfectant, anesthetic, contrast material, medications, or to latex if latex gloves, catheter, or tourniquet will be used in the procedure.

Organ/Disease Panels (with CPT Codes)

Acute Hepatitis Panel 80074 (serum in 5-mL red- or tiger-top tube):

> Hepatitis A antibody, IgA 86709
> Hepatitis B core antibody, IgM 86705
> Hepatitis B surface antigen 87340
> Hepatitis C antibody 86803

Arthritis Panel 80072 (serum in 3- or 5-mL red- or tiger-top tube; whole blood in 5-mL lavender- or gray-top tube):

> Erythrocyte sedimentation rate, nonautomated 85651
> Rheumatoid factor, qualitative 86430
> Screen for noninfectious agent, each antibody (such as antinuclear antibody or antistreptolysin O antibody) 86255
> Uric acid 84550

Basic Metabolic Panel 80048 (serum in 3- or 5-mL red- or tiger-top tube or plasma in 3- or 5-mL green-top tube):

> Calcium 82310
> Carbon dioxide 82374
> Chloride 82435
> Creatinine 82565
> Glucose 82947
> Potassium 84132
> Sodium 84295
> Urea nitrogen 84520

Comprehensive Metabolic Panel 80053 (serum in 3- or 5-mL red- or tiger-top tube or plasma in 3- or 5-mL green-top tube):

> Albumin 82040
> Aminotransferase, alanine (ALT) 84460
> Aminotransferase, aspartate (AST) 84450
> Bilirubin, total 82247
> Calcium 82310
> Carbon dioxide 82374
> Chloride 82435
> Creatinine 82565
> Glucose 82947
> Phosphatase, alkaline 84075
> Potassium 84132
> Protein, total 84155
> Sodium 84295
> Urea nitrogen 84520

Electrolyte Panel 80051 (serum in 3- or 5-mL red- or tiger-top tube or plasma in 3- or 5-mL green-top tube):

> Carbon dioxide 82374
> Chloride 82435
> Potassium 84132
> Sodium 84295

General Health Panel 80050 (serum in 3- or 5-mL red- or tiger-top tube or plasma in 3- or 5-mL green-top tube; whole blood in 3- or 5-mL lavender-top tube):

Comprehensive metabolic panel
80053
Hemogram, and platelet count,
automated, and automated
complete WBC differential 85025
Hemogram, automated and manual
WBC 85022; or
Thyroid-stimulating hormone 84443

Hepatic Function Panel 80076 (serum
in 3- or 5-mL red- or tiger-top tube or
plasma in 3- or 5-mL green-top tube):

Albumin 82040
Aminotransferase, alanine (ALT)
84460
Aminotransferase, aspartate (AST)
84450
Bilirubin, direct 82248
Bilirubin, total 82247
Phosphatase, alkaline 84075
Protein, total 84155

Lipid Panel 80061 (serum in 5-mL red-
or tiger-top tube):

Cholesterol, HDL 83718
Cholesterol, total 82465
Triglycerides 84478

Obstetric Panel 80055 (serum in 5-mL
red- or tiger-top tube for serology;
whole blood in 3- or 5-mL lavender-top
tube for hemogram; serum in 5-mL red-
top tube for blood bank; whole blood in
5-mL lavender-top tube for blood
bank):

Antibody, rubella 86762
Antibody screen, RBC 86850
Blood type, ABO 86900; and
Blood typing, Rh 86901
Hemogram, automated and manual
WBC 85022; or
Hemogram, and platelet count,
automated, and automated
complete WBC differential 85025
Hepatitis B surface antigen 87340
Syphilis test, qualitative 86592

Renal Function Panel 80069 (serum
in 3- or 5-mL red- or tiger-top tube
or plasma in 3- or 5-mL green-top
tube):

Albumin 82040
Calcium 82310
Carbon dioxide 82374
Chloride 82435
Creatinine 82565
Glucose 82947
Phosphorus, inorganic 84100
Potassium 84132
Sodium 84295
Urea nitrogen 84520

TORCH Antibody Panel 80090 (serum
in 5-mL red- or tiger-top tube):

Antibody, CMV 86644
Antibody, herpes simplex 86694
Antibody, rubella 86762
Antibody, *Toxoplasma* 86777

Potential Nursing Diagnoses Associated with Laboratory and Diagnostic Testing

Pretest Phase

Anxiety related to undiagnosed health problems

Anxiety related to perceived threat to health status

Anxiety and fear related to anticipated diagnostic results

Anxiety and fear related to perception of diagnostic procedure as frightening or embarrassing

Powerlessness related to unfamiliar procedure, equipment, environment, or personnel

Knowledge deficit related to lack of information or possible misinterpretation of information provided about the procedure

Knowledge deficit related to legal implications of testing

Potential for noncompliance with test protocols related to inability to understand or follow instructions

Potential for noncompliance to test protocols related to presence of high anxiety, confusion, or denial

Potential for noncompliance to test protocols related to lack of knowledge or appropriate instruction

Potential for noncompliance to test protocols related to confusion, weakness, and other individual factors

Intratest Phase

Risk for injury related to developmental age, psychological factors, and test procedures

Risk for infection or allergic reaction related to altered immune function, history of chronic illness, allergens, or infectious agent

Risk for latex allergy response associated with test equipment

Pain, nausea, vomiting, or diarrhea related to laboratory and diagnostic procedures

Injury, actual or risk for, related to invasive procedure associated with laboratory or diagnostic testing

Risk for infection related to invasive procedures

Risk for bleeding associated with altered bleeding tendencies related to invasive procedures

Fatigue related to diagnostic procedure

Anxiety and fear related to arterial puncture or venipuncture

Risk for injury, bleeding, hematoma, or infection related to arterial puncture or venipuncture

Pain related to arterial puncture or venipuncture

Risk for impaired skin integrity

Potential impairment of gas exchange associated with test procedure

Post-Test Phase

Knowledge deficit related to significance of test results and potential need for further testing

Knowledge deficit related to test outcome deviation that may necessitate medication or lifestyle alterations

Anxiety and fear related to test outcome deviation that may necessitate medication or lifestyle alterations

Ineffective coping related to test outcome and potential for other interventional techniques or procedures

Anticipatory grieving related to test outcomes

Anticipatory or actual grieving related to perceived loss of health or threat of death associated with diagnostic outcomes

Decisional conflict related to test outcome and potential for interventional procedures

Potential alteration in tissue perfusion: cerebral, cardiopulmonary, or peripheral

Knowledge deficit related to care after procedure

Guidelines for Age-Specific Communication

Effective communication between the health care giver and patient is influenced by the patient's cognitive abilities, sensory development or deprivation, level of stress, and environment. Effective communication with individuals at any stage of life is possible if one recognizes that it is essential to employ age-specific communication techniques based on an understanding of the continuum of human development as highlighted here.

Infants (Birth to 1 year)

Physical

Rapid gains in height and weight
Gradual shift from reflexive movements
   to intentional actions

Motor and Sensory

Responds to light and sound
Progresses to raising and turning head,
   bringing hand to mouth, rolling over,
   sitting upright, and standing

Cognitive

Learns by imitation
Progresses to recognize familiar objects
   and people
Advances to speaking three or four words

Psychosocial

Significant persons are parents or
   primary caregivers
Develops sense of trust and security if
   needs are met

May show fear of strangers
May exhibit separation anxiety

Interventions

Keep a parent or primary caregiver in
   view
Involve significant persons in care if
   appropriate
Provide consistency in health care staff
   to limit the number of strangers
Face the infant when providing care
Use soothing nonverbal communication,
   such as holding, rocking, and
   cuddling
Assess immunizations
Maintain safety and keep crib side rails
   up at all times

Toddler (1 to 4 years)

Physical

Learning bladder and bowel control
Temporary teeth erupt
Physiologic systems mature

Motor and Sensory

Developing a higher level of manual dexterity (builds towers with blocks)

Progresses to walking, jumping, and climbing

Loves to experiment

Cognitive

Has a short attention span

Understands simple directions and requests

Psychosocial

Significant persons are parents

Asserts independence

Understands ownership

Attached to security objects

Knows own gender

Plays simple games

Interventions

Face the toddler during interactions

Give one direction at a time

Tie words to action (toddlers learn by example)

Use firm, direct approach; avoid harsh/excited words or actions

Use distraction techniques

Use soothing nonverbal communication, such as rocking, cuddling, and holding

Communicate through play (dolls, puppets, music)

Prepare shortly before a procedure

Allow choices when possible

Encourage mother or parent to stay with the child as appropriate

Encourage parents to participate in care as appropriate

Maintain safety and keep crib side rails up at all times

Child (5 to 12 years)

Physical

Growth is slow and regular

Permanent teeth erupt

Pubescent changes start

May experience growing pains

May experience fatigue

Motor and Sensory

Skips and hops

Dresses and undresses independently

Throws and catches a ball

Uses common utensils and tools

Draws, paints, and likes quiet as well as active games

Cognitive

Major cognitive skill is communication

Understands numbers and can count

Constructs sentences and asks questions

Capable of logical thinking and can reason

Takes pride in accomplishments

Develops increased attention span

Psychosocial

Significant persons are parents, siblings, peers, teachers (prefers friends to family)

Increases independence and begins to assert self (may be physically aggressive)

Masters new tasks and acquires new skills

Behavior can be modified by rewards and punishment

Works hard to be successful

Interventions

Clearly define and reinforce behavior limits

Tell jokes and play games with rules
Check for special words used to identify
parents, body parts, or body functions
Explain procedures in advance using
correct terminology
Use dolls or puppets for explanations
when performing procedures
Provide privacy
Involve whenever possible
Allow to have some control
Promote independence
Praise for good behavior
Acknowledge fear, pain, or family
separation

Adolescent (13 to 18 years)

Physical

Growth in skeletal size is rapid
Reproductive system matures
Vital signs approximate those of an adult

Motor and Sensory

Easily fatigued
May need more rest and sleep in early
adolescence
Awkwardness in gross motor activity
Demonstrates improving fine motor
skills

Cognitive

Increased ability to use abstract thought
and logic
Able to handle hypothetical situations
and thoughts
Shows growth in self-esteem but is
challenged by bouts of insecurity
Avoids asking questions for fear of
appearing unintelligent

Psychosocial

Develops sexual identity
Shows interest and confusion with own
development

Develops concern with physical
appearance
Establishes critical need for privacy
Values belonging to peer group
Perceives self as invincible
Identity is threatened by hospitalization

Interventions

Likes to be treated like an adult
Do not talk to others about the patient
in front of him or her
Do not ask questions about drugs, sex,
or use of tobacco in front of parents
Provide information about routines and
therapy
Provide privacy
Supplement information with rationale
Encourage questions
Allow to maintain control
Involve in decision making and care
Allow for expression of fear, such as
bodily injury and loss of control

Adult (19 to 65 years)

Physical

Reaches physical and sexual maturity
Prone to health problems related to an
inability to cope with new
responsibilities
Health care needs related to preventive
medicine
Adjustment to menopause (women) and
sexual dysfunction (men) in middle
adulthood

Motor and Sensory

Skills are fully developed

Cognitive

Focus on time constraints and want to
learn only what is practical for them
May be dual caregivers (i.e., parents and
children)

Psychosocial

Experience emotional stress secondary to mate selection, vocational selection, assuming occupational roles, marriage, childbearing, financial pressure, and independence

Interventions

Involve family in patient's care and education

Explain benefits of adhering to treatment plan

Be honest and supportive

Respect personal values

Provide privacy

Keep a hopeful attitude

Focus on strength/not limitations

Recognize that unknown factors may affect behavior

Encourage patient to ask questions and talk about concerns

Provide information and support to make health care decisions

Geriatric (65 and older)

Physical

Ages gradually and individually

Experiences decreased tolerance to heat/cold

Encounters declining cardiac and renal function

Experiences skeletal changes (bones become more prominent, shrinkage in vertebral discs, stiff joints)

Becomes subject to increased susceptibility to infection, increased susceptibility to high blood pressure

Undergoes skin changes

Motor and Sensory

Experiences decrease in mobility, visual acuity, ability to respond to stimuli, hearing, and motor skills

Cognitive

Experiences decrease in memory, slowing of mental functions, slowness in learning, and drop in performance

Psychosocial

Encounters lifestyle changes secondary to children leaving home, children providing grandchildren, re-establishing a relationship as a couple, and retirement/hobbies

Develops increased concern for health and financial security

Accepts concept of own mortality

Faces decreased authority and autonomy

Experiences depression related to decreased physical, motor, and cognitive abilities

Interventions

Explain instructions well to patient and family

Ask questions to verify understanding

Review important points repeatedly

Keep room clutter-free and call bell within reach

Control room temperature for comfort

Consider additional lighting at night

Watch for signs of drug toxicity

Give respect and provide privacy

Focus on strengths and not limitations

Avoid assuming loss of abilities

Seek information as necessary to deal with impairments

Include patient in conversation/activity to prevent social isolation

Encourage to talk about feelings

Use humor and stay positive

Provide information and support regarding end-of-life decisions

Provide teaching for safety

Provide teaching for medications and test preparations

Effects of Natural Products on Laboratory Values

The use of natural products has increased significantly, but to date, their preparation is unregulated. Their actions can affect normal and abnormal physiologic processes as well as interact with prescription medications. Their presence in the body, alone or in combination with over-the-counter products or prescription medications, may physiologically affect the intended target or cause analytical interference in such a way that the test result is affected. For this reason, it is important to note their use. The herbs listed here are contraindicated or are recommended for use with caution in patients with body system disorders or patients taking medications for these disorders. The requesting health care practitioner and laboratory should be advised if the patient is regularly using these products so that their potential effects can be taken into consideration when reviewing results.

This list is not all-inclusive. Questions regarding the potential benefits and contraindications of natural products should be referred to the appropriate health care practitioner. As a general recommendation, herbs and nutraceuticals are contraindicated during pregnancy and lactation.

Herbs That May Affect Cardiovascular Disorders or Interact with Therapeutics (Including Hypertension and Hypotension)

Adonis
Aloe
Buckthorn
Bromelain
Cascara
Chinese rhubarb
Coleus
Dong quai
Elder
Ephedra
Ergot
Frangula
Garlic
Ginseng
Golden seal
Green tea (with caffeine)
Henbane
Horsetail
Lily of the valley
Ma-huang
Reishi
Senna
Squill
Tylophora
Valerian
Yohimbe bark

Herbs and Nutraceuticals That May Affect Endocrine Disorders or Interact with Therapeutics

Herbs

Bitter melon
Bilberry
Bladderwrack
Blupleurum
Bugleweed
Echinacea
Ephedra
Fenugreek
Garcinia
Garlic
Ginseng
Goat's rue
Green tea (with caffeine)
Guggul
Licorice
Marshmallow
Olive leaf
Psyllium
Tylophora

Minerals

Chromium

Nutraceuticals

Alpha lipoic acid
Dehydroepiandrosterone
p-Aminobenzoic acid
Thyroid extract

Herbs and Nutraceuticals That May Affect Gastrointestinal Disorders or Interact with Therapeutics

Herbs

Bromelain
Cascara
Chinese rhubarb
Dandelion
Psyllium
Senna

Nutraceuticals

Betaine hydrochloride

Herbs and Nutraceuticals That May Affect Genitourinary Disorders or Interact with Therapeutics

Herbs

Aloe
Arabinoxylane
Bladderwrack
Buckthorn
Cascara
Chinese rhubarb
Dandelion
Echinacea
Ephedra
Ergot
Frangula
Ginseng
Guarana
Horse chestnut
Horsetail
Licorice
Parsley oil (high doses)
Saw palmetto
Senna
Stinging nettle
White oak
White willow

Nutraceuticals

Creatine
Modified citrus pectin

Herbs and Nutraceuticals That May Affect Bleeding Disorders or Interact with Therapeutics

Herbs

Arnica
Astragalus
Bilberry
Bromelian
Cat's claw

Cayenne
Coleus
Cordyceps
Devil's claw
Dong quai
Evening primrose
Feverfew
Garlic
Ginger
Gingko
Ginseng
Grape seed
Green tea (with caffeine)
Guggui
Horse chestnut
Papaya
Red clover
Red yeast rice
Reishi
Turmeric
White willow

Nutraceuticals

Docosahexaenoic acid (DHA)
Fish oils (EPA and DHA)

Herbs and Nutraceuticals That May Affect Hepatobiliary Disorders or Interact with Therapeutics

Herbs

Alkanet
Alpine ragwort
Coltsfoot
Comfrey
Dusty miller
Forget-me-not
Germander
Groundsel

Olive leaf
Parsley oil (large doses)
Peppermint
Pennyroyal
Ragwort
Red yeast rice
Sweet clover
White oak
White willow

Nutraceuticals

Creatine

Herbs and Amino Acids That May Affect Immune Disorders or Interact with Therapeutics

Herbs

Astragalus
Black cohosh
Echinacea
Saw palmetto

Amino Acids

Arginine

Herbs That May Affect Respiratory Disorders or Interact with Therapeutics

Artichoke
Cayenne
Chamomile
Cordyceps
Echinacea
Feverfew
Garlic
Peppermint oil
White willow

Standard Precautions (CDC Isolation Precautions)

Background and Summary

In January 1996, the Centers for Disease Control and Prevention (CDC) issued new guidelines for isolation precautions in hospitals. The guidelines, based on the latest epidemiologic information on transmission of infection in hospitals, are intended primarily for use in acute-care hospitals, although some of the recommendations may be applicable to subacute-care or extended-care facilities. The recommendations are not intended for use in day care, well care, or domiciliary care programs.

The revised guidelines contain two tiers of precautions. In the first, and most important, tier are precautions designed for the care of all patients in hospitals regardless of their diagnosis or presumed infection status. Implementation of these Standard Precautions is the primary strategy for successful nosocomial infection control. In the second tier are precautions designed only for the care of specified patients. These additional Transmission-Based Precautions are used for patients who are known or suspected to be infected or colonized with epidemiologically important pathogens that can be transmitted by airborne or droplet transmission or by contact with dry skin or contaminated surfaces.

Standard Precautions synthesize the major features of Universal (Blood and Body Fluid) Precautions (designed to reduce the risk of transmission of blood-borne pathogens) and Body Substance Isolation (designed to reduce the risk of transmission of pathogens from moist body substances). Standard Precautions apply to (1) blood; (2) all body fluids, secretions, and excretions *except sweat,* regardless of whether they contain visible blood; (3) nonintact skin; and (4) mucous membranes. Standard Precautions are designed to reduce the risk of transmission of recognized and unrecognized sources of infection in hospitals.

Transmission-Based Precautions are designed for patients documented or suspected to be infected or colonized with highly transmissible or epidemiologically important pathogens for which additional precautions beyond Standard Precautions are needed to interrupt transmission in hospitals. There are three types of Transmission-Based Precautions: Airborne Precautions, Droplet Precautions, and Contact Precautions. They may be combined for diseases that have multiple routes of transmission. When used either singly or in combination, they are to be used in addition to Standard Precautions.

Airborne Precautions are designed to reduce the risk of airborne transmission of infectious agents. Airborne transmission occurs by dissemination of either airborne droplet nuclei (small-particle residue [5 μm or smaller in size] of evaporated droplets that may remain suspended in the air for long periods) or dust particles containing the infectious agent. Microorganisms carried in this manner can be dispersed widely by air currents and may become inhaled by or deposited on a susceptible host within the same room or over a longer distance from the source patient, depending on environmental factors; special air handling and ventilation are required to prevent airborne transmission. Examples of diseases spread by airborne droplet nuclei include measles, varicella (including disseminated zoster), and tuberculosis.

Droplet Precautions are designed to reduce the risk of droplet transmission of infectious agents. Droplet transmission involves contact of the conjunctivae or the mucous membranes of the nose or mouth of a susceptible person with large-particle droplets (larger than 5 μm in size) containing microorganisms generated from a person who has a clinical disease or who is a carrier of the microorganism. Droplets are generated from the source person primarily during coughing, sneezing, or talking and during the performance of certain procedures such as suctioning and bronchoscopy. Transmission via large-particle droplets requires close contact between source and recipient persons because droplets do not remain suspended in the air and generally travel only short distances, usually 3 ft or less, through the air. Because droplets do not remain suspended in the air, special air handling and ventilation are not required to prevent droplet transmission. Examples of illnesses spread by large-particle droplets include invasive *Haemophilus influenzae* type B disease (including meningitis, pneumonia, epiglottitis, and sepsis); invasive *Neisseria meningitidis* disease (including meningitis, pneumonia, and sepsis); diphtheria (pharyngeal); mycoplasmal pneumonia; pertussis; pneumonic plague; streptococcal pharyngitis, pneumonia, or scarlet fever in infants and young children; adenovirus influenza; mumps; parvovirus B19; and rubella.

Contact Precautions are designed to reduce the risk of transmission of epidemiologically important microorganisms by direct or indirect contact. Direct-contact transmission involves skin-to-skin contact and physical transfer of microorganisms to a susceptible host from an infected or colonized person, such as occurs when personnel turn patients, bathe patients, or perform other patient care activities that require physical contact. Direct-contact transmission also can occur between two patients (e.g., by hand contact), with one serving as the source of infectious microorganisms and the other as a susceptible host. Indirect-contact transmission involves contact of a susceptible host with a contaminated intermediate object, usually inanimate, in the patient's environment. Examples of illnesses spread by direct contact include gastrointestinal, respiratory, skin, or wound infections or colonization with multidrug-resistant bacteria judged by the infection control program (based on current state, regional, or national recommendations) to be of special clinical and epidemiologic significance; enteric infections with a low infectious dose or prolonged environmental survival, including *Clostridium difficile*; for diapered or incontinent patients, enterohemorrhagic *Escherichia coli* O157:H7, *Shigella*, hepatitis A, or rotavirus; respiratory syncytial virus, parainfluenza virus, or enteroviral infections in infants and young children; viral/hemorrhagic conjunctivitis; viral hemorrhagic infections (Ebola, Lassa, or Marburg); and skin infections that are highly contagious or that may occur on dry skin, including:

- Diphtheria (cutaneous)
- Herpes simplex virus (neonatal or mucocutaneous)
- Impetigo
- Major (noncontained) abscesses, cellulitis, or decubiti
- Pediculosis

- Scabies
- Staphylococcal furunculosis in infants and young children
- Zoster (disseminated or in the immunocompromised host)

Standard Precautions

Use the following Standard Precautions, or the equivalent, for the care of all patients.

Hand Washing

Wash hands after touching blood, body fluids, secretions, excretions, and contaminated items, whether or not gloves are worn. Wash hands immediately after gloves are removed, between patient contacts, and when otherwise indicated to avoid transfer of microorganisms to other patients or environments. It may be necessary to wash hands between tasks and procedures on the same patient to prevent cross-contamination of different body sites.

Use a plain (nonantimicrobial) soap for routine hand washing.

Use an antimicrobial agent or a waterless antiseptic agent for specific circumstances (e.g., control of outbreaks or hyperendemic infections), as defined by the infection control program. (See Contact Precautions for additional recommendations on using antimicrobial and antiseptic agents.)

Gloves

Wear gloves (clean, nonsterile gloves are adequate) when touching blood, body fluids, secretions, excretions, and contaminated items.

Put on clean gloves just before touching mucous membranes and nonintact skin.

Change gloves between tasks and procedures on the same patient after contact with material that may contain a high concentration of microorganisms.

Remove gloves promptly after use, before touching noncontaminated items and environmental surfaces, and before going to another patient. Wash hands immediately to avoid transfer of microorganisms to other patients or environments.

Mask, Eye Protection, Face Shield

Wear a mask and eye protection or a face shield to protect mucous membranes of the eyes, nose, and mouth during procedures and patient care activities that are likely to generate splashes or sprays of blood, body fluids, secretions, and excretions.

Gown

Wear a gown (a clean, nonsterile gown is adequate) to protect skin and to prevent soiling of clothing during procedures and patient care activities that are likely to generate splashes or sprays of blood, body fluids, secretions, or excretions.

Select a gown that is appropriate for the activity and amount of fluid likely to be encountered.

Remove a soiled gown as promptly as possible. Wash hands to avoid transfer of microorganisms to other patients or environments.

Patient Care Equipment

Handle used patient care equipment soiled with blood, body fluids, secretions, and excretions in a manner that prevents skin and mucous membrane exposures, contamination of clothing, and transfer of microorganisms to other patients and environments.

Ensure that reusable equipment is not used for the care of another patient until it has been cleaned and reprocessed appropriately. Ensure that single-use items are discarded properly.

Environmental Control

Ensure that the hospital has adequate procedures for the routine care, cleaning, and disinfection of environmental surfaces, beds, bedrails, bedside equipment, and other frequently touched surfaces, and ensure that these procedures are being followed.

Linen

Handle, transport, and process used linen soiled with blood, body fluids, secretions, and excretions in a manner that prevents skin and mucous membrane exposures and contamination of clothing and that avoids transfer of microorganisms to other patients and environments.

Occupational Health and Blood-Borne Pathogens

Take care to prevent injuries when using needles, scalpels, and other sharp instruments or devices; when handling sharp instruments after procedures; when cleaning used instruments; and when disposing of used needles.

Never recap used needles or otherwise manipulate them using both hands or use any other technique that involves directing the point of a needle toward any part of the body; rather, use either a one-handed "scoop" technique or a mechanical device designed for holding the needle sheath.

Do not remove used needles from disposable syringes by hand, and do not bend, break, or otherwise manipulate used needle by hand.

Place used disposable syringes and needles, scalpel blades, and other sharp items in appropriate puncture-resistant containers, which are located as close as practical to the area in which the items were used, and place reusable syringes and needles in a puncture-resistant container for transport to the reprocessing area.

Use mouthpieces, resuscitation bags, or other ventilation devices as an alternative to mouth-to-mouth resuscitation methods in areas where the need for resuscitation is predictable.

Patient Placement

Place a patient who contaminates the environment or who does not (or cannot be expected to) assist in maintaining appropriate hygiene or environmental control in a private room. If a private room is not available, consult with infection control professionals regarding patient placement or other alternatives.

Transmission-Based Precautions

Airborne Precautions

In addition to Standard Precautions, use Airborne Precautions, or the equivalent, for patients known or suspected to be infected with microorganisms transmitted by airborne droplet nuclei (small-particle residue [5 μm or smaller in size] of evaporated droplets containing microorganisms that remain suspended in the air and that can be dispersed widely by air currents within a room or over a long distance).

Patient Placement

Place the patient in a private room that has (1) monitored negative air pressure in
  relation to the surrounding areas, (2) 6 to 12 air changes per hour, and (3)
  appropriate discharge of air outdoors or monitored high-efficiency filtration of
  room air before the air is circulated to other areas in the hospital.
Keep the room door closed and the patient in the room.
When a private room is not available, place the patient in a room with a patient who
  has active infection with the same microorganism unless otherwise recommended,
  but with no other infection. When a private room is not available and cohorting is
  not desirable, consultation with infection control professionals is advised before
  patient placement.

Respiratory Protection

Wear respiratory protection when entering the room of a patient with known or
  suspected infectious pulmonary tuberculosis.
Susceptible persons should not enter the room of patients known or suspected to
  have measles (rubeola) or varicella (chickenpox) if other immune caregivers are
  available. If susceptible persons must enter the room of a patient known or
  suspected to have measles or varicella, they should wear respiratory protection.
  Persons immune to measles or varicella need not wear respiratory protection.

Patient Transport

Limit the movement and transport of the patient from the room to essential
  purposes only. If transport or movement is necessary, minimize patient dispersal of
  droplet nuclei by placing a surgical mask on the patient, if possible.

Additional Precautions for Preventing Transmission of Tuberculosis

Consult CDC "Guidelines for Preventing the Transmission of Tuberculosis in Health-Care Facilities" for additional prevention strategies.[1]

---

[1]Employees who received training in the year preceding the effective date of the standard need only receive training pertaining to any provisions not already included.

Droplet Precautions

In addition to Standard Precautions, use Droplet Precautions, or the equivalent, for a patient known or suspected to be infected with microorganisms transmitted by droplets (large-particle droplets [larger than 5 μm in size] that can be generated during coughing, sneezing, talking, or the performance of procedures).

Patient Placement

Place the patient in a private room. When a private room is not available, place the patient in a room with a patient who has active infection with the same microorganism but with no other infection (cohorting). When a private room is not available and cohorting is not achievable, maintain spatial separation of at least 3 ft between the infected patient and other patients and visitors.
Special air handling and ventilation are not necessary, and the door may remain open.

Mask

In addition to Standard Precautions, wear a mask when working within 3 ft of the patient. (Logistically, some hospitals may want to implement the wearing of a mask to enter the room.)

Patient Transport

Limit the movement and transport of the patient from the room to essential purposes only.
If transport or movement is necessary, minimize patient dispersal of droplets by masking the patient, if possible.

Contact Precautions

In addition to Standard Precautions, use Contact Precautions, or the equivalent, for specified patients known or suspected to be infected or colonized with epidemiologically important microorganisms that can be transmitted by direct contact with the patient (hand or skin-to-skin contact that occurs when performing patient care activities that require touching the patient's dry skin) or indirect contact (touching) with environmental surfaces or patient care items in the patient's environment.

Patient Placement

Place the patient in a private room. When a private room is not available, place the patient in a room with a patient who has active infection with the same microorganism but with no other infection (cohorting).
When a private room is not available and cohorting is not achievable, consider the epidemiology of the microorganism and the patient population when determining patient placement. Consultation with infection control professionals is advised before patient placement.

Gloves and Hand Washing

In addition to wearing gloves as outlined under Standard Precautions, wear gloves (clean, nonsterile gloves are adequate) when entering the room.

During the course of providing care for a patient, change gloves after having contact with infective material that may contain high concentrations of microorganisms (fecal material and wound drainage).

Remove gloves before leaving the patient's environment and wash hands immediately with an antimicrobial agent or a waterless antiseptic agent. After glove removal and hand washing, ensure that hands do not touch potentially contaminated environmental surfaces or items in the patient's room to avoid transfer of microorganisms to other patients or environments.

Gown

In addition to wearing a gown as outlined under Standard Precautions, wear a gown (a clean, nonsterile gown is adequate) when entering the room if you anticipate that your clothing will have substantial contact with the patient, environmental surfaces, or items in the patient's room or if the patient is incontinent or has diarrhea, an ileostomy, a colostomy, or wound drainage not contained by a dressing.

Remove the gown before leaving the patient's environment. After gown removal, ensure that clothing does not contact potentially contaminated environmental surfaces to avoid transfer of microorganisms to other patients or environments.

Patient Transport

Limit the movement and transport of the patient from the room to essential purposes only.

If the patient is transported out of the room, ensure that precautions are maintained to minimize the risk of transmission of microorganisms to other patients and contamination of environmental surfaces or equipment.

Patient Care Equipment

When possible, dedicate the use of noncritical patient care equipment to a single patient (or cohort of patients infected or colonized with the pathogen requiring precautions) to avoid sharing between patients.

If use of common equipment or items is unavoidable, adequately clean and disinfect them before use for another patient.

Additional Precautions for Preventing the Spread of Vancomycin Resistance

Consult the Hospital Infection Control Practices Advisory Committee report on preventing the spread of vancomycin resistance for additional prevention strategies.

OSHA Blood-Borne Pathogens Standard

Who Is Covered?

The Occupational Safety and Health Administration (OSHA) standard protects employees who may be occupationally exposed to blood and other potential infectious materials, which includes but is not limited to physicians, physician's assistants, nurses, nurse practitioners, and other health care employees in clinics and physicians' offices;

employees of clinical and diagnostic laboratories; housekeepers in health care and other facilities; personnel in hospital laundries or commercial laundries that service health care or public safety institutions; tissue bank personnel; employees in blood banks and plasma centers who collect, transport, and test blood; freestanding clinic employees (e.g., hemodialysis clinics, urgent care clinics, health maintenance organization [HMO] clinics, and family planning clinics); employees in clinics in industrial, educational, and correctional facilities (e.g., employees who collect blood and clean and dress wounds); employees designated to provide emergency first aid; dentists, dental hygienists, dental assistants, and dental laboratory technicians; staff of institutions for the developmentally disabled; hospice employees; home health care workers; staff of nursing homes and long-term care facilities; employees of funeral homes and mortuaries; human immunodeficiency virus (HIV) and hepatitis B virus (HBV) research laboratory and production facility workers; employees handling regulated waste; custodial workers required to clean up contaminated sharps or spills of blood or other potentially infectious material (OPIM); medical equipment service and repair personnel; emergency medical technicians, paramedics, and other emergency medical service providers; firefighters, law enforcement personnel, and correctional officers (employees in the private sector, the federal government, or a state or local government in a state that has an OSHA-approved state plan); maintenance workers, such as plumbers, in health care facilities; and employees of substance abuse clinics.

Blood means human blood, blood products, or blood components (plasma, platelets, and serosanguineous fluids [e.g., exudates from wounds]). Also included are medications derived from blood, such as immune globulins, albumin, and factors 8 and 9. Other potentially infectious materials include human body fluids, such as saliva in dental procedures; semen; vaginal secretions; cerebrospinal, synovial, pleural, pericardial, peritoneal, and amniotic fluids; body fluids visibly contaminated with blood; unfixed human tissues or organs; HIV-containing cell or tissue cultures; and HIV-containing or HBV-containing culture media or other solutions.

Occupational exposure means a "reasonably anticipated skin, eye, mucous membrane, or parenteral contact [human bites that break the skin, which are most likely to occur in violent situations such as may be encountered by prison personnel and police and in emergency departments or psychiatric wards] with blood or other potentially infectious materials that may result from the performance of the employee's duties." The term *reasonably anticipated contact* includes the potential for contact and actual contact with blood or OPIM. Lack of history of blood exposures among designated first aid personnel of a particular manufacturing site, for instance, does not preclude coverage. *Reasonably anticipated contact* includes, among others, contact with blood or OPIM, including regulated waste, as well as incidents of needle sticks. A compliance officer may document incidents in which an employee observes uncapped needles or contacts other regulated waste to substantiate occupational exposure.

Federal OSHA authority extends to all private sector employers with one or more employees, as well as federal civilian employees. In addition, many states administer their own occupational safety and health programs through plans approved under section 18(b) of the Occupational Safety and Health Act. These plans must adopt standards and enforce requirements that are at least as effective as federal requirements. Of the current 25 states and territories with plans, 23 cover the private and public (state and local governments) sectors and 2 cover the public sector only.

Determining occupational exposure and instituting control methods and work practices appropriate for specific job assignments are key requirements of the standard. The required written exposure control plan and methods of compliance show how employee exposure can be minimized or eliminated.

Exposure Control Plan

A written exposure control plan is necessary for the safety and health of workers. At a minimum, the plan must include the following:

Identify job classifications in which there is exposure to blood or other potentially infectious materials.

Explain the protective measures currently in effect in the acute-care facility or a schedule and methods of compliance to be implemented, including hepatitis B vaccination and postexposure follow-up procedures, how hazards are communicated to employees, personal protective equipment (PPE), housekeeping, and record keeping.

Establish procedures for evaluating the circumstances of an exposure incident.

The schedule of how and when the provisions of the standard will be implemented may be a simple calendar with brief notations describing the compliance methods, an annotated copy of the standard, or a part of another document, such as the infection control plan. The written exposure control plan must be available to workers and OSHA representatives and updated at least annually or whenever changes in procedures create new occupational exposures.

Who Has Occupational Exposure?

The exposure determination must be based on the definition of occupational exposure without regard to personal protective clothing and equipment. Exposure determination begins by reviewing job classifications of employees within the work environment, and then making a list divided into two groups: classifications in which all of the employees have occupational exposure and classifications in which some of the employees have occupational exposure.

Where all employees are occupationally exposed, it is not necessary to list specific work tasks. Some examples include phlebotomists, laboratory technicians, physicians, nurses, nurse's aides, surgical technicians, and emergency department personnel.

Where only some of the employees have exposure, specific tasks and procedures causing exposure must be listed. Examples include ward clerks or secretaries who occasionally handle blood or infectious specimens and housekeeping staff who may be exposed to contaminated objects or environments some of the time.

When employees with occupational exposure have been identified, the next step is to communicate the hazards of the exposure to the employees.

Communicating Hazards to Employees

The initial training for current employees must be scheduled within 90 days of the effective date of the blood-borne pathogens standard, at no cost to the employee, and during working hours.[1] Training also is required for new workers at the time of their initial assignment to tasks with occupational exposure or when job tasks change, causing occupational exposure, and annually thereafter.

Training sessions must be comprehensive in nature, including information on blood-borne pathogens as well as on OSHA regulations and the employer's exposure control plan. Although HBV and HIV are specifically identified in the standard, the term *blood-borne pathogen* includes any pathogenic microorganism that is present in human blood or other potentially infectious materials and can infect and cause disease in persons who are exposed to blood containing the pathogen. Pathogenic microorganisms also can cause diseases such as hepatitis C, malaria, syphilis, babesiosis, brucellosis, leptospirosis, arboviral infections, relapsing fever, Creutzfeldt-Jakob disease, adult T-cell leukemia/lymphoma (caused by human T-cell leukemia/lymphoma virus [HTLV-I]), HTLV-I-associated myelopathy, diseases associated with HTLV-II, and viral hemorrhagic fever. The person conducting the training must be knowledgeable in the subject matter as it relates to acute care facilities.

Specifically, the training program must do the following:

- Explain the regulatory text and make a copy of the regulatory text accessible.
- Explain the epidemiology and symptoms of blood-borne diseases.
- Explain the modes of transmission of blood-borne pathogens.
- Explain the employer's written exposure control plan.
- Describe the methods to control transmission of HBV and HIV.
- Explain how to recognize occupational exposure.
- Inform workers about the availability of free hepatitis B vaccinations, vaccine efficacy, safety, benefits, and administration.
- Explain the emergency procedures for and reporting of exposure incidents.
- Inform workers of the postexposure evaluation and follow-up available from health care professionals.
- Describe how to select, use, remove, handle, decontaminate, and dispose of personal protective clothing and equipment.
- Explain the use and limitations of safe work practices, engineering controls (controls that isolate or remove the blood-borne pathogens hazard from the workplace; examples include needleless devices, shielded needle devices, blunt needles, plastic capillary tubes), and PPE.
- Explain the use of labels, signs, and color coding required by the standard.
- Provide a question-and-answer session on training.

In addition to communicating hazards to employees and providing training to identify and control hazards, other preventive measures must be taken to ensure employee protection.

Preventive Measures

Preventive measures such as hepatitis B vaccination, universal precautions, engineering controls, safe work practices, PPE, and housekeeping measures help reduce the risks of occupational exposure.

Hepatitis B Vaccination

The hepatitis B vaccination series must be made available within 10 working days of initial assignment to every employee who has occupational exposure. The hepatitis B vaccination must be made available without cost to the employee, at a reasonable time and place for the employee, by a licensed health care professional,[2] and according to recommendations of the U.S. Public Health Service, including routine booster doses.[3] The health care professional designated by the employer to implement this part of the

---

[2]Licensed health care professional is a person whose legally permitted scope of practice allows him or her to perform independently the activities required under paragraph (f) of the standard regarding hepatitis B vaccination and postexposure and follow-up.

[3]Health care professionals can call the CDC disease information hotline (404) 332-4555, extension 234, for updated information on hepatitis B vaccination.

standard must be provided with a copy of the blood-borne pathogens standard. The health care professional must provide the employer with a written opinion stating whether the hepatitis B vaccination is indicated for the employee and whether the employee has received the vaccination.

Employers are not required to offer hepatitis B vaccination (1) to employees who have previously completed the hepatitis B vaccination series, (2) when immunity is confirmed through antibody testing, or (3) if vaccine is contraindicated for medical reasons. Participation in a prescreening program is not a prerequisite for receiving hepatitis B vaccination. Employees who decline the vaccination may request and obtain it at a later date, if they continue to be exposed. Employees who decline to accept the hepatitis B vaccination must sign a declination form, indicating that they were offered the vaccination but refused it. For more information, refer to "Immunization of Health-Care Workers: Recommendations of ACIP and HICPAC," *Morbidity and Mortality Weekly Report,* vol 46, no. RR-18, 1997.

Universal Precautions

The most important measure to control transmission of HBV and HIV is to treat all human blood and other potentially infectious materials *as if they were* infectious for HBV and HIV. (Coverage under this definition also extends to blood and tissues of experimental animals who are infected with HIV or HBV.) Application of this approach is referred to as *universal precautions. Blood and certain body fluids from all acute-care patients should be considered as potentially infectious materials.*[4] These fluids cause *contamination,* defined in the standard as "the presence or the reasonably anticipated presence of blood or other potentially infectious materials on an item or surface."

Alternative concepts in infection control are called *Body Substance Isolation and Standard Precautions.* These methods define all body fluids and substances as infectious. These methods incorporate not only the fluids and materials covered by this standard, but also expand coverage to include all body fluids and substances. These concepts are acceptable alternatives to universal precautions, provided that facilities using them adhere to all other provisions of this standard.

Methods of Control

Engineering and Work Practice Controls

Engineering and work practice controls are the primary methods used to control the transmission of HBV and HIV in acute-care facilities. Engineering controls isolate or remove the hazard from employees and are used in conjunction with work practices. Personal protective equipment also is used when occupational exposure to blood-borne pathogens remains even after instituting these controls. Engineering controls must be examined and maintained, or replaced, on a scheduled basis. Some engineering controls that apply to acute-care facilities and are required by the standard include the following:

- Use puncture-resistant, leak-proof containers, color-coded red or labeled, according to the standard (see table) to discard contaminated items such as needles, broken glass, scalpels, or other items that could cause a cut or puncture wound.

---

[4]See also "Recommendations for Prevention of HIV Transmission in Health-Care Settings," *Morbidity and Mortality Weekly Report,* vol 36(2S), August 21, 1987.

- Use puncture-resistant, leak-proof containers, color-coded red or labeled to store contaminated reusable sharps until they are properly reprocessed.
- Store and process reusable contaminated sharps in a way that ensures safe handling. Use a mechanical device to retrieve used instruments from soaking pans in decontamination areas.
- Use puncture-resistant, leak-proof containers to collect, handle, process, store, transport, or ship blood specimens and potentially infectious materials. Label these specimens if shipped outside the facility. Labeling is not required when specimens are handled by employees trained to use universal precautions with all specimens and when these specimens are kept within the facility.

Labeling Requirements

Item	No Label Needed If Universal Precautions Are Used and Specific Use of Container Is Known to All Employees	Biohazard Label	Red Container
Regulated waste container (e.g., contaminated sharps container)		X or	X
Reusable contaminated sharps container (e.g., surgical instruments soaking in a tray)		X or	X
Refrigerator/freezer holding blood or other potentially infectious material		X	
Containers used for storage, transport, or shipping of blood		X or	X
Blood/blood-borne products for clinical use	X		
Individual specimen containers of blood or other potentially infectious materials remaining in facility	X or	X or	X

(Continued on the following page)

Item	No Label Needed If Universal Precautions Are Used and Specific Use of Container Is Known to All Employees	Biohazard Label	Red Container
Contaminated equipment needing service (e.g., dialysis equipment, suction apparatus)		X Plus a label specifying where the contamination exists	
Specimens and regulated waste shipped from the primary facility to another facility for service or disposal		X or	X
Contaminated laundry	* or	X or	X
Contaminated laundry sent to another facility that does not use universal precautions		X or	X

* Alternative labeling or color coding is sufficient if it permits all employees to recognize containers as requiring compliance with universal precautions.

Similarly, work practice controls reduce the likelihood of exposure by altering the manner in which the task is performed. All procedures minimize splashing, spraying, splattering, and generation of droplets. Work practice requirements include the following:

- Wash hands when gloves are removed and as soon as possible after contact with blood or other potentially infectious materials.
- Provide and make available a mechanism for immediate eye irrigation, in the event of an exposure incident.
- Do not bend, recap, or remove contaminated needles unless required to do so by specific medical procedures or the employer can show that no alternative is feasible. In these instances, use mechanical means, such as forceps or a one-handed technique, to recap or remove contaminated needles.
- Do not shear or break contaminated needles.
- Discard contaminated needles and sharp instruments in puncture-resistant,

leak-proof, red or biohazard-labeled containers[5] that are accessible, maintained upright, and not allowed to be overfilled.
- Do not eat, drink, smoke, apply cosmetics, or handle contact lenses in areas of potential occupational exposure. (*Note:* Use of hand lotions is acceptable.)
- Do not store food or drink in refrigerators or on shelves where blood or potentially infectious materials are present.
- Use red, or affix biohazard labels to, containers to store, transport, or ship blood or other potentially infectious materials, such as laboratory specimens (Fig. A–6).
- Do not use mouth pipetting to suction blood or other potentially infectious materials; it is prohibited.

FIGURE Appendix F–1

Additional Information on Engineering Controls

Effective Engineering Controls ECRI: Contact:
   www.healthcare.ecri.org/site/whatsnew/press.releases/980724hdneedle.html. ECRI (formerly Emergency Care Research Institute), designated as an evidence-based practice center by the Agency for Healthcare Research and Quality, is a nonprofit international health services research organization. This web site discusses the June 1998 issue of ECRI's *Health Devices,* which evaluated 19 needle stick–prevention devices, and provides information on how to obtain this document.
Food and Drug Administration (FDA) Safety Alert: Needlestick and other risks from hypodermic needles on secondary IV administration sets—piggyback and intermittent IV. Contact: www.fda.gov/cdrh/safety.html. Warns of the risk of needlestick injuries from the use of hypodermic needles as a connection between two pieces of intravenous (IV) equipment. Describes characteristics of devices that have the potential to decrease the risk of needle stick injuries.
International Health Care Worker Safety Center, University of Virginia: Contact:
   www.people.virginia.edu/epinet/products.html. Features a list of safety devices with manufacturers and specific product names.

---

[5]Biohazard labeling requires a fluorescent orange or orange-red label with the biologic hazard symbol as well as the word *Biohazard* in contrasting color affixed to the bag or container.

National Institute for Occupational Safety and Health (NIOSH): Sharps disposal
containers. Contact: www.cdc.gov/niosh/sharps1.html. Features information on
selecting, evaluating, and using sharps disposal containers.

Occupational Safety and Health Administration (OSHA): Glass capillary tubes: Joint
Safety Advisory about potential risks. Contact:
www.oshaslc.gov/OshDoc/Interpdata/I19990222.html. Describes safer alternatives
to conventional glass capillary tubes.

Occupational Safety and Health Administration (OSHA): Needlestick injuries.
Contact: www.osha-slc.gov/SLTC/needlestick/index.html. Features recent news,
recognition, evaluation, controls, compliance, and links to information on
effective engineering controls.

Safety Sharp Device Contract: Contact: www.va.gov/vasafety/osh-
issues/needlesafety/safetysharpcontracts.htm. Features safety sharp devices on
contract with the U.S. Department of Veterans Affairs (VA).

SHARPS Injury Control Program: Contact: www.ohb.org/sharps.htm. Established
by Senate Bill 2005 to study sharps injuries in hospitals, skilled nursing facilities,
and home health agencies in California. Features a beta version of Safety
Enhanced Device Database Listing by Manufacturer.

Training for Development of Innovative Control Technologies (TDICT) Project:
Contact: www.tdict.org/criteria.html. Features safety feature evaluation forms for
specific devices.

Personal Protective Equipment

In addition to instituting engineering and work practice controls, the standard requires
that appropriate PPE be used to reduce worker risk of exposure. Personal protective
equipment is specialized clothing or equipment used by employees to protect against
direct exposure to blood or other potentially infectious materials. Protective equipment must not allow blood or other potentially infectious materials to pass through to
workers' clothing, skin, or mucous membranes. This equipment includes, but is not
limited to, gloves, gowns, laboratory coats, face shields or masks, eye protection, and
resuscitator devices. Hypoallergenic gloves, glove liners, powderless gloves, or other
similar alternatives must be readily available and accessible at no cost to employees who
are allergic to the gloves normally provided.

The employer is responsible for providing, maintaining, laundering, disposing,
replacing, and ensuring the proper use of PPE. The employer is responsible for ensuring that workers have access to the protective equipment, at no cost, including proper
sizes and types that take allergic conditions into consideration.

An employee may temporarily and briefly decline to wear PPE under rare and
extraordinary circumstances and when, in the employee's professional judgment, it
prevents the delivery of health care or public safety services or poses an increased or
life-threatening hazard to employees. In general, appropriate PPE is expected to be
used whenever occupational exposure may occur.

The employer also must ensure that employees observe the following precautions
for safely handling and using PPE:

- Remove all PPE immediately after contamination and on leaving the work area
  and place in an appropriately designated area or container for storing, washing,
  decontaminating, or discarding.

- Wear appropriate gloves when contact with blood, mucous membranes, non-intact skin (e.g., skin with dermatitis, hangnails, cuts, abrasions, chafing, acne), or potentially infectious materials is anticipated; when performing vascular access procedures[6]; and when handling or touching contaminated items or surfaces.
- Provide hypoallergenic gloves, liners, or powderless gloves or other alternatives to employees who need them.
- Replace disposable, single-use gloves as soon as possible when contaminated or if torn, punctured, or barrier function is compromised.
- Do not reuse disposable (single-use) gloves.
- Decontaminate reusable (utility) gloves after each use and discard if they show signs of cracking, peeling, tearing, puncturing, deteriorating, or failing to provide a protective barrier.
- Use full face shields or face masks with eye protection, goggles, or eyeglasses with side shields when splashes of blood and other bodily fluids may occur and when contamination of the eyes, nose, or mouth can be anticipated (e.g., during invasive and surgical procedures).
- Also wear surgical caps or hoods and shoe covers or boots when gross contamination may occur, such as during surgery and autopsy procedures.

Remember: The selection of appropriate PPE depends on the quantity and type of exposure expected.

Housekeeping Procedures

Equipment

The employer must ensure a clean and sanitary workplace. Contaminated work surfaces must be decontaminated with a disinfectant on completion of procedures; when contaminated by splashes, spills, or contact with blood or other potentially infectious materials; and at the end of the work shift. Surfaces and equipment protected with plastic wrap, foil, or other nonabsorbent materials must be inspected frequently for contamination; these protective coverings must be changed when found to be contaminated.

Waste cans and pails must be inspected and decontaminated on a regularly scheduled basis. Broken glass should be cleaned up with a brush or tongs; never pick up broken glass with hands, even when wearing gloves.

Waste

Waste removed from the facility is regulated by local and state laws. Special precautions are necessary when disposing of contaminated sharps and other contaminated waste and include the following:

- Dispose of contaminated sharps in closable, puncture-resistant, leak-proof, red or biohazard-labeled containers (see table earlier).

---

[6]Phlebotomists in volunteer blood donation centers are exempt in certain circumstances. See section (d)(3)(ix)(D) of the standard for specific details.

- Place other regulated waste[7] in closable, leak-proof, red or biohazard-labeled bags or containers. If outside contamination of the regulated waste container occurs, place it in a second container that is closable, leak-proof, and appropriately labeled.

Laundry

Laundering contaminated articles, including employee laboratory coats and uniforms meant to function as PPE, is the responsibility of the employer. Contaminated laundry is handled as little as possible with minimum agitation. This can be accomplished through the use of a washer and dryer in a designated area on-site, or the contaminated items can be sent to a commercial laundry. The following requirements should be met with respect to contaminated laundry:

- Bag contaminated laundry as soon as it is removed and store in a designated area or container.
- Use red laundry bags or those marked with the biohazard symbol unless universal precautions are in effect in the facility, and all employees recognize the bags as contaminated and have been trained in handling the bags.
- Clearly mark laundry sent off-site for cleaning, by placing it in red bags or bags clearly marked with the orange biohazard symbol; use leak-proof bags to prevent soak-through.
- Wear gloves or other protective equipment when handling contaminated laundry.

What to Do If an Exposure Incident Occurs

An exposure incident is the specific eye, mouth, or other mucous membrane, nonintact skin, or parenteral contact with blood or other potentially infectious materials that results from the performance of an employee's duties. An example of an exposure incident is a puncture from a contaminated sharp.

The employer is responsible for establishing the procedure for evaluating exposure incidents. When evaluating an exposure incident, immediate assessment and confidentiality are crucial issues. Employees should report exposure incidents immediately to enable timely medical evaluation and follow-up by a health care professional as well as a prompt request by the employer for testing of the source individual's blood for HIV and HBV. The "source individual" is any patient whose blood or body fluids are the source of an exposure incident to the employee.

At the time of the exposure incident, the exposed employee must be directed to a health care professional. The employer must provide the health care professional with a copy of the blood-borne pathogens standard; a description of the employee's job duties as they relate to the incident; a report of the specific exposure, including route of exposure; relevant employee medical records, including hepatitis B vaccination

---

[7]Liquid or semiliquid blood or other potentially infectious materials; items contaminated with these fluids and materials, which could release these substances in a liquid or semiliquid state, if compressed; items caked with dried blood or other potentially infectious materials that are capable of releasing these materials during handling; contaminated sharps; and pathologic and microbiologic wastes containing blood or other potentially infectious materials.

status; and results of the source individual's blood tests, if available. At that time, a baseline blood sample should be drawn from the employee, if he or she consents. If the employee elects to delay HIV testing of the sample, the health care professional must preserve the employee's blood sample for at least 90 days.[8]

Testing the source individual's blood does not need to be repeated if the source individual is known to be infectious for HIV or HBV; testing cannot be done in most states without written consent.[9] The results of the source individual's blood tests are confidential. As soon as possible, however, the test results of the source individual's blood must be made available to the exposed employee through consultation with the health care professional.

After postexposure evaluation, the health care professional provides a written opinion to the employer. This opinion is limited to a statement that the employee has been informed of the results of the evaluation and told of the need, if any, for any further evaluation or treatment. The employer must provide a copy of the written opinion to the employee within 15 days. This is the only information shared with the employer after an exposure incident; all other employee medical records are confidential.

All evaluations and follow-up must be available at no cost to the employee and at a reasonable time and place, performed by or under the supervision of a licensed physician or another licensed health care professional, such as a nurse practitioner, and according to recommendations of the U.S. Public Health Service guidelines current at the time of the evaluation and procedure. In addition, all laboratory tests must be conducted by an accredited laboratory and at no cost to the employee.

Record Keeping

There are two types of records required by the blood-borne pathogens standard: medical and training. A medical record must be established for each employee with occupational exposure. This record is confidential and separate from other personnel records. This record may be kept on-site or may be retained by the health care professional who provides services to employees. The medical record contains the employee's name, social security number, hepatitis B vaccination status including the dates of vaccination, and the written opinion of the health care professional regarding the hepatitis B vaccination. If an occupational exposure occurs, reports are added to the medical record to document the incident and the results of testing after the incident. The postevaluation written opinion of the health care professional is also part of the medical record. The medical record also must document what information has been provided to the health care provider. Medical records must be maintained 30 years past the last date of employment of the employee.

Emphasis is on confidentiality of medical records. No medical record or part of a medical record should be disclosed without direct, written consent of the employee or as required by law.

Training records document each training session and are to be kept for 3 years. Training records must include the date, content outline, trainer's name and qualifications, and names and job titles of all persons attending the training sessions.

---

[8]If, during this time, the employee elects to have the baseline sample tested, testing is performed as soon as feasible.

[9]If consent is not obtained, the employer must show that legally required consent could not be obtained. Where consent is not required by law, the source individual's blood, if available, should be tested and the results documented.

If the employer ceases to do business, medical and training records are transferred to the successor employer. If there is no successor employer, the employer must notify the Director of the National Institute for Occupational Safety and Health, U.S. Department of Health and Human Services, for specific directions regarding disposition of the records at least 3 months before disposal.

On request, medical and training records must be made available to the Assistant Secretary of Labor of Occupational Safety and Health. Training records must be available to employees on request. Medical records can be obtained by the employee or anyone having the employee's written consent. Additional record keeping is required for employers with 11 or more employees (see OSHA's "Recordkeeping Guidelines for Occupational Injuries and Illnesses" for more information.)

Other Sources of OSHA Assistance

Consultation Programs

Consultation assistance is available to employers who want help in establishing and maintaining a safe and healthful workplace. Largely funded by OSHA, the service is provided at no cost to the employer. Primarily developed for smaller employers with more hazardous operations, the consultation service is delivered by state government agencies or universities employing professional safety consultants and health consultants. Comprehensive assistance includes an appraisal of all mechanical, physical work practice, and environmental hazards of the workplace and all aspects of the employer's present job safety and health program. No penalties are proposed or citations issued for hazards identified by the consultant.

Voluntary Protection Programs

Voluntary protection programs and on-site consultation services, when coupled with an effective enforcement program, expand worker protection to help meet the goals of the Occupational Safety and Health Act. The three voluntary protection programs — Star, Merit, and Demonstration—are designed to recognize outstanding achievement by companies that have incorporated comprehensive safety and health programs successfully into their total management system. They motivate others to achieve excellent safety and health results in the same outstanding way, and they establish a cooperative relationship between employers, employees, and OSHA.

Employee Training

All employees who have occupational exposure to blood-borne pathogens should receive training on the epidemiology, symptoms, and transmission of blood-borne pathogen diseases. In addition, the training program covers, at a minimum, the following elements:

- A copy and explanation of the standard
- An explanation of the Engineering Control Plan and how to obtain a copy
- An explanation of methods to recognize tasks and other activities that may involve exposure to blood and other potentially infectious materials, including what constitutes an exposure incident
- An explanation of the use and limitations of engineering controls, work practices, and PPE

- An explanation of the types, uses, location, removal, handling, decontamination, and disposal of PPE
- An explanation of the basis for PPE selection
- Information on the hepatitis B vaccine, including information on its efficacy, safety, method of administration, the benefits of being vaccinated, and that the vaccine will be offered free of charge
- Information on the appropriate actions to take and persons to contact in an emergency involving blood or OPIM
- An explanation of the procedure to follow if an exposure incident occurs, including the method of reporting the incident and the medical follow-up that will be made available
- Information on the postexposure evaluation and follow-up that the employer is required to provide for the employee after an exposure incident
- An explanation of the signs and labels or color coding required by the standard and used at this facility
- An opportunity for interactive questions and answers with the person conducting the training session

For more information on grants and training and education, contact the OSHA Training Institute, Office of Training and Education, 1555 Time Drive, Des Plaines, IL 60018, (708) 297-4810. For more information on AIDS, contact the Centers for Disease Control National AIDS Clearinghouse, (800) 458-5231.

OSHA References for Hepatitis C and HIV

Occupational Exposure to Bloodborne Pathogens OSHA Instruction, Field Inspection Manual. The current CDC recommendation for HCV is found in "Recommendations for Prevention and Disease Control of Hepatitis C Virus (HCV) Infection and HCV-Related Chronic Disease," *Morbidity and Mortality Weekly Report,* vol 47, no. RR-19, 1998. Contact: www.cdc.gov/epo/mmwr/preview/mwrhtml/00055154.htm. The most current HIV postexposure follow-up recommendations for an exposure incident made applicable by the blood-borne pathogens standard are found in the CDC: "Public Health Service Guidelines for the Management of Health-Care Worker Exposures to HIV and Recommendations for Postexposure Prophylaxis," *Morbidity and Mortality Weekly Report,* vol 47, no. RR-7, 1998. Contact: www.cdc.gov/epo/mmwr/preview/mmwrhtml/00052722.htm.

SOURCE: Bloodborne Pathogens and Acute Care Facilities (OSHA 3128), Occupational Safety and Health Administration, Washington, DC, 1992.

BIBLIOGRAPHY

2000 Test Catalog. Mayo Medical Laboratories, Rochester, Minn., 1999.

Abbott Axsym System CK-MB: Abbott Laboratories Product Literature. Abbott Laboratories, Chicago, 1999.

Abbott Axsym System Troponin I: Abbott Laboratories Product Literature. Abbott Laboratories, Chicago, 1997.

Abrams, C: ADH-associated pathologies. Medical Laboratory Observer 25:25, 2000.

Ahmed, A: Autoantibody detection in autoimmune diseases. Advance for Administrators of the Laboratory Oct:68, 1998.

Alter, M, et al: Testing for Viral Hepatitis. Abbott Diagnostics Educational Services, Chicago, 1992.

American Diabetes Association: Clinical practice recommendations 1998. Diabetes Care 21:S23, 1998.

Arky, R, et al (eds): Physician's Desk Reference, ed 50. Medical Economics Company, Montvale, N.J., 1996.

Ballinger, P, and Frank, E: Merrill's Atlas of Radiographic Positions and Radiologic Procedures, ed 9. Mosby, St. Louis, Mo., 1999.

Banez, E, et al: Laboratory monitoring of heparin therapy—the effect of different salts of heparin on the activated partial thromboplastin time. Am J Clin Pract Oct:569, 1980.

Bard, BTA: Bard Diagnostic Sciences, Redmond, Wash., 1996.

Baskin, L, and Hsu, R: Laboratory evaluation of proteinuria. Medical Laboratory Observer Nov:30, 1999.

Berkow, R, et al (eds): The Merck Manual of Diagnosis and Treatment, ed 14. Merck Sharp & Dohme Research Laboratories, Rahway, N.J., 1982.

Bishop, ML, et al: Clinical Chemistry Principles, Procedures, Correlations. Lippincott Williams & Wilkins, Philadelphia, 2000.

Bladder cancer and biochemical assays. Clinical Laboratory Strategies 5:3, 2000.

Bodor, G: New gold standard in cardiac markers. Advance for the Laboratory Jul:43, 1998.

Bounameaux, H: D-dimer testing in suspected venous thromboembolism—An update. QJM 90:437, 1997.

Boyd, R, and Hoerl, B: Basic Medical Microbiology. Little, Brown, Boston, 1977.

Braunstein, G: HCG Testing Volume I: A Clinical Guide for the Testing of Human Chorionic Gonadotropin. Abbott Diagnostics Educational Services, Chicago, 1993

Braunstein, G: HCG Testing Volume II: Answers to Frequently Asked Questions about HCG Testing. Abbott Diagnostics Educational Services, Chicago, 1991.

Bringing homocysteine into your lab. Clinical Laboratory Strategies 3:1, 1998.

Burtis, C, and Ashwood, E (eds): Tietz Textbook of Clinical Chemistry, ed 2. WB Saunders, Philadelphia, 1994.

Beutler, E, et al (eds): Williams Hematology, ed 5. McGraw-Hill, New York, 1995.

Carpinito, G: Product technology brief, enzyme immunoassay for bladder cancer. Clinical Lab Products Apr:32, 1999.

Castellone, D: Coagulation the good, the bad and the unacceptable. Advance for Medical Laboratory Professionals Nov:53, 1999.

Cavanaugh, B: Nurses' Manual of Laboratory and Diagnostic Tests, ed 3. FA Davis, Philadelphia, 1999.

Chernecky, C, and Berger, B: Laboratory Tests and Diagnostic Procedures, ed 2. WB Saunders, Philadelphia, 1997.

Ciesla, B: Targeting the thalassemias. Advance for Medical Laboratory Professionals Apr:12, 2000.

Christenson, R: The basics of bone. Clinical Laboratory News May:10, 1998.

Christenson, R: Biochemical cardiac markers present and future. Medical Laboratory Observer Sept:26, 1999.

Colombraro, G: Pediatrics, Core Content at a Glance. Lippincott-Raven, Philadelphia, 1998.

Constantinescu, M, and Hilman, B: The sweat test for quantitation of electrolytes. Lab Med 27:472, 1996.

Corbett, J: Laboratory Tests and Diagnostic Procedures with Nursing Diagnosis, ed 5. Prentice-Hall Health, Upper Saddle River, N.J., 2000.

Corbett, J: Laboratory Tests and Diagnostic Procedures with Nursing Diagnoses, ed 4. Appleton & Lange, Stamford, Conn., 1996.

Corning Clinical Laboratories. The 1996/1997 Reference Manual. Author, Teterboro, N.J.

Cunningham, V: A review of disseminated intravascular coagulation. Medical Laboratory Observer July:42, 1999.

Davidsohn, I, and Henry, J (eds). Todd-Sanford: Clinical Diagnosis by Laboratory Methods, ed 15. WB Saunders Company, Philadelphia, 1994.

Doshi, M: Blood Gas and Electrolyte Regulation. Colorado Association for Continuing Medical Laboratory Education, Denver, 1997.

Dubin, D: Rapid Interpretation of EKGs. C.O.V.E.R. Publishing, Tampa, Fla., 1989.

Falk, RA, and Miller, S: Clinical evaluation of osteoporosis. Advance for Administrators of the Laboratory, May:57, 1999.

First blood test for congestive heart failure wins FDA clearance. Clinical Laboratory Strategies 5:1, 2000.

Fischbach, F: A Manual of Laboratory and Diagnostic Tests, ed 6. Lippincott Williams & Wilkins, Philadelphia, 2000.

Fischbach, F: Nurses' Quick Reference to Common Laboratory and Diagnostic Tests, ed 2. Lippincott-Raven, Philadelphia, 1998.

Gantzer, M: The value of urinalysis, an old method continues to prove its worth. Clinical Laboratory News Jan:14, 1998.

Gerson, M: Cardiac Nuclear Medicine, ed 3. McGraw-Hill, New York, 1997.

Gill, K: Abdominal Ultrasound, a Practioner's Guide. WB Saunders, Philadelphia, 2001.

Golish, J: Diagnostic Procedure Handbook

with Key Word Index. Lexi-Company, Cleveland, Ohio, 1992.

Green, R: Macrocytic and marrow failure anemias. Lab Med 30:595, 1999.

Gruenwald, J, et al (eds): PDR for Herbal Medicines, ed 2. Medical Economics Company, Montvale, N.J., 2000.

Hennerici, M, and Neiserberg-Heusler, D: (1998). Vascular Diagnosis with Ultrasound. Thieme Medical Publishers, New York, 1998.

Hicks, J, and Boeckx, R: (1984). Pediatric Clinical Chemistry. WB Saunders, Philadelphia, 1984.

Hoeltke, L: Phlebotomy: The Clinical Laboratory Manual Series. Delmar Thomson Learning, Albany, N.Y., 1995.

Hopfer Deglin, J, and Hazard Vallerand, A: Davis's Drug Guide for Nurses. FA Davis, Philadelphia, 1999.

Homocysteine vs cholesterol, competing views or a unifying explanation of arteriosclerotic cardiovascular disease. Lab Med 29:410, 1998.

Howard, V: Age Specific Guidelines. Champlain Valley Physicians Hospital Medical Center, Plattsburgh, N.Y., 2000.

hs-CRP Detecting the Inflammation of Silent Atherosclerosis. Dade Behring Inc, Newark, N.J., 1999.

hs-CRP to Improve Cardiac Risk Assessment. Dade Behring Inc, Newark, N.J., 1999.

The Importance of Urinalysis: Lab Notes. Becton Dickinson Vacutainer Systems, Franklin Lakes, N.J., 1996.

Jacobs, D, et al: Laboratory Test Handbook, ed 4. Lexi-Comp, Hudson, Ohio, 1996.

Jaffe, M, and McVan, B: Davis's Laboratory and Diagnostic Test Handbook. FA Davis, Philadelphia, 1997.

Kandarian, P: ThinPrep imaging follows ThinPrep PAP to market. Clinical Laboratory Products, May:37, 2000.

Kaplan, L, and Sawin, C: Laboratory Support for the Diagnosis and Monitoring of Thyroid Disease. The National Academy of Clinical Biochemistry, Washington, D.C., 1996.

Kee, J: Handbook of Laboratory and Diagnostic Tests with Nursing Implications, ed 3. Appleton & Lange, Stamford, Conn., 1998.

Kee, J: Laboratory and Diagnostic Tests with Nursing Implications, ed 5. Appleton & Lange, Stamford, Conn., 1999.

King, D: New Methods Facilitating Down's

Syndrome Screening. Advance for Laboratory Professionals May:8, 2000.

Kirschner, C, et al: Current Procedural Terminology 2001. AMA Press, Chicago, 2000.

Koepke, J: Update on reticulocyte counting. Lab Med 30:339, 1999.

Landicho, H: Product technology brief, urine assay quantitates bladder tumor antigen. Clinical Lab Products May:46, 2000.

LaValle, J, et al: Natural Therapeutics Pocket Guide. Lexi-Comp, Hudson, Ohio, 2000.

Lehman, C: Saunders Manual of Clinical Laboratory Science. WB Saunders, Philadelphia, 1998.

Lewis, S, et al: Medical Surgical Nursing Assessment and Management of Clinical Problems, ed 5. Mosby, Philadelphia, 2000.

Liu, N, and Garon, J: A new generation of thyroid testing. Advance for Administrators of the Laboratory, Nov:29, 1999.

Lott, J: Clinical laboratory testing in hepatobiliary diseases. Advance for Medical Laboratory Professionals Jan:24, 2000.

Lutz, C, and Przytulski, K: Nutrition and Diet Therapy. FA Davis, Philadelphia, 1997.

Malarkey, L, and McMorrow, M: Nurses's Manual of Laboratory Tests and Diagnostic Procedures, ed 2. WB Saunders, Philadelphia, 2000.

Malarkey, L, and McMorrow, ME: Nurses's Manual of Laboratory Tests and Diagnostic Procedures. WB Saunders, Philadelphia, 1996.

Marking time with bone markers: New tests aid in managing osteoporosis. Clinical Laboratory Strategies Jul:3, 1998.

Masood, H: Menopause, hormones, and osteoporosis. Advance for Administrators of the Laboratory Feb:64, 2000.

Massey, L: Error free urinalysis. Advance for Medical Laboratory Professionals Mar:19, 2000.

McCall, R, and Tankersly, C: Phlebotomy Essentials. JB Lippincott, Philadelphia, 1993.

McEvoy, G, et al (eds): American Hospital Formulary Service: AHFS Drug Information. American Society of Hospital Pharmacists, Bethesda, Md., 1991.

McMorrow, ME, and Malarkey, L. Laboratory and Diagnostic Tests, a Pocket Guide. WB Saunders, Philadelphia, 1998.

MLO clinical laboratory reference. Medical Laboratory Observer 31:10, 1999.

Meredith, J, and Rosenthal, N: Differential diagnosis of microcytic anemias. Lab Med 30:538, 1999.

Miale, J: Laboratory Medicine, ed 5. CV Mosby, St. Louis, Mo., 1997.

Miller, S: Preventing and detecting neural tube defects. Medical Laboratory Observer May:32, 1999.

Montgomery, J: Improvements in prostate cancer detection. Advance for Administrators of the Laboratory Oct:66, 1999.

Moving toward a more precise definition of myocardial infarction. Clinical Laboratory Strategies 5:1, 2000.

MRI Registry Review Program. Medical Imaging Consultants, West Paterson, N.J., 1999.

Nageotte MP, et al. fFN testing high risk asymptomatic women. Am J Obstet Gynecol 177:13, 1997.

NCEP Issues Major New Cholesterol Guidelines. National Institutes of Health, Bethesda, Md., 2001.

Nester, E, et al: Microbiology Molecules, Microbes, and Man. Holt, Reinhart, & Winston, New York, 1973.

A new era in newborn screening. Clinical Laboratory Strategies 5:1, 2000.

New thyroid testing guidelines. Clinical Laboratory Strategies 6:2, 2001.

The next evolution in chest pain evaluation. Clinical Laboratory Strategies 4:1, 1999.

Nutritional Assessment of the Hospitalized Patient. Diasorin, Stillwater, Minn., 1998.

Olds, S, et al: Maternal Newborn Nursing, ed 6. Prentice-Hall, Upper Saddle River, N.J., 2000.

Pagana, K, and Pagana, T: Diagnostic Testing and Nursing Implications, a Case Study Approach, ed 5. Mosby, Philadelphia, 1999.

Pagana, K, and Pagana, T: Mosby's Diagnostic and Laboratory Test Reference, ed 4. Mosby, St. Louis, Mo., 1999.

Palkuti, H: International Normalized Ratio (INR) Clinical Significance and Applications. BioData Corporation, Horsham, Penn., 1995.

Peaceman AM, et al: fFN testing women with signs and symptoms of preterm labor. Am J Obstet Gynecol 170:20, 1994.

Peter, J: Use and Interpretation of Tests in Clinical Immunology, ed 8. Specialty Labs Inc., Santa Monica, Calif., 1991.

Peter, J: Use and Interpretation of Tests in Infectious Disease, ed 4. Specialty Labs Inc., Santa Monica, Calif., 1996.

Peter, J, and Reyes, H: Use and Interpretation of Tests in Allergy and Immunology. Specialty Labs Inc., Santa Monica, Calif., 1992.

Peterson, P, and Cornacchia, M: Anemia: Pathophysiology, clinical features, and laboratory evaluation. Lab Med 30:463, 1999.

Petrillo, M, and Sanger, S: Emotionalized Care of Hospitalized Children, an Environmental Approach, ed 2. JB Lippincott, Philadelphia, 1980.

Quinley, ED: Immunohematology Principles and Practice, ed 2. Lippincott-Raven, Philadelphia, 1998.

Quinn, D, et al: D-dimers in the diagnosis of pulmonary embolism. Am J Respir Crit Care Med 159:1445, 1999.

Reber, G, et al: Comparison of two rapid DDi assays for the exclusion of venous thromboembolism. Blood Coagul Fibrinolysis 9:387, 1998.

Re-examining the ADA criteria for diagnosing diabetes. Clinical Laboratory Strategies Mar:3, 2000.

Remaley, A, et al: Point of care testing of parathyroid hormone during the surgical treatment of hyperparathyroidism. Medical Laboratory Observer Apr:21, 1999.

Ringel, M: Bladder tumor markers: Where do they fit in disease management? Clinical Laboratory News May:18, 1998.

Rodak, B: Diagnostic Hematology. WB Saunders, Philadelphia, 1995.

Runge, V: Contrast-Enhanced Clinical Magnetic Resonance Imaging. The University Press of Kentucky, Lexington, 1996.

Sainato, D: C-reactive protein and cardiovascular disease. Clinical Laboratory News Jun:1, 2000.

Sandrick, K: Teasing out the value of new C-reactive protein test. CAP Today Jan:43, 2000.

Schull, P: Illustrated Guide to Diagnostic Tests, ed 2. Springhouse Publishing, Springhouse, Penn., 1998.

Seeram, E: Computed Tomography Physical Principles Clinical Application and Quality Control, ed 2. WB Saunders, Philadelphia, 2001.

Sharp, P, et al: Practical Nuclear Medicine, ed 2. Oxford Medical Publications, New York, 1998.

Shimeld, LA: Essentials of Diagnostic Microbiology. Delmar Thomson Learning, Albany, N.Y., 1999.

Soldin, S, et al: Pediatric Reference Ranges, ed 3. AACC Press, Washington, D.C., 1999.

Soloway, M, et al: Use of a new tumor marker, urinary NMP22, in the detection of occult or rapidly recurring transitional cell carcinoma of the urinary tract following surgical treatment. J Urol 156:363, 1996.

Steine-Martin, EA, et al: Clinical Hematology Principles, Procedures, Correlations. Lippincott-Raven, Philadelphia, 1998.

Strasinger, S: Urinalysis and Body Fluids, ed 3. FA Davis, Philadelphia, 1989.

Strasinger, S, and Di Lorenzo, M: Phlebotomy Workbook for the Multiskilled Healthcare Professional. FA Davis, Philadelphia, 1996.

Sutton, I: Monitoring anticoagulation therapy. Advance for Medical Laboratory Professionals Jan:10, 2000.

Thomas, C (ed): Taber's Cyclopedic Medical Dictionary, ed 14. FA Davis, Philadelphia, 1981.

Tamul, K: Determining fetal-maternal hemorrhage with flow cytometry. Advance for Laboratory Professionals June:18, 2000.

Testing Services for Hereditary Motor Sensory Neuropathy. Athena Diagnostics, Worcester, Mass., 2000.

Thelan, L, et al: Critical Care Nursing, Diagnosis and Management, ed 3. Mosby, St. Louis, Mo., 1998.

Tietz, N: Clinical Guide to Laboratory Tests. AACC Press, Washington, D.C., 1995.

Tilkian, S, et al: Clinical and Nursing Implications of Laboratory Tests, ed 5. Mosby, St. Louis, Mo., 1995.

Torres, L: Basic Medical Techniques and Patient Care in Imaging Technology, ed 5. Lippincott-Raven, Philadelphia, 1997.

Tressler, K: Clinical Laboratory and Diagnostic Tests Significance and Nursing Implications, ed 3. Appleton & Lange, Norwalk, Conn., 1995.

Twiname, BG, and Boyd, S: (1999). Student Nurse Handbook, Difficult Concepts Made Easy. Appleton & Lange, Stamford, Conn., 1995.

Using FISH for prenatal diagnosis. Clinical Laboratory Strategies Mar:2, 2000.

Van Dyne, R: Diagnosing common bleeding disorders. Advance for the Administrators of the Laboratory Oct:74, 1998.

Van Leeuwen, A, and Perry, E: Basic Principles of Chemistry, Techniques Using Alternate Measurements. Colorado Association for Continuing Medical Laboratory Education, Denver, 2000.

Vitros Chemistry System Test Methodology Manual. Ortho-Clinical Diagnostics, Rochester, N.Y., 1999.

Von Schulthess, G: Clinical Positron Emission Tomography. Lippincott Williams & Wilkins, Philadelphia, 2001.

Wentz, P: Chelation therapy, conventional treatments. Advance for Administrators of the Laboratory May:74, 2000.

Wentz, P: Homocyst(e)ine the bad amino acid. Advance for the Laboratory May:71, 1999.

Wentz, P: Megaloblastic anemias: Laboratory screening and confirmation. Advance for Administrators of the Laboratory Nov:57, 1999.

Widman, FK, and Ittani, CA: An Introduction to Clinical Immunology and Serology. FA Davis, Philadelphia, 1998.

Wilson, D: Nurses' Guide to Understanding Laboratory and Diagnostic Tests.

Lippincott Williams & Wilkins, Philadelphia, 1999.

Winter, W: Evaluating calcium disorders. Advance for Administrators of the Laboratory Jul:30, 2000.

Winter, W: Real time monitoring of diabetes. Clinical Laboratory News June:12, 2000.

Wolf, P: Cardiac infarction markers: Do we need another one? ASCP Spring Teleconferences, Chicago, 1999.

Wong, D, and Hess, C: Wong and Whaley's Clinical Manual of Pediatric Nursing, ed 5. Mosby, Philadelphia, 2000.

Wright, M, and Dearing, L: The role of HLA testing in autoimmune disease. Advance for Administrators of the Laboratory Apr:81, 2000.

Wu, J: Prostate cancer progress. Advance for Administrators of the Laboratory Jul:25, 1998.

Yeomans, E, et al: Umbilical cord pH, pCO_2, and bicarbonate following uncomplicated term vaginal deliveries. Am J Obstet Gynecol Mar:798, 1985.

Young, D: Effects of Drugs on Clinical Laboratory Tests, ed 4. AACC Press, Washington, D.C., 1995.

INDEX